DIFFERENTIAL DIAGNOSIS *of* ORAL LESIONS

DIFFERENTIAL DIAGNOSIS *of* ORAL LESIONS

NORMAN K. WOOD, D.D.S., M.S., Ph.D.

Dean and Professor of Oral Biology and Stomatology
Faculty of Dentistry
University of Alberta
Edmonton, Alberta, Canada

PAUL W. GOAZ, B.S., D.D.S., S.M.

Professor, Department of Oral Diagnosis and Oral Radiology
Baylor Dental College
Dallas, Texas

FOURTH EDITION
with 1336 illustrations, plus 4 full-color plates

Mosby Year Book

St. Louis   Baltimore   Boston   Chicago   London   Philadelphia   Sydney   Toronto

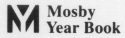

Mosby
Year Book
Dedicated to Publishing Excellence

Editor: Robert W. Reinhardt
Assistant editor: Melba Steube
Production editor: Mary McAuley
Designer: Laura Steube

FOURTH EDITION

Mosby–Year Book, Inc.
11830 Westline Industrial Drive
St. Louis, Missouri 63146

Library of Congress Cataloging in Publication Data

Wood, Norman K. (Norman Kenyon)
  Differential diagnosis of oral lesions / Norman K. Wood, Paul W. Goaz.—4th ed.
    p.   cm.
  Includes bibliographical references.
  Includes index.
  ISBN 0-8016-5846-2
  1. Mouth—Diseases—Diagnosis.   2. Diagnosis, Differential.
I. Goaz, Paul W.   II. Title.
  [DNLM: 1. Diagnosis, Differential.   2. Mouth Diseases—diagnosis.
WU 140 W877d]
RC815.W66   1991
616.3′1075—dc20
DNLM/DLC
for Library of Congress   90-5978
                                                                 CIP

C/MY/MY   9 8 7 6 5 4 3 2 1

Contributors

CHARLES G. BAKER, D.M.D., M.Sc.D., F.R.C.D.(C)

Assistant Dean, Clinical Affairs; Professor and Chairman, Department of Stomatology, Faculty of Dentistry, University of Alberta, Edmonton, Alberta, Canada

BRUCE F. BARKER, D.D.S.

Professor of Oral Pathology, Department of Oral Pathology, University of Missouri–Kansas City, School of Dentistry, Kansas City, Missouri

RONALD J. BARR, M.D.

Professor, Departments of Dermatology and Pathology; Director, Section of Dermal Pathology, University of California, Irvine, California

ROLLEY C. BATEMAN, D.D.S.

Professor Emeritus, Department of Radiology, Loyola University of Chicago, School of Dentistry, Maywood, Illinois

GEORGE G. BLOZIS, D.D.S., M.S.

Professor Emeritus, Section of Diagnostic Services, The Ohio State University College of Dentistry, Columbus, Ohio

HENRY M. CHERRICK, D.D.S., M.S.D.

Dean, School of Dentistry, University of California at Los Angeles Center for Health Sciences, Los Angeles, California

HENRY M. DICK, D.D.S., M.Sc., F.R.C.D. (C)

Associate Dean for Academic Affairs, Faculty of Dentistry, University of Alberta, Edmonton, Alberta, Canada

THOMAS E. EMMERING, D.D.S., F.I.C.D.

Visiting Professor, Department of Dental Radiology, Loyola University of Chicago, School of Dentistry, Maywood, Illinois

STUART L. FISCHMAN, D.M.D.

Professor of Oral Medicine, School of Dental Medicine, State University of New York at Buffalo; Director of Dentistry, Erie County Medical Center, Buffalo, New York

RONALD E. GIER, D.M.D., M.S.D.

Professor, Department of Oral Diagnosis and Oral Radiology, University of Missouri–Kansas City, Kansas City, Missouri

MARIE C. JACOBS, D.D.S.

Professor, Department of Oral Diagnosis, Pathology, and Radiology, Loyola University of Chicago, School of Dentistry, Maywood, Illinois

JERALD L. JENSEN, D.D.S., M.S.

Oral Pathologist, Laboratory Service, Veterans Administration Medical Center, Long Beach, California; Associate Clinical Professor of Pathology, University of California, Irvine, California

ROGER H. KALLAL, D.D.S., M.S.

Professor, Clinical Orthodontics, Department of Orthodontics, Northwestern University Dental School; Attending Oral and Maxillofacial Surgeon, Northwestern Memorial Hospital; Private Practice of Oral Surgery and Maxillofacial Surgery, Chicago, Illinois

JAMES F. LEHNERT, D.D.S.

Associate Professor, Department of Oral Diagnosis, Pathology, and Radiology; Director, Division of Oral Diagnosis, Loyola University of Chicago, School of Dentistry, Maywood, Illinois; Attending, Foster McGaw Hospital, Maywood, Illinois.

THOMAS M. LUND, D.D.S., M.S.

Professor and Director of Radiology, Northwestern University Dental School, Chicago, Illinois

RUSSELL J. NISENGARD, D.D.S., Ph.D.

Professor of Periodontology and Microbiology, State University of New York at Buffalo, Schools of Dental Medicine and Medicine, Buffalo, New York

DANNY R. SAWYER, D.D.S., Ph.D.

Professor and Chairman, Department of Oral Diagnosis, Pathology, and Radiology, Loyola University of Chicago, School of Dentistry, Maywood, Illinois

ORION H. STUTEVILLE, D.D.S., M.D.S., M.D.

Professor Emeritus of Surgery and Former Chief, Section of Plastic Surgery, Loyola University of Chicago, School of Medicine, Maywood, Illinois

RAYMOND L. WARPEHA, D.D.S., M.D., Ph.D.

Professor and Chairman, Division of Plastic Surgery, Loyola University of Chicago, School of Medicine, Maywood, Illinois

This effort is dedicated
to those who wage the battle against
oral disease in the private office,
clinic, and dental school—may it facilitate their
endeavors, as theirs have inspired ours.

Preface

Although "much study wearies the body" (Eccles. 12:12), the teacher and author must lead students to that point at which they discover that study is a "delight . . . [that becomes more satisfying] . . . in proportion to the application which one bestows upon it. Thus what [is] at first an exercise, becomes at length an entertainment" (Addison). Such was the intention of the first edition of *Differential Diagnosis of Oral Lesions:* to aid the student, neophyte and professional alike, to gain knowledge that will focus observational behavior and result in a more decisive and rewarding clinical experience. To perpetuate this intent and as a result of new developments, new data and statistics, and old omissions, the preparation of the fourth edition was in order.

Although books on various aspects of oral pathosis have been and are available, this and the earlier editions have been an effort to present the clinician with enough information to deal with all the steps necessary to recognize, understand, and identify the more commonly encountered oral pathoses.

Several definitive changes have been made in this edition. As a result of watching students confront lesions and the diagnostic process for the first time, we became convinced while organizing the first edition that a considerable benefit was to be gained from grouping similar-appearing lesions as components of unifying collections: this organization facilitated the development of a differential diagnosis. Consequently, two new chapters have been added: Chapter 9, "Red and White Lesions," and Chapter 18, "Interradicular Radiolucencies." These additions seemed appropriate and in keeping with the general plan of the book, since these categories represent relatively common groups of lesions that we have neglected in the past.

Although it has been a concern in earlier editions to list the entities included in a particular chapter in the order of their incidence, we have in this edition also reordered the chapters in Part II, "Soft Tissue Lesions," so that the groups, too, are organized in such a hierarchy of occurrence. For example, the chapter on white lesions appeared first in the earlier editions, whereas here we have placed the chapter on red lesions first, since we believe that these are more commonly encountered in practice. The other groups in the section on soft tissue lesions have also been appropriately repositioned.

Another improvement concerns the material on AIDS, which has been expanded, made current, further illustrated, and placed as Appendix D.

The material in Chapter 2, "History and Examination of The Patient," has been completely rewritten, and it contains new illustrations. Appendix B, "Normal Values for Laboratory Tests," has also been completely revised and expanded.

For the preparation of this fourth edition we are indebted to colleagues and students, the readers of the earlier editions, who submitted helpful suggestions, criticisms, corrections, and occasionally a compliment. We greatly appreciated this input, which was instructive and carefully considered. We were fortunate to be able to incorporate most of these suggestions into the text, which will surely make it a more effective educational tool. For this edition we earnestly enlist the help of clinicians and educators in identifying inaccuracies that, regardless of the care exercised, are bound to occur.

Again we wish to express our deep appreciation to our families for suffering through a period of neglect. We acknowledge the expertise of Carole Wood in completing some new line drawings and the cheerful diligence of Beth Cook, who typed the majority of the new manuscript.

Norman K. Wood
Paul W. Goaz

Contents

PART IV

LESIONS BY REGION

1

Introduction

The objective of this text is to present a systematic discussion of the differential diagnosis of oral lesions, based on a classification of lesions, which are grouped according to their similar clinical or radiographic appearances.

Part I consists of three *preparatory chapters*. Chapter 2 is devoted to a review of pertinent steps and modalities to follow in the examination of the patient. Chapter 3 explains on a functional and histologic basis the clinical and radiographic features of lesions discovered during the clinical examination. Chapter 4 outlines the diagnostic sequence we prefer, commencing with the detection of the lesion and progressing through intermediate steps until a final diagnosis is established.

Parts II and III make up the *differential diagnosis section* of the text, which deals with the specific disease entities. Part II is devoted primarily to the soft tissue lesions (Chapters 5 to 14), and Part III deals with lesions that originate in bone (Chapters 15 to 30). In each part the individual entities are classified into groups consisting of similar-appearing lesions, and each group forms the subject of a chapter.

Part IV is devoted to the presentation and discussion of lesions according to specific anatomic location. Thus Chapters 31 to 34 deal with masses in the neck, lesions of the facial skin, lesions of the lips, and intraoral lesions by anatomic region.

Although our text is primarily for the clinician, the microscopic picture is also discussed, but the microscopic picture is stressed only when it contributes to the recognition and comprehension of the clinical or radiologic features. This approach evolved from our observation of dental students entering the clinic and encountering great difficulty as they attempted to relate their knowledge of histopathology to the clinical features of lesions. Apparently students experience this difficulty because, first, they are not adequately instructed in the simple but meaningful correlations between the histologic and clinical pictures. Second, they lack experience in the grouping of lesions according to clinical appearances, which is necessary before a usable differential diagnosis can be developed.

Of course, there are several excellent textbooks of oral pathology that might be expected to complement the clinical study of oral lesions, but these books classify and discuss lesions according to etiology, tissue of origin, microscopic nature, or areas of occurrence. Although such an approach has proved to be effective for presenting a course in pathology, in our experience it has been cumbersome for the fledgling clinician. In an attempt to alleviate this problem, we group and discuss lesions according to their clinical appearance. Regardless of etiology or area of occurrence, *all similar-appearing lesions are grouped together* and discussed in the same chapter. Not only has the usefulness of our approach been demonstrated in practice, but the efficiency of our effort might well be anticipated, since the associations used for teaching the classification and recognition of clinical entities parallel the mental gymnastics one routinely employs in attempting to perceive and identify an unfamiliar object. Consequently the necessity of mentally reorganizing the material for effective recall is obviated.

The classic idea of the differential diagnosis seems to embody this natural ordering of information, and the same nature and sequential presentation of information may be successfully used in any endeavor to teach students to clinically apprehend and identify. We have attempted in the following chapters to arrange the presentation of what we consider the pertinent information in the same sequential manner.

Although our particular ranking of lesions in the ensuing pages may occasion the objection of some experts in various fields, no inerrant authority is claimed. We have attempted only to rank the entities in each category according to *frequency of occurrence*—with the discussion of the most common being first. The very rare lesions are simply listed. This particular arrangement is qualified as an impression that has developed from our personal experience and study as well as from our assessment of other authors' statistics.* It is not intended to be an authoritative statement but merely an aid to the clinician in the development of a differential diagnosis.

Our particular position regarding the ranking of lesions must be taken in the general context of this book, since different frequency rates occur in different age-groups and are modified by socioeconomics as well as by cultural and geographic factors. Also, when new cases are reported with each new issue of a journal, the rankings change, but we doubt that these changes will detract significantly from the usefulness of the arrangement presented here.

Those pathoses whose features are pathognomonic, and consequently do not generally present a problem in differential diagnosis, have not been included in this text, since they do not, by their nature, fall within its objectives and are adequately discussed elsewhere.

Pathoses of the dental hard tissues, gingivitis, temporomandibular joint problems, and nonspecific facial and oral pain have been excluded, since they also are adequately discussed elsewhere. In some cases entire books

---

*In this regard we are particularly indebted to Drs. Charles Halstead and Dwight Weathers of Emory University who have graciously made available to us statistical rankings from their extensive computerized study on the differential diagnosis of oral lesions.

have been devoted to these difficult and sometimes unresolved diagnostic problems.

At the same time it seems pertinent to point out that none of the discussions of entities included in this text are intended to be exhaustive descriptions of any disease but are intended only to present pertinent points that will help minimize confusion and contribute to the development of a differential diagnosis. Specifically we have not engaged in the detailed discussion of controversial questions concerning etiology and tissue origin when these subjects are in doubt, since they likewise have been exhaustively discussed in other sources and contribute little that is clinically useful to the inexperienced clinician.

Also the discussions of the features of particular lesions have not been specifically subdivided on the basis of clinical, radiographic, and histologic characteristics. On the contrary, these have been blended together in an attempt to illustrate how the three disciplines interrelate and aid in the explanation of the features found in each.

Again the primary aim of this book is to provide the clinician with the pertinent features of relatively common oral diseases that we consider necessary to the differentiation of similar-appearing lesions.

The diagnoses that appear in the descriptions of the reproduction of the clinical pictures and radiographs have been determined by microscopic examination in the vast majority of cases.

Part I

General principles of differential diagnosis

2

History and examination of the patient

PAUL W. GOAZ

Collecting the information necessary to determine the cause of a patient's complaint is accomplished by determining the patient's medical and dental history and performing a physical examination. Properly performed, the history and physical examination are frequently the most definitive of the diagnostic procedures. Without the information provided by the history and physical examination the diagnostic process is reduced to hazardous speculation. These diagnostic procedures include the following:

Recording the identifying data
History
  Chief complaint
  Present illness
  Past medical history
    Family history
    Social history
    Occupational history
    Dental history
  Review of symptoms by systems
  Physical examination
    Radiologic examination
  Differential diagnosis
  Working diagnosis
    Medical laboratory studies
    Dental laboratory studies
    Biopsy
      Incisional
      Excisional
      Fine needle aspiration
      Exfoliative cytology
    Toluidine blue staining
    Consultation
  Final diagnosis
  Treatment plan

HISTORY

A complete medical history is probably not necessary for most patients, but for certain patients, whose lives may be jeopardized by routine dental procedures, a carefully drawn history may disclose facts not otherwise identified or considered. Consequently, with training and experience able examiners will discern the nec-

essary areas of inquiry and produce histories that, although brief, will permit them to integrate their knowledge and experience with their observations and reach the appropriate conclusion.

It should not be overlooked that during this early contact, as the history is being determined and recorded and the physical examination is being conducted, a rapport with the patient is also being established. If the examiner demonstrates a genuine and sympathetic attitude at this time, the identity as the patient's "doctor" is developed. At the same time, valuable insight into the patient's psyche can be gained that will help the examiner evaluate the patient's reactions to questions and descriptions of symptoms.

Recording the identifying data

The following administrative information can usually be obtained by a receptionist. If this person is cordial, the patient is likely to develop a positive attitude about the practice, which in turn will facilitate successful treatment.

1. Name and address
2. Birth date
3. Sex
4. Principal racial or ethnic backgrounds
5. Occupation and address
6. Name and address of
   a. Informant, if other than the patient
   b. Referring source
   c. Family physician
   d. Family dentist or former dentist
   e. Third party health care provider
7. Other data (This may be tailored to a particular practice that will contribute to the health management of the patient. Medicolegal release and consent forms may be completed as the active therapy progresses.)

Some doctors and hospitals have the new patient sign a blanket consent for any procedure that may be determined necessary. However, it is recommended that the patient sign consent for only specific operations and that the consent be stated in terms that the patient understands, including the risks.

Chief complaint

The chief complaint is the patient's response to the dentist's question, "What problem brought you to see me?" It should be recorded briefly, in the patient's own words (within quotation marks*) if possible, and the duration of the disorder noted. In some cases the patient will indicate that he or she was referred by another dentist.

If there are two or more complaints, all should be recorded, whether they are related or not. The major complaint should be listed first, and the history of all complaints should be pursued. The successful management of the chief complaint will usually result in the successful treatment of the patient.

Present illness

Using the patient's own words, describe the chronologic order of the development of the primary (chief) complaint(s). Include the onset of the problem, its course, signs and symptoms, diagnostic studies and treatment received during the intervening period, and the current status of the problem. Help ensure a complete account of the patient's symptoms and an accurate description of the development of the disease by giving attention to the following topics.

ONSET

State in terms of time (days, weeks, months before the current appointment) when the primary complaint was first noted. Also determine what if anything in the patient's experience may have precipitated the signs and symptoms.

COURSE

A statement that describes the course of the chief complaint since its onset should be included. The symptoms may be described as intermittent, recurrent, constant, increasing, or decreasing in severity. Aggravating and alleviating factors should be noted. If pain is the major complaint, permit the patient to describe it in familiar terms. If necessary, a number of terms may be suggested to permit adequate

_____
*Quotation marks preclude the examiner's arriving at a premature diagnosis by translating the patient's comments into a pathological entity.

verbalization. Adjectives that may describe pain include:

throbbing	aching	burning
pounding	sharp	cramping
splitting	lancinating	constricting
bursting	stabbing	squeezing
exploding	cutting	gripping
heavy	bright	tight
dull	boring	scorching
pressing	gnawing	searing

PREVIOUS TREATMENT

Determine what was done, when, where, why, by whom, and note the outcome of previous treatment. Note the patient's attitude toward earlier treatment and any associated complaints. It is usually more revealing if the patient can be encouraged to provide this information with a minimum of direction or prompting.

Past medical history

Previous episodes of illness, their treatment, and the patient's response to treatment are detailed in the past medical history. This information can be elicited directly, in an interview by the doctor, or indirectly, by the use of forms on which the patient supplies the requested information. (Examples of such health questionnaires can be found in Rose and Kaye, 1990, and Seidel et al., 1987.) Each episode for which there was a previously established diagnosis should be recorded under this section. Dates of occurrence and details of severity or complications should be included. The examining doctor should expand those areas that he or she feels require amplification by directly questioning the patient during the subsequent review of symptoms by systems (see p. 6). The patient's responses and the assessment of the written responses on the health questionnaire should constitute an adequate past medical history and system review.

FAMILY HISTORY

The family history is important in the case of patients who are suspected of having inherited diseases that have familial patterns and in the case of those who may have been exposed to communicable disease. Family history is especially apropos when patients have had or are suspected of having, or have been exposed to, diabetes, hemophilia, cancer, one of the anemias, allergic disorders, cardiovascular-respiratory diseases, diseases of the nervous, renal, digestive, and musculoskeletal systems, tuberculosis, hepatitis, or acquired immunodeficiency syndrome (AIDS).

SOCIAL HISTORY

The social history will help the examiner differentiate between psychosomatic and somatic symptoms that may be described by a patient. Insight into the patient's habits, occupation, and personality, coupled with an awareness of such symptoms as sleep or appetite disturbance, constipation or diarrhea, low back pain, fatigue, decreased pleasure, oral mucosal inflammations and ulcerations, burning tongue, xerostomia, and altered taste, will help the examiner identify the individual with psychic maladies.

Of course, active therapy for an imagined or magnified complaint in a psychosomatically disabled patient will probably fail. Consultation with the family physician, psychiatrist, or psychologist is usually indicated when such psychologically troubled patients are encountered.

OCCUPATIONAL HISTORY

The occupational history of the patient is important, since some fields expose workers (cobblers, chemical workers, farmers, miners, and others) to hazardous physical environments that may be responsible for (sometimes characteristic) skeletal or oral lesions.

DENTAL HISTORY

How the patient interprets his or her dental history may or may not reveal the success of previous dental treatment (best assessed by the examiner). However, the patient's interpretation may well foretell how he or she will evaluate anticipated treatment.

Review of symptoms by systems

Although a variety of strategies have been proposed to facilitate the completion of this portion of the health history, a direct review of symptoms, system by system, is the most logical and efficient. In essence this method is based on the patient's response to either verbal or written questions about symptoms in each major body system. The method's aim is to identify problems the patient did not include in his or her chief complaint and to ensure a complete assessment of the patient's health questionnaire. By incorporating questions about the information from the health questionaire, the review checks the accuracy and completeness of the patient's past history and lessens the possibility of overlooking a particular area of the body and its correspondingly important symptoms. The review of systems also helps the examiner determine where he or she must concentrate the remainder of the examination. There is another potential benefit of the review. By talking to the dentist during the review, patients may learn something about themselves such as how an illness relates to recent changes in their lives (Bates, 1987). Such information may in turn provide the examiner with an additional diagnostic perception of a patient's condition. Lists of systems and symptoms that should be included in the review are given in Rose and Kaye (1990), Bates (1987), and Seidel et al. (1987). As the clinician's skill in posing the appropriate questions increases, experience deepens his or her understanding of what the symptoms may imply.

PHYSICAL EXAMINATION

The clinical examination of the oral and maxillofacial structures (or of any part of the body) is accomplished by using the examination techniques of observation (inspection); the sense of touch by feeling and pressing upon a part of the body (palpation); the detection of sounds from within the body produced by striking an area with a finger or hand (percussion); and the detection of functional sounds produced within the body (auscultation). The detection of odors of body and breath may also give the examiner important diagnostic clues. For a detailed description and discussion of the application of these techniques, see Chapter 3.

Although the patient's history usually directs the examiner's attention to a specific part of the body, the examination must be extended to exhaust the possibility that other body systems or parts are involved. To ensure that the examination is performed methodically and thoroughly and that important parts of the body are not overlooked, it is customary, even for the most skilled clinicians, to use an outline such as those shown in Rose and Kaye (1990), Bates (1987), and Seidel et al. (1987).

Radiologic examination

The use of diagnostic radiology should depend on the examiner's clinical judgment as to whether it will contribute to the diagnosis. Thus the decision to perform a radiographic examination should follow the completion of the history and physical examination. Only at this time can the views that will contribute to the recognition of the malady be identified and ordered. Although many unsuspected pathoses are discovered by routine radiography, the primary role of radiographs is to confirm clinical impressions. (See discussion of features obtained by palpation in Chapter 3.) In addition, the following strict admonition should be noted: Radiographs should never be accepted as the sole criterion for the selection of a treatment.

Most routine examinations may require one or more of the following radiographic projections:

I. Intraoral radiographic examinations; periapical, interproximal (bitewing), and occlusal projections.
II. Extraoral radiographic examinations* of oral and perioral areas
    A. Panoramic projection
    B. Lateral oblique projection
       1. Mandibular (anterior or posterior) body projection
       2. Mandibular ramus projection
    C. Skull projections
       1. Posteroanterior (anteroposterior) projection
       2. Lateral skull (cephalometric) projection
    D. Facial projections
       1. Waters' projection
       2. Submentovertex projection
       3. Reverse Towne projection
    E. Temporomandibular joint projection
       1. Transpharyngeal (infracranial) projection
       2. Transorbital (Zimmer)
       3. Facial projections

For a description of the structures these technical procedures demonstrate and how they are performed, see Goaz and White (1987).

Panoramic radiography. Panoramic radiography is available in many dental offices. This procedure provides a single image of the mandible, the lower portions of the maxilla, and their supporting structures. The resolution of the panoramic image is not as high as that of an intraoral film, and the image incorporates geometric and size distortion, superimposition of the structures imaged, and extensive blurring of possibly important structures outside its plane of focus. However, it does provide a view of a broad anatomic area. Panoramic radiography may be used for those patients who cannot open their mouths, and, although this should not be a compelling consideration, it is rapid and convenient for both the operator and the patient. For a detailed description of the physical principles of panoramic radiography,

as well as how to interpret the panoramic image, see Gratt (1987) and Langland et al. (1989).

CLASSICAL TOMOGRAPHY

In projection radiography, shadows of the object are cast on the image receptor (film). However, the image is of a large volume of the object and the structures within this object are usually superimposed, which causes the image of one internal structure to interfere with the recognition of low-contrast details that may be of diagnostic importance. Although it is not always a disadvantage to view the complete object in a single image, sometimes it is more advantageous to eliminate this superimposition so that particular anatomic sections can be clearly seen. At such times the radiographic technique of *tomography* (conventional tomography, laminography, body-section radiography) may be used. Tomography selectively images a layer of an object so that it may be clearly seen, while overlying and underlying structures are blurred or not imaged at all.

In tomography's simplest application an image of a "slice" of an object is generated by moving the x-ray source and the film reciprocally and linearly about a fulcrum fixed at a certain level within the object. This coordinated motion causes the selected plane within the object to remain stationary in relation to the image receptor (film). However, if the motion of the tube and film is linear, the result is an uneven density across the film. Because the ideal blurring of the image occurs when there is multidirectional movement of both tube and film, machines that can achieve the more mechanically difficult multidirectional movements have been developed. The basic principle applied in conventional tomography is also used in computed tomography (CT), sonography, single photon emission tomography, positron emission tomography, and magnetic resonance imaging (MRI). For a more detailed description of the physical principles involved in tomography, see Barrett and Swindell (1981).

In general, motion tomography finds its major application in imaging fine-detail, high-contrast objects. In dentistry, tomography is frequently used for the demonstration of the temporomandibular joint (Fig. 2-1) and for the identification and location of facial fractures. Tomograms in straight anteroposterior and lateral views assess more accurately than plain films the extent of both soft tissue disease and bony destruction of the paranasal sinuses (Som, 1984).

---

*Most extraoral radiographic projections that are appropriate for the examination of the oral and perioral structures can be made with the conventional dental x-ray machine and the proper combination of 5 × 7-inch-screen film and intensifying screens in a cassette.

Fig. 2-1. Multidirectional tomography of temporomandibular joint. (Courtesy Dan Waite, DDS, Dallas.)

Computer-assisted imaging

Although the traditional imaging modalities mentioned in the preceding section still play the principal role in the acquisition of information from patients with head and neck disease, developments and refinements in imaging technology have appeared with the advent of scanning and digital computer techniques. These developments have markedly expanded the limited capabilities of x-ray projection procedures. As a consequence of this new potential to discriminate between small differences in physical densities (such as those encountered in soft tissue disease) and to eliminate the confusion in interpretation caused by collapsing a three-dimensional object onto a two-dimensional image, an extended spectrum of examination is now possible. These new imaging technologies have also provided access to lesions in such areas as the pharyngeal space and the pterygopalatine fossa that were not easily evaluated by conventional x-ray transmission imaging. Some of the modern imaging procedures that have been applied with variable success to the diagnosis of head and neck disease are described here to acquaint and familiarize the newcomer with the general terms, methods, and extended diagnostic capabilities of

such extraordinary technologies as digital radiography, subtraction radiography, CT, radionuclide scanning, MRI, and ultrasound imaging. Because some understanding of the physical principles involved in these procedures is necessary if the examiner is to select the most cost-effective and rewarding imaging procedure in a particular setting, these principles are also discussed.

DIGITAL RADIOGRAPHY

Digital radiography (digital x-ray imaging) is a technique that is fundamental to CT, MRI, diagnostic ultrasound, nuclear medicine, and even film radiography. In digital radiography the remnant beam of x rays is directed onto a phosphor screen instead of a film. The screen is scanned by a television-type camera, the output of which is directed into a data acquisition system (digital computer). The contribution of the computer program to this technique is to digitize the image, that is, to divide the image into small areas, or pixels, and assign a number to each pixel, proportional to the intensity of the light at that pixel. These numbers can be stored in the computer and used to reconstruct the original image on a TV monitor by converting the numbers to light of appropriate intensity. The computer or digital processor performs a variety of functions, including (1) image acquisition control, (2) image reconstruction, (3) image storage and retrieval, (4) image processing, and (5) image analysis. Unlike the other techniques to be described here, the digital imaging equipment does not provide a cross-sectional image.

The image from a conventional radiograph can also be digitized, improved, and stored for future viewing. To improve the quality of an image, the operator manipulates its pixel numbers, thereby changing the density and contrast of selected areas or of the entire image (Fig. 2-2).

Subtraction radiography. Subtraction radiography is an extension of digital radiography. To subtract images the computer digitizes two radiographs of the same area and electronically subtracts the numbers representing the intensity of light at each pixel of the second radiograph from the numbers in analogous locations on the first radiograph. If the two films were made with the identical projection geometry and contrast, the subtraction image will appear uniformly gray. If, however, one image was made before and one after an event such as injection of contrast material or bone loss in an

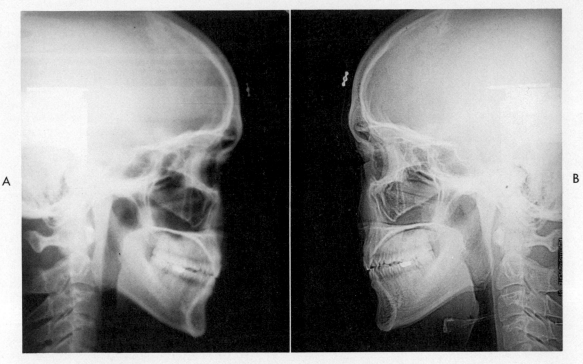

Fig. 2-2. Comparison of **A,** a conventional lateral cephalometric projection with **B,** a view of the video conversion of its digitized image, illustrating the increase in detail achieved by contrast modification.   (Courtesy Peter H. Buschang, PhD, Dallas.)

area, the area of change will be the only image that is clearly apparent without superimpositions on the subtracted image.

One of the major applications of this technique is to angiographic procedures. The greatest efforts to exploit subtraction techniques for dentistry are being applied to the detection of changes in alveolar bone (Hausmann et al., 1988). Although small changes in bone mass can be detected by this technique under ideal conditions of projection geometry (in the laboratory), comparable pairs of radiographs are difficult to obtain in the clinical setting. Although this technique is currently receiving considerable attention in the literature, it may best be described as a subject for research rather than a routine methodology for the evaluation of changes in the periodontal apparatus.

COMPUTED TOMOGRAPHY

CT, originally termed computerized axial tomography or computer-assisted tomography, has since been referred to as computerized reconstruction tomography, computed tomographic scanning, axial tomography, and computerized transaxial tomography. The acronym "CAT," or "CAT scan," appears in the litera-

ture. However, CT is now the preferred abbreviation in the diagnostic radiographic literature (Grossman et al., 1987).

In CT, a fan-shaped x-ray beam is rotated around the patient, and a ring of detector elements that also encircle the object detects the remnant radiation. The detectors convert the radiation to electric impulses that are in turn fed into a digital computer, which then constructs an image of the "slice" through which the fan-shaped beam was projected. This image may be projected onto a TV display, stored on magnetic tape, or converted to a hard copy (Fig. 2-3). The primary advantage of this system is that it eliminates superimposition of structures. Another important feature of CT scanning is that it can distinguish between tissues that differ in physical density by less than 1%, in contrast to the 10% difference required by conventional radiology (Redington and Beninger, 1981): such tissues as normal and clotted blood, cerebrospinal fluid, gray and white matter, bone, normal soft tissues, and tumors all appear in CT as separate entities (Thawley, Gado, and Fuller, 1978). Although computer scanning of the oral cavity is not practical because of the artifacts caused by dental restora-

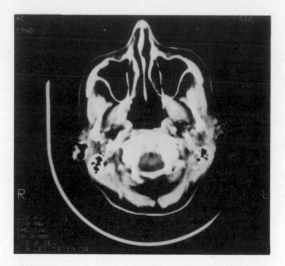

Fig. 2-3. Axial computed tomography scan. Such features as the nasal cavity and septum, nasopharynx, maxillary sinus, zygoma, mandibular ramus, lateral pterygoid muscles, mastoid processes, and air cells can be seen.

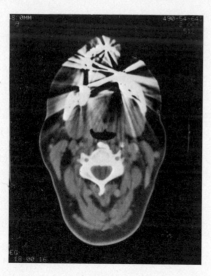

Fig. 2-4. Axial computed tomography scan illustrating artifacts produced by metal dental restorations.

tions (Fig. 2-4), it is frequently useful in determining how far a lesion may have extended from the oral cavity into the base of the skull, cervical spine, or paranasal sinuses (Nakagawa and Wolf, 1977).

A more detailed image of the paranasal sinuses, the nasopharynx, or the base of the skull and surrounding area is possible with CT than with conventional tomography (Carter and Bankoff, 1983). CT has been described by some

as the method of choice for evaluating salivary masses (Rabinov, 1984). It is also more reliable for the evaluation of tumor extent, but it does not image in the sagittal plane nor does it readily distinguish between tumor and inflammatory change in the sinuses (Lee and Van Tassel, 1989). For a detailed description of the physical principles of CT, as well as how to interpret the CT image, see Sprawls (1987) and Valvassori et al. (1988).

RADIONUCLIDE IMAGING

Radionuclide imaging takes advantage of the propensity of particular substances to concentrate selectively in certain "target" tissues and organs. These substances can be chemically tagged with radionuclides, and in some cases the ionic form of a nuclide selectively concentrates at the "target." The radionuclides used for this procedure are gamma ray producers with relatively short half-lives (a few hours to a day). These "radiopharmaceuticals" are injected or ingested. The gamma rays from the isotope that has concentrated at a particular area in the body are then detected by a gamma camera that converts the energy to electric impulses that are used by a computer to form an image on a cathode ray tube, transfer it to a film (Polaroid or x-ray), or store it for future viewing (Grossman et al., 1987).

The radionuclide imaging techniques that produce anatomic images actually assess function as well. In fact, the anatomic images are manifestations of function, delineating areas of increased or decreased metabolism (Fig. 2-5). The technique, however, is not specific. To determine the cause of the altered function, the clinician must qualify the information provided by the isotope scan with other diagnostic tests and clinical deductions. Despite these apparent drawbacks this technique demonstrates abnormalities in tissue and the extent of these changes even before they are demonstrable on routine radiographs (Beirne and Leake, 1980; Epstein et al., 1981).

In contrast to radionuclide imaging, a nuclear medicine technique for the measurement of bone-seeking radiopharmaceutical uptake is used to detect the alterations in diseases of bone resorption and formation such as bony metastases, primary bone tumors, infections, metabolic bone diseases, and stress fractures (Mettler and Guiberteau, 1983). Bone-seeking pharmaceutical uptake has been used as an indication of the rate of alveolar crest bone loss, and the results are verifiable by sequential radiographic examinations. This examination de-

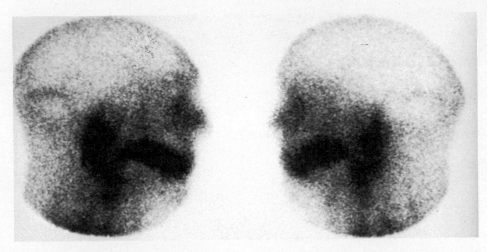

Fig. 2-5. Right and left radionuclide image of head showing more intense uptake in right parotid caused by chronic parotitis with accompanying abscess formation in this gland. The accumulation of activity in oral cavity is due to gingival inflammation and the appearance of the isotope in the saliva.   (Courtesy Byron W. Benson, DDS, Dallas.)

livers a radiation dose of less than 0.5 rem to the individual (Jeffcoat et al., 1987).

A variation of this nuclear imaging is *positron emission tomography*, in which the radiopharmaceuticals are labeled with positron-emitting isotopes ($^{11}C, ^{18}F, ^{13}N, ^{15}O$) and the gamma camera is moved around the patient. The information from the camera is analyzed by a computer, which constructs sectional images using the same mathematical models used in computed tomography (Phelps and Mazziotta, 1983).

MAGNETIC RESONANCE IMAGING (ZEUGMATOGRAPHY)

Chemical elements with nuclei that have an odd number of nucleons have a magnetic moment and a characteristic resonant frequency (in the FM radio range) when these magnetic nuclei are placed in a magnetic field. This frequency is unique to each element (nuclei) and varies with the strength of the magnetic field. If such elements are subjected to electromagnetic radiation (EMR) when they are in a magnetic field, they absorb energy and radiate it when the EMR is terminated. Since hydrogen represents at least 60% of the atoms in the body and hydrogen has the strongest MRI signal, most MRI systems are tuned to the resonant frequency of hydrogen (Bushong, 1988). It is these radio signals from hydrogen, detected by an antenna (field coil[s]), from which the MR image is constructed by a computer, using a mathematical model similar to that used to construct the CT image. The image is dis-

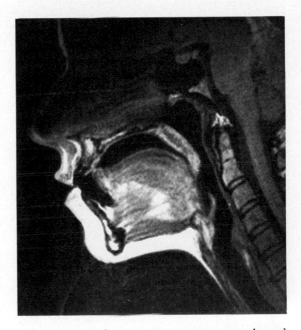

Fig. 2-6. Sagittal magnetic resonance scan through tongue and surrounding structures showing the mandible, hyoid bone, geniohyoid and genioglossus muscles, epiglottis, oropharynx, hard and soft palate, nasal turbinate, sphenoid sinus, pons, and medulla oblongata.   (Courtesy Dan Waite, DDS, Dallas.)

played on a TV screen that is also similar to that used by the CT scanner. It may also be recorded on film or magnetic tape for later interpretation.

MRI is being adapted for use in the diagnosis of almost all body organs and systems. MRI of head and neck pathoses is superior to CT in that its images of normal and abnormal tissues have better contrast and resolution (Fig. 2-6). Because of these improved image characteristics, tumor margins in the nasopharynx, oropharynx, and base of the skull are more sharply represented. MRI has proved useful for demonstrating the oral cavity, temporomandibular joint, and salivary glands. It can also differentiate between muscles, tonsils, mucosa, and lymph nodes. In contrast to CT, there is an absence of artifact degradation of the MR image by dental restorations. In CT, these artifacts frequently obscure regions of the oropharynx. Also, major blood vessels can be visualized in MRI without contrast medium, and images of transverse, coronal, and sagittal sections can be produced without repositioning the patient as is necessary with CT.

A disadvantage of MRI is its poor visualization of air spaces, of subtle osseous abnormalities, and of bone. The low concentration of magnetic nuclei in air and the rigid fixation of hydrogen in the bony matrix (precluding resonance) cause MRI to produce weak signals and no image. However, in contrast to the benefits of improved soft tissue contrast and the capacity to image exact tumor borders (Fig. 2-7), this disadvantage is minimal.

For a detailed description of the physical principles of MRI, and for how to interpret the MR image, see Sprawls (1987) and Mills et al. (1988).

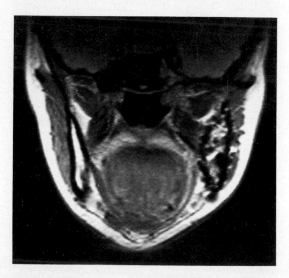

Fig. 2-7. Magnetic resonance image in coronal plane demonstrating a mass (desmoplastic fibroma) in the left ramus and angle of the mandible. (Courtesy Dan Waite, DDS, Dallas.)

SONOGRAPHY

Ultrasonic examination does not use any form of electromagnetic radiation. Instead high-frequency sound pulses (of approximately 1×10^{-6}/sec) are directed into the body (500 pulses/sec) from a hand-held transducer in contact with the skin. The sound is reflected by tissue interfaces, and the resulting echoes are detected by the same transducer, which then converts them to electrical signals that are fed into a computer. The time between transmission and receipt of the echo is proportional to the depth of the reflecting interface. If the sound is directed at the interfaces from different directions, the computer can use the echoes to create a map (image) that relates the reflecting surfaces to their three-dimensional distributions in the body. This three-dimensional image is called a B scan (brightness), or B-mode. If only the depth of a structure is determined (by keeping the transducer stationary), the image is referred to as an A-mode scan (amplitude display). A motion, or M-mode, image is produced when the transducer is stationary in relation to the body and records motion of internal body structures. Real-time scanning is produced by electronically sweeping the sound through an area of interest, which instantaneously produces a moving image of the internal structures. The images can be recorded like a moving picture and stored, or they can be viewed in real time on a TV monitor (Fig. 2-8).

Air and bone and other heavily calcified materials absorb almost all of the sound and are less echogenic than soft tissue. Fluid transmits sound so well that it is echo free, but it transmits echoes from structures opposite the transducer. Consequently ultrasound can be used to determine whether a structure is solid or cystic. The walls of a cyst produce good echoes, but the cystic fluid does not. A cyst can also act as an acoustic enhancer, causing an amplification of the echoes from the tissues behind it. On the other hand, a stone causes a great reduction of echoes from the tissues behind it, producing a definitive acoustic shadow. Ultrasound has proved useful for the examination of salivary glands (in some cases providing more definitive information than CT [DeClerk et al., 1988]), tumors (demonstrating consistency and size in different planes), cysts, and similar processes in the soft tissue of the cervicofacial region (Hell, 1989). Sonography only images structures, so assessments of physiology or pathologic changes are possible only when ar-

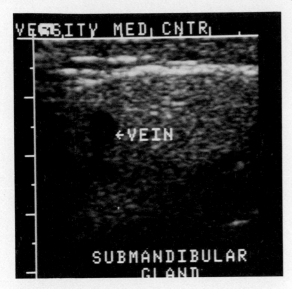

Fig. 2-8. Ultrasound image of a portion of normal submandibular gland. Note lack of internal echoes from the vein. The bright line at the top of the illustration is from fat on the surface of gland, which is more reflective than the salivary parenchyma. (Courtesy Robert Burpo, MD, Dallas.)

chitecture is affected. The reliability of an examination depends on the examiner's experience. Piette et al. (1987) found that results are more reliable when the maxillofacial surgeon performs the sonography.

To date, no harmful effects of this relatively inexpensive ultrasound examination have been documented. For a detailed description of the physical principles of sonography, as well as how to interpret the ultrasound image, see Sprawls (1987) and Yoshida et al. (1987).

DIFFERENTIAL DIAGNOSIS

The chief complaint and its history, a general medical history, and the physical and radiographic examinations provide a general clinical picture of the patient's problem. The clinician, on the basis of his or her knowledge and experience, ability to elicit information, and skills of observation, then compares the immediate complex of details with similar clinical pictures of various disease states. The list of similar clinical pictures, ordered according to the probable identity of the condition at hand, is the differential diagnosis. When equivocal cases are encountered, this list narrows the possibilities, reduces the number and cost of additional tests required to make a positive diagnosis, and provides a basis for an appropriate treatment plan.

Often the features of the disease process will be specific, and their signs pathognomonic, so a conclusive diagnosis can be established by evaluating pertinent information obtained from the history and examinations. However, when the diagnosis cannot be established and confirmed on the basis of the historical data and the clinical and radiographic examinations, its recognition may depend on positive and significant results from additional appropriate tests: a reappraisal of the information gathered to that date, laboratory studies, biopsy, and consultation.

Working diagnosis

Following a reappraisal of the diagnostic details at hand, including those from a follow-up examination, which may seem necessary and which may provide new, relevant findings, and including results from any additional diagnostic procedures, the working diagnosis should become apparent as the disease or condition that best satisfies all the data, or, if this is impossible, several diseases that satisfy most of the data. It must be emphasized that this working diagnosis is not a definitive diagnosis, since the definitive diagnosis may depend on further biochemical or hematologic tests or a histopathologic examination. However, the working diagnosis does narrow the differential diagnosis to the clinician's first-ranked choice and is certain enough that therapy may be initiated. Some diseases may be encountered whose identities are difficult to establish on the basis of historical data, clinical picture, and laboratory tests, but their response to specific therapy (*therapeutic diagnosis*) will be definitive.

Medical laboratory studies

Those clinical entities whose identities remain obscure following the patient's history and physical examination may be identified by the results from certain pertinent laboratory tests. Such tests are useful, however, only if the clinician is aware of what tests to order and how to interpret the results. For a description of the bewildering array of laboratory procedures available, their technical aspects, the circumstances in which they are appropriate, and the possibilities of both error and false reports, and for lists of substances that interfere with certain laboratory tests and the clinical application of test results, see Ravel (1979). Only a few of the numerous tests available are discussed here because, in general, only a few are essential in the dental setting. In addition to these procedures, bacteriologic culturing* (Doku, 1974) and antibiotic sensitivity testing† (Newan and Nisengard, 1988) may be necessary in certain circumstances.

COMPLETE BLOOD COUNT

The complete blood count usually includes a red blood cell count, hematocrit, or packed cell volume (PCV), hemoglobin content of whole blood (Hbg), red blood cell volume, hemoglobin concentration, and white blood cell and differential white blood cell counts. The mean corpuscular volume (MCV) of the red blood cells, the mean corpuscular hemoglobin (MCH) content of the individual red blood cell, and the mean corpuscular hemoglobin content in 1 dl of packed red blood cells (MCHC) can be calculated.‡ (See Appendix B for normal values.)

Red blood cell count

The red blood cell count gives the number of erythrocytes per cubic millimeter in the circulating blood and also gives an indirect estimate of the hemoglobin in the blood. The red blood cell count and hemoglobin content are determined with a manual red blood cell counting chamber (hemocytometer) or with electronic partial counting instruments, which provide more accurate results. The cardinal signs and symptoms of the hematologic diseases affecting the erythrocytes are the anemias, in which there is a significant decrease in red corpuscles or hemoglobin. The anemias may be due to a decrease in red cell production, an increase in red cell destruction, or blood loss. Polycythemia is defined as an increase in the number of circulating red cells that may be primary (idiopathic) or secondary to hypoxemia or dehydration. For a more detailed description of the laboratory procedures involved in the examination of the cellular elements of the blood, see Ravel (1989).

TOTAL ERYTHROCYTE COUNT. The total erythrocyte count is reduced in some anemias and fluid overload, and increased in polycythemia and dehydration.

HEMATOCRIT. The PCV is the measure of the volume percent of packed red blood cells in whole blood. This value is increased in primary and secondary polycythemia and dehydration and decreased in anemia. (Increases and decreases are affected by the same conditions that affect hemoglobin, below.)

HEMOGLOBIN CONCENTRATION. An increase in the concentration of hemoglobin is found in primary and secondary polycythemia and dehydration, and a decrease is found in anemia. The erythrocyte count and hemoglobin concentration do not always rise and fall proportionately.*

Elective general anesthesia should not be carried out when the hemoglobin level is less than 12 g/dl, but if surgery is imperative, it is justifiable if blood volume can be maintained. Normal blood volume is more important than normal hemoglobin.

Average (or mean) volume of the red blood cells. The average volume of the red blood cells is decreased in microcytic anemia and increased in macrocytic anemia.

Hemoglobin content of the individual RBC. The hemoglobin content of the individual RBC is decreased in microcytic anemia and increased in macrocytic anemia.

Average (or mean) amount of hemoglobin in 1 dl of packed red blood cells. The average amount of hemoglobin in 1 dl of packed red blood cells is reduced in hereditary spherocytosis and decreased in microcytic anemia.

White blood cell count

The white blood cell count (total leukocyte count) is the total number of cells per cubic millimeter of circulating blood. (See Appendix B for normal values.) To determine the number of white blood cells, a small amount of blood is mixed with a diluting solution that lyses the red blood cells. The diluted sample is placed in a chamber of known volume, and all the apparent cells are counted and multiplied by a diluting factor. The count may also be done with an automated cell counter. See Ravel (1989) for the details of the laboratory procedures. An elevation in the number of leukocytes (leukocyto-

---

*Microbiologic (bacteriologic) culturing should be undertaken when there is a failure to respond to an initial course of antibiotics, when there are systemic signs of infection before initiation of antibiotic therapy, in the case of pharyngeal lesions, when the patient is receiving immunosuppressant therapy, or when there is significant underlying disease.

†The susceptibility of bacteria to antimicrobial agents cannot always be anticipated, so testing the effects of antibiotics on pathogens isolated from the patient is required.

‡MCV = PCV × 10/red blood cells in 1 cubic micrometer; MCH = Hbg × 10/red blood cells in 1 micromicrogram; MCHC = Hbg × 100/PCV in grams per deciliter.

---

*In iron deficiency (microcytic) anemia the hemoglobin concentration is more reduced than the red blood cell count, and in pernicious (macrocytic) anemia the erythrocyte count is more reduced than the hemoglobin concentration.

sis) is most likely due to an infection, but it also occurs in inflammation, leukemia,* tissue destruction (trauma), exercise, pregnancy, and after general anesthesia. The WBCs of infants and children up to 3 years of age may be considerably higher than those of adults. A decrease in the white blood cell count may also be seen in aplastic anemia, certain viral and bacterial infections, early leukemia, depression of bone marrow by medications, drug and chemical toxicoses, and shock, or may occur from unknown causes.

Differential leukocyte count

The differential leukocyte count, taken from a blood smear stained with Wright's stain, determines the percentages of the different kinds of white blood cells present in the blood. Automated counters are also used to determine a limited differential in percentage and numbers, and these instruments produce more consistent results than manual differential cell counts (Ravel, 1989). This test significantly expands the information provided by the white blood cell count by delineating more specific indications for leukocytosis, leukopenia, or potential bleeding disorders. (See Appendix B for normal values.)

NEUTROPHILS. The neutrophil (polymorphonuclear leukocyte, polymorph, or PMN) is the most common of the leukocytes. The primary function of this cell is phagocytosis of bacteria and cell debris. The number of PMNs is increased in pregnancy, exercise, infection (a twofold to fivefold increase), inflammation, leukemia, a variety of neoplasms, severe hemorrhage, hemolysis, and corticosteroid therapy. A decrease in PMNs may be seen in some infections, aplastic anemia, cyclic neutropenia, drug-induced myelosuppression, and early leukemia.

LYMPHOCYTES. The lymphocytes play important roles in the immune response: the B-lymphocytes are concerned with the synthesis of circulating antibodies and the T-lymphocytes are responsible for cell-mediated immunity. The number of lymphocytes is increased in some infections (usually viral), bowel disease, and leukemia.

MONOCYTES. The monocytes survive for a short time in the peripheral blood (1½ days). From there, they migrate into various organs (liver, spleen, bone marrow, lungs, etc.) where they differentiate into mature tissue macrophages. Here they survive for months and constitute the reticuloendothelial system. In contrast to the polymorphs, which provide the major defense against the pyogenic bacteria, the macrophages play a valuable defensive role in phagocytosis of those bacteria, viruses, and protozoa that are capable of living in the cells of the host. An increase in the circulating monocytes (monocytosis) is relatively unusual, but it is encountered in patients with malignant tumors, autoimmune diseases, malaria, and such infections as acute bacterial endocarditis, tuberculosis, and brucellosis. A decrease in monocytes is observed in acute stressful illnesses, aplastic anemia, and acute leukemia.

EOSINOPHILS. The eosinophils disappear even more rapidly than the monocytes from the circulating blood (within 4 hours). They migrate into the tissues, where their life span is relatively long (7 to 10 days). Patients with certain parasitic infections, allergic diseases, or drug reaction dermatoses (pemphigus, pemphigoid, and atrophic dermatitis) show eosinophilia (increased number of eosinophils). Eosinopenia (decreased number of eosinophils) is found in some immune defects, in acute stress, or following the injection of adrenocorticotropic hormone or hydrocortisone.

BASOPHILS. The numbers of basophils in the circulating blood are so low that they are hard to locate. Although the function of the basophil is unknown, it resembles the connective tissue mast cell in many ways, so some regard it as a circulating form of the mast cell. (The granules of both contain histamine and heparin.) The percentage of basophils in the peripheral white blood cell count is increased in chronic myelogenous leukemia, myelofibrosis, and polycythemia vera. The basophils are degranulated by histamine-liberating drugs and discharge their granules in sensitized individuals who are exposed to the antigen.

PLATELETS. The platelets, the megakaryocytes, are fragments of a white blood cell. They play a role in hemostasis by forming platelet thrombi at the site of vessel (endothelial) injury and by supplying platelet clotting factors (platelet thromboplastin activity, factor V–like activity, and antiheparin activity). A thrombocytosis is seen in myeloproliferative diseases and trauma. Thrombocytopenia is the most common platelet abnormality. It may be induced by an immune reaction or drug or found following transfusions, bone marrow deficiency, or hypersplenism. A platelet count of less than 100,000 platelets/mm^3 indicates moderate

---

*A white blood cell count of 30,000 cells/mm^3 or higher that is not readily explained by an acute bacterial infection is referred to as a leukemoid reaction.

thrombocytopenia, and a count of less than 50,000 platelets/mm^3 indicates severe thrombocytopenia.

The platelet count can be evaluated reliably from a Wright-stained peripheral blood smear. The thrombocytes in the distal ends of the smear are counted in a number of oil-immersion fields (from 5 to 25). These numbers are averaged and multiplied by 20,000 to obtain a reliable estimate of the numbers of platelets per cubic millimeter. A more accurate procedure, employing a standard hemocytometer and whole blood, uses ethylenediaminetetraacetate (EDTA) as the anticoagulant and a diluting solution that contains brilliant cresyl blue. If a phase-contrast microscope is used, the technique has an error rate of approximately 8%, in contrast to the 10% to 20% error range of a conventional microscope. The most accurate platelet count is obtained with a platelet-counting machine.

EVALUATION OF HEMOSTATIC MECHANISMS

Hemostasis depends on the integrity of the vascular (occasionally), platelet, and coagulation systems. Although the patient's history and physical examination usually provide some indication as to the presence and nature of bleeding dyscrasias, four tests can be used to screen for specific hemostatic defects. These coagulation tests are bleeding time, clotting time, partial thromboplastin time, and prothrombin time. (See Appendix B for normal values.)

BLEEDING TIME. The bleeding time test assesses vessel reaction to injury and the adequacy of platelet number and function. This test measures the time it takes for a standard wound in the fingertip or earlobe to stop bleeding. That is, it measures the time required for a hemostatic plug to form. A lack of any of several of the clotting factors and especially platelet abnormalities can prolong this time. Although prolonged bleeding time is not diagnostically definitive, a dental patient with a prolonged bleeding time should receive a more detailed series of coagulation tests.

CLOTTING TIME. Clotting time is determined by filling several capillary tubes with blood from a finger puncture and then measuring the time required for fibrin to form, by breaking off small pieces of the tubes every 30 seconds. The endpoint is indicated when a fine thread of fibrin can be seen running from one fragment to the other. The clotting time depends on so many variables that a high degree of standardization is necessary to obtain accurate results.

The clotting time is prolonged in diseases affecting stages II and IV of the coagulation scheme and in severe deficiencies of any of the intrinsic factors. Clotting time is prolonged in cirrhosis, hemophilia A and B, factor XI deficiency, hypofibrinogenemia, and heparin and dicumarol anticoagulant therapy.

PARTIAL THROMBOPLASTIN TIME. The partial thromboplastin time (PTT) is the time in seconds that it takes for a clot to form in a sample of oxylated plasma to which an incomplete thromboplastin reagent and calcium chloride are added. The PTT, like the prothrombin time (PT) (see following discussion), is affected by abnormalities in the common pathway factors. Unlike the PT, however, the PTT also detects defects in the intrinsic clotting mechanism (factors VIII, IX, XI, XII) and reflects the activity of all the clotting factors except platelet factor 3, factor XII, and factor VII. This test is sensitive to defects in stage II. In hemophilia A and B, the PTT is increased although the PT is normal.

PROTHROMBIN TIME. PT is a test used to detect abnormalities not only in the common (prothrombin, factors V and X, and fibrinogen) but also in the extrinsic (factor VII) pathways. The test measures the time in seconds that it takes for fibrin threads to form in citrated or oxylated plasma when excess tissue thromboplastin and calcium chloride are added. Because the test is susceptible to subtle variables, a control test of normal plasma must be run concomitantly. A prolonged PT is generally caused by defects in stage III of the coagulation cascade—usually a prothrombin (factor II) deficiency. Deficiencies in factors I, V, VII, and X also prolong the PT. Anticoagulant therapy is usually the cause for stage III defects. Increased PT is also encountered in liver disease, when aspirin, antihistamines, steroids, or barbiturates are being used, and in vitamin K deficiency. The PT is shortened when antibiotics, hydroxyzine, sulfonamides, or oral contraceptives are being used.

If a patient has a clotting problem, surgical procedures should be avoided. A procedure that prompts bleeding of any kind can result in hemorrhage that may be difficult to control and may lead to the patient's death. In such cases discretion is to be observed. Dental treatment should be coordinated with a hematologist and may require the patient's hospitalization.

Blood glucose

Patients with a disorder in glucose metabolism pose problems as dental patients. They are prone to infection and in general are poor surgical risks with longer than normal convalescent periods. Diabetes is such a disease of glucose metabolism further characterized by disturbances in fat and protein metabolism. The medical history will have prompted the suspicion of diabetes based on the patient's description of weight loss, polyuria, polydipsia, and polyphagia. Clinically hypoglycemia and glycosuria are present.

Many manual and automated methods are used to determine blood glucose values. The clinician should be aware that certain technical differences and interferences by medications and metabolic substances can account for nonuniformity of test results and may affect interpretations. Although most laboratories provide ranges of normal values with the results, glucose values from plasma or serum are 10% to 15% higher than those from whole blood. Most automated equipment uses serum. If ranges of normal values are consulted, it should be confirmed that they refer to serum, plasma, or whole blood.

Semiquantitative paper strip methods are available to determine blood glucose.* A drop of blood, plasma, or serum is placed on the strip and the color that develops is compared with a reference color chart. Small electronic readout meters substantially improve the method's accuracy. With experience this method produces results that are within ±5% of standard laboratory values. (See Appendix B for normal values.)

Blood urea nitrogen

The blood urea nitrogen (BUN) test is useful for evaluating kidney (and liver) function. Urea is a nitrogenous waste product of protein metabolism that is synthesized in the liver and excreted by the kidney. Increase in the BUN level is associated with renal failure, congestive heart failure, protein catabolism (starvation), hyperthyroidism, dehydration, changes in plasma volume, hemorrhage (bleeding gastric ulcer), and shock. Decrease in the BUN level is seen in liver cirrhosis, nephrotic syndrome, and pregnancy. The clearance of urea is affected by the rate of urine flow, and there is a diurnal fluctuation.

The BUN is measured biochemically and enzymatically. Screening methods that use reagent strip tests are also available for BUN.† Recommended only for emergency screening, reagent strip tests permit the recognition of

normal BUN levels, mild azotemia, and high BUN levels. (See Appendix B for normal values.)

Urinalysis

The standard urinalysis may uncover disease present anywhere in the urinary tract, afford a semiquantitative assessment of renal function, and yield clues to the cause of dysfunction and to certain systemic diseases that may cause alterations in urine without directly affecting the kidneys. The laboratory report will indicate the appearance of the sample, pH, specific gravity, protein semiquantitation, presence or absence of glucose, ketones, and microscopic examination of the centrifuged sediment for white blood cell and red blood cell counts, casts, crystals, and squamous epithelial cells. With the exception of the microscopic examination these tests can be performed separately or in the various combinations available on dipsticks.* Instruments that read the dipsticks are available. The results of these tests are reliable, reproducible, and available in 30 seconds. (See Appendix B for normal values.)

APPEARANCE. The appearance of urine is not usually reported unless it is abnormal. A reddish, smoky appearance indicates concentration, or the presence of blood. Brown urine may be due to acid hematin (constituent of hemoglobin), alkaptonuria (on standing),† or melanin (urine may be brown and turn black on standing). White may indicate the presence of pus, whereas dark orange may indicate the presence of bile or a urinary tract infection.

pH. In general, pH is a measure of the exchange of hydrogen (H^+) for sodium (Na^+) by the renal tubules. The pH of freshly voided urine (normally 5 to 6) is decreased in diabetic acidosis, fevers, diarrhea, and dehydration. A sample left standing at room temperature will increase in pH (bacterial growth). The urine will be persistently alkaline in chronic glomerulonephritis and urinary tract infections (usually *Proteus*, which splits urea to form ammonia). In general, pH determination is of minor importance.

SPECIFIC GRAVITY. The test for the specific gravity of urine measures the kidney's ability to concentrate urine. A decrease in specific gravity is not only an indicator of tubular function. Kidneys with normal tubules may not be able

---

*Dextrostix, Ames Division, Miles Laboratories, Inc., Elkhart, Ind.
†Ames Division, Miles Laboratories, Inc.

*Labstix, for pH, protein, glucose, ketone, and occult blood values, Ames Division, Miles Laboratories, Inc., Elkhart, Ind.
†The urine contains alkapton bodies that are mostly homogentisic acid. It may not be indicative of pathosis, or it may be associated with ochronosis or arthritic symptoms.

to concentrate urine in diseases such as diabetes insipidus, hyperthyroidism (occasionally), and sickle cell anemia. The specific gravity of urine is important not only because of its association with disease but also because it may affect other urine tests. For example, a concentrated specimen may give higher results on the protein test. If the dipstick method is used to test the specific gravity of urine, moderate changes in pH and protein may affect the results.

PROTEIN. Most of the relatively large protein molecules are not passed into the urine. A great variety of conditions that alter the physiology alter glomerular filtration and may increase protein excretion in the urine. Albumin tends to be the dominant constituent in proteinuria because it is a relatively small molecule. The proteins found in the urine are those that constitute normal plasma. Some abnormal proteins such as Bence Jones* may be found.

Proteinuria may be produced by functional mechanisms (severe muscular exertion, pregnancy, and orthostatic proteinuria [associated with prolonged standing that causes renal passive congestion]), or associated with organic causes (fever, venous congestion [heart failure caused by intra-abdominal compression of the renal artery], renal hypoxia, severe dehydration, shock, severe acidosis, acute cardiac decompensation, or severe anemias). It is one of the most important indicators of renal disease. Although dipstick methods† are only semi-quantitative and are affected by a number of variables, most laboratories now use them rather than the older biochemical methods to detect protein in the urine. The dipstick methods do not react with other substances that might give false positives (except hemoglobin) but a number of variables (amount of protein in sample, length of time urine is in contact with dipstick, etc.) affect test results.

KETONE BODIES IN THE URINE. Under abnormal conditions, such as carbohydrate restriction or impaired carbohydrate metabolism (diabetes), fat is improperly oxidized for energy. This results in excess amounts of ketone bodies‡ in the urine (and the blood) producing

the condition known as ketosis, a type of acidosis. Few if any ketone bodies are found in the normal blood or urine of children or adults. Ketonuria can be caused by starvation, alcoholism, normal pregnancy, severe dehydration (vomiting, diarrhea, severe infection), or a noncarbohydrate diet of more than a few days' duration. Ketone bodies also occur in the urine of persons with maple syrup urine disease, renal glycosuria, or diabetes. Although ketonuria is found in so many abnormal conditions, it is of real diagnostic importance only in diabetes. Reagent tablet formulations (placed in specimen,* dipstick methods,† and biochemical (enzymatic) methods are used to detect ketone bodies. The tablet method can be used for plasma, serum, and urine, while use of the dipstick method is recommended only for urine.

Dental laboratory studies

The fabrication and analysis of articulated models of the dental arches and the attendant records are an integral part of the examination of many patients. Metabolic diseases, neoplasms, odontogenic diseases, congenital deformities, developmental malformations, and acquired maladies affecting the configurations of the oral cavity are often well visualized in properly prepared models.

Biopsy

Biopsy is the term used to describe the process of surgically removing tissue from a patient for histopathologic examination. The procedure is undertaken as the most accurate means of establishing a definitive diagnosis (confirming the working diagnosis) before the initiation of therapy. Biopsy should be pursued in the case of oral ulcers that persist for 2 to 3 weeks beyond the elimination of their suspected cause, persistent red and white lesions on the oral mucosa, suspected neoplasms, or any unidentified tissue mass or any pathologic mass that has been removed.

There are at least four types of biopsy: excisional biopsy, incisional biopsy, fine needle aspiration, and exfoliative cytology.

EXCISIONAL BIOPSY. An excisional biopsy is a therapeutic as well as a diagnostic procedure performed when the lesion is no larger than 1 cm in diameter and when its removal does not necessitate a major surgical procedure. Exci-

---

*Bence Jones protein is found in the urine of 50% of patients with multiple myeloma. It is soluble at room and body temperatures. Upon heating, it precipitates at between 45° and 60° C and then redissolves when the urine is further heated to 100° C.
†Albustix, Uristix, Multistix, and reagent tablet tests such as Acetest, Clinitest, Ames Division, Miles Laboratories, Inc., Elkhart, Ind.
‡Two acids, β-hydroxybutyric acid, and acetoacetic acid and acetone.

---

*Acetest reagent tablet test, Ames Division, Miles Laboratories, Inc., Elkhart, Ind.
†Ketostix, Multistix, Ames Division, Miles Laboratories, Inc., Elkhart, Ind.

sional biopsy has the advantage that only one surgical encounter is required.

INCISIONAL BIOPSY. An incisional biopsy is indicated if the lesion is too large for an excisional procedure. However, it may require that more than one tissue sample be removed for examination (serial biopsy). The sample, taken from the most suspect area, which toluidine blue staining may help identify (see p. 33), should be relatively large and deep and should include the junction with surrounding normal tissue. The sample should not be crushed, nor should electrosurgery be used to remove it.

The specimen should be placed in a solution of 5% to 10% formalin and fixed immediately. If there are two or more samples, each should be placed in a separate container. Each container should then be identified with the patient's name, the physician's name, and the measurements and location of the lesion from which the sample came. An adequate patient history should also be included with the specimen.

For more detailed discussions of the indications for a biopsy and the mechanics of the techniques, see Bernstein (1978) and Sabes (1979).

FINE NEEDLE ASPIRATION. In fine needle aspiration (FNA, fine needle biopsy, aspiration biopsy) a fine needle (21- to 23-gauge) is inserted into a tissue or suspected lesion. The needle may be guided with a fluoroscope or with ultrasound to ensure that an exact area of tissue is sampled (Ravel, 1989). A minute piece of tissue is sucked into the needle tip, expressed onto a glass slide, dried, and rapidly stained (Boccato, 1983). The cytomorphology of the aspirated tissue is then studied. The main advantages of FNA are simplicity of technique (it can be easily performed on an outpatient basis using a local anesthetic), greater patient acceptance and less risk of delayed wound healing and infection than with incisional or excisional biopsy, rapid diagnosis, and economy (it avoids hospitalization, saves operating room time, and avoids tissue processing). Another advantage is that different areas within a mass can easily be sampled to ensure that representative material has been obtained (Raju et al., 1988). The risk of seeding the needle track with cancer cells that accompanies the use of a large needle is unlikely with FNA (Scher et al., 1988). A 90% to 100% accuracy range for the technique has been reported in lymph node aspiration (for metastatic carcinoma and melanoma, Hodgkin's and non-Hodgkin's lymphoma), salivary glands and the head and neck region (oral cav-

ity, maxillary antrum, oropharynx, and nasopharynx), and other neck swelling (Feldman et al., 1983; Frable and Frable, 1983). The positive predictive value of FNA for malignancy in the head and neck is considered to be 100% for patients with or without a prior history of malignancy. It is considered the definitive diagnostic technique and allows the clinician to begin treatment. A negative, unsatisfactory, or suspect FNA diagnosis should be considered an indication for open biopsy to confirm the nature of the lesion. FNA is a safe, reliable method of diagnosing suspect lesions in the head and neck area and greatly aids and speeds the implementation of appropriate treatment.

EXFOLIATIVE CYTOLOGY. The technique for the cytologic examination of exfoliated cells scraped from suspect oral lesions is similar to that used for the detection of uterine cervix cancer. However, it has not provided the same level of reliability in the diagnosis of oropharyngeal malignancy. The lesion is scraped with a moistened tongue blade or a cement spatula and the cells obtained are smeared evenly over a glass slide, fixed, stained, and examined under the microscope for the presence of malignant-appearing cells (Barrett et al., 1986). The oral exfoliative technique has a tendency to produce a false-negative result an average of 37% of the time (Scher et al., 1988). Most of these false-negative reports, however, are associated with hyperkeratotic lesions in which the well-differentiated surface cells do not reflect the dysplastic or anaplastic changes in the deeper layer. Therefore, unless a keratotic lesion is associated with an adjacent ulcerated or erythroplastic area, exfoliative cytology is not indicated. In addition, some of the oral and nasopharyngeal lesions are nonepithelial or located submucosally. The technique is unsuitable for them. It is primarily for epithelial lesions. Oral exfoliative cytology is recommended as an adjunct to open biopsy, for prebiopsy assessment, and for the evaluation of patients following definitive treatment. Since the false-negative rate is too high to make this a practical screening procedure and the reliability rate depends on the specific site being examined, it is not considered a definitive diagnostic procedure (Folsom et al., 1972). However, the presence of malignant cells on a smear should prompt a search for primary tumor.

Toluidine blue staining

Most epithelial surfaces stain blue after the application of a 1% toluidine blue solution, but the stain is lost after application of a 1% acetic acid solution to a normal epithelial surface or to benign erythematous lesions on oral mucosa. In contrast, malignant erythematous lesions are not decolorized by the acetic acid. Toluidine blue is not a specific stain for cancer cells but is an acidophilic, metachromatic nuclear dye that selectively stains acid tissue components, particularly nucleic acids such as DNA and RNA. It is believed to have greater affinity for nucleic DNA than for cytoplasmic RNA (Herlin et al., 1983), and dysplastic and anaplastic cells contain more DNA than normal cells. Vital staining of mucous membranes with toluidine blue has been effective in demonstrating dysplastic and early malignant lesions not otherwise clinically recognizable on most of the mucous membrane surfaces and linings of the body, including the oral cavity (Hix and Wilson, 1987). The technique is useful for differentiating the small dysplastic erythroplakia that requires biopsy from small erythematous lesions caused by infection, inflammation, or trauma. It has also been observed that benign ulcerations usually have a well-defined uptake of dye at the margins whereas a diffuse marginal pattern is characteristic of the dysplastic or malignant lesion (Silverman et al., 1984). Nearly all false-positive staining (persistent blue color, no carcinoma) occurs (in 8% to 10% of cases) in keratotic lesions and at the regenerating edges of erosions and ulcerations. It follows that if all keratotic and erosive lesions are excluded, the test is highly sensitive and specific for dysplastic mucosal epithelium (Mashberg, 1980). False negatives (no persistent blue staining, carcinoma present in 6% to 7% of cases) may occur in dysplasia with severe parakeratosis, which prevents penetration of the stain so the dye does not reach submucosal extensions of a tumor (Mashberg, 1981). Although some contend that preoperative toluidine blue staining more reliably indicates the border of a lesion and serves as a guide for its surgical excision than does clinical examination alone (Eliezri, 1988), this contention must be qualified with the warning that the technique cannot show tumor that is present under normal epithelium (Bengel et al., 1989). When the edges of recent or small erosive mucosal lesions stain positively, a biopsy may be temporarily postponed while the cause of the erosion is considered. If it is inferred to be the result of infection or trauma, a short course of conservative therapy can be initiated. In the event that the erosion heals, the toluidine blue test can be repeated. If positive staining occurs, biopsy is in order (Lundgren et al., 1979).

Toxic effects of toluidine blue have been described but are not associated with the minute doses incurred during vital staining of mucosal surfaces (Registry of Toxic Effects of Chemical Substances, 1975).

Test for hepatitis (serology of hepatitis)

The diagnosis of hepatitis B is based on the examination of serum by means of radioimmunoassays and enzyme immunoassays. Five "markers" are of particular importance to this diagnosis: HBsAg (Australian antigen, the virion surface antigen [coat]); the antibody to the surface antigen (anti-HBs); the DNA viral polymerase, a core antigen (HBeAg); the anti-HBe, the antibody to the e-core antigen of the hepatitis B virus (HBV); and anti-HBc, the antibody to another core antigen (the HBc antigen that is never found in the serum). The HBsAg is not normally present in a patient with or without a history of hepatitis, but a serum that is positive for HBsAg is potentially infectious. The presence of HBeAg indicates circulating Dane particles (hepatitis virus) and a very infectious state. As the level of HBeAg declines, it is replaced with anti-HBe and the individual is less likely to be infectious. (A few carriers with anti-HBe are known to have transmitted the disease.) The anti-HBc is the first antibody to appear, even before symptoms develop. It increases rapidly to a high titer and persists indefinitely, with a subsequent, slow decrease in titer. The titer level can be used to estimate whether the infection is recent or remote. In some individuals with a level of HBsAg production too low to be detected, the presence of anti-HBc may be the only evidence of exposure to hepatitis B virus and may indicate a carrier state. For a detailed description of the sequence of the clinical and laboratory findings in hepatitis B, see White and Fenner (1986) and Gallo (1988). Viral hepatitis is described in detail in Appendix C.

Acquired immunodeficiency syndrome antibody test

Although the control of human immunodeficiency virus (HIV) infection is a major concern for the dental profession, testing to detect the HIV-infected individual is controversial, and the application of testing to different social and clinical situations is not well defined. However, as the accuracy of the tests improves, their use will probably be extended to more and larger population groups. Thus a few comments relative to the testing procedure seem appropriate to this discussion of laboratory studies.

The diagnosis of AIDS is based on the identification of the HIV antibody in the serum. A number of techniques identify the antibodies (immunofluorescent assay [IFA]), Western blot, radioimmunoprecipitation [RIP] tests), but an enzyme-linked immunosorbent assay (ELISA) is the most often used. It is low in cost and simple to perform and can be used for large-scale screening. The sensitivity and specificity* of the test are 95% to 99%, and its predictive value is close to 100% in a population with a high incidence of infection (homosexual men). It may give negative values for serum from individuals who have been infected for only 8 to 12 weeks. One percent of healthy, uninfected blood donors show positive albeit weak test reactions. When this happens, a second "confirmation" test is performed using one of the other techniques. A seropositive result is not reported unless the results from two techniques are positive. For a detailed discussion of the serologic tests for HIV infection, see Sandler et al. (1989). AIDS is described in detail in Appendix D.

Consultation

Before considering a consultation the clinician should be satisfied that he or she, by taking a reliable history and conducting a thorough physical examination, has made an effort to solve the problem. Reasonable consideration should also be given to the identity of an appropriate consultant. There should be a written form of the request for consultation, which includes a brief summary of the patient's history and physical examination, a description of the problem, and an indication of the nature of the request: advice, treatment of the patient, or transfer of the patient. Finally, when the report from the consultant is received, it should always be placed in the patient's record along with the consultant's name and address.

FINAL DIAGNOSIS

The final diagnosis is a statement that a precise diagnosis has been made on the basis of all required observations: the identification of definitive symptoms, the pathologist's report, and the patient's response to therapy.

TREATMENT PLAN

In-depth accounts of treatment planning (Wood, 1978, and Barsh, 1981) should be consulted for a description of the detailed procedures involved in developing a course of treatment for any of the wide variety of problems the clinician will encounter. During the diagnostic process the clinician acquires and organizes the disclosures from the patient's medical and dental history, clinical and radiographic examinations, and laboratory tests, with the intent of establishing a digest of the individual's state of health. This appraisal is necessary if an effective and comprehensive treatment plan is to be developed, although the diagnosis does not always suggest a particular method of treatment that will necessarily restore the health of the diseased area (dentition). The formulation of an appropriate treatment plan will depend on both the knowledge, experience, and competence of the clinician and the nature and extent of the treatment facilities available. The treatment plan cannot be an inflexible set of procedures identified by impersonal circumstances. Its design must be qualified by all the personal characteristics of the patient, and long-range follow-up care or monitoring or both must often be considered. The conscientious practitioner aims to design a treatment plan that is as individual as the patient and the person treating the patient. The characteristics of a particular case may even occasion the referral of the patient as the most judicious course.

REFERENCES

Barrett AP, Greenberg ML, Earl MJ, et al: The value of exfoliative cytology in the diagnosis of oral herpes simplex infection in immunosuppressed patients, Oral Surg 62:175-178, 1986.

Barrett HH and Swindell W: Radiological imaging: the theory of image formation, detection, and processing, vols 1 and 2, New York, 1981, Academic Press, Inc.

Barsh LI: Dental treatment planning for the adult, Philadelphia, 1981, WB Saunders Co.

Bates B: A guide to physical examination and history taking, ed 4, New York, 1987, JB Lippincott Co.

Beirne OR and Leake DL: Technetium 99m pyrophosphate uptake in a case of unilateral condylar hyperplasia, Oral Surg 38:385-386, 1980.

Bengel W, Veltman G, Loevy HT, et al: Differential diagnosis of diseases of the oral mucosa, Chicago, 1988, Quintessence Publishing Co, Inc.

Bernstein ML: Biopsy techniques: the pathological considerations, J Am Dent Assoc 96:438-443, 1978.

Boccato P: Rapid staining techniques employed in fine needle aspiration, Acta Cytol 27:82, 1983.

Bushong SC: Radiologic science for technologists, ed 4, St. Louis, 1988, The CV Mosby Co.

Carter BL and Bankoff MS: Facial trauma: computed versus conventional tomography. In Littleton JS and Durizch ML, editors: Sectional imaging methods: a comparison, Baltimore, 1983, University Park Press.

DeClerk LS, Corthouts R, Francx L, et al: Ultrasonography and computer tomography of the salivary glands in the evaluation of Sjögren's syndrome: comparison with parotid sialography, J Rheumatol 15:1777-1781, 1988.

---

*Sensitivity is the ability to detect low levels of target molecule; specificity is the ability to detect the target molecule exclusively.

Doku HC: Basic clinical bacteriologic techniques of importance to dentists, Dent Clin North Am 18:209-227, 1974.

Eliezri YD: The toluidine blue test: an aid in the diagnosis and treatment of early squamous cell carcinomas of mucous membranes, J Am Acad Dermatol 18:1339-1349, 1988.

Epstein JB, Hatcher DC, and Graham M: Bone scintigraphy of fibro-osseous lesions of the jaw, Oral Surg 51:346-350, 1981.

Feldman PS, Kaplan MJ, Johns ME, et al: Arch Otolaryngol Head Neck Surg 109:735-742, 1983.

Folsom TC, White CP, Bromer L, et al: Oral exfoliative study: review of the literature and report of a three-year study, Oral Surg 33:61-74, 1972.

Frable MAS and Frable WJ: Fine needle aspiration biopsy revisited, Laryngoscope 92:1414-1418, 1982.

Gallo RC: Retroviruses that cause human disease. In Wyngaarden JB and Smith LH Jr: Cecil text book of medicine, vol 2, ed 18, Philadelphia, 1988, WB Saunders Co.

Goaz PW and White SC: Oral radiology principles and interpretation, St. Louis, 1987, The CV Mosby Co.

Gratt BM: Panoramic radiography. In Goaz PW and White SC: Oral radiology principles and interpretation, ed 2, St. Louis, 1987, The CV Mosby Co.

Grossman LD, Chew FS, Ellis DA, and Brigham SC: The clinician's guide to diagnostic imaging: cost effective pathways, ed 2, New York, 1987, Raven Press.

Hausmann E, Dunford R, Christersson L, et al: Crestal alveolar bone changes in patients with periodontitis as observed by subtraction radiography: an overview, Adv Dent Res 2:378-381, 1988.

Hell B: B-scan sonography in maxillofacial surgery, J Craniomaxillofac Surg 17:39-45, 1989.

Herlin P, Marnay J, Jacob JH, et al: A study of the mechanism of the toluidine blue dye test, Endoscopy 15:4-7, 1983.

Hix WR and Wilson WR: Toluidine blue staining of the esophagus, Arch Otolaryngol Head Neck Surg 113:864-865, 1987.

Jeffcoat MK, Williams RC, Kaplan ML, and Goldhaber P: Nuclear medicine techniques for the detection of active alveolar bone loss, Adv Dent Res 1:80-84, 1987.

Langland OE, Langlis RP, McDavid WD, and DelBalso AM: Panoramic radiology, ed 2, Philadelphia, 1989, Lea & Febiger.

Lee Y and Van Tassel P: Craniofacial chondrosarcomas: imaging findings in 15 untreated cases, AJNR 10:165-170, 1989.

Lundgren J, Olofasson J, and Hellquist H: Toluidine blue: an aid in the microlaryngoscopic diagnosis of glottic lesions? Arch Otolaryngol Head Neck Surg 105:169-174, 1979.

Mashberg A: Reevaluation of toluidine blue application as a diagnostic adjunct in the detection of asymptomatic oral squamous carcinoma: a continuing prospective study of oral cancer, III, Cancer 46:758-763, 1980.

Mashberg A: Tolonium (toluidine blue) rinse—a screening method for recognition of squamous carcinoma: continuing study of oral cancer, IV, JAMA 245:2408-2410, 1981.

Mettler FA and Guiberteau, MJ: Essentials of nuclear medicine imaging, New York, 1983, Grune & Stratton, Inc.

Mills CM, de Groot J, and Posin JP: Magnetic resonance imaging: atlas of the head, neck, and spine, Philadelphia, 1988, Lea & Febiger.

Nakagawa H and Wolf B: Delineation of lesions of the base of the skull by computed tomography, Radiology 124:75-80, 1977.

Newan MD and Nisengard R: Oral microbiology and immunology, Philadelphia, 1988, WB Saunders Co.

Phelps ME and Mazziotta JC: Cerebral positron computed tomography. In Newton TH and Potts DG, editors: Advanced imaging techniques, San Anselmo, Calif, 1983, Clavadel Press.

Piette EJ, Lendoir L, and Reychler H: The diagnostic limitations of ultrasonography in maxillofacial surgery, J Craniomaxillofac Surg 15:297-305, 1987.

Rabinov K: CT of salivary glands, Radiol Clin North Am 22:145-149, 1984.

Raju G, Kakar PK, Das DK, et al: Role of fine needle aspiration biopsy in head and neck tumors, J Laryngol Otol 102:248-251, 1988.

Ravel R: Clinical laboratory medicine: clinical application of laboratory data, Chicago, 1989, Year Book Medical Publishers, Inc.

Redington RW and Beninger WH: Medical imaging systems, Physics Today 34:36-44, 1981.

Registry of Toxic Effects of Chemical Substances, Pub No 76-191, Rockville, Md, National Institute for Occupational Safety and Health, June 1975.

Rose LF and Kaye D: Internal medicine for dentistry, ed 2, St. Louis, 1990, The CV Mosby Co.

Sabes WR: The dentist and clinical laboratory procedures, St. Louis, 1979, The CV Mosby Co.

Sandler SG, Dodd RY, and Fang CT: Diagnostic tests for HIV infection: serology. In DeVita VT Jr, Hellman S, and Rosenberg SA, editors: AIDS: etiology, diagnosis, treatment, and prevention, ed 2, Philadelphia, 1989, JB Lippincott Co.

Scher RL, Oostingh PE, Levine PA, et al: Role of fine needle aspiration in the diagnosis of lesions of the oral cavity, oropharynx and nasopharynx, Cancer 62:2602-2606, 1988.

Seidel HM, Ball JW, Dains JE, et al: Mosby's guide to physical examination, St. Louis, 1987, The CV Mosby Co.

Silverman S, Migliorati C, and Barbosa J: Toluidine blue staining in the detection of oral precancerous and malignant lesions, Oral Surg 57:379-382, 1984.

Som PM: The paranasal sinuses. In Bergeron RT, Osborn AG, and Som PM, editors: Head and neck imaging: excluding the brain, St Louis, 1984, The CV Mosby Co.

Sprawls P: Physical principles of medical imaging, Rockville, Md, 1987, Aspen Publishers, Inc.

Thawley SE, Gado H, and Fuller TR: Computerized tomography of head and neck lesions, Laryngoscope 88:451-459, 1978.

Valvassori GE, Buckingham RA, Carter BL, et al: Head and neck imaging, New York, 1988, Thieme Medical Publishers, Inc.

White DO and Fenner DO: Medical virology, ed 3, Orlando, Fla, 1986, Academic Press, Inc.

Wood NK, editor: Treatment planning: a pragmatic approach, St Louis, 1978, The CV Mosby Co.

Yoshida H, Akizuki H, and Michi K: Intraoral ultrasonic scanning as a diagnostic aid, J Craniomaxillofac Surg 15:306-311, 1987.

3

Correlation of gross structure and microstructure with clinical features

NORMAN K. WOOD
PAUL W. GOAZ

IMPORTANCE OF NORMAL ANATOMY AND HISTOLOGY TO THE DIAGNOSTICIAN

The diagnosis of oral lesions is fundamentally an exercise in clinical pathology, which, in turn, is a study of changes. Usually such changes are precipitated by pathogenic or disease-producing agents. If the clinician is going to recognize and describe these changes, however, he or she must have a reference by which the altered states can be measured and compared.

For the clinical oral diagnostician this reference state is, of course, the state of oral health; it follows that a thorough and basic knowledge of the normal oral cavity and surrounding regions is fundamental to the detection of oral disease.

In addition, it is quite apparent that the physical characteristics of a tissue cannot be appreciated without an awareness of the tissue's microstructure. This is because the microanatomy of the tissue correlates extremely well with the clinical features on which the diagnostician bases his judgments. The low-magnification photomicrograph of a tissue quite adequately illustrates the tissue architecture and so clearly provides a basis for the interpretation of the tissue's physical features that the conscientious clinician cannot afford to ignore.

Oral and perioral systems

The mucous membrane that lines the oral cavity consists of a layer of stratified squamous epithelium and a subepithelial layer, the lamina propria, which consists of a fibrous connective tissue and contains capillaries, nerves, and the minor salivary glands (Fig. 3-1).

The skin, like the mucous membrane, also possesses two layers—the epidermis and the underlying corium with its associated appendages, the sweat and sebaceous glands and the hair follicles (Fig. 3-2).

The remaining glandular systems of the perioral region of direct concern to the clinician are the major salivary glands and the thyroid and parathyroid glands. Either these glands are directly identified by the examiner, or the effects of their pathologic involvement come to his or her attention when an adequate examination of the head and neck is completed.

The bones of the region include the maxilla, the mandible, the zygoma and vomer, and the palatine, sphenoid, hyoid, and temporal bones, as well as the cervical vertebrae. Inasmuch as these become especially apparent in any radiographic examination of their areas, the examiner must know their morphology and their relationship to each other and must be able to anticipate and interpret the bizarre forms their shadows may assume on the radiograph.

Other systems with which the oral examiner must be well informed are the teeth, larynx, trachea, and esophagus and the blood and lymphatic systems. Aberrations of these also occur in his area of responsibility and must be recognized.

The muscle systems with which the oral diagnostician must be familiar are those of facial expression, mastication, and swallowing, as well as those involved in movements of the head. Not only do these muscles, along with the bony and cartilaginous structures and vessels, provide landmarks that facilitate an effective examination; they also, with the fascial planes, tend to mechanically obstruct or guide invading and spreading disease processes such as infections and neoplasms. Consequently the examiner must be aware of the exact location and plane of each muscle and the extent of its normal movements during function.

Oral and perioral tissues

The epithelial tissues of the oral and perioral region include the following:

1. Stratified squamous epithelial lining
2. Mucous, serous, and sebaceous glandular units
3. Enamel

The connective tissues, located beneath the surface epithelium, including the following:

1. Fibrous, adipose, and loose connective tissue
2. Muscle (skeletal and smooth) and nerves
3. Cartilage and bone
4. Dentin, cementum, and dental pulp

A well-defined layer of loose connective tissue is usually present beneath the skin or mucous membrane and permits these superficial layers to move over the deeper, firmer tissues such as muscle and bone. If this loose connective tissue layer is absent, the superficial layer

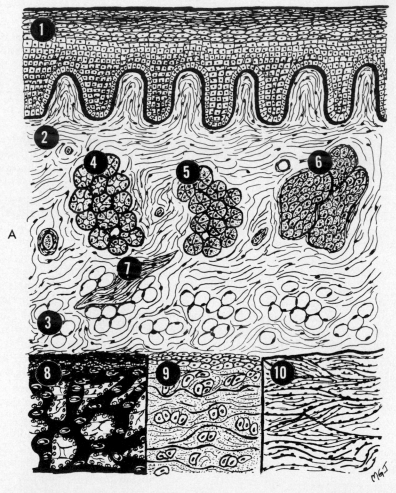

Fig. 3-1. **A,** Diagram of the oral tissues, illustrating the component tissues and their relative positions: *1,* stratified squamous epithelium; *2,* lamina propria; *3,* loose connective tissue; *4,* mucous glands; *5,* serous glands (occasionally); *6,* sebaceous glands (Fordyce's granules); *7,* nerve; *8,* bone; *9,* cartilage; *10,* skeletal muscle. Fortunately, a firm platform of muscle, bone, or cartilage is present beneath the superficial tissues. This facilitates examination and palpation of oral lesions.

is bound to the deep layer and cannot be moved separately from the underlying structures. Such a situation is normally found on the anterior hard palate and on the attached gingivae. Loose connective tissue contains blood and lymphatic vessels, nerves, adipose tissue, myxomatous tissue, sparse fibrous tissue, reticular fibers (precollagen fibers), elastic fibers, undifferentiated mesenchymal cells, and blast cells of many varieties.

Only through a thorough understanding of these tissues, their specific natures, their physical relationships to each other, how they support or fail to support each other when subjected to the deforming pressures of the examiner's fingers, and even the characteristic sensations the examiner can feel when palpating them will a full appreciation of the precepts of a physical examination be obtained.

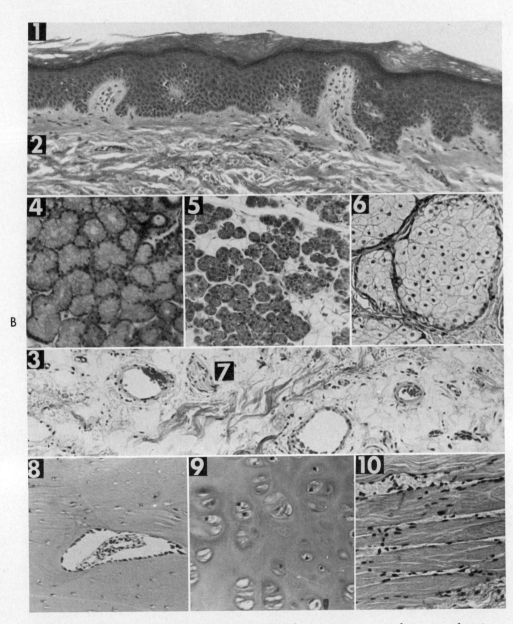

Fig. 3-1, cont'd. **B**, Composite photomicrographs of tissue components diagrammed in **A**.

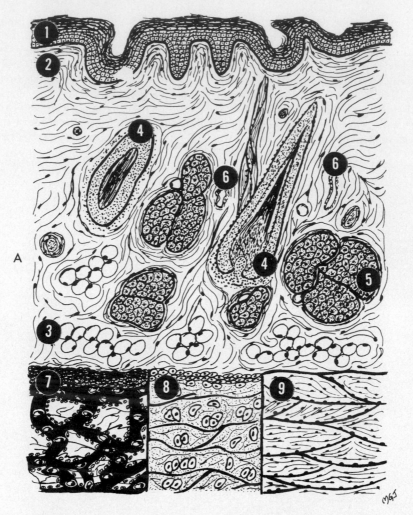

Fig. 3-2. A, Diagram of the skin and deeper tissues, illustrating the component tissues and their relative positions: *1,* keratinizing stratified squamous epithelium; *2,* corium; *3,* loose connective tissue; *4,* hair follicle; *5,* sebaceous glands; *6,* sweat glands; *7,* bone; *8,* cartilage; *9,* skeletal muscle. The firm platform below the oral tissues is also present beneath these dermal structures.

EXPLANATION OF CLINICAL FEATURES IN TERMS OF NORMAL AND ALTERED TISSUE STRUCTURE AND FUNCTION

Features obtained by inspection

The examiner can only visualize the surface tissue and its topography, including contours, color, and texture. For a more critical evaluation of irregularities, he or she must rely on other procedures.

CONTOURS

The diagnostician must, of course, be familiar with the normal tissue contours in and around the oral cavity to be able to detect any disorder that might alter the usual configuration of the area. Changes in contour, however, are not in themselves specifically diagnostic, since so many vastly different types of pathoses can produce similar alterations in contour.

COLOR

The examiner must be familiar with the normal characteristic color of each region in the oral cavity. He or she must be aware of the normal variations in color and shadings these tissues can assume, and certainly the examiner must be able to recognize the color changes that signal abnormal conditions in a particular area.

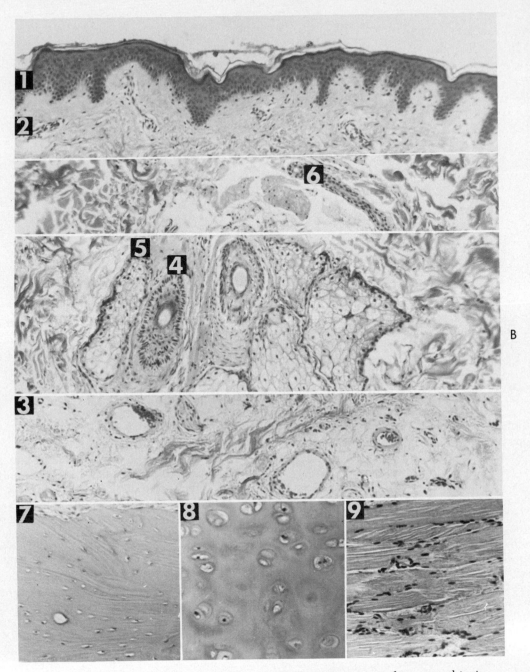

Fig. 3-2, cont'd. **B,** Composite photomicrographs of tissue components diagrammed in **A.**

Pink. The normal color of the oral mucosa in whites is pink, because healthy stratified squamous epithelium is semitransparent and hence the red color of the blood in the extensive capillary bed beneath, although somewhat muted, shows through. The oral mucosa is *not* uniformly pink throughout, however, but has a deeper shade in some regions and a lighter shade in others. This is illustrated by the con-

trast between the darker red vestibular mucosa and the lighter pink gingiva.

Certain normal variations in the tissue that are related to function are known to influence this spectrum of pink and thus to shift the color toward the red or, in the opposite direction, toward a lighter pink. One of the two main factors that induce a transition to a whiter appearance is an increase in the thickness of the epi-

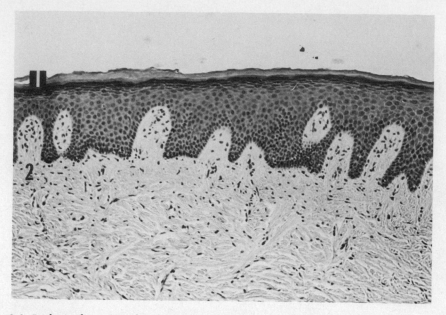

Fig. 3-3. Light pink region of oral mucosa. Photomicrograph of mucosa taken from the hard palate. The generous keratin layer, *1*, is combined with, *2*, the dense fibrous and quite avascular lamina propria. *2*. This combination accounts for the lighter coloration seen clinically on the hard palate and attached gingivae.

thelial layer, which makes the epithelium more opaque and is normally the result of an increased retention of keratin (Fig. 3-3). The other modification responsible for a more blanched appearance of the mucosa is a less generous vascularity of the subepithelial tissues concomitant with a denser collagen component. These two modifications are often found simultaneously (Fig. 3-3), and the effective clinician must be able to correlate them with observed variations in microstructure as well as be able to interpret them as alterations caused by function, variations in function, or trauma.

For example, regions in the oral cavity that receive the greatest mechanical stimulation from mastication (the *masticatory mucosa*) react by developing a thicker layer of keratin for protection and also a denser, less vascular lamina propria and so appear a light pink in color. These regions are the hard palate, the dorsal surface of the tongue, and the attached gingivae. On the other hand, regions such as the buccal mucosa, vestibule, floor of the mouth, and ventral surface of the tongue are not normally subjected to vigorous masticatory stimulation, so they require only a thin layer of stratified squamous epithelium, which retains little keratin and consequently permits the very vascular submucosa to show through and impart

the redder color (Fig. 3-4). These areas are said to be covered with *lining mucosa*.

White. Because of the many white lesions that may occur in the oral cavity, not only must the clinician inspect the color of the soft tissues carefully but he or she must also become intimately familiar with the normal color variations from region to region. These pathologic white lesions are discussed in detail in Chapter 8.

For example, although a chronic mild irritation may act as a stimulus and induce the changes necessary to cause the mucosa to take on a lighter pink color, a more acute intense irritation will produce a thinning of the stratified squamous epithelium and a consequent inflammation of the subepithelial tissues. Thus such an involved area of the mucosa changes from pink to red because of (1) a thinning of the epithelial covering combined with (2) an increased vascularity and (3) a dissolution of part of the collagen content of the subepithelial tissue.

Yellow. A yellowish cast is frequently seen in areas of the oral mucosa. The soft palate in many persons appears quite yellow. The explanation for this can be readily found in the histologic features of the area, which reveal a moderate distribution of adipose tissue contained in the connective tissue just beneath the

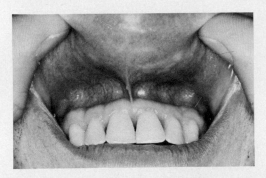

Fig. 3-4. This clinical picture illustrates the darker color of vestibular mucosa as contrasted with the lighter color of the attached gingivae. The histologic difference between the two regions explains these color differences.

basement membrane. Fordyce's granules, occurring in the buccal mucosa of most adults, are yellow, colored directly by the sebaceous material within the glandular units just beneath the epithelium.

Brownish, bluish, or black. Lesions of these colors are discussed in Chapter 12. It is appropriate to point out here, however, that the basis for the apparent clinical color of these lesions is frequently well demonstrated by histologic study whether the color is induced by melanin, hemosiderin, or heavy metals.

SURFACES

Normal mucosa is smooth and glistening except for the area of the rugae and the attached gingiva, which frequently demonstrates stippling and pebbling.

The surface of a pathologic mass may be smooth, papillomatous, ulcerated, eroded, keratinized, necrotic, or bosselated.

Masses that arise in tissues *beneath* the stratified squamous lining are, almost without exception, smooth surfaced. They may originate from mesenchyme, the salivary glands, a purulent infection, or an embryonic rest. As the nest of cells enlarges below and presses against the stratified squamous epithelium, the epithelium responds by a combination of stretching and minimal mitotic activity. Hence, as the mass becomes larger and bulges into the oral cavity, it is covered with a smooth epithelial surface. Examples of such masses are fibromas, osteomas, chondromas, hemangiomas, intradermal and compound nevi, many of the minor salivary gland tumors, cysts, retention phenomena, lipomas, myomas, schwannomas, neurofibromas, space abscesses, subepithelial bul-

lae of erythema multiforme, bullous lichen planus, and bullous pemphigoid (Fig. 3-5).

Even the malignant counterparts of such tumors often have smooth surfaces, especially in their early phases, but when these bulging lesions are situated in a region subjected to repeated trauma, they of course become ulcerated and necrotic and their smooth surfaces become roughened. Some exceptions to the rule that smooth-surfaced elevations originate below the epithelium are the intraepithelial vesicles and blebs seen in pemphigus and certain viral lesions.

As a general rule, however, masses that originate *in* the stratified squamous epithelium almost invariably have corrugated or papillomatous surfaces. Examples of these are papillomas, verrucae vulgari (warts), seborrheic keratoses, keratoacanthomas, verrucous carcinomas, and exophytic and ulcerative squamous cell carcinomas (Fig. 3-6). Exceptions would be the less than rough but pebbly surfaces sometimes seen overlying a granular cell myoblastoma and a lymphangioma. The granular cell myoblastoma often induces a pseudoepitheliomatous hyperplasia in the overlying epithelium, and this sometimes is severe enough to produce a pebbly surface (Fig. 3-7). The superficial lymphangioma frequently has dilated lymphatic spaces that extend right to the basement membrane, and these produce folds in the surface epithelium (Fig. 3-8).

The smooth-surfaced and rough-surfaced masses are categorized in Table 3-1.

Flat and raised entities. A macule is the result of a localized color change produced by the deposition of pigments or slight alterations in the local vasculature or other minimal local changes. This is a nonelevated lesion, since there is usually no significant increase in the number (hyperplasia) or size (hypertrophy) of the cells. Significant hyperplasia and hypertrophy always result in an elevation, which may take the shape of a papule, a nodule, a polypoid mass, or a papillomatous mass.

For example, an ephelis or freckle is a brownish macule that on histologic examination represents only an increased production of melanin by the normal number of melanocytes. On the other hand, an intradermal or intramucosal nevus on histologic examination shows a significantly increased number of nevus cells producing melanin and an increased amount of collagen in the subepithelial area. Hence both hypertrophy and hyperplasia are present and the lesion appears clinically to be pigmented and elevated (Fig. 3-9).

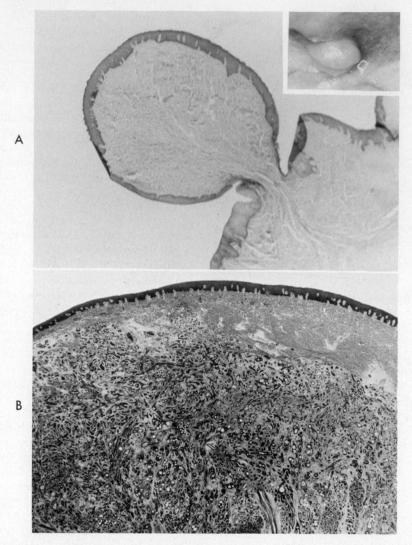

Fig. 3-5. Smooth-surfaced masses usually arise in tissues beneath the surface epithelium. **A,** Fibroma. **B,** Adenoid cystic carcinoma.

ASPIRATION

Some clinicians consider aspiration to be an extension of the visual examination, so its discussion is included here. Its primary value is to investigate the fluid contents of soft, cheesy, or rubbery masses whose characteristics suggest that they may contain fluid. An awareness therefore of the nature of the material contained in a mass will contribute significantly to the formulation of the appropriate differential diagnosis.

To aspirate masses indiscriminately, however, is generally considered unwise. Most clinicians recommend that a mass not be subjected to aspiration until just before surgery because of the danger of introducing bacteria

from the surface flora and thus secondarily infecting the mass. If the mass does contain fluid, the fluid may be an excellent medium for the growth of bacteria; if the mass does become infected, it may be necessary to delay surgery until the infection has resolved. Even then the tissue in the immediate area that was infected will prove difficult to dissect because of poor texture and postinflammatory fibrosis. If the mass is aspirated immediately before surgery, the introduction of organisms will not pose such a problem, since the mass will have been enucleated before the potential bacterial infection could attain clinical significance.

The preoperative aspiration of a fluid-filled mass is a worthwhile precautionary procedure,

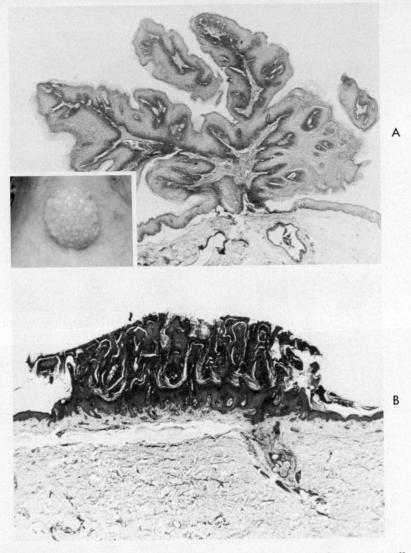

Fig. 3-6. Rough-surfaced masses usually arise within the surface epithelium. **A,** Papilloma. **B,** Seborrheic keratosis.

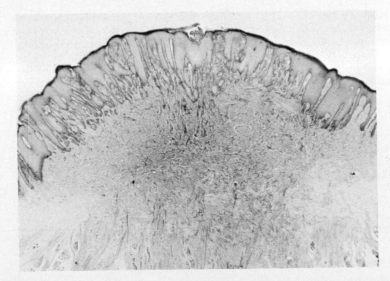

Fig. 3-7. Pebbly surfaced mass (granular cell myoblastoma). Note the presence of the pseudoepitheliomatous hyperplasia, which is often severe enough in these lesions to produce a pebbled surface.

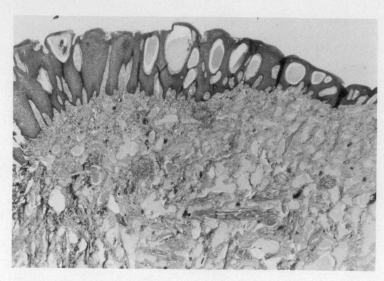

Fig. 3-8. Pebbly surfaced mass (lymphangioma). Note the numerous lymphatic channels throughout the tissue and especially those extending into the surface epithelium. A roughened surface frequently results from such extensions.

Table 3-1. Smooth-surfaced and rough-surfaced masses

Lesions	Exceptions
SMOOTH SURFACE*	
Benign and malignant mesenchymal tumors	Highly malignant varieties
	Late stages of less malignant varieties
	Traumatized lesions
	Superficial lymphangiomas
Embryonal rests	Draining cysts with sinuses
Cysts and nevi	Some raised nevi with roughened surfaces
Space abscesses	Draining abscesses and parulides
Subepithelial bullae	
Erythema multiforme, bullous lichen planus, bullous pemphigoid, and epidermolysis bullosa	Ruptured bullae
Inflammatory hyperplasias	
Hormonal tumors, epulides fissurata, epulides granulomatosa, papillary hyperplasias, and fibrous hyperplasias	Pyogenic granulomas
	Epulides fissurata occasionally
Benign minor salivary gland tumors	Traumatized lesions
Early malignant salivary gland tumors	
Retention phenomena	Traumatized lesions
Mucoceles and ranulas	
ROUGH SURFACE†	
Papillomas	None
Verrucae vulgares	None
Seborrheic keratoses	None
Keratoacanthomas	None
Verrucous carcinomas	None
Exophytic carcinomas	None
Ulcerative carcinomas	None
Condyloma latum	None

*All smooth-surfaced lesions, with the exception of intraepithelial bullae, originate *beneath* the surface epithelium.
†All rough-surfaced lesions, with the exception of those that were smooth surfaced and became roughened because of trauma, infection, or malignancy, originate *in* the surface epithelium.

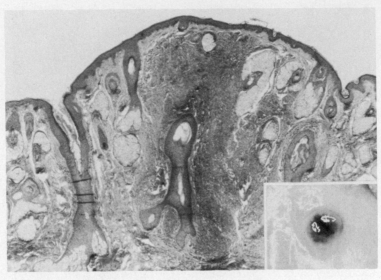

Fig. 3-9. Raised lesion (intradermal nevus). The large number of nevus cells present in the dermis produces the elevation of the lesion above the surface.

however, because, if carried out properly, it eliminates the unpleasant surprise of opening an innocuous-appearing lesion that proves to be a dangerous vascular tumor.

Aspirate. Examination of the fluid withdrawn at aspiration is the essential, indeed the only, step in this aspect of the visual examination.

A straw-colored fluid may be yielded on aspiration of odontogenic and some fissural cysts (e.g., midpalatal cysts) and occasionally from cystic ameloblastomas. These generally have cholesterol crystals in their walls that are frequently shed into the lumen of the cyst and may be seen as small shiny particles when the syringe containing the aspirated fluid is transilluminated (Fig. 3-10). The crystals, which have a characteristic needlelike shape, may be studied in more detail under the microscope by placing a few drops of fluid on a slide under a coverslip.

Other types of cysts, such as epidermoid, sebaceous, and dermoid, which feel firmer on palpation than do odontogenic cysts, yield more viscous aspirates and thus require at least a 15-gauge needle for successful aspiration.

1. The lumina of the epidermoid cyst and the keratocyst are filled with exfoliated keratin, and the aspirate is a *thick, yellowish white, granular fluid* (Fig. 3-11).
2. The sebaceous cyst yields sebum, which is *thick, homogeneous,* and *yellowish to gray.*
3. The walls of the dermoid cyst may contain most of the dermal appendages, including

stratified, squamous, keratinizing epithelium with sebaceous and sweat glands and hair follicles. Thus the aspirate from this cyst is the *thickest of all, a yellowish, cheesy substance that can be aspirated only with difficulty* because it consists of keratin, sebum, sweat, and exfoliated squamous cells.

A dark, amber-colored fluid on aspiration may indicate a thyroglossal duct cyst (Fig. 3-12).

Lymph fluid may be aspirated from cystic hygromas and lymphangiomas. It is colorless, has a high lipid content, and thus appears cloudy and somewhat frothy.

Bluish blood is aspirated from early hematomas, hemangiomas, and varicosities, whereas the blood from an aneurysm or an arteriovenous shunt is brighter red, reflecting the higher ratio of oxygenated to reduced hemoglobin of arterial blood (Fig. 3-13).

When a vascular lesion is suspected, care must be taken to use a needle of as small a gauge as possible to minimize postaspiration hemorrhage.

The aspiration of painful, warm, fluctuant swellings usually yields pus. If the infectious organism is staphylococcal, and a significant percentage of pyogenic infections of odontogenic origin are, the color of the pus usually is yellow or yellowish white. A superinfection with *Pseudomonas aeruginosa* produces greenish blue pus.

Usually, aspirating a streptococcal infection, such as Ludwig's angina, is futile because most

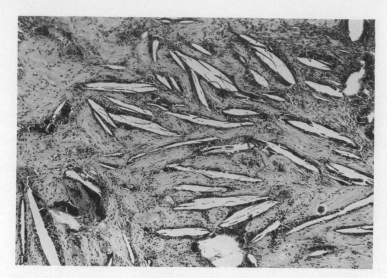

Fig. 3-10. Cholesterol clefts. The cholesterol crystals that occupy these clefts migrate to the luminal surface, are suspended in the cyst fluid, and may be subsequently discovered in the aspirate.

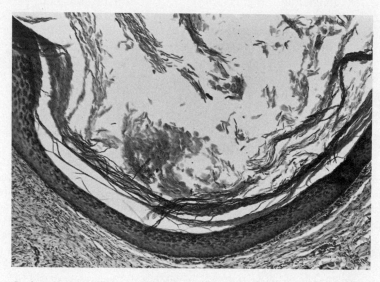

Fig. 3-11. Thick yellowish white cyst aspirate. Note the large quantity of keratin that occupies the lumen of this epidermoid cyst and produces a viscous yellowish cystic fluid that would require a large-gauge needle for aspiration.

streptococcal organisms are not pyogenic and do not localize. Instead they produce spreading factors (e.g., the enzymes hyaluronidase, streptokinase, streptodornase, and coagulase), which facilitate their rapid dispersal through the tissues. Streptococcal organisms produce a red serosanguineous fluid, but usually not in large enough quantities to pool or be aspirated or to demonstrate fluctuance. Also, in contrast to staphylococcal infections, the streptococcal va-

riety is more often associated with painful regional lymphadenitis.

Actinomycosis in its early stage is indicated by firm red swellings. Later, pus pools under the surface and produces fluctuance. At this intermediate stage, aspiration often yields a yellowish white pus with a few firm yellow granules in it. These are the "sulfur granules," thought to be composed of mycelia and material produced as a by-product of the natural de-

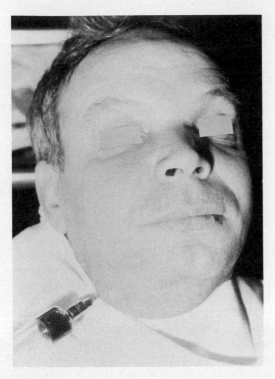

Fig. 3-12. Aspiration of a thyroglossal duct cyst. Note the unusual displacement of this particular cyst to the right of the midline.

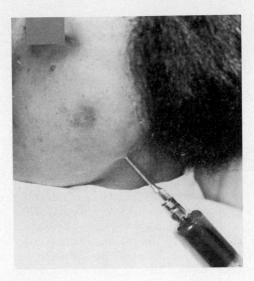

Fig. 3-13. Aspiration of a deep cavernous hemangioma of the face.

fenses of the host. Any aspirate from an infection should be sent to the laboratory for routine bacterial culture and sensitivity tests. If actinomycosis is suspected, special anaerobic cultures should be requested.

A sticky, clear, viscous fluid is yielded on aspiration of retention phenomena (mucoceles and cysts of the glands of Blandin and Nuhn and of the sublingual gland [ranula]) and sometimes from tumors of the minor salivary glands. This pooled liquid is a concentrated mucous secretion from which water is resorbed by the cells lining the cyst. Occasionally a low-grade mucoepidermoid tumor produces enough mucus to clinically resemble a mucocele and yields mucus on aspiration.

The papillary cystic adenoma and papillary cystadenoma lymphomatosum (their names indicate they are cystic) are often fluctuant and contain a thin, straw-colored liquid that can be aspirated.

Subcutaneous emphysemas and laryngoceles are soft masses that are filled with air, as are the rare pockets of carbon dioxide and hydrogen produced by *Clostridium perfringens* in gas gangrene. The former two entities can be completely deflated by aspiration.

NEEDLE BIOPSY

Needle biopsies can be performed with a special biopsy needle; this procedure can be advantageous in the biopsy of deeper structures such as the lymph nodes. The needle biopsy technique has the disadvantage of yielding a small-sized sample, and there is the added danger of lacerating some large blood vessels in the area (see Chapter 2, p. 18).

Features obtained by palpation

The knowledgeable examiner is able to distinguish the various tissues encountered in and around the oral cavity by palpation. He or she is able to do this because, first, the examiner is familiar with the normal gross anatomy of the structures and knows where these tissues and organs are situated, their extent, in which plane they lie, and their anatomic relationship to each other. Second, he or she can visualize the microscopic structures of these tissues, which correlate so well with the tactile sensations elicited by the palpation of these structures and tissues.

Palpation is actually a "third eye"—the most informative method of clinically examining the tissues lying beneath the surface. Fortunately for the examiner, the soft tissues of the body lie over bones, cartilages, or skeletal muscles; hence the superficial tissues can be palpated against a sturdy base.

SURFACE TEMPERATURE

Before attempting to make a judgment relative to the level of the surface temperature of a region or part, the examiner should first establish the patient's systemic temperature as indicated on an oral thermometer. A rise in surface temperature of the skin is simple to detect. The examiner merely places the fingers of one hand on the skin in the area of concern and the fingers of the other hand on the skin on the contralateral spot of the body. Thus relatively subtle differences in temperature may be rapidly and comfortably detected and can frequently contribute significantly to arriving at the diagnosis.

The skin generally has an increased temperature when it is inflamed or when it overlies an inflamed or infected region. The increased metabolic rate of the inflamed tissue, together with the increased vascularity of the area, is responsible for the increased local temperature of the part. The surface temperature of the skin overlying superficial aneurysms, arteriovenous shunts, and relatively large recent hematomas may also be elevated, since the higher deep body temperature is carried by the blood to the skin overlying these areas. The estimation of normal surface temperature is a useful test on the skin, but trying to transfer such a reference to the oral cavity is of little value, since the oral mucosa has a higher normal temperature than the skin. Although the examiner may be able to detect slight variations in temperature with fingers over his or her own skin surface (being the same as that in the normal reference area on the patient), when the reference temperature to be evaluated is somewhat greater than the skin temperature of the examiner's fingers (as it is in the oral cavity), he or she is unable to detect subtle differences.

ANATOMIC REGIONS AND PLANES INVOLVED

In addition to knowing the microscopic anatomy of a region being inspected, the examiner must be thoroughly familiar with the gross anatomy of the region. Since many of the structures in the head and neck region can be at least partly palpated through the skin or oral mucosa or both, it becomes imperative that normal structures be anticipated and recognized.

For example, if the diagnostician locates a firm mass high in the submandibular space, he or she must be aware that the submaxillary gland is peculiar to that area and must then establish whether the mass is discrete from the salivary gland. If he or she can determine that the mass is separate from the gland, pathoses of this gland will be deemphasized in the differential diagnosis. If this cannot be determined,

the diagnostician must consider salivary gland pathoses as a probable diagnosis.

Although it is important for the examiner to know what organs and tissues occur in an involved anatomic space, it is also essential that he or she be able to detect, identify, and evaluate their condition by manual examination. The acquisition of such a capability requires not only the basic anatomic knowledge but also considerable experience examining the area.

Sometimes, however, the information gained by palpation is limited, and the palpation itself may be difficult—especially if the area is swollen, because the swelling will tend to obscure the definitive structures. Furthermore, if the area is painful, the patient does not permit a thorough palpation of the region and the mass. The clinician must keep in mind that sometimes a complete palpation is not possible until the patient is anesthetized.

Initially the examiner must determine whether a mass in question is located superficially or deep. If it is superficial, he or she must then verify whether it involves the skin over the subcutaneous or fascial layer and also whether it involves a muscle or a muscle layer. If it involves a muscle layer, the examiner must ascertain which muscles and whether regional organs (glands, vessels) or bones are associated with the mass.

MOBILITY

Once the examiner has defined a mass in terms of its location in an anatomic plane and the tissue and organ involved, he or she will determine whether the mass is mobile or fixed with regard to its neighboring tissues. By palpation the examiner can establish whether the mass is freely movable in all directions. If it is freely movable, it is most likely a benign, possibly encapsulated, process originating in the loose subcutaneous or submucosal tissue (such as epidermoid or dermoid cyst or lymph node) (Fig. 3-14).

The mobility can be illustrated by fixing the mass with the fingers of one hand while moving the skin or mucosa over the mass with the other hand. Next an attempt is made to move the mass independent of its underlying tissue. This demonstrates whether it is freely movable in all directions. If the mass is found to be fixed to the skin, that is, the skin cannot be moved independent of the mass but is not fixed to the underlying tissue, this is an important clue and limits the differential diagnosis.

For instance, epidermoid and dermoid cysts would be regarded as unlikely alternatives be-

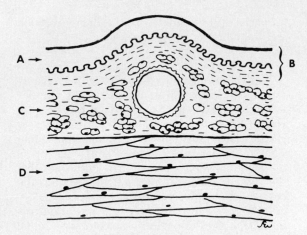

Fig. 3-14. Diagram of a freely movable mass. An example of this type of mass is the epidermoid cyst, which can be moved freely in all directions by digital pressure. *A*, Stratified squamous epithelium; *B*, mucosa or skin; *C*, loose connective tissue layer; *D*, skeletal muscle.

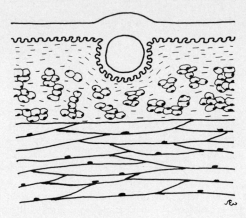

Fig. 3-15. Diagram of a mass attached to the skin. An example of this type of mass is the sebaceous cyst, which cannot be moved independent of the skin but is not attached to the deeper structures. This type of cyst thus can be moved as a unit with the skin.

cause, although they are not fixed to the underlying tissues, they are not bound to skin but are freely movable in all directions (unless fibrosis has resulted from a previous infection). These two cysts originate in nests of epithelium that have been trapped in the subcutaneous layer either during embryonic formation or as a result of a traumatic incident in which surface epithelial fragments were driven deep to the subepithelial layer.

On the other hand, sebaceous cysts would be high on the list of possibilities since they are freely movable over underlying tissues but are bound to the skin. This diagnosis is logical if one considers that sebaceous cysts form when sebaceous units of the skin become blocked but retain their continuity with the cystic glandular elements and the skin (Fig. 3-15).

A contrary set of circumstances might be observed when the skin is found to be freely movable over the mass but the mass is bound to the deeper structures. This situation then poses a question relative to the structures to which the mass is bound. It could be attached to muscle, bone, cartilage, fat, salivary gland, or thyroid gland. The tissue or organ to which the mass is most intimately attached will most often prove to be the tissue of origin (Fig. 3-16). For example, if the mass is located in or bound to the parotid gland, the most likely possibility is that it is of salivary gland origin.

If the mass is bound to the skin or mucosa and also to the underlying structures, however, there are only four possibilities:

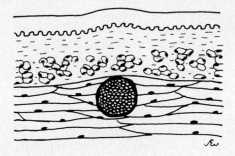

Fig. 3-16. Diagram of a mass attached to muscle. A rhabdomyoma is an example of this type of mass, which cannot be moved independent of the involved muscle but is not fixed to the skin or mucous membrane.

1. Fibrosis after a previous inflammatory episode
2. An infiltrating malignant tumor that originated in the skin or mucous membrane and has invaded the deep structures (Fig. 3-17)
3. A malignancy that originated in a deep structure and has invaded the subcutaneous or submucosal tissue and the skin or mucosa
4. A malignancy that originated in the loose connective tissue and has invaded both the superficial and the deep layers

When examining the oral cavity, the diagnostician should remember that under normal conditions the mucosa covering the hard palate and the gingivae is bound tightly to the under-

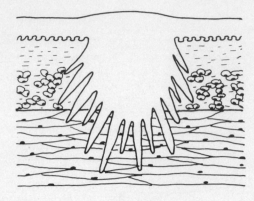

Fig. 3-17. Diagram of an epithelial mass—fixed to all layers of tissue. An invasive squamous cell carcinoma at this stage fixes the skin or mucous membrane to the deeper tissues.

lying bone. In addition, the loose submucosal layer under the papillated, keratinized, stratified squamous epithelium of the dorsal surface of the tongue is very thin and frequently nonexistent; the epithelial layer is therefore actually bound closely to the underlying tongue musculature. Hence the mucosa of the dorsal surface cannot normally be moved independent of the deeper muscular part. In the remaining regions of the oral cavity, however, there is a substantial loose submucosal layer, which, in the absence of disease, permits the surface epithelial layer to be moved independent of the deeper tissues and structures.

The palpation of a mass during function frequently reveals whether the mass is fixed to deeper structures—and if so, which ones. The mass in question is palpated while the patient demonstrates the normal movements of the region. For example, if a fluctuant mass in the anterior midline of the neck moves up and down as the patient swallows, it may be diagnosed as part of, or attached to, the hyoid bone, larynx, trachea, thyroid or parathyroid gland, or intervening muscles. If it elevates when the patient protrudes his tongue, the examiner may suspect that it is a thyroglossal cyst and that a persistent epithelial or fibrous cord or a fistula is leading to the tongue. (These are not always present in patients with thyroglossal cysts, however, so if a mass does not elevate on protrusion of the tongue, a thyroglossal duct cyst is not necessarily ruled out.)

In some cases a mass may encroach on adjacent moving structures and impair or limit movement. For example, a chondroma or hyperplasia of the condyle may produce deviation and limitation of jaw movements.

EXTENT

The determination of the foregoing characteristics by palpation is important not only for masses located below the surface but also for visible superficial lesions.

Clinicians must always bear in mind that what is visible may represent just the "tip of the iceberg." Consequently it is important that the tissue surrounding and underlying the bases of these apparent surface lesions be carefully palpated to determine the maximum extension of the lesion into adjacent tissues. Of course, positive identification of small cellular areas of penetration into the surrounding tissue can be made only by microscopic examination, but the surgeon must grossly estimate the extent of penetration of the surrounding tissue by palpation before surgery.

Whether a mass will have poorly defined, moderately defined, or well-defined borders, as determined by palpation, will depend on four factors:
1. Border characteristics of the mass
2. Relative consistency of the surrounding tissues
3. Thickness and nature of the overlying tissue
4. Sturdiness of the underlying tissue

Borders of the mass. Malignancies usually have ill-defined borders that are extremely difficult to detect by palpation. This observation is readily evident if we consider two features characteristic of these disorders:
1. Malignant tumors often infiltrate adjacent tissue by extending many *processes of tumor* into the surrounding normal tissue.
2. Malignant tumors also produce a *scirrhous reaction* in the infiltrated tissue.

The processes of the tumor are irregular in size, shape, and distribution. The result is an irregular and vague outline. These extensions also anchor the neoplasm to neighboring tissue and thus preclude the possibility that the tumor may be moved manually independent of its surroundings.

The tumor, with its extensions, elicits an inflammatory reaction in the adjacent tissue that is somewhat similar to an allergic or foreign body reaction. This inflammatory reaction results in the sequela of fibrosis. The fibrosis develops in the irregular and diffuse areas that are inflamed and results in a more tenacious binding of the tumor to the adjacent tissues, by an ill-defined fibrous attachment whose limits are impossible to perceive by manipulation of the mass.

One exception involves some of the slow-growing malignancies that develop definable fibrous borders. The borders are composed of (1) connective tissue from the stroma of the dislodged normal tissue and (2) fibrous tissue newly formed in response to the tumor. These masses have borders that may be detected and delineated by palpation.

Inflammation occurs much more frequently as a response to other insults than as a response to malignant tumors, and it usually has poorly defined borders regardless of etiology.

Inflammation in a nonencapsulated organ or tissue seldom develops a smooth, well-defined border, and the subsequent scarring in the areas of resolved inflammation will duplicate the limits of the inflammatory process, which are vague and irregular. On the contrary, if the inflammation of an encapsulated organ or tissue is confined within the capsule, the margins of the affected tissue will possess the well-defined characteristics of the encapsulated organ.

Also the resolution of the inflammation as well as reparative scarring within the capsule (e.g., a lymph node, the parotid gland) will result in a mass with a well-defined detectable border. This, of course, is a consequence of the enclosing and restricting action of the capsule. If the inflammation breaks through the capsule and involves the surrounding tissue, however, the resultant extracapsular fibrosis will render the mass fixed to the surrounding tissue and the borders may then be ill defined. The postinflammatory fixed lymph node would be an example of such a process.

Whether the limits of a pathologic process can be well defined by palpation will depend significantly on the shape of the lesion as well as on the nature of its borders. Of course, to determine the exact extent of a thin lesion or any lesion with a flattened, feather-edged border is difficult. On the other hand, the limits of a plump lesion (e.g., spherical mixed tumor) are relatively easy to detect.

CONSISTENCY OF SURROUNDING TISSUE

The consistency or the degree of firmness of a lesion, in contrast to that of its surrounding tissue, will also affect the ease with which the lesion itself or its borders may be identified by palpation.

For example, the borders of a firm dermoid cyst occurring in loose subcutaneous tissue can be readily determined, whereas to ascertain the borders of a relatively soft lipoma when it occurs in the same type of loose connective tissue is difficult, if not impossible.

The same relative situation often pertains in the case of a firm mass occurring on or around the borders of a muscle. If the surrounding normal tissue is of the same consistency as the pathologic mass, the borders cannot by determined. Again the determination of the exact proportions of firm masses or lesions in the oral cavity that are situated over bone, and especially where mobility over the bone cannot be demonstrated, will prove to be extremely difficult by palpation. Regardless of the physical circumstance attending the palpation of a lesion in or over bone, determining the extent of bony involvement without a radiograph is impossible.

When a radiograph indicates some degree of bone loss, identifying the site of origin as being soft tissue or bone itself without a biopsy may be difficult and often impossible. Even when the microscopic diagnosis is fibrosarcoma, the clinician still cannot be certain of the origin of the mass. If an adequate radiographic examination does not reveal a radiolucency in the bone, the clinician can proceed on the assumption that the lesion in question most likely has originated in the soft tissue.

THICKNESS OF OVERLYING TISSUE

Clearly, to determine by palpation the physical characteristics of a superficial mass is much easier than to make a similar determination of a deep mass. Also it is apparent that overlying dense fibrous tissue or tensed muscle tissue will obscure and may even obliterate the characteristic features of a lesion.

As an example, the borders of a branchial cleft cyst lying superficial to the sternocleidomastoid muscle may be readily delineated and the mass is soft and fluctuant. In contrast, if the cyst lies beneath the sternocleidomastoid muscle, its borders may not be defined by palpation and the cystic mass feels firm and nonfluctuant. A covering of bone or cartilage, of course, precludes the palpation of an underlying mass, although if the mass has expanded the bone or cartilage, its presence may be suspected.

STURDINESS OF UNDERLYING TISSUE

If the tissue underlying a mass is bone, cartilage, dense fibrous tissue, or tensed muscle, the true physical characteristics of the mass are more readily determined and the margins, if discrete, easier to delineate by the palpation. On the other hand, soft tissue platforms that fail to support a mass for adequate manipulation may confuse the examiner concerning the characteristics of the mass. Fortunately, firm platforms for palpation are present in most regions of the body.

SIZE AND SHAPE

The examiner determines the size and shape of a protuberant lesion by inspecting it or measuring it with a millimeter rule. In addition, a careful history frequently indicates the duration of the growth; on the basis of the present size, the growth rate can be approximated, which information may be of significant value. Likewise, the history helps to establish whether a lesion is increasing in size at a steady rate, whether it is paroxysmal and predictable (like a retention phenomenon of the parotid gland, which enlarges just before eating), or whether it drains intermittently (like a rupturing abscess, which periodically decreases in size).

When masses are located within a tissue, however, palpation is necessary to determine their approximate size and shape. Round or ovoid masses are generally cysts, early benign tumors, or enlarged lymph nodes. Primary malignant tumors of lymph nodes and also early metastatic tumors of lymph nodes are usually round or ovoid with a smooth border. As indicated, irregularly shaped masses are most likely to be inflammatory fibrotic conditions or malignant tumors.

CONSISTENCY

Consistency provides one of the most important clues to the identification of the tissue, organ, or pathosis that the examiner may encounter during the physical examination. Since the examiner must be as familiar with the texture and compressibility of normal tissue as with those of abnormal tissue, a description of the normal is given in Table 3-2.

The following terms are commonly used to define the consistency of tissue: soft, cheesy, rubbery, firm, and bony hard. The term *soft* is associated with easily compressible tissue such as a lipoma or a mucocele. Cysts filled with thin fluid are generally soft, but if they are under tension, they are rubbery. *Cheesy* indicates a somewhat firmer tissue that gives a more granular sensation but no rebound. *Rubbery* describes a tissue that is firm but can be compressed slightly and rebounds to its normal contour as soon as the pressure is withdrawn, such as skin. *Firm* identifies a tissue, such as fibrous tissue, that cannot be readily compressed. *Bony hard* is self-explanatory.

Needless to say, there are examples in each category that are borderline and appear to overlap adjacent categories, so it may not always be possible to explicitly describe a consistency with one of these terms. However, they are universally employed and, in general, connote a similar meaning to most individuals.

At least three different factors can modify the consistency of a tissue or mass as perceived by palpation:

1. A thick layer of overlying tissue, especially muscle or fibrous tissue, will appreciably modify or mask the true nature of a mass.
2. Soft glandular tissue surrounded by a dense connective capsule will be perceived firmer than it otherwise would be and is.
3. The depth in the tissue will alter the consistency sensed by palpation; that is, a soft mass will seem firmer if it is deeper in the tissue than it would feel if it were situated more superficially.

Table 3-2. Consistency of normal tissues and organs*

Consistency	Tissues or organs
Soft	Adipose tissue
	Fasciae
	Veins
	Loose connective tissue
	Glandular tissue, minor salivary glands, and sublingual salivary gland
Cheesy	Brain tissue
Rubbery	Skin
	Relaxed muscle
	Glandular tissue with capsule
	Arteries and arterioles
	Liver
Firm	Fibrous tissue
	Tensed muscle
	Large nerves
	Cartilage†
Bony hard	Bone
	Enamel
	Dentin
	Cementum
	Cartilage†

*Many normal tissues and organs, e.g., dental pulp, thyroid and parathyroid glands, lymph nodes, and lymphatic vessels, usually cannot be palpated under normal conditions, so they have not been categorized here.

†Cartilage is difficult to classify; it seems to fall into an intermediate category, being too firm to be included in the firm group and not firm enough to be placed in the bony hard group.

Each tissue's consistency correlates so well with its microstructure that the examiner should at least be familiar with the microstructure as revealed by histologic examination. To demonstrate the close correlation between texture and histology, the microscopic anatomies of examples from each group of consistencies are shown together in Fig. 3-18 for comparison.

Once the examiner has become familiar with the location and consistency of normal tissues and organs, he or she will be quite capable of differentiating between normal and abnormal tissue when a consistency is detected that contrasts with the expected consistency of the tissue being palpated.

The consistency of abnormal tissue can be described with the same terms as those used for characterizing normal tissue: soft, cheesy, rubbery, firm, and bony hard. Representative segments of pathologic masses have been selected and categorized according to consistency in Table 3-3. Again, in an effort to underscore the correlation between microstructure and physical consistency, photomicrographs of pathologic tissues and similar consistencies have been grouped together in Fig. 3-19.

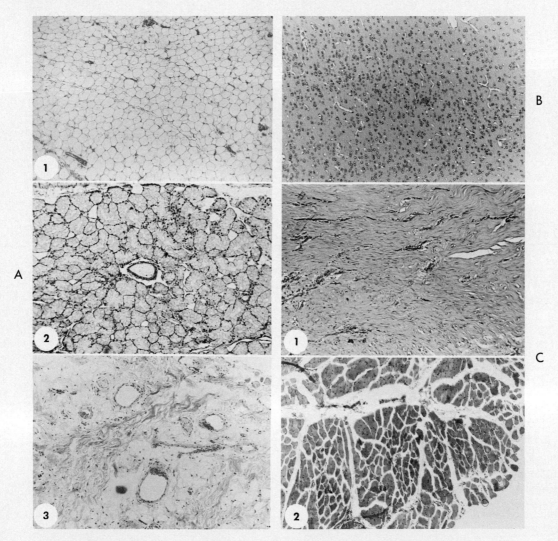

Fig. 3-18. Normal tissues categorized according to consistency. The general appearance of the following normal tissues at low magnification reflects the consistency of the tissue to palpation. **A,** Tissues with soft consistency: *1,* adipose tissue; *2,* unencapsulated mucous glands; *3,* loose connective tissue; note the presence of thin-walled vessels. **B,** Tissue with cheesy consistency: brain tissue. **C,** Tissues with firm consistency: *1,* fibrous tissue; *2,* skeletal muscle; tensed muscle feels firm whereas relaxed muscle feels rubbery.

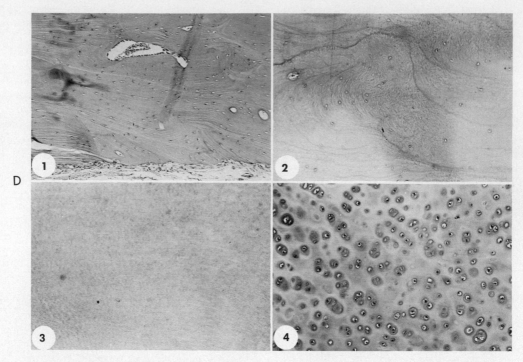

Fig. 3-18, cont'd. D, Tissues with bony hard consistency: *1,* bone; *2,* cementum; *3,* dentin; *4,* cartilage.

Table 3-3. Consistency of pathologic masses

Lesions	*Exceptions*
SOFT	
Cysts	Cysts under tension—rubbery
	Infected and fibrosed cysts—firm
	Sebaceous cysts, keratocysts, and dermoid cysts—cheesy
Warthin's tumors and papillary cystic adenomas	Occasionally sclerosed types firm in some areas
Vascular tumors and phenomena	Sclerosing types—firm
Hemangiomas, lymphangiomas, varicosities, and cystic hygromas	Hemangioendotheliomas—firm
	Hemangiosarcomas—firm
Fatty tumors	Sclerosing types of liposarcoma—firm
Lipomas, hibernomas, xanthomas, and liposarcomas	
Myxomas	None
Plexiform neurofibromas	None
Inflammatory hyperplasias (granulomatous stage)	Fibrosed types—firm
Emphysemas	None
Laryngoceles	None
Retention phenomena	If high tension, rubbery
Mucoceles and ranulas	If fibrosed, firm
CHEESY	
Cysts	Infected and fibrosed types—firm or alternate areas
Sebaceous, dermoid, and epidermoid	of cheesiness and firmness
Tuberculous nodes	Early or late tuberculosis nodes—firm

Table 3-3. Consistency of pathologic masses—cont'd

Lesions	Exceptions
RUBBERY	
Cysts with contents under tension	None
Lymphomas	None
Myomas	None
Myoblastomas	Those with severe pseudoepitheliomatous hyperplasia—firm
Aneurysms	None
Pyogenic space infection	Early stages—firm
Edematous tissue	None
Early hematomas	If not much tension, soft
FIRM	
Infection Streptococcus, early staphylococcus, early actinomycosis, and histoplasmosis	None
Benign tumors of soft tissue Fibromas, neurofibromas, schwannomas, and amputation neuromas	Fatty tumors, plexiform neurofibromas, myxomas, and hemangiomas
Malignancies of soft tissues Squamous cell carcinomas, melanomas, fibrosarcomas, and sclerosing liposarcomas	None
Osteosarcomas	Occasionally bony hard
Chondrosarcomas	Occasionally bony hard
Metastatic carcinomas	Occasionally (osteoblastic, metastatic, and prostatic carcinomas) bony hard
Benign and malignant salivary gland tumors	Warthin's tumors and papillary cyst adenomas—soft Occasionally mucoepidermoid tumors with alternate soft and firm areas
Inflammation and infection of parotid and submaxillary salivary glands	None
Inflammation and infection of lymph nodes	Caseous or liquefied nodes—soft and cheesy
BONY HARD	
Osteomas	None
Exostoses	None
Osteogenic sarcomas	Undifferentiated—firm
Pleomorphic adenomas occasionally	Usually firm
Chondromas	Occasionally firm
Chondrosarcomas	Occasionally firm
Osteoblastic, metastatic, and prostatic carcinomas, occasionally	Usually firm

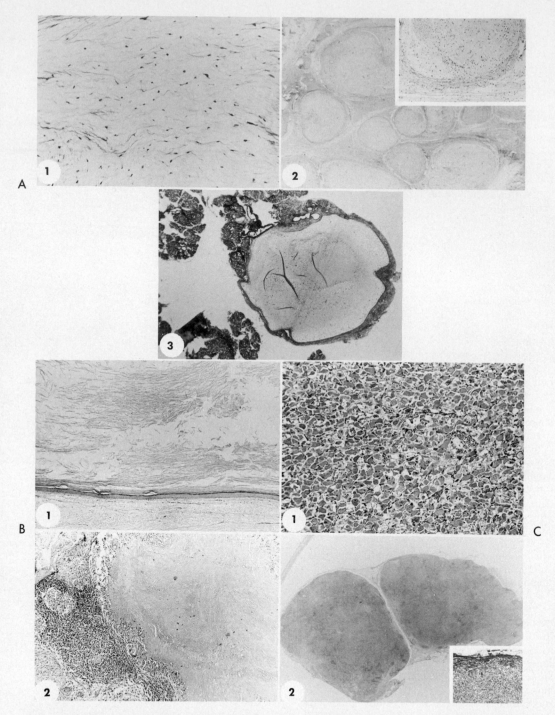

Fig. 3-19. Pathologic tissues categorized according to consistency. The general appearance of each of the following pathologic tissues at low magnification reflects the consistency of the tissue to palpation. **A,** Soft consistency: *1,* myxoma; *2,* plexiform neurofibroma (low and high magnifications); *3,* ranula. **B,** Cheesy consistency: *1,* epidermoid cyst; note that the lumen is filled with keratin, which imparts the cheesy consistency; *2,* tuberculous node; the large amorphous area is caseation necrosis, which imparts the cheesy consistency. **C,** Rubbery consistency: *1,* rhabdomyoma; *2,* lymphoma; the lymph node capsule helps to impart the rubbery consistency to this entity.

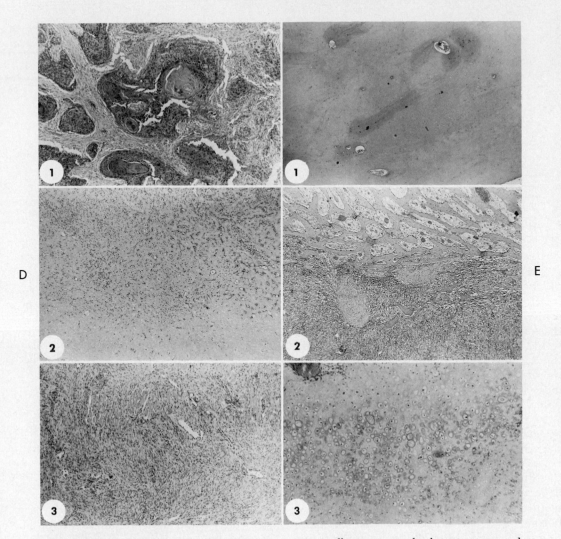

Fig. 3-19, cont'd. **D,** Firm consistency: *1*, squamous cell carcinoma; the keratin nests and surrounding fibrous tissue contribute to the firmness of this lesion; *2*, pleomorphic adenoma; the generous amount of hyaline in this tissue is responsible for the firmness; occasionally cartilage and bone are present in this type of tumor and impart a bony hardness to some areas; *3*, fibrosarcoma; the amount of dense fibrous tissue imparts the firmness to this lesion. **E,** Bony hard consistency: *1*, torus; *2*, osteogenic sarcoma; frequently new bone formation and the production of fibrous tissue contribute to the consistency of this tumor; *3*, chondrosarcoma.

FLUCTUANCE AND EMPTIABILITY

All soft, cheesy, or rubbery lesions or masses over 1 cm in diameter should be tested for fluctuance. This is done by placing the sensing fingers of one hand on one side of the mass and gently pressing on the mass with the probing fingers of the other hand. If the sensing fingers can detect a wave or force passing through the lesion, the mass is said to be fluctuant (Fig. 3-20). The following four factors determine whether fluctuance can be perceived in a soft, cheesy, or rubbery lesion (Table 3-4):

1. *The mass must contain liquid or gas in a relatively enclosed cavity* (Fig. 3-20). Examples of such fluctuant masses are cysts, mucoceles, ranulas, pyogenic space abscesses, early hematomas, subcutaneous emphysemas, varicosities, Warthin's tumors, papillary cyst adenomas, lipomas, and plexiform neurofibromas (Fig. 3-21). Although a lipoma and a plexiform neurofibroma do not have a true lumen containing a fluid, the high liquid content of the cells and interstitial tissue is apparently sufficient to produce fluctuance in these tumors.

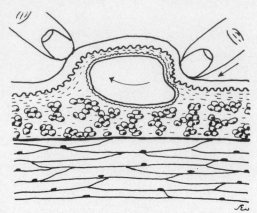

Fig. 3-20. Diagram illustrating fluctuance in a cyst-like lesion.

2. *The mass must be located in a superficial plane.* If the mass is covered by a thick layer of relatively inflexible tissue or a structure such as a muscle, it cannot be palpated in a manner that might demonstrate fluctuance. An example would be a branchial cleft cyst situated under the sternocleidomastoid muscle. In this position its fluctuance would be obscured, as might most of its other characteristics that could be determined by palpation (Fig. 3-22).

3. *The mass must be in a fluctuant stage.* Many clinical lesions represent a fluctuant stage in a multiphasic disease process. Earlier, however, in the development of the disorder, the fluid-filled cavity may not have formed; later, during the resolution, the required architecture on which fluctuance depends may have become altered or obliterated. This may be either the natural history of the disease or the result of treatment. For example, an odontogenic staphylococcal infection that has broken through the cortical plates and commenced to involve the adjacent soft tissue is tender, red, and firm. As the process continues, pus produced by the typical staphylococcal space infection results in a soft, fluctuant, painful, nonemptiable mass. As the abscess resolves, regardless of the treatment, the fluctuant stage gives way to a firm stage and the firm stage may either disappear completely or leave a small area of fibrosis. Actinomycosis often demonstrates the same cycle, as do infected cysts to some extent.

4. *Developing fibrosis around the mass may obscure the fluctuance.* Chronically infected cysts that flare up from time to time often lose their fluctuance and become hard and tender. This is an example in which inflammation and the resulting fibrosis around a fluid-filled cavity can mask fluctuance. Occasionally the epithelial lining and the lumen are completely de-

Table 3-4. Characteristics of soft, cheesy, or rubbery masses

Lesions	Fluctuant	Emptiable
Cysts	Yes	No
Abscesses	Yes	No
Mucoceles	Yes	No
Ranulas	Yes	No
Early hematomas	Yes	No
Subcutaneous emphysemas	Yes	No
Lipomas	Yes	No
Plexiform neuro-fibromas	Yes	No
Myxomas	Yes	No
Papillary cystic adenomas	Yes	No
Warthin's tumors	Yes	No
Varicosities	Variable	Variable
Cystic hygromas	Variable	Variable
Laryngoceles	Variable	Variable
Capillary hemangiomas*	Variable	Variable
Lymphangiomas	Usually	Usually not
Cavernous hemangiomas	Usually not	Usually
Aneurysms	No	Yes
Draining cysts	No	Yes
Draining abscesses	No	Yes
Inflammatory hyperplasias	No	No

*Capillary hemangiomas are often less than 1 cm in diameter and are usually too small for fluctuance to be accurately detected.

stroyed, so the basic requirement for fluctuance, a fluid-filled cavity, is lost.

Lesions demonstrating variable fluctuance. A large group of the soft and rubbery lesions demonstrate variable fluctuance. This is almost always related to the degree of emptiability that a particular lesion has. In other words, some lesions are fluctuant whereas others of the same variety are not. All soft, cheesy, or rubbery lesions can be classified according to emptiability.

1. Some cannot be emptied at all by digital pressure (Fig. 3-23).
2. Others, such as hemangiomas, cystic hygromas, lymphangiomas, and laryngoceles, may show fluctuance or emptiability, depending on the individual structural characteristics of the specific lesion.
3. Still others, including aneurysms, most cavernous hemangiomas, draining cysts, and draining space abscesses, are usually nonfluctuant and completely emptiable with ease. They rarely develop an architecture that results in fluctuance.

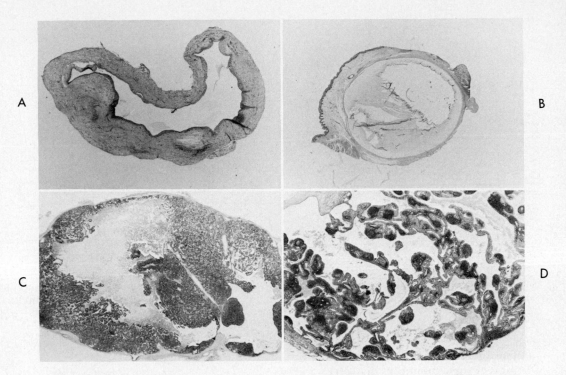

Fig. 3-21. Fluctuant pathologic masses. **A,** Radicular cyst. **B,** Mucocele. **C,** Papillary cyst adenoma. **D,** Warthin's tumor (papillary cystadenoma lymphomatosum).

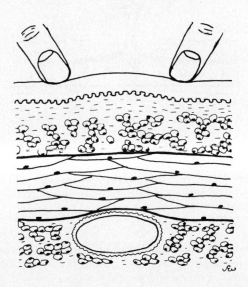

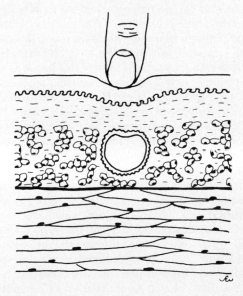

Fig. 3-22. Diagram of muscle overlying a cyst and masking its characteristics.

Fig. 3-23. Diagram illustrating a nonemptiable cyst-like lesion.

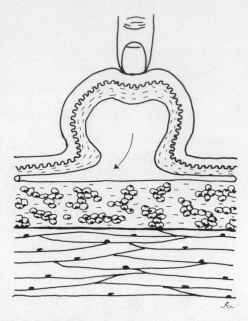

Fig. 3-24. Diagram illustrating complete emptiability in an aneurysm-like lesion.

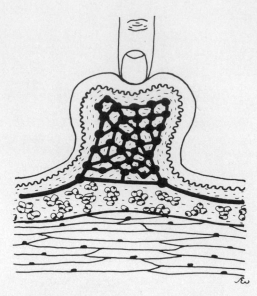

Fig. 3-25. Diagram illustrating the difficulty encountered in attempting to completely empty a capillary hemangioma, which has many small channels and few exit vessels.

A number of factors influence the emptiability of a mass: course, number, diameter, and position of exit vessels or channels. Also the width of the base of a lesion relates to the ease with which the lesion can be emptied.

Fig. 3-24 shows a diagram of an aneurysm. Note that the aneurysm could be readily emptied by digital pressure. The usual cavernous hemangioma is similar in this respect. The cavernous spaces are large but few. The exit channels are large, and the base of the lesion is sessile. Such a hemangioma would not demonstrate fluctuance, since it has all the features that permit rapid and complete emptying.

Fig. 3-25, by contrast, is a diagram representing a capillary hemangioma with many blood sinuses connected by small vessels. Note that the exit vessels are few and small and the base is somewhat pedunculated. A hemangioma of this type would probably not be readily emptied by digital pressure, since the slight pressure that would deform the lesion would also tend to occlude the small exit vessels. Thus the lesion would consequently be partially fluctuant and partially emptiable.

Fig. 3-26 is also an illustration of a capillary hemangioma that probably could not be emptied at all. The laryngocele, a developmental pouch projecting from the larynx, is inflated with air when the patient coughs. Frequently the connecting channel to the larynx is small

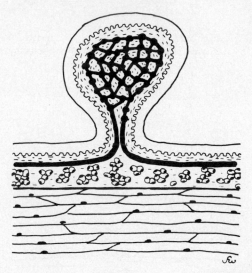

Fig. 3-26. Diagram illustrating a pedunculated capillary hemangioma, which would be nonemptiable by digital pressure.

and easily occluded, and although the laryngocele usually shows fluctuance, it can be slowly emptied by careful digital pressure. A cyst also would be fluctuant but not emptiable since a channel for the egress of the fluid is not a usual feature of this lesion.

Position or location of the examiner's finger or fingers is important in determining whether

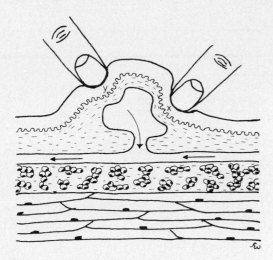

Fig. 3-27. Diagram illustrating the importance of finger position when attempting to empty a lesion with this configuration. Careful pressure applied at point Y would readily empty the lesion, whereas rapid pressure applied at point X would tend to occlude the exit channel and render the lesion nonemptiable.

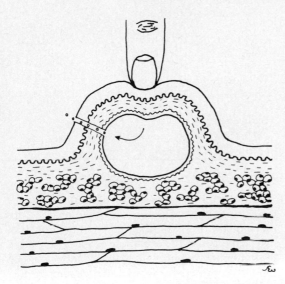

Fig. 3-28. Diagram illustrating the presence of a sinus draining a cyst or abscess. This causes a usually fluctuant lesion to become nonfluctuant and emptiable.

a lesion can be emptied or not. In Fig. 3-27 the examiner's finger at point X would block the efferent channel and mask the fact that the lesion is really emptiable. This lesion would empty readily, however, with digital pressure if the finger were positioned at point Y.

The reason for the emptiability of a draining cyst or abscess is obvious and is illustrated in Fig. 3-28. Such a lesion generally is not fluctuant unless the opening is quite small.

PAINLESS, TENDER, OR PAINFUL

During the digital examination it becomes apparent whether a mass is painless, tender, or painful. This information aids greatly in arranging a suitable list of diagnostic possibilities. In the development of a working diagnosis, it is helpful if the painful mass is evaluated on the basis of the following possible etiologies (Table 3-5):

1. *Pain because of inflammation.* The painful effect of an increase in the fluid content of a tissue by a pathologic agent is intensified when the tissue is confined within rigid or semirigid walls (dental pulp, lymph node, submaxillary or parotid salivary glands). The increased internal pressure that results from the interstitial accumulation of fluid is intensified by the external pressure of the examiner's fingers and is registered as pain or an increase in pain.

The most frequently encountered example is, of course, an inflammatory process resulting from mechanical trauma or infection. Occasionally a tumor, especially of the malignant variety, indirectly causes pain by infiltrating a major duct of a major salivary gland—thereby inducing a retention phenomenon and an enlarged salivary gland that is tender or painful because of the markedly increased internal pressure. Occasionally also a tumor confined by adjacent normal tissue will become secondarily infected and thus change from a painless to an inflamed and painful lesion.

2. *Painful tumors.* Some neural tumors (e.g., the amputation neuroma, which actually is not a true neoplasm but represents an overexuberant misdirected repair process in a severed nerve) are commonly painful to palpation. As a general rule, however, benign and malignant tumors are painless masses unless they are traumatized or secondarily infected.

3. *Pain because of sensory nerve encroachment.* Masses otherwise painless but located near relatively large sensory nerves may elicit pain when they rapidly enlarge and encroach on the nerve space. This most frequently happens when the nerve pathway is bone as opposed to soft tissue; in soft tissue, especially when the process is slow growing, the nerve is pushed ahead of the mass and pain is not elicited until an unyielding tissue is encountered. Occasionally a rapidly growing malignant tumor, such as an osteosarcoma growing within the bone, will cause pain because it expands more rapidly than the bone can be resorbed.

Table 3-5. Painless, tender, and painful masses

Lesions	Exceptions
PAINLESS	
Benign and malignant tumors	Amputation neuromas
	Adenoid cystic carcinomas
	Chondrosarcomas within bone occasionally
	Infected tumors
	Traumatized tumors
	Tumors pressing nerves
Cysts	Traumatized lesions
Benign hyperplasias	Traumatized lesions
Vascular phenomena, aneurysms, etc.	Traumatized lesions
Laryngoceles	Traumatized lesions
Late hematomas	Traumatized lesions
Sarcoidosis and tuberculosis	Traumatized lesions
Retention phenomena in nonencapsulated glands	Traumatized lesions
TENDER	
Low-grade inflammations or infections	None
Mild physical trauma	
Retention phenomena in encapsulated glands	
Bacterial, viral, fungal, and rickettsial infections	
Mononucleosis	Occasionally nontender
Early hematomas	Occasionally nontender
Subcutaneous emphysemas	Occasionally nontender
Mikulicz's disease	Occasionally nontender
Sjögren's syndrome	Occasionally nontender
PAINFUL	
Acutely inflamed tissue	None
Severe physical trauma and acute infections	
Infected cysts	Those with draining sinuses
Infected tumors	None
Tumors	
Amputation neuromas	Early stage
Adenoid cystic carcinomas	Early stage
Chondrosarcomas	Peripheral

Hence the pressure on the surrounding bone and nerve tissue evokes pain.

Usually, however, the pain produced by the encroachment of a malignant tumor on a sensory nerve is of short duration, since the rapidly growing tumor causes its early destruction. An exception is the adenoid cystic carcinoma, which frequently spreads through the perineural space. Pain is usually of long duration with these untreated tumors because they may travel along the periphery of but seldom invade the nerve.

Tenderness in a mass usually indicates the presence of a low-grade inflammation and internal pressure, which in practice are frequently induced by the repeated manipulation of a painless mass by a series of examiners. Frequently, however, a tender mass indicates the presence of a chronic infection.

The degree of pain that a mass produces often varies, depending on the stage of development of the mass or the type of infection that may have caused the pain. For example, a retention phenomenon of major glands may be tender in the early stages but become exquisitely painful as the situation worsens. Untreated bacterial infections are typically tender in the early stage, painful in the acute phase, and tender during resolution. Fungal, spirochetal, tuberculous, rickettsial, and viral infections, on the other hand, are more typically chronic in their nature and are tender only throughout the course of their development and resolution. Hence an infection of a node that demonstrates the same level of tenderness for a prolonged period is unlikely to be bacterial, especially if the patient has not received treatment. On the contrary, the tender node that becomes acutely painful and then resolves is frequently an example of a bacterial infection.

The foregoing discussion notwithstanding, a bacterial infection of a tissue caused by a virulent resistant organism that is being unsuccessfully treated may remain tender for a prolonged period.

UNILATERAL OR BILATERAL

Whether a lesion is unilateral or bilateral can be determined by inspection and palpation. When a clinician encounters pathosis, he or she should investigate the contralateral region of the body for the purpose of determining whether the condition is bilateral. As a general rule, if similar masses are present bilaterally and in the same locations, they are most likely normal anatomic structures. The carotid bulb in the bifurcation of the artery, the mastoid process, the lateral processes of the cervical vertebrae, and the wings of the hyoid bone are such bilaterally occurring anatomic structures that are frequently mistaken for pathologic masses. Bilateral palpation coupled with a knowledge of anatomy is obligatory if these normal structures are to be differentiated from pathologic masses.

SOLITARY OR MULTIPLE

A solitary lesion nearly always indicates a local benign condition or an early malignancy. Multiple lesions, on the other hand, must alert the examiner to the following possibilities:

Addison's disease
Blood dyscrasias
Hodgkin's disease
Infectious mononucleosis
Multiple fungal infections
Multiple metastases
Paget's disease
Reticuloendotheliosis

The syndromes with multiple lesions should also be considered:

Albright's syndrome
Basal cell nevus syndrome
Gardner's syndrome
Peutz-Jeghers syndrome
Syndrome of multiple neuromas, carcinoma of the thyroid, and pheochromocytoma
von Recklinghausen's disease

A more complete list is presented at the beginning of Chapter 10.

Features obtained by percussion

Percussion is the act of tapping a part of the body to evaluate the quality of the echo produced. The physician routinely percusses the chest to determine the outline of the heart and also to evaluate the lung fields. The dentist frequently percusses teeth to determine whether they have adequate bone support and to determine whether they are sensitive. Percussion is not particularly useful, however, for the examination of the lesions discussed in this text.

Features obtained by auscultation

Auscultation is the act of listening with or without the aid of a stethoscope to sounds produced inside the body. The physician routinely auscultates the chest to evaluate heart and lung sounds. The dentist may auscultate the temporomandibular joint to detect crepitus. Auscultation of pathologic masses is to be encouraged because this method detects the presence of bruits, which are a characteristic of aneurysms and arteriovenous shunts.

BIBLIOGRAPHY

Dolby AE: Oral mucosa in health and disease, Oxford, Eng., 1975, Blackwell Scientific Publications.

Whitten JB: Cytologic examination of aspirated material from cysts or cystlike lesions, Oral Surg 25:710-716, 1968.

4

The diagnostic sequence

NORMAN K. WOOD

PAUL W. GOAZ

It is of paramount importance that the clinician confronted by a lesion initiate a precisely formulated diagnostic sequence. Such an established approach to the perception, examination, and conception of a set of circumstances helps to ensure two safeguards: first, when a definite and methodical diagnostic procedure is formulated and followed, *all the pertinent features* will be identified; second, by adapting and following a routine, the dentist accomplishes the total procedure *rapidly as well as effectively*.

Some authorities argue that the experienced diagnostician does not rely on such a cumbersome and formal procedure, since he or she is apparently able to diagnose a lesion after only a brief inspection. This is seldom if ever the case, however, because generally expertise is based not on instant recognition but on the rapid and effective use of a diagnostic sequence perfected through experience. Of course, the astute diagnostician has seen many lesions on numerous occasions and is thus able to anticipate the nature of a familiar disorder and still maintain an excellent "batting average."

We have found the following diagnostic sequence to be both effective and practical:

Detection and examination of the patient's lesion
Examination of the patient
  Chief complaint(s)
  Onset and course
Reexamination of the lesion
Classification of the lesion
Listing the possible diagnoses
Developing the differential diagnosis
Developing the working diagnosis (operational
  diagnosis, tentative diagnosis, clinical impression)
Formulating the final diagnosis (proved by
  biopsy, culture, and/or response to treatment)

DETECTION AND EXAMINATION OF THE PATIENT'S LESION

Obviously a lesion must be detected before it is examined. Most lesions are discovered during routine examination, but in some cases, especially when pain or discomfort is a symptom, the patient is the first to become aware of the disorder and initiates its examination.

Once the clinician has recognized or at least suspects that an abnormal change is at hand, he or she proceeds to examine it using the modalities described in Chapters 2 and 3. These include visual examination in combination with palpation, percussion, and auscultation. The findings are noted and mentally evaluated. As a matter of personal preference, the clinician may elect to perform a cursory or a thorough examination of the lesion at this time, although the situation may dictate a thorough examination immediately. The importance of first examining the lesion is that the clinician can gain information that will alert him or her to look especially for possible related findings in the remainder of the patient examination.

EXAMINATION OF THE PATIENT

Patient examination has been discussed in depth in Chapters 2 and 3. Although the specific steps of examination of the patient are not detailed here, the sections of the interview dealing with the patient's chief complaint(s) and the onset and course of the present problem should be emphasized because they often yield particularly helpful diagnostic clues.

Chief complaint(s)

Common chief complaints related to oral diseases include sores, burning sensation, bleeding, loose teeth, recent occlusal problems, delayed tooth eruption, dry mouth, too much saliva, a swelling, bad taste, halitosis, paresthesia, and anesthesia.

PAIN

The patient should be encouraged to describe the main characteristics of the pain, its nature (sharp or dull), severity, duration, and location, and the precipitating circumstances.

The following entities may produce oral and facial pain:

1. Teeth
   a. Pulpal disease
   b. Pulpoperiapical disease
   c. Gingival and periodontal disease
2. Mucous membrane disease
3. Tongue conditions
4. Salivary gland inflammations and/or infection
5. Lesions of the jawbones
6. Lymph node inflammations and infections
7. Temporomandibular joint diseases
8. Myofascial pain syndrome
9. Maxillary sinus disease
10. Ear diseases
11. Psychoses
12. Angina pectoris
13. Tonsillar disease
14. Pretender (e.g., drug addict trying to obtain narcotics)
15. Central nervous system diseases
16. Neuralgias
17. Neuritis
18. Vasculitis
19. Berry aneurysms
20. Diaphragmatic hernia
21. Esophageal diverticulum
22. Eagle's syndrome (calcification of stylohyoid ligament)
23. Trotter's syndrome (pain caused by carcinoma of pharynx)

SORES

When a patient uses the term "sore" or "a sore" to describe a complaint, this may indicate the presence of mucosal inflammations or ulcers from any cause except early ulcerative malignancies (which are usually painless).

BURNING SENSATION

A burning sensation is usually felt in the tongue and is often caused by a thinning or erosion of the surface epithelium. The following disease states may produce a burning sensation:

1. Idiopathic burning tongue
2. Psychosis
3. Neurosis
4. Viral infection
5. Fungal infection
6. Chronic bacterial infection
7. Geographic tongue
8. Fissured tongue
9. Generalized oral mucositis diseases
10. Xerostomic conditions
11. Anemia
12. Achlorhydria
13. Multiple sclerosis
14. Vitamin deficiencies

A generalized burning sensation in the mouth is also frequently found to be associated with an increased interalveolar space.

BLEEDING

Intraoral bleeding may be caused by these disturbances:

1. Gingivitis and periodontal disease
2. Traumatic incidents, including surgery
3. Inflammatory hyperplasias
4. Allergies
5. Tumors (traumatized tumors and tumors that are very vascular, e.g., hemangiomas)
6. Diseases that cause or are associated with deficiencies in hemostasis

LOOSE TEETH

Loss of supporting bone or the resorption of roots may result in loose teeth and may indicate the presence of any of the following:

1. Periodontal disease
2. Trauma
3. Normal resorption of deciduous teeth
4. Pulpoperiapical lesions
5. Malignant tumors
6. Benign tumors that may induce root resorption (chondromas, myxomas, hemangiomas)
7. Histiocytosis X
8. Hypophosphatasia
9. Familial hypophosphatemia
10. Papillon-Lefèvre syndrome
11. Acquired immunodeficiency syndrome (AIDS)

RECENT OCCLUSAL PROBLEM

When a patient complains that "recently the teeth don't bite right" or "recently some teeth are out of line," the clinician must consider overcontoured restorations or the following:

1. Periodontal disease
2. Traumatic injury (fracture of bone or tooth root)
3. Periapical abscess
4. Cysts or tumors of tooth-bearing regions of the jaws
5. Fibrous dysplasia

DELAYED TOOTH ERUPTION

Delayed eruption of a tooth may be related to any of the following:

1. Malposed or impacted teeth
2. Cysts
3. Odontomas
4. Sclerosed bone
5. Tumors
6. Maldevelopment

If there is a generalized delay, the clinician should consider the possibilities of anodontia, cleidocranial dyplasia, or hypothyroidism.

DRY MOUTH (XEROSTOMIA)

A dry mouth may result from the following disorders:

1. Local inflammation
2. Infection and fibrosis of major salivary glands
3. Dehydration states
4. Drug therapy
   a. Tranquilizers
   b. Antihistamines
   c. Anticholinergics
5. Autoimmune diseases
   a. Mikulicz's disease
   b. Sjögren's syndrome
6. Chemotherapy
7. Postradiation changes
8. Psychosis

TOO MUCH SALIVA

The complaint of excessive saliva may be related to psychosomatic problems. It may be associated with the insertion of new dentures; if it continues, it may indicate a decreased or an increased vertical dimension.

A SWELLING

When a patient's chief complaint is a swelling, all of the following entities must be considered as a probable cause:

1. Inflammations and infections
2. Cysts
3. Retention phenomena
4. Inflammatory hyperplasias
5. Benign and/or malignant tumors

BAD TASTE

A complaint of bad taste may result from any of the following:

1. Aging changes
2. Heavy smoking
3. Poor oral hygiene
4. Dental caries
5. Periodontal disease
6. Acute necrotizing ulcerative gingivitis
7. Diabetes
8. Hypertension
9. Medication
10. Psychoses
11. Neurologic disorders
12. Decreased salivary flow
13. Uremia
14. Intraoral malignancies

HALITOSIS

Although this is more frequently classified as an objective symptom, we have included it here because of its close relationship to bad taste.

1. Poor oral hygiene
2. Periodontal disease
3. Third molar opercula
4. Decayed teeth
5. Acute necrotizing ulcerative gingivitis
6. Oral cancer
7. Spicy food
8. Tobacco use
9. Nasal infection
10. Sinus infection
11. Tonsillitis
12. Pharyngeal infections or tumors
13. Gastric problems
14. Diabetes
15. Uremia

PARESTHESIA AND ANESTHESIA

Such changes in sensation may be caused by any of the following:

1. Injury to regional nerves
   a. Anesthesia needles
   b. Jawbone fractures
   c. Surgical procedures
2. Malignancies
3. Medications
   a. Sedatives
   b. Tranquilizers
   c. Hypnotics
4. Diabetes
5. Pernicious anemia
6. Multiple sclerosis
7. Acute infection of the jawbone (unusual cause)
8. Psychoses

Onset and course

The following classification of onsets and courses related to the growth rate of specific masses has proved helpful to us:

1. Masses that increase in size just before eating
   a. Salivary retention phenomena
2. Slow-growing masses (duration of months to years)
   a. Reactive hyperplasias
   b. Chronic infections
   c. Cysts
   d. Benign tumors
3. Moderately rapid growing masses (weeks to about 2 months)
   a. Chronic infections
   b. Cysts
   c. Malignant tumors
4. Rapidly growing masses (hours to days)
   a. Abscesses (painful)
   b. Infected cysts (painful)
   c. Aneurysms (painless)
   d. Salivary retention phenomena (painless)
   e. Hematomas (painless but sting on pressure)
5. Masses with accompanying fever
   a. Infections
   b. Lymphomas

REEXAMINATION OF THE LESION

At this point in the examination, unanswered questions frequently occur to the clinician, who may want to reexamine the lesion to reevaluate the original findings or to complete more detailed observations. For example, if the lesion is found to be soft, he or she may wish to determine whether it (1) is fluctuant, (2) can be emptied, (3) blanches on pressure, (4) pulsates, or (5) produces a gas or liquid on aspiration and what the nature of the aspirate is. On the other hand, if the lesion is firm, the clinician may want to determine its extent, whether it is freely movable, whether it is fixed to the mucosa or the underlying tissue, and so on.

CLASSIFICATION OF THE LESION

By the time the clinician has reached this point in the diagnostic sequence, he or she should be able to classify the lesion according to whether it has originated in soft tissue or bone. Having arrived at a conclusion, he or she must next describe the lesion in terms of its clinical or radiographic appearance.

For example, the soft tissue lesions will be subclassified as white, exophytic, ulcerative, and so on, whereas the bony lesions may be categorized as periapical radiolucencies, cystlike radiolucencies, multiple radiopacities, and so on. Since the lesions in the ensuing pages of this text have been classified and the chapters organized on the basis of similar clinical or radiographic appearances, the clinician can use the same scheme to describe the lesion he or she encounters and thus facilitate reference between patient and book.

LIST OF THE POSSIBLE DIAGNOSES

When most of the available appropriate data have been collected, a list of all the lesions that may produce a similar clinical or radiographic picture should be compiled. Initially the order of the list is not important, since the primary objective of this step is merely to include every entity that is clinically and/or radiographically similar to the condition under study.

At this point in the diagnostic exercise, the clinician may find it convenient to refer to the list that begins each chapter. These previews are compilations of the entities that could fit into the general descriptive category of each chapter; they form, in turn, the chapter titles.

DEVELOPMENT OF THE DIFFERENTIAL DIAGNOSIS

The process of developing a differential diagnosis may be defined briefly in this discussion as the rearranging of the list of possible diagnoses, with the most probable lesion ranked at the top and the least likely at the bottom.

The actual process of ranking the lesions may become complicated as the clinician attempts to match the features of the lesion being examined with the usual (or characteristic) features of the specific lesions in his or her list. To become competent in the art of differential diagnosis, therefore, not only must the clinician be familiar with the signs and symptoms produced by a great many diseases but also he or she must possess some statistical knowledge relative to the incidence of each disease entity. It is particularly important that the clinician be aware of the relative incidences of individual lesions because in the completed differential diagnosis the most commonly occurring lesion will usually be ranked above the least commonly occurring unless other features prompt a modification of this ranking. The following researchers have reported on the frequency of lesions: Bouquot (1986), Goltry and Ryer (1986), and Weir et al. (1989).

Consequently, we strongly recommend that in developing the differential diagnosis, the clinician first rank the lesions in order of their *relative frequency of occurrence*, as they are in the list at the beginning of each chapter; however, he or she must realize that many conditions modify the general frequency: age, sex, race, country of origin, and anatomic location.

Age

The age of a patient will greatly modify the rankings. For example, an ulcer occurring in the floor of a 50-year-old man's mouth indicates a high probability of squamous cell carcinoma, but such a diagnosis would be unlikely if an ulcer occurred in a 10-year-old boy's mouth. Boxes on p. 56 and p. 57 group the soft tissue and bony lesions that tend to occur in patients within particular age spans. Hand and Whitehill (1987) discussed the prevalence of oral mucosal lesions in one elderly patient.

Sex

The fact that certain lesions occur more frequently in males or in females also contributes to the ranking of the lesions in the differential diagnosis. For example, squamous cell carcinoma affects males two to four times more often than females. On the other hand, about 80% of periapical cementomas occur in women over 30 years of age. Boxes on p. 58 group the soft tissue and bony lesions that show a predilection for occurring in female or male patients.

Predilection of soft tissue lesions for special age-groups

INFANTS

Candidiasis*
Eruption cyst
Hemangioma (85% by 1 year of age)
Lingual thyroid
Lymphangioma
Neuroectodermal tumor (before 6
  months of age)
White sponge nevus

CHILDREN

Albright's disease (ages 6-10)
Childhood infectious diseases
Eruption cyst
Infectious mononucleosis
Juvenile melanoma
Pulp polyps
White sponge nevus

PERSONS UNDER AGE 40

Albright's disease (ages 6-10)
ANUG (ages 15-35; rare below age 12)
Benign salivary gland tumor (ages 30-39)
Brachial cyst
Candidiasis
Childhood infectious diseases
Cystic hygroma
Dermoid or epidermoid cyst
Eruption cyst
Erythema multiforme
Hemangioma (85% by 1 year of age)
Hodgkin's disease (ages 20-40)
Infectious mononucleosis
Juvenile melanoma
Lingual thyroid
Lymphangioma (88% before age 3)
Mucocele (65% before age 30)
Neuroectodermal tumor (before 6
  months)

Palatal tori (peak before age 30)
Papilloma
Peripheral giant cell granuloma (over age
  30)
Peripheral fibroma with calcification
  (peak at age 25)
Plasma cell gingivitis
Pulp polyps
Pyogenic granuloma (60%)
Recurrent aphthous ulcer
Thyroglossal cyst
White sponge nevus

PERSONS OVER AGE 40

Benign mucous membrane pemphigoid
Candidiasis†
Denture stomatitis
Desquamative gingivitis
Epulis fissuratum
Hemochromatosis
Inflammatory papillary hyperplasia
Keratoacanthoma
Leukoedema
Leukoplakia (90%)
Lichen planus
Lipoma
Lymphoma
Malignant salivary gland tumors (ages
  40-60)
Melanoma
Metastatic carcinoma
Metastatic carcinoma to cervical nodes
Pemphigus (seldom under age 30)
Radiation mucositis
Squamous cell carcinoma
Verrucous carcinoma (ages 60-80)

*Also common in persons over age 40.
†Also common in infants.

Predisposition of bony or calcified lesions for special age-groups

INFANTS

Caffey's disease (birth to 2 years of age)
Letterer-Siwe disease (ages 1-3)
Osteopetrosis (malignant)
Rickets
Stafne's cyst?
Thalassemia major

CHILDREN

Acute leukemia
Basal cell nevus syndrome (ages 5-30)
Burkitt's tumor (ages 2-14)
Central hemangioma (ages 10-20)
Cherubism
Fibrous dysplasia (ages 10-20)
Follicular cyst (ages 10-20)
Garré's osteomyelitis (ages 5-12)
Hand-Schüller-Christian disease (ages 1-10)
Multilocular cyst (over age 15)
Osteoid osteoma
Osteopetrosis (malignant)
Rickets
Stafne's cyst
Thalassemia major

PERSONS UNDER AGE 30

Acute leukemia
Adenomatoid odontogenic tumor (peak at age 16)
Ameloblastic fibroma (peak at age 16)
Aneurysmal bone cyst (under age 20)
Basal cell nevus syndrome (ages 5-30)
Burkitt's tumor (ages 2-14)
Caffey's disease (birth to 2 years of age)
Cancer
    Ewing's sarcoma (peak at ages 14-18)
    Osteogenic sarcoma of jaws (ages 10-40, peak at age 27)
    Reticulum cell sarcoma of bone (70% under age 40)
Cementifying and ossifying fibroma (young adults)
Cementoblastoma (under age 25)
Central giant cell granuloma (60% under age 20)
Central hemangioma (ages 10-20)
Cherubism
Developing tooth crypt (under age 20)
Eosinophilic granuloma
Fibrous dysplasia (ages 10-20)
Follicular cyst (ages 10-20)

Garré's osteomyelitis (under age 25)
Hand-Schüller-Christian disease (ages 1-10)
Letterer-Siwe disease (ages 1-3)
Multilocular cyst (over age 15)
Mural ameloblastoma (ages 18-30)
Odontogenic fibroma (under age 25)
Odontogenic keratocyst (ages 10-20)
Odontoma in developing stages (under age 20)
Osteoblastoma (75% under age 20)
Osteoid osteoma
Osteopetrosis (malignant)
Parulis
Primordial cyst (ages 10-30)
Rickets
Sickle cell anemia
Stafne's cyst
Thalassemia major
Thalassemia minor
Traumatic bone cyst (under age 25)

PERSONS OVER AGE 30

Ameloblastoma (ages 20-50, peak at age 40)
Cementoma
Chondrosarcoma (ages 20-60, peak in 50s)
Osteopetrosis (benign)
Pindborg tumor (ages 28-48)
Primary hyperparathyroidism (ages 30-60)
Residual cyst (peak at age 52)
Sclerosing cemental masses

PERSONS OVER AGE 40

Artery calcification
Calcified node
Cancer
    Chondrosarcoma (ages 20-60; peak in 50s)
    Metastatic carcioma
    Minor salivary tumor
    Multiple myeloma (ages 40-70)
    Squamous cell carcinoma (peripheral)
Osteomalacia
Osteomyelitis
Paget's disease
Postextraction sockets
Secondary hyperparathyroidism (ages 50-80)
Sialolith

Sex predilection of soft tissue lesions (ratios or percents are given in parentheses)

MALE

Cancer (except minor salivary gland tumors and metastatic carcinoma from distant sites)
  Lymphoma (2:1)
  Melanoma (2:1)
  Metastatic carcinoma to cervical nodes
  Squamous cell carcinoma (4:1 to 2:1)
    Buccal (10:1)
    Floor (93%)
    Lip (98%)
    Tongue (75%)
  Verrucous carcinoma (3:1)
Erythema multiforme
Hemochromatosis
Keratoacanthoma (2:1)
Leukoplakia
Lymphoepithelial cyst (3:1)
Median rhomboid glossitis
Mucocele
Radiation mucositis

FEMALE

Benign mucous membrane pemphigoid (2:1)
Desquamative gingivitis
Geographic tongue (2:1)
Hemangioma
Lichen planus (2:1)
Lipoma (7:1 or equal)
Palatal tori (2:1)
Peripheral giant cell granuloma (2:1)
Peripheral fibroma with calcification
Plasma cell gingitivis
Pyogenic granuloma (3:1)
Ranula
Recurrent aphthous ulcers
Salivary gland tumors (2:1)

Sex predisposition of bony lesions

MALE

Cancer
  Chondrosarcoma
  Ewing's sarcoma (2:1)
  Lymphoma (2:1)
  Melanoma (2:1)
  Multiple myeloma (2:1)
  Osteogenic sarcoma
  Squamous cell carcinoma
    Central (2:1)
    Peripheral (4:1 to 2:1)
Cherubism
Eosinophilic granuloma (2:1)
Hand-Schüller-Christian disease (2:1)
Incisive canal cyst (3:1)
Osteoblastoma
Osteoid osteoma (2:1)
Osteomyelitis (5:1)
Residual cyst (2:1)
Traumatic bone cyst

FEMALE

Cancer
  Metastatic carcinoma
  Minor salivary gland tumors
Cementoma
Central giant cell granuloma (2:1)
Central hemangioma (2:1)
Osteoporosis
Primary hyperparathyroidism (7:1)
Sclerosing cemental masses
Secondary hyperparathyroidism (2:1)
Stafne's cyst

Race

The importance of racial (and hereditary) influences on the incidence of some diseases is illustrated by the well-known fact that a preponderance of patients with sickle cell anemia are black. Also, diffuse cementosis (sclerosing cemental masses) occurs predominantly in black women over 30 years of age.

Country of origin

Information concerning the country of origin or residence may be an important clue for identification of the disease. Burkitt's lymphoma seldom affects people of non-African origin. Also the greater use of chewing tobacco and snuff in the southeastern section of the United States is related to the increased incidence of intraoral verrucous carcinoma observed in that region.

Anatomic location

The extent to which the anatomic location of the lesion may affect the lesion's ranking in the differential diagnosis is illustrated by the following examples:
1. Although the lower lip is a common site for the development of a mucocele but a rare location for a minor salivary gland tumor, both these lesions may be in the same list of possible diagnoses.

Jawbone and regional predilection of bony lesions

MANDIBLE AND PREDOMINANT REGION

Ameloblastic fibroma (molar, premolar)
Ameloblastoma (80%; posterior, 70%)
Aneurysmal bone cyst (much more common in molar)
Benign nonodontogenic tumors (molar, ramus)
Caffey's disease
Calcifying odontogenic cyst (70%)
Cancer
   Acute leukemia (molar)
   Ewing's sarcoma
   Metastatic carcinoma (95%; molar, premolar)
   Osteogenic sarcoma (body)
   Reticulum cell sarcoma (molar, angle, ramus)
   Squamous cell carcinoma
      Peripheral (3:1, molar)
      Central (2:1)
Cementifying and/or ossifying fibroma (molar, premolar)
Cementoblastoma (first molar, premolar)
Cementoma (90%; incisor)
Central giant cell granuloma (65%; two thirds are anterior to molar)
Central hemangioma (65%; ramus, premolar)
Cherubism (ramus, third molar)
Complex odontoma

Condensing osteitis
Eosinophilic granuloma
Follicular cyst
Garré's osteomyelitis
Odontogenic fibroma
Odontogenic keratocyst (65%)
Odontogenic myxoma (molar, premolar)
Osteomyelitis (7:1; body)
Pindborg tumor (2:1; molar, premolar)
Postextraction sockets
Primordial cyst (third molar)
Sclerosing cemental masses

MAXILLA AND PREDOMINANT REGION

Adenomatoid odontogenic tumor (canine)
Chondrosarcoma (2:1)
Compound odontoma
Fibrous dypslasia (4:3)
Paget's disease (20:3)
Residual cyst (65%)

RARE IN MAXILLA

Caffey's disease
Cementifying and/or ossifying fibroma
Ewing's sarcoma
Garré's osteomyelitis
Osteomyelitis
Reticulum cell sarcoma
Traumatic bone cyst

---

2. The posterior region of a hard palate is a characteristic location for a minor salivary gland tumor but is an uncommon location for a mucocele.
3. Although the posterior hard palate is a characteristic site for a salivary gland tumor, this lesion is almost never found in the anterior hard palate and gingivae.

The box on this page groups the various bony lesions that show a preference for either the maxilla or mandible and also for specific sites within these bones. Parapharyngeal masses are not discussed in this book. However, Pedlar and Ravindranathan (1987) discussed the differential diagnosis of these lesions. Frommer (1982) discussed differential diagnosis of lesions seen on pantograms.

• • •

It is important to emphasize that the preceding pertinent facts are just a few examples from a large body of general information concerning the natural behavior of lesions that the clinician acquires from clinical experience in addition to the knowledge provided by formally structured courses.

After the ranking has been adjusted for incidence, the next step is to compare pertinent information, signs, symptoms, or other findings gained from examination of the patient with the usual features of the lesions in the list. The lesion showing the most correlation with the present findings should be ranked highest, and the lesion showing the least correlation should be ranked lowest. Thus the earlier ranking on a frequency basis is modified at this time. Halstead and Weathers did an extensive differential diagnosis of soft tissue lesions in 1977.

TWO OR MORE LESIONS PRESENT

From time to time clinicians examine patients with various combinations of lesions. Perhaps one patient will present with two lesions in the oral cavity. Another patient may have a lesion in the oral cavity and another in the neck. In still another patient the examination may reveal a lesion in the oral cavity and another in a more distant site, for example, the lung. After some thought, it becomes obvious that it is necessary to develop the differential diagnosis along distinctly contrasting lines in each of these cases.

Basically when two or more lesions are present, seven possibilities or propositions must be considered (modified from Mitton et al., 1976):

1. Lesions are related
   a. Lesion A and lesion B are identical (two aphthous ulcers)
   b. Lesion B is secondary to lesion A (metastatic tumor and primary tumor)
   c. Lesion A is secondary to lesion B (metastatic tumor and primary tumor)
   d. Lesion A and lesion B are both secondary to a third lesion, which may be occult (metastatic tumors and primary tumor)
   e. Lesion A and lesion B are manifestations of systemic disease (infections, histiocytosis X, disseminated malignancy)
   f. Lesion A and lesion B form part of a syndrome (café-au-lait spots and multiple neurofibromas in von Recklinghausen's disease)
2. Lesions are completely unrelated to each other and occur together only as a matter of chance

DEVELOPING THE WORKING DIAGNOSIS (OPERATIONAL DIAGNOSIS, TENTATIVE DIAGNOSIS, CLINICAL IMPRESSION)

Although the clinician has completed a differential diagnosis, he or she is not yet completely prepared to treat the lesion. He or she must now recheck the *credibility* of these top choices. This is done by further examination of the lesion, by asking the patient more definitive questions to expand the history, by perhaps ordering additional tests, and finally by reevaluating all the assembled pertinent data. Once their validity has been supported, the top choices will be referred to as the working diagnosis or clinical impression. The clinician may, in some cases, be so confident of the first-ranked entity that he or she excludes all the others from the working diagnosis.

The *working diagnosis* must indicate the proper management, especially if the management is to include surgery, because it will aid the surgeon in planning any operation—how long to reserve the operating room, what instrument setups to have prepared, whether to do an incisional or an excisional biopsy or a frozen section, whether to have blood available and, if so, how much and what type.

Before the surgery commences, the surgeon may choose to do one last test, such as aspiration of the lesion. This is an excellent precaution in certain instances and will rule out or identify vascular tumors, thereby avoiding the dangerous surprise that awaits the unsuspecting surgeon who encounters an unrecognized vascular tumor at surgery.

FORMULATING THE FINAL DIAGNOSIS

The final diagnosis in most cases of oral pathoses is provided by the oral pathologist who evaluates a biopsy in the light of all the available clinical data. In some instances the microscopic picture is quite diagnostic. In other cases, however, the microscopic picture may be so equivocal that the pathologist must depend heavily on the accompanying clinical symptoms in establishing the final diagnosis. In still other cases (e.g., an empty traumatic bone cyst) the clinician must establish the final diagnosis at the time of the surgery, since there may not be a specimen available for microscopic examination.

REFERENCES

Bouquot JE: Common oral lesions found during a mass screening examination, J Am Dent Assoc 112:50-57, 1986.

Frommer HH: Differential diagnosis from pantomograms, Dent Radiogr Photogr 55:25-36, 1982.

Goltry RR and Ayer WA: Head, neck, and oral abnormalities in dentists participating in the health assessment program, J Am Dent Assoc 112:338-341, 1986.

Halstead CL and Weathers DR: Differential diagnosis of oral soft tissue pathoses: site unit(s)-3379: instructional materials for health professional education, National Library of Medicine/National Medical Audiovisual Center, US Department of Health Education and Welfare, Washington, DC, 1977.

Hand JA and Whitehall JM: The prevalence of oral mucosal lesions in an elderly population, J Am Dent Assoc 112:73-76, 1987.

Mitton VA, Eversole LR, Kramer HS, and Stern M: Clinical-Pathological Conference: case 16, part 1 and part 2. Stafne's bone cyst of the mandible and concurrent pulmonary coccidioidomycosis, J Oral Surg 34:616-617, 715-716, 1976.

Pedlar J and Ravindranathan N: Differential diagnosis and surgical management of parapharyngeal masses: review and an unusual illustrative case, Oral Surg 63:412-416, 1987.

Weir JC, Davenport WD, and Skinner RL: A diagnostic and epidemiologic survey of 15,783 oral lesions, J Am Dent Assoc 115:439-442, 1987.

Part II

Soft tissue lesions

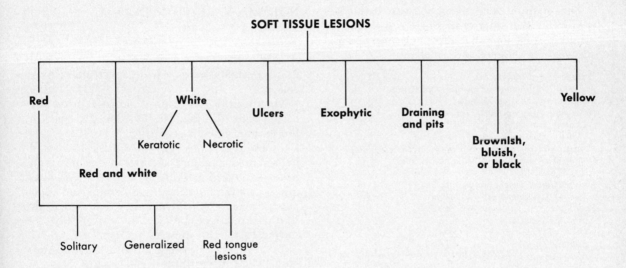

5

Solitary red lesions

NORMAN K. WOOD
GEORGE G. BLOZIS
PAUL W. GOAZ

This chapter deals primarily with pathologic conditions that appear as single red lesions or else diffuse lesions that affect only one mucosal surface. These are listed as follows:

Pathologic red lesions
Traumatic erythematous macules and erosions
Purpuric macules (early stage)
Inflammatory hyperplastic lesion
  (granulomatous stage)
Reddish ulcers or ulcers with red halos
Nonpyogenic soft tissue odontogenic infection (cellulitis)
Chemical or thermal erythematous macule
Nicotine stomatitis
Erythroplakia, carcinoma in situ, and red
  macular squamous cell carcinoma
Exophytic, red squamous cell carcinoma
Atrophic candidiasis
  Denture stomatitis
  Angular cheilitis
  Acute atrophic candidiasis
Macular hemangioma and telangiectasias
Allergic macules
Herald lesion of generalized stomatitis or
  vesiculobullous disease
Metastatic tumors
Kaposi's sarcoma (AIDS)
Rarities
  Actinomycosis
  Anemia (solitary red patch)
  Amyloidosis
  Angiosarcoma
  Blastomycosis
  Candidiasis endocrinopathy syndrome
  Coccidioidomycosis
  Erysipelas
  Exfoliative cheilitis
  Gonococcal infection
  Herpangina
  Histoplasmosis
  Hyperemic oral tonsils
  Plasma cell gingivitis
  Lupus erythematosus
  Ludwig's angina
  Sarcoidosis
  Secondary syphilis
  Tuberculosis

NORMAL VARIATION IN ORAL MUCOSA
Masticatory and lining mucosa

As discussed in Chapter 8, the normal oral mucosa demonstrates a wide spectrum of pink colors.

The healthy masticatory mucosa (over the hard palate, the gingiva, and dorsal surface of the tongue) is light pink (Fig. 5-1). These surfaces are exposed to heavy mechanical forces of friction and pressure during mastication and have adapted to meet these stresses by producing (1) a protective layer of keratin and (2) a subepithelial connective tissue that is densely fibrous, relatively avascular, and firmly attached to bone or muscle.

In contrast, the lining mucosa (the oral mucosa over the vestibule, cheeks, lips, floor of the mouth, and ventral surface of the tongue) is not subjected to such intense mechanical and chemical stimulations, so similar tissue modification does not occur in these areas. As a consequence of this different morphology, the color from the underlying vasculature is transmitted through the more transparent overlying tissue and imparts a more reddish color to the surface in comparison to the pinkish hue of the masticatory mucosa.

Palatoglossal arch region

In a significant number of individuals, areas of apparently normal mucosa covering the palatoglossal arch region are a deep dusky red in contrast to the light red color of the surrounding tissues (Fig. 5-2).

These entirely painless red macular bands are usually present bilaterally, and although the size and shape of the areas in the same individual may not be uniform, they persist un-

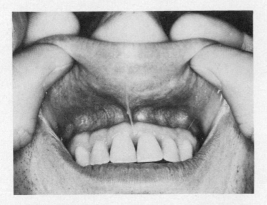

Fig. 5-1. Clinical view showing the paler pink of the attached gingiva (masticatory mucosa) in contrast to the deeper pink of the vestibular mucosa (lining mucosa).

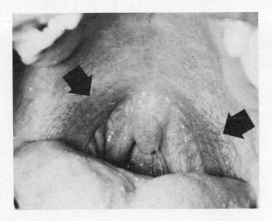

Fig. 5-2. Note the red appearance of the palatoglossal arch *(arrows)* in this healthy asymptomatic patient.

changed. In some cases bands are also found on the mucosa lining the tonsillar fossa, particularly in individuals who have had tonsillectomies some years before. It seems to us that these regions have a richer blood supply than the surrounding tissues and may be associated with Waldeyer's ring. Although this entity must be considered an individual variation that is normal, it is important that the clinician be familiar with the condition because it is often misdiagnosed as "sore throat."

Pathologic red lesions

The red color of a lesion is, to some extent, usually the result of increased vascularity in the underlying tissues. The loss of part or all of the covering epithelium also contributes to the measures of color developed; a thick membrane obscures the underlying red color, whereas more color is transmitted through a thin one. The degree of redness is also, in part, a function of the amount of the pigment hemoglobin present in the area and the extent of its oxygenation. Red lesions frequently have a thin mucosa that covers numerous dilated and engorged vessels and as a consequence frequently hemorrhage after minimal trauma.

A red color can also be imparted to the tissues by another pigment, melanin. This color may vary from light brown to a reddish brown to a bluish black. The reddish brown color is seen infrequently in melanin-producing lesions.

When the surface of a red lesion is smooth, presumptive evidence exists that the epithelium is uniformly atrophic and somewhat edematous. When some irregularities are present on the surface, the epithelium often shows variable degrees of hyperplasia or surface keratinization or both, and these changes are responsible for a granular or papillary appearance. Sloughing white patches, representing necrotic tissue and fibrinous exudate, may also appear in areas where the mucosa is erythematous.

In summary, the basic tissue changes or causes that produce abnormal red conditions are as follows:

I. Marked increase in hemoglobin concentration of circulating blood (polycythemia)
II. Vascular dilatation from:
    A. Inflammation (erythema)
        1. Mechanical trauma (e.g., cheek biting, ill-fitting denture)
        2. Thermal trauma (e.g., hot food)
        3. Chemical trauma (strong mouthwashes, iatrogenic spills)
        4. Infection (cellulitis, Ludwig's angina)
        5. Allergy or autoimmune disease (e.g., Sjögren's syndrome)
        6. Ulcer with inflamed rim (e.g., recurrent herpetic lesion)
    B. Congenital defects (e.g., hemangioma)
III. Extravasation of blood (e.g., trauma or hemostatic disease or both)
IV. Atrophy or thinning of mucosa (e.g., atrophic candidiasis [inflammatory component usually present too])

TRAUMATIC ERYTHEMATOUS MACULES AND EROSIONS

Mechanical trauma to the oral mucosa can produce a variety of clinical lesions depending on the nature and circumstances of the insult.

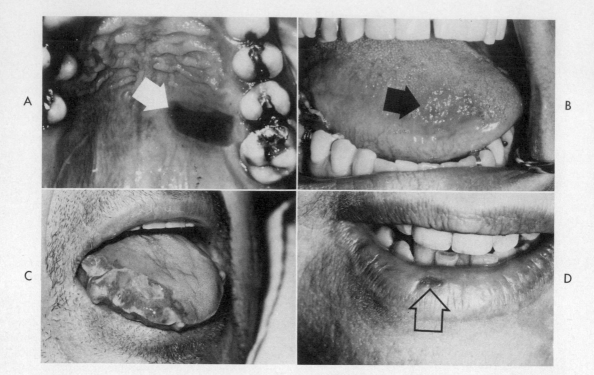

Fig. 5-3. Traumatic erythematous macules. These red patches all blanched on digital pressure. **A,** Palatal lesion caused by ill-fitting palatal connector of a partial denture. **B,** Red lesion at anterolateral border of tongue caused by a carious tooth with a sharp edge. **C,** Red and white traumatic lesion of the tongue caused by the patient chewing his tongue while it was anesthetized. The darker areas (red) are erythematous, and the white areas are necrotic. **D,** Small red macule on lip of middle-aged woman who repeatedly touched this spot with the incisal edge of her maxillary incisor.

The following are some of the clinical lesions that may be produced: (1) a keratotic lesion (increased retention of keratin), (2) a necrotic white lesion (necrosis of the epithelium and possibly the subepithelial tissue to some extent), (3) a reddish erythematous macule (an area of inflammation), (4) a purpuric macule (subepithelial hemorrhage within the tissue spaces), (5) a bleb (a pooling of tissue fluid in the tissue), (6) an erosion, (7) an ulcer, and (8) an exophytic lesion (inflammatory hyperplasia). Three of these, the erythematous macule and erosion, the purpuric macule, and the granulomatous stage of the inflammatory hyperplastic lesion, are essentially red and are discussed in this chapter.

Traumatic erythematous macules are produced by a low-grade, usually chronic physical insult. A more intense degree of brief trauma would be expected to produce a purpuric macule, an erosion, or a frank ulcer, in order of increasing severity. Common causes include sharp margins of teeth or restorations and ill-fitting prostheses. Self-inflicted trauma such as cheek biting or other habits also may produce traumatic erythematous macules.

Features

The usual sites for erythematous macules are on the anterior and lateral borders of the tongue, the floor of the mouth, the posterior palate, buccal mucosa, and mucosal surfaces of the lips. The macule may show considerable variation in the intensity of its red color. The size of the red zone corresponds closely to the size of the traumatic agent. Consequently size and shape may vary considerably. The margins of macular lesions are not usually sharply defined but may be in some instances (Fig. 5-3). Symptoms may vary from mild tenderness to considerable pain. The causative agent is usually easily identified through either the history or the clinical examination. The lesion generally regresses quickly after the cause is removed; however, if the lesion is located on the tongue it may persist for several weeks and heal as a bald pink area devoid of papillae.

Microscopic changes include an inflamed lamina propria covered with perhaps a slightly thinned or eroded stratified squamous epithelium that is completely nonkeratinized. Because this lesion is basically inflammatory, it may blanch when digital pressure is applied.

Differential diagnosis

For a discussion of the differential diagnosis of traumatic erythematous macules and erosions refer to the differential diagnosis section under purpuric macules.

Management

The mechanical irritant should be identified and eliminated and the lesion kept under surveillance until it disappears. Healing usually takes place in 3 or 4 days. If the lesion does not disappear soon, additional workup should be done. If the suspicion index is high, a biopsy should be performed to rule out more serious conditions such as erythroplakia, squamous cell carcinoma, and fungal diseases such as candidiasis and histoplasmosis.

PURPURIC MACULES (EARLY STAGE)

The purpuric macule is produced by a blunt traumatic insult to the mucosa or skin of sufficient force to cause the superficial extravasation of blood. If the patient is examined soon after the traumatic incident has occurred, petechial (small pinpoint) or ecchymotic (larger) areas are observed, which are quite red. If sufficient time has lapsed to permit some breakdown of the hemoglobin pigment, the "bruise" is bluish, undergoing the color changes from green to yellow described in Chapter 12.

Features

The size of the purpuric macule varies according to the size and force of the physical agent inflicting the damage. Usually the borders are poorly demarcated, blending almost imperceptibly with the surrounding normal tissue (Fig. 5-4). The lesion does not usually blanch on pressure because the red blood cells are within the tissues rather than in vessels. Nevertheless, purpuric macules may also have an accompanying inflammatory component, and in such cases the clinician may observe some blanching on palpation. Virtually any of the oral surfaces may be involved, but in our experience the palate, buccal mucosa, and floor of the mouth are the most common sites.

Frequently, reddish elliptic purpuric macules occurring on the palatal mucosa near the junction of the hard and soft palate may result from oral sexual practices and are caused by the repeated bumping of the male organ on the soft tissue in this region (Fig. 5-4). In such a case the lesion disappears within 2 or 3 days only to return again when the act is repeated (Giansanti et al., 1975). A judicious history taken in a confidential setting frequently reveals the true identity of such a lesion.

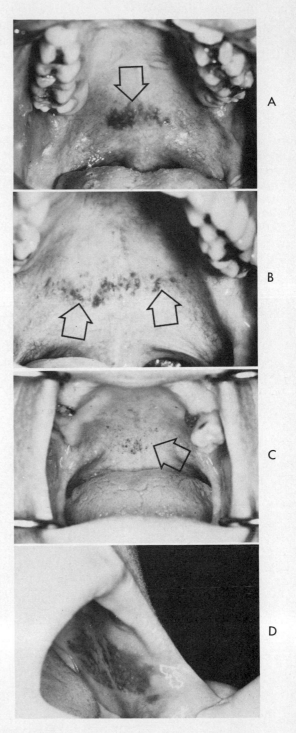

Fig. 5-4. Red purpuric macules. These lesions either blanched minimally or did not blanch at all to digital pressure. **A,** Palatal ecchymosis caused by fellatio. **B,** Palatal petechiae apparently caused by violent coughing, although a history of fellatio was not satisfactorily ruled out. **C,** Palatal petechiae in a patient with hemophilia. **D,** Reddish ecchymotic patch of the buccal mucosa following an oral surgical procedure.

Differential diagnosis

When transient reddish macules are observed near the junction of the hard and soft palate, the following entities should be considered: traumatic erythematous macule, purpuric macule of oral sex, palatal bruising because of severe coughing or severe vomiting, macular hemangioma, atrophic candidiasis, mononucleosis, and herpangina. The first four lesions are usually painless, and a careful history establishes the occurrence of a traumatic incident. Hemangiomas seldom occur on the posterior palate, and both the erythematous macule and the hemangioma blanch somewhat on pressure. In contradistinction to the purpuric macule and the erythematous macule, the hemangioma is not transient.

Management

Once the diagnosis of purpuric macule has been established, the patient should be advised of its nature. He or she should be seen at a later date to ensure that the diagnosis was correct and that the lesion has disappeared. In cases where erythema is the main component, a smear for *Candida albicans* should be performed (Damm et al., 1981). If candidal organisms are present, nystatin or amphotericin therapy should be instituted.

If several purpuric areas are present, the patient should be asked if he or she has always bruised excessively and how extensive the trauma was. If the correlation is unsatisfactory, the patient should be tested for the presence of a bleeding diathesis.

INFLAMMATORY HYPERPLASTIC LESIONS (GRANULOMATOUS STAGE)

Inflammatory hyperplastic lesions are discussed in considerable detail in Chapter 10. They are similar in cause to the traumatic erythematous macule and the purpuric macule except that the precipitating insults are invariably chronic irritants such as calculus, ragged margins of cavities, overhanging restorations, overextended denture flanges, sharp spicules of bone, or chronic biting of the cheek or lip. Such prolonged chronic insults stimulate the production of granulation tissue. A list of inflammatory hyperplastic lesions includes pyogenic granuloma, hormonal tumor, traumatic hemangioma, fibroma, epulis fissuratum, epulis

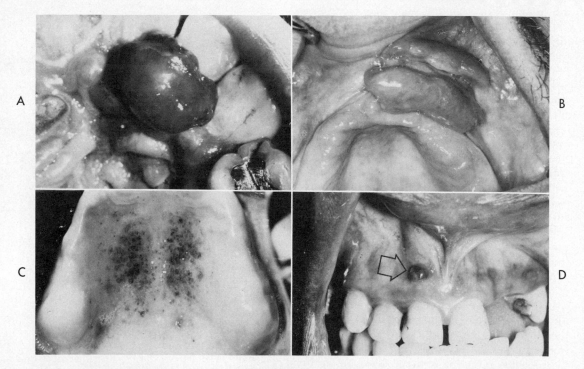

Fig. **5-5.** Reddish inflammatory hyperplastic lesions. All these lesions contained a large inflammatory component. **A,** Red pyogenic granuloma of the lingual gingiva caused by the sharp edges of a large carious lesion on the lateral incisor. **B,** Large red epulis fissuratum. **C,** Red papillary hyperplasia in its earliest stages, caused by an ill-fitting upper denture. **D,** Red parulis on the labial mucosa in an early stage of development. The lesion occurred at the opening of a sinus that was draining the infected periapical region of the maxillary right central incisor.   (**A** courtesy E. Seklecki, DDS, Tucson, Ariz.)

granulomatosum, papillary hyperplasia, peripheral giant cell granuloma, parulis, and the peripheral fibroma with calcification.

In the life cycle of one of these lesions the entity initially develops as a mass of inflamed granulation tissue and so clinically appears quite soft and very red. Later, when fibrous tissue is laid down, the lesion becomes firmer and less red. If the irritant is eliminated at this stage, the remainder of the inflammation disappears and the lesion shrinks noticeably, becomes firm, and takes on a pale hue. This endpoint lesion is a "garden-variety" fibroma.

Features

Features of inflammatory hyperplastic lesions are discussed in detail in Chapter 10. In the stage being considered here, the lesions are quite red, moderately soft, polypoid or nodular masses (Fig. 5-5).

Microscopy of the early hyperplastic lesions reveals granulomatous tissue covered with an intact layer of stratified squamous epithelium that is nonkeratinized. If the surface becomes traumatized, a white necrotic area usually develops in the region of the injury and the lesion becomes a pyogenic granuloma.

Differential diagnosis

The early inflammatory hyperplastic lesion must be differentiated from hemangioma, a metastatic tumor, a primary malignant tumor, a papilloma, condylomas, and verrucae. In the case of most inflammatory hyperplastic lesions in their early stages of development, a precipitating irritant is usually identifiable. This strengthens the impression and supports a working diagnosis.

However, if such an irritant is not apparent, the possibility that the lesion is either a primary or secondary malignant tumor beginning below a normal epithelium is given more consideration in the differential diagnosis. In turn a history of treatment or symptoms of a primary tumor elsewhere prompts the ordering of these possibilities in favor of a metastatic tumor (see Fig. 5-21). Primary malignant tumors of the oral soft tissue are rare. Likewise, it is rare for a squamous cell carcinoma to appear as a small exophytic red lesion with a smooth unulcerated surface.

In the case of gingival lesions juxtaposed with unrelated alveolar bony changes, it is most important to differentiate the inflammatory hyperplastic lesions from malignant tumors.

A congenital *hemangioma* is present from birth, whereas a traumatic (acquired) hemangi-oma is really a type of inflammatory hyperplastic lesion.

Papillomas, condylomas, and verrucae are included for the sake of completeness. However, since the inflammatory hyperplastic lesions are red and have a basically smooth, evenly contoured surface, they should be readily differentiated from these epithelial growths that are frequently white with a cauliflower-like surface. The pyogenic granuloma may have an area on its otherwise smooth surface that is white, but this is necrotic material and can be easily removed, leaving a raw bleeding surface.

Management

Excisional biopsy in combination with elimination of the irritant is the treatment of choice for lesions of substantial size. Small red lesions may shrink to a size that precludes treatment when the irritant is eliminated.

ULCERS WITH RED HALOS

Solitary ulcers are discussed at length in Chapter 11. They are included here for completeness because ulcerative conditions frequently are first manifested as erythematous macules, for example, the recurrent herpetic lesion and the recurrent aphthous ulcer. Furthermore, in these conditions, when the reddish area ultimately ulcerates, the defect frequently has a reddish border (Fig. 5-6). Such an observation might prompt the clinician to classify such an entity as a red lesion; however, experience has demonstrated that for the purpose of a differential diagnosis it is more beneficial to classify such lesions as ulcers.

Differential diagnosis

The differential diagnosis of the various oral ulcers is covered in Chapter 11.

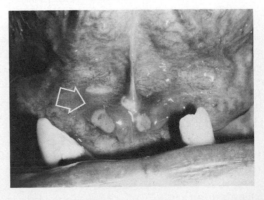

Fig. 5-6. Reddened mucosa surrounding three recurrent aphthous ulcers in the floor of the mouth.

NONPYOGENIC SOFT TISSUE ODONTOGENIC INFECTION (CELLULITIS)

This section includes a discussion of soft tissue odontogenic infections that either are caused by nonpyogenic bacteria or represent prepyogenic or postpyogenic infections. That is, the causative bacteria may be nonpyogenic, or else the infection has not reached the pus-forming or pus-pooling stage. Odontogenic infection may originate in three sites: the canals and the periapex of pulpless teeth, the gingiva in periodontal disease, and the gingival operculum over an erupting tooth.

Features

In most of these cases a suitable history and clinical and radiographic examinations coupled with pulp testing usually clearly indicate the diagnosis of dental infection (Fig. 5-7).

The alveolar mucosa and gingiva are the most frequent sites of dental infection, but if the infection is permitted to spread, a number of the oral mucosal surfaces, as well as the overlying skin, may become involved. Various degrees of swelling show a hot, red, tender to painful surface. However, pus that has formed and pooled near the surface of the swollen tissue imparts a yellowish white color to the central region of the swelling and renders the swelling rubbery and fluctuant to the touch (see Chapter 3).

Ludwig's angina is an unusual example of a reddish soft tissue infection that is produced by a mixed infection of nonspecific microorganisms, but a nonpyogenic strain of streptococcus is almost invariably present. This condition causes a sudden swelling of the floor of the mouth and also of the submental and submaxillary spaces, often of such a magnitude that obstruction of the airway is threatened. In most cases a very red, moderately firm, painful swelling of the floor of the mouth produces an elevation of the tongue. The skin of the neck overlying the swollen submental and submaxillary spaces is usually also red and feels hot on palpation (Fig. 5-8).

Cervical or intraoral actinomycosis is a specific infection that frequently occurs as a tender, reddish swelling (Fig. 5-8).

Differential diagnosis

When a patient has a reddish painful swelling of the oral soft tissues with an accompanying tender cervical lymphadenitis, the diagnosis of infection is reasonably certain. An extremely high percentage of these infections are

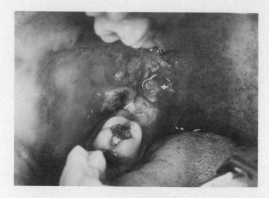

Fig. 5-7. Cellulitis of the mucosa of the cheek and surrounding pterygomandibular region originating from a pericoronitis involving the erupting third molar tooth. The white necrotic material represents a localized ANUG. (Courtesy G. Blozis, DDS, Columbus, Ohio.)

odontogenic in origin and hence bacterial in etiology. However, the clinician should also at least consider the unlikely possibilities of actinomycosis, tuberculosis, and various fungal infections such as histoplasmosis, coccidioidomycosis, and blastomycosis.

Management

When a diagnosis of odontogenic infection has been established, the associated dental problem should be eliminated by root canal therapy, extraction, curettage, excision, or incision and drainage. In addition, we recommend concomitant systemic administration of an appropriate antibiotic.

Patients with infections that are or may become a threat to their airway should be hospitalized so that any respiratory complication can be managed properly.

CHEMICAL OR THERMAL ERYTHEMATOUS MACULE

The cause of a chemical or thermal erythematous macule is usually a caustic drug or hot foods or beverages. Obviously the severity of the tissue damage varies with the intensity and duration of the insult, so several different clinical appearances may be produced. Caustic or hot agents may produce a coagulation necrosis of the superficial tissue that appears whitish and can be scraped off. Fig. 8-43 illustrates such a change precipitated by aspirin. Still more intense or prolonged insults may result in frank ulceration or stripping of the mucosa. Milder agents or briefer applications of strong agents produce the mildest clinically detectable

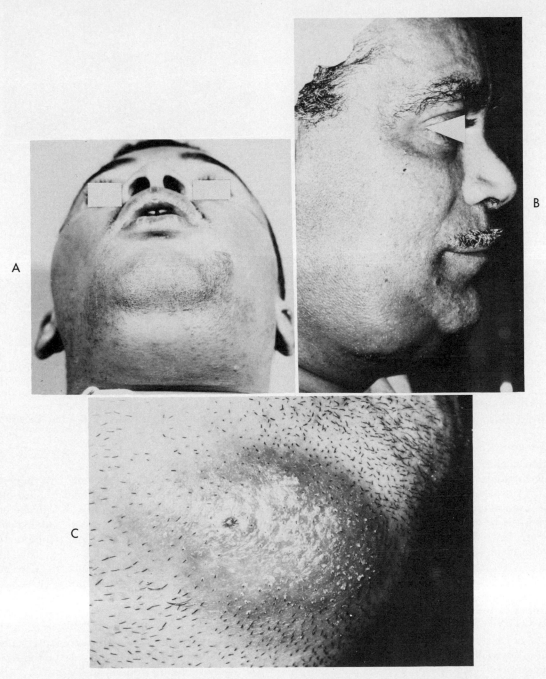

Fig. 5-8. Red infectious lesions. **A,** Ludwig's angina. Note the swelling of the submental and submandibular spaces. Unfortunately the redness of the overlying skin does not show in this black-and-white photo. The patient also had a red painful sublingual swelling. **B** and **C,** A case of actinomycosis in the submandibular space of a 56-year-old man. **C** shows the redness of the lesion.   (**B** and **C** courtesy E. Seklecki, DDS, Tucson, Ariz.)

reaction, an *erythema* of the superficial tissues, which explains why this condition is included in this chapter (Fig. 5-9). Sometimes a mixed reaction is produced, so the clinical lesion may appear as necrotic white dots or patches on an erythematous base (Fig. 5-9).

Features

The red area is tender to painful, may blanch somewhat on pressure, and usually bleeds on the slightest manipulation. The size and shape corresponds to the area of contact with the caustic agent. The buccal and palatal mucosa are the sites most commonly affected. Mild aspirin burns are good examples as are mild palatal burns from hot food (Fig. 5-9). A careful history elicits the facts concerning the causative agent in almost all cases.

Differential diagnosis

Many of the lesions discussed in this chapter should be considered in the differential diagnosis: erythema from mechanical trauma, purpuric macule, cellulitis (nonpyogenic odontogenic infection), allergic manifestations, erythroplakia, atrophic candidiasis (formerly known as atrophic candidosis), herald spot of disseminated red conditions, and fungal infections. A recent history of chemical or thermal injury along with uncomplicated resolution of the lesion in question eliminates these possibilities and establishes the correct diagnosis.

Management

The majority of these cases are mild and relatively painless. If pain is a problem, systemic analgesics and topical applications of hydrocortisone in an emollient base (Kenalog in Orabase) can be used. If any doubt persists as to the correct diagnosis or if the injury appears to be superimposed on a serious lesion, surveillance is required and a biopsy should be performed if the lesion in question does not resolve.

NICOTINE STOMATITIS

Nicotine stomatitis is discussed at length as a white lesion of the palate in Chapter 8. This lesion is included in the present chapter because it is a red lesion in its earliest stage, before keratosis has been produced (Shafer et al., 1984). Also, in the later keratotic stage the inflamed minor salivary duct openings appear as small red dots in the center of low flat nodules of hyperplastic tissue. Nicotine stomatitis is seen primarily on the palate of pipe smokers.

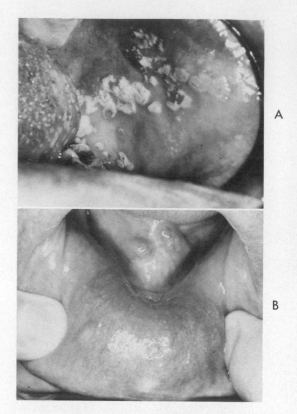

Fig. 5-9. Reddish lesions caused by chemical burns. **A,** Red and white acetaminophen (Tylenol) burn. **B,** Reddish area on mucosa of lower lip represents a stage in healing of lesion caused by the overzealous use of Listerine mouthwash.   (**B** from Bernstein M: Oral Surg 46:781-789, 1978.)

Differential diagnosis

The following conditions particularly have to be considered as somewhat similar clinical pictures when nicotine stomatitis is suspected: multiple papillomatosis, denture stomatitis, and atrophic candidiasis. Multiple papillomatosis and denture stomatitis can be quickly excluded if the condition is on the hard palate because nicotine stomatitis does not occur under a denture as the former two entities do. A smear quickly identifies atrophic candidiasis. A history of pipe smoking and the relatively greater prevalence of nicotine stomatitis cause it to be a more likely possibility in the differential diagnosis than atrophic candidiasis.

ERYTHROPLAKIA, CARCINOMA IN SITU, AND RED, MACULAR SQUAMOUS CELL CARCINOMA

The term "erythroplakia" is used in this book as a clinical term for a specific red lesion much as "leukoplakia" is used for white lesions of a

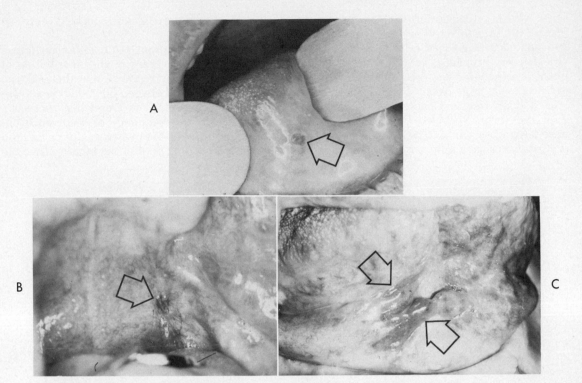

Fig. 5-10. Homogeneous erythroplakia. **A,** Very small red lesion on ventral surface of tongue, which showed invasion microscopically. This 52-year-old woman had had two previous oral squamous cell carcinomas removed from other locations. **B,** Small red lesion on the soft palate at upper extent of pterygomandibular raphe. Lesion was barely discernible until the tissue was dried with a gauze. **C,** Red macule involving the sublingual papilla on the right side. Excisional biopsy revealed early invasion in some sections and carcinoma in situ in others.   (**B** courtesy R. Lee, DDS, Findlay, Ohio.)

specific spectrum. Thus an "erythroplakic" lesion can be defined as a persistent velvety red patch that cannot be identified as any other specific red lesion such as inflammatory erythemas or those produced by blood vessel anomalies. Mashberg (1989) made the point that red patches are much more likely to become malignant than are leukoplakic lesions and advocated the use of toluidine blue rinse for their detection. Mashberg and Morrisey (1973) and Mashberg (1978) identified erythroplasia (erythroplakia) as the earliest sign of asymptomatic cancer and reported that invasion may occur in small lesions of less than 1 cm in diameter. Indeed the term "erythroplakia" carries a more serious implication than its white counterpart "leukoplakia" because almost all erythroplakias show malignant changes. In a study of 58 cases by Shafer and Waldron (1975) 51% were invasive carcinoma and 41% were carcinoma in situ or severe epithelial dysplasia.

These authors reported that on microscopic examination the lesion's reddish color results from the absence of a surface keratin layer and also occurs because the connective tissue papillae, containing enlarged capillaries, project close to the surface. They also described a general failure of the epithelial cells to achieve significant maturation (keratinization). Their work showed that when actual invasion occurs, cellular maturation may commence.

Features

Erythroplakia usually appears as a velvety red or granular red macule (patch) that may be slightly raised (Fig. 5-10). The painless lesion varies greatly in size; the borders may be well circumscribed or may blend imperceptibly with the surrounding normal mucosa. Small lesions are easily overlooked, but the chances for their detection are greatly enhanced by first drying the mucosa with a gauze, since this intensifies the red color. The use of toluidine blue rinse highlights the lesion (see Chapter 2).

Three different clinical appearances were described by Shear (1972): (1) the *homogenous form*, which is completely red in appearance (Fig. 5-10); (2) *patches* of erythroplakia and leukoplakia occurring together (Fig. 5-11); and (3) *speckled* erythroplakia, in which small leukoplakic specks are scattered over an area of erythroplakia (Fig. 5-12). The term "speckled leukoplakia" used in Chapter 8 is synonymous with the term "speckled erythroplakia" used here. Amagasa et al. (1985) confirmed that erythroplakias generally are much more aggres- sive than leukoplakias or speckled erythroplakias.

Shafer and Waldron (1975) found no difference between the sexes in the distribution of erythroplakia. They reported that the peak age of occurrence fell between 50 and 70 years. Interestingly these authors found that there is a difference in the frequency of occurrence between men and women when anatomic location is considered. The floor of the mouth proved to

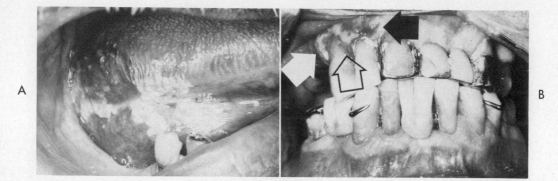

Fig. 5-11. Erythroplakic patches and leukoplakic patches in the same lesion. **A,** Lateral border of the tongue in a 64-year-old man. The red patch showed carcinoma in situ. **B,** Facial gingiva in a 57-year-old man. Some of the red areas showed invasive squamous cell carcinoma.   (**A** courtesy R. Crum, DDS, Hines, Ill. **B** courtesy E. Seklecki, DDS, Tucson, Ariz.)

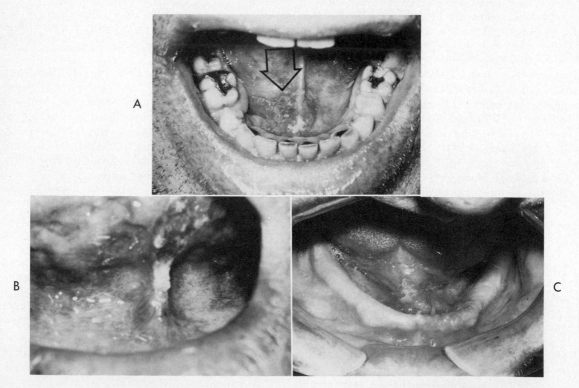

Fig. 5-12. Speckled erythroplakia of the oral floor. All lesions proved to be invasive squamous cell carcinoma on biopsy.   (**A** courtesy J. Lehnert, DDS, Minneapolis. **B** courtesy R. Lee, DDS, Findlay, Ohio.)

be the most common site affected in men, whereas the mandibular gingival and alveolar mucosa and mandibular sulcus make up the most common site in women. The retromolar region was the second most common site in both sexes.

Differential diagnosis

Although all the red macular lesions listed in this chapter should be considered in a differential diagnosis of an erythroplakic lesion, the lesions that are obviously macular hemangiomas and telangiectasias can be readily eliminated on the basis of their characteristic features. In a similar way the traumatic lesions, odontogenic infections, and allergies can be given a low ranking on the basis of their transient nature, their pain, and often obvious events in the history. The traumatic erythematous macules of the tongue are often more difficult to differentiate because these may persist for weeks after the irritant has been eliminated. Also red lesions of atrophic candidiasis may be indistinguishable clinically. In cases of candidiasis, features in the history are often suggestive of susceptibility and a smear is diagnostic. Tuberculosis and fungal lesions such as histoplasmosis should be considered (Shear, 1972), but their probability is low on the basis of incidence alone.

Erythroplakic areas on the gingiva may be overlooked or misinterpreted as local areas of gingivitis. Torabinejad and Rick (1980) and Gallagher and Svirsky (1984) reported cases of erythroplakic squamous cell carcinoma of the gingiva that had been initially considered to be periodontal disease. If a red area of the gingiva has no apparent cause or else does not respond to the usual periodontal therapeutic measures, it should be considered to be an erythroplakic lesion until proved otherwise.

Management

We concur with Mashberg and Morrissey's recommendation (1973) that if a red lesion persists for more than 14 days after all local trauma and infectious foci have been eliminated, a biopsy is mandatory. Obviously, if the suspicion index is high, arrangements should be made for immediate biopsy and further care. It is the senior author's experience that unless laser surgery is used to avoid seeding a superficial cancer or carcinoma in situ deeper into the tissue, incisional biopsies should not be performed on erythroplakic lesions. Horch et al. (1986) discussed the use of laser surgery with oral premalignant lesions.

EXOPHYTIC, RED SQUAMOUS CELL CARCINOMA

Exophytic squamous cell carcinoma is discussed in Chapter 10 without emphasis on color. Macular, red squamous cell carcinomas are discussed under erythroplakia earlier in this chapter. To further develop the differential picture it is necessary to include and describe an additional clinical lesion: the exophytic, red squamous cell carcinoma. Fig. 5-13 illustrates two examples of this entity.

Features

The lesions of exophytic squamous cell carcinoma nicely illustrate the rule of thumb (Chapter 10 that holds that a mass that arises in the covering epithelial surface has a rough surface and contour. These exophytic, red squamous cell carcinomas usually have a broad base and are usually domelike or nodular. The surface may vary considerably in roughness from lesion to lesion and also from area to area on the same lesion (Fig. 5-13). The surface may range from granular to pebbly to deeply creviced. The lesion may be completely red, or the red surface may be sprinkled with white necrotic or white keratotic foci. The lesion itself is firm to palpa-

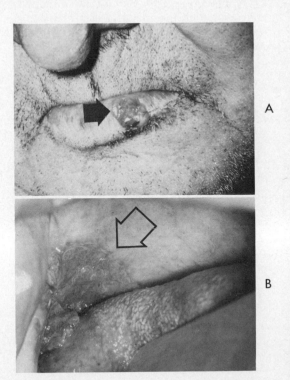

Fig. 5-13. Red exophytic squamous cell carcinoma. **A,** Small lesion on the lower lip. **B,** Large red lesion in the retromolar region.   (**A** courtesy James Love, DDS, Raleigh, N.C.)

tion, and the base usually shows induration and fixation to the deeper structures such as the periosteum. Pain is seldom a complaint.

Differential diagnosis

All red exophytic lesions such as inflammatory hyperplasias (granulomatous stage), hemangiomas, minor salivary tumors, primary mesenchymal tumors, metastatic tumors, amelanotic melanoma, and rare proliferating lesions such as tuberculosis, gummas, actinomycosis, and histoplasmosis must be considered.

Red inflammatory hyperplastic lesions are more common than exophytic squamous cell carcinoma and are considerably softer to palpation. In almost all cases the mechanical irritant is evident.

Many of the *hemangiomas* empty or partially empty on digital pressure, which is accompanied by a similar degree of blanching. Consequently these lesions are usually readily identified.

Because approximately 90% of all oral malignancies are primary squamous cell carcinomas, the chance of the red lesion being either a *metastatic tumor* or a *primary mesenchymal tumor* is unlikely, but it must be considered. However, in contrast to the exophytic squamous cell carcinoma the majority of primary mesenchymal tumors, as well as minor salivary gland tumors, have a smooth nonulcerated surface in the early stages of development.

Management

A good working recommendation to follow is to promptly perform a biopsy of any red exophytic lesion of the oral cavity that does not appear to be an infection, an inflammatory hyperplastic lesion, or a hemangioma. If it is not one of these lesions, it is likely a malignant lesion or else a rare proliferative infectious disorder. Strong et al. (1979) reported using with some success carbon dioxide laser therapy on localized carcinoma of the oral cavity. The treatment of oral squamous cell carcinoma is discussed in detail in Chapter 11, p. 207.

ATROPHIC CANDIDIASIS

Atrophic candidiasis is an interesting clinical variant of the candidal infection that produces a red appearance rather than the better known white pseudomembranous lesion that is discussed in Chapter 8. The red color is produced by a thinning or even a complete erosion of the surface epithelium with an accompanying inflammation of the underlying connective tissue.

Denture stomatitis

The diffuse redness of the palate seen under dentures has posed a diagnostic dilemma for many years. The tissue reaction has often been attributed to an allergic response to the denture base material, but that particular association has seldom been substantiated. Current studies offer strong evidence that the lesion is the result of a chronic infection by *Candida albicans*. The redness is not the typical change described in candidiasis, however, but represents a tissue response that has been labeled "chronic atrophic candidiasis." *Candida* organisms are almost always found in smears from the red lesions of these patients.

Of specific interest is the observation that the *Candida* organisms can be identified in larger quantities on the denture base material than on the palatal mucosa. This observation has prompted the suggestion that *Candida* organisms are residents on or in the denture base and the clinical lesion is a result of extremely irritating toxins produced by the fungus (Davenport, 1970). Phelan and Levin (1986) did not find an increased incidence of denture stomatitis in diabetic patients. Also Koopmans et al. (1988), reporting on plaque sampling in denture stomatitis, suggested the need to consider bacteria, as well as *Candida*, an etiologic factor. On the other hand, Segal et al. (1988) did show that various *Candida* species do adhere to acrylic surfaces.

FEATURES

Denture stomatitis occurs under either complete or partial dentures and is found more frequently in women. The lesions are almost always confined to the palate and seldom if ever involve the mandibular ridge. In approximately 50% of the patients, there is an associated angular cheilitis with or without an inflammatory papillary hyperplasia of the palate. A significantly high correlation has also been established between the occurrence of this condition and the wearing of dentures at night. There is some question as to what role trauma by ill-fitting dentures plays in the pathogenesis of the lesions. Chronic injury may predispose the tissue to infection by *Candida* organisms, which are considered to be normal inhabitants of the oral cavity. Greenspan (1983) discussed the possible causes of the inflammatory reaction: (1) tissue invasion by organisms, (2) effect of fungal toxins, or (3) hypersensitivity to fungus. Samaranayake et al. (1983) suggested that the carboxylic acids produced by the microflora of denture plaque may be a causative factor in the inflammation. At times there is an underlying chronic debilitating disease that predisposes patients to infection by *Candida* organisms.

The lesions may be totally asymptomatic, or the patient may complain of a soreness and dryness of the mouth. This soreness may also be described as a burning sensation. The palatal tissue is bright red, somewhat edematous, and granular. Only the tissue covered by the denture is involved. The redness usually involves the entire area covered by the denture but may be focal in its distribution (Fig. 5-14).

When seen microscopically, the lesion is rather nonspecific. The epithelium is atrophic and may be ulcerated in areas. An intense chronic inflammatory infiltrate is present in the lamina propria and also involves the epithelium. Usually the *Candida albicans* organism is not found in tissue specimens. The most accurate diagnostic test is a smear from the area of the lesion stained with periodic acid–Schiff reagent. This shows the yeast and hyphal forms of *Candida*. Cultures are not as useful, however, since they are also positive in patients who are carriers but do not have lesions.

DIFFERENTIAL DIAGNOSIS

The clinical picture of denture stomatitis is rather specific; few if any other diseases appear the same. Infections by other organisms, however, could be responsible for a similar diffuse redness.

MANAGEMENT

Currently, at least two effective antifungal agents for the local treatment of oropharyngeal candidiasis are available: troches containing clotrimazole (Myclex) and nystatin (Mycostatin) pastilles. These antifungal preparations should be dissolved in the mouth four or five times a day, after meals and at bedtime. These medicaments are pleasantly flavored, unlike the ill-tasting vaginal tablets that were taken as lozenges (and were undoubtedly responsible for poor patient compliance [Martin et al., 1986]). Although both agents are effective against Candida, an antifungal concentration is maintained in the saliva significantly longer after the clotrimazole troche dissolves than after the dissolution of the nystatin pastille. Dentures may be placed in nystatin solution during the night and covered by a nystatin ointment while being worn during the day. It is interesting that Walker et al. (1981) reported that denture stomatitis can be treated as effectively with a hydrogen peroxide denture cleaner as with antifungal agents.

Angular cheilitis

Angular cheilitis is usually a reddish ulcerative or proliferative condition marked by one or a number of deep fissures spreading from the corners of the mouth. The lesions are bilateral, usually do not bleed, and are restricted to the skin surface (Fig. 5-15). Although such factors as decreased vertical dimension of dentures, anemia, and vitamin B deficiencies may be predisposing factors or at least be associated

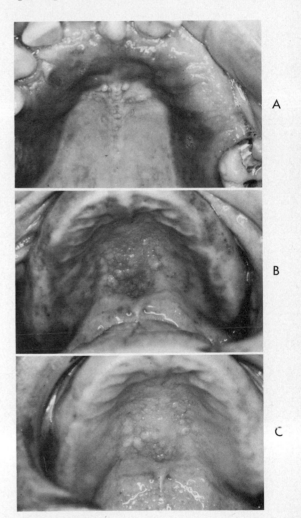

Fig. 5-14. Denture stomatitis. **A,** Only the palatal tissue contacted by an acrylic transitional partial denture is inflamed. Smears containing *Candida* were obtained from both the palatal tissue and the denture. **B,** Patchy redness covers the entire palate in a patient who wears a full denture. An exfoliative cytologic smear was positive for *Candida*. **C,** Same patient after therapy with nystatin for 1 week.

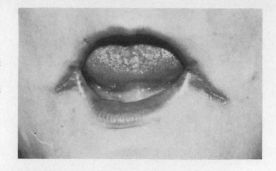

Fig. 5-15. Red lesions of angular cheilitis. *Candida albicans* had secondarily infected this condition, which was primarily caused by wearing dentures with decreased vertical dimension.

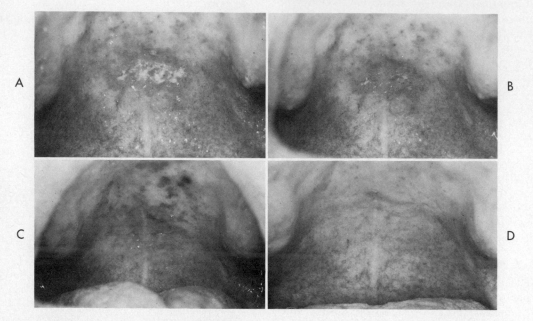

Fig. 5-16. Candidiasis. **A,** Palatal lesion of acute pseudomembranous candidiasis. **B,** Same area after the white plaque was removed by means of a tongue blade. **C,** Same area 1 week after the plaque was removed. An exfoliative cytologic smear of the palatal tissue was positive for *Candida*. The lesions are typical of acute atrophic candidiasis. **D,** Same area after therapy with nystatin for 1 week.

with the development of this lesion, infection with *C. albicans* and in some cases with a mixture of other microorganisms seems to represent a major cause. Ohman et al. (1986), in a study of 64 patients, isolated *Staphylococcus aureus* in cultured specimens of 40 patients and *C. albicans* in cultured specimens of 45. Konstantinidis and Hatziotis (1984) reported on their findings of 156 cases. Thus the lesions usually persist even though the predisposing factors have been eliminated, unless they are treated with an antifungal ointment such as nystatin.

Acute atrophic candidiasis

The lesion of acute atrophic candidiasis represents another though less common form of a *Candida* infection. It usually is the sequela of the typical lesion of *Candida*, the acute pseudomembranous candidiasis. When the white plaque of pseudomembranous candidiasis is shed or removed, a red, atrophic, and sore mucosa is often left (Fig. 5-16). At times the lesion may be asymptomatic. It may resolve spontaneously or require treatment with nystatin (Lehner, 1964, 1967).

FEATURES

The lesions are seen in essentially the same types of patients—persons who are prone to acute pseudomembranous candidiasis. Included are individuals who are taking broad-spectrum antibiotics, steroids, or immunosuppressive agents. In addition, the lesions occur during pregnancy and may accompany diabetes, hypothyroidism, and other debilitating diseases. They are also found in apparently healthy individuals.

Tissue sections show an atrophic epithelium that may contain a few hyphae in the superficial layers. The lamina propria usually has a mild acute inflammatory infiltrate and increased vascularity. An exfoliative cytologic smear of the lesion is most useful in establishing a diagnosis.

DIFFERENTIAL DIAGNOSIS

Frequently the red lesions of acute atrophic candidiasis are seen in association with those of the pseudomembranous type and do not pose a diagnostic problem. When discovered as isolated red lesions, they are rather nonspecific in appearance. Lesions produced by chemical burns, drug reactions, and other organisms have a similar clinical appearance but can usually be excluded or included on the basis of the history.

MANAGEMENT

The lesions of acute atrophic candidiasis respond well to either an oral suspension of nystatin or nystatin vaginal tablets used as oral troches. However, Barrett (1984) indicated that nystatin was of little use in eliminating oropharyngeal *Candida* in immunosuppressed patients.

MACULAR HEMANGIOMAS AND TELANGIECTASIAS

The majority of the oral hemangiomas of soft tissue are exophytic and bluish and so are discussed in Chapters 10 and 12. However, red macular hemangiomas and exophytic red hemangiomas occur both as nonsyndrome entities and as syndrome manifestations (Figs. 5-17 and 5-18). Red hemangiomas are usually of the capillary rather than the cavernous variety, which are usually more bluish. These reddish macular hemangiomas are also known as port-wine stains or nevus flammeus on the skin. People who have Sturge-Weber syndrome usually have both facial and intraoral macular hemangiomas (Fig. 5-18), although the intraoral hemangiomas may also be of the exophytic variety. An additional characteristic is the "tramline" calcifications seen in lateral skull radiographs.

The macular hemangiomas are readily differentiated from erythemas by their history of long duration, by their nontenderness, and by the fact that an inflammatory component is not present. They can be differentiated from red purpuric macules by the absence in the history of a recent traumatic episode and the transience of the latter condition.

Telangiectasias represent permanently enlarged end-capillaries that are located superficially just under the skin or mucosa. They are red, are seldom over 5 mm in diameter, and blanch readily on digital pressure, which easily and rapidly differentiates them from red petechiae. They may occur as solitary red macular or multiple lesions; as such they are usually a manifestation of the Rendu-Osler-Weber syndrome, also known as hereditary telangiectasia.

Management

Woods and Tulumello (1977) listed the following methods of treatment for the oral hemangioma: conscientious observation, use of radiation, steroids, embolization, antimetabolites, sclerosing solutions, surgical removal, or a combination of sclerosing agents and surgery.

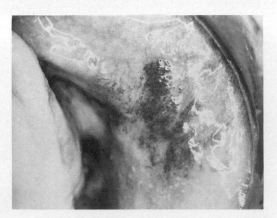

Fig. 5-17. Red macular hemangioma on the buccal mucosa, which had been present since birth.

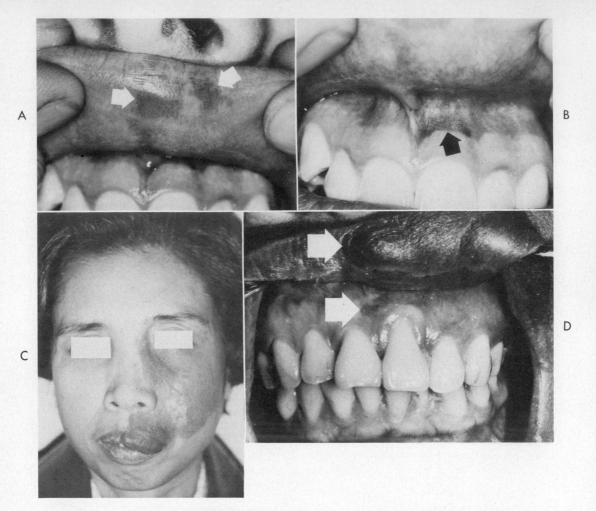

Fig. 5-18. Red macular hemangiomas associated with Sturge-Weber syndrome. **A** and **B,** Macular hemangiomas on the lip and alveolar mucosa in a 17-year-old patient who also had a port-wine stain on the left side of the face. The intraoral lesions blanched readily on digital pressure. **C** and **D,** Another patient with Sturge-Weber syndrome. **C,** Full-face view showing large superficial hemangioma (port-wine stain) on the left side of the face and upper lip terminating at the midline. **D,** Intraoral view of same patient showing the large red macular hemangioma that has involved the maxillary alveolar and gingival mucosa on the left side of the midline. The lip involvement on the left side can also be seen. (Courtesy S. Raibley, DDS, Maywood, Ill.)

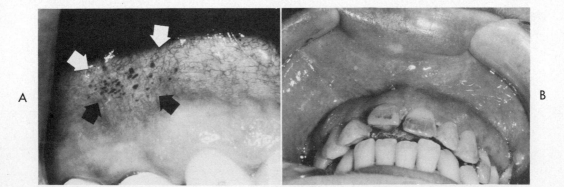

Fig. 5-19. Red allergic manifestations. **A,** Petechiae in red patch *(arrows)*, which was allergic reaction to topical anesthetic (unfortunately the red patch is not clearly visible in this black-and-white picture). **B,** Allergic reaction to agents in periodontal dressing. Note the deep mostly uniform color of all the mucosa in this picture. (**A** courtesy E. Rainieri, DDS, Maywood, Ill.)

ALLERGIC MACULES

Allergic manifestations in the oral cavity usually occur as a generalized eruption. Occasionally, solitary lesions occur, generally as the result of a contact allergy, and hence have to be differentiated from the other solitary red lesions (Fig. 5-19). When appearing as a red lesion they may be either an erythema or an ulcer. Usually the offending allergen can be identified by taking a careful history. Shepherd et al. (1983) reported an allergic contact stomatitis from a gold alloy. Cohen and Hoffman (1981) reported a case of allergy to rubber products, and Barkin et al. (1984) described an allergic reaction to eugenol. Dunlap et al. (1989) reported a case of allergic reaction to orthodontic wire.

HERALD LESION OF GENERALIZED STOMATITIS OR VESICULOBULLOUS DISEASE

Vesiculobullous disease and other conditions that may cause a generalized stomatitis are discussed in Chapter 6. Occasionally such conditions occur first as a solitary lesion (erythema, bleb, or ulcer) perhaps one or several months before a full-blown attack occurs. Examples of this occurrence are patients who have had occasional, single, recurrent aphthous ulcers and then suddenly experience a widespread involvement of their oral mucosal membranes, that is, a recurrent aphthous stomatitis.

Fig. 5-20, *A*, illustrates the case of a woman who originally was seen with two small blebs on the buccal mucosa. These soon disappeared, but several months later the woman was seen with a full-blown attack of pemphigus.

The solitary lesion illustrated in Fig. 5-20, *B*, illustrates a herald lesion of erosive lichen planus. When the 45-year-old woman first came for diagnosis and treatment, only the one lesion was found. Several months later she was seen with a severe attack of erosive lichen planus.

METASTATIC TUMORS

Exophytic metastatic tumors are discussed in Chapter 10. It is helpful to reiterate that this group of lesions includes those that arise in bone and extend into the soft tissue, as well as those that begin in the soft tissue. A number of reports suggest that the more common locations of the primary tumors that metastasize to the jaws (listed in descending order of frequency) are the breast, lung, kidney, gastrointestinal tract, thyroid, and prostate.

Metastatic tumors in the oral cavity are uncommon lesions, representing about 1% of all oral malignancies (Clausen and Poulsen, 1963; Meyer and Shklar, 1965). The vast majority are located in bone, although some of these central lesions involve the oral soft tissue by extension (Hatziotis et al., 1973). In Meyer and Shklar's series (1965) 92% arose in jawbone, compared to 8% in the oral soft tissue; 85% of these secondary bone tumors occurred in the mandible. It is interesting that 70% of their cases were adenocarcinomas. Metastatic carcinoma of the gingiva is even more rare, as evidenced by the sparsity of reports (Ellis et al., 1977; Sanner et al., 1979; Sato et al., 1978).

Features

Exophytic metastatic tumors are usually rapidly growing nodular or polypoid masses. The

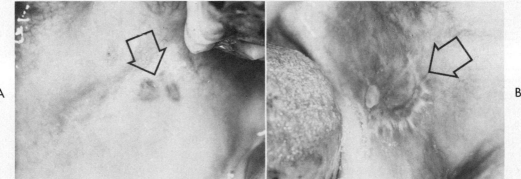

Fig. 5-20. Herald lesion of generalized stomatitis. **A,** Two vesicles with red rims on the buccal mucosa of a patient. These soon disappeared, but a full-blown case of pemphigus developed in the patient several months later. **B,** Solitary reddish lesion with a keratotic white component that was observed in a 45-year-old woman. Several months later a severe disseminated attack of erosive lichen planus was observed in the patient.

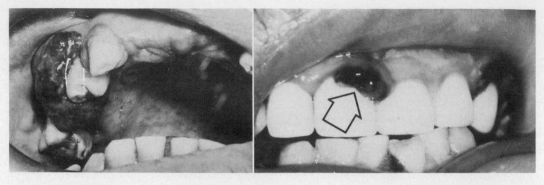

Fig. 5-21. Red metastatic tumors. **A,** Mass of 3 cm on the right maxillary gingiva of a 58-year-old man, which proved to be a metastatic adenocarcinoma from the lung. **B,** Reddish granuloma-like mass on the anterior gingiva of a 27-year-old man, which proved to be metastatic synovial sarcoma. (**A** and **B** from Ellis GL, Jensen J, Reingold IM, and Barr RJ: Oral Surg 44:238-245, 1977.)

surfaces may be smooth and covered with intact mucosa, which varies from light pink to normal mucosal pink to red, depending on the integrity of the covering epithelium, the vascularity, and the amount of inflammation present (Fig. 5-21). When the lesions become larger, they frequently develop an ulcerated surface as a result of chronic trauma from mastication, and the appearance varies from one of red and white patches to part or complete ulceration of the entire surface, which has a tendency to bleed easily.

The location of metastatic lesions varies considerably, but most occur in the lower half of the oral cavity. The premolar-molar region of the mandible is the most commonly involved site. Other areas of involvement in the oral soft tissue and bone are the alveolus, body of the jawbone, ramus, lip, tongue, and gingiva.

Although the diagnostic features of metastatic tumors may vary, the following should add to the suspicion index: paresthesia, rapid swelling or expansion of the jaws, pain, loose or extruded teeth without apparent cause, or failure of an extraction site to heal (Birkholz and Reed, 1979).

Osseous involvement is usually quite evident in radiographs and may present a wide spectrum of possible appearances: (1) solitary, ragged, poorly marginated radiolucency, (2) cystlike radiolucency, (3) multilocular radiolucency, (4) multiple separate radiolucencies, (5) mixed radiolucency and radiopacity, and (6) complete radiopacity.

Differential diagnosis

The lesions that should be included in the differential diagnosis are inflammatory hyperplasia, primary mesenchymal malignant tumors, traumatized minor salivary tumors, and amelanotic melanoma.

Inflammatory hyperplastic lesions are the most common by far. They can usually be tentatively identified by the identification of a chronic irritant.

Minor salivary tumors are almost never red, but if the red exophytic tumor in question is located in the posterolateral hard palate, the possibility of a tumor of the minor salivary glands would have to be considered.

Primary malignant mesenchymal tumors represent less than 1% of all oral malignancies; they are less common than the metastatic variety. Nevertheless, some of these primary tumors are red, especially the vascular variety, and must be considered, although they are assigned a low ranking in differential diagnosis.

Amelanotic melanoma of the oral cavity is a very rare tumor but can be indicated by a pink or reddish exophytic lesion (Fig. 10-30, *A*), so it cannot be completely dismissed.

The suspicion of *metastatic tumor* is enhanced by symptoms of a primary tumor elsewhere or a history of previous treatment of such a tumor. However, it is important to consider that the metastatic oral lesion may be the first indication of the presence of a primary tumor.

Management

Treatment of individual cases of metastatic carcinoma in the oral cavity may be careful observation, palliative measures, or aggressive measures, depending on the general condition of the patient. If the patient is dying as a result of disseminated tumor, observation or palliative measures are the management of choice. On the other hand, if the oral lesion appears to

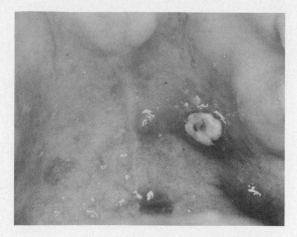

Fig. 5-22. Kaposi's sarcomas. Note the four red nodular lesions on the soft palate of a male with AIDS. One of the more anterior lesions has a white necrotic surface.   (Courtesy S. Silverman, DDS, San Francisco, Calif.)

be the only existing metastatic lesion, attempts should be made to eradicate it.

KAPOSI'S SARCOMA (AIDS)

Acquired immunodeficiency syndrome and associated Kaposi's sarcoma are discussed in Chapter 12 and in Appendix D. A red color is one of the frequent characteristics of Kaposi's sarcoma. Fig. 5-22 illustrates several nodular red Kaposi's sarcomas on the soft palate of a patient with AIDS.

RARITIES

The following intraoral conditions are rare but nevertheless must be considered when a red lesion is detected:

Actinomycosis
Amyloidosis
Anemia (solitary red patch)
Angiosarcoma
Blastomycosis
Candidiasis endocrinopathy syndrome
Coccidioidomycosis
Erysipelas
Exfoliative cheilitis
Gonococcal infection
Herpangina
Histoplasmosis
Hyperemic oral tonsils
Plasma cell gingivitis
Ludwig's angina
Lupus erythematosus
Sarcoidosis
Secondary syphilis
Tuberculosis

REFERENCES

Amagasa T, Yokoo E, Sato K, et al: A study of the clinical characteristics and treatment of oral carcinoma in situ, Oral Surg 60:50-55, 1985.

Barkin ME, Boyd JP, and Cohen S: Acute allergic reaction to eugenol, Oral Surg 57:441-442, 1984.

Barrett AP: Evaluation of nystatin in prevention and elimination of oropharyngeal *Candida* in immunosuppressed patients, Oral Surg 58:148-151, 1984.

Birkholz H and Reed JH: Bronchogenic carcinoma metastatic to the lip and the mandible, J Am Dent Assoc 98:414-416, 1979.

Clausen F and Poulsen H: Metastatic carcinoma to the jaws, Acta Pathol Microbiol Immunol Scand 57:361-374, 1963.

Cohen DM and Hoffman M: Contact stomatitis to rubber products, Oral Surg 52:491-494, 1981.

Damm DD, White DK, and Brinker CM: Variations of palatal erythema secondary to fellatio, Oral Surg 52:417-421, 1981.

Davenport JC: The oral distribution of *Candida* in denture stomatitis, Br Dent J 129:150-156, 1970.

Dunlap CL, Vincent SK, and Barker BF: Allergic reaction to orthodontic wire: report of case, J Am Dent Assoc 118:449-450, 1989.

Ellis GL, Jensen JL, and Barr RJ: Malignant neoplasms metastatic to gingivae, Oral Surg 44(2):238-245, 1977.

Gallagher CS and Svirsky JV: Misdiagnosis of squamous cell carcinoma as advanced periodontal disease, J Oral Med 39:35-38, 1984.

Giansanti JS, Craner JR, and Weathers DR: Palatal erythema: another etiologic factor, Oral Surg 40:379-381, 1975.

Greenspan JS: Infectious and non-neoplastic diseases of the oral mucosa, J Oral Pathol 12:139-166, 1983.

Hatziotis JC, Constantinido H, and Papanayotto PH: Metastatic tumors of the oral soft tissues, Oral Surg 36(4):544-550, 1973.

Horch HH, Gerlach KL, and Schaefer HE: CO_2 laser surgery of oral premalignant lesions, Int J Oral Maxillofac Surg 15:19-24, 1986.

Konstantinidis AB and Hatziotis JH: Angular cheilosis: an analysis of 156 cases, J Oral Med 39:199-206, 1984.

Koopmans ASF, Kippow N, and de Graaff J: Bacterial involvement in denture-induced stomatitis, J Dent Res 67:1246-1250, 1988.

Lehner T: Oral thrush, or acute pseudomembranous candidiasis, Oral Surg 18:27-37, 1964.

Lehner T: Oral candidosis, Dent Pract 17:209-216, 1967.

Martin MV, Farrelly PJ, and Hardy P: An investigation of the efficacy of nystatin for the treatment of chronic atrophic candidosis (denture sore mouth), Br Dent J 160:201-204, 1986.

Mashberg A: Erythroplasia: the earliest sign of asymptomatic oral cancer, J Am Dent Assoc 96:615-620, 1978.

Mashberg A and Morrissey JB: A study of the appearance of early asymptomatic oral squamous cell carcinoma, Cancer 32:1436-1445, 1973.

Mashberg A and Samit AM: Early detection, diagnosis and management of oral and oropharyngeal cancer, CA 39:67-88, 1989.

Meyer I and Shklar G: Malignant tumors metastatic to mouth and jaws, Oral Surg 20(3):350-362, 1965.

Ohman SC, Dahlen G, Moller A, and Ohman A: Angular cheilitis: a clinical and microbial study, J Oral Pathol 15:213-217, 1986.

Phelan JA and Levin SM: A prevalence study of denture stomatitis in subjects with diabetes mellitus or elevated plasma glucose levels, Oral Surg 62:302-305, 1986.

Samaranayake LP, Weetman DA, Geddes DAM, et al: Carboxylic acids and pH of dental plaque in patients with denture stomatitis, J Oral Pathol 12:84-89, 1983.

Sanner JR, Ramin JE, and Yang C: Carcinoma of the lung metastatic to the gingiva: review of the literature and report of case, J Oral Surg 37:103-106, 1979.

Sato M, Nishio J, Yoshida H, et al: Metastatic choriocarcinoma involving the gingiva, Int J Oral Surg 7:182-196, 1978.

Segal E, Lehrman O, and Dayan D: Adherence in vitro of various *Candida* species to acrylic surfaces, Oral Surg 66:670-673, 1988.

Shafer WG, Hine MK, and Levy BM: A textbook of oral pathology, ed 4, Philadelphia, 1984, WB Saunders Co.

Shafer WG and Waldron CA: Erythroplakia of the oral cavity, Cancer 36:1021-1028, 1975.

Shear M: Erythroplakia of the mouth, Int Dent J 22:460-473, 1972.

Shepherd FE, Moon PC, Grant GC, et al: Allergic contact stomatitis from a gold alloy-fixed partial denture, J Am Dent Assoc 106:198-199, 1983.

Strong MS, Vaughan CW, Healy GB, et al: Transoral management of localized carcinoma of the oral cavity using the CO_2 laser, Laryngoscope 89:897-905, 1979.

Torabinejad M and Rick GM: Squamous cell carcinoma of the gingiva, J Am Dent Assoc 100:870-872, 1980.

Walker DM, Stafford GD, Huggett R, et al: The treatment of denture induced stomatitis: evaluation of two agents, Br Dent J 151:415-419, 1981.

Woods WR and Tulumello TN: Management of oral hemangioma, Oral Surg 44:39-44, 1977.

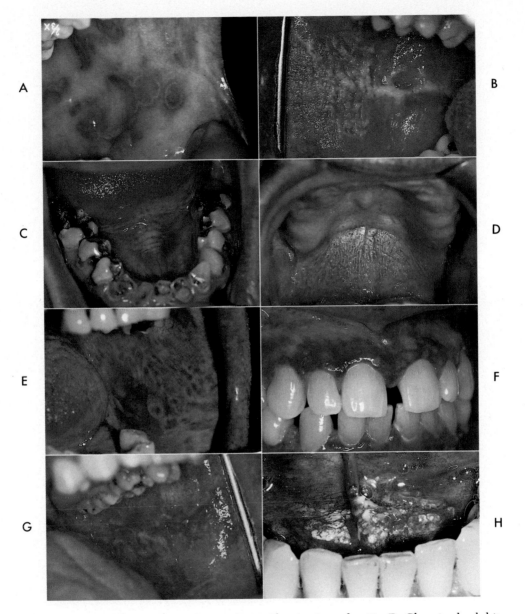

Plate 1. **A,** Migratory stomatitis in a patient with migratory glossitis. **B,** Chronic cheek biting. **C,** Keratotic and erythematous lesion of the oral floor due to sharp anterior teeth. **D,** Nicotine stomatitis of the soft palate. **E,** Lichen planus, reticular and atrophic. **F,** Lichen planus, atrophic and plaquelike. **G,** Lichen planus, erosive. **H,** Speckled leukoplakia in the oral floor. Biopsy revealed squamous cell carcinoma. (**A** courtesy S. Fischman, DDS, Buffalo)

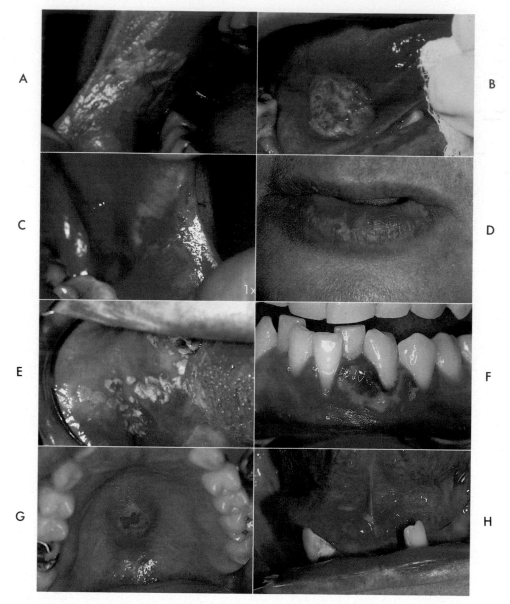

Plate 2. **A,** Erythroleukoplakia at the commissure. **B,** Squamous cell carcinoma on the lateroventral surface of the tongue. **C,** Candidiasis, atrophic and hypertrophic, at the commissure. **D,** Lupus erythematosus on the lower lip. **E,** Red (erythematous) and white (necrotic) acetaminophen burn on the cheek mucosa. **F,** Cocaine-induced changes on the gingiva. **G,** Burn on the palate from hot food. **H,** Recurrent aphthous stomatitis. (**A** courtesy O.H. Stuteville, DDS, MD, St. Joe, Ark. **B** courtesy V. Saunders, DDS, Richmond, Vir. **F** courtesy A. Gargiulo, DDS, Westchester, Ill.)

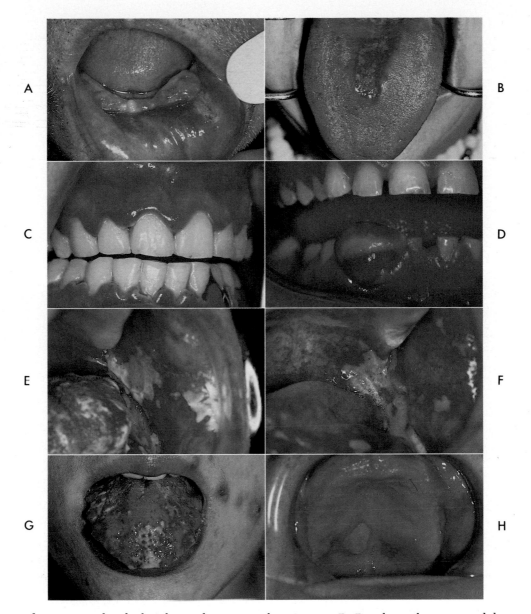

Plate 3. **A,** Red and white lesion due to a crushing trauma. **B,** Pseudomembranous candidiasis on the dorsal surface of the tongue. **C,** Acute necrotic ulcerative gingivitis. **D,** Pyogenic granuloma. **E,** Allergic mucositis caused by cold tablets. **F,** Radiation mucositis. **G,** Primary herpetic gingivostomatitis. **H,** Benign mucous membrane pemphigoid. (**D** courtesy T. Nading, DDS, Chicago, Ill. **E** and **F** courtesy G. Blozis, DDS, Columbus, Ohio.)

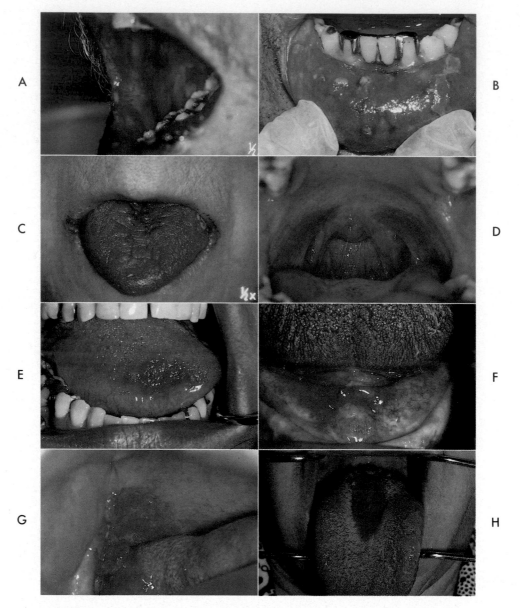

Plate 4. **A,** Erythema multiforme. **B,** Pemphigus. **C,** Xerostomia following radiation. **D,** Normal red band over the palatoglossal arch bilaterally. **E,** Contact allergy to temporary restoration on the lateral border of the tongue. **F,** Erythroplakia on the anterior section of the right sublingual ridge. **G,** Red exophytic squamous cell carcinoma. **H,** Median rhomboid glossitis. (**A** and **C** courtesy S. Fischman, DDS, Buffalo. **B** courtesy M. Lehnert, DDS, Minneapolis, Minn. **G** courtesy G Blozis, DDS, Columbus, Ohio.)

6

Generalized red conditions and multiple ulcerations

STUART L. FISCHMAN
RUSSELL J. NISENGARD
GEORGE G. BLOZIS

This chapter deals primarily with the diffuse red conditions and multiple ulcerations that occur in the oral cavity and affect several oral surfaces simultaneously. The majority of these occur as multiple ulcerations distributed over erythematous mucosal surfaces. They include:

Recurrent aphthous stomatitis and Behçet's syndrome
Primary herpetic gingivostomatitis
Erosive lichen planus
Erythema multiforme
Acute atrophic candidiasis
Benign mucous membrane pemphigoid
Pemphigus
Desquamative gingivitis
Radiation and chemotherapy mucositides
Xerostomia
Plasma cell gingivitis
Stomatitis areata migrans
Allergies
Polycythemia
Lupus erythematosus
Rarities
  Actinomycosis
  Acute gangrenous stomatitis
  Agranulocytosis
  Amyloidosis
  Bullous pemphigoid
  Cheilitis granulomatosa (Melkersson-Rosenthal syndrome)
  Crohn's disease
  Darier's disease
  Diabetic ulcerations
  Epidermolysis bullosa
  Gonococcal stomatitis
  Graft-versus-host disease

Granulomatous disease of the newborn
Hand-foot-mouth disease
Heavy metal poisoning
Hereditary mucoepithelial dysplasia
Hereditary telangiectasia
Herpangina
Herpes zoster (primary and secondary)
Histoplasmosis
Impetigo
Job's syndrome
Kaposi's sarcoma (multiple)
Leukemia
Major aphthous ulcerations (Sutton's disease)
Maple syrup urine disease
Measles
Metastatic hemangiosarcomas
Mycosis fungoides
Pernicious anemia
Polyarteritis nodosa
Psoriasis
Psoriasis variants
  Pustular psoriasis
  Acrodermatitis continua
  Impetigo herpetiformis
  Pyostomatitis vegetans
Reiter's syndrome
Scurvy
Streptococcal stomatitis
Thermal and chemical burns (mild, recent)
Ulcerative colitis
Uremic stomatitis

Varicella
Vincent's angina

Vitamin B deficiencies (severe)

Chapter 5 is devoted to the solitary red lesions. In contrast, this chapter discusses those diseases that simultaneously produce multiple red lesions and multiple ulcerations on several oral mucous membranes. The lesions may also appear on other mucous membranes and on the skin. Also included are those vesicular lesions that appear red both before the eruption of the vesicles and after their rupture.

For a variety of reasons, these conditions represent the most difficult challenge to clinical diagnosis. In many instances the specific cause is unknown, and frequently laboratory and biopsy results are nonspecific. Many of these conditions are relatively uncommon. Even the specialist may not have the opportunity to study a sufficient quantity of cases to gain expertise. There is a wide variation in the degree of severity of individual cases.

Although the initial clinical appearance of the diseases varies, they all appear similar in their later stages. For example, the vesiculobullous group is quite distinctive in the early stages, but after the "blisters" rupture and disappear, the resultant ulcerative stomatitis is quite nonspecific in appearance.

The vesicular diseases are a particular enigma because the "blisters" may form and rupture within 24 hours; hence the clinician and patient may be unaware that vesicles were even present in a given case. Presentation, remission, and recurrence make up the frequent course of many of these diseases. Treatment is palliative for the vast majority of them.

An overview of the various conditions reveals a considerable divergence; for instance, polycythemia is present as a painless, deep, dusty red color of the mucosa usually without inflammation, blisters, or ulcerations. The stomatitis accompanying xerostomia does not produce bullae and is otherwise nonspecific except for the decrease in salivary pooling. The bullous diseases are similar in that vesicles or blebs are the first lesions to appear; however, these soon rupture to form ulcers on inflamed mucosal surfaces. Diseases such as lichen planus, lichenoid drug reaction, lupus erythematosus, stomatitis areata migrans, and psoriasis may form a fifth group frequently demonstrating both white (keratotic) and red lesions.

These conditions have in common the generalized reddened appearance of the oral mucosa. Pain is usually a symptom.

ETIOLOGY

The spectrum of causes of generalized red conditions is especially broad and varied. It includes the following (unfortunately, the specific cause is unknown in many conditions):

    Hereditary conditions
    Allergic conditions
    Autoimmune conditions
    Infections (bacterial, fungal, viral)
    Altered host state (e.g., diabetes, uremia)
    Altered local resistance (e.g., xerostomia)
    Trauma
    Iatrogenic conditions
    Neoplasia
    Gastrointestinal conditions
    Deficiency states (e.g., vitamin deficiencies)
    Idiopathic conditions

RECURRENT APHTHOUS STOMATITIS AND BEHÇET'S SYNDROME

Solitary recurrent aphthous ulcers (RAU) are discussed in detail in Chapter 11. Their characteristic history and clinical picture permit ready recognition. However, a patient occasionally is seen with multiple aphthous ulcers distributed over several inflamed mucosal surfaces (Fig. 6-1 and Plate 2). The differential diagnosis of this condition, known as recurrent aphthous *stomatitis*, should therefore include those diseases that appear as generalized red ulcers.

The cause of this condition is unknown. Miller et al. (1980) demonstrated a hereditary component. Wray et al. (1981) suggested mechanical trauma as a precipitating cause. There are excellent data suggesting that immunologic factors (humoral immune response, cell-mediated immune responses, and immune com-

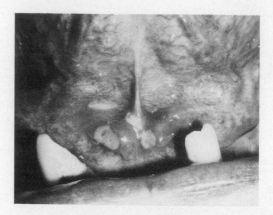

Fig. 6-1. Recurrent aphthous stomatitis. This middle-aged woman had many ulcers scattered throughout the oral mucosa. Note the characteristic reddened (darker) mucosa surrounding these ulcers in the sublingual region.

plexes) play an important role in recurrent aphthous ulceration (Antoon and Miller, 1980; Graykowski and Hooks, 1978; Lehner, 1968). Eversole et al. (1982) and Hay and Reade (1984) studied the effect of diet on exacerbation of RAU. The former obtained negative results, whereas the latter were able to demonstrate a correlation with certain foods.

Features

The ulcers of recurrent aphthous stomatitis are basically round or ovoid, have yellowish necrotic bases, and are surrounded by a region of inflamed mucosa. When the lesions are less than 1 cm they are referred to as "minor" ulcers; if larger than 1 cm they are referred to as "major" ulcers. The lesions are multiple and invariably painful, and they occur most frequently on the labial or buccal mucosa, floor of the mouth, and soft palate (Fig. 6-1). The recurrent attacks each last for about 10 days. If major aphthous ulcers are present, they may persist for months. The patient then enjoys a disease-free period varying from a few weeks to several months before having a recurrence of aphthous stomatitis. As with all of the other stomatitides a painful lymphadenitis may accompany each ulcerative episode.

If extraoral problems accompany recurrent aphthous stomatitis, the diagnosis of Behçet's syndrome may be made (Lehner and Barnes, 1979). Behçet's syndrome is characterized by oral and genital ulcers and ocular inflammation. At least two of these symptoms are required to establish the diagnosis. Behçet's syndrome is further classified as mucocutaneous (oral, genital, or skin lesions, or all three), arthritic (arthritis in addition to mucocutaneous lesions), and neuro-ocular (neurologic or ocular symptoms or both in addition to the mucocutaneous and arthritic signs).

Differential diagnosis

All the ulcerative mucositides listed at the beginning of this chapter should be considered. The absence of vesicles and blebs rules out *benign mucous membrane pemphigoid* and *pemphigus* and partially eliminates *erythema multiforme*. The ulcers in recurrent aphthous stomatitis are quite uniform in appearance and also somewhat similar in size. This uniformity differentiates this condition from the lesions of erythema multiforme, which vary greatly from one another in appearance: erythematous macules, blebs, ulcers, and crusted lesions on the lip. The presence of crusted lesions on the vermilion border is not compatible with a diagnosis of recurrent aphthous ulceration. The absence of a white (keratotic) component tends to rule out *lichen planus, lichenoid drug reaction, lupus erythematosus,* and *psoriasis.*

Atrophic candidiasis may also appear red, but the clinician expects to discover predisposing conditions in the patient evaluation. Most cases of candidiasis, even the atrophic type, pass through a white necrotic phase or have a minor keratotic component. Negative results on a cytologic test for *Candida albicans* rules out this possibility.

Primary herpetic gingivostomatitis must be differentiated from recurrent aphthous stomatitis. Herpetic gingivostomatitis is a systemic viral infection. The patient usually has a fever and complains of malaise and often nausea. Small vesicles precede herpetic ulceration. The vesicles and subsequent ulcers are pinpoint size, and the attached gingivae are almost invariably involved. In recurrent aphthous stomatitis the gingivae are seldom involved. A history of contact with an active lesion on another person can often be established in primary herpetic infection.

Herpetiform ulcers are characterized by recurrent crops of as many as 100 small (1 to 2 mm) painful ulcers that may involve any part of the oral mucosa. They probably do not represent a herpesvirus infection.

Management

The cause of the lesion is currently obscure, and there is no specific treatment. Patients are generally given supportive therapy, including the use of systemic analgesics and topical anesthetic agents. In especially severe cases the use of topical or systemic steroids should be considered. Tetracycline mouth rinse has been reported to be effective in reducing the severity of lesions of recurrent aphthous ulcerations (Graykowski and Hooks, 1978). Tyldesley (1983) reported that 9.5% of his patients with recurrent oral ulceration (ROU) had lowered serum folate or B_{12} levels without iron deficiency. Thus he advocated a full blood screening for ROU patients in order to identify these cases. Olson et al. (1982) reported opposite findings and suggested that these extra tests are not warranted. Hay and Reade (1984) obtained encouraging results with the use of an elimination diet in a significant number of patients. Wray (1982) found that the administration of systemic zinc sulfate was not helpful.

PRIMARY HERPETIC GINGIVOSTOMATITIS

Primary infections with herpes simplex virus (herpesvirus hominis) are a relatively common cause of multiple oral ulcerations.

Features

Approximately 80% of Americans have antibodies to type 1 herpesvirus, presumptive evidence of a prior infection. The initial infection with the herpesvirus may be subclinical or may be heralded by the appearance of a vesicular lesion on the vermilion border. The primary infection is occasionally characterized by the acute onset of a systemic illness. Following an incubation period of 5 to 10 days, the patient complains of malaise, irritability, headache, and fever, and within a few days the mouth becomes very painful. Oral examination reveals a widespread inflammation of the marginal and attached gingivae. Numerous small vesicles are seen throughout the oral mucosa and on the lips (Fig. 6-2 and Plate 3). These vesicles soon rupture and become pinpoint ulcers, and secondary infection generally occurs. Ulcers on the lips may become bloody and crusted, and saliva may "drool" from the oral cavity. Cervical lymphadenopathy is also a frequent finding. In young children the diagnosis of the infection may be missed: the symptoms may be assumed to result from teething.

Dental personnel should be aware of the possibility of implantation of the virus on the hands. This is one of many reasons to take uniform infection control precautions, including the routine use of gloves. Herpetic whitlow is a primary infection of the finger with this virus. It may be seen in dental personnel who examine mouths of patients with primary herpetic

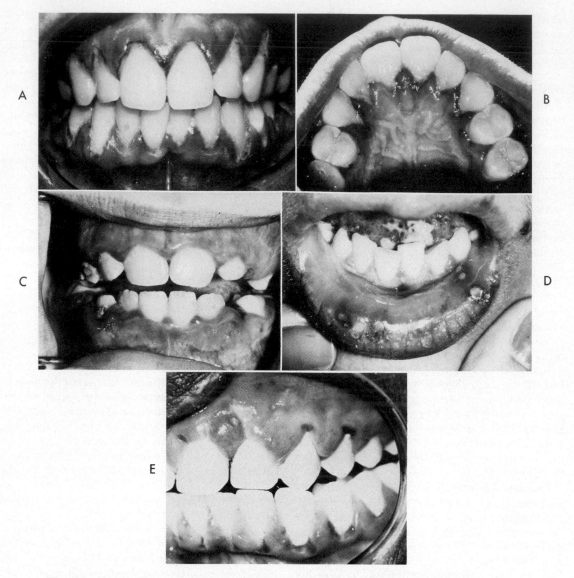

Fig. 6-2. Primary herpetic gingivostomatitis. **A** and **B,** Example in a woman. Note the inflamed gingivae and the ragged appearance with a faint whitish pattern. Close inspection revealed that the ragged white appearance was produced by the rupture and ulceration of the many pinpoint vesicles. **C,** Example in a 9-year-old boy; the primary infection was mostly confined to the gingivae. **D,** Case in which the prominent manifestations involved the mucosa of the lip and the anterior portion of the tongue in a 13-year-old girl. **E,** Gingival inflammation and swelling in leukemia. The ragged appearance with the multiple pinpoint ulcerations is not present in this disease.   (**A** and **B** courtesy E. Ranieri, DDS, Maywood, Ill. **E** courtesy P. Akers DDS, Evanston, Ill.)

gingivostomatitis or in patients who have a habit of biting the cuticle.

Recurrent herpetic infections develop in about one third of those patients who have had a primary infection. Herpes labialis is the most frequent type of recurrent infection. It usually is seen as a cluster of vesicles appearing around the lips after a systemic illness or other stress-ful situation. Ultraviolet light and mechanical stimuli may also produce recurrences.

Differential diagnosis

The differential diagnosis of primary herpetic gingivostomatitis has been reviewed in the differential diagnosis section of recurrent aphthous stomatitis. In addition, *hand-foot-mouth disease* (viral etiology) needs to be considered because multiple pinpoint oral vesicles and ulcers, as well as fever, are common signs. The absence of lesions on the palms and soles eliminates hand-foot-mouth disease from consideration. *Herpangina* (coxsackievirus) can generally be identified by the limited distribution of the small vesicles and ulcers to the soft palate and oropharynx.

Occasionally a very severe intraoral manifestation of *recurrent herpes* occurs (e.g., small pinpoint vesicles and ulcers covering the whole palate). It is important to note that only one surface is involved in the recurrence, whereas multiple surfaces are involved in primary herpetic gingivostomatitis.

ESTABLISHMENT OF DIAGNOSIS

The diagnosis of primary herpetic gingivostomatitis is usually made on a clinical basis. The patient has a number of vesicles or small painful ulcers throughout the oral cavity. A history of systemic signs and symptoms of a viral illness helps to establish the diagnosis.

Confirmation of the viral infection by laboratory methods is available but not routinely used. The virus may be isolated in tissue culture if fluid can be obtained from an intact vesicle. Primary infections are associated with an increase in antibody titer, and paired acute and convalescent sera may be studied. Histologic and cytologic examination of tissue may be done, but the examination does not permit identification of the specific virus (Burns, 1980).

There are two types of herpes simplex virus that cause disease in humans. The type 1 virus is primarily associated with infections of the skin and oral mucous membrane, and type 2 with infections of the genitalia (although the converse can and does occur). Epidemiologic studies have suggested a relationship between carcinoma of the uterine cervix and herpes simplex virus type 2; however, a relationship between oral infection with the type 1 virus and oral carcinoma has not been demonstrated. The frequency of oral herpesvirus infection is so high that these relationships are statistically difficult to demonstrate (Scully, 1983; Shillitoe and Silverman, 1979).

Management

There is no specific treatment for primary herpetic gingivostomatitis. Acyclovir (Zovirax) is effective in the management of initial herpes genitalis. It is also useful in treating non-life-threatening mucocutaneous herpes simplex virus infections in immunocompromised patients (Myers et al., 1982; Whitley et al., 1982). In these patients a decrease in the duration of viral shedding has been reported. There is no reported clinical evidence of benefit in treating herpes labialis in nonimmunocompromised patients.

The usual supportive measures for an acute viral infection should be instituted. These include maintenance of proper oral hygiene, adequate fluid intake to prevent dehydration, and the use of systemic analgesics for control of pain. Antipyretic agents are also prescribed when fever is a symptom. In severe cases it may be necessary to use a topical anesthetic mouth rinse such as viscous lidocaine or elixir of diphenhydramine. The patient is often able to tolerate cold liquids, and they may aid in preventing dehydration. Secondary bacterial infection of the many small punctate ulcers invariably is a major contributor to the pain after the vesicles rupture.

EROSIVE LICHEN PLANUS

The lesions of lichen planus may take several different forms and have been classified into the following types: keratotic, vesiculobullous, atrophic, and erosive (Shklar, 1972). The lesions of the atrophic and erosive forms are somewhat distinct, but they are discussed under the common heading of erosive lichen planus. The cause of the disease is obscure, but some studies have implicated emotional stress.

Features

The keratotic form of lichen planus (discussed in Chapter 8 as a white lesion) has been considered the most common, but one report suggests that the erosive form may be seen more often (Silverman and Griffith, 1974). The disease occurs about twice as often in women as in men. The initial lesion usually does not occur in patients under 40 years of age; the average age of the patient is 50 years.

Lichen planus is primarily a disease of whites and is seldom reported in blacks or Orientals. The most common site of involvement is the buccal mucosa, but the tongue, gingiva, palate, lip, and floor of the mouth (in decreasing order of frequency) are also involved. Reports of concurrent skin involvement are quite variable, in the range of 20%. A spontaneous remission has been reported in many cases, and the oral lesions are especially prone to recurrence and remission.

Although the keratotic form of lichen planus is usually asymptomatic, the patient with the atrophic or erosive variety almost always complains of a burning sensation or pain. The atrophic lesions appear smooth and erythematous and may have a feathery, white, keratotic border. In the erosive form the surface is usually granular and bright red and tends to bleed when traumatized. A pseudomembrane composed of necrotic cells and fibrin covers the more severe areas of erosion. The patterns of involvement change from week to week. However, almost invariably a white keratotic component is clinically apparent in a reticular, feathery, or plaque pattern (Fig. 6-3 and Plate 1).

Cases have been reported in which lichen planus was associated with a squamous cell carcinoma, and as a consequence, it has been speculated that lichen planus might be a premalignant lesion (Fulling, 1973; Silverman and Griffith, 1974). In recent follow-up studies, however, the number of patients with lichen planus in whom squamous cell carcinoma developed ranged from less than 1% to 2.5%. (Please refer to p. 128 in Chapter 8.) These results do not confirm the previous reports and leave the question unresolved (Drinnan and Fischman, 1990). As a matter of precaution,

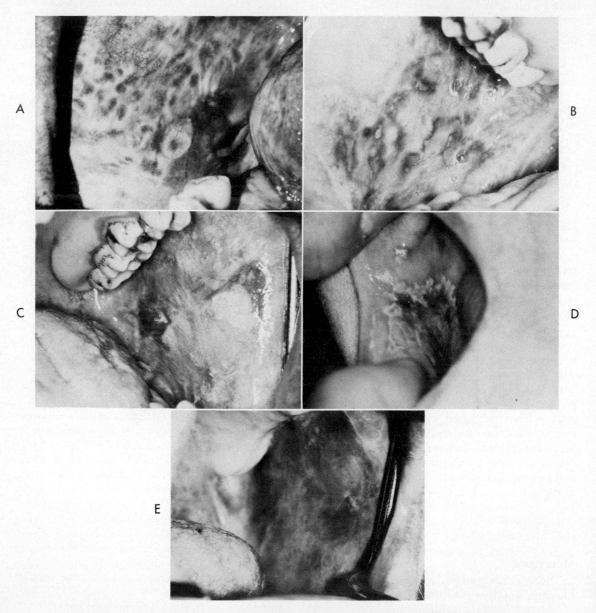

Fig. 6-3. Erosive lichen planus. **A** and **D,** Four cases of erosive lichen planus. Note the various proportions of keratotic and erythematous involvement in each. **E,** Case of erosive lichen planus in which almost no keratotic component was present. Two weeks later a considerable keratotic component was observed in this same case.

such patients should be observed carefully so that any changes can be detected early and investigated.

On histopathologic study, the atrophic form shows a thinned epithelium with hydropic degeneration in the basal cell layer. A dense bandlike infiltrate of lymphocytes is confined to the area immediately beneath the epithelium. In the erosive form either the epithelium is completely missing or only remnants of epithelial tissue are seen. The underlying lymphocytic inflammatory infiltrate becomes mixed with polymorphonuclear leukocytes and loses its distinctive bandlike pattern. The diagnosis of lichen planus can be confirmed only by a biopsy.

In the atrophic lesions, in which the epithelium is still intact, the changes are usually characteristic. Unfortunately, an intact epithelium does not exist in erosive lesions and the diagnosis may be difficult if not impossible. A biopsy specimen from the edge of an erosive lesion is usually more helpful than one from the erosive central area in establishing a diagnosis. When more typical lesions are present on other areas of the mucosa or skin, it may be assumed that the red lesions represent lichen planus (Fig. 6-3). However, if the lesions are clinically suggestive of squamous cell carcinoma, biopsy is imperative.

Differential diagnosis

Other diseases that contain a clinically apparent keratotic component in combination with a mucositis and so present lesions similar to those of lichen planus are speckled leukoplakia, squamous cell carcinoma, lichenoid drug reaction, electrogalvanic mucosal lesions, psoriasis, stomatitis areata migrans, atrophic candidiasis with a keratotic border, and discoid lupus erythematosus. An extensive discussion may be found on p. 130 in Chapter 8.

When red lesions are confined to the gingiva, it is virtually impossible to distinguish atrophic or erosive lichen planus from benign mucous membrane pemphigoid and desquamative gingivitis on the basis of clinical and histologic examination. Immunofluorescence findings in gingival biopsies are diagnostic of benign mucous membrane pemphigoid and some forms of desquamative gingivitis. Kippi et al. (1988) summarized the use of this technique.

SPECIAL DIAGNOSTIC PROCEDURES

In lichen planus, immunofluorescence studies of biopsies reveal characteristic but not diagnostic findings (Table 6-1). Globular deposits, sometimes called cytoid bodies or Civatte

Table 6-1. Immunofluorescence findings important in the diagnosis of red conditions

Disease	Serum		Tissue		
	Types of antibodies	Findings	Pattern of staining	Findings	Significance
Benign mucous membrane pemphigoid or cicatricial pemphigoid	Basement membrane antibodies	- or + (<25%)	Basement membrane	+	Diagnostic
Bullous pemphigoid	Basement membrane antibodies	+(80%)	Basement membrane zone	+(100%)	Diagnostic
Lichen planus	Negative		Globular deposits or cytoid bodies in dermis and epidermis; fibrin deposits along dermoepidermal junctions	+(97%)	Characteristic
Pemphigus, all forms	Intercellular antibodies of epithelium	+(>95%)	Intercellular epithelial deposits	+(100%)	Diagnostic
Discoid lupus erythematosus	Negative or low titer of antinuclear antibodies		Dermoepidermal deposits of immunoglobulins and complement: lesion only	+(80%)	Highly characteristic
Systemic lupus erythematosus	High titer of antinuclear antibodies	+(90%-100%)	Dermoepidermal deposits of immunoglobulins and complement: lesion and normal tissue	+(>90%)	Diagnostic

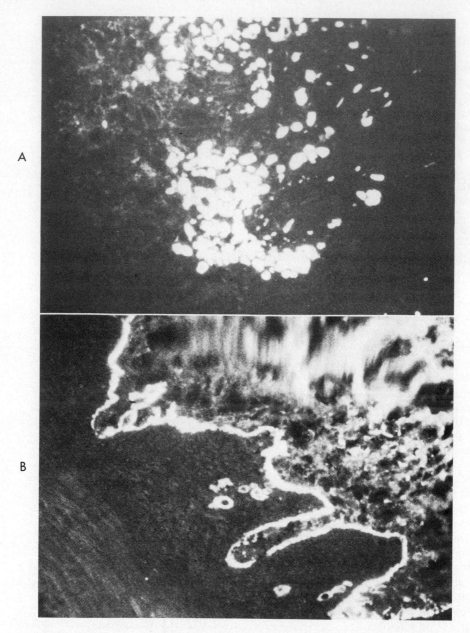

Fig. 6-4. A, Direct immunofluorescence test on oral biopsy specimen from patient with lichen planus demonstrating IgG deposits in cytoid or globular pattern in the dermis. Similar deposits of IgA, IgM, fibrin, and complement can also be seen. Such findings are characteristic. **B,** Direct immunofluorescence test on oral biopsy specimen from patient with lichen planus demonstrating fibrin deposits in a granular pattern along the dermoepidermoid junction.

bodies, contain immunoglobulins, fibrin, or complement and are observed in the papillary dermis along the dermoepidermal junction (Fig. 6-4). Cytoid bodies are more often seen in active stages of the disease and are more common in lesions than in normal tissue. Although cytoid bodies are neither disease specific nor diagnostic, their identification can be helpful when routine histopathologic studies

are inconclusive. Cytoid bodies are seen in biopsy specimens in 97% of lichen planus, 41% of systemic lupus erythematosus, 70% of discoid lupus erythematosus, 75% of dermatomyositis, 50% of erythema multiforme, 50% of pemphigoid, 40% of pemphigus, and 40% of normal specimens. The findings in lichen planus can be partially differentiated from the other diseases and the normal specimens on the basis of size and number of cytoid bodies and other immunologic findings. In addition to revealing cytoid bodies, immunofluorescence studies also reveal fibrin deposits along the basement membrane. Fibrin deposits, found in later stages of lesions, are not disease specific and occur in other diseases. Diagnostic immunofluorescence findings can also be seen in biopsy specimens of lupus erythematosus, pemphigus, and pemphigoid (Table 6-1). In normal biopsy specimens, smaller and fewer cytoid bodies are observed.

Management

It is necessary to establish a firm diagnosis of erosive lichen planus. In particular, lichenoid drug reactions should be considered. Because of the increased incidence of lichen planus in diabetic patients, it is important to examine the patient for the possibility of this disease. If the patient is shown to have diabetes, prompt stabilization of the condition by the medical colleague is beneficial to management of the oral condition.

A specific and uniformly successful treatment for erosive lichen planus is not available. Nevertheless the suffering patient can usually be greatly helped. It is almost always possible to reduce the degree of pain and produce regression of the lesions with extended drug therapy. Generally when a remission has been induced and drug therapy has been discontinued for a variable period of weeks or months, the painful lesions recur and drug therapy has to be reinstituted.

Milder cases may be managed successfully with the application of steroid salves such as Lidex or Kenalog in Orabase after meals and before sleep.

For more severe cases the standard treatment has been the oral administration of adequate doses of prednisone for 2 weeks. If the lesions are well into remission by this time, the dosage of systemic corticosteroids may be tapered off and discontinued. If small isolated lesions are still present, these can be managed with the topical application of corticosteroid pastes such as Lidex or Kenalog in Orabase. In many cases, when the systemic administration of corticosteroids must be continued for several months, the complications of extended corticosteroid therapy must be considered.

Zegarelli (1983) described an approach that combined three modalities of corticosteroid therapy: topical application, lesion injection, and systemic administration. Silverman (1984) and Lozada (1981) advocated a combination of systemic prednisone and azathioprine. This short course of azathioprine therapy permitted a lower dosage of prednisone to be used.

Solberg et al. (1983) reported significant success using vitamin A analogues for a 6-month period.

Recently griseofulvin has shown promise in the treatment of erosive lichen planus. However, many months of continued administration of this drug are required, and the serious potential side effects require periodic monitoring of the patient. Aufdemorte et al. (1983) discussed their experience with this modality of treatment.

ERYTHEMA MULTIFORME

Erythema multiforme is a disease of unknown etiology that has many different manifestations; however, when seen in its classic form, it is easily recognized. Although it is a vesiculobullous disease, vesicles and bullae usually are present for only a limited time.

Although an attack of erythema multiforme usually occurs without apparent reason, certain agents have been identified as precipitating the disease. The most common is a herpes simplex infection (Nesbit and Gobetti, 1986), but other infections and many drugs have also been implicated.

Features

The disease occurs primarily in young adults, usually men. It has a sudden onset and runs a course of 2 to 6 weeks. Recurrences are common. In many cases lesions are limited to the oral mucosa and involve, in descending order of frequency, the buccal mucosa, lips, palate, tongue, and fauces (Fig. 6-5 and Plate 4). The gingivae are rarely involved.

Sloughing of the mucosa and diffuse redness are the most frequent clinical features. The initial lesions are small red macules that may enlarge and show a whitish center. The macules progress to form bullae that soon rupture, leaving a sloughing mucosal surface. A bright red, raw surface is seen when the tissue is lost. In time the denuded surface becomes covered with a pseudomembrane of fibrin and cells and assumes a grayish appearance. Involvement of the oral tissues may be limited to merely a diffuse redness.

Skin lesions of erythema multiforme are pathognomonic. They may accompany the oral condition, or there may be cutaneous manifestation without oral involvement. Skin lesions have a characteristic "bull's eye" or "target" appearance (Fig. 6-5). Although the palms of the

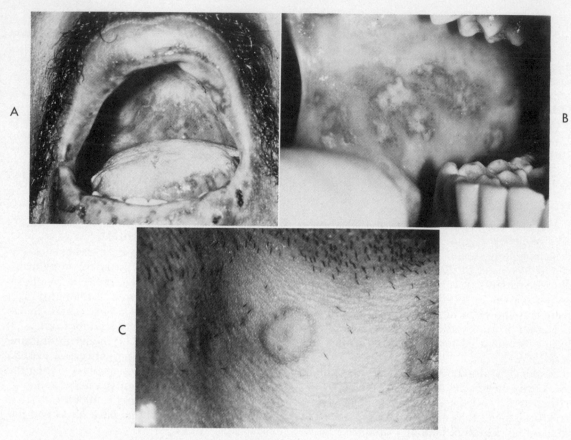

Fig. 6-5. Erythema multiforme. **A,** Extensive lesions of the lips and oral mucous membranes in a 26-year-old man. **B,** A milder case with erythematous patches, blebs, erosions, and ulcers restricted to the mucosa of the cheeks. **C,** Target lesion on the skin of another patient with erythema multiforme.   (**A** courtesy W. Heaton, DDS, Chicago.)

hands are a classic location, these lesions may occur anywhere on the skin.

A microscopic examination of vesicles and bullae reveals a subepithelial cleft. The underlying connective tissue contains a mixed inflammatory infiltrate with numerous eosinophils. The light microscopic changes and immunologic findings seen in immunofluorescence examination of biopsy specimens are not diagnostic but can be used to rule out other diseases. Buchner et al. (1980) reported on the histologic spectrum of oral erythema multiforme. There are no useful laboratory studies.

The diagnosis is made on the basis of clinical information. Obviously this can pose a problem if the lesions are limited to the oral cavity. A history of previous attacks that involved other mucous membranes or the skin is most useful in making the diagnosis. Stevens-Johnson syndrome is a severe episode of erythema multiforme that involves the mucosa, conjunctiva, and skin. Nazif and Ranalli reviewed 14 cases in 1982.

Differential diagnosis

Similar oral lesions may be seen in pemphigus vulgaris, benign mucous membrane pemphigoid, allergic reactions, erosive lichen planus, primary herpetic gingivostomatitis, and xerostomia. All of these diseases must be considered in a differential diagnosis. Oral lesions resulting from drug reactions may appear similar to those of erythema multiforme and may vary from focal or diffuse areas of erythema to areas of erosion and ulceration. At times it may be difficult to decide whether the drug precipitated an attack of erythema multiforme or the lesions resulted from drug allergy.

Management

Since erythema multiforme is a self-limiting disease, usually only supportive care is necessary. When areas other than the oral cavity are involved, the patient is best managed through a cooperative effort of physician and dentist. If the oral cavity is severely involved, systemic corticosteroids usually bring about prompt and

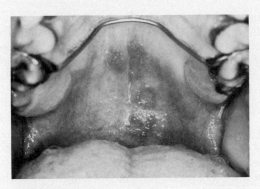

Fig. 6-6. Erythematous papules of candidiasis that were an incidental finding and resolved without treatment. An exfoliative cytologic smear was positive for *Candida*.

dramatic relief. Lozada (1981) reported that if 50 to 100 mg of azathioprine were combined with prednisone, a lower dosage of prednisone could be used. A corticosteroid in oral suspension used as a mouthwash may provide symptomatic relief in mild cases.

ACUTE ATROPHIC CANDIDIASIS

The lesions of acute atrophic candidiasis (formerly known as acute atrophic candidosis) represent a less common form of *Candida* infection. They usually are the sequelae to the typical lesions of acute pseudomembranous candidiasis. When the white plaque of pseudomembranous candidiasis is shed or removed, often a red, atrophic, and painful mucosa remains (Fig. 6-6 and Plate 3). At times the lesion may be asymptomatic.

Features

The lesions are seen in the same types of patients who are prone to acute pseudomembranous candidiasis, for example, those taking broad-spectrum antibiotics, steroids, or immunosuppressive agents. In addition, the lesions occur in patients with diabetes, hypothyroidism, and other debilitating diseases and during pregnancy. They are also sometimes found in apparently healthy individuals.

Tissue sections show an atrophic epithelium that may contain a few hyphae in the superficial layers. The lamina propria usually has a mild acute inflammatory infiltrate and increased vascularity. An exfoliative cytologic smear of the lesions may be useful in establishing a diagnosis.

Differential diagnosis

Frequently the red lesions of acute atrophic candidiasis are seen in association with those of the pseudomembranous type and so do not pose a diagnostic problem. When present as multiple red lesions, they are rather nonspecific in appearance. Lesions produced by chemical burns, drug reactions, and other organisms have a similar clinical appearance, as may the predominantly red lesions of erosive lichen planus, mild cases of erythema multiforme, and discoid lupus erythematosus.

Management

The lesions of acute atrophic candidiasis respond well to a dosage of either nystatin oral suspension or nystatin troches. A typical therapeutic regimen includes the use of nystatin troches four or five times daily. Treatment should be continued for at least 15 days. Barrett (1984) indicated that nystatin was of little use in eliminating oropharyngeal *Candida* in immunosuppressed patients. Fluconazole (Diflucan) is an effective alternative treatment in these patients (Chuck and Sande, 1989).

Ketoconazole (Nizoral) is a systemic antifungal agent useful in treating chronic mucocutaneous candidiasis. In patients whose disease does not respond to topical therapy, a daily administration of one 200-mg tablet for 2 weeks has been effective. Maintenance therapy may be required. Ketoconazole has been associated with hepatic toxicity, and patients receiving this drug should be closely monitored (Kirkpatrick, 1980; Peterson, 1980).

Clotrimazole (Mycelex) is available in troche form for the treatment of oropharyngeal candidiasis. Reports indicate that one 10-mg troche used 5 times a day is highly effective in the treatment of chronic oral candidiasis (Kirkpatrick and Alling, 1978; Yap, 1979).

BENIGN MUCOUS MEMBRANE PEMPHIGOID

The cause of benign mucous membrane pemphigoid, or cicatricial pemphigoid, is unknown.

Features

Benign mucous membrane pemphigoid (cicatricial pemphigoid) is seen twice as frequently in women as in men. The disease affects older individuals, with the highest incidence occurring in the late 50s. It has rarely been reported in other than whites. Lesions are found primarily on the mucous membranes, with infrequent involvement of the skin. The mucous membranes of the oral cavity and eyes are most often involved. Lesions occur on the gingiva, buccal mucosa, and palate.

The gingiva, the most common site (Silverman et al., 1986), becomes edematous and bright red—a striking feature of the disease (Plate 3). This involvement may be patchy or diffuse. Subsequent to bulla formation or trauma, the surface epithelium may be lost, leaving a raw, red, bleeding surface. The vesic-

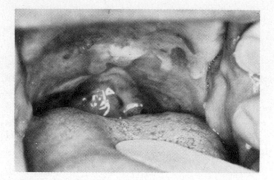

Fig. 6-7. Benign mucous membrane pemphigoid. This illustration shows whitish areas of intact and collapsed bullae and some erythematous and ulcerated areas.

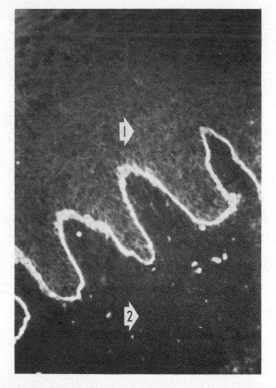

Fig. 6-8. Direct immunofluorescence test on oral biopsy specimen from patient with benign mucous membrane pemphigoid revealing complement deposits along the basement membrane zone in a linear pattern (1, epithelium; 2, lamina propria). Similar deposits of IgG and other immunoglobulins also occur. These findings are diagnostic.

ulobullous lesions in other areas of the oral cavity do not appear as red, nor do they bleed as readily. The ulcers that result from the collapse of bullae are surrounded by a zone of erythema (Fig. 6-7) and are relatively asymptomatic. Unless treated, the disease follows a chronic course of partial remission and exacerbation.

The histologic changes are only characteristic if the epithelium is intact. Frequently the roof of the subepithelial bulla is lost and the histologic changes become nonspecific, characterized by a chronic inflammatory infiltrate of the connective tissue. If the surface is intact, direct immunofluorescence study of the biopsy is particularly important, since the immunofluorescence findings are diagnostic. The basement membrane zone contains a deposition of immunoglobulins and complement (Fig. 6-8). The immunofluorescence findings can also be observed in the adjacent clinically normal mucosa. The biopsy site of choice for immunofluorescence is actually the perilesional or clinically normal mucosa, since these areas have dermal-epidermal relationships necessary for evaluation (see Table 6-1). In approximately 25% of the cases, low titers of serum antibodies to the basement membrane are also observed. When these occur, they are also diagnostic of pemphigoid.

Immunofluorescence is an important and useful diagnostic technique because it can help differentiate the gingival lesions of benign mucous membrane pemphigoid from those of erosive lichen planus and desquamative gingivitis. A clinical feature common to these three diseases is the production of a gingival bleb by a strong jet of air. This occurs because of the defect in the basement membrane region. Manton and Scully (1988) emphasized the necessity of using a combination of clinical, histologic, and immunostaining examinations to establish a diagnosis of mucous membrane pemphigoid.

Differential diagnosis

Other diseases that should be considered in a differential diagnosis of benign mucous membrane pemphigoid are pemphigus vulgaris, bullous pemphigoid, bullous lichen planus, and early cases of erythema multiforme.

Benign mucous membrane pemphigoid and *bullous pemphigoid* are clinically and histologically similar but differ in sites of involvement. Benign mucous membrane pemphigoid characteristically involves the mucous membranes, most commonly the oral cavity and secondly the conjunctiva. Skin lesions are infrequently observed. In bullous pemphigoid, the usual site of involvement is the skin. In approximately 30% of cases the oral mucosa is involved. The immunofluorescence pathologic findings in both diseases are identical, showing immune deposits along the basement membrane. However, the two diseases differ in the incidence and titer of basement membrane zone antibodies in sera. In bullous pemphigoid, basement membrane zone antibodies, generally of high titer (greater than 1:80), occur in approximately 97% of patients. In benign mucous membrane pemphigoid, antibody titers (usually less than 1:40) occur in only approximately 20% to 25% of patients.

Management

The patient with benign mucous membrane pemphigoid may be extremely difficult to treat. Corticosteroids have been the only useful form of therapy, but their side effects must be considered. The use of corticosteroids on alternate days has been somewhat successful, as a way to prevent these complications.

Recently, Rogers et al. (1982) recommended topical corticosteroids for mild cases and dapsone for more symptomatic cases. Dapsone therapy must be carefully monitored, since it can cause hemolysis and methemoglobulinemia, particularly in patients with glucose 6-phosphate dehydrogenase deficiency. Dapsone, however, appears to be the most effective treatment of benign mucous membrane pemphigoid. Because the mucous membranes of the eyes are often involved, patients with benign mucous membrane pemphigoid are at risk for blindness and should be referred to an ophthalmologist for examination.

PEMPHIGUS

Pemphigus is a vesiculobullous disease of unknown cause that may affect mucous membranes and skin. The four major forms of pemphigus are pemphigus vulgaris, pemphigus vegetans, pemphigus foliaceus, and pemphigus erythematosus. They have similar immunologic findings, which are diagnostic (see Table 6-1).

Features

Pemphigus affects the sexes approximately equally, and the vast majority of patients are white. In a report by Rosenberg et al. (1976) 74% of the patients with the vulgaris or vegetans type were Jewish people; approximately 98% of the patients were over 31 years of age at the time of onset; 80% of cases of the vulgaris variety (by far the most common type) first occurred intraorally. In this 20-year follow-up study, the mortality rate was reported at 32% with more than half of the deaths occurring within 12 months of the onset of the disease. Laskaris and Stoufi (1990) have reviewed the rare cases of pemphigus vulgaris in children.

The lesions of pemphigus vulgaris may appear as areas of erosion, but more often they are seen as ulcers, bullae, or areas of sloughing mucosa or skin (Fig. 6-9 and Plate 4). Diffuse erythematous involvement of the gingiva has been reported but is not the typical manifestation of the disease. In approximately half the cases, initial lesions occur orally, followed by skin lesions.

The histologic study of intact vesicles or bullae reveals that the basic defect is intraepithelial. The individual cells separate from one another and a pooling of fluid occurs. The basal layer of epithelial cells remains in position on the basement membrane.

Differential diagnosis

All the vesiculobullous conditions listed at the beginning of this chapter should be considered in the differential diagnosis. As a general rule, the pemphigus bulla is smaller than the bulla in benign mucous membrane pemphigoid and considerably larger than those seen in the viral diseases such as herpes and hand-foot-mouth disease.

SPECIAL DIAGNOSTIC PROCEDURES

Immunofluorescence studies of sera and biopsy specimens reveal a diagnostic finding of antibodies confined to the intercellular substance of epithelium and intercellular deposits of IgG (Fig. 6-9). The sera from more than 95% of pemphigus patients with active disease contain intercellular epithelial antibodies. During early stages of the disease or during remission, the antibody titers may be low or negative. The significance of the antibody titer must be considered together with the clinical and histologic findings. Low titers (10 to 20) are significant when there are typical clinical and histologic findings. Low titers of intercellular antibodies with atypical clinical and histologic findings may be termed "pemphigus-like" antibodies rather than true pemphigus antibodies. Pemphigus-like antibodies may occur as a result of extensive burns and following some drug eruptions but do not bind in vivo as those in true pemphigus do.

The intercellular antibody titer frequently relates to disease activity by rising and falling with exacerbations and remissions. In many

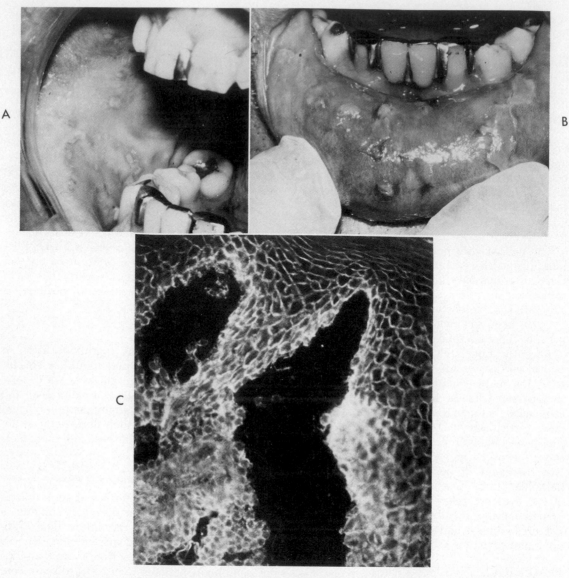

Fig. 6-9. Pemphigus. **A** and **B,** Clinical views of the same case. The mucosa of the lower lip is much more severely involved than the buccal mucosa. **C,** Direct immunofluorescence test on oral biopsy specimen from patient with pemphigus revealing IgG deposits intercellularly in the epithelium. Epithelial intercellular antibodies are also seen in the serum. Both are diagnostic.   (**A** and **B** courtesy M. Lehnert, DDS, Minneapolis.)

cases, titer changes of two or more doubling dilutions precede clinical changes and provide a prognostic test for control of drug therapy. Sera should be tested every 2 to 4 weeks until the patient is in remission and then every 1 to 6 months.

Almost all the patients with active pemphigus have intercellular deposits of IgG and sometimes IgA, IgM, and complement in biopsy specimens. These findings are diagnostic. Biopsies of oral lesions should be taken from the periphery of the lesion, where the epithelium is still intact (Daniels and Quadra-White,

1981). Laskaris (1981) gave a detailed report of an immunofluorescence study that included 58 cases of oral pemphigus. Handlers et al. (1982) advocated immunoperoxidase techniques as an alternative method to immunofluorescence as a diagnostic aid in cases of pemphigus.

Management

Corticosteroid therapy is the preferred treatment for severe pemphigus. Other modes of treatment include alternate-day steroid and gold therapy and immunosuppressive treatment with methotrexate or azathioprine

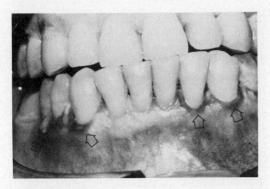

Fig. 6-10. Desquamative gingivitis. Note areas of erosion on the gingiva *(arrows)*. (Courtesy E. Ranieri, DDS, Maywood, Ill.)

(Rosenberg et al., 1976). Lozada et al. (1982) reported favorable results with a combination of levamisole and prednisone, in which lower dosages of prednisone were effectively used.

DESQUAMATIVE GINGIVITIS

There is some question as to whether desquamative gingivitis is a specific disease entity or a clinical manifestation of several different diseases. In a study of 40 patients with clinical desquamative gingivitis, McCarthy and Shklar (1964) histologically identified 17 cases of benign mucous membrane pemphigoid, two cases of pemphigus, and four cases of lichen planus. The remainder were considered hormonal, idiopathic, or abnormal responses to local factors. In an immunofluorescence study of 100 patients with clinical desquamative gingivitis, 35 were identified as having benign mucous membrane pemphigoid, three were identified as having pemphigus, and one patient was identified as having psoriasis. Of the remaining 61, 28 had findings consistent with lichen planus (Nisengard and Neiders, 1981). Although the cause of desquamative lesions of the gingivae is not always known, it is generally considered to represent a degenerative pathosis of the gingivae. Because it occurs more frequently in postmenopausal women, there may also be an underlying hormonal factor.

Features

Desquamative gingivitis is seen in both sexes but is far more prevalent in women (Glickman and Smulow, 1964). Usually it occurs after the age of 40, but it may occur at any age after puberty. The gingivae become bright red and edematous. The changes are usually confined to the labial gingivae. The palatal and lingual surfaces are not often involved. Changes may be limited to a few small areas of the palate (Fig. 6-10), or they may be diffuse and extend throughout the gingivae. The epithelium is quite friable and can be easily removed from the underlying connective tissue, leaving a red surface that bleeds readily after minimal trauma. Patients may complain of a burning sensation but often are asymptomatic.

On histologic examination, the epithelium is thin and atrophic. The rete ridges are blunted, and there may be clefting below the basement membrane. Edema and a mild chronic inflammatory infiltrate are seen in the underlying connective tissue. The microscopic findings are not diagnostic and serve only to exclude other diseases. Immunofluorescence studies of gingival biopsy specimens are especially valuable to determine if the underlying cause is benign mucous membrane pemphigoid, pemphigus, or lichen planus. The diagnosis is made on the basis of a careful history, physical examination, and laboratory tests.

Differential diagnosis

As previously mentioned, the other diseases that produce similar lesions are erosive lichen planus, benign mucous membrane pemphigoid, bullous pemphigoid, and, rarely, pemphigus vulgaris.

Management

Treatment of desquamative gingivitis is directed at providing symptomatic relief. It is important that all possible local irritating factors be removed. Different drugs such as estrogens and steroids have been applied topically and do provide variable degrees of improvement. Systemic steroids are also indicated (Nisengard and Rogers, 1987).

RADIATION AND CHEMOTHERAPY MUCOSITIDES

The diagnosis of the mucositis occurring as a result of radiation or chemotherapy should be readily established from the patient history. Kolbinson et al. (1988) discussed the early oral changes following chemotherapy and radiation therapy. The dental management of the patient with cancer has been reviewed by Fischman (1983).

Radiation mucositis
FEATURES

Radiation therapy produces characteristic and dramatic changes. During the course of therapy, which may continue for 6 weeks, a diffuse inflammatory change develops in the mucosa. The amount of tissue involved is determined by the portal used for the radiation therapy.

Tissue changes do not become apparent until the last part of the first week or the beginning of the second week. Distinct blebs may be produced, or a whitish area resulting from decreased cellular division and retention of squamous cells is seen. In subsequent weeks the surface layers are lost and a thin erythematous mucosa is present. Focal areas may ulcerate and then become covered with a tan-yellow, fibrous exudate (Fig. 6-11 and Plate 3). The tissue response varies considerably among patients. Profound changes resolve a few weeks after therapy is completed, but there is some residual redness for variable periods of time.

MANAGEMENT

Symptomatic relief is necessary for these patients because the pain can be severe, especially when eating. Topical anesthetics such as elixir of diphenhydramine or lidocaine can be combined with milk of magnesia, Maalox, or Kaopectate and used as mouthwash. Analgesics may be necessary.

Chemotherapy mucositis

FEATURES

Oral lesions resulting from chemotherapy may occur during and following the course of therapy. Initially, patients may complain of a burning sensation. Lesions may or may not be associated with this burning sensation. The lesions begin as focal areas of redness that may persist and ultimately ulcerate (Plate 3). Infrequently the ulcerations become numerous and large.

MANAGEMENT

Treatment is directed toward providing symptomatic relief. If the lesions become debilitating, it may be necessary to interrupt chemotherapy briefly. When secondarily infected, the lesions respond well to an oral suspension of tetracycline used as a mouthwash and then swallowed. Chlorhexidine mouth rinses are excellent for prophylaxis and therapy.

XEROSTOMIA

Dryness of the mouth is not a disease but a sign of reversible or irreversible impaired function of the salivary glands. Infectious lesions of the salivary glands such as mumps produce a transient xerostomia. When the primary disease resolves, the flow of saliva returns to normal. Diseases such as Mikulicz's disease or Sjögren's syndrome produce irreversible

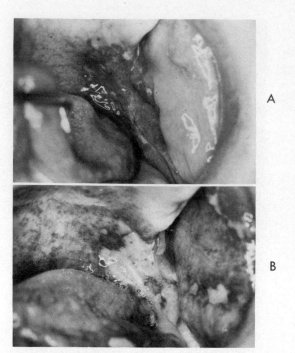

Fig. 6-11. Radiation mucositis. **A,** Squamous cell carcinoma appearing clinically as a large area of erythroplakia in the retromolar and soft palate region. **B,** Same patient approximately midway through radiation therapy. Note the areas of erythema and the fibrinous exudate.

changes that result in a progressive decrease in the production of saliva. Radiation to the head and neck area causes atrophy of the glands and a decrease in the amount of saliva secreted. Dehydration and senile atrophy of the glands reduce the amount of saliva produced by the glands. Many widely used medications decrease salivary gland activity. Ganglionic blocking agents used to control hypertension, many psychotherapeutic agents (tranquilizers and antidepressants), and antihistamines have this side effect. Eisenberg (1978) discussed the causes of xerostomia in considerable detail.

Features

In mild short-term cases of xerostomia, the patient may be asymptomatic and the mucosa appears normal. In moderately severe cases, the patient may complain of a dry mouth or burning sensation. When these symptoms are intense, patients experience difficulty with speech, mastication, and the retention of artificial appliances. Patches of mucosa appear very atrophic and take on a dark, dusty red appearance (Plate 4). In severe xerostomia, erosion and ulceration of the inflamed mucosa occurs.

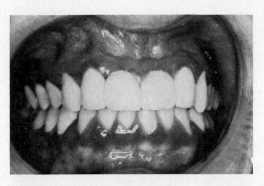

Fig. 6-12. Diffuse and striking erythematous changes of plasma cell gingivitis are confined to the gingiva.

The combined features of decreased salivary and lacrimal production suggest a diagnosis of Mikulicz's disease. In Sjögren's syndrome xerostomia, conjunctivitis sicca, rhinitis sicca, and arthritis are seen.

Differential diagnosis

A lack of saliva is the symptom that enables the clinician to differentiate the mucositis of xerostomia from the other types listed in this chapter.

Historical evidence is useful in establishing the type of xerostomia. A history of radiation treatment, antisialagogue medication, and combinations of features suggesting one of the syndromes associated with xerostomia are clues that direct the clinician to the correct diagnosis.

Management

Artificial saliva preparations are helpful. Hatton et al. (1987) discuss these in detail.

PLASMA CELL GINGIVITIS

Plasma cell gingivitis is a disease that was recognized as a distinct entity in 1968. It has also been reported under the name of atypical gingivostomatitis. Studies indicate that the lesions may be caused by some ingredient in chewing gum, and the disease has been suggested as a type of allergic response (Kerr et al., 1971; Perry et al., 1973). Although this condition was frequently seen in the 1960s and early 1970s, it has been seen much less frequently since then (Silverman and Lozada, 1977).

Features

Plasma cell gingivitis occurs much more frequently in women and is seen predominantly in young adults. The patient complains of a sore or burning mouth. The most striking and characteristic feature of the disease is the gingival involvement. The entire free and attached gingivae are edematous and bright red (Fig. 6-12). Frequently, there are associated lesions of the lips, tongue, and buccal mucosa, a scaling of the lips, and an angular cheilitis. The tongue is erythematous and devoid of filiform papillae. The patient may state that the problem has been present for as long as 3 years.

The most spectacular microscopic changes are seen in the lamina propria, which is densely infiltrated by plasma cells. The other changes are nonspecific. A diagnosis is made primarily on the basis of the clinical appearance of the lesions and is supported by a biopsy.

Differential diagnosis

The clinical features of plasma cell gingivitis are distinctive and are not simulated by other diseases. However, early leukemic infiltrate of the gingiva may appear somewhat similar, as may allergies to toothpaste ingredients.

Management

The patient usually shows a marked improvement shortly after he or she stops chewing gum or changes brands of toothpaste. Complete remission of the disease takes approximately 4 weeks.

STOMATITIS AREATA MIGRANS

Stomatitis areata migrans is a recently recognized disorder that is also known as migratory mucositis or ectopic geographic tongue.

Features

Most frequently the lesions of geographic tongue are confined to the dorsal surface and lateral borders of the tongue. Occasionally, similar lesions have been reported on other mucosal surfaces of the oral cavity (Weathers et al., 1974). These lesions are considered a more extensive involvement of the same process. The basic appearance is that of red patches of various sizes and shapes surrounded by white (keratotic), raised rims (Fig. 6-13 and Plate 1). The white rims may show a radiating, feathery appearance as they fade into the surrounding normal mucosa. The patterns change continuously and finally fade completely as the condition enters a remission. Stomatitis areata migrans is usually asymptomatic and found on routine oral examination.

The histopathologic study of stomatitis areata migrans shows a thinning of the surface epithelium in some areas and an epithelial hyperplasia in others. The epithelium may show spongi-

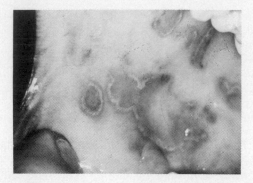

Fig. 6-13. Stomatitis areata migrans on the buccal mucosa.

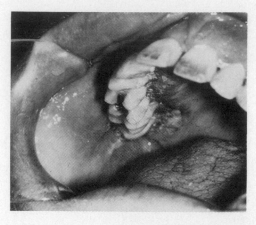

Fig. 6-14. Reaction to periodontal dressing. Note erythematous reaction on superior aspect of buccal mucosa where it was in contact with the dressing. Note severe tissue destruction on lingual gingiva. Plate 4 shows another view of this case.

osis and infiltration by acute and chronic inflammatory cells, often in focal arrangement (Munro's abscesses).

Differential diagnosis

Lesions that should be differentiated from stomatitis areata migrans are lichen planus, psoriasis, lupus erythematosus, Reiter's syndrome, and electrogalvanically induced lesions (Bánóczy et al., 1979).

Management

Most cases of stomatitis areata migrans are asymptomatic. Patients who complain of burning tenderness or pain should be placed on a bland diet and use diphenhydramine mouth rinses until the condition becomes asymptomatic.

ALLERGIES

Diffuse erythematous lesions may be seen on the oral mucosa as a result of allergies or as a toxic effect from drugs. These lesions take a variety of forms and have been classified as "erythema multiforme caused by medication" (stomatitis medicamentosa) or as "lichenoid drug reaction" (lichen planus caused by medication). The clinical presentation is identical to that of erythema multiforme and lichen planus, and the diagnosis is made from a careful history. Cessation of drug therapy, with the concurrent administration of antihistaminic agents, usually results in prompt resolution.

Reactions to topical agents used in the oral cavity are relatively unusual. Individual idiosyncracies to agents used in preparations such as surgical dressings, mouth rinses, toothpaste, and chewing gums have been reported (Fig. 6-14). A careful history is usually of assistance in making the diagnosis. The patient frequently reports changing from one brand of oral product to another immediately before development of the symptoms. Prompt withdrawal of the etiologic agent is usually both therapeutic and diagnostic.

Patients and clinicians frequently confuse the irritating effects of poorly fitting prosthetic appliances with allergy to a denture base material. Denture base materials are rarely allergenic, but poorly fitting appliances may produce such pathologic changes as papillary hyperplasia. Appliances that are not kept clean may be associated with an increased incidence of intraoral candidiasis. Improperly cured acrylic materials and improperly used denture relining materials can also cause injury to the oral mucosa, but this injury is a "burn" rather than a true allergy.

POLYCYTHEMIA

Polycythemia is a chronic and sustained elevation in the number of erythrocytes and level of hemoglobin. Both primary and secondary polycythemias occur. Primary polycythemia (polycythemia vera) is a neoplastic condition of the erythropoietic system analogous to leukemia. Transition between polycythemia and myelogenous leukemia has been reported. Secondary polycythemia is a sustained elevation of erythrocytes and hemoglobin, usually resulting from bone marrow stimulation caused by living at high altitudes or by chronic pulmonary diseases such as emphysema. It is also seen in untreated congenital heart disease.

The entire oral mucosa of patients with polycythemia has a deep red or purple color. This discoloration is particularly noticeable in the gingivae and soft palate. The gingivae usually are prone to easy bleeding, and petechial hemorrhages may be seen on the palate and labial mucosa. These changes are much more frequently seen in polycythemia vera. Infarcts may occur in the smaller vessels because of increased viscosity of the blood and may result in multiple ulcers in the red mucosa. Laboratory tests indicating a marked increase in erythrocytes, hemoglobin concentration, and hematocrit values quickly establish the general diagnosis of polycythemia and thus separate this condition from the other mucositides.

LUPUS ERYTHEMATOSUS

Lupus erythematosus (LE) is a connective tissue disease of unknown cause. Because nearly every organ in the body runs the risk of involvement, the disease produces a vast array of signs and symptoms. The term "discoid LE" has been applied to cases in which there is only skin involvement; this is usually a benign disease with a good prognosis. Chances of conversion of discoid lupus to systemic lupus are small. Skin lesions may also accompany systemic lupus.

Features

Lupus erythematosus occurs predominantly in adult females, and most are affected before the age of 40. Oral manifestations of discoid lupus erythematosus (DLE) occur in about 20% of patients. The oral lesions may occur with or without skin involvement, before skin lesions develop, after skin lesions develop, or simultaneously with the skin lesions. Oral lesions may also be seen in patients with systemic lupus erythematosus (SLE) (Plate 2).

Schiødt et al. (1978) studied 32 patients (26 females, 6 males) with LE lesions of the oral mucosa. The age of the patient at onset of the oral lesions ranged from 6 to 75 years with a mean age of 41 years. The mean duration of the oral lesions was 4.2 years. Symptoms such as discomfort, burning, and pain associated with hot spicy food were present in 75% of the patients. The lesions were most often located on the buccal mucosa, gingiva, labial mucosa, and vermilion border. The oral lesions were infected by yeast in more than half the patients.

In Schiødt's study, early lesions were characterized by erythema without striae. The classic well-developed discoid lesions appeared as an area of central erythema with white spots and a 2 to 5 mm wide border of white striae radiating from the center. Some lesions were white plaques, as in leukoplakia, and still others had areas of Wickham's striae as in lichen planus, usually on a reddish base.

On microscopic examination the epithelium shows hyperorthokeratosis or parakeratosis or both, acanthosis, and pseudoepitheliomatous hyperplasia interspersed with atrophy. The basal layer shows liquefaction degeneration, and keratin plugs can be found. A lymphocytic infiltrate is present beneath the epithelial layer. It may concentrate around vessels and extend deeply into the subepithelial tissue. In some cases the microscopic study of lesions may be inconclusive. Schiødt and Pindborg (1976) completed a blind study of oral lesions from 21 patients with LE and 21 patients with oral lichen planus and leukoplakia. The correct histologic diagnosis was made in less than half the cases. In one third of the cases differentiation could not be made between DLE and lichen planus.

Differential diagnosis

Multiple lesions on several surfaces are the rule in lupus erythematosus. When the lesions are mostly of the red variety, conditions that should be considered are lichen planus, lichenoid drug reaction, ectopic geographic tongue, psoriasis, diffuse leukoplakia with erythroplakic components, and electrogalvanic lesions. Oral lesions of LE may be differentiated from lichen planus on the basis of immunofluorescence studies of sera and biopsy specimens (Table 6-1).

Management

Treatment of lupus erythematosus consists of the administration of systemic corticosteroids or antimalarials. Topical steroids may be used on symptomatic intraoral lesions.

RARITIES

The following generalized red conditions occur more rarely:

Actinomycosis
Acute gangrenous stomatitis
Agranulocytosis
Amyloidosis
Bullous pemphigoid
Cheilitis granulomatosa (Melkersson-Rosenthal syndrome)
Crohn's disease
Darier's disease
Diabetic ulcerations
Epidermolysis bullosa
Gonococcal stomatitis
Granulomatous disease of the newborn
Hand-foot-mouth disease
Heavy metal poisoning

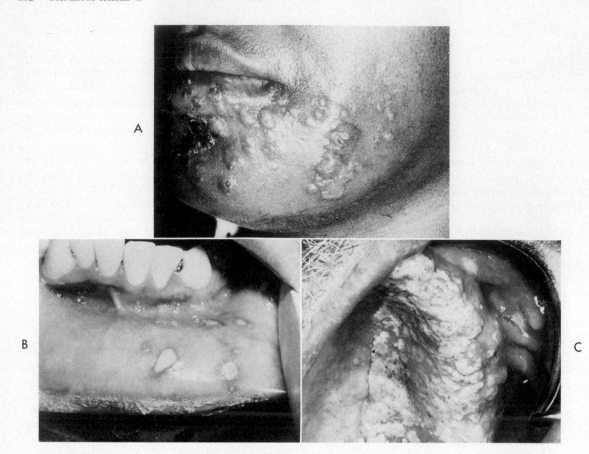

Fig. 6-15. Herpes zoster. **A** and **B,** Same case showing involvement of the skin and mucous membrane in area innervated by the mandibular branch of the trigeminal nerve. **C,** Another case of herpes zoster. Note white vesicles on an erythematous base and the sharp demarcation at the midline.   (Courtesy A.C.W. Hutchinson collection, Northwestern University Dental School Library, Chicago.)

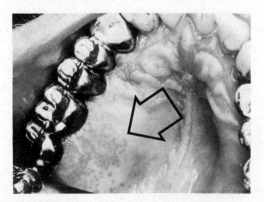

Fig. 6-16. Psoriasis (red macular areas) on palate. (From White DK, Leis HJ, and Miller AS: Oral Surg 41(2):174-181, 1976.)

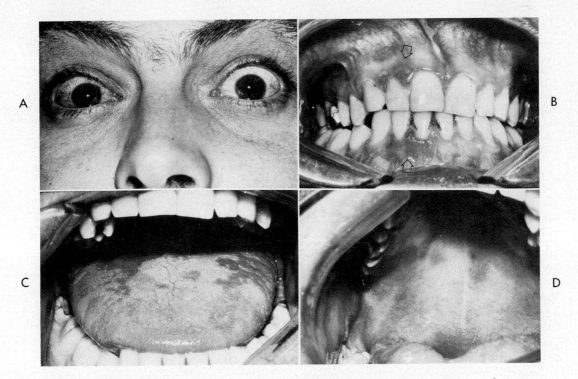

Fig. 6-17. Reiter's syndrome. **A,** Erythema involving the sclera. **B,** Anterior intraoral view. Note small erythematous patches *(arrows).* **C,** View showing reddish macules on tongue. **D,** View of palate showing reddish patches.   (Courtesy M. Lehnert, DDS, Minneapolis.)

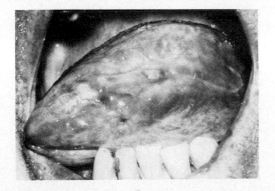

Fig. 6-18. Uremic stomatitis. Note erythematous and eroded areas on the lateral border of the tongue. (Courtesy M. Lehnert, DDS, Minneapolis.)

Hereditary mucoepithelial dysplasia
Hereditary telangiectasia
Herpangina
Herpes zoster (primary and secondary) (Fig. 6-15)
Histoplasmosis
Impetigo
Kaposi's sarcoma (multiple)
Leukemia
Major aphthous ulcerations (Sutton's disease)
Measles
Metastatic hemangiosarcomas
Mycosis fungoides
Pernicious anemia
Polyarteritis nodosa
Psoriasis (Fig. 6-16)
Psoriasis variants
　　Pustular psoriasis
　　Acrodermatitis continua
　　Impetigo herpetiformis
Pyostomatitis vegetans
Reiter's syndrome (Fig. 6-17)
Scurvy
Streptococcal stomatitis
Thermal and chemical burns (mild, recent)
Ulcerative colitis
Uremic stomatitis (Fig. 6-18)
Varicella
Vincent's angina
Vitamin B deficiencies (severe)

REFERENCES

Antoon JW and Miller RL: Aphthous ulcers—a review of the literature on etiology, pathogenesis, diagnosis and treatment, J Am Dent Assoc 101:803-808, 1980.

Aufdemorte TB, De Villez RL, and Gieseker DR: Griseofulvin in the treatment of three cases of oral erosive lichen planus, Oral Surg 55:459-462, 1983.

Bánóczy J, Roed-Petersen B, Pindborg JJ, and Inovay J: Clinical and histologic studies on electrogalvanically induced oral white lesions, Oral Surg 48:319-323, 1979.

Barrett AP: Evaluation of nystatin in prevention and elimination of oropharyngeal *Candida* in immunosuppressed patients, Oral Surg 58:148-151, 1984.

Buchner A, Lozada F, and Silverman S: Histological spectrum of oral erythema multiforme, Oral Surg 49:221-228, 1980.

Burns J: Diagnostic methods for herpes simplex infection: a review, Oral Surg 50:346-349, 1980.

Chuck SL and Sande MA: Infections with cryptococcus neoformans in the acquired immunodeficiency syndrome, N Engl J Med 321:794-799, 1989.

Daniels DE and Quadra-White C: Direct immunofluorescence in oral mucosal disease: a diagnostic analysis of 130 cases, Oral Surg 51:38-47, 1981.

Drinnan A and Fischman S: Controversies in oral medicine, Dent Clin North Am 34:159-169, 1990.

Eisenberg E: Medical considerations: cardiovascular, respiratory, gastrointestinal, and hematologic systems, xerostomia, and irradiation. In Wood NK, editor: Treatment planning: a pragmatic approach, St Louis, 1978, The CV Mosby Co, pp 122-128.

Eversole LR, Shopper TP, and Chambers DW: Effects of suspected food stuff challenging agents in the etiology of recurrent aphthous stomatitis, Oral Surg 54:33-38, 1982.

Fischman S: The patient with cancer. In Symposium on patient with increased medical risks, Dent Clin North Am 27:235-246, 1983.

Fulling HJ: Cancer development in oral lichen planus: a follow-up study of 327 patients, Arch Dermatol 108:667-669, 1973.

Glickman I and Smulow JB: Chronic desquamative gingivitis: its nature and treatment, J Periodontol 35:397-405, 1964.

Graykowski E and Hooks J: Summary of workshop on recurrent aphthous stomatitis and Behçet syndrome, J Am Dent Assoc 97:599-602, 1978.

Handlers JP, Melrose RJ, Abrams AM, and Taylor CR: Immunoperoxidase technique in diagnosis of oral pemphigus vulgaris: an alternative method to immunofluorescence, Oral Surg 54:207-212, 1982.

Hatton MN, Levine MJ, Margarone JE, and Aquirre A: Lubrication and viscosity features of human saliva and commercially available saliva substitutes, J Oral Maxillofac Surg 45:496-499, 1987.

Hay KD and Reade PC: The use of an elimination diet in the treatment of recurrent aphthous ulceration of the oral cavity, Oral Surg 57:504-507, 1984.

Kerr BA, McClatchey KD, and Regezi JA: Idiopathic gingivostomatitis, Oral Surg 32:402-423, 1971.

Kippi AM, Rich AM, Radden BG, and Reade PC: Direct immunofluorescence in the diagnosis of oral mucosal diseases, Int J Oral Maxillofac Surg 17:6-10, 1988.

Kirkpatrick C and Alling DW: Treatment of chronic oral candidiasis with clotrimazole troches, N Engl J Med 299:1201-1203, 1978.

Kirkpatrick C et al: Treatment of chronic mucocutaneous candidiasis with ketoconazole: preliminary results of a controlled double-blind clinical trial, Rev Infect Dis 2:599, 1980.

Kolbinson DA, Schubert MM, Flournoy N, and Truelove EL: Early oral changes following bone marrow transplantation, Oral Surg 66:130-138, 1988.

Laskaris G: Oral pemphigus vulgaris: an immunofluorescent study of fifty-eight cases, Oral Surg 51:626-631, 1981.

Laskaris G and Stoufi E: Oral pemphigus vulgaris in a 6-year-old girl, Oral Surg 69:609-613, 1990.

Lehner T: Autoimmunity in oral diseases, with special reference to recurrent oral ulceration, Proc R Soc Med 61:515-524, 1968.

Lehner T and Barnes C, editors: Behçet's syndrome, London, 1979, Academic Press, Inc.

Littner M, Dayan D, Kaffe I et al.: Acute streptococcal gingivostomatitis, Oral Surg 53:144-147, 1982.

Lozada F: Prednisone and azathioprine in the treatment of patients with vesiculoerosive oral diseases, Oral Surg 52:257-260, 1981.

Lozada F: Levamisole in the treatment of erythema multiforme: a double-blind trial in fourteen patients, Oral Surg 53:28-31, 1982.

Lozada F, Silverman S, and Cram D: Pemphigus vulgaris: a study of six cases treated with levamisole and prednisone, Oral Surg 54:161-165, 1982.

Manton SL and Scully C: Mucous membrane pemphigoid: an elusive diagnosis? Oral Surg 66:37-40, 1988.

McCarthy PL and Shklar G: Disease of the oral mucosa: diagnosis, management and therapy, New York, 1964, McGraw-Hill, Inc., pp 183-191.

Miller MF, Garfunkel AA, Ram CA et al: The inheritance of recurrent aphthous stomatitis: observations on susceptibility, Oral Surg 49:409-412, 1980.

Myers J et al: Multicenter collaborative trial of intravenous acyclovir for treatment of mucocutaneous herpes simplex virus infection in the immunocompromised host, Am J Med 73(1A):229-235, 1982.

Nazif MM and Ranalli DN: Stevens-Johnson syndrome: a report of fourteen pediatric cases, Oral Surg 53:263-266, 1982.

Nesbit SP and Gobetti JP: Multiple recurrence of oral erythema multiforme after secondary herpes simplex: report of case and review of literature, J Am Dent Assoc 112:348-352, 1986.

Nisengard RJ and Neiders M: Desquamative lesions, J Periodontol 52:500-510, 1981.

Nisengard RJ and Rogers RS: The treatment of desquamative gingival lesions, J Periodontol 58:167-172, 1987.

Olson J, Feinberg I, Silverman S et al: Serum vitamin B_{12}, folate, and iron levels in recurrent aphthous ulceration, Oral Surg 54:517-520, 1982.

Perry HO, Deffner NF, and Sheridan PJ: Atypical gingivostomatitis, Arch Dermatol 107:872-878, 1973.

Peterson E et al: Treatment of chronic mucocutaneous candidiasis with ketaconazole: a controlled clinical trial, Ann Intern Med 93:791-797, 1980.

Rogers RS, Seehafer JR, and Perry HO: Treatment of cicatricial (benign mucous membrane) pemphigoid with dapsone, J Am Acad Dermatol 6:215-223, 1982.

Rosenberg FR, Sanders S, and Nelson CT: Pemphigus: a 20-year review of 107 patients treated with corticosteroids, Arch Dermatol 112:962-970, 1976.

Schiødt M, Halberg P, and Hentzer B: A clinical study of 32 patients with oral discoid lupus erythematosus, Int J Oral Surg 7:85-94, 1978.

Schiødt M and Pindborg JJ: Histologic differential diagnostic problems for oral discoid lupus erythematosus, Int J Oral Surg 5:250-252, 1976.

Scully C: Viruses and cancer: herpesviruses and tumors in the head and neck, Oral Surg 56:285-292, 1983.

Shillitoe E and Silverman S: Oral cancer and herpes simplex virus—a review, Oral Surg 48:216-224, 1979.

Shklar G: Lichen planus as an oral ulcerative disease, Oral Surg 33:376-388, 1972.

Silverman S: Chronic mucosal ulcerations of the oral mucosa, C.E. course at annual meeting of the American Academy of Oral Pathology, Boston, 1984.

Silverman S Jr, Gorsky M, Lozada-Nur F, and Liu A: Oral mucous membrane pemphigoid, Oral Surg 61:233-237, 1986.

Silverman S Jr and Griffith M: Studies on oral lichen planus. II. Follow-up on 200 patients, clinical characteristics and associated malignancy, Oral Surg 37:705-710, 1974.

Silverman S and Lozada F: An epilogue to plasma-cell gingivostomatitis (allergic gingivostomatitis), Oral Surg 43:211-217, 1977.

Solberg K, Hersle K, Mobacken H, and Thilander H: Severe oral lichen planus: remission and maintenance with vitamin A analogues, J Oral Pathol 12:473-477, 1983.

Tyldesley WR: Stomatitis, and recurrent oral ulceration: is a full blood screen necessary? Br J Oral Surg 21:27-30, 1983.

Weathers DR, Baker G, Archard HO, and Burkes J: Psoriasiform lesions of the oral mucosa (with emphasis on "ectopic geographic tongue"), J Oral Pathol 37:872-888, 1974.

Whitley R et al: Mucocutaneous herpes simplex virus infections in immunocompromised patients, Am J Med 73(1A):236-240, 1982.

Wray D: A double blind trial of systemic zinc sulfate in recurrent aphthous stomatitis, Oral Surg 53:469-472, 1982.

Wray D, Graykowski EA, and Notkins AL: Role of mucosal injury in initiating recurrent aphthous stomatitis, Br Med J 283:1569-1570, 1981.

Yap B et al: Oropharyngeal candidiasis treated with a troche form of clotrimazole, Arch Intern Med 139:656-657, 1979.

Zegarelli D: Multimodality steroid therapy of erosive and ulcerative oral lichen planus, J Oral Med 38:127-130, 1983.

7

Red conditions
of the tongue

NORMAN K. WOOD
GEORGE G. BLOZIS
PAUL W. GOAZ

The red conditions discussed in this chapter are the following:

Migratory glossitis
Median rhomboid glossitis
Deficiency states
Xerostomia
Rarities

All the single red lesions of the oral mucosa discussed in Chapter 5 have been reported to occur on the tongue. Likewise all the generalized reddish conditions of the oral mucosa (Chapter 6) may involve the tongue. In some cases the tongue is involved first, in others different mucosal surfaces are initially affected, and in some patients one or more mucosal surfaces and the tongue are involved simultaneously.

However, this chapter discusses red conditions that occur only on the tongue or else have a predisposition for that structure. Such conditions usually produce one or more bald reddish patches or affect the entire dorsal surface and margins of the tongue.

MIGRATORY GLOSSITIS

A plethora of terms (erythema migrans, glossitis areata migrans, glossitis areata exfoliativa, geographic tongue, wandering rash of the tongue, and annulus migrans) has been used to describe this condition. Although the cause is unknown, emotional stress may be one of several factors involved in the onset or exacerbation of this lesion (Redman et al., 1966; Sumner and Shklar, 1973). Marks and Czarny (1984) proposed "sensitivity to the environment" as a possible cause.

Features

Migratory glossitis is a relatively common condition, occurring in 1% to 2% of the population. The lesions are usually asymptomatic and are discovered as an incidental finding during a routine examination. The patient may complain of a burning sensation that is made worse by spicy foods or citrus fruits. Migratory glossitis occurs most commonly in young or middle-aged adults but has been seen in patients ranging in age from 5 to 84 years. There is a reported predilection for females. The lesions are found more frequently on fissured tongues (Gorlin and Goldman, 1970).

Although the lesions of migratory glossitis have a typical appearance, they may be extremely variable in size and duration. Initially they appear as small, erythematous, nonindurated, atrophic areas bordered by a slightly elevated, distinct rim that varies from gray to white to light yellow (Fig. 7-1). Loss of the filiform papillae produces a pink to red, relatively smooth, shiny surface, except for the residual fungiform papillae. A more intense redness may be present near the advancing margin of a lesion.

Single or multiple lesions may occur in migratory glossitis, and when multiple they frequently coalesce to produce large areas of involvement that encompass much of the tongue. They appear as irregular circinate areas that gradually widen, change shape, and migrate over the tongue (Fig. 7-1). The progression of the lesions is usually quite rapid, with the pattern changing in a few days, or the lesions may remain relatively static. The duration of an attack is also variable, ranging from a few weeks to months; on rare occasions it may continue for years. However, recurrent episodes of involvement are the general pattern.

Most frequently the lesions are confined to the dorsal surface and lateral borders of the tongue, but they may extend to the ventral surface. Lesions similar to those seen on the tongue have been seen occasionally on other mucosal surfaces of the oral cavity (Weathers et al., 1974). These lesions are considered a more extensive involvement by the same process and have been referred to as stomatitis areata migrans or ectopic geographic tongue (Fig. 6-14). Brooks and Balciunas reviewed the literature on this condition and reported on five cases in 1987.

The histopathology of the lesions shows a loss of the filiform papillae and a variable thinning of the mucosa. In some areas there is an epithelial hyperplasia. The epithelium shows spongiosis and infiltration by acute and chronic inflammatory cells.

Differential diagnosis

A diagnosis of migratory glossitis is made on the basis of the clinical appearance and history of the lesion. Similar-appearing lesions are reported in psoriasis, Reiter's syndrome, ectopic geographic tongue, and occasionally pityriasis rubra pilaris (Dawson, 1974; O'Keefe et al., 1973; Weathers et al., 1974). These authors report that the clinical and histologic appearances of these conditions are often identical to those of geographic tongue. Thus the possibility must be considered that these conditions may be closely related. As far as the diagnostic aspects are concerned, if the classic tongue lesions are the only finding, the clinician is correct in establishing a working diagnosis of migratory glossitis. However, he or she should be alert to the possibility that this isolated finding could be the first manifestation of the more generalized diseases included in the preceding differential diagnosis.

Thus in cases in which skin, ocular, tongue, and urethral lesions occur with arthritis, the most likely diagnosis is Reiter's syndrome.

On the other hand, if the patient has skin lesions of psoriasis (particularly of the generalized pustular type), the tongue changes may represent intraoral psoriasis. Likewise if the patient has skin lesions of pityriasis rubra pilaris, the possibility that the "geographic tongue" might really be a manifestation of this disease must be considered.

Lichen planus may occasionally produce reddish patches on the tongue, which in the healing phase may resemble geographic tongue (Fig. 7-2). The absence of raised whitish yellow rims in lichen planus helps to differentiate these lesions from geographic tongue. In addition, it is unusual for lichen planus to affect only the tongue. Moreover, at least one white

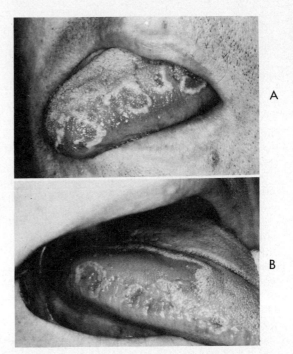

Fig. 7-1. Migratory glossitis. **A,** Multiple lesions with distinct borders and an inflamed atrophic mucosa. **B,** A larger, more diffuse lesion with less inflammatory change and residual fungiform papillae.

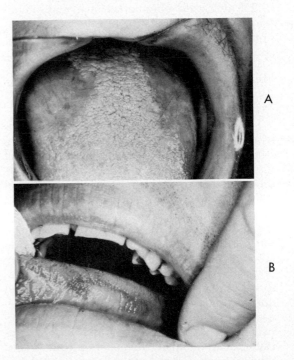

Fig. 7-2. Lesions resembling migratory glossitis. **A,** Bilateral areas of atrophic lichen planus. **B,** Focal red and white areas on the lateral border of the tongue of an anemic patient.

keratotic area can almost always be found on one of the oral mucosal surfaces in lichen planus.

The use of strong mouthwash can produce a variety of clinical lesions, one of which resembles geographic tongue (Kowitz et al., 1976). The history of frequent use of mouthwash followed by the disappearance of the lesions when the use of mouthwash is discontinued permits the clinician to differentiate this condition from geographic tongue.

Anemic conditions that produce a patchy baldness of the tongue may be confused with geographic tongue (Fig. 7-2). Again the absence of the characteristic raised yellowish white border from the red patches of anemia differentiates these conditions from geographic tongue. Careful blood studies demonstrate whether the patient is anemic.

Management

Usually, all that is required in the management of migratory glossitis is to reassure the patient that the problem is not serious. If there is some discomfort, bland diets and topical corticosteroids provide symptomatic relief while the lesions run their usual course and resolve. Helfman (1979) advocated the use of topical retin-A solution for very sensitive cases. Bánóczy (1982) advocated elimination of irritants, mild symptomatic treatment, and psychologic reassurance. On rare occasions, painful cases that are refractory to treatment are encountered.

MEDIAN RHOMBOID GLOSSITIS (CENTRAL PAPILLARY ATROPHY OF THE TONGUE)

For years median rhomboid glossitis has been generally considered a developmental defect resulting from an incomplete descent of the tuberculum impar and entrapment of a portion of it between the fusing lateral halves of the tongue. However, it has been noted that there is not a single report of this entity in a child (Baughman, 1971). Guggenheimer and Verbin (1985) reported a case that occurred in a 5-year-old girl, which was said to have been observed when she was 10 months old, although the nature of the lesion at that time had not been documented. The clinical photograph used in their paper, however, showed an appearance not compatible with that usually associated with median rhomboid glossitis. Thus other causes have been offered. Baughman (1971) suggested the possibility of inflammatory infections (*Candida*) or degenerative causes. Wright's study (1978) strongly supported a the-

ory that implicated a chronic candidal infection. Farman et al. (1977), using the term "central papillary atrophy of the tongue" (CPA), suggested that this condition represents only a clinical appearance and that the underlying disease process may not be identical in all cases. Van der Waal et al. (1979) support this concept suggesting the possibility of several different etiologies. Farman (1976) showed that there was an increased incidence of CPA in diabetes and in 1977 postulated that in some cases of CPA the defective microvasculature, which is commonly found in diabetic patients, may predispose the patient to candidal infection and the resultant tongue lesion. Wright and Fenwick (1981) cast doubt on this concept. Van der Wal and van der Waal (1986) and van der Wal et al. (1986) discussed the possible roles of smoking and *Candida*. Fig. 7-3, *A*, shows an interesting, ulcerative, white necrotic lesion from which smears showed abundant clumps of *Candida*. The lesion was treated with applications of nystatin ointment. Within a week the lesion became asymptomatic and by 2 weeks was almost completely healed, assuming the reddish macular appearance of median rhomboid glossitis (Fig. 7-3, *B*).

Features

Although most reports have indicated that median rhomboid glossitis occurs more frequently in males (Baughman, 1971; van der Wal et al., 1986), in Wright's study of 28 cases (1978) 23 were in women and five were in men. It has been reported in patients ranging in age from 15 to 84 years. The lesion is located on the dorsal surface of the tongue in the midline and anterior to the circumvallate papillae (Figs. 7-4 and 7-5). The surface is dusky red, completely devoid of filiform papillae, and usually smooth; however, nodular or fissured surfaces have been noted (see Fig. 11-17, *E*). Rarely there may be some keratosis. The size and shape of the lesion are somewhat variable, at times causing confusion as to the diagnosis. The lesions are generally asymptomatic, but pain and ulceration have been reported.

The histologic changes include an epithelium devoid of filiform papillae and slightly thickened and elongation and branching of the rete ridges. The underlying connective tissue shows increases vascularity and a chronic inflammatory infiltrate.

Differential diagnosis

Median rhomboid glossitis is easily recognized by its usual asymptomatic nature and its

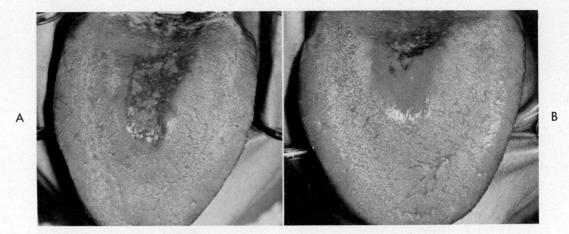

Fig. 7-3. A, Tongue of a middle-aged woman with pseudomembranous candidiasis of the dorsal surface. After 2 weeks of nystatin applications the candidal lesion had almost completely healed as shown in **B.** In 3 weeks the white appearance had completely resolved and the resultant picture was that of median rhomboid glossitis.

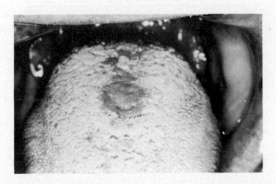

Fig. 7-4. A small but relatively typical lesion of median rhomboid glossitis.

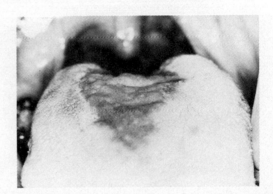

Fig. 7-5. Classic appearance of median rhomboid glossitis.

characteristic location. Nevertheless, according to the foregoing discussion the clinician should consider the possibility that such a patient may have diabetes.

Such a lesion also could be a squamous cell carcinoma or could represent another type of glossitis.

Management

The completely asymptomatic lesion that looks smooth and is not indurated requires no treatment but should be checked periodically in case of change.

Burning or painful lesions should be investigated for the presence of candidal organisms, and if these are found, the lesion should be treated with nystatin ointment.

DEFICIENCY STATES

It has been recognized for years that certain deficiency states can produce a glossitis of ei-

ther a completely bald or a patchy bald type. Diagnosticians of bygone years prided themselves in their ability to diagnose the specific deficiency by recognizing minute differences in appearance. Now it is generally agreed that the glossal changes induced by specific deficiencies are so similar that a definitive diagnosis based on their differentiation is at least unlikely, if not impossible.

Features

Symptoms vary from tender to burning tongue to extreme glossodynia. Frequently the tongue is initially intensely red and then becomes smooth as either the filiform or both types of papillae atrophy (Fig. 7-6). In some instances normal papillation returns when the patient's basic problem is successfully treated (Basker et al., 1978).

The deficiency states that have been reported to produce the type of glossitides being

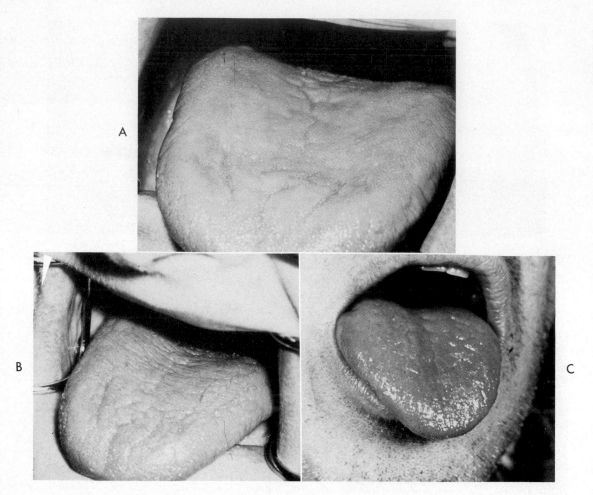

Fig. 7-6. Generalized glossitis. **A,** Patient with iron deficiency anemia. **B,** Patient had an untreated case of pernicious anemia. **C,** This man was severely malnourished and had several vitamin deficiencies.   (**A** and **B** courtesy M. Lehnert, DDS, Minneapolis. **C** courtesy J. Lavieri, DDS, Maywood, Ill.)

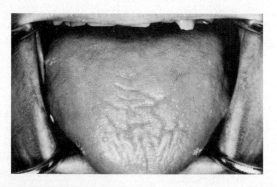

Fig. 7-7. Xerostomia. Tongue changes in a patient with Sjögren's syndrome. The tongue appears dry and is almost completely devoid of papillae.

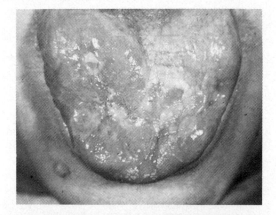

Fig. 7-8. Syphilitic glossitis.   (Courtesy R. Gorlin, DDS, Minneapolis.)

discussed here are iron deficiency anemia, pernicious anemia, Plummer-Vinson syndrome, sprue, and vitamin B complex deficiencies, especially thiamine, riboflavin, nicotinic acid, pyridoxine, panthothenic acid, and B_{12} (cyanocobalamin).

Differential diagnosis

If the tongue in question is completely bald, the only other condition that needs to be considered is the bald tongue of xerostomia (Fig. 7-7). Xerostomia can usually be readily recognized by noting the absence of a salivary pool in the floor of the mouth or the sticking of a tongue blade to the oral mucosa during the oral examination.

If the tongue in question shows partial or patchy baldness, all the conditions mentioned previously should be considered: migratory glossitis, psoriasis, Reiter's syndrome, pityriasis rubra pilaris, changes caused by the use of mouthwash, atrophic lichen planus, and median rhomboid glossitis. The differential diagnosis of these entities may be reviewed under the differential diagnosis section of median rhomboid glossitis. A thorough discussion of the differential aspects of all the deficiency states that may produce a glossitis is well beyond the intended scope of this text.

Management

Once the deficiency state or states have been identified, specific measures may be undertaken for their correction if such are available.

XEROSTOMIA

The oral changes found in cases of xerostomia are discussed in Chapter 6, "Generalized Red Conditions." The red tongue of xerostomia (Fig. 7-7) is rather easily differentiated from the other causes by the absence of the formation of a salivary pool in the floor of the mouth.

RARITIES

A host of specific infectious diseases can effect superficial red changes in the surface of the tongue, but these are very rare examples indeed. Fig. 7-8 illustrates a case of syphilitic glossitis.

REFERENCES

Bánóczy J: Oral leukoplakia, The Hague, 1982, Martinus Nijhoff Publishers, p 51.

Basker RM, Sturdee DW, and Davenport JC: Patients with burning mouths: a clinical investigation of causative factors, including the climacteric and diabetes, Br Dent J 145:9-16, 1978.

Baughman RA: Median rhomboid glossitis: a developmental anomaly? Oral Surg 31:56-65, 1971.

Brooks JK and Balciunas GA: Geographic stomatitis: review of the literature and report of five cases, J Am Dent Assoc 115:421-424, 1987.

Dawson TAJ: Tongue lesions in generalized pustular psoriasis, Br J Dermatol 91:419-424, 1974.

Farman AG: Atrophic lesions of the tongue: a prevalence study among 175 diabetic patients, J Oral Pathol 5:255-264, 1976.

Farman AG: Atrophic lesions of the tongue among diabetic outpatients: their incidence and regression, J Oral Pathol 6:396-400, 1977.

Farman AG, Van Wyk CW, Staz J, et al: Central papillary atrophy of the tongue, Oral Surg 43:48-58, 1977.

Gorlin RJ and Goldman HM: Thoma's oral pathology, ed 6, St. Louis, 1970, The CV Mosby Co, p 31.

Guggenheimer J and Verbin RS: Median rhomboid glossitis in an infant, J Oral Med 40:110-111, 1985.

Helfman RJ: The treatment of geographic tongue with topical retin-A solution, Cutis 24(2):179-180, 1979.

Kowitz GM, Lucatorto FM, and Chernick HM: Effects of mouthwashes on the oral soft tissues, J Oral Med 31:47-50, 1976.

Marks R and Czarny D: Geographic tongue: sensitivity to the environment, Oral Surg 58:156-159, 1984.

O'Keefe E, Braverman IM, and Cohen I: Annulus migrans: identical lesions in pustular psoriasis, Reiter's syndrome, and geographic tongue, Arch Dermatol 107:240-244, 1973.

Redman RS, Vance FL, Gorlin RJ et al: Psychological component in the etiology of geographic tongue, J Dent Res 45:1403-1408, 1966.

Sumner MS and Shklar G: Stomatitis areata migrans, Oral Surg 36:28-33, 1973.

Van der Waal I, Bessmster G, and van der Kwast WAM: Median rhomboid glossitis caused by Candida, Oral Surg 47:31-35, 1979.

Van der Wal N, van der Kwast WAM, and van der Waal I: Median rhomboid glossitis: a follow-up study of 16 patients, J Oral Med 41:117-120, 1986.

Van der Wal N and van der Waal I: Candida albicans in median rhomboid glossitis: a postmortem study, Int J Oral Maxillofac Surg 15:322-325, 1986.

Weathers DR, Baker G, Archard HO, and Burkes JE: Psoriasiform lesions of the oral mucosa (with emphasis on "ectopic geographic tongue"), Oral Surg 37:872-888, 1974.

Wright BA: Median rhomboid glossitis: not a misnomer, Oral Surg 46:806-814, 1978.

Wright BA and Fenwick F: Candidiasis and atrophic tongue lesions, Oral Surg 51:55-61, 1981.

8

White lesions of the oral mucosa

NORMAN K. WOOD
PAUL W. GOAZ

Following is a list of white lesions of the oral mucosa:

Keratotic white entities
Leukoedema
Linea alba buccalis
Leukoplakia
  Nicotine stomatitis or
    smoker's palate
  Snuff dipper's lesion
  Cigarette smoker's lip
    lesion
Benign migratory glossitis
  and mucositis
Peripheral scar tissue (not
  keratotic)
Lichen planus and
  lichenoid reactions
Electrogalvanic white
  reactions
White hairy tongue
Papilloma
Verruca vulgaris
Verrucous carcinoma
Hyperplastic (hypertrophic
  candidiasis)
White hairy leukoplakia
White sponge nevus
Skin grafts
Rarities
  Acanthosis nigricans
  Bohn's nodule (Epstein's
    pearl)
  Candidiasis
    endocrinopathy
    syndrome
  Clouston's syndrome
  Condyloma acuminatum
  Condyloma latum
  Cysts—keratin-filled and
    superficial
    Epidermoid
    Dermoid
    Lymphoepithelial
  Darier's disease
  Dermatitis herpetiformis
  Dyskeratosis congenita
  Focal epithelial
    hyperplasia

  Focal palmoplantar and
    marginal gingival
    hyperkeratosis
  Grinspan's syndrome
  Hereditary benign
    intraepithelial
    dyskeratosis
  Hyalinoses cutis et
    mucosae
  Hypersplenism and
    leukoplakia oris
  Hypovitaminosis A
  Inverted papilloma
  Juvenile juxtavermilion
    candidiasis
  Koplik's spots
  Lupus erythematosus
  Molluscum contagiosum
  Pachyonychia congenita
  Pityriasis rubra pilaris
  Porokeratosis
  Pseudoepitheliomatous
    hyperplasia
  Pseudoxanthoma
    elasticum
  Psoriasis
  Scleroderma
    (nonkeratotic)
  Squamous acanthoma
  Submucous fibrosis
    (non-keratotic)
  Superficial sialolith of
    minor glands
    (nonkeratotic)
  Syndrome of dyskeratosis
    congenita, dystrophia
    unguium, and aplastic
    anemia
  Syphilitic interstitial
    leukoplakial glossitis
  Verruciform xanthoma
  Warty dyskeratoma

Sloughing,
pseudomembranous,
necrotic white lesions

Plaque
Traumatic ulcer
Pyogenic granuloma
Chemical burns
Acute necrotizing
  ulcerative gingivitis
Candidiasis
Necrotic ulcers of systemic
  disease
Diffuse gangrenous
  stomatitis
Rarities
  Candidiasis
    endocrinopathy
    syndrome
  Syndrome of familial
    hypoparathyroidism,
    candidiasis, and
    retardation

  Syndrome of idiopathic
    hypoparathyroidism,
    Addison's disease,
    and candidiasis
  Congenital insensitivity
    to pain syndrome
  Diphtheria
  Eosinophilic granuloma
  Heavy metal mucositis
  Henoch-Schönlein
    purpura
  Noma
  Superficial abscess
  Syphilitic chancre and
    mucous patch
  Tuberculosis

Vesicles and bullae
(discussed in Chapter 6)

White lesions of the oral mucosa may be conveniently divided into two groups: those that cannot be scraped off with a tongue blade (most are keratotic) and those that can be scraped off with a tongue blade (sloughing, pseudomembranous necrotic types). This chapter is likewise divided into two such parts—the first dealing with the keratotic entities (which as a group are the more commonly encountered white lesions) and the second reviewing the sloughing types.

A third type, vesiculobullous lesions, almost invariably have a white or grayish white appearance and so must be considered as white lesions, particularly during the examination process (Fig. 8-1). Touyz and Hille (1984) described such a case: an extensive white lesion of the gingiva that would not be scraped off. It was caused by excessive use of mouthwashes and acidic fruit juices. The white appearance was produced by a hyperplasia of the epithelium, marked intracellular edema, and much microvesicular formation in the prickle cell layer.

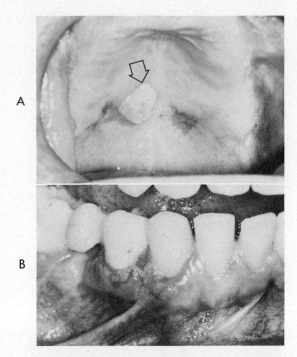

A

B

Fig. 8-1. **A,** Benign mucous membrane pemphigoid; arrow indicates white bullous lesion. Two ulcers, one on each side of the bullous lesion, were produced when previous bullae ruptured. Although vesicular and bullous lesions are white, they are more suitably grouped with generalized reddish conditions (see Chapter 6). **B,** Recurrent herpetic lesion on the buccal gingiva. Note that in this case the predominant clinical change is white, although careful scrutiny reveals pinpoint ulcers in the center of the white areas.

However, when advancing to the differential diagnosis process, the clinician finds it much more suitable to group these lesions by themselves or as generalized reddish conditions (see Chapter 6). We introduce this information at the onset of this chapter particularly to alert students to the fact that such lesions are white both when the blisters are intact and for a day or two after they rupture.

Keratotic white entities

To the inexperienced clinician the oral mucosa may appear only pink.

As experience increases and observation becomes more acute, however, the clinician will discover the wide spectrum of pinks that are characteristic of the normal oral mucosa, varying from a dark pink (reddish) to a very pale pink (almost white). In addition, he or she will become familiar with the mucosal locations in the oral cavity where these different shades

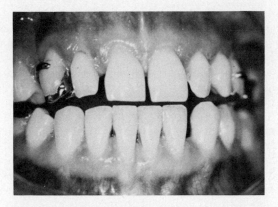

Fig. 8-2. The attached gingiva is a paler pink than the vestibular mucosa because of the keratinized surface and less vascularity.

may normally be found. Furthermore, the clinician will be able to comprehend the variations on the basis of microscopic structure and function.

The various colors and hues and the morphologic structure of the oral mucous membrane are related, in part, to the mechanical influences of mastication.

Surfaces exposed to vigorous stimulation by the mastication of hard and rough foods respond by forming a thicker epithelium with perhaps a heavier keratin covering and usually a denser, fibrous, less vascular subepithelial connective tissue. These surfaces compose the *masticatory* mucosa and appear white—the mucous membrane on the hard palate, the fixed gingiva, and the dorsal surface of the tongue (Fig. 8-2).

On the other hand, protected surfaces form very little keratin, have a less fibrous, more vascular subepithelial layer, and are of a darker pink or more reddish hue—the vestibule, floor of the mouth, ventral surface of the tongue, and retromolar regions. These surfaces are said to be *lining* mucosa.

Individual variations in the color of the oral mucosa will be apparent and are probably an expression of one or more genetically controlled factors; that is, some people readily form keratin as a result of minor stimuli, whereas others require a strong stimulus to produce minimal keratinization. The clinician must also know that a patient's hemoglobin concentration will affect the shade of pink. For example, the patient with polycythemia will have a redder mucosa than will the patient with anemia.

In some regions normal keratinization or epithelial thickening or both may be so marked as to appear pathologic. Leukoedema and linea alba are such examples.

LEUKOEDEMA

Leukoedema is a common variation of the normal oral mucosa. It appears as a diffuse, filmy, milky opalescence on the buccal mucosa. Although its cause is unknown, leukoedema may develop as a result of masticatory function and has been shown to be related to poor oral hygiene (Martin and Crump, 1972). Studies have failed to demonstrate that its formation is related to tobacco use, syphilis, or malocclusion, but an increased incidence and severity have been shown to occur with age. Martin and Crump reported that about 50% of black teenagers and children have this normal variation, and it is a common observation in 90% of black adults. Although the percentage of whites affected is reported to be approximately 45%, Durocher et al. (1972) showed that under good lighting conditions leukoedema could be found in 93% of the whites they examined. Von Wyk (1985) reported from a study of almost 2000 black high school students that leukoedema was found in 26% of the students and occurred more often in male students. He concluded that smoking does not cause the condition but may aggravate it. Current consensus holds that this entity does not undergo malignant changes.

Features

Leukoedema is totally asymptomatic and is usually found during routine oral examination. Although frequently discovered on the buccal mucosa, it also occurs on the labial mucosa and soft palate. The degree of severity varies from a faint, filmy appearance, which requires close inspection for detection, to a much denser opalescence with wrinkling or folding of the surface (Figs. 8-3 and 8-4). Leukoedema cannot be removed with a tongue blade.

Microscopic studies show an increased thickness of the epithelium can be observed usually with marked intracellular edema (ballooning) in the prickle cell layer. A hyperparakeratosis (hyperkeratosis with retention of nuclei) of varying thickness may be present (Fig. 8-3).

Differential diagnosis

The commonly occurring lesions that may be confused with leukoedema are *leukoplakia, cheek-biting lesion,* and *white sponge nevus.* A discussion of the differential diagnosis of these lesions is presented under the differential diagnosis of leukoplakia (p. 121).

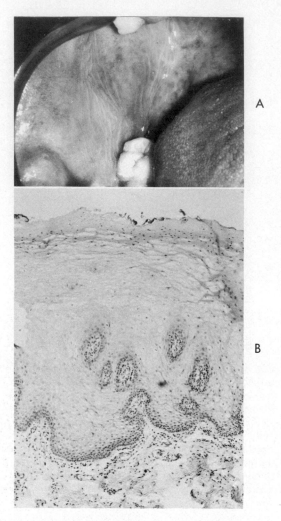

Fig. 8-3. Leukoedema. **A,** The white wrinkled appearance of the buccal mucosa, present bilaterally, occurred in a 45-year-old black man. **B,** Photomicrograph showing acanthosis, ballooning in the prickle cells, and parakeratosis.

Management

Since leukoedema is a normal variant, its recognition is important and no treatment is required.

LINEA ALBA BUCCALIS

Linea alba (white line) is a streak on the buccal mucosa at the level of the occlusal plane extending horizontally from the commissure to the most posterior teeth. It is usually seen bilaterally and may be quite prominent in some people (Fig. 8-5). Because it occurs at the occlusal plane and conforms to the space between the teeth, it is thought to result from slight occlusal trauma to the buccal mucosa.

This impression is strengthened by the observation that a linea alba is frequently more

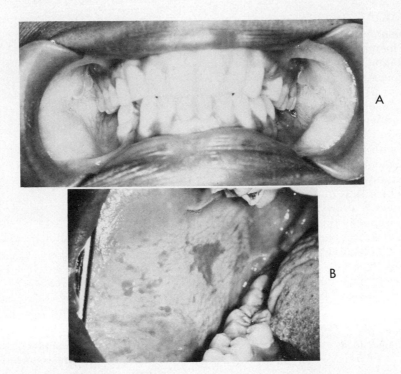

Fig. 8-4. Leukoedema. **A,** Milky wrinkled appearance was present bilaterally in this 52-year-old black woman. **B,** Red eroded areas in this example of leukoedema were caused by cheek biting. Stretching the tissue eliminated the white appearance in both cases.   (**A** courtesy S. Smith, DDS, Chicago.)

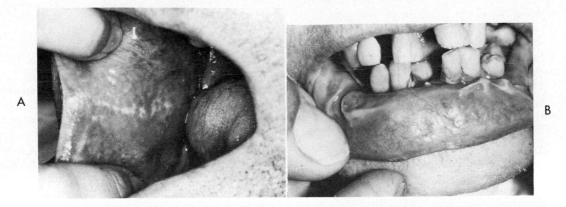

Fig. 8-5. Linea alba. **A,** Prominent example in classic location. **B,** Unusual location and appearance of linea alba on mucosal surface of lower lip. Patient habitually sucked the tissue in against his anterior teeth.

prominent in people with little overjet of the molars and premolars. The prominence of the linea alba varies greatly from one individual to another, being especially marked in some people and completely absent in others (Fig. 8-5).

Histologically an increased thickness or hyperorthokeratosis (hyperkeratosis without retention of nuclei) is seen.

Management requires only the recognition of linea alba as a normal variation.

LEUKOPLAKIA

Leukoplakia* is a keratotic plaque occurring on mucous membranes; its immediate cause is chronic irritation. The World Health Organization defined leukoplakia in these words: "It is a white patch or plaque that cannot be characterized clinically or pathologically as any other disease" (Pindborg, 1982).

As with other keratotic lesions, it cannot be scraped off with a tongue blade. Although definitive statements on the role of genetics and systemic conditions that predispose the oral mucosa to leukoplakia must await further investigations, much is already known about the local or direct causes of this condition. For example, a variety of local chronic irritations, acting alone or in combination, will produce leukoplakial lesions in certain individuals.

The following have been suggested to be of etiologic importance in leukoplakia:

Tobacco products
Cold temperatures
Hot and/or spicy foods
Alcohol
Occlusal trauma
Sharp edges of prostheses or teeth
Actinic radiation
Syphilis
Candida albicans

The role of smoking and drinking in relation to oral cancer was summarized by Blot et al. (1988). These authors showed that increased smoking increased the risk of oral cancer, as did increased consumption of alcohol. Also, combined use of tobacco and alcohol was shown to markedly increase the risk of oral cancer. Squier et al. (1986) demonstrated that the presence of ethanol enhanced the penetration of carcinogens in both the gingival and the floor-of-the-mouth mucosa of pigs.

The fact that the presence of these factors cannot be documented in approximately 20% of oral cancer patients (Ballard et al., 1978) has produced a search for additional causative factors. Recent studies have suggested a possible relationship between viruses (papilloma, herpesvirus) and oral premalignant and malignant lesions (Eskinazi, 1987; Greer et al., 1988; Kassim and Daley, 1988; Loning et al., 1984; Scully et al., 1988; Syrjänen et al., 1988).

---

*At one time a significant number of pathologists used the term "leukoplakia" to describe a specific histopathologic picture. Today most pathologists use "leukoplakia" only to describe a keratotic white patch that cannot be diagnosed as any other disease, caused by chronic irritation on a mucous membrane; only thus is the term used in this book.

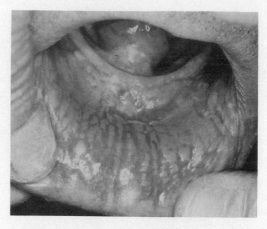

Fig. 8-6. Keratotic condition of the oral mucosa produced by holding Listerine mouthwash in the mouth for 15 minutes once a day.   (From Bernstein ML: Oral Surg 46(6):781-785, 1978.)

Weaver et al. (1979) reported interesting findings from a study of 200 patients with squamous cell carcinoma of the head and neck. These investigators reported that 11 of these patients had never used alcohol or tobacco, but all but one of these 11 had used mouthwash containing 25% alcohol many times daily for more than 20 years. In this context Bernstein (1978) reported and illustrated diffuse keratotic changes (leukoplakia type, we would presume) in the oral mucosa because of the use of Listerine mouthwash (Fig. 8-6). These changes disappeared soon after discontinuation of the mouthwash.

The chronic irritation, regardless of type, must be intense enough to induce the surface epithelium to produce and retain keratin but not so intense as to cause a breakdown of the tissue with resulting erosion or ulcer formation. Obviously genetic and systemic factors play a role in preconditioning the mucosa because some people develop a leukoplakial lesion as the result of a relatively minor insult whereas others either show no reaction to the same or more prolonged and severe stimulus or suffer tissue destruction and an inflammatory lesion.

Leukoplakia, then, likely commences as a protective reaction against a chronic irritant. This reaction produces a dense layer of keratin, which is retained for the purpose of insulating the deeper epithelial components from the deleterious effects of the irritant.

When clinical leukoplakial lesions are studied microscopically, they can be seen to embrace a spectrum of histologic changes from an innocuous lesion that shows only increased keratosis to invasive squamous cell carcinoma.

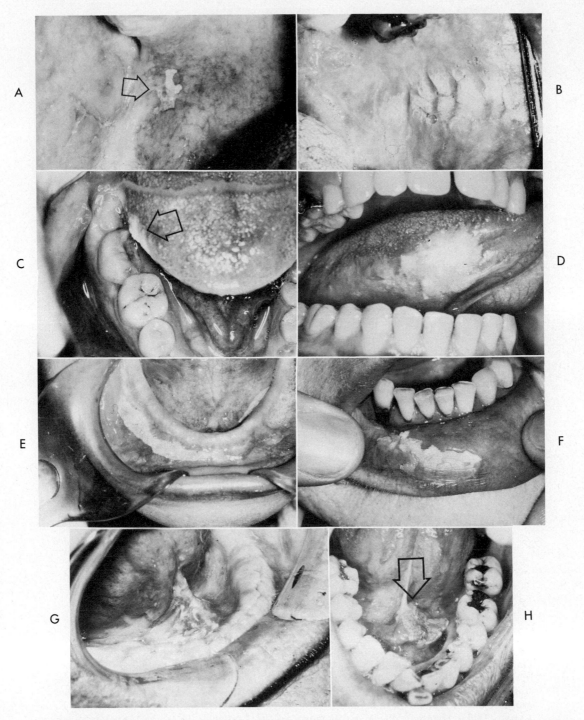

Fig. 8-7. Leukoplakia. **A** and **B,** Both patients smoked heavily. When the patients stopped smoking, the lesions did not regress, so they were excised. Neither showed dysplastic change. **C** and **D,** Lesion in 17-year-old boy caused by irritation from sharp edges of second molar. Lesion regressed after tooth was restored. **E,** Lesion in vestibule caused by denture irritation. **F,** Prominent lesion on lower lip caused by biting habit and sharp incisal edges of lower anterior teeth. **G** and **H,** Microscopy showed squamous cell carcinoma. **G,** Speckled sublingual leukoplakia or speckled erythroplakia. **H,** Elevated firm mass with induration of the base.   (**G** courtesy J. Lehnert, DDS, Minneapolis. **H** courtesy S. Smith, DDS, Chicago.)

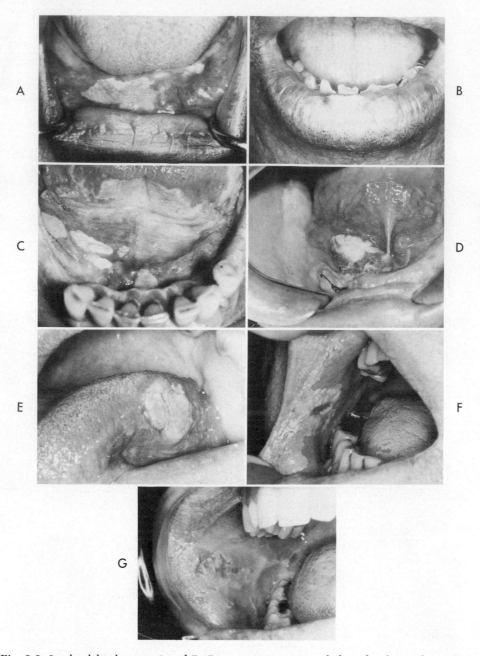

Fig. 8-8. Leukoplakic lesions. **A** and **B,** Biopsy specimen revealed no dysplastic changes. **C,** One of the prominent white areas showed moderate dysplastic changes, whereas the remainder showed only acanthosis and hyperkeratosis. **D** to **F,** These lesions proved to be squamous cell carcinoma. **G,** Although this lesion on the buccal mucosa appears suspect because of the ulcerations, it is a benign condition caused by cheek biting.   (**D** courtesy E. Kasper, DDS, Maywood, Ill.; **E** and **F** courtesy O.H. Stuteville, DDS, MD, St. Joe, Ark.)

These differences cannot be detected clinically, so to establish the specific diagnosis the lesion must be examined microscopically.

Leukoplakial lesions are characteristically asymptomatic and are most often discovered during a routine oral examination. Leukoplakia is a common lesion as shown by the fact that 6.2% of all tissue specimens submitted to two large oral pathology laboratories were leukoplakia (Waldron and Shafer, 1975). The greater percentage of patients with these lesions are between 40 and 70 years of age, and the lesions are seldom found in individuals under 30 years of age. Bouquot and Gorlin (1986) reported that approximately 3% of white Americans over 35 years of age had leukoplakic lesions. Sites by frequency in their study were the lip vermilion, buccal mucosa, mandibular gingiva, tongue, oral floor, hard palate, maxillary gingiva, lip mucosa, and soft palate. The lesions may vary greatly in size, shape, and distribution (Figs. 8-7 and 8-8). The borders may be either distinct or indistinct and smoothly contoured or ragged.

Lesions may be divided into four basic clinical appearances: (1) *homogeneous* white plaques have no red component but have a fine, white, grainy texture or a more mottled, rough appearance (Fig. 8-7, *A, B, D, E,* and *F,* and Fig. 8-8, *A* and *B*); (2) *speckled* leukoplakias are composed of white and red flecks of either fine or coarse variety (see Fig. 8-11, *B,* and Fig. 5-12); (3) *combination white* and *red patches* demonstrate segregation of the red and white components and are basically erythroleukoplakic lesions (Fig. 8-7, *A*); and (4) *verrucous leukoplakias* possess a red and white component also but the white component is much thicker and protrudes above the surface mucosa (Fig. 8-11, *A*).

Bánóczy (1982, pp. 60-62) presented impressive evidence that each of these clinical types has some potential to change from one type to another and so they should not be considered as totally separate entities.

Red components of leukoplakias represent dysplasias, carcinomas in situs, and invasive carcinomas, providing that the red component is not a traumatic erosion or traumatic ulcer. If the lesion is malignant, enlarged cervical nodes may signal the occurrence of metastatic spread. The lesions may be solitary, or multiple plaques may be scattered through the mouth.

The cause may be obvious from the location of the lesion (for example, a white patch on an edentulous ridge directly beneath an occluding maxillary molar, in direct line with the course of the smoke from a pipe held in the smoker's favorite position, or in the area where the individual prefers to hold the quid of tobacco or dip of snuff).

Waldron (1970) stated that leukoplakias may be histologically divided into two main categories (Fig. 8-9): those that show no atypia (dysplasia) and those that show different degrees of atypia.

In Bánóczy and Csiba's study of oral leukoplakia in Hungry (1976) 24% of their subjects showed dysplasia. Waldron and Shafer's study

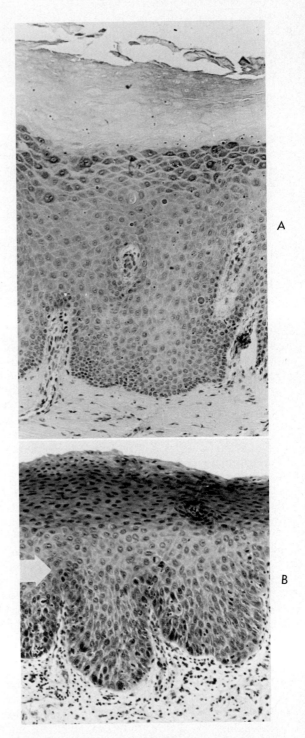

Fig. 8-9. Leukoplakia. **A,** Photomicrograph of a completely benign leukoplakic lesion showing acanthosis and hyperkeratosis but no dysplasia (atypia). **B,** Photomicrograph of a leukoplakic lesion that has undergone moderate dysplasia. Dysplastic cells are present in the lower portion of the epithelium. Arrow indicates the approximate superior extent of the dysplastic change.

(1975) revealed a similar figure (20%). A lesion may show severe atypia with malignant change throughout the depth of the epithelial layer, but its basement membrane may still be intact. Such a lesion is identical with carcinoma in situ or intraepithelial carcinoma (Fig. 8-10).

When an intraepithelial carcinoma breaks through the basement membrane, it becomes a frank invasive squamous cell carcinoma. The investigator must study microscopic sections from various areas of a biopsy of leukoplakia, since the complete spectrum of histopathologic features from increased keratosis to invasive squamous cell carcinoma may be found in the surgical specimen from one lesion.

Leukoplakia may also be divided into two types according to whether or not it spontaneously disappears after the chronic irritant has been eliminated. Those lesions that disappear are referred to as *reversible* leukoplakias, whereas the remaining lesions are termed *irreversible* leukoplakias.

Pindborg et al. (1968) reported that 20% of the leukoplakial lesions in their study disappeared completely, 18% diminished in size, and 45% did not decrease in size. On this basis 62% of the lesions could then be classified as completely or partially irreversible. Obviously reversible leukoplakias are not malignant, but a significant number of irreversible leukoplakias are premalignant or frankly malignant.

It has been tempting to speculate that reversible leukoplakia would not show dysplastic changes histologically. In this regard it is informative that both Pindborg et al. (1977) and Mincer et al. (1972) showed that some of these lesions that show dysplastic changes within the epithelium do regress spontaneously after elimination of the causative factor.

Concerning malignancy in leukoplakic lesions Waldron and Shafer reported in 1975 that 3.1% of their series were infiltrative squamous cell carcinomas. It is currently believed that there is an overall malignant transformation rate of 3% to 6% for oral leukoplakia (Kramer, Lucas, Pindborg, and Sobin, 1978). Bouquot and Gorlin (1986) reported that almost 7% of leukoplakias from their study demonstrated carcinoma or severe dysplasia. Bánóczy and Sugár (1972) stated that if the following features are present there is a higher risk of malignant transformation in oral leukoplakial lesions:

1. Persistence of the lesion for some years
2. Female patient
3. Lesion situated on the margin or base of the tongue
4. Combination of these first three factors
5. Erosive lesion

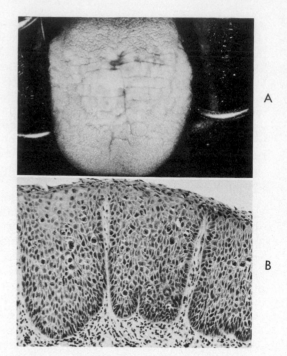

Fig. 8-10. Leukoplakic lesions. **A,** The ulcer in the leukoplakic lesion on the dorsal surface of the tongue proved to be a carcinoma in situ. **B,** Photomicrograph of the ulcerated area in **A** showing malignant changes throughout the epithelium. The basement membrane is still intact.

The consensus of pathologists is that the speckled variety of leukoplakia (with small red velvety areas dispersed through the white lesion, Figs. 8-8, *B,* and 8-11) is much more likely to be malignant than the more homogeneous variety. Also, if the lesion has cracks or erosions or ulcers in the absence of mechanical trauma, this is an ominous sign (Fig. 8-8, *F*).

Recently it has been recognized that leukoplakias occurring in the floor of the mouth and ventral surface of the tongue have a much greater chance of undergoing malignant transformation. Kramer et al. (1978), referring to this lesion as *sublingual keratotis,* reported that 27% of their lesions were carcinoma at the time of initial biopsy and that 24% showed malignant change in the follow-up period. Pogrel's study (1978) corroborated this trend; he reported that 16% of the leukoplakias he studied from this region showed malignant transformation within 5 years. Waldron and Shafer (1975) reported that 42% of the floor of the mouth leukoplakias they studied showed dysplasia as compared with 20% of all the leukoplakias studied. Browne and Potts (1986) warned of the possibility of dysplasia in salivary gland ducts in

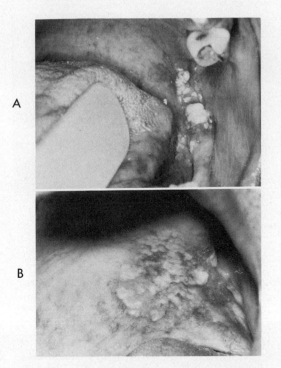

Fig. 8-11. **A,** Verrucous leukoplakia in the retromolar region. **B,** Speckled leukoplakia on the posterior palate. Both lesions proved to be squamous cell carcinoma. (**B** courtesy J. Lehnert, DDS, Minneapolis.)

cases of sublingual leukoplakia and erythroplakia. They reported on five such cases.

Bánóczy (1982, pp. 15-27) reported on 520 leukoplakial lesions that she followed for an average of 8.7 years. None of the homogeneous leukoplakias transformed to malignancy, whereas 28% of the leukoplakias that had a red component or had fissures showed malignant transformation. It was interesting that her study showed that 12.7% of the leukoplakias transformed from one clinical type of leukoplakia to another. Some of these took on a more worrisome appearance while some improved, that is, changed to a less worrisome (homogeneous) appearance (1982, pp. 60-62).

Concerning site or location of the lesion and malignant change Bánóczy (1982, pp. 15-27) reported the following: lesions of the margins or root of the tongue (including floor of the mouth, we presume) showed the most frequent malignant transformation (38.8%). Lesions of the lip were next (16.2%). The study revealed that of the 17 leukoplakias of the tongue that occurred in females, 8 showed malignant transformation (47%).

Silverman et al. (1984) reported on a follow-up study of 257 patients with leukoplakia. The patients were studied for an average period of 7.2 years; squamous cell carcinoma developed in the leukoplakic lesions of 17.5% of these patients. Other results of this study strongly support the concept that leukoplakias with red components (speckled leukoplakias and combination leukoplakic and erythroplakic patches) and also verrucous leukoplakias showed a somewhat higher rate of malignant change (23.4%) than did the homogeneous type (6.5%). Malignant changes in the lesions that possessed a red component demonstrated a fourfold increase over the homogeneous type. Also 36.4% of lesions with dysplastic changes at the initial biopsy showed malignant transformation later. It is instructive that 90% of the dysplastic cases had an associated red component. Patients with leukoplakic lesions who had never smoked were found to be at increased risk for developing squamous cell carcinoma.

Differential diagnosis

When a white lesion is encountered, the clinician should determine whether it can be easily removed by scraping. If it cannot, all the sloughing pseudomembranous types can be eliminated and the following keratotic varieties should especially be considered in the differential diagnosis: electrogalvanic current lesion, cheek-biting lesion, lupus erythematosus, lichen planus, verrucous carcinoma, verruca vulgaris, hairy leukoplakia, leukoedema, and white sponge nevus.

White sponge nevus is the most uncommon of the group. In addition, it occurs soon after birth or at least by puberty and is usually widely distributed over the oral mucous membrane. In contrast, leukoplakia is seen mostly in patients over 40 years of age and usually is not disseminated throughout the oral cavity. White sponge nevus, furthermore, shows a familial pattern not so characteristic for leukoplakia.

Leukoedema is usually easily differentiated from leukoplakia because it classically occurs on the buccal mucosa, frequently covering most of the oral surface of the cheeks and extending onto the labial mucosa with a faint milky opalescence. Thus the definite whiteness that characterizes the leukoplakial lesion is not a feature of the mild case of leukoedema. The characteristic folded and more prominent wrinkled pattern (eliminated by stretching) of the leukoedema, furthermore, distinguishes it from the leukoplakial lesion.

Hairy leukoplakia is a corrugated leukoplakic lesion that occurs usually on the lateral or ventral surfaces of the tongue in patients with

AIDS or AIDS-related complex (Fig. 8-12). The associated features of these serious diseases are usually evident. AIDS tests are helpful in making a definitive diagnosis as is biopsy of the oral leukoplakic lesion in question.

Verruca vulgaris must be differentiated from the verrucous type of leukoplakia; this is usually possible because the verruca vulgaris, which does not commonly occur in the oral cavity, is a small, raised, white lesion seldom more than 0.5 cm in diameter. Verrucous leukoplakia, on the other hand, tends to be much larger and is usually circumscribed by a border of inflamed mucosa, a feature not usually found in the verruca vulgaris. In addition, if chronic trauma to the area can be identified, the diagnosis of leukoplakia is further favored.

Since *verrucous carcinoma* may develop from a leukoplakial lesion, the clinician must decide whether the lesion's fronds are elevated (exophytic) enough to be suspected as a verrucous carcinoma.

Lichen planus may appear as a plaquelike lesion, and in such instances it may be confused with leukoplakia. In contrast to leukoplakia, however, which is more often a solitary lesion, lichen planus usually occurs as several lesions distributed throughout the oral cavity. Also the lesions of lichen planus may develop several different configurations simultaneously in the same mouth (e.g., white plaques, Wickham's striae,* bullae, erosions). When such a variety of lesions is present, distinguishing between these two diseases is greatly facilitated. If reddish white skin lesions accompany the oral lesions, this also favors a diagnosis of lichen planus.

Oral discoid lupus erythematosus lesions are more common than generally thought. They occur frequently in patients who have discoid lupus lesions of the skin and in patients with systemic lupus erythematosus (Schiødt, 1984a). Oral discoid lesions may initially appear as isolated lesions in a significant number of patients who do not show evidence of having either discoid lupus or systemic lupus (Schiødt, 1984b).

The oral discoid lesions share much in common with leukoplakia and lichen planus. The mean patient age at onset is 40 years. Like lichen planus these lesions occur much more frequently in women. Buccal mucosa is the most common site of oral discoid lupus lesions, and the gingiva, labial mucosa, and vermilion border are the next most common sites. Also the

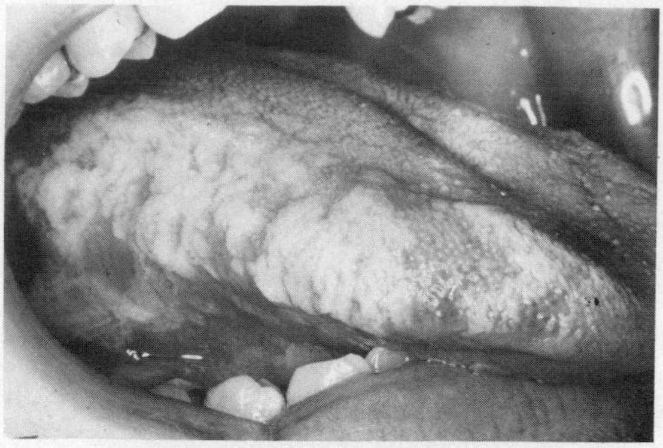

*Fine grayish white lines arranged in a lacelike pattern.

Fig. 8-12. White hairy leukoplakia.   (Courtesy S. Silverman, DDS, San Francisco.)

lesions are frequently bilateral. In certain cases the clinical appearance of oral discoid lesions may be identical to a leukoplakia or a lichen planus lesion (Fig. 8-13).

It is not uncommon for early lesions to be completely red, but after many years these may slowly change into leukoplakia-like lesions. Oral discoid lesions frequently have a red and white appearance and as such often mimic lichen planus lesions, which have an atrophic, erosive, or ulcerative component (Fig. 8-13). When an oral discoid lesion has typical appearance, it is readily identified. Schiødt (1984a) described the classic oral discoid lesion as "having four outstanding clinical features: (1) a central atrophic area with (2) small white dots and a slightly elevated border zone of (3) irradiating white striae and (4) telangiectasis." However, this researcher explained that considerable variation occurs in about one third of the cases. Some of this latter group mimic leukoplakias, white and red lichen planus lesions, lichenoid drug reactions, and electrogalvanic lesions.

Identifying the *cheek-biting lesion* may be a problem for the clinician. In the chronic cheek chewer the buccal mucosa takes on a whitish cast because of the increased thickness of the epithelium and keratin. In special periods of heightened stress, the patient may actually chew away small bits of tissue, producing a plaquelike whitish lesion with a ragged eroded surface that may cause the inexperienced clinician to suspect squamous cell carcinoma (Fig. 8-8, *G*). Paradoxically, true erythroplakic patches characteristically have smoothly contoured borders. Careful questioning of the patient usually elicits the cause and promote the proper diagnosis. Careful follow-up reveals the

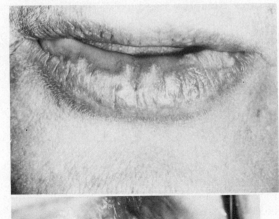

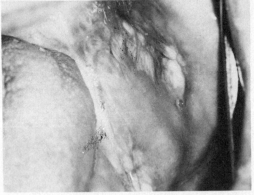

A

B

Fig. 8-13. Lupus erythematosus. Oral discoid lesions in a woman with systemic lupus. Note characteristic feathery edges of keratotic patches, which have a red component. **A,** Vermilion border. **B,** Buccal mucosa.

regression of the erosions when the habit is modified or eliminated.

Electrogalvanic white lesions as described by Bánóczy et al. (1979) perhaps should be considered as an entity separate from leukoplakia. The two types of clinical lesions that a microgalvanic current from dissimilar metal restorations can produce on adjacent tongue or buccal mucosa are (1) keratotic plaque lesions like leukoplakia and (2) a variation that mimics lichen planus. In Bánóczy's study the vast majority of these lesions disappeared when the different metal restorations were replaced with composites or when the teeth were extracted. This is a practical approach to use in differentiating these electrogalvanic white lesions from the true leukoplakic lesion, providing the suspicion index is low (no erythroplakic or verrucal component). Of course, if the suspicion index is high for dysplasia or malignancy, the lesion should be completely excised and studied microscopically, in addition to replacement of the dissimilar metal restorations.

Management

Paramount to proper management of a specific clinical lesion that the clinician considers to be a leukoplakia is the understanding that not all leukoplakias are the same. Current knowledge permits the alert clinician to develop a "suspicion index" or "risk quotient" for each lesion, which is based for the most part on the following:

1. Leukoplakias occurring in the following sites are much more likely to be malignant or to undergo malignant transformation in the near future than those that occur in other oral sites—tongue, floor of the mouth, lips, and gingiva.
2. Leukoplakias with a red component or verrucous appearance are much more likely to be malignant than are homogeneous leukoplakias.
3. Leukoplakias that show dysplastic changes are more likely to develop into squamous cell carcinoma than are those that show no dysplasia.
4. Leukoplakias in patients who have never smoked have a greater propensity for malignant change.
5. Erythroplakic lesions of carcinoma in situ are more agressive than those with leukoplakic components (Amagasa et al., 1985).
6. Leukoplakic tongue lesions in women have a significantly higher malignant transformation rate than those in men.

Thus a patient who has one of the preceding characteristics is at risk for malignancy. If a particular lesion has two or more of these features, it should be assigned a high-risk quotient. In turn, aggressive excision should be done promptly and a careful periodic follow-up planned to detect and treat the earliest recurrence.

For leukoplakic lesions with a low-risk quotient, a conservative approach is generally indicated. This approach is described as follows: the clinician must make every effort to identify the local chronic irritants that may have induced its development. All these irritants must then be eliminated and the patient reexamined every week to determine whether the lesion is regressing. If evidence of regression is not detectable within 2 weeks (color photographs are useful as records for comparison), the lesion should be completely excised. This is a simple procedure for small lesions but is a relatively complicated operation if the lesions are large or involve many surfaces.

If the lesions are large or widespread, stripping procedures must be used—in stages with free grafts or else with allowance for the denuded surface to epithelialize by secondary healing. Since longitudinal studies by Silverman and Rosen (1968) and Bánóczy and Sugár (1972) showed that approximately 6% of the irreversible leukoplakial lesions underwent malignant transformation to squamous cell carcinoma, there seems to be little doubt that irreversible leukoplakial lesions should be completely excised. In any case careful postsurgical follow-up is essential. If the microscopic diagnosis is squamous cell carcinoma, the patient should be referred to a clinician who is competent in treating oral cancers. The management of intraoral squamous cell carcinoma is discussed in more detail in Chapter 11. Abdel-Salam et al. (1988) reported success in predicting malignant transformation by image cytometry.

The preceding management approaches are most suitable for relatively small, single lesions. However, when large lesions or widely disseminated lesions (which are basically superficial) are encountered, complete surgical excision leaves a large surgical wound. This wound is usually difficult to close and frequently causes the patient a great deal of discomfort, as well as some mutilation and some loss of function. Skin grafts are used to close some of these wounds, but this procedure requires a second surgery, which is complicated and uncomfortable, and the results are frequently less than desirable.

Cryosurgical procedures have been used to treat large leukoplakic lesions with apparently good results. Pertinent studies have been published by Al-Drouby (1983), Carpenter and Snyder (1979), Frame (1984), Gongloff et al. (1980), Gongloff and Gage (1983), Tal et al. (1982), and Bekke and Baart (1979).

Laser surgery has been used for the removal of oral lesions, including leukoplakia. The advantage of laser over blade surgery is that laser surgery eliminates the risk of seeding the surgical wound with cancer cells during incisional biopsies of early lesions or during an attempt to excise the lesion. Pecaro and Garehime (1983) reported on their experiences with this method. Others reporting on the use of this technique are Abt et al. (1987), Frame (1985), and Horch et al. (1986). Maxson et al. (1989) discussed the use of both topical 5-fluorouracil and laser surgery in the same patients. Hong et al. (1986) reported on leukoplakial response to 13-cis retinoic acid, whereas Hammersley et al. (1985) used topical bleomycin.

Nicotine stomatitis or smoker's palate

Nicotine stomatitis is a specific type of leukoplakia seen mostly in men who are pipe smokers. It occurs on the palate, and in most cases the whole mucosal surface of the hard palate is affected. It begins as a reddish stomatitis of the palatal mucosa, and as the irritation is continued, keratotic changes occur and the lesion becomes slightly opalescent and finally white in color. Classically it is described as having a parboiled appearance because of its many transecting wrinkles and fissures, which divide the white mucosal surface into small nodular areas (Fig. 8-14). A red dot is usually situated in the middle of each nodule and represents the inflamed orifice of a minor salivary gland duct. The lesion usually disappears rapidly after the habit is discontinued. Nicotine stomatitis seldom if ever becomes malignant.

Nicotine stomatitis must be differentiated from all the other conditions of the oral cavity that produce multiple papules: papillary hyperplasia, Darier's disease (Fig. 8-15), focal epithelial hyperplasia, Goltz syndrome, Cowden's syndrome, acanthosis nigricans, multiple neuroma syndrome, multiple oral fibromas in tuberous sclerosis, multiple papillomas and ver-

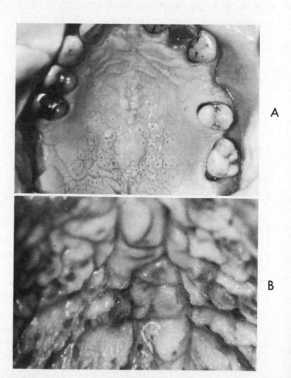

Fig. 8-14. **A,** Nicotine stomatitis. Both patients were pipe smokers. **B,** Close-up view.   (**B** courtesy P.D. Toto, DDS, Maywood, Ill.)

rucae (no syndrome), and multiple condylomas (modified from Buchner and Sandbank, 1978).

Papillary hyperplasia and nicotine stomatitis are the only entities that have a marked predilection for the palate. The small centrally placed dots in nicotine stomatitis differentiate this condition from papillary hyperplasia, which occurs under an acrylic denture.

Snuff dipper's lesion

Christen et al. (1982) summarized the history of use of smokeless tobacco in the United States. Its use was much more frequent in the South, but this has changed recently. The reported sales of snuff and chewing tobacco have been increasing at an alarming annual rate of 11% since 1974 (Anderson et al., 1979; Lindemeyer et al., 1981). Presumably this is partly because of the public awareness of the link between smoking and lung cancer. Christen (1980) attributed much of the increase in use to mass media advertising, much of which is directed toward the youth population. A few years ago the extensive use of chewing tobacco and snuff was mostly limited to senior citizens and athletes. Now the use of these agents has become a fad in the younger population as observed in various locales around the country (Wood, 1988).

Greer and Poulson (1983) documented the frequency of use in the young people of Den-

ver, Colorado, and reported four specific clinical lesions: (1) hyperkeratotic or erythroplakic lesions of the oral mucosa, (2) gingival or periodontal inflammation, (3) a combination of (1) and (2), and (4) cervical erosions of the teeth. Baughman (1984) advised of the trend in the young people in Florida as did Offenbacker and Weathers (1984) in the young people of Georgia.

This leukoplakia-type lesion occurs on the mucosal surface where the snuff is habitually held. The mandibular vestibule, in both the incisor and the molar regions, is the most prevalent site. The resultant leukoplakic lesion usually has a wrinkled appearance (Fig. 8-16). If the habit is eliminated, the majority of the lesions completely disappear in about 2 weeks. Those that remain should be completely excised and examined microscopically. Roed-Petersen and Pindborg (1973) were unable to demonstrate a statistical difference between the percentage of snuff dipper's lesions that showed atypias and the percentage of other leukoplakias that showed atypias. Long expo-

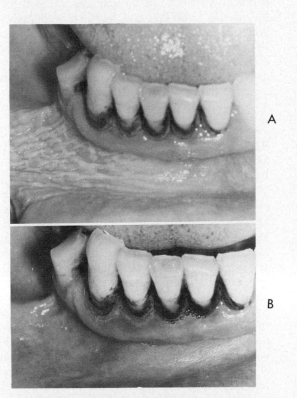

Fig. 8-16. Snuff dipper's leukoplakia. **A,** Note the parboiled appearance of the white lesion in the vestibule where the patient held his snuff. **B,** The lesion disappeared 2 weeks after discontinuance of the habit.

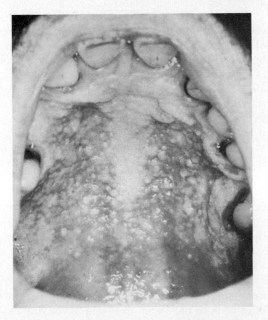

Fig. 8-15. Darier's disease. These multiple firm papules were present on various oral surfaces and the skin.   (Courtesy M. Bernstein, DDS, Louisville.)

sure to snuff is usually required, however, to induce malignant changes, and when carcinoma does develop, the lesions are usually low-grade malignancies.

Hirsch et al. (1982) reported on a clinical, histomorphologic, and histochemical study of snuff-induced lesions of varying severity. Sundström et al. (1982) described the clinical and histologic features of 23 oral carcinomas that were associated with snuff dipping: a spectrum of types of oral carcinomas were observed.

Cigarette smoker's lip lesion

Cigarette smoker's lip lesion is an interesting entity that has only recently been recognized. Berry and Landwerlen (1973) reported it in about 11% of the inpatients at a neuropsychiatric hospital. Early lesions showed increased redness and stippling of the lip in a localized area and were typically flat or slightly raised with elliptical, circular, irregular, or triangular borders. More advanced lesions appeared pale to white and were slightly elevated with a nodular or papillary shape. Berry and Landwerlen reported that 62% of the patients affected had lesions on both lips and most showed associated finger burns. The authors theorized that the sedation these psychiatric patients received increased their pain threshold and consequently they repeatedly suffered low-grade thermal damage to the lips and fingers. Berry and Landwerlen reported that biopsy did not reveal malignant change in any of the lesions.

BENIGN MIGRATORY GLOSSITIS AND MUCOSITIS (GEOGRAPHIC TONGUE, ECTOPIC GEOGRAPHIC TONGUE)

Geographic tongue occurs in 1% to 2% of children and adults. Although its cause is unknown, psychologic influences are suspected. Marks and Czarny (1984) found a significantly higher incidence of this condition in extrinsic asthma and rhinitis. On clinical examination, irregularly shaped red patches and white patterns resembling a map are distributed over the dorsal and ventral surfaces and borders of the tongue (Fig. 8-17). The red patches are initially quite small and surrounded by a small white rim. These red patches, which are areas of desquamated filiform papillae, enlarge and regress—thus changing the pattern from week to week. Eventually they disappear entirely for a time.

Pogrel and Cram (1988) reported an increased incidence of geographic tongue, ectopic geographic tongue, and periodontal disease in patients with severe cutaneous psoria-

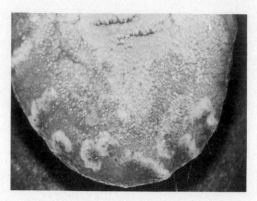

Fig. 8-17. Geographic tongue.   (Courtesy P. Akers, DDS, Chicago.)

sis. Wysocki and Daley (1987) reported an increased incidence of geographic tongue in juvenile diabetics.

The condition is usually asymptomatic, but occasionally a patient complains of burning sensation, tenderness, and pain. In our experience, instituting a bland diet and coating the denuded surface with triamcinolone in Orabase at bedtime relieve the discomfort until the painful desquamated areas regress.

Benign migratory glossitis is usually not a diagnostic problem, although some atypical cases have been diagnosed as *leukoplakia* by inexperienced clinicians. The differential diagnosis of benign migratory glossitis is discussed in greater detail in Chapter 7.

Recently situations have been described in which the condition also affected other regions of the oral mucosa. These cases have been referred to under different names, one of which is ectopic geographic tongue (Weathers et al., 1974). Brooks and Balciunas (1987) reviewed the literature on this condition and reported five cases of their own. They identified a male predominance ratio of 2.6:1 in patients with an average age of 35 years. Fifty-nine percent of the patients were under 40 years of age. Fissured tongue was seen in 41% of cases. The most frequent sites of occurrence were the buccal and labial mucosa and vestibules. Ralls and Warnock (1985) reported a case affecting the gingiva.

PERIPHERAL SCAR TISSUE

Peripheral scar tissue (a nonkeratotic lesion) involving the subepithelial layer or the epithelium or both has been observed in the oral cavity. The condition is not common because oral tissue is so vascular that the superficial tissue destroyed by a pathologic process is usually completely replaced by normal tissue. In some

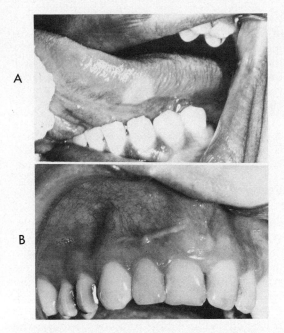

Fig. 8-18. Fibrosed areas appearing as white lesions. **A,** Posttraumatic scar on the lateral border of the tongue. **B,** Scar at the site of a root resection incision.

instances, however, the healing of surgical wounds, large traumatic ulcers, giant aphthae in Sutton's disease, or other conditions may result in the formation of dense scar tissue. Although the scar tissue does not become as light in color as most keratotic lesions, it does appear pale and may not be recognized by the student, especially if the lesion is plaquelike (Fig. 8-18).

Usually scars may be identified by relating to pertinent points in the patient's history or by the location of the entity (e.g., a linear pale mark on the labial alveolus that corresponds to an incision for root resection, Fig. 8-18). Some patients show a tendency toward keloid formation on the skin, and a few patients are also prone to oral keloid formation although the oral cases are usually not so pronounced.

Oral scars may be solitary entities but are multiple in cases of Sutton's disease and submucous fibrosis.* The area of the scar is firm to palpation, and in some cases the deeper layers are bound to the mucosa. Intraoral scar tissue is usually not a diagnostic or management

---

*Submucous fibrosis is a chronic disease affecting any part of the oral and sometimes the pharyngeal mucosa. It is considered to be precancerous and may simulate scleroderma inasmuch as ultimately there is a stiffening of certain areas of the oral mucosa. The mucosa eventually becomes blanched and opaque.

problem although adhesions after major surgery may have to be excised.

LICHEN PLANUS AND LICHENOID REACTIONS

Lichen planus is a complex mucocutaneous disease of unknown origin that occurs in the oral cavity. When the cause is identified, the condition is termed a "lichenoid reaction" (Lovas, 1989). It occurs with a variety of different-appearing lesions, some of which are white. There are four basic types of lesions: keratosis, bullae, iatrophic lesions, and erosions. The disease affects less than 1% of the population. Bouquot and Gorlin's 1986 study revealed a prevalence of the disease of 1.2:1000 people. Lichen planus does not appear to be related to the use of tobacco and is not restricted to any particular ethnic group; a familial pattern has not been identified, although Watanabe et al. (1986) suggested that genetic factors may be involved. Some clinicians believe that psychologic problems may play an etiologic role (Hampf et al., 1987; Lowenthal and Pisanti, 1984). On the other hand, studies by Allen et al. (1986) showed that patients with lichen planus did not exhibit a greater tendency to anxiety or stress than those without the condition.

It has long been considered that lichen planus may represent an autoimmune, generalized, or localized immunologic disorder. Lacy et al. (1983) suggested from their studies that lichen planus may be a predetermined condition (or diathesis), which is more likely to have a genetic basis than to be a simple cause and effect disorder. In other words these patients possess the genetic tendency to have lichen planus, but perhaps lesions do not appear until stress, mechanical irritations, drugs, galvanic currents, or emotional crises occur to precipitate their arrival. Also some factors could increase the severity of lesions in patients who have them already. Nonsteroidal anti-inflammatory drugs and many other medications, as well as materials such as amalgam, have given rise to lichenoid reactions (Allen and Blozis, 1988; Chau et al., 1984; Colvard et al., 1986; Ferguson et al., 1984; Firth and Reade, 1989; Glenert, 1984; James et al., 1987; Lovas, 1989; Potts et al., 1987).

Several reports have indicated that oral lichen planus may be associated with diabetes mellitus (Grinspan et al., 1966; Howell and Rick, 1973; Smith, 1977). It is interesting that Christensen et al., (1977) found no difference in glucose tolerance test results between lichen planus patients and patients without lichen planus. Lundström (1983), in a study of 40 Swedish patients with oral lichen planus, reported that 43% proved to be diabetics (two were of the latent type). Since 3% of the general population without mucosal changes of any type had diabetes, the findings of this study supported the concept of a higher incidence of diabetes in lichen planus patients. Lozada-Nur et al. (1985) did not support this association. On another topic, del Olmo et al. (1989) reported an increased incidence of chronic liver disease and cirrhosis in patients with lichen planus.

Many reports indicate that squamous cell carcinoma can arise in oral lichen planus lesions. However, the question as to whether there is an increased rate of malignancy in cases of oral lichen planus is more difficult to answer. The results of most studies are inconclusive, showing a slightly increased risk of malignancy, some of which may be related to tobacco use (Krutchkoff et al., 1978; Murti et al., 1986; Neumann-Jensen and Pindborg, 1977; Silverman et al., 1985a). In 1988, Holmstrup et al. reported a 50-fold increase in malignancy in patients with oral lichen planus and concluded that oral lichen planus is a premalignant condition. Kaugers et al. (1988), studying epithelial dysplasia, found that cases associated with lichen planus usually occurred on the buccal mucosa and were a mild degree of dysplasia. Pursuing a different line of thought, Krutchkoff and Eisenberg (1985) proposed the term "lichenoid dysplasia," which they applied to lichenoid lesions that showed dysplasic areas. These authors used specific histologic criteria to differentiate epithelial dysplasia, oral lichen planus, and other oral inflammatory conditions. Additionally Eisenberg et al. (1987) demonstrated that nonspecific lichenoid stomatitis and lichen planus exhibited strong involucrin reactivity whereas lichenoid dysplasia did not. These authors concluded that these findings supported prior evidence that lichen planus and lichenoid dysplasia are biologically distinct lesions. Lovas et al. (1989) supported the distinction of lichenoid dysplasia and contended that "some, if not most, cases of apparent malignant transformation of lichen planus likely represent red and white lesions that were dysplastic from their inception, but that mimic oral lichen planus both clinically and histologically."

The characteristic microscopic picture reveals a hyperparakeratosis or hyperorthokeratosis with an acanthosis. The rete ridges are often saw-toothed in appearance, there is an eosinophilic acellular ribbonlike layer in the connective tissue, and there is a bandlike distribution of dense chronic inflammation below the basement membrane, which is usually restricted to the lamina propria. The basal cell layer frequently undergoes hydropic and vacuolar degeneration and may be entirely missing (Fig. 8-19).

If degeneration is severe and restricted to small foci, bullae may form, but if the process is severe and more disseminated, erosions develop because of the loss of surface epithelium.

Features

Bánóczy (1982, pp. 147-155) recognized six different clinical types of oral lichen planus lesions, as follows, along with the various percentages of occurrence in her patient population: (1) reticular type—51.5%, (2) erosive type—27.6%, (3) atrophic and (4) papular types—12.6%, and (5) bullous type—8.3%. In this chapter, discussion of the various lesions is restricted to the white keratotic varieties: the reticular, papular, and annular types. Those with a red component, atrophic, erosive, and bullous types are discussed in Chapter 5, "Solitary Red Lesions" and Chapter 6, "Generalized Red Conditions and Multiple Ulcerations." This separation is made on the basis of clinical appearance and not because this latter group represents a different disease process. However, they are more intense and are usually painful, in contrast to the purely keratotic types, which are usually asymptomatic. It is important to recognize too that various types can transform into other types and that various types of clinical lesions may be present in the same mouth at the same time (Fig. 8-20, D).

The reticular type with a lacework of intersecting and meandering white lines (Wickham's striae) is a characteristic and common appearance (Fig. 8-19). Annular lesions are variations and appear as a round or ovoid white outline with either a pink or a reddish pink center (Fig. 8-20, A and B). Various picturesque and interesting patterns may form. Papular lesions are solid, white lesions with a slight elevation that are round or else have a wide, short, linear pattern. Occasionally, plaquelike lesions that resemble leukoplakia form, but these usually have a reticular or feathery pattern at the margins.

Bánóczy (1982, pp. 147-155) reported that more than 86.5% of her patients were over 40 years of age and that lichen planus occurred most frequently in patients between 50 and 59 years of age; 62.6% of the patients were women. In Tyldesley's series (1974) 98.4% of

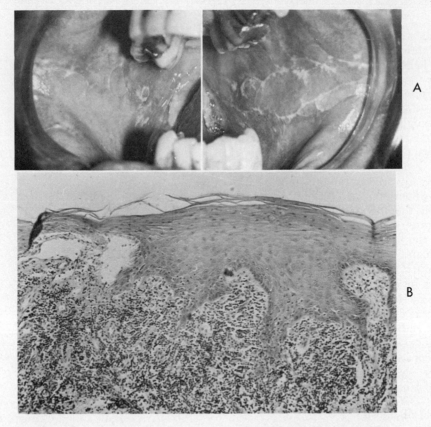

Fig. 8-19. Lichen planus. **A,** Wickham's striae on the right and left buccal mucosa of a 45-year-old woman. **B,** Photomicrograph of lichen planus showing the sawtooth rete ridges and chronic inflammation, which is limited to the upper segment of the lamina propria. Note the early formation of microbullae just beneath the epithelium on the left side of the photomicrograph.

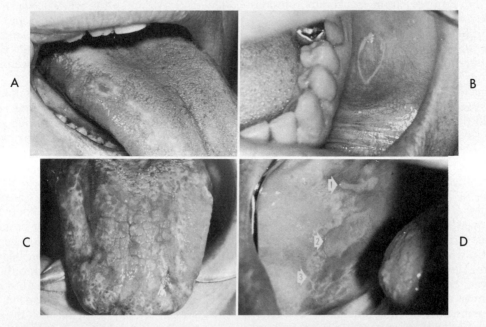

Fig. 8-20. Lichen planus. **A** and **B,** Annular lesions on the tongue and vestibular mucosa, respectively. Note that papular lesions are also present on the tongue in **A. C,** Extensive involvement of the dorsal surface of the tongue. **D,** Three types of lesions on the buccal mucosa: *1,* bullous type; *2,* erosion; *3,* Wickham's striae. (**B** courtesy P.D. Toto, DDS, Maywood, Ill.)

the patients were over 30 years old. The average age of those affected is 52 years. The initial lesions of lichen planus may appear on either the skin or the oral mucous membrane. In a series studied by Silverman and Griffeth (1974), about 25% of the patients with oral lesions had accompanying skin lesions. Thirty-five percent of Tyldesley's intraoral cases also had skin lesions; 19.3% of Bánóczy's patients had concurrent skin lesions. Although there does not seem to be any area of the oral mucosa that is immune, Silverman and Griffeth (1974) reported that the following sites (listed in descending order of frequency) were most often involved: the buccal mucosa (85%), gingiva, tongue, palate, floor of the mouth, and vermilion border.

The skin lesions are small, flat papules that may coalesce to form larger, flat plaques or nodules (Fig. 8-21). The borders are smoothly contoured and sharply demarcated from the surrounding skin. They are reddish purple and are often covered with a semitransparent, thin scale. Fine grayish lines (Wickham's striae) may be present on their surfaces.

Differential diagnosis

Leukoplakia, electrogalvanic mucosal lesions, lichenoid drug reactions, unusual examples of linea alba, cheek-biting lesions, leukoedema, ectopic geographic tongue, lupus erythematosus, and white sponge nevus must all be differentiated from the keratotic lesions of lichen planus.

The differential diagnosis of the *bullous* and *erosive types* is taken up with the discussion of the other mucositides in Chapter 6. As with the other keratotic lesions in this group, the fact that the white lesions cannot be removed with a tongue blade eliminates from consideration all the sloughing white lesions, which are discussed in the latter half of this chapter (p. 142).

White sponge nevus can be eliminated from consideration because it is usually manifested at birth or at the latest by puberty, whereas 98% of the lichen planus lesions occur in patients over 30 years of age.

Lupus erythematosus may be indicated by keratotic white lesions with or without a surrounding area of erythematous oral mucosa. However, these keratotic lesions are not in a thin linear reticular pattern but have a much broader dimension. In addition, the characteristic flaky or feathery appearance of these lupus lesions is helpful for diagnosis (see Fig. 8-13). Nevertheless some atypical lesions may look

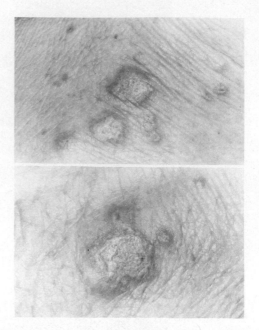

Fig. 8-21. Skin lesions of lichen planus.   (Courtesy N. Thompson, DDS, Maywood, Ill.)

identical to lichen planus. In systemic lupus the characteristic blood changes are diagnostic.

Ectopic geographic tongue may be distinguished by the fact that its lesions have a red center with a slightly raised white border (see Figs. 8-17 and 6-14) that is rapidly altered, producing a noticeable change in pattern within a few days. Although the white lesions of lichen planus may occur in a variety of shapes and distributions and these characteristics may change, such changes take place relatively slowly and usually require a few weeks before they become apparent.

Leukoedema is easily recognized, but if wrinkles are present, these may be interpreted as Wickham's striae by the inexperienced clinician. Stretching the tissue, however, will eliminate the wrinkles or folds in leukoedema and permit the distinction between it and lichen planus.

Cases in which *cheek biting* is superimposed on a leukoedema may be easily confused with lichen planus, and a biopsy may be necessary to correctly identify the condition. The fact that the whiteness of leukoedema can be made to completely disappear by stretching the buccal mucosa is a helpful differentiating test.

Unusual examples of *linea alba* may mimic lichen planus. Some patients suck their cheeks into tight contact with their teeth, and this may produce linea alba patterns that resemble Wickham's striae on the buccal mucosa where

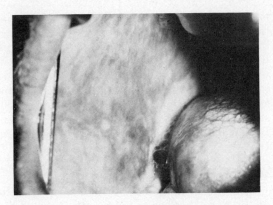

Fig. 8-22. Lichenoid drug reaction in a 64-year-old woman receiving antihypertensive medication. Patient had a diffuse stomatitis. Distinct small regions of white reticular patterns can be seen.

the mucosa contacts the crowns of the teeth (see Fig. 8-5, *B*).

Lichenoid drug reactions have been reported with increasing frequency. In such cases drugs have induced changes that resemble the Wickham's striae of lichen planus.

Various degrees of severity occur, ranging from painless keratotic lesions to painful, severely erosive cases (Fig. 8-22). The following drugs have been implicated: thiazides, methyldopa, bismuth, chloroquine, gold derivatives, meprobamate, para-aminosalicylic acid, and quinacrine.

Apparently the best way to differentiate between painful cases of erosive lichen planus and lichenoid drug reaction is to initiate a course of systemic administration of cortisone. If no improvement is observed within 2 weeks, lichenoid drug reaction should be considered the working diagnosis. Then, under the physician's direction the drugs the patient is taking should be discontinued or substituted for. With such an approach lichenoid drug lesions slowly heal, but 4 to 6 months may be required before complete remission occurs (Burry and Kirk, 1974). Severe cases of lichenoid drug reaction could appear similar clinically to allergic manifestations such as erythema multiforme. As with bona fide lichen planus one would expect improvement of allergic states after the systemic administration of cortisone.

Electrogalvanic white lesions are discussed on p. 132.

Leukoplakia is frequently the lesion that is the most difficult to differentiate from lichen planus. When skin lesions of lichen planus are present, the distinction is easy; if the white intraoral lesions of lichen planus take the form of

Wickham's striae, the diagnosis is also readily discernible. If, however, as sometimes happens, the lichen planus is a solitary plaquelike lesion, the disturbance may be incorrectly diagnosed as leukoplakia, since leukoplakia most often occurs as a solitary plaquelike lesion. Because both diseases usually affect patients over 40 years of age, the differentiation is rendered more difficult. Leukoplakia more often affects men, whereas lichen planus occurs more frequently in women; this distinction provides a hint as to the nature of the lesion. If, after a thorough investigation, a chronic irritant cannot be identified and an area characteristic of Wickham's striae is discovered, no matter how small, the probability that the lesion is lichen planus is increased. Cases such as these, however, frequently must be identified by a biopsy. In addition, cases of disseminated intraoral leukoplakia in which several areas of the oral mucosa are involved may be easily mistaken for lichen planus, but again biopsy will usually distinguish between the two.

Management

The vast majority of patients with only *keratotic* oral lesions of lichen planus are asymptomatic. These patients do not require active treatment. However, the diagnosis should be established and the patient informed about the nature of the disease. Zegarelli (1981) has described a simple and reliable biopsy technique. Patients should be reexamined every 6 months to check on the course of the disease so that treatment can be instituted promptly if painful atrophic, erosive, or bullous lesions appear. Because malignancy may develop, it behooves the clinician to place each patient with oral lichen planus on a carefully monitored recall system so that if malignant change does occur, the lesion can be detected and managed at the earliest possible moment.

If the lesions are present on the gingiva or lateral borders of the tongue or the buccal mucosa and seem to be associated with dissimilar metals, consideration should be given to possible replacement with similar restorative materials. Likewise if the patients are taking medications that are known to have the potential to produce lichenoid drug reactions, the diagnosis of the lichenoid drug reaction must be considered. If the physician thinks it is feasible to change the medication, this should be accomplished and disappearance of the lesions should be anticipated in a significant number of cases.

Patients with localized painful lesions of oral lichen planus will find relief with the generous application of topical salves or pastes containing cortisone, three or four times a day. The management of severe cases of disseminated painful types of lichen planus is discussed in Chapter 5.

In our experience oral lichen planus cases that are in reality lichenoid drug reactions respond less favorably to systemic administration of cortisone. Should this experience occur and should the patient be taking drugs known to cause lichenoid reactions, the patient's physician should substitute other drugs for those in question, and the course of the lesions should be followed. Improvement may not be evident immediately but may require up to 9 months following withdrawal of the drug.

Likewise if contact allergy to dental restorative materials is suspected, the patient should be patch tested for allergy to those materials. If test results are positive, the materials should be eliminated. If there is a suspicion of galvanic action present (the lesions are in contact with dissimilar metals, or adjacent restorations reveal a blackened corrosive state), this possibility should be eliminated. In addition, if there is a gold restoration adjacent to the lesion, a last possibility should be considered: that of radioactive gold. Cases of skin lesions caused by radioactive gold jewelry have been documented, and it is possible that some radioactive gold may have inadvertently been used as dental gold!

ELECTROGALVANIC WHITE LESIONS

Electrogalvanic white lesions have been reported for some time. Such lesions may be leukoplakic, lichenoid, or like oral discoid lupus erythematosus lesions. Bánóczy et al. (1979) reported on their series of 1128 patients with oral leukoplakia and 326 patients with oral lichen planus. Thirty-six of their patients showed white lesions of the oral mucosa that could have been attributed to electrogalvanism. In their series, 31 of the 36 lesions disappeared completely when the metals were changed or the teeth were extracted.

Bánóczy (1982, pp. 37-42) expressed the opinion that white lesions caused by electrogalvanism would reverse if the causative metal restorations were replaced. However, the lesion would not regress in cases where the restoration had been present for over a decade.

Lundström (1984) reported on his series of 48 oral lichen planus patients. Clinical signs of corrosion (black, discolored amalgams) were much more common in his lichen planus group

than in his control group (72%/28%). In addition, he found that corrosion was much more frequently observed in the erosive type than in the reticular type (83%/46%). He found that the presence of mixed gold and amalgam restorations was not higher in the oral lichen planus group. The Council on Dental Materials, Instruments and Equipment of the American Dental Association reviewed these concerns in 1987.

WHITE HAIRY TONGUE

White hairy tongue is a condition that occurs on the dorsal surface of the tongue and is of little clinical significance. Its cause is still unknown. It results from an elongation of the filiform papillae because of the increased retention of keratin. It is much more common in men and seldom produces symptoms or causes clinical problems. On occasion, patients may become alarmed when they suddenly detect its presence. The length of the papillae may vary from short to relatively long (Fig. 8-23). When the papillae are extremely long, patients may complain of gagging. Under the influences of a varying diet, this lesion may take on different colors. Farman (1977) reported that patients with malignant neoplasia are much more prone to this condition.

White hairy tongue does not present a diagnostic problem, and careful frequent brushing of the dorsal surface of the tongue is the preferred treatment for milder cases. When the papillae have reached an extreme length, clipping followed by tongue brushing is an effective control measure.

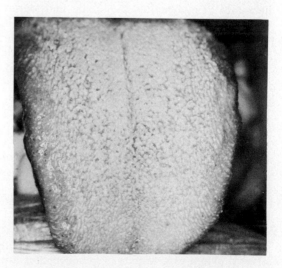

Fig. 8-23. White hairy tongue.

PAPILLOMA

The papilloma is classified as a benign tumor of epithelium. It is a relatively infrequent lesion of the oral cavity. Some investigators consider it to be caused by a papilloma virus, which is the same virus that is found in warts. The virus has been difficult to identify, and electron microscopy is necessary to find these small viruses and small viral subunits. Specific antibody techniques have been used to identify the presence of human papilloma virus antigens in papillomas (Loning et al., 1984). Recently DNA hybridization studies have been used successfully to show nucleic acids of the virus. Not all studies yield positive findings.

Features

The patient may complain of a small tab or mass on the mucosa, or the papilloma may be an incidental finding during an oral examination. It is an exophytic lesion with a characteristic papillomatous shape; that is, the lesion is almost always pedunculated and has a rough, cauliflower-like, pebbly surface caused by the presence of deep clefts that extend well into the lesion from the surface (Figs. 8-24 and 8-25). The intraoral papilloma is seldom larger than 1 cm in diameter but may occasionally grow to several centimeters. It is either pink or white.

In a review of 110 lesions, Greer and Goldman (1974) reported that, although it may occur anywhere on the mucosa, the papilloma is most frequently seen on the tongue; these authors found 33% of the lesions in their study at this site. In descending order of frequency, the following were sites where a papilloma was found: the tongue, palate, buccal mucosa, gingiva, lips, mandibular ridge, and floor of the mouth. Greer and Goldman also reported that most of the cases occurred in persons aged 21 through 50 years and that the average age was 38 years. The majority of tumors in their study varied in size from 2 × 2 mm to 1.0 × 1.5 cm, with a few measuring as large as 2.5 to 3 cm in diameter. A narrow stalk was characteristic of these lesions.

Because no dysplastic areas were found in any of the 110 papillomas in their series, Greer and Goldman concluded that malignant change in oral papillomas must be very rare, if indeed it occurs at all.

Microscopically a narrow connective tissue core extends from the tissue beneath the lesion and branches into numerous folds; the folds are covered by epithelium that characteristically shows acanthosis. A surface layer of keratin may or may not be present, depending on the amount of irritation to the surface, and this determines whether the lesion is white or pink. Superficial vacuolated cells are usually present, and it is the nuclei of these cells that showed specific binding of human papilloma virus antibodies (Loning et al., 1984).

Differential diagnosis

The lesions that must be differentiated from the papilloma are verruca vulgaris, papillary squamous cell carcinoma, verrucous carcinoma, condyloma acuminatum, condyloma latum, and pseudoepitheliomatous hyperplasia.

The *verruca vulgaris*, although common on the skin, is not frequent in the oral cavity. It almost always has a relatively sessile base, whereas the papilloma is pedunculated. On microscopic examination the verruca vulgaris often has round eosinophilic bodies in the cells of the upper part of the prickle cell layer and in the granular cell layer; these are thought to be viral inclusion bodies and are not found in papillomas. Actually the clinical distinction between verruca vulgaris and papilloma is not critical, since both are managed identically. Some pathologists do not even distinguish between verruca vulgaris and papilloma.

The *papillary squamous cell carcinoma* is a "garden-variety" exophytic squamous cell carcinoma that possesses basically a polypoid shape and a surface that is white and pebbly or relatively smooth (Fig. 8-26). In contrast to the papilloma, its base is not as pedunculated, the lesion grows much more rapidly, and it soon exceeds the usual 0.5 to 2.0 cm size of the papilloma. Its rapid growth and narrower base differentiate the papillar squamous cell carcinoma from the verrucous carcinoma, which has a very broad base and usually achieves much less vertical growth into the oral cavity.

Verrucous carcinoma characteristically is seen in patients in their 60s and 70s and is mostly associated with smoking or chewing tobacco or snuff. It usually covers a much wider surface area, has a base that is almost as wide as the lesion, and does not achieve much vertical height (Fig. 8-27).

Condyloma latum and *condyloma acuminatum* (Fig. 8-28) may look identical to the papilloma clinically. However, they are much less common and a careful history would frequently reveal that the patient has practiced oral sex with an infected individual, although autoinoculation is possible.

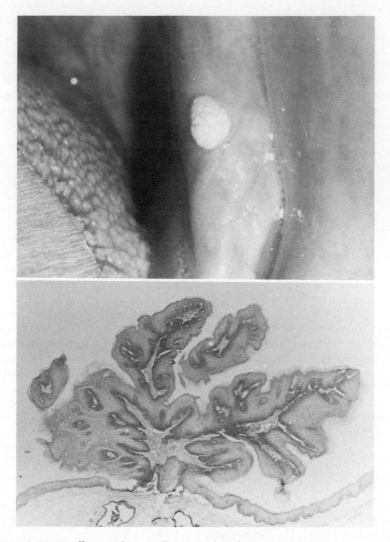

Fig. 8-24. Papilloma. This papilloma is white because of its keratotic surface.

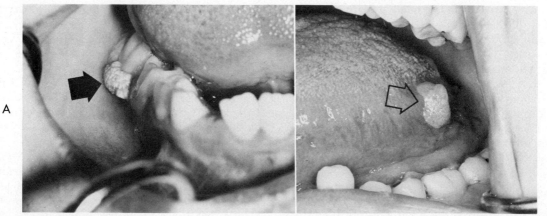

A

B

Fig. 8-25. Papillomas. Both lesions were pedunculated.   (**B** courtesy S. Smith, DDS, Chicago.)

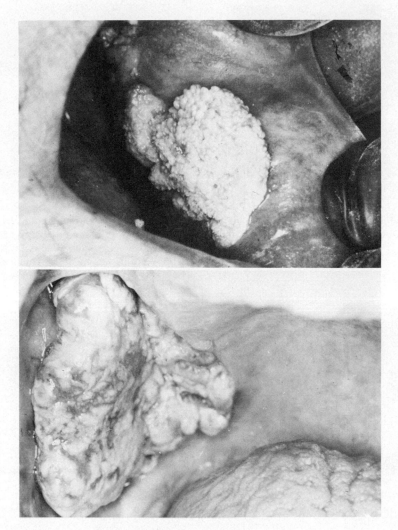

Fig. 8-26. Papillary squamous cell carcinomas.

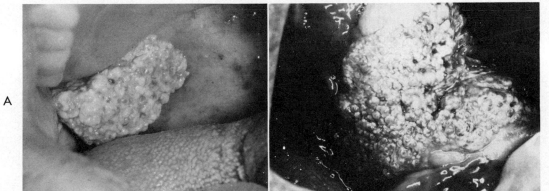

A

B

Fig. 8-27. Verrucous carcinomas.   (**A** from Claydon PJ and Jordan JE: J Oral Surg 36:564-567, 1978. Copyright by the American Dental Association. Reprinted by permission. **B** courtesy R. Lee, DDS, Findlay, Ohio.)

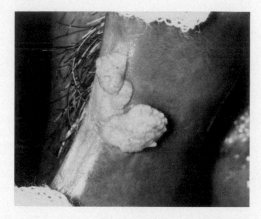

Fig. 8-28. Condyloma acuminatum at the angle of the mouth. (Courtesy E. Seklecki, DDS, Tucson, Ariz.)

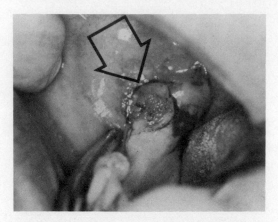

Fig. 8-29. Pseudoepitheliomatous hyperplasia on the surface of a peripheral ameloblastoma in the edentulous third molar region. Photograph was taken after initial incision was made for removal of hyperplasia. (Courtesy R. Latronica, DDS, Albany, N.Y.)

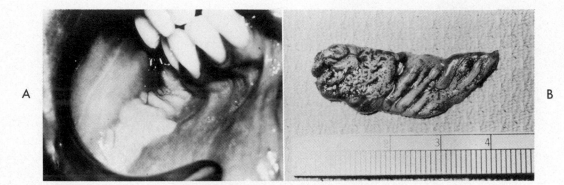

Fig. 8-30. Verruciform xanthoma. **A,** Intraoral view showing white lesion in buccal mucosa. **B,** View of surgical specimen showing corrugated surface. (From Graff S et al: Oral Surg 45:762-767, 1978.)

Pseudoepitheliomatous hyperplasias are surface epithelial changes that may occur in lesions such as fungal infections, syphilis, granular cell myoblastomas, and peripheral ameloblastomas. The papillary changes may be severe enough to produce a pebbly surface usually of a broad nature, but sometimes they occur as a smaller lesion (Fig. 8-29). However, in almost every case these epithelial proliferations have a sessile base. Thus the lesion should not be confused with a papilloma.

The *verruciform xanthoma* is a white keratotic lesion that occurs with some frequency on the skin but rarely occurs in the oral cavity. Its whitish, corrugated surface is illustrated in Fig. 8-30. It is similar to the verrucous carcinoma in that it has a broad base and vertical projection into the oral cavity is minimal. However, it has a much softer consistency than verrucous carcinoma because there is much less keratin in the

former lesion. Also the corrugations are much more shallow and more regular in the verruciform xanthoma. Eversole and Papanicolaou (1983) have developed an extensive differential diagnosis of papillary and verrucous lesions of oral mucous membranes.

Management

The papilloma must be excised by means of an elliptic incision in the tissue underlying the lesion. Excision through the stalk usually results in recurrence. The excised tissue must always be examined microscopically to ensure the final diagnosis.

VERRUCA VULGARIS

Verruca vulgaris is an exophytic growth of the epithelium that is a common lesion of the skin but seldom occurs orally. It has been convincingly shown to be caused by a virus

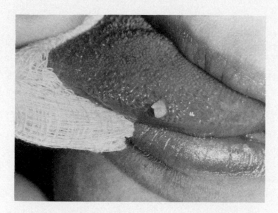

Fig. 8-31. Small verruca vulgaris on the border of the tongue.

(Wysocki and Hardie, 1979). It is possible that a papilloma is the same lesion as a wart: the wart occurring on the skin and the papilloma on the mucous membrane.

Features

The verruca vulgaris has been found on the skin, on the vermilion border, and infrequently on the labial or buccal mucosa or tongue. It is a mass with a rough, coarse, pebbly surface and a broad base. Although it cannot always be differentiated from papilloma, its surface clefts and depressions are characteristically much more shallow and the mass more sessile. It will vary in whiteness according to the degree of surface keratinization (Fig. 8-31). Multiple lesions may occur, and these most likely represent examples of autoinoculation.

On microscopic examination the verruca has a broad base, usually only slightly narrower than the greatest diameter of the lesion, with a relatively thicker connective tissue core than is found in the papilloma. The core ramifies into the epithelium-covered papillae. The connective tissue branches of the core tend to slant upward and outward from the center of the base. Eosinophilic viral inclusion bodies are frequently seen in the superficial part of the prickle cell layer and in the granular cell layer. The degree of surface keratinization varies from lesion to lesion.

Differential diagnosis

The differentiating aspects of verruca vulgaris are discussed under the differential diagnosis of papilloma (p. 133).

Management

Complete excision with microscopic study of the specimen is the proper treatment for a sol-itary oral lesion of verruca vulgaris. Dermatologists frequently use fulguration for the removal of multiple verrucae on the skin.

VERRUCOUS CARCINOMA

Verrucous carcinoma is a type of slow-growing, low-grade carcinoma of the oral cavity and upper aerodigestive tract. It is a superficial carcinoma that invades the connective tissue with an indolent pushing front rather than in an infiltrating manner. The clinical and microscopic appearances are quite characteristic. It should be considered a clinical pathologic entity distinct from "garden variety" squamous cell carcinoma of the oral cavity because of its unique biologic behavior (McCoy and Waldron, 1981). Verrucous carcinoma usually occurs in persons who smoke or use snuff or chewing tobacco. This lesion was first defined as a separate entity by Ackerman in 1948.

Features

Verrucous carcinoma most often occurs in the buccal mucosa, alveolar ridge and gingiva, tongue, floor of the mouth, and palate of elderly patients. In Shafer's study (1972) men and women were affected with approximately equal frequency, the average age for men being 64.7 years and for women, 71 years. In Jacobson and Shear's paper (1972) ten were women and five were men. McCoy and Waldron's series (1981) also showed a slight female preponderance (60%). In Slootweg and Müller's series (1983) 77.7% of the lesions occurred in men. Tornes et al. (1985) reported a female preponderance.

Clinical appearance is that of a large, broad lesion with minimal to extensive elevation above the surface mucosa (Fig. 8-27, *B*). A few lesions are small and even somewhat pedunculated (Fig. 8-27, *A*). Generally the lesions appear initially as a broad-based, warty, fungating mass. The surface is rough, pebbly, and cauliflower-like with deep crevices in some instances separating distinct, mamillated folds (Fig. 8-27). The surface may be white, red, or red and white depending on the degree of surface keratinization, and ulceration may be present. Verrucous carcinoma is frequently associated with leukoplakia at its periphery. Clinically the margins are usually well defined and characteristically show a rim of slightly elevated normal mucosa where the tumor has pushed under the edge of the normal tissue and has undermined it slightly.

Microscopically the lesion is deceptively benign. The tumor epithelium is greatly thickened with papillary projections outward and with downward projections of broad, blunt, rete ridges into the connective tissue. The basement membrane is intact. These down growths of epithelium into the connective tissue demonstrate a "pushing border" rather than showing small, thin, invasive extensions. Often the rete ridges reach the same level and form a "broad front." There is characteristically a sharp margin of demarcation at the borders of the tumor between the lesion and normal tissue. Frequently the tumor retracts a margin of normal epithelium down with it into the connective tissue. An abundance of keratin is generally seen on the surface and will dip down with the invaginating epithelium and be seen as keratin plugs. Generally there is a marked chronic inflammatory cell infiltrate, which is predominantly lymphocytic in the connective tissue directly under the invading rete ridges. Characteristically, the verrucous carcinoma lacks the cytologic criteria for malignancy. It is noteworthy that Batsakis et al. (1982) found areas of less well-differentiated carcinoma in three of seven laryngeal verrucous carcinomas.

Concerning biologic behavior, verrucous carcinoma has classically been thought to be a slow-growing progressive neoplasm with a clinical phase that lasts several years. Metastasis has been considered to occur rarely if ever. However, recent information reveals that verrucous carcinoma has the potential to transform into squamous cell carcinoma and to adopt a much more aggressive behavior (Batsakis et al., 1982). In addition, several studies have shown that verrucous carcinomas coexist or are associated with squamous cell carcinoma or epithelial dysplasia in a significant number of cases (Slootweg and Müller, 1983). From their own study these workers reported that there was an associated or coexisting premalignant or malignant condition in 48% of cases of verrucous carcinoma. These other lesions formed part of the verrucous carcinoma or occurred separately from the verrucous neoplasm.

VERRUCOUS HYPERPLASIA VS VERRUCOUS CARCINOMA

In 1980 Shear and Pindborg introduced the concept of "verrucous hyperplasia," describing how this differed from verrucous carcinoma in their opinion. They described "verrucous hyperplasia" as a proliferative epithelial lesion with the epithelial hyperplastic folds extending *above* the margins of the surrounding mucosa, whereas in verrucous carcinoma the folds invade down into the connective tissue and hence below the surrounding normal mucosal margins. They believed that "verrucous hyperplasia" may develop into verrucous or squamous carcinoma. Other authorities believe that "verrucous hyperplasia" and "verrucous carcinoma" are really the same lesion (Batsakis et al., 1982; Slootweg and Müller, 1983). Hansen et al. (1985) introduced an umbrella term, "proliferative veruccous leukoplakia," to describe a continuum of lesions that includes leukoplakia verrucous hyperplasia, verrucous carcinoma, and papillary squamous cell carcinoma.

Differential diagnosis

The differential diagnosis of verrucous carcinoma is discussed under the differential diagnosis of papilloma (p. 133).

Management

It is paramount to establish a correct diagnosis. Toward this end, it is helpful to have the reporting pathologist examine the lesion clinically. Bohmfalk and Zallen (1982) recommended multiple deep biopsies to avoid the problem of underdiagnosis. Wide surgical excision has been the recommended treatment for many years. Close and continued postsurgical surveillance is obligatory to effect early identification of recurrences resulting from inadequate excision or to find new carcinomas arising from the neighboring mucosa.

For many years radiation therapy has been frowned on as a treatment modality for verrucous carcinoma because of reports of induced anaplastic change. Recently this danger has been given less consideration, since it has become recognized that verrucous carcinomas, on their own, may undergo anaplasia. McDonald et al. (1982) in reviewing the world literature identified six cases of verrucous carcinoma that did so. In addition, it is now well understood that the surrounding mucosa frequently shows epithelial dysplasia or early squamous cell carcinoma. Thus many of these "anaplasia transformation cases" may actually have arisen independent of the radiation therapy. In line with this finding, Schwade et al. (1976) concluded from their study that radiation therapy of verrucous carcinoma did not induce anaplastic changes, and McClure et al. (1984) suggested that large oral lesions of verrucous carcinoma may benefit from a combination of surgery and radiation therapy. Chemotherapy has also been used with some success as a palliative measure or to shrink the tumor before excision (Kapstad and Bang, 1976).

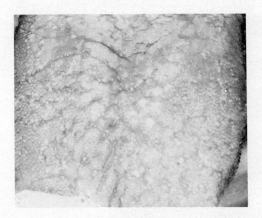

Fig. 8-32. Chronic keratotic (hyperplastic) candidiasis of long standing, on the dorsal surface of the tongue. It could not be scraped off.

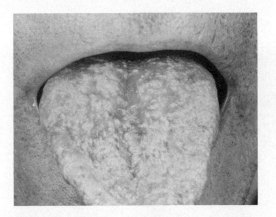

Fig. 8-33. Hyperplastic candidiasis of the dorsal surface of the tongue.

HYPERTROPHIC AND HYPERPLASTIC CANDIDIASIS

Chronic hyperplastic candidiasis (moniliasis) is a keratotic lesion that has been described by some pathologists as differing from the usual picture of candidiasis insofar as it cannot be scraped off. In cases of very low-grade chronic infections by *Candida albicans*, the yeast products may not be sufficiently concentrated to coagulate the surface epithelium but rather may stimulate the production or retention of keratin. The resultant lesion in such cases is then actually a type of leukoplakia (Figs. 8-32 and 8-33). Then too it must be realized that candidal organisms frequently are present in lesions that are primarily leukoplakias. Krogh et al. (1987) reported that 82% of leukoplakias in their study demonstrated *Candida*.

Microscopically the pseudohyphae of *Candida albicans* can be identified in the superficial layers of the keratin. Whether the *Candida* organisms initiated the hyperkeratosis or were secondary invaders of a leukoplakial lesion is not positively known. The more common pseudomembranous type of candidiasis is discussed later in this chapter in the section on sloughing pseudomembranous white lesions.

Cases of chronic hyperplastic candidiasis occurring at the angles of the mouth (angular cheilitis) and the vermilion border are reported from time to time. These may occur as chronic mucocutaneous candidiasis (Collins and Van Sickles, 1983) or as a feature of chronic multifocal candidiasis (Holmstrup and Besserman, 1983). Recently Bouquot and Fenton (1988) reported another mucocutaneous form, "juvenile juxtavermilion candidiasis," which affects the lip vermilion.

These lesions are usually keratotic and show varying degrees of keratinization so that clinically the lesions range from slightly white to a dense white. Cracks and fissures may be present. Such lesions are very difficult to treat and require prolonged regimens of antifungal drugs (Lamey et al., 1989). Bjorlin and Palmer (1983) discussed the benefits of surgical treatment of angular cheilosis.

WHITE HAIRY LEUKOPLAKIA

Hairy leukoplakia is a keratotic white lesion that frequently occurs in the mouths of patients with AIDS or AIDS-related complex. This entity is discussed in Appendix D.

WHITE SPONGE NEVUS

White sponge nevus is a hereditary condition in which white lesions occur on various mucous membranes of the body (e.g., the mucosa of the oral cavity, vagina, and pharynx). It has an autosomal dominant inheritance pattern, and the lesions may be present at birth or may begin or become more intense at puberty.

Features

White sponge nevus is a mucous membrane abnormality that varies considerably in its severity of involvement. Sometimes the white lesions, which have a rough, wrinkled surface, occur only on the buccal mucosa; at other times they may be widespread and include almost the entire oral mucosa (Fig. 8-34). The lesions are asymptomatic and do not show a tendency toward malignant change.

Microscopically the epithelium is greatly thickened because of an acanthosis and a hyperparakeratosis. Marked spongiosis (intracellular edema) occurs throughout the prickle cell layer.

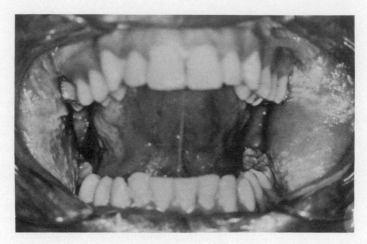

Fig. 8-34. White sponge nevus. The lesions are easily seen bilaterally on the buccal mucosa. The patient stated they had been present all his life.   (Courtesy J. Jacoway, DDS, Chapel Hill, N.C.)

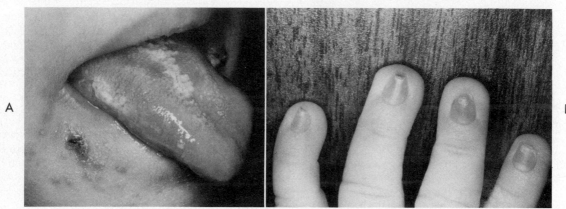

Fig. 8-35. Pachyonychia congenita. **A,** Intraoral view showing keratotic lesions on the tongue. Lesions had been present from infancy. Skin lesions were also present. **B,** Characteristic malformation of the nails.   (From Maser ED: Oral Surg 43:373-378, 1977.)

Differential diagnosis

Clinically the white sponge nevus must be differentiated from leukoedema, leukoplakia, lichen planus, pachyonychia congenita, and hereditary benign intraepithelial dyskeratosis.

If the clinician is able to establish that the lesions have been present since birth or at least since early life, this will almost completely eliminate *lichen planus* and *leukoplakia* because these lesions are quite unusual in patients under 30 years of age.

Leukoedema is found with some regularity in children, although it usually is not pronounced and is only a milky opalescence, whereas white sponge nevus has a rough, granular, somewhat leathery surface. Furthermore, stretching the tissue frequently obliterates leukoedema but does not affect the appearance of white sponge nevus.

The intraoral picture of *pachyonychia congenita* might be easily confused with white sponge nevus because the keratotic white lesions may look quite similar and may be present from birth in both diseases (Fig. 8-35). However, the presence of the nail anomalies as well as the skin lesions in pachyonychia congenita distinguish this entity from white sponge nevus.

Hereditary benign intraepithelial dyskeratosis (HBID) may be indicated by similar whitish keratotic oral lesions, but this entity is seen only in a triracial population in North Carolina.

Microscopically there may be a tendency to confuse the white sponge nevus with leukoedema, hereditary benign intraepithelial dyskeratosis, and pachyonychia congenita; however, further discussion of this problem is beyond the scope of this text.

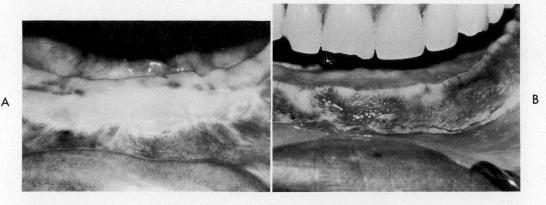

Fig. 8-36. Intramucosal skin grafts. **A,** White man. **B,** Black man. (Courtesy P. Akers, DDS, Chicago.)

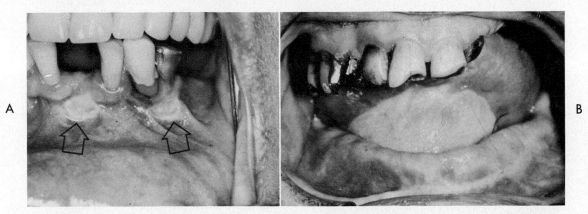

Fig. 8-37. Intraoral skin grafts. **A,** Two small skin grafts *(arrow)* placed in treatment for periodontal disease. **B,** Large skin graft on ventral surface of the tongue placed in ridge-deepening procedure. (Courtesy P. O'Flaherty, DDS, Downers Grove, Ill.)

Management

Usually proper identification is all that is required, since the white sponge nevus is benign. Occasionally a raw surface results from the desquamation of the thickened epithelium, and various palliative procedures are necessary to relieve the burning and tenderness.

SKIN GRAFTS

Although intraoral skin grafts are easily recognized by most clinicians who have seen them, they may be misdiagnosed as leukoplakic lesions by the uninitiated (Figs. 8-36 and 8-37). This is especially true with white patients because the skin graft appears white, and after some months its borders may not be clearly defined. In black patients the abundance of melanin in the skin graft usually precludes confusion with leukoplakia (Fig. 8-36, *B*). Mistaking a skin graft for a lesion is not likely because the nature of the area becomes evident during the patient interview (history).

RARITIES

The following diseases may occur rarely as white lesions of the oral mucosa that cannot be removed by scraping with a tongue blade (Figs. 8-38 to 8-40):

Acanthosis nigricans
Bohn's nodule (Epstein's pearl)
Candidiasis endocrinopathy syndrome
Clouston's syndrome
Condyloma acuminatum
Condyloma latum
Cysts—keratin filled and superficial
   Epidermoid
   Dermoid
   Lymphoepithelial
Darier's disease
Dermatitis herpetiformis
Dyskeratosis congenita
Focal epithelial hyperplasia
Focal palmoplantar and marginal gingival hyperkeratosis
Grinspan's syndrome
Hereditary benign intraepithelial dyskeratosis

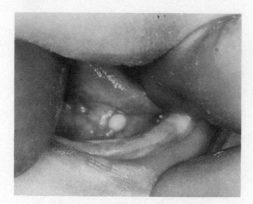

Fig. 8-38. Superficial keratin-filled lymphoepithelial cyst in the sublingual area of an infant.

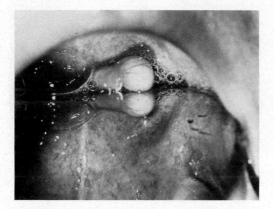

Fig. 8-39. Small epidermoid cyst attached to the uvula. The keratin-filled lumen in this superficial cyst produces the white color.

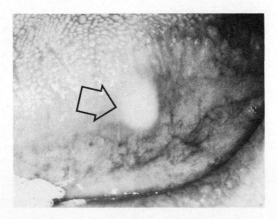

Fig. 8-40. Granular cell lesion, which had a yellowish white cast.

Hyalinosis cutis et mucosae
Hypersplenism and leukoplakia oris
Hypovitaminosis A
Inverted papilloma
Koplik's spots
Lupus erythematosus
Molluscum contagiosum
Pachyonychia congenita
Pityriasis rubra pilaris
Porokeratosis
Pseudoepitheliomatous hyperplasia
Pseudoxanthoma elasticum
Psoriasis
Scleroderma (nonkeratotic)
Squamous acanthoma
Submucous fibrosis (nonkeratotic)
Superficial sialolith of minor glands (nonkeratotic)
Syndrome of dyskeratosis congenita, dystrophia unguium, and aplastic anemia
Syphilitic interstitial glossitis leukoplakia
Verruciform xanthoma
Warty dyskeratoma

Sloughing, pseudomembranous, necrotic white lesions

The sloughing, pseudomembranous, necrotic white lesions, in contrast to the keratotic lesions, *may be scraped off the mucosa* with a tongue blade, leaving a raw, bleeding surface. The white material may be necrotic or coagulated surface epithelium or a mixture of necrotic epithelium, plasma proteins, blood cells, and microorganisms.

PLAQUE (MATERIA ALBA)

Plaque, or materia alba, is included in this group for completeness and because it may be mistaken for a lesion. In some mouths exhibiting particularly poor hygiene a mixture of food debris and bacteria may be seen as white plaques on the gingiva and alveolar mucosa and on the teeth (Fig. 8-41).

The clinician may notice a slightly inflamed mucosal surface beneath the plaque after the plaque has been removed with a gauze.

TRAUMATIC ULCER

On occasion, oral mucosa that has been crushed by mechanical trauma will appear as a sloughing white lesion (Fig. 8-42). A history of such a traumatic event is diagnostic. Pattison (1983) reviewed 49 published cases of self-inflicted gingival injury. Shiloah et al. (1984) reported on a patient's reddish white lesion that was self-inflicted in an effort to secure narcotic drugs. Clinicians must learn that in a patient whose resistance is lowered by systemic disease, secondary infections or gangrene may de-

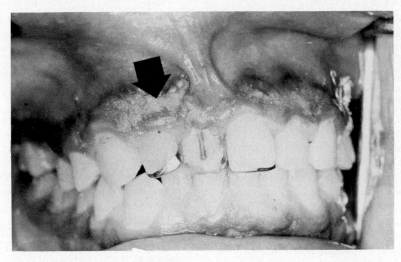

Fig. 8-41. Arrow indicates white plaque (materia alba) that can be easily removed.

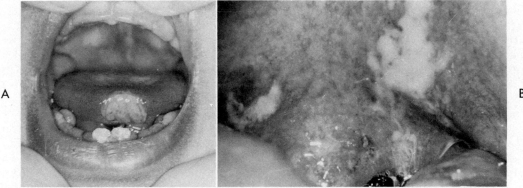

Fig. 8-42. Sloughing traumatic lesions. A, Traumatic lesion on the tip of the tongue caused by neonatal incisors. B, Sloughing white lesion on the palate produced during a traumatic orotracheal intubation.   (Courtesy G. MacDonald, DDS, Belleville, Ill.)

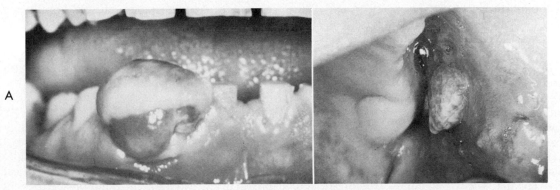

Fig. 8-43. Pyogenic granuloma. A, On labial gingiva. B, On buccal mucosa. Note the white necrotic material on the surfaces of both lesions.   (B courtesy A.C.W. Hutchinson collection, Northwestern University Dental School Library, Chicago.)

velop in these injured areas. Thus, if the severity of a traumatic lesion seems to be out of proportion to the intensity of the precipitating trauma, underlying systemic disease should be suspected.

PYOGENIC GRANULOMA

The pyogenic granuloma is discussed in considerable detail in Chapter 10 with the other exophytic lesions. We make brief mention of it here because this particular variety of inflammatory hyperplastic lesion almost invariably has a white area of varying size on its surface (Fig. 8-43). This white material is necrotic tissue that can be removed easily with a gauze or a tongue blade. The necrosis is produced by recurrent mechanical trauma and superficial infection of this exophytic lesion.

CHEMICAL BURNS

Chemical burns most often result from the patient applying analgesics, such as aspirin or acetaminophen, to the mucosa adjacent to an aching tooth. Other cases may result, however, from the dentist's inadvertently applying caustic medicaments to the mucosa. These types of lesions are now being seen in patients who use recreational drugs, such as cocaine, by applying them to a favored location in the oral mucous membrane.

We have frequently seen an interesting, mild, white, filmy desquamation on the oral mucosa of new patients who apply for dental care in the dental school clinic. Invariably, when questioned, these patients admit to the vigorous use of mouthwash and dentifrice just before coming to the clinic. Evidently they are trying to cover up their neglect of dental hygiene with a concentrated last-minute effort. It seems to us that the strong concentration of various agents has caused a superficial "burn" to the mucosa. Kowitz et al. (1976) and Rubright et al. (1978) reported this type of mild sloughing precipitated by the use of mouthwashes and dentifrices, respectively.

The clinical appearance of these burns in most cases depends on the severity of the tissue damage. Chronic mild burns usually produce keratotic white lesions, whereas intermediate insults cause a localized mucositis. More severe burns coagulate the surface of the tissue and produce a diffuse white lesion. If the coagulation is severe, the tissue can be scraped off—leaving a raw, bleeding, painful surface (Fig. 8-44).

The identification of these lesions is best accomplished by determining, through the history, that medicaments or drugs have been applied to the oral mucosa.

The sloughing of the surface mucosa caused by excessive use of mouthwash or dentifrice would be much milder and more disseminated than the more localized reaction to an analgesic tablet.

The treatment for chemical burns is the application of a protective coating such as Orabase and the initiation of a bland diet.

Systemic analgesics may be administered if pain is a problem. The patient should be advised that analgesic tablets are to be swallowed and not to be used topically.

ACUTE NECROTIZING ULCERATIVE GINGIVITIS (VINCENT'S INFECTION, TRENCH MOUTH)

Acute necrotizing ulcerative gingivitis (ANUG) is a moderately common inflammatory disorder of the gingiva, which produces a necrotic ulcerative destruction of the free margin, crest, and interdental papillae. Since a discussion of gingivitis and periodontitis has not been included in the text, we have accordingly abbreviated the description of ANUG and include it here only because it complements the group of white lesions that are the subject of this section of the chapter.

The untreated lesions are almost always covered by a grayish white membrane that can be readily scraped off, leaving a raw bleeding surface. The etiology of ANUG is complex. There seems to be little doubt that predisposing conditions are essential for the development of this disease and that the most important predisposing condition is a decreased resistance to infection. Some presumptive evidence exists that gingivitis and periodontitis (poor oral hygiene) may predispose an individual to ANUG. The lowered resistance could, in turn, be the result of one or a combination of stress-producing conditions that would permit the overgrowth of or superinfection by components of the normal oral flora. Such a synergistic combination of anaerobic oral fusiform bacilli and spirochetes is usually incriminated.

Features

The patient with ANUG frequently complains of tenderness, discomfort, or increasingly intense pain in the gingiva. Lassitude, bad taste, a fetid odor, and an inability to eat properly are also frequent symptoms. A patient may state that this problem has recurred several times. Clinical examination often discloses that one or more, or all, of the crests—or per-

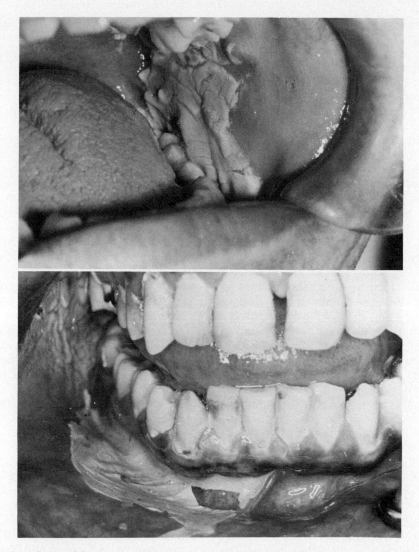

Fig. 8-44. Chemical burns. Both lesions were caused by the topical use of aspirin to relieve toothache. The white material could be removed.

A 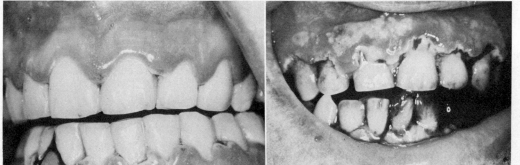 B

Fig. 8-45. Acute necrotic ulcerative gingivitis. **A,** The tips of the interdental papillae are destroyed first. **B,** Severe case in which necrotizing process has extended to the remaining marginal gingiva and to the alveolar mucosa.   (**B** courtesy J. Keene, DDS, Downers Grove, Ill.)

haps the complete interdental papillae—have been destroyed by an ulcerative process and are covered by a necrotic grayish white pseudomembrane (Fig. 8-45). Erupting teeth are often seen in cases of ANUG.

Although removal of the pseudomembrane may be painful for the patient, this maneuver is usually easily accomplished and leaves a raw bleeding surface. In severe cases the process may spread, causing destruction of the marginal gingivae between the papillae and producing extensive ulcers.

The ANUG patient may have an increased temperature and usually a painful regional lymphadenopathy. The disease can occur at any age, but the majority of cases affect patients between 17 and 35 years of age. ANUG does not show a predilection for either sex.

Cogen et al. (1983) reported the findings of their study of 100 ANUG patients referred to the periodontal clinic. They found that the patients were young with a mean average age of 23.9 years and that only one of the 100 patients was black, whereas 40% of the general clinic population was black. Urine tests showed that ANUG patients had higher levels of free cortisol in the urine. Other tests also suggested depressed immune function. In 1982 Cogen et al. demonstrated significantly depressed PMN responsiveness in ANUG patients in both chemotaxis and phagocytosis. Also there was a decreased DNA synthesis by ANUG patients' lymphocytes upon stimulation by a nonspecific mitogen (Con A). The fact that the ANUG patients also had significantly higher stress and anxiety test scores is suggestive that stress may be having a deleterious effect on the immune responses in ANUG patients. Cogen believed that altered host susceptibility as well as genetic factors may be implicated in other periodontal diseases also.

Differential diagnosis

The picture of destructive lesions that have produced punched-out defects of the interdental papillae is practically pathognomonic for ANUG, so long as the process has not affected other areas of the mucous membrane.

Somewhat similar lesions may occur in *sickle cell anemia*, but this disease may be readily identified by a special sickle cell blood preparation or by the electrophoretic examination of the hemoglobin.

If the necrotic gangrenous process has involved other regions of the oral mucosa in addition to the interdental papillae and marginal gingivae, then the diagnosis is *diffuse gangrenous stomatitis*—whose presence is suggestive of an underlying debilitating systemic disease.

Management

Treatment of ANUG is directed toward the features of the etiology: (1) superinfection by the anaerobic fusiforms and spirochetes and other oral microorganisms, (2) the underlying gingival or periodontal problem, and (3) the patient's lowered resistance to infection.

The acute phase may be managed by any of the following procedures, either singly or in combination:

1. Administration of penicillin (500 mg 4 times a day) for at least 5 days
2. Careful scaling, curettement, and debridement (NOTE: This can be accomplished with considerably less discomfort to the patient if it is postponed 24 to 48 hours after the institution of antibiotic therapy.)
3. Oral rinsing with a solution of 3% hydrogen peroxide in saline (1:3) 12 times a day (It is important that the patient understand the role lowered resistance has played in gum infection.)

Recontouring of the gingiva after regression of the disease may be necessary.

CANDIDIASIS (CANDIDOSIS, MONILIASIS, THRUSH)

Candidiasis is an infection by a dimorphic yeastlike fungus, *Candida*. Although there are several species, *albicans* is the most frequent cause of disease (Kolnick, 1980). The saprophytic yeast phase of this microorganism is a component of the normal oral flora of a significant number of normal patients. Berdicevsky et al. (1984) reported from a study of 140 healthy children that 45% of 3- to 5½-year-olds and 65% of 6- to 12-year-olds were *Candida* carriers. In an earlier study Berdicevsky et al. (1980) demonstrated that 52% of normal adults were carriers. *Candida* exists in a probable antipathetic symbiotic relationship* with many of the other oral microorganisms.

Because *C. albicans* has such low virulence in the yeast phase, some changes must take place in the local environment to produce conditions favorable to its relative overgrowth and tissue invasion. Two such changes have been identified: (1) a reduction or a proportional

---

*An association between dissimilar groups of organisms that is advantageous to one but disadvantageous to the other.

change in the competitive flora predisposes a person to candidiasis, and (2) a drastic reduction in the resistance of the tissues also favors this infection. These alterations may be effected by either local or systemic factors and may be related to age, hormonal status, and genetics.

Changes in the physical nature of the local tissue surfaces that permit penetration and afford a compatible medium for the growth of the organism are frequently present. Thrush in infants and candidiasis in patients receiving long-term broad-spectrum antibiotic therapy are examples of candidiasis caused by an altered oral flora.

Secondary *Candida* infections in angular cheilosis, denture mucositis, erythema multiforme, leukoplakia, and ruptured bullous lesions are examples of a candidiasis resulting from a lowered resistance of the local tissues as well as from the altered epithelial surface— providing the proper soil for proliferation of the organism. In such instances the candidiasis may mask the initial disease process. Candidiasis in terminal patients or in patients who have leukemia or other severe and often debilitating diseases is probably an example of a *Candida* infection resulting from lowered systemic resistance.

Patients who are receiving chemotherapy or immunosuppressive drugs or irradiation form another susceptible group. Dreizen et al. (1983) reported that almost 70% of chemotherapy-associated oral infections in patients with solid tumors were caused by *C. albicans*. Al-Tikriti et al. (1984) concluded that there were sharp increases in fungal colony counts from a period extending from shortly after treatment to as long as 6 months in 22 patients with oral or circumoral carcinomas that were irradiated. Moskow et al. (1972) discussed some aspects of severe oral infection associated with prolonged steroid therapy. Epstein and Komiyama (1986) studied the relationship between oral topical steroids and secondary oral candidiasis. They reported that secondary oral candidiasis developed in 31% of those patients who were using oral topical steroids. Candidiasis did not develop in a high percentage (88%) of those patients who were carriers.

The clinician also needs to be aware that asthmatic adults who use cortisone nebulizers as a prophylactic measure may contract candidiasis of the soft palate, fauces, and pharynx. Several studies have failed to show this effect on children (Ben-Aryeh et al., 1985). Patients predisposed to candidiasis are infants and debilitated geriatric patients; those with carcinoma, rheumatoid disease, lupus erythematosus, iron deficiency anemia, pernicious anemia or hypoparathyroidism; those receiving systemic or topical corticosteroid therapy or broad-spectrum antibiotic therapy, wearing dentures, or exhibiting lichen planus; irradiated patients; those receiving chemotherapy or immunosuppressive drugs; those with syndrome of familial hypoparathyroidism, candidiasis, and retardation; and those with syndrome of idiopathic hypoparathyroidism, Addison's disease, and candidiasis (Holbrook and Rogers, 1980). Samaranayake (1986) reviewed the connection between nutritional factors and oral candidiasis. Greenspan (1983) nicely summarized the current consensus on oral candidiasis.

There are three basic types of clinical lesions: pseudomembranous white lesions, hypertrophic or hyperplastic (keratotic) white lesions, and atrophic red lesions. Hypertrophic or hyperplastic candidiasis is discussed earlier in this chapter with keratotic lesions. Atrophic candidiasis is discussed in Chapter 5, "Solitary Red Lesions." Pseudomembranous candidiasis is the subject of this section.

Features

The patient with candidiasis may complain of a burning sensation, tenderness, or sometimes pain in the area of the affected mucosa. Spicy foods will cause occasional discomfort because of the increased sensitivity of the affected mucosa. Zegarelli and Zegarelli-Schmidt (1987) reported from their study that these infections were more common in women and in patients over 40 years of age. Fifty percent of their patients came to them with a chief complaint of oral burning. The patient may report having been on a prolonged course of broad-spectrum antibiotics for a sore throat or other infection.

The pseudomembranous oral infection may show as fine whitish deposits on an erythematous patch of mucosa or as more highly developed small, soft, white, slightly elevated plaques that closely resemble to milk curds (Figs. 8-46 and 8-47). The disease may range in severity from a solitary region to a diffuse whitish involvement of several or all the mucosal surfaces. The mucosa adjacent to, or between, these whitish plaques appears red and moderately swollen. The plaques or pseudomembranes may be stripped off the mucosa, leaving a raw bleeding surface. When solitary restricted sites are involved, the buccal mucosa

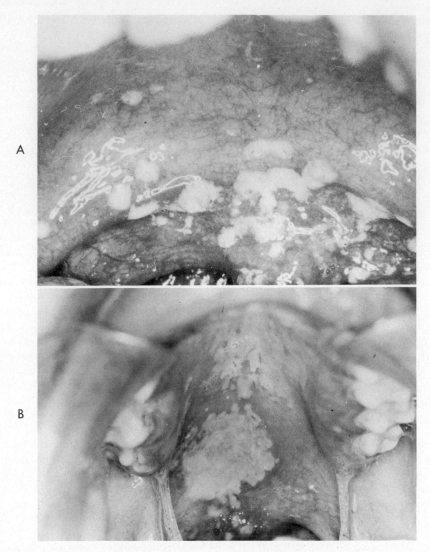

Fig. 8-46. Candidiasis. **A,** Typical milk curd lesion on the soft palate of a man receiving prolonged broad-spectrum antibiotic therapy. **B,** Lesions on the palate of a leukemic patient.

and vestibule are the most frequent regions affected—followed by the tongue, palate, gingivae, floor of the mouth, and lips.

A convincing diagnosis can be made by microscopically examining some of the pseudomembrane or plaque material. In cases of candidiasis, several species of oral flora are present in the scrapings along with coagulated surface epithelium and significantly great masses of both yeast forms and mycelial filaments. Culturing *C. albicans* is a less sensitive diagnostic procedure; since this microorganism can be obtained from a large percentage of healthy mouths, its isolation is of little pathologic significance.

It is important to remember that any oral lesion with surface debris may harbor candidal organisms even to the extent that a secondary candidiasis may become established. Nystatin treatment in such cases would produce some improvement, but full remission must await successful treatment for the primary lesion.

Differential diagnosis

As a rule all the keratotic lesions discussed in the first part of this chapter may be readily eliminated from consideration, since they cannot be easily removed by scraping with a tongue blade.

Necrotic white lesions that must be considered in the differential diagnosis are chemical burns, gangrenous stomatitis, superficial bacterial infections, traumatic ulcers, necrotic ulcers of systemic disease, and the mucous patch.

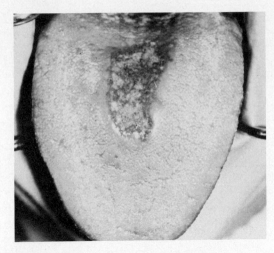

Fig. 8-47. Candidiasis on the dorsal surface of the tongue.

The *mucous patch* of syphilis is usually a discrete, small, white necrotic lesion on the tongue, palate, or lips (Fig. 8-48), whereas candidiasis is usually much more diffuse. The accompanying skin lesions of secondary syphilis and the positive serologic findings readily differentiate the mucous patch from candidiasis.

Necrotic ulcers and *gangrenous stomatitis* of debilitating systemic disease may be difficult to differentiate from candidiasis because the latter entity is usually also found in patients with debilitating secondary disease. These lesions are discussed in Chapter 11 (see Fig. 11-11). As a general rule, if the ulcer is deep then candidiasis would not be the primary cause, although such an ulcer could indeed be secondarily infected with *C. albicans.*

Traumatic ulcers with necrotic surfaces can in almost all instances be related to a history of specific trauma.

Superficial bacterial infections may occur in patients with debilitating disease and indeed may mimic pseudomembranous candidiasis. Tyldesley et al. (1979) described such lesions occurring in renal transplant patients who were receiving combined steroid and immunosuppressive drug therapy. Previously some of these lesions were believed to be antibiotic-resistant candidiasis. Culture of these lesions yielded abundant bacteria such as staphylococci, *Neisseria,* coliform bacteria, and lactobacilli. On the other hand, if removable white plaques filled with yeast forms and pseudohyphae are present, the diagnosis is either primary or secondary candidiasis.

Because its oral lesions are also covered by pseudomembranes, *gangrenous stomatitis* may

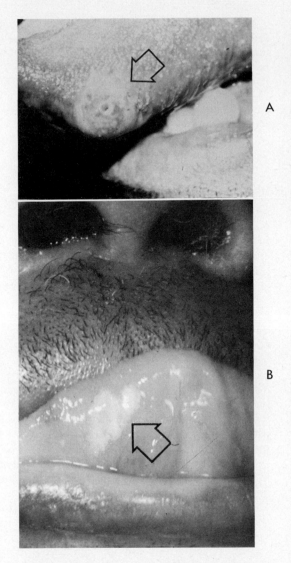

Fig. 8-48. Syphilitic lesions. **A,** Chancre on the anterolateral border of the tongue. It is unusual for a chancre to have a white necrotic surface. **B,** Mucous patch on the tongue of a patient with secondary syphilis.   (**A** courtesy T. Wall, DDS, Chicago. **B** courtesy R. Gorlin, DDS, Minneapolis.)

be confused with candidiasis. Its plaques or pseudomembranes are not raised above the mucosa, however, but cover an ulcerating lesion that may extend to bone. Also its pseudomembranes are usually a dirty gray color, in contrast to the whiteness of those that develop in candidiasis. Gangrenous stomatitis may carry a much graver prognosis than does candidiasis, since the patient may be seriously ill with an uncontrolled debilitating disease; however, candidiasis also affects terminally ill patients.

Chemical burns in some instances closely mimic candidiasis. The distinction is usually made by an accurate history, disclosing that a medicament has been applied to the mucosa.

Management

The management of patients with oral candidiasis is twofold: (1) attempts to identify, correct, or eliminate predisposing or precipitating factors and (2) antifungal therapy.

ELIMINATION OF PREDISPOSING CONDITIONS

The diagnosis and management of underlying systemic conditions, such as diabetes, malnutrition, anemia, and the discontinuation of broad-spectrum antibiotics with substitution of a drug with a more selective spectrum, illustrate some of the approaches that should be considered in this important phase of management. Local resistance can be improved by good oral hygiene and by leaving dentures out as much as possible.

ANTIFUNGAL THERAPY

The six drugs that are chiefly used for antifungal therapy are gentian violet, nystatin, amphotericin B, miconazole, clotrimazole, and ketoconazole. Painting with gentian violet was used a great deal before the development of the modern antifungal drugs. Although it possesses a general antifungal activity it has fallen into disuse because of its unsightly appearance and the availability of better drugs.

Nystatin and amphotericin have been the standard drugs used for oral candidal infections for the last 25 years. Each of these drugs is absorbed poorly from the gastrointestinal tract but is excellent for topical use on mucous membrane and skin lesions. Also these drugs are indicated for the treatment of intestinal candidiasis and are ingested orally for this purpose. Indeed oral antifungal topical agents should be supplemented with the oral ingestion of these drugs if the clinician thinks that the intestines are serving as a reservoir of candidal organisms and thus prolonging the oral lesions. Nystatin is not given parenterally. Amphotericin B infusion is reserved for severe systemic fungal infections because of the many, serious side effects.

The usual dosage for nystatin is 250 mg tablets or troches three times a day for 2 weeks followed by 1 troche per day for a third week. The troches are placed in the mouth and permitted to dissolve completely. Nystatin suspension preparations may be substituted, but it is generally thought that the dissolving of troches permits a more prolonged period of contact between the drug and microorganism. Salves and ointments (nystatin) may be applied concurrently to the commissures or vermilion border if angular cheilosis is present. Dentures should be placed in nystatin solution at night. Barrett (1984) indicated that nystatin was of limited use in eliminating oropharyngeal *Candida* in immunosuppressed patients.

Amphotericin B is available as ointments and lozenges and may be used in exactly the same fashion as nystatin. The usual dosage is one lozenge (10 mg) four times a day for 14 days followed by one lozenge a day for another 14 days. Kolnick (1980) stated that amphotericin B has a greater antifungal spectrum than nystatin, has been shown to be more active in vitro against *C. albicans*, and has a more pleasant taste.

Miconazole and clotrimazole are among the more recent drugs that appear to have given encouraging results. Used topically these drugs are effective and harmless, but oral ingestion must be monitored carefully because of the potential for many and varied systemic side effects, the most worrisome of which is hepatic damage.

Ketoconazole, the most recently introduced of all these agents, shows promise as an effective drug in the treatment of *Candida* infection. It can be administered systemically, and minimal side effects have been reported (Jones et al., 1984; Jorizzo, 1982). Nevertheless, toxic effects on the liver do occur (Svedhem, 1984; Lewis, 1984). Ketoconazole is much more expensive than nystatin but is easily absorbed after oral ingestion. Use of this drug should be reserved for serious fungal infections.

Various papers stress the importance of continuing antifungal therapy at least 2 weeks following disappearance of signs and symptoms of oral lesions lest residual organisms produce a recurrence (Epstein et al., 1981; Kolnick, 1980). Holbrook and Rogers (1980) reported that 13% of their treated candidal patients required anticandidal therapy for more than 1 year.

NECROTIC ULCERS OF SYSTEMIC DISEASE

Necrotic ulcers may occur in debilitating systemic diseases such as leukemia, sickle cell anemia, and uremia. The ulcers are usually deep craters with a white necrotic surface (Fig. 8-49). In most instances they commence as small mucosal injuries that become chronically infected because of the decreased resistance of the patient. These lesions are discussed and illustrated in Chapter 11.

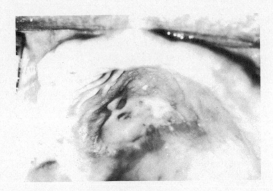

Fig. 8-49. Necrotic ulcer on the palate of a patient with mycosis fungoides. (Courtesy M. Sneed, DDS, Los Angeles.)

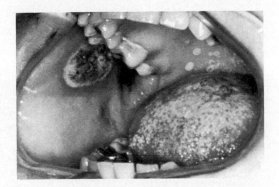

Fig. 8-50. Noma on the buccal mucosa of a patient terminally ill with acute myelogenous leukemia. (From Weinstein RA et al: Oral Surg 38:10-14, 1974.)

DIFFUSE GANGRENOUS STOMATITIS

Diffuse gangrenous stomatitis is also an oral disease in which a pseudomembrane is formed. Its cause is almost identical to that of ANUG, but it occurs in extremely debilitated patients. It must be differentiated from localized gangrenous stomatitis (cancrum oris or noma), a single localized and very destructive lesion (Fig. 8-50) seldom encountered in the United States. Griffin et al. (1983) described two cases that occurred in young children.

Features

Diffuse gangrenous stomatitis is usually found in patients with severe debilitating diseases, such as advanced diabetes, uremia, leukemia, blood dyscrasias, malnutritional states, or heavy metal poisoning. The patient complains of sensitive or painful oral lesions and a very unpleasant odor. The lesions are multiple, affecting several mucosal surfaces, and are surrounded by a thin inflamed margin. The lesions are covered by a dirty gray to yellow pseudomembrane that can be readily removed,

leaving a raw, bleeding, painful surface. They may be elliptic, linear, or angular. A tender to painful cervical lymphadenopathy is invariably present.

Differential diagnosis

Differential aspects of diffuse gangrenous stomatitis are discussed under the differential diagnosis of candidiasis (p. 148).

Management

Local treatment of diffuse gangrenous stomatitis is similar to the regimen described for ANUG—systemic penicillin and hydrogen peroxide rinses many times a day. This condition has a much graver prognosis than does ANUG because of the serious predisposing systemic conditions present. Unless the systemic problems can be improved, the oral lesions may be difficult to eliminate completely.

RARITIES

The following either are rare disease entities or seldom occur as white sloughing lesions of the oral mucosa:

Candidiasis endocrinopathy syndrome
    Syndrome of familial hypoparathyroidism, candidiasis, and retardation
    Syndrome of idiopathic hypoparathyroidism, Addison's disease, and candidiasis
Congenital insensitivity to pain syndrome
Diphtheria
Eosinophilic granuloma
Heavy metal mucositis
Henoch-Schönlein purpura
Noma
Superficial abscess
Syphilitic chancre and mucous patch
Tuberculosis
Vesicles and bullae (discussed in Chapter 6)

Although these are rare lesions, the examining clinician must be cognizant of them while developing a differential diagnosis. Unless specific characteristics of the lesion in question indicate otherwise, however, they should be assigned a low rank on his or her list of probable entities.

REFERENCES

Abdel-Salam M, Mayall BH, Chew K, et al: Prediction of malignant transformation in oral epithelial lesions by image cytometry, Cancer 62:1981-1987, 1988.

Abt E, Wigdor H, Lobraico R, et al: Removal of benign intraoral masses using the CO_2 laser, J Am Dent Assoc 115:729-731, 1987.

Ackerman LV: Verrucous carcinoma of the oral cavity, Surgery 23:670-678, 1948.

Al-Drouby HAL: Oral leukoplakia and cryotherapy, Br Dent J 155:124-125, 1983.

Allen CM, Beck FM, Rossie KM, and Kaul TJ: Relation of stress and anxiety to oral lichen planus, Oral Surg 61:44-46, 1986.

Allen CM and Blozis GC: Oral mucosal reactions to cinnamon-flavoured chewing gum, J Am Dent Assoc 116:664-667, 1988.

Al-Tikriti V, Martin MV, and Bramley PA: A pilot study on the clinical effects of irradiation on the oral tissues, Br J Oral Maxillofac Surg 22:77-86, 1984.

Amagasa T, Yokoo E, Sato K, et al: A study of the clinical characteristics and treatment of oral carcinoma in situ, Oral Surg 60:50-55, 1985.

Anderson H et al: A tobacco boom with no smoke, Newsweek 94:67-68, 1979.

Ballard BR, Sues GR, Pickren JW, et al: Squamous cell carcinoma of the floor of the mouth, Oral Surg 45:568-579, 1978.

Bánóczy J: Oral leukoplakia, The Hague, 1982, Martinus Nijhoff Publishers.

Bánóczy J and Csiba A: Occurrence of the epithelial dysplasia in oral leukoplakia, Oral Surg 42:766-774, 1976.

Bánóczy J, Roed-Petersen B, Pindborg JJ, and Inovay J: Clinical and histologic studies on electrogalvanically induced oral white lesions, Oral Surg 48:319-323, 1979.

Bánóczy J and Sugár L: Longitudinal studies in oral leukoplakia, J Oral Pathol 1:265-272, 1972.

Barrett AP: Evaluation of nystatin in prevention and elimination of oropharyngeal Candida in immunosuppressed patients, Oral Surg 58:148-151, 1984.

Batsakis JG, Hybels R, Crissman JO, et al: The pathology of head and neck tumors: verrucous carcinoma. Part 15, Head Neck Surg 5:29-35, 1982.

Baughman R: Personal communication, 1984.

Bekke JPH and Baart JA: Six years experience with cryosurgery in the oral cavity, Int J Oral Surg 8:251-270, 1979.

Ben-Aryeh H, Berdicevsky I, Zinmann P, et al: Salivary composition and oral candida in asthmatic children and the effect of inhaled drugs, J Oral Med 40:123-126, 1985.

Berdicevsky I, Ben-Aryeh H, Szargel R, et al: Oral candida in asymptomatic denture wearers, Int J Oral Surg 9:113-115, 1980.

Berdicevsky I, Ben-Aryeh H, Szargel R, et al: Oral candida in children, Oral Surg 57:37-40, 1984.

Bernstein ML: Oral mucosal white lesions associated with excessive use of Listerine mouthwash, Oral Surg 46:781-785, 1978.

Berry HH and Landwerlen JR: Cigarette smokers lip lesion in psychiatric patients, J Am Dent Assoc 86:657-662, 1973.

Bjorlin G and Palmer B: Surgical treatment of angular cheilosis, Int J Oral Surg 12:137-140, 1983.

Blot WJ, McLaughlin JK, Winn DM, et al: Smoking and drinking in relation to oral and pharyngeal cancer, Cancer Res 48:3282-3287, 1988.

Bohmfalk C and Zallen RD: Verrucous carcinoma of the oral cavity, Oral Surg 54:15-20, 1982.

Bouquot JE and Fenton SJ: Juvenile juxtavermilion candidiasis: yet another form of an old disease? J Am Dent Assoc 116:187-192, 1988.

Bouquot JE and Gorlin R: Leukoplakia, lichen planus, and other keratoses in 23,616 white Americans over the age of 35 years, Oral Surg 61:373-381, 1986.

Brooks JK and Balciunas BA: Geographic stomatitis: review of the literature and report of five cases, J Am Dent Assoc 115:421-424, 1987.

Browne RM and Potts AJC: Dysplasia in salivary gland ducts in sublingual leukoplakia and erythroplakia, Oral Surg 62:44-48, 1986.

Buchner A and Sandbank M: Multiple fibroepithelial hyperplasias of the oral mucosa, Oral Surg 46:34-39, 1978.

Burry JN and Kirk J: Lichenoid drug reaction from methyldopa, Br J Dermatol 91:475-476, 1974.

Carpenter RJ and Snyder GG: Cryosurgery: theory and application to head and neck neoplasia, Head Neck Surg 2:129-141, 1979.

Chau NY, Reade CP, Rich AM, and Hay KD: Allopurinol-amplified lichenoid reactions of the oral mucosa, Oral Surg 58:397-400, 1984.

Christen AG: The case against smokeless tobacco: five facts for the health professional to consider, J Am Dent Assoc 101:464-469, 1980.

Christen AG, Swanson BZ, Glover ED, et al: Smokeless tobacco: the folklore and social history of snuffing, sneezing, dipping, and chewing, J Am Dent Assoc 105:821-829, 1982.

Christensen E, Holmstrup P, Wiberg-Jørgesen, F, et al: Glucose tolerance in patients with oral lichen planus, J Oral Pathol 6:143-151, 1977.

Clayton JR and Jordon JE: Verrucous carcinoma, J Oral Surg 36:564-567, 1978.

Cogen RB, Stevens AW Jr, Cohen-Cole S, et al: Leukocyte function in the etiology of acute necrotizing gingivitis, J Periodontol 54:402-407, 1982.

Cogen RB, Stevens AW, and Cohen-Cole SA: Stressed whites especially prone to "trench mouth," study finds, Medical News, JAMA 249:157-158, 1983.

Collins JR and Van Sickles JE: Chronic mucocutaneous candidiasis, J Oral Maxillofac Surg 41:814-818, 1983.

Colvard MD, Nadimi H, and Gargiulo AV: Ativan (lorazepam) lichenoid reaction of the human attached gingiva: case report, Periodont Case Reports 8:69-70, 1986.

Council on Dental Materials, Instruments, and Equipment: American Dental Association status report on the occurrence of galvanic corrosion in the mouth and its potential effects, J Am Dent Assoc 115:783-787, 1987.

del Olmo JA, Bagan JV, Rodrigo JM, et al: Oral lichen planus and hepatic cirrhosis: letter to the editor, Ann Intern Med 110:666, 1989.

Dreizen S, Bodey GP, and Valdivieso M: Chemotherapy-associated oral infections in adults with solid tumors, Oral Surg 55:113-120, 1983.

Durocher RT, Thalman R, and Fiore-Donno G: Leukoedema of the oral mucosa, J Am Dent Assoc 85:1105-1109, 1972.

Eisenberg E, Murphy GF, and Krutchkoff DJ: Involucrin as a diagnostic marker in oral lichenoid lesions, Oral Surg 64:313-319, 1987.

Epstein JB, Komiyama K, and Duncan D: Oral topical steroids and secondary oral candidiasis, J Oral Med 41:223-227, 1986.

Epstein JB, Pearsall NP, and Truelove EL: Oral candidiasis: effects of antifungal therapy upon clinical signs and symptoms, salivary antibody, and mucosal adherence of Candida albicans, Oral Surg 51:32-36, 1981.

Eskinazi DP: Oncogenetic potential of sexually transmitted viruses with special reference to oral cancer, Oral Surg 64:35-40, 1987.

Eversole LR and Papanicolaou SJ: Papillary and verrucous lesions of oral mucous membrane, J Oral Med 38:3-13, 1983.

Farman AG: Hairy tongue (lingua villosa), J Oral Med 32:85-91, 1977.

Ferguson MM, Wiesenfeld D, and MacDonald DG: Oral mucosal lichenoid eruption due to Fenclofenac, J Oral Med 39:39-40, 1984.

Firth NA and Reade PD: Angiotensin-converting enzyme inhibitors implicated in oral mucosal lichenoid reactions, Oral Surg 67:41-44, 1989.

Frame JW: Removal of oral soft tissue pathology with the CO_2 laser, J Oral Maxillofac Surg 43:850-855, 1985.

Frame JW: Treatment of sublingual keratosis with the CO_2 laser, Br Dent J 156:243-346, 1984.

Glenert V: Drug stomatitis due to gold therapy, Oral Surg 58:52-56, 1984.

Gongloff RK and Gage AA: Cryosurgical treatment of oral lesions: report of cases, J Am Dent Assoc 106:47-52, 1983.

Gongloff RK, Samit AM, Greene GW, et al: Cryosurgical management of benign and dysplastic intraoral lesions, J Oral Surg 38:671-676, 1980.

Graff SG, Burk JL, and McKean TW: Verruciform xanthoma, Oral Surg 45:762-767, 1978.

Greenspan JS: Infections and non-neoplastic disease of the oral mucosa, J Oral Pathol 12:139-166, 1983.

Greer RO and Goldman HM: Oral papillomas, Oral Surg 38:435-440, 1974.

Greer RO and Poulson TC: Oral tissue alterations associated with the use of smokeless tobacco by teen-agers. I. Clinical findings, Oral Surg 56:275-284, 1983.

Greer RO, Schroeder KL, and Crosby L: Morphologic and immunohistochemical evidence of human papillovirus capsid antigen in smokeless tobacco keratoses from juveniles and adults, J Oral Maxillofac Surg 46:919-929, 1988.

Griffin JM, Bach DE, Nespeca JA, et al: Noma: report of two cases, Oral Surg 56:605-607, 1983.

Grinspan D, Diaz J, Villapol LO, et al: Lichen ruber planes de la muquese buccale son association a un diabete, Bull Soc Fr Dermatol Syphiligr 72:721, 1966.

Hammersley N, Ferguson MM, and Rennie JS: Topical bleomycin in the treatment of oral leukoplakia: a pilot study, Br J Oral Maxillofac Surg 23:251-258, 1985.

Hampf BGC, Malmstrom MJ, Aalberg VA, et al: Psychiatric disturbance in patients with oral lichen planus, Oral Surg 63:429-32, 1987.

Hansen LS, Olson JA, and Silverman S Jr: Proliferative verrucous leukoplakia, Oral Surg 60:285-298, 1985.

Hirsch JM, Heyden G, and Thilander H: A clinical, histomorphological and histochemical study on snuff-induced lesions of varying severity, J Oral Pathol 11:387-398, 1982.

Holbrook WP and Rogers GD: Candidal infections: experience in a British dental hospital, Oral Surg 49:122-125, 1980.

Holmstrup P, Thorn JJ, Rindum J, and Pindborg JJ: Malignant development of lichen planus–affected mucosa, J Oral Pathol 17:219-225, 1988.

Holmstrup P and Bessermann M: Clinical, therapeutic, and pathogenic aspects of chronic oral focal candidiasis, Oral Surg 56:388-395, 1983.

Hong WK, Endicott J, Loretta MI, et al: 13-cis retinoic acid in the treatment of oral leukoplakia, N Engl J Med 315:1501-1505, 1986.

Horch HH, Gerlach KL, and Schaefer HE: CO_2 laser surgery of oral premalignant lesions, Int J Oral Maxillofac Surg 15:19-24, 1986.

Howell FV and Rick GM: Oral lichen planus and diabetes: a potential syndrome, J Calif Dent Assoc 1:58-59, 1973.

Jacobson S and Shear M: Verrucous carcinoma of the mouth, J Oral Pathol 1:66-75, 1972.

James J, Ferguson MM, Forsyth A, et al: Oral lichenoid reactions related to mercury sensitivity, Br J Oral Maxillofac Surg 25:474-480, 1987.

Jones PG, Kauffman CA, McAuliffe LS, et al: Efficacy of ketoconazole V nystatin in prevention of fungal infections in neutropenic patients, Arch Intern Med 144:549-551, 1984.

Jorizzo JL: Chronic mucocutaneous candidiasis: an update, Arch Dermatol 118:963, 1982.

Kapstad B and Bang G: Verrucous carcinoma of the oral cavity treated with bleomycin, Oral Surg 42:588-590, 1976.

Kassim KH and Daley TD: Herpes simplex virus type 1 proteins in human oral squamous cell carcinoma, Oral Surg 65:445-448, 1988.

Kaugars GE, Burns JC, and Gunsolley JC: Epithelial dysplasia of the oral cavity and lips, Cancer 62:2166-2170, 1988.

Kolnick JR: Oral candidosis: report of a case implicating *Candida paropsilosis* as a pathogen, Oral Surg 50:411-415, 1980.

Kowitz GM, Lucatorto FM, and Cherrick HM: Effects of mouthwashes on the oral soft tissues, J Oral Med 31:47-50, 1976.

Kramer IRH, El-Labbon N, and Lee KW: The clinical features and risk of malignant transformation in sublingual keratosis, Br Dent J 144:171-180, 1978.

Kramer IRH, Lucas RB, Pindborg JJ, and Sobin LH: Definition of leukoplakia and related lesions: an aid to studies on oral precancer, WHO Collaborating Centre for Oral Precancerous Lesions, Oral Surg 46:518-539, 1978.

Krogh P, Holmstrup P, Thorn JJ, et al: Yeast species and biotypes associated with oral leukoplakia and lichen planus, Oral Surg 63:48-54, 1987.

Krutchkoff DJ, Cutler L, and Laskowski S: Oral lichen planus: the evidence regarding potential malignant transformation, J Oral Pathol 7:1-7, 1978.

Krutchkoff DJ and Eisenberg E: Lichenoid dysplasia: a distinct histopathologic entity, Oral Surg 30:308-315, 1985.

Lacy MF, Reade PC, and Hay KD: Lichen planus: a theory of pathogenesis, Oral Surg 56:521-526, 1983.

Lamey PJ, Lewis MAO, and MacDonald DG: Treatment of candidal leukoplakia with fluconazole, Br Dent J 166:296-298, 1989.

Lewis JH: Hepatic injury associated with ketoconazole therapy, Gastroenterology 86:503-513, 1984.

Lindemeyer RG, Baum RH, Hsu SC, et al: In vitro effect of tobacco on the growth of oral cariogenic streptococci, J Am Dent Assoc 103:719-722, 1981.

Loning Th, Reichart P, Staquet MJ, et al: Occurrence of papilloma-virus structural antigens in oral papillomas and leukoplakias, J Oral Pathol 13:155-165, 1984.

Lovas JGL: Lichenoid reaction to amalgam or lichen planus? A clinicopathologic analysis. Paper presented at the American Academy of Oral Pathology Meeting, Savannah, Ga, April 1989.

Lovas JGL, Harsanyi BB, and El Geneidy AK: Oral lichenoid dysplasia: a clinicopathologic analysis, Oral Surg 68:57-63, 1989.

Lowenthal U and Pisanti S: Oral lichen planus according to the modern medical model, J Oral Med 39:224-226, 1984.

Lozada-Nur F, Luangjarmekorn L, Silverman S Jr, and Karam J: Assessment of plasma glucose in 99 patients with oral lichen planus, J Oral Med 40.60-61, 1985.

Lundström IMC: Incidence of diabetes mellitus in patients with oral lichen planus, Int J Oral Surg 12:147-152, 1983.

Lundström IMC: Allergy and corrosion of dental materials in patients with oral lichen planus, Int J Oral Surg 13:16-24, 1984.

Marks R and Czarny D: Geographic tongue: sensitivity to the environment, Oral Surg 58:156-159, 1984.

Martin JL, and Crump EP: Leukoedema of the buccal mucosa in Negro children and youth, Oral Surg 34:49-58, 1972.

Maxson BB, Scott RF, and Headington JT: Management of oral squamous cell carcinoma in situ with topical 5-fluorouracil and laser surgery, Oral Surg 68:44-48, 1989.

McClure DL, Gullane PJ, Slinger RP, et al: Verrucous carcinoma—changing concepts in management, J Otolaryngol 13:7-12, 1984.

McCoy JM and Waldron CA: Verrucous carcinoma of the oral cavity: a review of 49 cases, Oral Surg 52:623-629, 1981.

McDonald JS, Crissman JD, and Gluckman JL: Verrucous carcinoma of the oral cavity, Head Neck Surg 5:22-28, 1982.

Mincer HH, Coleman SA, and Hopkins KP: Observations on the clinical characteristics of oral lesions showing histologic epithelial dysplasia, Oral Surg 33:389-399, 1972.

Moskow BS and Wheaton EA: Severe oral infection associated with prolonged steroid therapy, Oral Surg 34:590-602, 1972.

Murti PR, Daftary DK, Bhonsle RB, et al: Malignant potential of oral lichen planus: observations in 722 patients from India, J Oral Pathol 15:71-77, 1986.

Neumann-Jensen BJ and Pindborg JJ: Smoking habits of 611 patients with oral lichen planus, Oral Surg 43:410-415, 1977.

Offenbacker S and Weathers D: Personal communication, 1984.

Pattison GL: Self-inflicted gingival injuries: literature review and case report, J Periodontol 54:299, 1983.

Pecaro BC and Garehime WJ: The CO_2 laser in oral and maxillofacial surgery, J Oral Maxillofac Surg 41:725-728, 1983.

Pindborg JJ: Oral precancer. From Evans PHR, Robin PE, and Fielding JWL: Head and neck cancer, New York, 1982, Alan R Liss, Inc.

Pindborg JJ, Daftary DK, and Mehta FS: A follow-up study of sixty-one oral dysplastic precancerous lesions in Indian villagers, Oral Surg 43:383-390, 1977.

Pindborg JJ, Jolst O, Renstrup G, and Roed-Petersen B: Studies in oral leukoplakia, a preliminary report on the period prevalence of malignant transformation in leukoplakia based on a follow-up study of 248 patients, J Am Dent Assoc 78:767-771, 1968.

Pogrel MA: Sublingual keratosis and malignant transformation, J Oral Pathol 8:176-178, 1978.

Pogrel MA and Cram D: Intraoral findings in patients with psoriasis with a special reference to ectopic geographic tongue (erythema circinata), Oral Surg 66:184-189, 1988.

Potts AJC, Hamburger J, and Scully C: The medication of patients with oral lichen planus and the association of nonsteroidal antiinflammatory drugs with erosive lesions, Oral Surg 64:541-543, 1987.

Ralls SA and Warnock GR: Stomatitis areata migrans affecting the gingiva, Oral Surg 60:197-200, 1985.

Roed-Petersen B and Pindborg JJ: A study of Danish snuff-induced oral leukoplakia, J Oral Pathol 2:301-313, 1973.

Rubright WC, Walker JA, Karlsson UL, and Diehl DL: Oral slough caused by dentifrice detergents and aggravated by drugs with antisialic activity, J Am Dent Assoc 97:215-220, 1978.

Samaranayake LP: Nutritional factors and oral candidosis, J Oral Pathol 15:61-65, 1986.

Schiødt M: Oral discoid lupus erythematosus. II. Skin lesions and systemic lupus erythematosus in sixty-six patients with 6 year follow up, Oral Surg 57:177-180, 1984a.

Schiødt M: Oral manifestations of lupus erythematosus, Int J Oral Surg 13:101-147, 1984b.

Schwade JG, Wara WM, Dedo HH, et al: Radiotherapy for verrucous carcinoma, Radiology 120:677-679, 1976.

Scully C, Cox MF, Prime SS, et al: Papillomaviruses: the current status in relation to oral disease, Oral Surg 65:526-532, 1988.

Shafer WG: Verrucous carcinoma, Int Dent J 22:451-459, 1972.

Shear M and Pindborg JJ: Verrucous hyperplasia of the oral mucosa, Cancer 46:1855-1862, 1980.

Shiloah J, Lee WB, and Binkley LH: Self-inflicted oral injury to secure narcotic drugs, J Am Dent Assoc 108:977-978, 1984.

Silverman S, Gorsky M, and Lozada-Nur F: A prospective follow-up study of 570 patients with oral lichen planus: persistence, remission, and malignant association, Oral Surg 60:30-34, 1985.

Silverman S, Gorsky M, and Lozada F: Oral leukoplakia and malignant transformation: a follow-up study of 257 patients, Cancer 53:563-568, 1984.

Silverman SJ and Griffeth M: Studies on oral lichen planus. II. Follow-up on 200 patients, clinical characteristics, and associated malignancy, Oral Surg 37:705-710, 1974.

Silverman SJ and Rosen RP: Observations on the clinical characteristics and natural history of oral leukoplakia, J Am Dent Assoc 76:772-777, 1968.

Slootweg PJ and Müller H: Verrucous hyperplasia or verrucous carcinoma: an analysis of 27 patients, J Oral Maxillofac Surg 11:13-19, 1983.

Smith MJA: Oral lichen planus and diabetes mellitus: a possible association, J Oral Med 32:110-112, 1977.

Squier CA, Cox P, and Hall BK: Enhanced penetration of nitrosonornicotine across oral mucosa in the presence of ethanol, J Oral Pathol 15:276-279, 1986.

Sundström B, Mornstad H, and Axell T: Oral carcinomas associated with snuff dipping, J Oral Pathol 11:245-251, 1982.

Svedhem A: Toxic hepatitis following ketoconazole treatment, Scand J Infect Dis 16:123-125, 1984.

Syrjänen SM, Syrjänen KJ, and Happonen RP: Human papillomavirus (HPV) DNA sequences in oral precancerous lesions and squamous cell carcinoma demonstrated by in situ hybridization, J Oral Pathol 17:273-278, 1988.

Tal H, Cohen MA, and Lemmer J: Clinical histological changes following cryotherapy in a case of widespread oral leukoplakia, Int J Oral Surg 11:64-68, 1982.

Tornes K, Bang G, Koppang HS, and Pedersen KN: Oral verrucous carcinoma, Int J Oral Surg 14:485-492, 1985.

Touyz LZG and Hille JJ: A fruit-mouthwash chemical burn: report of a case, Oral Surg 58:290-292, 1984.

Tyldesley WR: Oral lichen planus, Br J Oral Surg 11:187-206, 1974.

Tyldesley WR: Malignant transformation in oral lichen planus, Br Dent J 153:329-330, 1983.

Tyldesley WR, Rotter E, and Sells RA: Oral lesions in renal transplant patients, J Oral Pathol 8:53-59, 1979.

Von Wyk CW: An investigation into the association between leukoedema and smoking, J Oral Pathol 14:491-499, 1985.

Waldron CA: Oral epithelial tumors. In Gorlin RJ and Goldman HM, editors: Thoma's oral pathology, ed 6, St. Louis, 1970, The CV Mosby Co., p. 813.

Waldron CA and Shafer WG: Leukoplakia revisited, Cancer 36(4):1386-1392, 1975.

Watanabe T, Ohishi M, Tanaka K, and Sato H: Analysis of HLA antigens in Japanese with oral lichen planus, J Oral Pathol 15:529-533, 1986.

Weathers DR, Baker G, Archard HO, and Burkes EJ: Psoriasiform lesions of the oral mucosa (with emphasis on "ectopic geographic tongue"), Oral Surg 37:872-888, 1974.

Weaver A, Fleming SM, and Smith DB: Mouthwash and oral cancer: carcinogenic or coincidence? J Oral Surg 37:250-253, 1979.

Wood NK: Smokeless tobacco and oral cancer: a summary, Ill Dent J 57:334-336, 1988.

Wysocki GP and Daley TD: Benign migratory glossitis in patients with juvenile diabetes, Oral Surg 63:68-70, 1987.

Wysocki GP and Hardie J: Ultrastructural studies of intraoral verruca vulgaris, Oral Surg 47:58-62, 1979.

Zegarelli DJ: Lichen planus: a simple and reliable biopsy technique, J Oral Med 36:18-20, 1981.

Zegarelli DJ and Zegarelli-Schmidt EC: Oral fungal infections, J Oral Med 42:76-79, 1987.

9

Red and white lesions

NORMAN K. WOOD
HENRY M. DICK

Solitary red lesions, generalized red conditions, and white lesions compose the spectrum of conditions discussed in Chapters 5, 6, and 8. This chapter, to provide a broad approach to differential diagnosis, categorizes, illustrates, and briefly describes a significant group of mixed red and white lesions that affect the oral mucosa.

Mixed red and white lesions can be separated into three distinct clinical groups depending on whether the white component is keratotic, necrotic, or vesiculobullous. The red component is produced by thinning or loss of the surface epithelium (atrophy, erosion, or ulceration), by increased capillary blood supply just beneath the epithelium, or by combinations of these (inflammation, congenital hyperplasia, hypertrophy, and hemangioma). These lesions may be categorized as follows:

Red with keratotic component
Migratory glossitis
Chronic mechanical trauma
Nicotine stomatitis
Erosive lichen planus and lichenoid reaction
Speckled leukoplakia and erythroleukoplakia
Squamous cell carcinoma
Hyperplastic candidiasis
Lupus erythematosus
Rarities
  Darier's disease
  Migratory stomatitis
  Papilloma
  Snuff lesions
  Verrucous carcinoma

Red with necrotic component
Chemical and drug burns
Thermal burns
Aphthous ulcers and stomatitis
Crushing types of trauma
Pseudomembranous candidiasis
Acute necrotic ulcerative gingivitis
Pyogenic granuloma
Allergic mucositis
Xerostomia
Radiation mucositis
Chemotherapy mucositis

Rarities
Actinomycosis
Agranulocytosis
Anemia (severe)
Gangrenous stomatitis
Inflamed soft tissue around denuded bone
Leukemic
Midline granuloma
Mucous patch
Mycotic lesions
Cyclical neutropenia
Nonspecific ulcers

Vesiculobullous lesions
Primary and secondary herpes simplex
Benign mucous membrane pemphigoid
Erythema multiforme
Pemphigus
Radiation mucositis
Rarities
  Childhood viral diseases
  Drug allergies
  Hand-foot-mouth disease
  Herpangina
  Herpes zoster
  Stevens-Johnson syndrome

RED AND WHITE LESIONS WITH A KERATOTIC COMPONENT

Lesions in this group have a white component that cannot be removed with a tongue blade.

Migratory glossitis is usually identified by its classical features: location on the tongue, red patches with raised whitish rims, the changing patterns, and its usual asymptomatic course (see Figs. 7-1 and 8-17). On rare occasions migratory stomatitis accompanies this condition with lesions involving various mucosal surfaces in addition to the tongue (Plate 1, A).

Mechanical trauma of a chronic and mild nature produces whitish leukoplakial patches. Chronic cheek or lip chewing is a good example. Periodically the chewing habit may become more severe, perhaps as a result of increased stress, and small bites may be taken out of the white patch, thus producing a red and white lesion (see Fig. 8-8, *G,* and Plate 1, *B* and *C*). The condition may look quite worrisome and reminiscent of speckled leukoplakia. However, close inspection reveals the rough tissue tags that surround the red areas. These tissue tags are not characteristic of speckled leukoplakia.

Nicotine stomatitis characteristically occurs on the hard palate of smokers, usually pipe smokers. This condition is painless. The white keratotic component may have a cobblestone appearance speckled with red dots that may be the size of pinpoints in some cases and much larger in others (Fig. 8-14). These red dots are the inflamed ducts of minor salivary glands. This appearance is pathognomonic for the condition. Occasionally the soft palate may also have an appearance similar to Wickham's striae of lichen planus with reddened mucosa between the striae (Plate 1, *D*). This appearance may be difficult to differentiate from speckled leukoplakia and atrophic or erosive lichen planus. A cobblestone appearance in any area of the lesion, most commonly near the junction of the hard palate, permits the diagnosis. A definitive diagnosis can be made if the lesion disappears on discontinuation of smoking.

Erosive lichen planus and lichenoid reaction in its classic presentation and in a bilateral or generalized distribution in the mouth is usually readily identifiable, although lupus erythematosus can mimic it (Plate 1, *E* to *G*). When this condition occurs as a single lesion, it can easily be confused with speckled leukoplakia. Biopsy usually is necessary to distinguish between them.

Speckled leukoplakia and *erythroleukoplakia* are, as the name implies, lesions with a mix of erythroplakia and leukoplakia (Plates 1, *H,* and 2, *A*). Considering that almost all erythroplakial lesions histologically demonstrate extensive dysplasia, carcinoma in situ, or early invasive carcinoma, diagnosis and treatment must be established quickly. In the authors' experience the red components are usually smoothly marginated, which distinguishes them from leukoplakias with roughly marginated red areas resulting from episodes of chronic trauma. The characteristic white feathering at the borders of lichen planus lesions is usually not seen in these lesions, nor do they exhibit the Wickham's striae of lichen planus.

Frank *squamous cell carcinoma* may have both a red and white component, as shown in Plate 2, *B.*

Hyperplastic candidiasis is a condition in which a leukoplakial lesion is associated with or caused by low-grade candidiasis. A red component is frequently part of the clinical picture. Hyperplastic candidiasis is most commonly seen at the oral commissures as angular cheilosis or mucocutaneous candidiasis (Plate 2, *C*).

Lupus erythematosus produces variable red and white lesions, which may be similar to lichen planus but usually adopt a broader, less linear pattern with a feathered border (Plate 2, *D*). Like lichen planus, these lesions have a wide distribution in the oral cavity and the lips and may involve the skin. Systemic workup and biopsy are usually necessary to establish the diagnosis.

RED LESIONS WITH NECROTIC COMPONENT

Chemical or drug burns may produce red and necrotic white areas on an erythematous background, depending on the severity of injury. Aspirin and acetaminophen burns, for example, are produced when patients hold these analgesics in their mouths to relieve toothache (Plate 2, *E*). Occasionally a clinician accidentally spills chemicals in a patient's mouth, and the chemicals produce burns. Some patients apply addictive drugs to the oral mucosa, and these drugs may produce red and white necrotic lesions (Plate 2, *F*). Facts from the patient's history establish the diagnosis.

Thermal burns may result when patients ingest food or beverages that are very hot (Plate 2, *G*). Depending on the severity of the burn the lesion may be red (erythematous) and white (deeply necrotic) or white (mildly necrotic).

Aphthous ulcers and stomatitis characteristically show ulcers with serofibrinous yellow or white necrotic centers with well-defined red borders. (Plate 2, *H*).

Crushing types of trauma produce various clinical appearances, one of which is a combined necrotic and erythematous reaction (Plate 3, *A*). Red patches or rims may be apparent when inflammation or gross loss of surface tissue occurs. Exophytic lesions are subject to trauma and may demonstrate surface necrosis.

Pseudomembranous candidiasis characteristically shows a necrotic surface with red inflammatory components surrounding the necrotic pseudomembrane. Red bleeding areas occur when the necrotic curds are stripped away (Plate 3, *B*).

Acute necrotic ulcerative gingivitis involves principally the interdental papillae and the marginal gingiva. Although necrosis is the most prominent aspect of the condition, varying degrees of erythema (redness) are seen around the necrotic margins (Plate 3, *C*).

The *pyogenic granuloma* is frequently reddish with a necrotic white patch of variable size on the surface (Plate 3, *D*). Identifying a chronic irritant usually helps to establish the working diagnosis.

In mild to moderate cases, *allergic mucositis*, shows as an inflammatory red plaque and in severe cases also has a necrotic white component (Plate 3, *E*).

Xerostomia varies in severity and may give rise to a generalized erythematous mucositis. In severe cases necrosis may occur and give a disseminated red and white appearance.

Radiation mucositis, also depending on stage and severity, may show erythematous and necrotic components disseminated as patches throughout the oral mucosa (Plate 3, *F*). Frank blebs that appear white before and after rupture may also be present. History is usually diagnostic.

Chemotherapy mucositis usually shows patches of red scattered throughout the mouth. Although necrosis may also be present, it is not usually as prominent in chemotherapy mucositis as in radiation mucositis.

VESICULOBULLOUS LESIONS

These lesions are discussed in detail in Chapter 6, "Generalized Red Conditions and Multiple Ulcerations." Originally surrounded by red rims, these lesions appear white while the vesicles, or blebs, are intact. When coalesced vesicles rupture, they may retain a white appearance for a while. When the blebs fully rupture and become emptied, their white appearance usually disappears, although the torn fragments of their roof tissue may persist as whitish flaps for a period of time. Some vesiculobullous conditions that the clinician might expect to see are herpes simplex, both primary and secondary, benign mucous membrane pemphigoid, erythema multiforme, pemphigus and its variants, and occasionally radiation mucositis (Plates 3, *G* and *H*, and 4, *A* and *B*).

10

Peripheral oral exophytic lesions

NORMAN K. WOOD
PAUL W. GOAZ

Peripheral exophytic structures and lesions of the oral cavity include the following:

Exophytic anatomic structures
Accessory tonsillar tissue
Buccal fat pads
Circumvallate papillae
Foliate papillae
Genial tubercles
Lingual tonsillar tissue
Palatal rugae
Palatine tonsils
Papilla palatina
Retrocuspid papilla
Retromolar papilla
Stensen's papillae
Sublingual caruncles
Tongue
Uvula

Exophytic lesions
Tori and exostoses
Inflammatory hyperplasias
    Fibroma
    Pyogenic granuloma
    Hormonal tumor
    Epulis fissuratum
    Parulis
    Inflammatory papillary
        hyperplasia
    Peripheral giant cell
        granuloma
    Pulp polyp
    Epulis granulomatosum
    Myxofibroma
    Peripheral fibroma with
        calcification, peripheral
        odontogenic fibroma,
        peripheral ossifying
        fibroma
Mucocele and ranula
Hemangioma,
    lymphangioma, and
    varicosity
Central exophytic lesions
Papilloma and verruca
    vulgaris
Exophytic squamous cell
    carcinoma

Verrucous carcinoma
Minor salivary gland
    tumors
Peripheral benign
    mesenchymal tumors
Nevus and melanoma
Peripheral metastatic
    tumors
Peripheral malignant
    mesenchymal tumors
Rarities
    Solitary lesions
        Actinomycosis
        Alveolar soft part
            sarcoma
        Ameloblastoma
            (peripheral)
        Angiolymphoid
            hyperplasia
        Antral neoplasms
        Benign lymphoid
            hyperplasia
        Blastomycosis
        Bohn's nodule
            (Epstein's pearl)
        Calcinosis
        Chondroma of soft
            tissue
        Choristoma
        Condyloma acuminatum
        Condyloma latum
        Congenital epulis of the
            newborn
        Early chancre
        Early gumma
        Eruption cyst
        Extraosseous
            odontogenic tumor
        Focal hyperplasia of the
            minor salivary glands
        Focal mucinosis
        Foreign body
            granuloma
        Giant cell fibroma
        Gingival cyst
        Glomus tumor
        Granular cell lesion

Granulomatous fungal
    disease
Hamartoma
Herpes proliferative
    lesion
Histiocytosis X
Juvenile
    nasopharyngeal
    angiofibroma
Juvenile
    xanthogranuloma
Kaposi's sarcoma
Kaposi's sarcoma
    (AIDS)
Keratoacanthoma
Lead poisoning
Leukemic enlargement
Lingual thyroid gland
Lymphoma
Median nodule of the
    upper lip
Median rhomboid
    glossitis (nodular
    variety)
Midline nonhealing
    granuloma
Molluscum contagiosum
Myxoma of soft tissue
    or oral focal
    mucinosis
Necrotizing
    sialometaplasia
    (nodular)
Neuroectodermal tumor
    of infancy
Nodular leukoplakia
Plasmacytoma of soft
    tissue
Pseudosarcomatous
    fasciitis
Pulse granuloma
Rhabdomyoma
Rhabdomyosarcoma
Rheumatoid nodule
Rhinoscleroma
Sarcoidosis
Sialolith
Spindle cell carcinoma
Squamous acanthoma
Sturge-Weber syndrome
Teratoma

Tuberculosis
Verruciform xanthoma
Multiple lesions
    Acanthosis nigricans
    Acrokeratosis
        verruciformis of Hope
    Amyloidosis
    Bohn's nodules
    Calcinosis
    Chronic granulomatous
        disease
    Condyloma acuminatum
    Condyloma latum
    Cowden's disease
    Crohn's disease
    Cysticercosis
    Darier's disease
    Eruption cysts
    Focal dermal
        hypoplasia (Goltz
        syndrome)
    Focal epithelial
        hyperplasia
    Gardner's syndrome
    Giant cell fibromas
    Hereditary
        telangiectasia
    Histiocytosis X
    Idiopathic gingival
        fibromatosis
    Kaposi's sarcoma
    Kaposi's sarcoma
        (AIDS)
    Lichenoides chronica
    Lymphangiomas of
        neonates
    Lymphomas
        (extranodal)
    Lymphomatoid
        papulosis
    Lymphoproliferating
        disease of the palate
    Maffucci's syndrome
    Melkersson-Rosenthal
        syndrome
    Molluscum contagiosum
    Multiple exophytic
        metastatic carcinomas
    Multiple exostoses
    Multiple fibroepithelial
        hyperplasias

Multiple gingival cysts
Multiple hamartoma
    neoplasia syndrome
Multiple lipomas
Multiple melanomas
Multiple mucoceles
Multiple myeloma
Multiple papillomas
Multiple peripheral
    brown giant cell
    lesions
    (hyperparathyroidism)
Multiple peripheral
    metastatic carcinomas
Multiple verrucae
Murray-Puretic-
    Drescher syndrome
Noonan's syndrome
Oral florid
    papillomatosis

Orodigitofacial
    syndrome (multiple
    hamartomas of the
    tongue)
Phenytoin hyperplasia
Pyostomatitis vegetans
Sarcoidosis
Syndrome of multiple
    mucosal neuromas,
    pheochromocytoma,
    and carcinoma of the
    thyroid
Syphilitic papules
Thrombocytopenic
    purpura
Urticaria pigmentosa
von Recklinghausen's
    disease
Xanthoma
    disseminatum

The term "exophytic lesion" in the context of the following discussion means *any pathologic growth that projects above the normal contours of the oral surface.*

Hypertrophy, hyperplasia, neoplasia, and the pooling of fluid are four mechanisms by which exophytic lesions may be produced. *Hypertrophy* refers to an enlargement caused by an increase in the size but not in the number of cells. *Hyperplasia* is generally defined as an enlargement caused by an increase in the number of normal cells. *Neoplasia* is defined as the

formation of a *neoplasm*, which is identical with a *tumor* and may be either benign or malignant.

In our opinion a sharp distinction as to whether a particular exophytic lesion is the result of hypertrophy or hyperplasia or a combination of these two processes cannot often be made. Because this distinction does not usually contribute to the clinical recognition of a lesion, it is not stressed in the discussion that follows.

The terms used to describe the shapes of exophytic lesions are often confusing. The descriptive terms used in this discussion to identify the specific shapes are as follows: *papillomatous, verrucous, papule, nodule* (a papule more than 0.5 cm in diameter), *dome shaped, polypoid,* and *bosselated* (Fig. 10-1). As a general rule exophytic lesions with a papillomatous or verrucous shape originate in the surface epithelium (for example, verrucae vulgares, papillomas, verrucous carcinomas, and keratoacanthomas), whereas those with a smoothly contoured shape originate in the deeper tissues and are beneath and separate from the stratified squamous epithelium (for example, tori, fibromas, lipomas, and early malignant mesenchymal tumors.)*

---

*This concept is discussed in detail in Chapter 3.

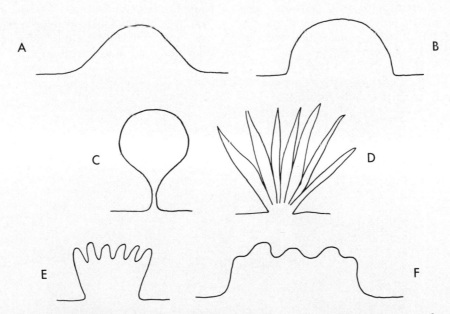

Fig. 10-1. Various shapes of exophytic lesions. **A,** Nodular. (A papular mass is a nodule measuring less than 0.5 cm.) **B,** Dome shaped. **C,** Polypoid. **D,** Papillomatous. **E,** Verrucous. **F,** Bosselated.

The surfaces of the lesions may become eroded (red), keratinized (white), or ulcerated, depending on the reaction of the epithelial surface to varying degrees of trauma. Mild trauma may cause the epithelial surface to become either eroded or keratinized, whereas severe trauma may cause the surface to become ulcerated.

When an exophytic lesion is found on an area of oral mucosa that is overlying bone, it must be identified as originating in either the soft tissues or the bone. Such a distinction is extremely important in developing the differential diagnosis. Careful visual, digital, and radiographic examinations usually indicate whether the origin is in soft tissue or bone.

If the lesion and accompanying soft tissues can be moved over the underlying bone and a radiograph fails to show bony changes, the lesion probably originated in the soft tissue. The examiner must realize, however, that the mucosa over the anterior hard palate and alveolar gingivae cannot normally be moved independent of the underlying bone. Thus in these locations, determining tissue mobility does not help the clinician identify whether the lesion originated in tissue or bone. In other locations, the examiner may have difficulty identifying the tissue of origin when there are changes in both tissues. This circumstance prompts the inclusion of a large number of possibilities in the differential diagnosis and multiple entities in the working diagnosis.

Lesions originating centrally (in bone) may become exophytic lesions, but these are not detailed in this chapter, since they are discussed in Part III of the text.

Bouquot and Gundlach (1986) studied oral exophytic lesions in 23,616 white Americans over 35 years of age and reported an incidence of 6.1% in this population.

Exophytic anatomic structures

Although exophytic anatomic oral structures are not likely to be confused with pathologic lesions, the following are listed to complete the series:

Accessory tonsillar tissue
Buccal fat pads (Fig. 10-2)
Circumvallate papillae
Foliate papillae
Genial tubercles
Lingual tonsillar tissue
Palatal rugae
Palatine tonsils
Papilla palatinae
Retrocuspid papilla
Retromolar papilla
Stensen's papillae
Sublingual caruncles
Tongue
Uvula

Occasionally some of these structures attain such a size that they are not recognized by the student but are mistaken for pathoses. The anatomic location of the structures, however, usually enables the experienced clinician to immediately recognize them. Nevertheless, since some normal structures are occasionally mistaken for exophytic lesions, the location and appearance of the foliate papillae, genial tubercles, lingual tonsillar tissue, and accessory tonsillar tissue are described here.

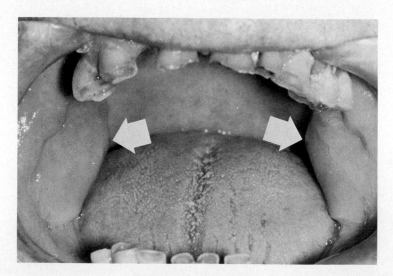

Fig. 10-2. Buccal fat pads.

The *foliate papillae* are located on the posterolateral borders of the tongue. They vary greatly in size, being absent in some patients and prominent in others. Frequently they are nodular with deep vertical fissures appearing to divide them into several closely associated exophytic projections (Fig. 10-3). They are normally pink unless traumatized, and they have approximately the same consistency as the rest of the tongue. The great variation in size and occasionally appearance is frequently troublesome for the inexperienced clinician. Furthermore, lingual tonsillar tissue is also frequently seen in the area of the foliate papillae and may be confused with the foliate papillae or similar-appearing pathoses.

The *genial tubercles* may become exophytic in patients who have experienced extreme resorption of their edentulous mandibular ridges. In some cases the genial tubercles project into the anterior floor of the mouth under the mucosa just posterior to the lingual surface of the mandible; in others they project superiorly above the level of the anterior portion of the ridge. If an exophytic mass is bony hard to palpation and is attached to the lingual surface of the mandible in the midline, it should be recognized as the genial tubercles; if the genial tubercles interfere with the construction of dentures, they should be surgically reduced.

Lingual tonsillar tissue forms part of Waldeyer's ring, which is composed of the pharyngeal tonsil (adenoids), the palatine tonsil, and the lingual tonsil. These large aggregates of lymphatic tissue are linked together by isolated tonsillar nodules; thus they encircle the entrance to the oropharynx. The lingual tonsillar tissue is on the pharyngeal surface of the tongue and frequently extends over the pos-

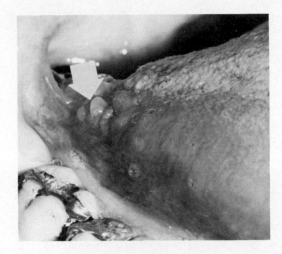

Fig. 10-3. Foliate papillae.

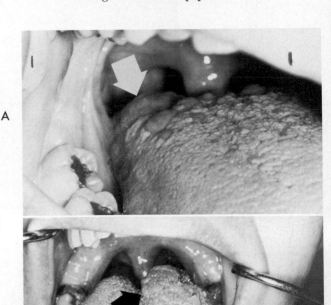

A

B

Fig. 10-4. Lingual tonsillar tissue. **A,** Classic position for the tonsil *(arrow).* **B,** Unusually large tonsil located more anterior than usual.

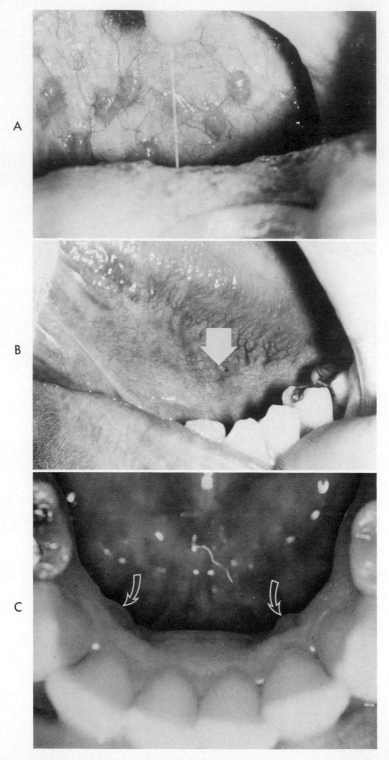

Fig. 10-5. Accessory tonsillar tissue. **A,** several nodules on the posterior pharyngeal wall. **B,** Small deposit of tonsillar tissue on the ventral surface of the tongue *(arrow).* **C,** Retrocuspid papillae situated bilaterally *(arrows)* on the lingual gingiva.   (**C** courtesy D. Weathers, DDS, Atlanta, Ga.)

terolateral borders into, or just posterior to, the location of the foliate papillae (Fig. 10-4, A).

The portion of the lingual tonsil that is apparent in the area of the foliate papillae may vary greatly in size. It may be just a small deposit of tonsillar tissue appearing as a single discrete pink papule or nodule with a smooth yellowish pink glossy surface, or it may be larger accumulations of tonsillar tissue giving the appearance of an aggregation of papules and thus recognizable as a nodular or dome-shaped mass with a coarse, pebbly (papular) surface (Fig. 10-4). In some cases the grooves between the individual papules are deep and impart a papillomatous appearance to the structure (Fig. 10-4). Lingual tonsillar tissue is usually moderately firm to palpation.

Accessory tonsillar tissue may occur in various locations in the oral cavity (floor of the mouth, ventral surface of the tongue, soft palate, and most often, posterior pharyngeal wall) (Fig. 10-5). Some patients seem to have a relative abundance of lymphoid tissue; these are the people in whom the small, usually smooth-surfaced papules and nodules are most commonly found, in various sites throughout the oral cavity. The glossy yellowish pink sheen often permits the ready identification of small deposits of tonsillar tissue.

Studies indicate a higher prevalence of accessory oral tonsil tissue than was previously believed (Adkins, 1973; Knapp, 1970a). Knapp examined 503 randomly selected young men for the presence of oral tonsil tissue. He reported that 21% of the patients had tonsil aggregates on the soft palate, 12% had tonsil aggregates on the floor of the mouth, and 5% had them on the ventral surface of the tongue. These nodules varied from 1 to 3 mm in size, and their number in individual patients ranged from 1 to 25.

Concerning pathosis of oral tonsil tissue, Adkins described in some detail the changes observed in lymphoid hyperplasia. In a more comprehensive study, Knapp (1970b) described three types of pathosis most commonly found in these aggregates: hyperplasia—pink, pseudocyst—yellow (lymphoepithelial cyst), and hyperemia—red. Knapp stressed the importance of including these entities in the differential diagnosis of exophytic, yellow, and red lesions.

• • •

The *retrocuspid papilla* is a small papule that is present in some patients. It occurs on the lingual gingiva by the mandibular cuspid tooth (Fig. 10-5, C). This normal variation usually occurs bilaterally, measures approximately 0.4 cm in width, and has a normal mucosal pink color. Gorsky et al. (1986), in a study of Israeli Jews, reported finding this structure in 38.5% of individuals from 6 to 17 years of age and in 11.3% of those ranging in age from 18 to 60 years. It is generally believed to be a developmental condition that has no pathologic significance.

The *retromolar papillae* are normal structures that are located just behind the most posterior molar teeth on the crest of the ridge of both arches. In the maxilla these structures correspond to the crestal mucosa covering the tuberosities. The retromolar papillae in the mandibular arch extend posteriorly from the free gingival margins of the most posterior molars to blend into the retromolar pads bilaterally.

Although each of the exophytic anatomic structures can undergo pathologic change, a discussion of every possibility is beyond the scope of this text.

Exophytic lesions

TORI AND EXOSTOSES

Tori and exostoses are the most common oral exophytic lesions and are discussed in detail in Chapters 27 to 29 as radiopacities of the jaws. They are readily recognizable, peripheral, benign, slow-growing bony protuberances of the jaws. They usually appear symmetrically as nodular or bosselated lesions having smooth contours and covered with normal mucosa. They are bony hard to palpation and are attached by a broad, bony base to the underlying jaw. Growth occurs mainly during the first 30 years of life.

Palatal tori are located on the hard palate usually in the midline (Fig. 10-6). They are seen in approximately 42% of females and 25% of males (King and Moore, 1976). Mandibular tori are found in about 12% of adults and are located on the lingual aspect of the mandible above the mylohyoid ridge, most often bilaterally in the premolar region (Fig. 10-6). No differences in occurrence between the sexes have been noted. King and Moore (1976) reported that patients from London have a markedly lower incidence and smaller-sized tori than do patients from the United States.

King and King (1981) reported on the results of a study of three population groups, Florida whites, Florida blacks, and Kentucky whites.

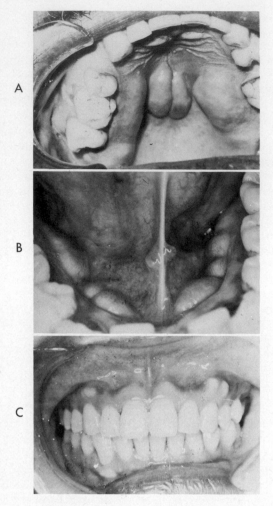

Fig. 10-6. **A,** Palatal tori and lingual exostoses. **B,** Mandibular tori. **C,** Buccal exostoses.

These investigators found no significant difference in incidence of maxillary tori among the three groups. However, maxillary tori were twice as common in females. Concerning mandibular tori, no sex preponderance was found, but Florida blacks had a lower incidence than Florida and Kentucky whites.

Similar bony protuberances that occur in other locations around the jawbones are termed "exostoses" (Fig. 10-6).

Differential diagnosis

Tori and exostoses are usually so readily identifiable that it does not seem necessary to discuss their distinguishing features. Ulcerated mucosa over these bony protuberances may pose a diagnostic problem. In almost all cases, however, the ulcers are traumatic in origin and the history and clinical examination disclose the cause.

Despite the foregoing, occasionally the following lesions may closely resemble a torus or exostosis on both clinical and radiologic examination: a mature cementifying or ossifying fibroma that has caused a bulge on the cortical palate (Fig. 28-2), an ossified subperiosteal hematoma, a nonresolved bony callus, an osteoma, and an early osteosarcoma or an early chondrosarcoma.

Management

Removal is usually considered unnecessary unless prompted by psychologic, prosthetic, phonetic, or traumatic considerations.

INFLAMMATORY HYPERPLASIAS

Inflammatory hyperplasias include a relatively large group of lesions that have an identical basic pathogenesis: chronic trauma. The spectrum of lesions is usually divided into separate entities according to the specific traumatic agent involved. Following is a list of these lesions, in the approximate descending order of frequency of occurrence:

Fibroma (inflammatory fibrous hyperplasia)
Pyogenic granuloma
Hormonal tumor
Epulis fissuratum
Parulis
Inflammatory papillary hyperplasia (palatal papillomatosis)
Peripheral giant cell granuloma
Pulp polyp (chronic hyperplastic pulpitis)
Epulis granulomatosum
Myxofibroma
Peripheral fibroma with calcification, peripheral odontogenic fibroma, and peripheral ossifying fibroma

Features

The initiating chronic injury, regardless of type, produces an inflammation, which in turn stimulates the formation of granulation tissue that consists of proliferating endothelial cells, a very rich patent capillary bed, chronic inflammatory cells, and a few fibroblasts (Fig. 10-7). The granulation tissue (granuloma) soon becomes covered with stratified squamous epithelium.

Clinically at this stage the lesion is asymptomatic and smoothly contoured or lobulated with a very red appearance because of the rich vascularity and transparency of the nonkeratinized epithelial covering. It is moderately soft and spongy and blanches on careful digital pressure. Most lesions are sessile (broad based).

If the recurring insult is eliminated at this stage, the lesion shrinks markedly as the inflammation subsides and the vascularity is reduced. If the insult is permitted to continue, however, the granulomatous lesion continues to increase in size, although some fibrosis may occur in the regions farthest removed from the areas being irritated. These fibrotic areas appear as pale pink patches on the reddish surface of the lesion. In time, the complete lesion may fibrose, resulting in a pale pinkish, smooth or lobulated firm lesion (a fibroma).

If the instigating factor is eliminated at the mixed stage, the decrease in size of the lesion is directly proportional to the amount of inflammation present—in other words, if the lesion is composed mostly of fibrous tissue, there is not much shrinkage, but if there is considerable granulation tissue and inflammation present, there is marked regression in size. Usually these lesions show a fairly consistent pattern of injury, healing, and reinjury.

Differential diagnosis

The inflammatory hyperplasias are not usually confused with other lesions because their locations are suggestive of the cause and the causative traumatic factors are easily identified. However, certain *benign* and *malignant tumors* that may mimic these lesions are discussed when the specific lesions are described.

Management

Management of the inflammatory hyperplastic lesions is prescribed on the basis of the clinical appearance of the specific lesion, which in turn is governed by the microstructure.

Basically, if the lesion is red and soft and the irritating cause can be eliminated, the clinician may expect to observe a significant reduction in size, perhaps even to the point of eliminating the need for excision. If excision is required, however, the procedure is much easier and less blood is lost if the lesion is permitted to regress (sclerose) before it is removed.

If, on the other hand, the lesion is pale pink and quite firm, almost no reduction can be expected because its bulk is probably fibrous tissue. Excision of such a lesion followed by microscopic examination of the specimen is the procedure indicated.

Fibroma (inflammatory fibrous hyperplasia)

Bouquot and Gundlach (1986) reported that the fibroma was the second most common oral exophytic lesion found in their study. The great majority of fibromas of the oral mucosa are not

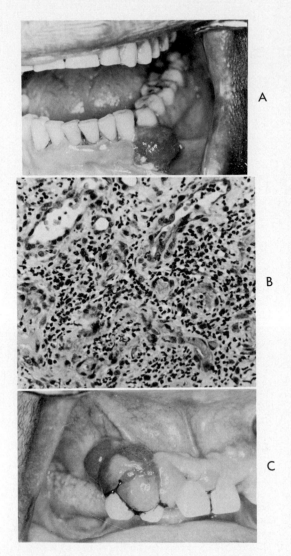

Fig. 10-7. Inflammatory hyperplasia. **A,** This lesion is composed of mostly granulation tissue and inflammatory components. **B,** Photomicrograph of granulation tissue showing the inflammatory components. **C,** This inflammatory hyperplastic lesion has some fibrosed regions that appear clinically as pale patches in the red lesion.   (**A** courtesy P.D. Toto, DDS, Maywood, Ill.)

generally believed to be true neoplasms but to represent endpoint inflammatory hyperplastic lesions, such as any of the 10 other types listed on p. 164. Thus they are really aggregates of scar tissue covered with a smooth layer of stratified squamous epithelium (Fig. 10-8).

The lesions are most often sessile or slightly pedunculated with a smooth contour, pale pink, and firm to palpation; they occur on the gingiva, tongue, buccal mucosa, and palate. An excisional biopsy is the indicated treatment.

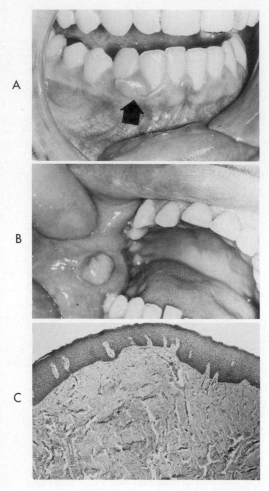

Fig. 10-8. Inflammatory fibrous hyperplasia (fibroma). **A,** This lesion represents a fibrosed pyogenic granuloma or hormonal tumor. **B,** Fibrosed lesion of inflammatory hyperplasia on the buccal mucosa. **C,** Photomicrograph of a fibroma. Note the dense avascular collagen.

DIFFERENTIAL DIAGNOSIS

The fibroma may be confused with such benign tumors as lipofibroma, myxofibroma, minor salivary gland tumors, neurofibroma, neurilemoma, rhabdomyoma, and leiomyoma.

The *lipofibroma* and *myxofibroma* may feel softer on palpation than the fibroma, but the *other benign tumors* noted here possess no distinguishing characteristics that would permit a differential diagnosis.

The giant cell fibroma is a small, firm, papular or polypoid lesion that occurs on the gingiva, tongue, buccal mucosa, and palate and is not more than 1 cm in diameter. These should be included in the differential diagnosis of fibroma (Weathers and Callihan, 1974).

The fibroma is ranked above any of these lesions, however, because of its relatively high incidence in the oral cavity.

Pyogenic granuloma

The pyogenic granuloma is a special type of inflammatory hyperplasia. Its surface becomes ulcerated, usually because of trauma during mastication, and this granulomatous lesion then becomes contaminated by the oral flora and liquids. As a result an acute inflammatory response occurs.

Clinically the necrotic ulcerated surface often appears to be composed of a white sloughy material. The fact that this necrotic material clinically resembles pus prompted early clinicians to refer to the lesion as a pyogenic granuloma; however, there is no pus in the lesion.

On microscopic examination clusters of polymorphonuclear leukocytes are present in some areas of the granuloma, especially areas adjacent to the necrotic or ulcerated surface (Fig. 10-9).

A pyogenic granuloma may also be produced by such chronic irritants as calculus, overhanging margins of crowns or other restorations, implantation of foreign bodies, and chronic biting of soft tissue.

FEATURES

Clinically the pyogenic granuloma is an asymptomatic papule, nodule, or polypoid mass usually with a rough, ulcerated necrotic surface (Figs. 8-42 and 10-9). In the granulomatous stage it appears red, feels moderately soft, and bleeds readily. If the lesion is of the mixed variety (granuloma with fibrous areas), it appears red with pink areas. If it is completely fibrosed, it is light pink and firm to palpation (a fibroma).

Angelopoulos (1971), reviewing a large series of pyogenic granulomas, reported that 65% to 70% occurred on the gingivae. Sites involved, in decreasing order of frequency, were the lips, tongue, buccal mucosa, palate, vestibule, and alveolar mucosa in edentulous regions. Angelopoulos also found that the maxillary labial gingiva was the most commonly involved region. The lesions occurred in patients of all ages, but 60% were in patients between 11 and 40 years of age. Females were affected more often than males. The average size of the lesions was 0.9 × 1.2 cm.

Eversole and Rovin (1972), reporting on a series of 166 pyogenic granuloma—gingival fibromatoid lesions, found that 56% involved the anterior segment of the dental arch. These au-

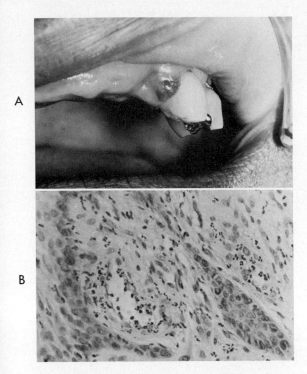

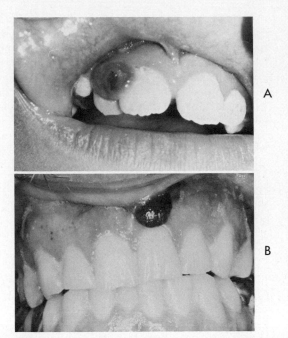

Fig. 10-9. Pyogenic granuloma. **A,** Clinical view. **B,** Photomicrograph. The polymorphonuclear leukocytes are distributed throughout the granulation tissue.

Fig. 10-10. **A,** Hormonal tumor. This inflammatory hyperplastic lesion was present in a girl at puberty. Poor hygiene was evident. **B,** Kaposi's sarcoma in the labial gingiva of a patient with AIDS. This reddish polypoid to nodular lesion mimics the clinical appearance of inflammatory hyperplastic lesions. (**B** courtesy S. Silverman, DDS, San Francisco, Calif.)

thors found a female-to-male incidence ratio of 4:1, with an average patient age of 35.1 years. Vilmann et al. (1986) reported that 35% of pyogenic granulomas in their study occurred on the marginal gingiva. Macleod and Soames (1987) divided lesions in their study into fibrous (64.5%), vascular (28.5%), and giant cell (7%) types and found that a greater percentage of the vascular types occurred in females.

DIFFERENTIAL DIAGNOSIS

We consider any of the other lesions of the inflammatory hyperplastic type with ulcerated surfaces to be examples of pyogenic granuloma. This consideration includes traumatized fibromas, hormonal tumors, epulis fissuratum and epulis granulomatosum, parulis, pulpitis aperta, myxofibroma, peripheral giant cell granuloma, and peripheral fibroma with calcification. Thus it is not necessary to discuss the distinguishing features of these lesions.

The pyogenic granuloma may be confused with an exophytic capillary hemangioma, small benign and malignant mesenchymal tumors that have become ulcerated because of trauma, and metastatic tumors. Correll et al. (1983) discuss the latter possibility in their differential

diagnosis of a large vascular pyogenic granuloma of the lateral palate and gingiva.

Small benign and malignant mesenchymal tumors with ulcerated surfaces may appear clinically identical to the pyogenic granuloma, although the much higher incidence of the granuloma should prompt the clinician to rank this lesion first in his or her differential diagnosis. However, if absolutely no evidence can be established to show the existence of a chronic irritant either present or past, the diagnostician is prompted to deemphasize the inflammatory hyperplasia lesions. Additional discussion of differential aspects is found in Chapter 5, p. 67. If the patient is suspected of having acquired immunodeficiency syndrome (AIDS), Kaposi's sarcoma should be considered (Fig. 10-10, *B*). AIDS is discussed in Appendix D.

An *exophytic capillary hemangioma* likewise may be indistinguishable from the pyogenic granuloma on both clinical and microscopic examination, especially when the surface of the former lesion is ulcerated. Actually the acquired (noncongenital, traumatic) capillary hemangioma may represent a type of inflammatory hyperplasia.

If its surface is ulcerated, a *peripheral giant cell granuloma* may also appear clinically identical to a gingival pyogenic granuloma. If the lesion is more bluish, however, there is a greater probability that it is a peripheral giant cell granuloma than if it is red to pink, in which case the diagnosis of pyogenic granuloma takes precedence.

The *peripheral fibroma with calcification,* which characteristically displaces the interdental papilla, also mimics the fibrosed pyogenic granuloma occurring on the gingiva (see Fig. 10-18). If a slightly underexposed radiograph shows small radiopaque foci within the shadow of the growth, the lesion is most likely a peripheral fibroma with calcification.

MANAGEMENT

Elimination of the causative trauma and the removal and microscopic study of the lesion itself are all that is required in most cases. If the lesion is small and reddish, elimination of the chronic irritating factor usually results in its regression to a point at which excision is not required.

Hormonal tumor

Some pathologists include hormonal tumors with the pyogenic granuloma. On the basis of the circumstances influencing the development of hormonal tumors, however, we are inclined to treat them as a somewhat different entity. They are inflammatory hyperplastic lesions of the gingivae (usually involving the interdental papillae) observed in patients who are experiencing the hormonal imbalances that occur during puberty, pregnancy, and menopause. The hormonal changes are thought to be responsible for an exaggerated response of the gingivae to local irritation. The causative irritants are usually calculus or overhanging margins of dental restorations (Fig. 10-10). The development of a differential diagnosis is the same as that described for the pyogenic granuloma.

Epulis fissuratum

Epulis fissuratum is an inflammatory hyperplastic type of lesion observed at the borders of ill-fitting dentures. In most instances the dental flanges are overextended, usually as a result of alveolar bone resorption.

FEATURES

The exophytic, often elongated epulis usually has at least one cleft into which the denture

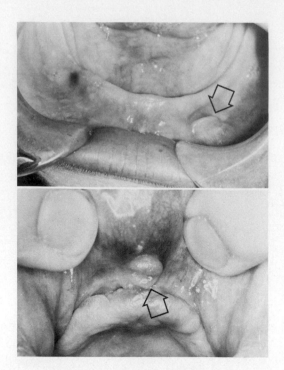

Fig. 10-11. Epulis fissuratum.

flange fits, with a proliferation of tissue on each side (Fig. 10-11).

Cutright (1974), reviewing a large series of these lesions, reported that most were asymptomatic, that there was a greater incidence in the maxilla than in the mandible, and that the anterior regions of both jaws were more often affected than the posterior regions. He also found that the lesions occurred most often under the buccal and labial flanges and were seen predominantly in female patients. Epulides fissurata were found in patients from childhood to old age but were seen more often in patients in their 40s and 50s. Budtz-Jørgensen (1981) preferred the term "denture irritation hyperplasia."

DIFFERENTIAL DIAGNOSIS

The frequency of occurrence of the epulis fissuratum so far exceeds that of any other exophytic lesion at the periphery of dentures that a discussion of differential diagnosis is not particularly helpful.

The slight possibility that a concurrent *malignant tumor* could be arising in the epulis fissuratum must be appreciated, however, and the microscopic examination of excised tissue is always imperative. In addition, on rare occasions squamous cell carcinomas, verrucous carcinomas, and malignant salivary gland tumors

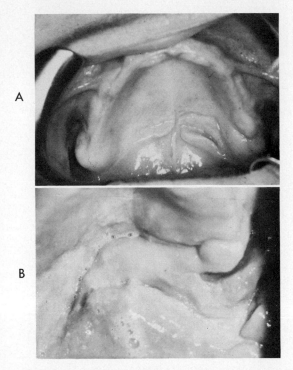

Fig. 10-12. Palatal growths posterior to denture flanges. **A,** Epulis fissuratum. **B,** Malignant salivary gland tumor.

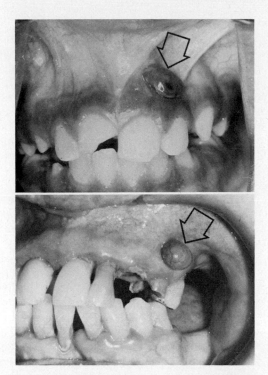

Fig. 10-13. Parulis. These inflammatory hyperplastic-type lesions occur at the mucosal draining site of a chronic alveolar abscess.

have arisen around denture flanges (Fig. 10-12) where there was no preexisting epulis fissuratum; hence, this slight possibility must always be borne in mind.

MANAGEMENT

If the lesion is small and composed mostly of inflamed tissue and if the denture flange is reduced, the hyperplastic growth may subside in 2 or 3 weeks without further treatment. When there are larger, more fibrosed lesions, excision combined with perhaps a sulcus-deepening procedure is necessary. In either case a new well-adapted denture should be fabricated, or at least the current appliance should be adjusted and rebased.

Parulis

A parulis is a small, inflammatory hyperplastic type of lesion that develops on the alveolar mucosa at the oral terminal of a draining sinus (Fig. 10-13). This lesion usually accompanies a draining chronic alveolar abscess in children. We have noted that the maxillary labial and buccal alveolar mucosa is the most frequent site, but the mandibular alveolar mucosa and palate may also be involved (Fig. 10-13).

Slight digital pressure on the periphery of a parulis may force a drop of pus from the sinus opening, and this is almost pathognomonic.

The lesion usually regresses spontaneously after the chronic odontogenic infection has been eliminated. If it is of considerable size and there is a substantial amount of fibrosis, however, the lesion regresses somewhat and then persists as a fibroma.

Rarely, a draining osteomyelitis or infected malignant tumor may produce a similar appearance.

Inflammatory papillary hyperplasia (palatal papillomatosis)

Inflammatory papillary hyperplasia occurs almost exclusively on the palate beneath either a complete or a partial removable denture. We have noted that it is more commonly associated with a flipper-type partial denture or a full denture. Approximately 10% of the people who wear dentures have this condition, and most of them wear their dentures continuously. Although its cause is not well understood, palatal papillomatosis appears to be related to the frictional irritation produced by loose-fitting dentures on the palatal tissue.

FEATURES

A small region in the vault or perhaps the whole palatal mucosa under the denture may be covered with numerous small painless polypoid masses that are seldom over 0.3 cm in diameter (Fig. 10-14). As with all the other inflammatory hyperplastic lesions, these masses are red and soft and bleed easily in the inflammatory or granulomatous stage. If they become fibrosed, however, they are firm and pale pink.

DIFFERENTIAL DIAGNOSIS

Since inflammatory papillary hyperplasia occurs almost exclusively on the palate under a full or partial removable denture, it can seldom be confused with other lesions.

Nicotine stomatitis may also feature small multiple nodules on the palate, which are reddish before a hyperkeratosis develops. The following observations aid in the differentiation of this condition from inflammatory papillary hyperplasia:

1. Nicotine stomatitis on the hard palate occurs almost exclusively in pipe smokers who are not wearing maxillary full dentures.
2. The lesions in nicotine stomatitis are more nodular and broader but less elevated.
3. The nodules in nicotine stomatitis have a characteristic red dot in their approximate center, which is not seen in papillary hyperplasia.

In unusual cases the clinician may consult the list of entities catalogued at the end of this chapter, in the column of rare multiple lesions.

MANAGEMENT

The patient must be persuaded to remove the denture at night to rest the tissues.

If the case is in the granulomatous stage, the placement of a soft tissue–conditioning liner in the denture may curb the inflammatory response and effect a reduction in the size and extent of the polypoid masses, possibly to such a degree that surgery is not necessary.

In fibrosed cases surgical removal is usually required, and the denture containing a surgical dressing may be used as a stent. Miller (1977) reviewed the suggested methods of removal: surgical curettage, electrosurgery, cryosurgery, and mucobrasion. A new denture that is well adapted to the oral tissues should then be fabricated.

Uohara and Federbusch (1968) described a procedure, loop-knife surgery, that requires a modified razor blade attached in a bow shape

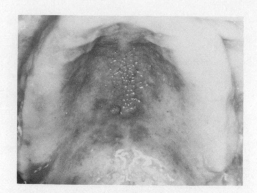

Fig. 10-14. Inflammatory papillary hyperplasia.

to a holder. The cutting edge is drawn from the back to the front of the site in continuous strokes, removing strips of hyperplastic tissue with clean incisions. Bergendal et al. (1980) reported excellent results using this same method. Rathofer et al. (1985) compared loop-knife surgery with electrosurgery and received equally good results from both techniques.

Although inflammatory papillary hyperplasia does not usually undergo malignant change, any excised tissue should be examined microscopically.

Peripheral giant cell granuloma

Some authors may object to including peripheral giant cell granuloma with the group of inflammatory hyperplastic lesions, but it seems appropriate to do so in the context of differential diagnosis because the two share several clinical characteristics. Although the cause of peripheral giant cell granuloma is unknown, trauma appears to play a role in many cases.

FEATURES

On microscopic examination, multinucleated giant cells are scattered throughout the granulation tissue. Extravasated erythrocytes and varying amounts of hemosiderin are observed. If a sufficient amount of hemosiderin exists near the periphery, the lesion is bluish. Otherwise it is red to pale pink, depending on the relative proportions of collagen and vascular component present.

The peripheral type occurs as an exophytic lesion on the gingivae and edentulous alveolar mucosa exclusively (Eversole and Rovin, 1972) (Fig. 10-15). The peripheral giant cell granuloma is most often nodular, but sometimes it is polypoid (base pedunculated rather than sessile). It may feel soft to hard, depending on the relative proportions of collagen and inflammatory component present.

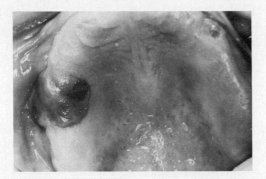

Fig. 10-15. Peripheral giant cell granuloma. The significant amount of hemosiderin in addition to the sluggish capillary flow through the extensive capillary network in this lesion produced a bluish color. (Courtesy S. Svalina, DDS, Maywood, Ill.)

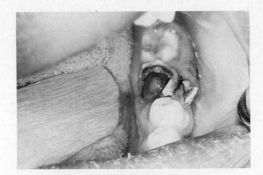

Fig. 10-16. Pulp polyp.

Bhaskar and Cutright (1971), reviewing a series of peripheral giant cell granulomas, reported that the lesions occurred most often in patients over 20 years of age, with an average age of approximately 45 years. These authors observed, furthermore, that the lesions were found predominantly in whites and on the mandible more often than on the maxilla.

In a series of 720 peripheral giant cell granulomas reviewed by Giansanti and Waldron (1969) a significantly greater number of women were affected, especially among 20- to 60-year-olds. The mean patient age was 31.3 years, 45% of the granulomas occurred on the maxillary gingiva or mucosa, and 55% were located on the mandibular gingiva or mucosa. This lesion accounted for 0.5% of all surgical accessions to their laboratory. Katsiteris et al. (1988) discussed 224 new cases and reviewed the findings on 956 lesions reported in the literature.

DIFFERENTIAL DIAGNOSIS

The differential diagnosis of pink or red lesions of the peripheral giant cell granuloma is identical to that of the *gingival pyogenic granuloma* (p. 167). The differential diagnosis for the bluish variety is discussed in Chapter 12 (p. 236).

MANAGEMENT

All tumors clinically identified as peripheral giant cell granulomas should be excised with a border of normal tissue, and the specimen should be examined microscopically. Since there is some inclination to suspect the role played by chronic trauma in the formation of this lesion, all chronic irritants should be eliminated. Because researchers have recently reported on peripheral giant cell lesions of hyperparathyroidism that manifest as exophytic giant cell granulomas (Burkes and White, 1989; Smith et al., 1988), hyperparathyroidism should be considered in the workup.

Pulp polyp (chronic hyperplastic pulpitis, pulpitis aperta)

A chronic hyperplastic proliferation of the pulp tissue occurs when caries have destroyed part or all of the tooth crown covering the pulp chamber (Fig. 10-16). The pulp polyp is an uncommon lesion observed mostly in the deciduous and permanent first molars of children and young adults. The lesion acquires a stratified squamous covering, apparently as the result of a fortuitous grafting of vital exfoliated epithelial cells from the adjacent oral mucosa. Its histologic characteristics are identical to those of the other types of inflammatory hyperplasias.

DIFFERENTIAL DIAGNOSIS

Occasionally a flap of *adjacent gingiva* extends into a large proximal carious lesion and appears to be a chronic hyperplastic pulpitis. Careful examination, however, discloses that the exophytic growth is continuous with the gingiva rather than the pulp. The occurrence of any other type of lesion growing from the pulp is too rare to be considered in this text.

MANAGEMENT

Two ways of treating a pulp polyp are conservation of the tooth through endodontic procedures followed by a full coverage and extraction of the tooth.

Epulis granulomatosum

Epulis granulomatosum is the specific inflammatory hyperplastic type of lesion that grows from a tooth socket after the tooth has been lost (Fig. 10-17). The precipitating cause

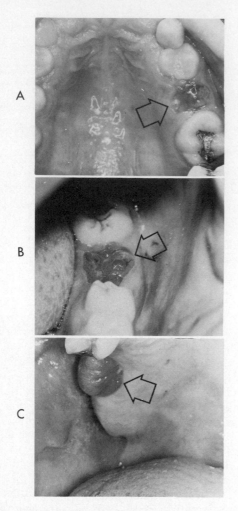

Fig. 10-17. Epulis granulomatosum. **A,** A retained deciduous root was the irritating factor in this case. **B,** Sharp bony spicules remaining in an extraction socket caused this lesion. **C,** This lesion proved to be an antral polyp that had extruded through a socket with an oroantral fistula.   (**B** courtesy P. Akers, DDS, Chicago. **C** courtesy P.D. Toto, DDS, Maywood, Ill.)

in almost every case is a sharp spicule of bone in the socket. The growth may become apparent in a week or two after the loss of the tooth, and the clinical characteristics are similar to those of the other inflammatory hyperplasias.

DIFFERENTIAL DIAGNOSIS

The two other lesions that might be confused with an epulis granulomatosum are an antral polyp protruding into the oral cavity through a maxillary molar or premolar socket and a malignant tumor growing from a recent extraction (Fig. 10-17). In most cases a radiograph helps the clinician identify either of these two entities.

In the case of a *malignant mesenchymal lesion* growing out of a recent extraction wound, a radiograph usually shows either bony destruction or a combined radiolucent-radiopaque lesion.

The oroantral fistula that permits the extrusion of an *antral polyp* often is evident as a well-defined loss of bone from the antral floor. If antral polyps are present, the patient should be referred to a surgical specialist for management and for confirmation that the "polyp" is not an antral malignancy.

MANAGEMENT

Careful inspection of the socket and removal of any bony spicules at the time the tooth is extracted prevent the formation of epulides granulomatosae. Treatment of an epulis granulomatosa requires the excision of the lesion and a careful curettement of the alveolus to ensure the elimination of irritating bony spicules. Because the growth might be malignant, the excised tissue should be examined microscopically.

Myxofibroma (fibroma with myxomatous change)

A myxofibroma is generally considered a variety of inflammatory fibrous hyperplasia in which some myxomatous tissue has developed or some area of the fibroma has undergone myxomatous degeneration. On microscopic examination regions of dense fibroblastic tissue are interspersed with pale myxomatous-appearing tissue.

FEATURES

A myxofibroma may occur anywhere in the oral cavity or on the lips. It most commonly occurs on the palate and gingiva, usually feels significantly softer than the fibroma, and often is less pale. Rapidis and Triantafyllou (1983) reviewed the literature on the oral myxoma and myxofibroma of the soft tissues. They reported that the clinical appearance of the lesion is not pathognomonic and can only be identified by histologic examination.

DIFFERENTIAL DIAGNOSIS

A myxofibroma may be confused with a lipofibroma, a plexiform neurofibroma, or some of the inflammatory hyperplastic lesions.

Both the *lipofibroma* and the *plexiform neurofibroma* are soft, spongy, and fluctuant. The myxofibroma is usually not so soft and occurs more commonly in the oral cavity than does the lipofibroma or the plexiform neurofibroma, so it is assigned a more prominent rank in the list of possible diagnoses.

An exception might occur when a patient with a moderately soft nodular or polypoid exophytic oral lesion has von Recklinghausen's disease. In this case the plexiform neurofibroma (the only soft, fluctuant, peripheral neural tumor) would be assigned the first rank in the differential diagnosis. Tomich (1974) discussed some of the rare lesions that should be differentiated from the myxofibroma.

MANAGEMENT

Complete excision followed by microscopic study of the tissue is the indicated treatment.

Peripheral fibroma with calcification, peripheral odontogenic fibroma, peripheral ossifying fibroma

The peripheral fibroma with calcification is a benign overgrowth of gingival tissue that most oral pathologists consider to be a type of inflammatory hyperplastic lesion. It is believed to involve the periodontal ligament superficially, and it often contains odontogenic epithelial nests and deposits of cementum, bone, and dystrophic calcification scattered throughout a background of fibrous tissue. If the calcified element is significant, radiopaque foci within the soft tissue tumor mass are observed on radiographs (Fig. 10-18). Gardner (1982) clearly described the lesion's typical histopathologic pattern that differentiates its characteristic features from those of the central odontogenic fibroma, which on rare occasions may occur peripherally. Buchner et al. (1987) stressed the need to distinguish between the more frequently occurring lesion (peripheral fibroma with calcification) and the more rare peripheral odontogenic fibroma (WHO-type).

King et al. (1979) reported that gingival tissue possesses unusually thin, stringy rete ridges (usually formed by two rows of basal cells) that extend a considerable distance into the underlying connective tissue. They reported seeing the same phenomenon in peripheral fibromas with calcification. These interesting findings raise the probability that the nests and strands of epithelial cells in the lesion represent isolated sections of this unique rete ridge system rather than odontogenic epithelium. This lesion is also included with the mixed radiolucent-radiopaque lesions in Chapter 25, in the section on the differential diagnosis of osteosarcoma.

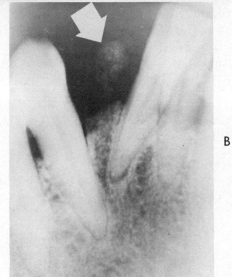

Fig. 10-18. Peripheral fibroma with calcification. **A,** The lesion (*arrow*) is causing the lateral incisor and canine to separate. **B,** Radiograph. The arrow indicates calcification within the mass.

FEATURES

The peripheral fibroma with calcification occurs exclusively on the free margin of the gingiva and usually involves the interdental papilla (Fig. 10-18). The lesion frequently causes a separation of the adjacent teeth, and occasionally minimal bone resorption can be seen beneath the lesion. Cundiff (1972) reviewed a series of 365 cases and found that 50% of the lesions occurred in patients between the ages of 5 and 25 years, with a peak incidence at 13 years. In addition, he reported that the female was more often affected than the male and that 80% of the lesions occurred anterior to the molar areas.

The lesion is usually asymptomatic and, although frequently discovered by the patient, comes to professional attention during a routine examination. In our experience it is often associated with irritation (overextended margins of faulty restorations, deposits of calculus, and the like), which indicates that it most likely represents a lesion of the inflammatory hyperplastic type such as a pyogenic granuloma or a hormonal tumor involving a segment of the periodontal ligament. Certainly it appears to pass through the same clinical stages as the inflammatory hyperplasias: the early lesions are soft, quite vascular, and red and bleed readily; the more mature lesions are firm, fibrous, and pale pink.

DIFFERENTIAL DIAGNOSIS

Other inflammatory hyperplastic lesions of the gingiva, osteogenic sarcoma, and chondrosarcoma should be included in the differential diagnosis for the peripheral fibroma with calcification.

The *chondrosarcoma* and *osteogenic sarcoma*, considered together, are less frequent gingival lesions than the peripheral fibroma with calcification. Although a slight bony resorption may occur beneath the peripheral fibroma with calcification, severe bony changes typically are seen when the lesion is malignant. A bandlike asymmetric widening of the periodontal ligaments of involved teeth is another expected finding with chondrosarcoma and osteogenic sarcoma but is not a feature of the peripheral fibroma with calcification (Fig. 21-11).

The common varieties of *gingival inflammatory hyperplastic lesions* (hormonal tumor, pyogenic granuloma) occur more often than the peripheral fibroma with calcification, but many identical clinical features occur with both. In contrast, the peripheral fibroma with calcification may cause a separation of the adjacent teeth, which does not frequently occur with the other inflammatory hyperplasias. Also, if calcified foci are present within the soft tissue overgrowth, the clinician should exclude the other inflammatory hyperplasias, since these foci suggest instead the peripheral odontogenic fibroma, the osteogenic sarcoma, and the chondrosarcoma.

MANAGEMENT

The peripheral fibroma with calcification should be excised and special care taken to remove the lesion's attachment in the periodontal ligament. As a rule, the adjacent teeth do not have to be extracted. These lesions occasionally recur (Mulcahy and Dahl [1985] indicated a 13% recurrence rate), but their management is not a problem. All excised tissue should be examined microscopically.

MUCOCELE AND RANULA

The mucocele and ranula are retention phenomena of the minor salivary glands and the sublingual (major) salivary glands, respectively. Although they are discussed in detail in Chapter 12 as bluish lesions, it is noteworthy that in a review of 63 oral mucoceles, Cohen (1965) observed 82% (52) on the lower lip and 8%, 2%, and 1% on the cheek, in the retromolar area, and on the palate, respectively.

Differential diagnosis

When the mucosal covering is thicker than usual, the lesion appears pink, is soft to rubbery in consistency, and is fluctuant but not emptiable.

In such instances it must be differentiated from a *superficial cyst, lipoma, plexiform neurofibroma, relatively deep cavernous hemangioma, lymphangioma,* and *mucus-producing salivary gland tumor.*

If aspiration of the lesion produces a sticky, viscous, clear, mucuslike fluid, all the foregoing lesions can be eliminated except the mucus-producing salivary gland tumors, and these are uncommon lesions.

Although retention phenomena should be initially considered as a possible mucus-producing malignant salivary gland tumor (mucoepidermoid tumor, mucous adenocarcinoma, for examples), these occur most often on the posterior hard palate, retromolar area, and posterolateral aspect of the floor of the mouth. An induration at the base of a retention phenomenon may be just fibrous tissue, but it should alert the clinician to the possibility of a malignant tumor.

Management

If the conservative approach of marsupialization is followed, the base of the lesion must be examined carefully for pathosis and a cautious periodic follow-up must be maintained. If the lesion is treated by complete excision, the specimen must be examined microscopically.

HEMANGIOMA, LYMPHANGIOMA, AND VARICOSITY

Hemangiomas, lymphangiomas, and varicosities are discussed as bluish lesions in Chapter 12.

If a hemangioma, lymphangioma, or varicosity is covered with a thicker than usual layer of oral mucosa, however, its bluish color is masked, and it is seen as a pink, smooth nodular or dome-shaped lesion.

The differential diagnosis of such lesions is similar to that of the mucocele and ranula, in that significant information can be obtained by sampling the material within the lesion by aspiration.

CENTRAL EXOPHYTIC LESIONS

Central lesions of the jawbones frequently produce exophytic masses as the result of expansion, erosion, or invasion. Thus, for the differential diagnosis of oral lesions, the possibility that an exophytic mass could be central in origin must always be considered. Usually a complete examination, including a history and clinical and radiographic surveys, indicates whether the lesion is central in origin. Since lesions of bone are discussed in detail in Part III

of this text, only the more common pathoses that may produce these exophytic growths are listed here (Fig. 10-19):

Benign tumors
Cysts
Infections
Malignant tumors
Odontogenic tumors

Soft tissue abscesses such as the foregoing, resulting from odontogenic infection, are central in origin, but because their peripheral manifestations are usually exophytic dome-shaped masses (Fig. 10-19), they must often be considered in the differential diagnosis of peripheral lesions. Actually such abscesses are readily recognized by their location, by the fact that they are rubbery, fluctuant, painful, and hot, and by the fact that they yield pus on aspiration.

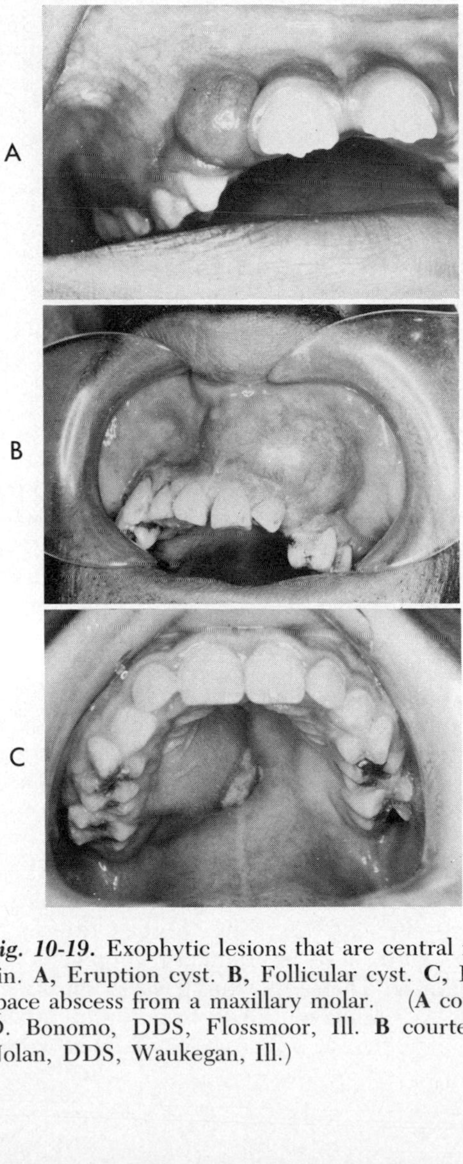

PAPILLOMA AND VERRUCA VULGARIS

The papilloma and verruca vulgaris are benign exophytic growths of the surface epithelium, as their rough surfaces indicate. Because their surfaces often retain a significant amount of keratin, these lesions are discussed with the white lesions in Chapter 8. Nevertheless, occa-

Fig. 10-19. Exophytic lesions that are central in origin. **A,** Eruption cyst. **B,** Follicular cyst. **C,** Palatal space abscess from a maxillary molar. (**A** courtesy D. Bonomo, DDS, Flossmoor, Ill. **B** courtesy R. Nolan, DDS, Waukegan, Ill.)

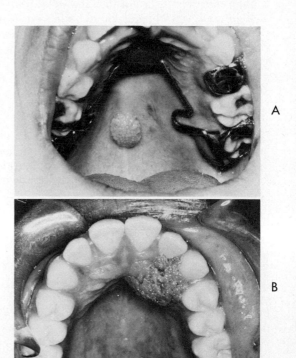

Fig. 10-20. Pink papilloma. **A,** Midline of the palate. **B,** Maxillary lingual alveolus. Both lesions were pedunculated.

sionally keratinization is not a feature and the lesions appear pink. Papillomas and verrucae vulgares seldom measure more than 1 cm in diameter (Fig. 10-20). Recent DNA hybridization studies reveal that human papillomavirus DNA is present in these lesions (Adler-Storthz et al., 1986; Eversole and Laipis, 1988; Syrjanen et al., 1986).

Differential diagnosis

Solitary examples of a lightly keratinized papilloma and verruca must be differentiated from a pyogenic granuloma, papillary squamous cell carcinoma, condyloma acuminatum, condyloma latum, and lesions such as peripheral ameloblastomas that may show extensive pseudoepitheliomatous hyperplasia. With the exception of the pyogenic granuloma the differentiating features of the other lesions are covered in Chapter 8 (p. 133).

The rounded smooth contours of the *pyogenic granuloma* (except for a possible area of ulceration), permit the differentiation between the pyogenic granuloma and the papilloma and verruca, as does the tendency for the pyogenic granuloma (in contrast to the papilloma and verruca) to readily bleed.

If several lesions are present, the examiner should consult the list of rare multiple lesions at the end of this chapter for additional entities that may be included in the list of possibilities. A detailed discussion of all these lesions is beyond the scope of the text.

EXOPHYTIC SQUAMOUS CELL CARCINOMA

Squamous cell carcinoma is discussed in Chapter 8 as a white lesion, in Chapter 11 as an ulcerative lesion, in Chapter 5 as a red lesion, and in Chapter 9 as a red and white lesion. In this chapter the exophytic variety of squamous cell carcinoma is described.

Verrucous carcinoma is not included in the discussion because although an exophytic lesion, it has markedly different characteristics.

Features

In our experience exophytic carcinoma occurs most often on the lateral borders of the tongue, the floor of the mouth, and the soft palate. Approximately 55% of all the squamous cell carcinomas of the tongue in a series reported by Whitaker et al. (1972) were exophytic-type lesions.

The lesions are firm to palpation, and their bases may be indurated because of infiltration of the underlying tissue. They may be nodular

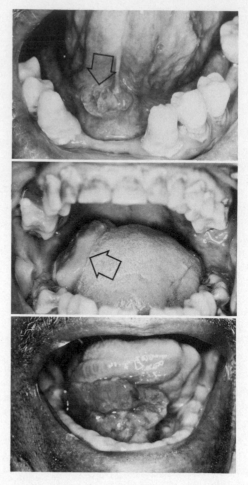

Fig. 10-21. Exophytic types of squamous cell carcinoma.

or polypoid, are usually somewhat pink to red, and invariably have at least one ulcerated patch on their surfaces (Figs. 10-21 and 10-22). In some cases the surfaces may be entirely necrotic and have a ragged whitish gray appearance. Pain and a tendency to bleed are not early characteristics.

It is generally believed that the majority of exophytic carcinomas are less aggressive than the ulcerative varieties, but all lesions must be evaluated on an individual basis. Cervical lymph node involvement is the usual route of metastatis.

Occasionally an exophytic squamous cell carcinoma has a polypoid shape and a papillated surface (Fig. 10-23). Such lesions are sometimes referred to as papillary squamous cell carcinomas. They represent a variation of exophytic carcinoma and need to be differentiated from papillomas, verrucae, condyloma acumi-

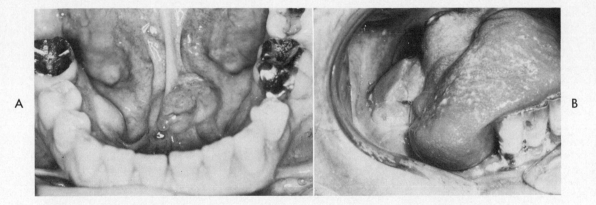

Fig. 10-22. Exophytic squamous cell carcinoma. **A,** Ulcerated exophytic lesion in a 54-year-old woman. **B,** Large exophytic lesion of the floor of the mouth, ridge, and lateral border of the tongue. (**B** courtesy M. Lehnert, DDS, Minneapolis.)

natum, condyloma latum, pseudoepitheliomatous hyperplasia, and verrucous carcinoma.

Differential diagnosis

The lesions that must be distinguished from the exophytic carcinoma are the pyogenic granuloma, verrucous carcinoma, malignant salivary gland tumors, peripheral malignant mesenchymal tumors, peripheral metastatic tumors, and amelanotic melanoma.

Amelanotic melanoma is a rare oral tumor which, when it becomes ulcerated, is clinically indistinguishable from an exophytic carcinoma. Because of its low frequency of occurrence, however, it has a low rank in the differential diagnosis.

Peripheral metastatic tumors in their early stages may be innocent-appearing, firm, and nodular, dome shaped, or polypoid with smoothly contoured surfaces and may be covered with normal-appearing mucosa. Later, when their surfaces become ulcerated, they may be indistinguishable from squamous cell carcinomas. Again, because this pathosis has such a low incidence, it is be assigned a low rank in the list of possible entities unless evidence from the history or examination suggests the presence of a parent tumor.

Peripheral malignant mesenchymal tumors (for example, fibrosarcoma, myosarcoma, neurosarcoma, liposarcoma) are also rare oral lesions. In their early stages, like most metastatic lesions, they are often firm, smooth surfaced, and nodular, dome shaped, or polypoid. The fact that their surfaces are smooth and covered with normal-appearing mucosa permits the differentiation between these early lesions and the rough-surfaced ulcerated squamous cell

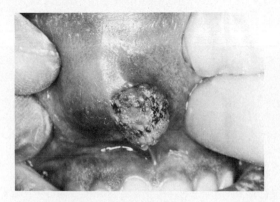

Fig. 10-23. Papillary squamous cell carcinoma. Early invasion of the underlying tissue was observed microscopically. The obvious swelling under the lesion was produced by a recent injection of local anesthetic solution, not by gross invasion.

carcinomas. Later, though, when these malignant mesenchymal tumors become ulcerated, they may appear similar to an exophytic squamous cell carcinoma. Evidence of metastatic involvement of cervical lymph nodes is unusual in most mesenchymal tumors and strongly supports a diagnosis of squamous cell carcinoma. A clinician must conclude, on the basis of the lesion's low incidence, that an ulcerated exophytic lesion is more likely a squamous cell carcinoma than a peripheral malignant mesenchymal tumor.

Malignant salivary gland tumors are second to squamous cell carcinoma as the most common oral malignancy. The firm types are under consideration here. The fluctuant mucus-producing varieties (for example, low-grade mucoepidermoid tumors, mucous adenocarcinomas) have necessarily been grouped in the differential diagnosis with the retention phenomena. Like the early secondary tumors and early peripheral malignant mesenchymal tumors, the malignant salivary gland tumors originate in tissue situated deep to and separate from the surface epithelium. Thus in their early stages they are nodular or dome shaped, have a smooth contour, and are covered with normal-appearing epithelium. Later, when their surfaces become ulcerated because of the trauma of mastication or biopsy, or perhaps as a result of the rupturing of retained fluid, they may appear to be malignant (that is, have ulcerated, necrotic, friable surfaces). At this stage the malignant salivary gland tumors may not be readily differentiated from exophytic squamous cell carcinomas. The following clues, however, are helpful:

1. Squamous cell carcinoma is not so common on the posterior hard palate as malignant salivary gland tumors.
2. Salivary gland tumors occur more frequently in women, whereas squamous cell carcinoma occurs two to four times as frequently in men. The significance of this difference between the two tumors must be modified, however, because approximately 95% of the oral malignancies are squamous cell carcinomas, whereas only about 4% are malignant minor salivary gland tumors.
3. Malignant minor salivary gland tumors frequently maintain their dome shape even after their surfaces become ulcerated.

The *verrucous carcinoma* is a more slowly growing lesion than the exophytic squamous cell carcinoma and is most often associated with the prolonged use of chewing tobacco or snuff. The sites frequently affected are the vestibule and buccal mucosa. The surface of the lesion is usually papillomatous and frequently white because of the retention of keratin. Exophytic squamous cell carcinoma, on the other hand, is most often observed on the lateral border of the tongue or floor of the mouth and frequently has a partly ulcerated surface that is not papillomatous or keratotic. The verrucous carcinoma seldom metastasizes; in contrast, the exophytic squamous cell carcinoma commonly spreads to the cervical lymph nodes.

The large *pyogenic granuloma* with an ulcerated surface may appear suspect. It is usually moderately soft to palpation and bleeds easily, however, whereas the exophytic carcinoma is firm and usually does not bleed when manipulated.

Many rare exophytic lesions such as the following may be confused with exophytic squamous cell carcinoma, but an in-depth discussion of these possibilities is beyond the scope of this text:

Condyloma acuminatum
Granulomatous fungal diseases
Gumma
Keratoacanthoma
Lethal midline granuloma
Sarcoidosis
Tuberculosis

Management

The management of intraoral squamous cell carcinomas is discussed in detail in Chapter 11.

VERRUCOUS CARCINOMA

Verrucous carcinoma is a specific kind of low-grade squamous cell carcinoma that occurs as a verrucous type of exophytic lesion (Fig. 10-24). It seldom metastasizes, is usually cured by adequate local excision, and carries a better prognosis than does regular squamous cell carcinoma. The lesion frequently has a white keratotic surface and is discussed in detail with the white lesions in Chapter 8.

On occasion, the surface of the verrucous carcinoma is not heavily keratinized and appears pink. The differential diagnosis in such cases is discussed in the differential diagnosis section of exophytic squamous cell carcinoma (p. 177).

MINOR SALIVARY GLAND TUMORS

Most of the minor salivary gland tumors are exophytic lesions, which explains their inclusion in this chapter. The intraoral minor salivary glands are predominantly of the mucous type and are normally distributed throughout the oral mucosa except for the anterior hard palate, attached gingivae, and anterior two thirds of the dorsal surface of the tongue. Unusual cases of salivary gland tumors occurring in these locations have been reported and are considered to have arisen in ectopic minor salivary glands.

The mucous glands are not attached to the surface mucosa except by the common ducts that drain a cluster of glands. These clusters of mucous glands are situated deep to the surface mucosa and usually lie just superficial to the loose connective tissue layer if such a layer is present. Thus as a tumor originates in these glands and enlarges, it becomes a nodular or dome-shaped exophytic mass with a smooth surface (Chapter 3).

Because of the great variety of neoplasms that occur in the salivary glands, the establishment and adoption of a uniform classification and nomenclature for these tumors have not yet been achieved. (With only one or two exceptions, all the tumors occurring in the major salivary glands are also found in the minor salivary glands.)

To establish some common order that contributes to a universal comprehension of descriptions and discussions of this homogeneous group of lesions, the World Health Organization (WHO) has introduced the following classification (Thackray and Sabin, 1972):

I. Epithelial tumors
   A. Adenomas
      1. Pleomorphic adenoma (mixed tumor)
      2. Monomorphic adenomas
         a. Adenolymphoma [Warthin's tumor, papillary cystadenoma lymphomatosum]*
         b. Oxyphilic adenoma [oncocytoma]*
         c. Other types
   B. Mucoepidermoid tumor
   C. Acinic cell tumor
   D. Carcinomas
      1. Adenoid cystic carcinoma [cylindroma]*
      2. Adenocarcinoma
      3. Epidermoid carcinoma
      4. Undifferentiated carcinoma
      5. Carcinoma in pleomorphic adenoma (malignant mixed tumor)
II. Nonepithelial tumors
III. Unclassified tumors

Most North American oral pathologists recommend some modification of the WHO classification, as illustrated by the minutes of an ESTOP† meeting at London, Ontario, on October 17, 1976. This group suggested the following modifications:

1. The term "adenolymphoma" for papillary cystadenoma lymphomatosum was unsatisfactory.
2. Papillary cystadenoma lymphomatosum should not be included under monomorphic adenoma, and possibly the same holds for oxyphilic adenoma.
3. Many oral pathologists thought that the term mucoepidermoid "tumor" was unacceptable because they believed that all of these lesions are carcinomas.
4. Most oral pathologists favored the term acinic cell "carcinoma" over acinic cell "tumor," for reasons similar to that given in (3).

As with other groups of lesions, the diagnostician would be aided considerably if there were certain clinical features of salivary gland

---

*Contents of brackets are ours.
†Eastern Society of Teachers of Oral Pathology.

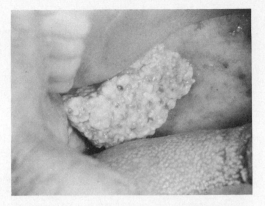

Fig. 10-24. Verrucous carcinoma. Note the pebbly white surface of this slow-growing lesion, which has a relatively sessile base.   (From Claydon RJ and Jordan JE: J Oral Surg 36:564-567, 1978. Copyright by the American Dental Association. Reprinted by permission.)

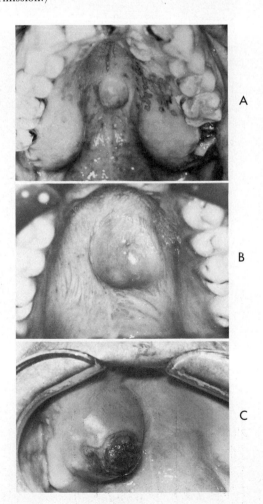

A

B

C

Fig. 10-25. Minor salivary gland tumors. **A** and **B,** Pleomorphic adenomas. **C,** Adenoid cystic carcinoma that became ulcerated after an incisional biopsy.   (**B** and **C** courtesy E. Kasper, DDS, Maywood, Ill.)

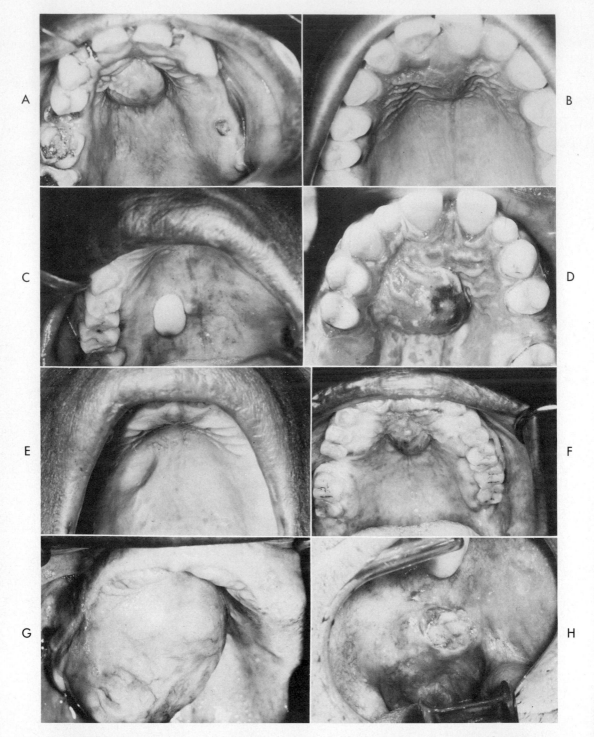

Fig. 10-26. Palatal masses. **A,** Palatal space abscess from infected lateral incisor tooth. **B,** Nasopalatine cyst. **C,** Fibroma. **D,** Palatal space abscess from periapical abscess of first premolar tooth. **E,** Pleomorphic adenoma. **F,** Small midline fissural cyst of palate. **G,** Large benign salivary tumor. **H,** Large squamous cell carcinoma of the soft palate.   (**B** and **E** courtesy W. Heaton, DDS, Chicago. **H** courtesy M. Lehnert, DDS, Minneapolis.)

tumors that would enable him or her to determine whether the tumors were malignant or benign. In our opinion, however, no distinctive clinical features of either malignant or benign minor salivary gland tumors have been found to signal their identity. The clinical appearances of both are so similar that in most cases a tumor cannot be ranked in the working diagnosis according to its malignancy or lack of malignancy.

One exception to this circumstance is the highly malignant tumor recognizable by its rapid growth.

Early minor salivary gland tumors, whether benign or not, are usually nodular or dome-shaped elevations with smooth contours, and the overlying mucosa either is normal or appears smoother and glossier because of the tension created by the underlying expanding tumor (Figs. 10-25 and 10-26). As the overlying mucosa becomes thinned by the expanding tumor and traumatized during mastication, or as the pooled mucus ruptures or a biopsy of the growth is made, an ulcer appears that is persistent and usually becomes necrotic. We have seen several benign tumors that have taken on the appearance of angry malignant-looking lesions as the result of an incisional biopsy or other traumatic episode. Consequently, although the more rapidly growing malignant varieties of minor salivary gland tumor may tend to ulcerate earlier, the number of benign tumors that ulcerate is high enough that this feature cannot be considered clinically useful in distinguishing between the types.

Likewise the firmness (induration) of a lesion is no better a prognostic sign than is surface ulceration for clinically distinguishing between the malignant and the benign salivary tumors, because the majority of both malignant and benign tumors are firm. The fact that some malignant salivary tumors and some benign ones are moderately soft and fluctuant, or have soft and firm areas, further emphasizes this point.

Although it is not possible to establish clinical guidelines that enable the examiner to determine whether a particular minor salivary gland tumor is malignant or benign, salivary tumors can be categorized into two clinical classes: those that are firm to palpation and those that are moderately soft and fluctuant.

The following tumors are almost categorically firm to palpation. They are ranked, as much as possible, in order of frequency of occurrence:

Pleomorphic adenoma (benign mixed tumor)
Adenoid cystic carcinoma
Mucoepidermoid tumor of high-grade malignancy

Carcinoma in pleomorphic adenoma (malignant mixed tumor)
Acinic cell carcinoma
Oncocytoma

The firmness in these tumors results from the presence of dense aggregates, nests, and cords of closely packed tumor cells, fibrous tissue, and hyaline areas, as well as cartilage-like and bonelike tissue (pleomorphic adenoma).

The following tumors, on the other hand, are moderately soft and frequently fluctuant. Again, an attempt has been made to arrange them in descending order of incidence:

Well-differentiated mucoepidermoid tumor
Papillary cyst adenoma
Mucus-producing adenocarcinoma
Warthin's tumor or papillary cystadenoma lymphomatosum

The softness of these tumors results from the fluid produced and the consequent retention phenomena; in other words, mucus is produced in well-differentiated mucoepidermoid tumors and in mucous adenocarcinomas, whereas cyst fluid is produced in the papillary cyst adenoma and in Warthin's tumor. The tumors in this group are fluctuant because of the enclosed fluid.

Features

Most of the intraoral minor salivary gland tumors occur on the posterior aspect of the hard palate (see Figs. 10-25 and 10-26). In a series studied by Soskolne et al. (1973), 66% of the tumors were found in this site, and in a review by Chaudhry et al. (1961), 57.7% of the tumors occurred on the palate. In a large series, Chaudhry et al. (1984) reported that approximately 56% of the minor salivary gland tumors occurred in the palate. In Pogrel's series (1979) 47% occurred on the palate. Isacsson and Shear reported in 1983 that 81% of benign tumors in their study occurred on the palate, whereas 60% of malignant tumors occurred on the palate. They reported that 74.6% of all minor salivary gland tumors occurred on the palate. The next most frequent sites, in approximate descending order of frequency, are the upper lip, buccal mucosa, retromolar region, tongue, and floor of the mouth. In the Canadian series reported by Main et al. (1976) the approximate percentage by location was as follows: palate, 53%; buccal mucosa, 17%; tongue, 8%; upper lip, 5%; gingiva, 4%; bone, 2.6%; unspecified, 7%. Concerning incidence of mixed tumors of the lips the Armed Forces Institute of Pathology series reported the ratio of occurrence in the upper lip to lower lip of 75:13 (Krolls and Hicks, 1973). The vast majority of malignant intraoral salivary gland tumors are mucoepidermoid carcinomas and adenoid cystic carcinomas (Chau and Radden, 1986). However, Waldron et al. (1988), reporting on a study of 426 intraoral minor salivary gland tumors, indicated that low-grade (terminal duct lobular, polymorphous) adenocarcinoma was the second most common malignancy, following mucoepidermoid carcinoma. Eveson and Cawson (1985), reporting on their study of 336 intraoral cases, indicated that adenoid cystic carcinoma was the most common minor salivary gland malignancy.

The incidence according to sex varies from series to series and from type to type, but most reports indicate a higher frequency in women. The peak patient age for the benign tumors is between 30 and 39 years, whereas for the malignant tumors it is between 40 and 49 years (Soskolne et al., 1973).

The ratio of benign to malignant lesions among minor salivary gland tumors slightly favors the benign variety, as illustrated by the series of Soskolne et al. (1973), in which 67% were benign, and by the series of Chaudhry et al. (1961), in which 60% were benign. Interestingly Main et al. (1976) reported that 62.2% of their series from Scottish patients were benign whereas only 34.7% of their series from Canadian patients were benign. The pleomorphic adenoma accounted for 60.9% of all tumors described by Soskolne's group and 55.7% of the tumors reviewed by Chaudhry's. Isacsson and Shear (1983) reported that 72.5% of their series were benign, whereas Chaudhry et al. (1984) reported that 52% of their series were benign.

These tumors may be present and tolerated for several months or even years because they are characteristically asymptomatic; consequently they usually come to professional attention only during routine examination. The adenoid cystic carcinoma, however, may be painful, especially if it has extended into a perineural space.

Benign salivary gland tumors may produce a well-defined saucerlike depression in the underlying bone. In contrast, malignant tumors may invade the bone and produce a ragged radiolucent defect with poorly defined borders (Fig. 21-9). Such tumors positioned on the lateral aspect of the posterior hard palate may destroy the alveolar bone and invade the maxillary sinus.

The malignant types may spread via lymphatic vessels to the cervical lymph nodes. The lungs are the most common site of distant metastasis. The adenoid cystic carcinoma frequently spreads along the perineural spaces, and other types also occasionally do this.

Comprehension of the histopathologic features of the minor salivary gland tumors is difficult because of the many varieties of tumors. The following have clear-cut histologic features, which makes their identification relatively easy:

Acinic cell carcinoma
Adenoid cystic carcinoma
Canalicular adenoma
Mucoepidermoid tumor
Papillary cyst adenoma
Pleomorphic adenoma
Oncocytoma
Warthin's tumor

Some of the unclassified adenocarcinomas are difficult to identify; in the case of the low-grade lesions, it is frequently difficult to determine whether the tumors are malignant or benign. Occasionally this also happens when a carcinoma occurs within a pleomorphic adenoma. Often many slides must be prepared from different areas of the specimen before a malignant change can be detected, and even then the changes may not be pronounced. A detailed discussion of the histopathology of the minor salivary gland tumors is beyond the scope of this text.

Differential diagnosis

Since the following tumors account for from 82% (Soskolne et al., 1973) to 94% (Chaudhry et al., 1961) of all minor salivary gland tumors the clinician is likely to encounter, they should initially be included in the differential diagnosis when the lesion seems likely to be a minor salivary tumor: pleomorphic adenoma, adenoid cystic carcinoma, unclassified or undifferentiated adenocarcinomas, mucoepidermoid tumor, and carcinoma in pleomorphic adenoma.

To facilitate the consideration of the differential diagnosis, the discussion has been divided into two sections: the first includes the firm tumors; the second includes the softer fluctuant ones. As previously noted, we do not believe that there are enough clinical differences between the lesions within each group to attempt a differentiation between the individual minor salivary tumors. Nevertheless, the following facts may be useful prognostic aids:

1. The pleomorphic adenomas make up about 60% of all minor salivary gland tumors.

2. The majority of intraoral adenoid cystic carcinomas and mucoepidermoid tumors occur on the posterolateral aspect of the hard palate.
3. An ulcerated minor salivary tumor, in the absence of a history of incisional biopsy or other traumatic incident, is more likely to be malignant.

FIRM MINOR SALIVARY GLAND TUMORS

Several lesions must be included in the differential diagnosis for a firm minor salivary tumor: mature lesions of inflammatory hyperplasia (fibromas), benign and malignant mesenchymal tumors, necrotizing sialometaplasia, focal hyperplasia of minor salivary glands, and the rare granulomatous lesions of tuberculosis, syphilis (gumma), and fungal infections.

The very low incidence of the last-mentioned *rare lesions of tuberculosis, syphilis,* and *fungal infections* would prompt a low ranking for these tumors.

Likewise, the relatively low incidence of oral *benign* and *malignant mesenchymal tumors* prompts the clinician to rank the minor salivary tumors above this group in the differential diagnosis, except in special cases (for example, von Recklinghausen's disease) (Fig. 10-27).

The *mature lesions of inflammatory hyperplasia (fibromas)* are much more common than the minor salivary tumors, but unlike the minor salivary tumors, they are seldom dome shaped. The fibromas are usually slightly polypoid or sessile. Also the agent causing the chronic irritation usually can be identified. In addition, the posterolateral aspect of the hard palate is not a common site for a solitary inflammatory hyperplastic lesion but is the most frequent site for a minor salivary tumor.

Metastatic cancers, lymphomas, and benign lymphoid hyperplasias of the palate, although not common, should be included in the differential diagnosis of firm swellings of the palate (Bradley et al., 1987).

SOFT MINOR SALIVARY GLAND TUMORS

Several lesions must be considered in the differential diagnosis for a soft fluctuant minor salivary gland tumor: mucoceles, superficial cavernous hemangiomas, submerged lipomas, and plexiform neurofibromas.

The *plexiform neurofibroma* is uncommon except in patients with von Recklinghausen's disease. It and the *submerged lipoma* cannot be differentiated from the minor salivary tumors in this group through palpation or visual examination. Aspiration, however, will be productive in the case of soft and fluctuant minor salivary gland tumors although not with plexiform neurofibromas or lipomas. The yellow color of the superficial lipoma will prompt the clinician to identify this lesion.

Superficial cavernous hemangiomas will be bluish, whereas deeper ones will be pink. Both are emptiable by carefully applied digital pressure, and this fact differentiates hemangiomas from mucoceles and soft salivary gland tumors.

Mucoceles are encountered much more often than are minor salivary gland tumors, but approximately 82% of them occur on the lower lip, which is not a common site for a minor salivary gland tumor (Cohen, 1965). In practical terms, mucoceles cannot be differentiated from some of the early malignant tumors containing

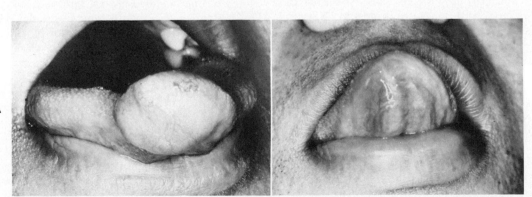

Fig. 10-27. Mesenchymal tumors. **A,** Leiomyoma of the tip of the tongue. **B,** Amputation neuroma on the ventral surface of the tongue. (From Kelly DE and Harriagan WF: J Oral Surg 35:316-318, 1977. Copyright by the American Dental Association. Reprinted by permission.)

mucus (e.g., mucoepidermoid tumor, mucus-producing adenocarcinoma). Thus it is important to do a biopsy of all mucoceles. The relative incidences of mucoceles and minor salivary gland tumors would prompt the diagnostician to conclude that a small superficial retention-phenomenon type of lesion is much more likely to be a mucocele than a salivary gland tumor.

ULCERATED MINOR SALIVARY GLAND TUMORS

The possible causes of a large ulcerated lesion or ulcerated exophytic lesion of the posterior hard palate include tumors of the minor glands, squamous cell carcinomas (usually commence on the soft palate), antral malignancies, major aphthous ulcers, gummas, necrotizing sialometaplasia, lethal midline granulomas, Wegener's granulomatosis, lymphomas, actinomycosis, blastomycosis, tuberculosis, rhinoscleroma, mucormycosis, and noma.

Other pathoses to be considered when soft masses on the hard palate are encountered are pyogenic granuloma, fibroma, palatal space abscess, cyst of the papilla palatina, mesenchymal tumors (benign and malignant), non-Hodgkin's lymphoma, benign lymphoproliferative disease, and hyperplasia of mucous salivary glands.

Non-Hodgkin's lymphoma may mimic a salivary gland tumor very closely as to firmness and frequent location on the posterolateral hard palate. Eisenbud et al. (1983) reported on 10 cases and Blok et al. (1979) described eight cases on the palate.

Wright and Dunsworth (1983) presented a case of a benign lymphoproliferative lesion of the posterolateral hard palate and discussed aspects of its differential diagnosis.

Hyperplasia of mucous salivary glands can occur anywhere on the oral mucosa. Nine out of 10 cases reported by Arafat et al. (1981) occurred on the hard palate. All were asymptomatic masses, lumps, or nodules. In the author's experience (N.K.W.), oftentimes careful examination shows the presence of a central pit that represents the opening of a common duct. Fig. 10-26 illustrates a variety of lesions that may occur as palatal swellings.

MANAGEMENT

The recurrence rates for the minor salivary gland tumors vary greatly from series to series but are relatively high even in the case of benign tumors. This is probably because the original tumor was incompletely excised. Although many of these benign tumors appear encapsulated, a few tumor cells frequently penetrate the pseudocapsule and escape excision (Clairmont et al., 1977; Krolls and Boyers, 1972). Thus it is expedient to include a wide margin of normal tissue in the removal of benign or malignant lesions. Frozen sections completed at surgery will help to indicate whether or not the margins are free of tumor and whether a wider excision should be undertaken. Pogrel (1979) reported that in his series, 67% of the adenoid cystic carcinomas recurred whereas 18% of the pleomorphic adenomas recurred. Malignant tumors are treated by surgery or a combination of surgery and radiation.

Close posttreatment surveillance should be maintained to detect early recurrences. In malignant cases, chest radiographs every 6 months are imperative to detect the earliest stage of possible pulmonary metastasis.

PERIPHERAL BENIGN MESENCHYMAL TUMORS

Individual types of oral peripheral mesenchymal tumors are uncommon lesions, but when considered as a group, they demonstrate a more impressive incidence. Such a group would include the following:

Lipomas
Myomas (rhabdomyoma and leiomyoma)
Peripheral nerve tumors (neurofibroma, plexiform type of neurofibroma, schwannoma, traumatic neuroma)

Features

All the peripheral benign mesenchymal tumors are nodular, polypoid, or dome shaped with smooth contours and are characteristically covered with normal mucosa unless chronically traumatized. They may be located on the tongue, buccal mucosa, lips, hard and soft palates, floor of the mouth, and vestibule. They usually are asymptomatic, grow slowly, and can be moved over the deeper tissue. When situated within loose connective tissue, they are often exceptionally movable.

The lipoma, although the most frequently occurring true peripheral mesenchymal tumor, is an uncommon oral lesion. It is soft, spongy, fluctuant, sessile, and usually nodular or dome shaped and asymptomatic. The superficial lesion will have a definite yellow color, and in the thinned mucoa over its surface there are often small red blood vessels that blanch on pressure (Fig. 10-28). The lipoma that is deeper in the tissue will have a normal pink mucosal color, however, and its margin may be so diffuse as to be difficult to define by palpation. This lesion is about equally distributed be-

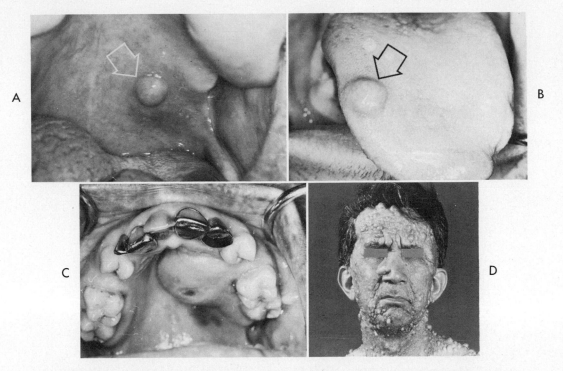

Fig. 10-28. Benign mesenchymal tumors. **A** and **B**, Lipomas. **C**, Neurofibroma on the palate. **D**, Multiple neurofibromatosis.   (**C** courtesy R. Nolan, DDS, Waukegan, Ill. **D** courtesy P.D. Toto, DDS, Maywood, Ill.)

tween the sexes and occurs most frequently on the buccal mucosa, but it may also be found in the mandibular retromolar area, the buccal sulci, tongue, lip, and floor of the mouth (de Visscher, 1982; Greer and Richardson, 1973; Hatziotis, 1971; MacGregor and Dyson, 1966).

The remainder of the benign mesenchymal tumors (i.e., myomas, schwannomas, firm neurofibromas, traumatic neuromas) are so different from the lipoma that they must be discussed separately. With the exception of the fibromas, most of which are actually mature inflammatory hyperplastic lesions, these other lesions seldom occur in the oral cavity, although some have been reported on the tongue, lip, buccal mucosa, floor of the mouth, and posterior palate (Figs. 10-27 and 10-28). They are invariably firm with discrete borders, and if situated in the loose connective tissue layer, they will be freely movable (Sist and Greene, 1981; Wright and Jackson, 1980).

Differential diagnosis

Since the lipoma is so different from the other benign mesenchymal tumors, its differential diagnosis is best discussed separately. Lesions that should be included in the differential diagnosis are dense focal aggregates of Fordyce's granules, the buccal fat pads, the superficial cavernous hemangioma, lymphangioma, myxomas, and varicosity, the superficial retention phenomena (e.g., mucoceles, ranulas, mucus-producing salivary gland tumors) as well as deeper vascular lesions, and the plexiform neurofibroma.

The *plexiform neurofibroma* may be difficult to distinguish from a nonyellow lipoma because both lesions are soft, fluctuant, and nonproductive on aspiration. Because of their rarer occurrence, however, the plexiform neurofibromas should follow the lipoma in the differential diagnosis, except in patients with von Recklinghausen's disease (Fig. 10-28, *C* and *D*).

Superficial retention phenomena (mucoceles, ranulas, mucus-producing minor salivary gland tumors) are bluish, whereas the *deeper lesions* are pink. Aspiration of a clear sticky viscous fluid (mucus) distinguishes the retention phenomena from the lipoma.

The *superficial cavernous hemangioma, lymphangioma,* and *varicosity* are also blue, so the clinician should be able to distinguish them from the yellow lipoma. When they are deeper and covered with normal pink mucosa, they may be differentiated from the lipoma by the fact that they are emptiable by pressure. Also

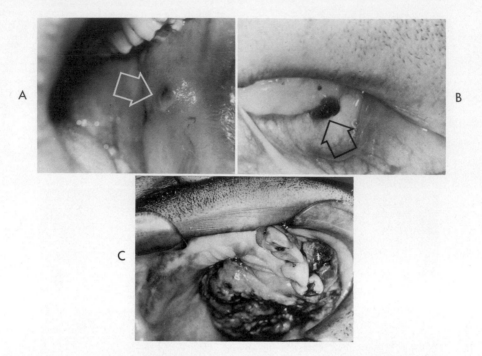

Fig. 10-29. Nevus and melanoma. **A,** Intramucosal nevus. **B,** Melanoma. **C,** Large melanoma. (**A** courtesy E. Kasper, DDS, Maywood, Ill. **B** courtesy D. Skuble, DDS, Hinsdale, Ill. **C** courtesy R. Oglesby, DDS, Chicago.)

aspiration of hemangiomas and varicosities produces venous blood and of lymphangiomas a frothy lymph fluid, whereas aspiration of a lipoma is nonproductive.

The *buccal fat pads* in some individuals may become so hypertrophied as to be mistaken for a lipoma by the inexperienced clinician. They should be recognized, however, by their characteristic bilateral position in the posterior cheek. They are usually symmetric in size, except when one has herniated after trauma or a surgical procedure.

If the lipoma is superficial, its yellow color distinguishes it from all the foregoing entities except the *dense focal aggregates of Fordyce's granules.* These should not pose a problem, though, since the accumulations of spots are seldom larger than a few millimeters in diameter, and the presence of individual granules scattered in the surrounding mucosa aids the clinician in recognizing them.

Since the myoma, schwannoma, firm neurofibroma, and traumatic neuroma have so many similar features and few if any distinguishing characteristics, they are difficult to discern from each other clinically, and attempts to make a differential diagnosis are not of any potential value.

Lesions that must be considered with this group include the *fibroma,* the *firm minor salivary gland tumors,* and the *granular cell myoblastoma.*

When a firm smoothly contoured lesion covered with normal pink mucosa is encountered on the oral mucosa, the examiner would normally conclude (on the basis of incidence) that it is a fibroma. If it is on the posterolateral aspect of the palate, he would likely consider it a minor salivary gland tumor. Finally, if it is on the dorsal surface or lateral border of the tongue, it could be a granular cell myoblastoma. In addition, Cherrick et al. (1973) found that the tongue is the most frequent intraoral site for a leiomyoma.

Management

The recommended treatment for the peripheral benign mesenchymal tumors is excision, microscopic examination of the tumor tissue, and postoperative surveillance to ensure the early detection of a recurrence.

NEVUS AND MELANOMA

Nevus and melanoma are uncommon intraoral tumors that are discussed in detail in Chapter 12 as macular and exophytic brownish,

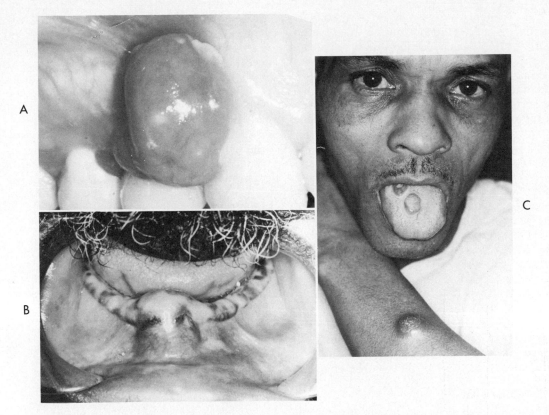

Fig. 10-30. Exophytic metastatic tumors. **A,** Metastatic melanoma. **B,** Metastatic adenocarcinoma from the lung. **C,** Three metastatic lesions from a carcinoma of the esophagus in a 46-year-old man.   (**A** from Mosby EL et al: Oral Surg 36:6-10, 1973. **B** courtesy R. Kallal, DDS, Chicago. **C** courtesy E. Robinson, DDS, Toledo, Ohio.)

bluish, or black lesions. If individual lesions are typical in appearance (i.e., pigmented and firm), the list of possibilities is restricted (Fig. 10-29).

If a lesion is amelanotic and is discovered in its early stage of development, however, it appears as a firm, smoothly contoured, nodular or somewhat polypoid mass covered with normal-appearing mucosa (Fig. 10-30, A). The list of possible lesions then must include fibromas and benign mesenchymal tumors, and if its surface is ulcerated as the result of trauma, it may mimic a pyogenic granuloma.

As the intraoral amelanotic melanoma grows and is traumatized, its surface ulcerates and becomes necrotic. At this stage it has the clinical appearance of a malignant tumor. Then, based on the incidence of similar-appearing lesions, the possible diagnoses would be ranked as follows: squamous cell carcinoma, malignant salivary gland tumor, peripheral metastatic tumor, malignant primary mesenchymal tumor, and amelanotic melanoma.

PERIPHERAL METASTATIC TUMORS

Intrabony metastatic tumors are much more common than peripheral metastatic tumors of the oral cavity (Hatziotis et al., 1973) and are discussed in detail in Chapter 21.

Much of what has been described for the central tumors is true for the peripheral variety, so this material will not be repeated here. In addition, peripheral metastatic tumors are discussed in Chapter 5 under solitary red lesions. The most common tumors to metastasize to the oral cavity originate in the kidney, lung, gastrointestinal tract, breast, and prostate gland.

Features

There may be a history of a primary tumor, or the symptoms of such a tumor may indicate its probable existence.

Bhaskar (1971) stated, however, that 33% of the oral secondary tumors he examined were the first recognized indication of the presence of the primary tumor.

The secondary lesion may be asymptomatic and thus be detected on routine examination, or the patient may describe any or all of the following as the chief complaint: intraoral swelling that may or may not relate to an ill-fitting denture, pain, or paresthesia. Although the secondary malignancy may occur anywhere on the oral mucosa, it is more frequently seen on the tongue and gingivae (Hatziotis et al., 1973).

Because the nests of tumor cells are expanding beneath the surface epithelium, the early lesions are usually nodules or dome-shaped masses—smooth surfaced and covered with normal-appearing mucosa. At this stage the lesions frequently appears deceptively benign (Fig. 10-30). Later, as a result of trauma, their surfaces may ulcerate and become necrotic. When this occurs, they appear clinically to be malignant.

As the tumor invades the deeper tissue, it becomes fixed. In some cases underlying bone is destroyed, and this circumstance causes the appearance of an ill-defined, ragged, saucerlike radiolucency on the periphery of the bone.

Differential diagnosis

The advanced ulcerated lesion of a peripheral metastatic tumor may appear similar to an *exophytic squamous cell carcinoma, malignant salivary tumors, malignant mesenchymal tumors*, and an *amelanotic melanoma*.

If the patient has a history of a tumor elsewhere, this would prompt the clinician to consider the possibility that the oral lesion is a metastatic tumor. If there is no history of a primary tumor or suggestive symptoms, however, the incidence of these tumors would prompt the clinician to pursue the possibility of the entities in foregoing groups in the indicated order. If the patient is less than 20 years old, the probability that the lesion is a squamous cell carcinoma or a malignant salivary gland tumor is considerably lessened.

Management

The rationale of the management of metastatic tumors is considered in Chapter 20.

PERIPHERAL MALIGNANT MESENCHYMAL TUMORS

Since reports of intraoral peripheral malignant mesenchymal tumors (for example, neurosarcomas, malignant schwannomas, fibrosarcomas, rhabdomyosarcomas, hemangiosarcomas, liposarcomas) are found only occasionally in the literature, it must be concluded that this group

of lesions is uncommon. The intraoral osteogenic sarcoma and chondrosarcoma occur relatively more frequently, but these usually are central in origin and consequently are discussed in Part III of the text.

There is very little that is distinctive about the mesenchymal tumors that would differentiate them from any of the clinically benign or malignant-appearing lesions, except possibly the age factor (Fig. 10-31). These tumors usually affect a considerably younger age-group than does squamous cell carcinoma.

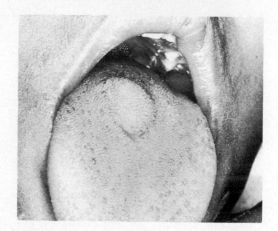

Fig. 10-31. Rhabdomyosarcoma of the dorsal surface of the tongue.   (Courtesy N. Choukas, DDS, Maywood, Ill.)

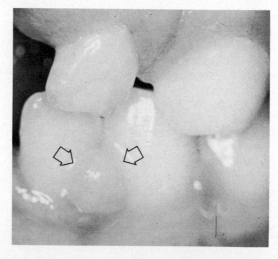

Fig. 10-32. Giant cell fibroma *(arrows)* situated on the interdental papilla area.   (Courtesy D. Weathers, DDS, Atlanta, Ga.)

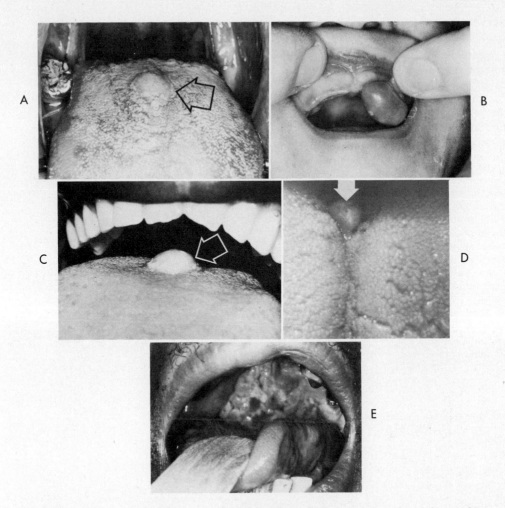

Fig. 10-33. Rare exophytic lesions. **A,** Granular cell myoblastoma. **B,** Epulis of the newborn. **C,** Lingual thyroid gland. **D,** Persistent tuberculum impar. **E,** Lymphosarcoma in the pharynx.   (**A** courtesy R. Kallal, DDS, Chicago. **C** and **D** courtesy E. Kaspar, DDS, Maywood, Ill. **E** courtesy E. Evans, DDS, St. Cloud, Minn.)

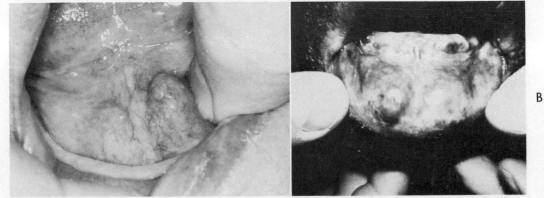

Fig. 10-34. Rare exophytic lesions. **A,** Sialolith in Wharton's duct. **B,** Two dome-shaped masses on lower lip are focal hyperplasias of minor salivary glands. Each aggregation of minor glands drained through one duct opening in the middle of each mass.

RARITIES
Solitary lesions

The rare solitary exophytic lesions represent a formidable number of entities (Figs. 10-32 to 10-34). In spite of the rarity of these lesions, the clinician must at least be aware of the possibilities they represent, when examining a specific lesion.

The circumstances and special characteristics may prompt the clinician to include one or more of these lesions in the differential list:

Actinomycosis
Alveolar soft part sarcoma
Ameloblastoma (peripheral)
Angiolymphoid hyperplasia
Antral neoplasms
Benign lymphoid hyperplasia
Blastomycosis
Bohn's nodule (Epstein's pearl)
Calcinosis
Chondroma of soft tissue
Choristoma
Condyloma acuminatum
Condyloma latum

Congenital epulis of the newborn
Early chancre
Early gumma
Eruption cyst
Extraosseous odontogenic tumor
Focal hyperplasia of the minor salivary glands
Focal mucinosis
Foreign body granuloma
Giant cell fibroma
Gingival cyst
Glomus tumor
Granular cell lesion
Granulomatous fungal disease
Hamartoma
Herpes proliferative lesion
Histiocytosis X
Juvenile nasopharyngeal angiofibroma
Juvenile xanthogranuloma
Kaposi's sarcoma
Kaposi's sarcoma (AIDS)
Keratoacanthoma
Lead poisoning
Lethal midline granuloma
Leukemic enlargement
Lingual thyroid gland

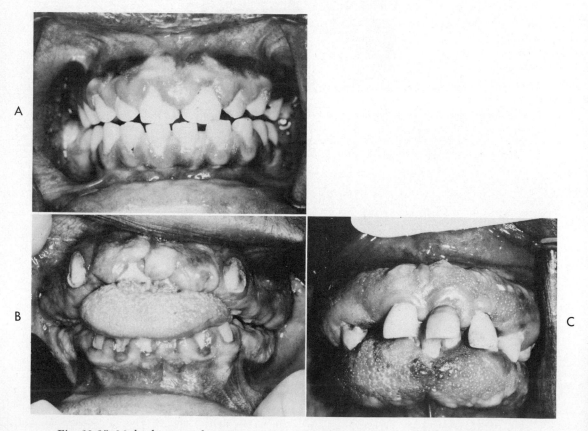

Fig. 10-35. Multiple gingival masses. **A,** Mouth-breathing gingivitis. **B,** Phenytoin (Dilantin) hyperplasia. **C,** Familial gingival fibromatosis. (**C** courtesy W. Heaton, DDS, Chicago.)

Lymphoma
Median nodule of the upper lip
Median rhomboid glossitis (nodular variety)
Midline nonhealing granuloma
Molluscum contagiosum
Myxoma of soft tissue or oral focal mucinosis
Necrotizing sialometaplasia (nodular)
Neuroectodermal tumor of infancy
Nodular leukoplakia
Plasmacytoma of soft tissue
Pseudosarcomatous fasciitis
Pulse granuloma
Rhabdomyoma
Rhabdomyosarcoma
Rheumatoid nodule
Rhinoscleroma
Sarcoidosis
Sialolith
Spindle cell carcinoma
Squamous acanthoma
Sturge-Weber syndrome
Teratoma
Tuberculosis
Verruciform xanthoma

Multiple lesions

As are the solitary rarities, the rare exophytic pathoses that occur as multiple lesions are almost impossible to rank according to frequency; they are listed therefore in alphabetical order (Figs. 10-35 and 10-36):

Acanthosis nigricans
Acrokeratosis verruciformis of Hope
Amyloidosis (Fig. 10-36, A)
Benign symmetric lipomatosis
Bohn's nodules
Calcinosis
Chronic granulomatous disease
Condyloma acuminatum
Condyloma latum (Fig. 10-36, C)
Cowden's disease
Crohn's disease
Cysticercosis
Darier's disease (Fig. 10-36, D)
Eruption cysts
Focal dermal hypoplasia (Goltz syndrome)
Focal epithelial hyperplasia (Fig. 10-37)
Gardner's syndrome

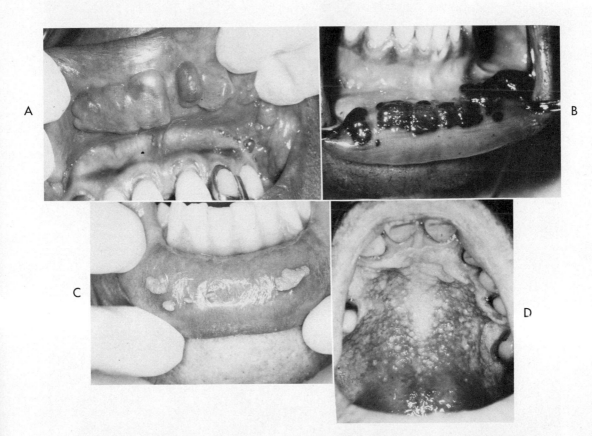

Fig. 10-36. Multiple exophytic masses. **A,** Amyloidosis in multiple myeloma. **B,** Multiple blood clots in heroin-induced thrombocytopenic purpura. **C,** Multiple condylomata lata of the lower lip. **D,** Multiple papules of palate in a patient with Darier's disease.   (**A** from Kraut RA, Buhler JE, LaRue JR, and Acevedo A: Oral Surg 43:63-68, 1977. **B** from Kraut RA and Buhler JE: Oral Surg 46:637-640, 1978. **C** courtesy S. Smith, DDS, Chicago. **D** courtesy M. Bernstein, DDS, Louisville.)

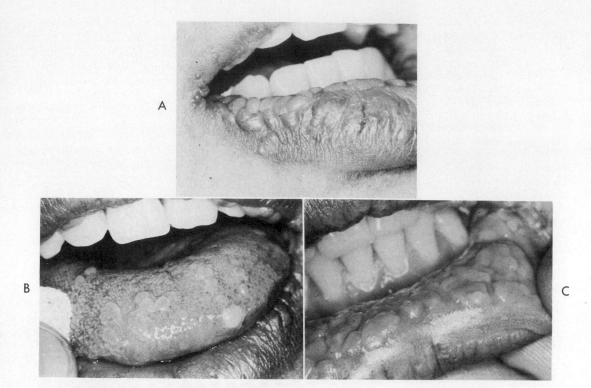

Fig. 10-37. Focal epithelial hyperplasia in an Israeli patient.   (From Buchner A: Oral Surg 46:64-69, 1978.)

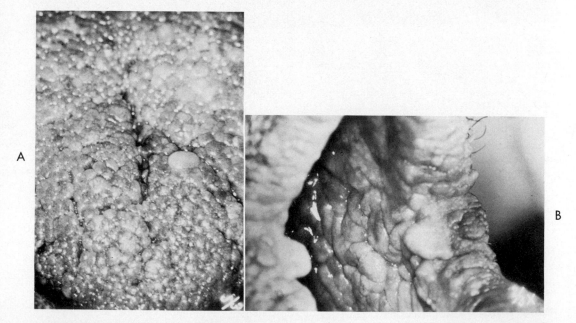

Fig. 10-38. Multiple fibroepithelial hyperplasia seen on the tongue, buccal mucosa, and lips of a patient.   (From Buchner A and Sandbank M: Oral Surg 46:34-39, 1978.)

Giant cell fibromas
Hereditary telangiectasia
Histiocytosis X
Hyperplasias (drug-induced)
Idiopathic gingival fibromatosis
Kaposi's sarcoma
Kaposi's sarcoma (AIDS)
Leukemia
Lichenoides chronica
Lymphangiomas of neonates
Lymphomas (extranodal)
Lymphomatoid papulosis
Lymphoproliferating disease of the palate
Maffucci's syndrome
Melkersson-Rosenthal syndrome
Molluscum contagiosum
Multiple exophytic metastatic carcinomas
Multiple exostoses
Multiple fibroepithelial hyperplasias (Fig. 10-38)
Multiple gingival cysts
Multiple hamartoma neoplasia syndrome
Multiple lipomas
Multiple melanomas
Multiple mucoceles
Multiple myeloma
Multiple papillomas
Multiple peripheral brown giant cell lesions (hyperparathyroidism)
Multiple verrucae
Murray-Puretíc-Drescher syndrome (juvenile hyaline fibromatosis)
Myelodysplastic syndrome
Noonan's syndrome
Oral florid papillomatosis
Orodigitofacial syndrome (multiple hamartomas of the tongue)
Pyostomatitis vegetans
Sarcoidosis
Syndrome of multiple mucosal neuromas, pheochromocytoma, and carcinoma of the thyroid
Syphilitic papules
Thrombocytopenic purpura
Urticaria pigmentosa
von Recklinghausen's disease
Xanthoma disseminatum

REFERENCES

Adkins KF: Lymphoid hyperplasia in the oral mucosa, Aust Dent J 18:38-40, 1973.

Adler-Storthz K, Newland JR, Tessin BA, et al: Identification of human papillomavirus types in oral verruca vulgaris, J Oral Pathol 15:230-233, 1986.

Angelopoulos AP: Pyogenic granuloma of the oral cavity: statistical analysis of its clinical features, J Oral Surg 29:840-847, 1971.

Arafat A, Brannon RB, and Ellis GL: Adenomatoid hyperplasia of mucous salivary glands, Oral Surg 52:51-55, 1981.

Bergendal T, Heindahl A, and Isacsson G: Surgery in the treatment of denture related inflammatory hyperplasia of the palate, Int J Oral Surg 9:312-319, 1980.

Bhaskar SN: Oral manifestations of metastatic tumors, Postgrad Med 49:155-158, 1971.

Bhaskar SN and Cutright DE: Giant cell reparative granuloma (peripheral): report of 50 cases, J Oral Surg 29:110-115, 1971.

Blok P, van Delden L, and van der Waal I: Non-Hodgkin's lymphoma of the hard palate, Oral Surg 47:445-452, 1979.

Bouquot JE and Gundlach KKH: Oral exophytic lesions in 23,616 white Americans over 35 years of age, Oral Surg 62:284-291, 1986.

Bradley G, Main JHP, Birt BD, and From L: Benign lymphoid hyperplasia of the palate, J Oral Pathol 16:18-26, 1987.

Buchner A, Ficcarra G, and Hansen LS: Peripheral odontogenic fibroma, Oral Surg 64:432-438, 1987.

Budtz-Jørgensen E: Oral mucosal lesions associated with the wearing of removable dentures, J Oral Pathol 10:65-80, 1981.

Burkes EJ and White RP: A peripheral giant cell granuloma manifestation of primary hyperparathyroidism: report of case, J Am Dent Assoc 118:62-63, 1989.

Chau MNY and Radden BG: Intraoral salivary gland neoplasms: a retrospective study of 98 cases, J Oral Pathol 15:339-342, 1986.

Chaudhry AP, Vickers RA, and Gorlin RJ: Intraoral minor salivary gland tumors, Oral Surg 14:1194-1226, 1961.

Cherrick HM, Dunlap CL, and King OH: Leiomyomas of the oral cavity, Oral Surg 35:54-66, 1973.

Clairmont AA, Richardson GS, and Hanna DC: The pseudocapsule of pleomorphic adenomas (benign mixed tumors), Am J Surg 134:242-243, 1977.

Cohen L: Mucoceles of the oral cavity, Oral Surg 19:365-372, 1965.

Correll RW, Wescott WB, and Siegel WM: Rapidly growing, nonpainful, ulcerated swelling on the posterolateral palate, J Am Dent Assoc 106:494-495, 1983.

Cundiff EJ: Peripheral ossifying fibroma: a review of 365 cases, MSD thesis, Indiana University, 1972. Cited in Shafer WG, Hine MK, and Levy BM: A textbook of oral pathology, ed 3, Philadelphia, 1974, WB Saunders Co.

Cutright DE: The histopathologic findings in 583 cases of epulis fissuratum, Oral Surg 37:401-411, 1974.

de Visscher JG: Lipomas and fibrolipomas of the oral cavity, J Maxillofac Surg 10:177-181, 1982.

Eisenbud L, Sciubba J, Mir R, et al: Oral presentations in thirty-one cases of non-Hodgkin's lymphoma. I. Data analysis, Oral Surg 56:151-156, 1983.

Eversole LR and Laipis PJ: Oral squamous papillomas: detection of HPV DNA by in situ hybridization, Oral Surg 65:545-550, 1988.

Eversole LR and Rovin S: Reactive lesions of the gingiva, J Oral Pathol 1:30-38, 1972.

Eveson JW and Cawson RA: Tumors of the minor (oropharyngeal) salivary glands: a demographic study of 336 cases, J Oral Pathol 14:500-509, 1985.

Gardner DG: The peripheral odontogenic fibroma: an attempt at clarification, Oral Surg 54:40-48, 1982.

Giansanti JS and Waldron CA: Peripheral giant cell granuloma: review of 720 cases, J Oral Surg 27:787-791, 1969.

Gorsky M, Begleiter A, Buchner A, and Harel-Raviv M: The retrocuspid papilla in Israeli Jews, Oral Surg 62:240-243, 1986.

Greer RO and Richardson JF: The nature of lipomas and their significance in the oral cavity: a review and report of cases, Oral Surg 36:551-557, 1973.

Hatziotis J: Lipoma of the oral cavity, Oral Surg 31:511-524, 1971.

Hatziotis J, Constantinidou H, and Papanayotou PH: Metastatic tumors of the oral soft tissues, Oral Surg 36:544-550, 1973.

Isacsson G and Shear M: Intraoral salivary gland tumors: a retrospective study of 201 cases, J Oral Pathol 12:57-62, 1983.

Katsiteris N, Kakarantza-Angelopoulou E, and Angelopoulos AP: Peripheral giant cell granuloma: clinicopathologic study of 224 new cases and review of 956 reported cases, Int J Oral Maxillofac Surg 17:94-99, 1988.

King DR and King AC: Incidence of tori in three population groups, J Oral Med 36:21-23, 1981.

King DR and Moore GE: An analysis of torus palatinus in a transatlantic study, J Oral Med 31:44-46, 1976.

King RE, Altini M, and Shear M: Basal extensions in human mucosa, J Oral Pathol 8:140-146, 1979.

Knapp MJ: Oral tonsils: location, distribution, and histology, Oral Surg 29:155-161, 1970a.

Knapp MJ: Pathology of oral tonsils, Oral Surg 29:295-304, 1970b.

Krolls SO and Boyers RC: Mixed tumors of salivary glands: long-term follow-up, Cancer 30:276-281, 1972.

Krolls SO and Hicks JL: Mixed tumors of the lower lip, Oral Surg 35:212-217, 1973.

MacGregor AJ and Dyson DP: Oral lipoma: a review of the literature and report of twelve new cases, Oral Surg 21:770-777, 1966.

Macleod RI and Soames JV: Epulides: a clinicopathological study of a series of 200 consecutive lesions, Br Dent J 163:51-53, 1987.

Main JHP, McGurk FM, McComb RJ, and Mock D: Salivary gland tumors: review of 643 cases, J Oral Pathol 5:88-102, 1976.

Miller EL: Clinical management of denture-induced inflammations, J Prosthet Dent 38:362-365, 1977.

Mulcahy JV and Dahl EC: The peripheral odontogenic fibroma: a retrospective study, J Oral Med 40:46-48, 1985.

Pogrel MA: Tumors of the salivary glands: a histological and clinical review, Br J Oral Surg 17:47-56, 1979.

Rapidis AD and Triantafyllou AG: Myxoma of the oral soft tissue, J Oral Maxillofac Surg 41:188-192, 1983.

Rathofer SA, Gardner FM, and Vermilyea SG: A comparison of healing and pain following excision of inflammatory papillary hyperplasia with electrosurgery and blade-loop knives in human patients, Oral Surg 59:130-135, 1985.

Sist TC and Greene GW: Traumatic neuroma of the oral cavity: report of thirty-one new cases and review of the literature, Oral Surg 51:394-402, 1981.

Smith BR, Fowler CB, and Svane TJ: Primary hyperparathyroidism presenting as a "peripheral" giant cell granuloma, J Oral Maxillofac Surg 46:65-69, 1988.

Soskolne A, Ben-Amar A, and Ulmansky M: Minor salivary gland tumors: a survey of 64 cases, J Oral Surg 31:528-531, 1973.

Syrjanen SM, Syrjanen KJ, and Lamberg MA: Detection of human papilloma virus DNA in oral mucosal lesions using in situ DNA hybridization applied on paraffin sections, Oral Surg 62:660-667, 1986.

Thackray AC and Sabin LH: International histological classification of tumors. No. 7. Histological typing of salivary gland tumors, Geneva, 1972, World Health Organization.

Tomich CE: Oral focal mucinosis: a clinicopathologic and histochemical study of eight cases, Oral Surg 38:714-724, 1974.

Uohara GI and Federbusch MD: Removal of papillary hyperplasia, J Oral Surg 26:463-466, 1968.

Vilmann A, Vilmann P, and Vilmann H: Pyogenic granuloma: evaluation of oral conditions, Br J Oral Maxillofac Surg 24:376-382, 1986.

Waldron CA, El-Mofty S, and Gnepp DR: Tumors of the intraoral salivary glands: a demographic and histologic study of 426 cases, Oral Surg 66:323-333, 1988.

Weathers DR and Callihan MD: Giant-cell fibroma, Oral Surg 37:374-384, 1974.

Whitaker LA, Lehr HB, and Askovitz SI: Cancer of the tongue, Plast Reconstr Surg 30:363-370, 1972.

Wright BA and Jackson D: Neural tumors of the oral cavity: a review of the spectrum of benign and malignant oral tumors of the oral cavity and jaws, Oral Surg 49:509-522, 1980.

Wright JM and Dunsworth AR: Follicular lymphoid hyperplasia of the hard palate: a benign lymphoproliferative process, Oral Surg 55:162-168, 1983.

11

Solitary oral ulcers and fissures

NORMAN K. WOOD
PAUL W. GOAZ

Ulcers and fissures of the oral cavity include the following:

Ulcers
Traumatic ulcer
Recurrent aphthous ulcer
  (canker sore) and
  intraoral recurrent ulcer
  of herpes simplex
Ulcers from odontogenic
  infections
Sloughing,
  pseudomembranous
  ulcers
Generalized mucositides
  and vesiculobullous
  diseases
Squamous cell carcinoma
Syphilis
  Chancre
  Gumma
Ulcers secondary to
  systemic disease
Traumatized tumors (types
  usually not ulcerated)
Minor salivary gland
  tumors
Rarities
  Actinomycosis
  Adenoid squamous cell
    carcinoma
  Basal cell carcinoma
  Basidiobolus haptosporus
  Botryomycosis hominis
  Cancrum oris
  Crohn's disease
  Foot-and-mouth disease
  Fungal infections
    (blastomycosis,
    coccidioidomycosis,
    cryptococcosis,
    histoplasmosis,
    sporotrichosis)
  Gonococcal stomatitis
  Granulomatous disease of
    the newborn

Hand-foot-mouth disease
Herpangina
Herpes zoster
Keratoacanthoma
Midline nonhealing
  granuloma (midline
  malignant reticulosis)
Leukemia
Lymphoma
Median rhomboid
  glossitis—ulcerative
  variety
Metastatic tumor
Mucormycosis
Mycosis fungoides
Necrotizing
  sialometaplasia
Neurotrophic ulcer
Phycomycosis
Sarcoidosis
Self-mutilation wounds
Sutton's disease
Syringomyelia
Tuberculosis
Waldenström's
  macroglobulinemia
Warty dyskeratoma

Fissures
Angular cheilosis
Congenital cleft
Epulis fissuratum
Fissured tongue
Median rhomboid
  glossitis—fissured variety
Melkersson-Rosenthal
  syndrome
Squamous cell
  carcinoma—fissured
  variety
Syphilitic rhagades

Ulcers

Oral ulcers represent a variable and impressive group of lesions. A cursory examination of

the foregoing list reveals that some of these lesions are caused by local influences (for example, traumatic ulcers), whereas others are manifestations of systemic problems (for example, the oral ulcers in sickle cell anemia).

Also, when attempting to characterize this group of lesions, the clinician is aided by considering Spouge's general description (1973, p. 371): some oral ulcers are *primary,* with early manifestations as erosions or ulcers, such as the traumatic ulcers; others are actually *secondary* because they are subsequent to other clinical forms, which after rupturing and sloughing become ulcerated (for example, vesicles and blebs).

Exophytic lesions frequently illustrate this secondary change when they become ulcerated from chronic mechanical injury or as the result of an incisional biopsy.

The terms "erosion" and "ulcer" are often confused and mistakenly used interchangeably. Spouge (1973, p. 371) defined an *erosion* as a shallow crater in the epithelial surface that appears on clinical examination as a very shallow erythematous area and implies only superficial damage. Spouge defined an *ulcer* as a deeper crater that extends through the entire thickness of surface epithelium and involves the underlying connective tissue.

Oral ulcers are unique: they have diverse causes but frequently show similar histologic changes and thus cannot be differentiated by routine microscopy. This uniformity on microscopic examination derives from the irritating effect of oral liquids and flora: as soon as an ulcer is formed in the oral mucosa it is subjected to irritating oral liquids and flora; consequently an acute or chronic inflammation is immediately initiated. The resultant inflammatory changes may mask the more characteristic and diagnostic histologic changes that are a feature of the basic pathosis.

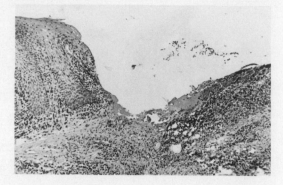

Fig. 11-1. Nonspecific ulcer. Photomicrograph reveals loss of both the surface epithelium and the upper portion of the lamina propria. Inflammatory cells are abundant.

The intraoral herpes simplex lesion is a good example of an oral ulcer that loses its microscopic identity because of secondary contamination. In its early vesicular stage pathognomonic features are the ballooning of the epithelial cells and the presence of giant cells in the vesicular fluid. After the vesicle ulcerates, these definitive features are soon lost and all that remains is the histologic picture of a nonspecific ulcer.

The following changes are inferred when the clinician encounters on microscopic examination a diagnosis of "nonspecific" ulcer:

1. The complete thickness of the surface epithelium is missing, and the exposed connective tissue often is necrotic on the surface and covered by a fibrinous exudate (Fig. 11-1).
2. Depending on its age and the circumstances relating to its development, the ulcer has acute inflammation with polymorphonuclear leukocytes in the connective tissue at its borders.
3. A less acute phase of the ulcer shows a greater concentration of chronic inflammatory cells, such as lymphocytes, plasma cells, and possibly macrophages with some fibroblastic proliferation.
4. In the healing phase of the ulcer, granulation tissue with fibroblastic proliferation predominates, and a few macrophages, plasma cells, and lymphocytes may also be present.

In spite of the foregoing, some of the ulcers discussed in this chapter can be diagnosed by routine light microscopy when they are stained with hematoxylin and eosin.

For example, histologic changes in squamous cell carcinoma and ulcerative mesenchymal mi-

nor salivary gland tumors are diagnostic as long as the biopsy actually includes a section of tumor underlying the ulcer. It is true that lesions such as chancres, herpetic ulcers, and tuberculous, sarcoid, and fungal lesions may produce tissue changes that indicate a definitive diagnosis, but usually special staining procedures, such as Gram's, silver, or PAS,* must be used to assist in making a definitive microscopic identification.

When attempting to complete a differential diagnosis of a clinical ulcer, the clinician should separate the oral ulcers into two groups: *short-term* ulcers (that is, those that persist no longer than 3 weeks and regress spontaneously) and *persistent ulcers* (those that last for weeks and months).

The majority of traumatic ulcers, recurrent aphthous ulcers (except major aphthae), recurrent intraoral herpetic ulcers, and chancres fall into the category of short-term ulcers.

Occasional traumatic ulcers, major aphthae, ulcers from odontogenic infection, malignant ulcers, gummas, and ulcers secondary to debilitating systemic disease are classified as persistent ulcers and may remain for months and even years. Persistent ulcers should be considered malignant till proved otherwise.

TRAUMATIC ULCER

The traumatic ulcer is by far the most common oral mucosal ulcer. The cause may be mechanical, chemical, or thermal; the traumatic incident may be accidentally self-inflicted or iatrogenic.

Features

The patient with a traumatic ulcer complains of tenderness or pain in the area of the lesion and usually is able to identify its cause. A variety of causes come to the inquiring clinician's attention: lip, tongue, and cheek biting (sometimes after the administration of a local anesthetic), a toothbrush that slipped, a child who was running with an object in his or her mouth and fell, or a mouth burned by hot liquids or toothache drops.

Schiødt (1981) described long-standing ulcerations of the attached gingiva that were caused by repeated trauma from toothbrushing. In 1983 Pattison reported a case of self-inflicted necrotic ulcerative lesion of the gingiva in a pa-

---

*The periodic acid–Schiff reaction is a widely used method that stains glycogen, epithelial mucus, neutral polysaccharides, and glycoproteins.

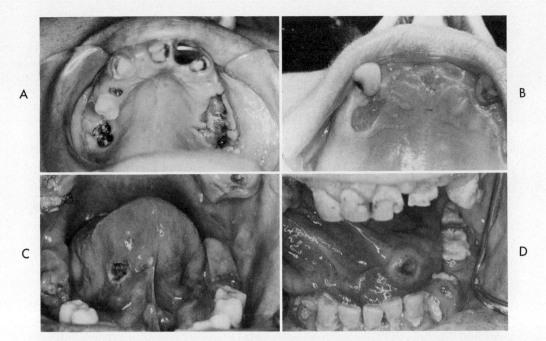

Fig. 11-2. Traumatic ulcers. **A,** Ulcer on the maxillary ridge caused by a traumatic extraction. **B,** Ulcer on the maxillary alveolus resulting from trauma from the lower canine. **C,** Traumatic ulcer on the ventral surface of the tongue resulting from a self-inflicted bite. **D,** Ulcer caused by a sharp premolar root. This lesion, which appeared on clinical examination to be a squamous cell carcinoma, proved on biopsy to be a traumatic lesion.   (**A** courtesy D. Bonomo, DDS, Flossmoor, Ill. **B** courtesy P.D. Toto, DDS, Maywood, Ill.)

tient who was seeking a prescription for narcotic drugs. Budtz-Jorgensen (1981) relayed the information that denture-induced traumatic ulcers were observed in 5.5% of a population aged 65 to 74 years. Peters et al. (1984) discussed the problem of self-inflicted trauma of the tongue in decerebrate and comatose patients. This author recommended the placement of a fixed acrylic tongue stent in some of these cases. Mader (1981) discussed the occurrence of a lingual frenum ulcer that resulted from orogenital sex.

Traumatic ulcers are most common on the tongue, lips, mucobuccal fold, gingiva, and palate. They may persist for just a few days or may last for weeks (especially ulcers of the tongue). They may vary greatly in size and shape but seldom are multiple or recurrent, unless they result from ill-fitting dentures. Their borders are somewhat raised and reddish, and their bases have a yellowish necrotic surface that can be readily removed (Figs. 11-2 and 11-3). Ulcers on the vermilion border, unlike those on the oral mucosa, usually have a crusted surface because of the absence of saliva. In some instances the ulcers conform nicely to the shape of a tooth cusp or a denture

flange, or they may be positioned against a sharp edge of a tooth.

The clinician must be certain of the cause-and-effect relationship not only to make a definitive diagnosis of traumatic ulcer but also to identify and eliminate the traumatizing agent. Frequently a tender or painful regional lymphadenitis occurs as a result of contamination of the ulcer by the oral flora.

Differential diagnosis

The history of the traumatic injury in most cases enables the clinician to identify the traumatic ulcer and establish a working diagnosis. The history of a traumatic incident may be misleading, however, and cause the true identity of a more serious lesion to be overlooked. Since traumatic ulcers may be either short-term or persistent, both varieties must be considered in the differential diagnosis. For a more thorough discussion, refer to the differential diagnosis section at the end of this chapter (pp. 215-219).

Management

Most traumatic ulcers become painless within 3 or 4 days after the injury-producing

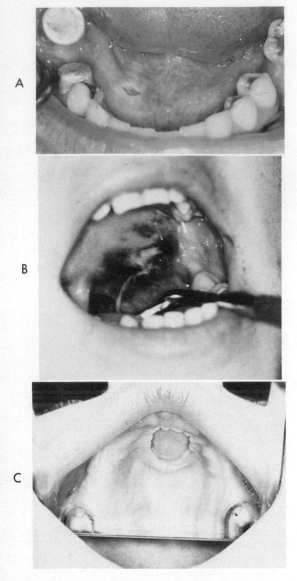

Fig. 11-3. Traumatic ulcers. **A,** Ulcer on the floor of the mouth caused by a rough temporary crown on the mandibular right second premolar tooth. **B,** Ulcerated and ecchymotic lesion on the posterior palate of a male who was holding a Popsicle stick in his mouth when he fell. **C,** Symmetric ulceration and hyperplastic reaction on the anterior palate that was caused by a suction cup on a denture.   (**C** courtesy A.C.W. Hutchinson collection, Northwestern University Dental School Library, Chicago.)

agent has been eliminated, and most heal within 10 days. Occasionally, however, a lesion persists for some weeks because of continued traumatic insults or continued irritation by the oral liquids or because of the development of a secondary infection. This last occasion often indicates the presence of a lowered resistance from an underlying systemic disease.

In our experience, coating the ulcerated surface of the persistent traumatic ulcers and the less serious varieties with triamcinolone acetonide in emollient (Kenalog in Orabase) before bedtime and after meals usually relieves the pain and hastens the healing. The Orabase protects the denuded connective tissue from continued contamination by the oral liquids, and the cortisone component tends to arrest the inflammatory cycle (which may become self-perpetuating).

Persistent ulcers not responding to the foregoing regimen should be surgically excised and closed primarily; the excised tissue must always be microscopically examined, since a persistent ulcer could very likely be a malignant lesion or one of the other benign lesions discussed in this chapter.

RECURRENT APHTHOUS ULCER (CANKER SORE) AND INTRAORAL RECURRENT ULCER OF HERPES SIMPLEX

Until the recent past, much confusion existed concerning recurrent aphthous ulcers (RAUs)* and intraoral recurrent herpes simplex (IRHS) ulcers, despite much research that described these entities. Some investigators consider that the lesions have a common cause and are identical because both share the following characteristics:

1. They are recurrent, painful, superficial oral ulcers that persist 8 to 14 days.
2. They are associated with a tender regional lymphadenopathy.
3. They heal spontaneously, usually without sequelae, in healthy patients.

It is generally agreed now, however, that RAU and IRHS are distinct and separate entities.

Several hypotheses as to the cause of RAU have been proposed; they include psychic, allergic, microbial, traumatic, endocrine, hereditary, and autoimmune mechanisms (Stanley, 1973). Antoon and Miller (1980) updated the knowledge on cause, pathogenesis, diagnosis, and treatment of aphthous ulcers. Wray et al. (1981) reported that mechanical trauma ap-

---

*Sutton's disease, in contrast to the aphthous ulcers, was at one time considered to be a separate entity, since the ulcers are larger and more persistent and characteristically cause scarring. Currently Sutton's disease is thought of as a more severe manifestation of RAU, and the lesions are frequently referred to as major aphthae (Stanley, 1973). In addition, the oral lesions of Behçet's and Reiter's syndromes may be identical with RAU, although they frequently involve the whole mucosa. Consequently these are listed as mucositides in Chapter 6.

peared to play a role in the precipitation of these ulcers. Eversole et al. (1982) reported on a study of patients with RAUs who were challenged with foods they thought might be causing their ulcers. No causative effect was found with regard to tomatoes, strawberries, or walnuts. Hay and Reade (1984) reported that the results of their study clearly indicated that some food components contributed to the cause of some cases of recurrent aphthous ulcers. The inheritance of recurrent aphthous ulcers was investigated by Miller et al. (1980). Their results showed that the incidence of the disease in children was significantly higher when RAUs were present in one or both parents. Ship (1966) reported that recurrent aphthous ulcers occurred more commonly in patients from higher socioeconomic groups.

Studies concerning the importance of routinely determining vitamin B_{12} and folate levels in these patients have yielded conflicting results. Tyldesley (1983) reported that he found several RAU patients with decreased folate levels. Olson et al. (1982) failed to find significantly lower serum levels of vitamin B_{12} or folate in RAU patients as compared with patients in control groups. Currently it seems likely that the RAUs develop as a result of several different mechanisms. Rennie et al. (1985) summarized the various possibilities concerning cause. Studies showing shifts in immune balance are numerous (Lindemann, 1985; Savage et al., 1985, 1986, 1988; Schroeder et al., 1984). Ferguson et al. (1984) reported that the highest incidence occurred in menstruating women.

In addition, it is generally agreed that the usual IRHS ulcers are secondary lesions produced by the herpesvirus and are the counterpart of herpes labialis. This means that patients have been primarily infected with the herpesvirus, and although a small percentage may experience the more severe primary herpetic stomatitis, the majority of the initial infections must be subclinical or minor manifestations. Although primary herpetic gingivostomatitis has been considered primarily a disease of children, Main (1989) has reported that IRHS ulcers are more prevalent during the third decade of life. In patients who have recurrent lesions only occasionally, the lesions recur in the same location, whereas in those who have frequent recurrences, the lesions recur in different locations (Davis et al., 1988). This disease is discussed in greater detail in Chapter 6.

Using serum complement fixation and neutralizing antibody techniques, Brooks et al. (1981) studied the prevalence of herpes simplex viral disease in a dental professional population. These authors reported that almost all the subjects with a history of herpetic infection did show antibodies to herpes simplex virus (HSV) and that 57% of those lacking such a history had a significant level of antibodies to HSV.

The *herpetic whitlow* is an occupational disease of practicing dentists and dental workers (Rowe et al., 1982; Merchant et al., 1983). This infection of the fingers with HSV may be contracted by working on a patient who has a herpetic lesion of the lips or oral cavity. Such infections of the fingers may be recurrent and may also spread to the rest of the hand (Merchant et al., 1983). As a preventive measure Rowe et al. (1982) recommended that dental treatment be delayed until the patient's active herpetic lesion is healed; if this is not possible, they advised use of a rubber dam and disposable rubber gloves and autoclaving of both these items before discarding. Safety glasses are commonly used to guard against herpetic infections of the eye.

Shillitoe and Silverman (1979) reviewed the literature on the question of HSV being a possible etiologic agent in oral cancer. Primary herpetic gingivostomatitis is discussed in Chapter 6.

Features

The RAU and IRHS ulcers may be clearly differentiated on a clinical basis by referring to the contrasting features summarized by Weathers and Griffin (1970) (Figs. 11-4 and 11-5, and Table 11-1).

The senior author (N.K.W.) has observed cases of IRHS that carry an atypical history. In the usual course of events the lesions appear, regress, and heal within 4 to 10 days. In these atypical cases, however, the lesions may appear without remission for as long as 2 or 3 months. In some of these cases the patient has reported that the lesions are constantly present but have shifted location during the course of the disease. Necrotic tissue and uncharacteristic ulceration are usually present in these cases, which characteristically occur on the attached gingiva. Actually, close scrutiny with a magnifying glass is required to observe one or several punched-out, pinpoint ulcerations. In such cases the lesions usually disappear within 2 weeks after the institution of a regimen of tetracycline mouthwash, which eradicates the secondary bacterial infection and permits healing. The patients are also requested not to brush their teeth in the lesional area until the lesions have completely regressed. We believe that these cases represent recurrent herpes infec-

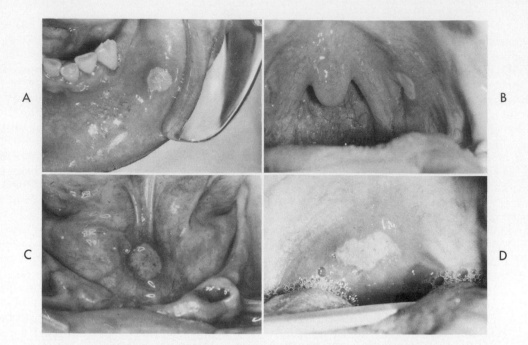

Fig. 11-4. Recurrent aphthous ulcers. **A** to **C**, Typical lesions that disappeared within 14 days. **D**, Major aphtha (Sutton's disease) that persisted for several months.

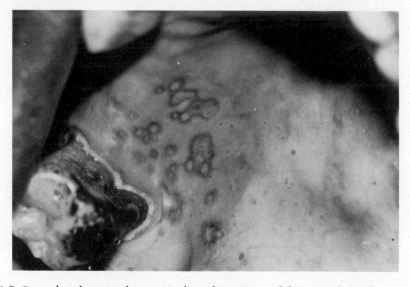

Fig. 11-5. Secondary herpetic lesions on the palate. Some of the several, small, punctate ulcers have coalesced to form larger ulcers.   (Courtesy P. Akers, DDS, Chicago.)

tions and that the prolonged uncharacteristic course occurs because the patient is carrying HSV from the original gingival lesion on the toothbrush and is infecting the neighboring gingiva. This process may be repeated several times. Actually, a protracted course of continual lesional development is occurring in these patients.

The features of IRHS described in the preceding paragraph are different from those described by Cohen and Greenberg (1985) in their study of immunocompromised patients. These researchers reported that IRHS in their patients featured ulcers with white vesicular borders. The ulcers continued to enlarge until treated. Barrett (1986), discussing the problem

Table 11-1. Comparison of features of recurrent aphthous ulcers (RAU) and intraoral recurrent herpes simplex (IRHS) ulcers

	RAU	*IRHS*
Age	Wide range	Any age but more common in middle and older age-groups
Location	On freely movable mucosa (nonkeratinized), lips, buccal mucosa, tongue, mucobuccal fold, floor of mouth, soft palate (Fig. 11-4)	On fixed mucosa; tightly bound to periosteum (keratinized), hard palate, gingiva, and alveolar ridge (Fig. 11-5)
Initial lesion	Erythematous macule or papule; undergoes central blanching followed by necrosis and ulceration	Cluster of small, discrete, gray or white vesicles without red erythematous halo; vesicles quickly rupture, forming small punctate ulcers 1 mm or less in diameter
Mature lesion	Shallow ulcer 0.5 to 2 or 3 cm in diameter; yellow necrotic center; regular border; constant erythematous halo	Shallow ulcer no larger than 0.5 cm in diameter; several lesions may coalesce to form large lesion, usually not larger than 0.5 cm in diameter
Number of lesions	Usually occur singly; occasionally two or three widely distributed (Fig. 11-4)	Usually several small, punctate ulcers in cluster in small localized area (Fig. 11-5); regular border, usually round; variable erythematous halo
Histology	Mature lesion: nonspecific ulcer	Early lesion: vesicular fluid contains epithelial cells with balloon degeneration, multinucleated giant cells, and virus particles Mature lesion: after third day, nonspecific ulcer

of infection with HSV in patients with acute leukemia, reported an incidence of 40% in those patients. Flaitz and Hammond (1988) reported that infection with HSV occurred in 80% of patients who received bone marrow transplants.

Patient history, clinical features, and results from laboratory tests contribute to the diagnosis of RAU and IRHS. Cytologic smears and viral cultures have been used routinely and are discussed by Barrett et al. (1986). Recently the use of monoclonal antibody typing systems (Fox et al., 1987) and cytologic smears in combination with immunoperoxidase techniques has been reported, and results are encouraging. The difficulty with all diagnostic techniques is that the viruses are shed quickly after vesicles rupture.

Differential diagnosis

Application of the criteria in Table 11-1 enables the clinician to differentiate between RAU and IRHS in most cases. Of course, if other body surfaces are involved, the various syndromes mentioned earlier must be considered.

Herpangina and hand-foot-mouth disease are two other conditions that must be differenti-ated from IRHS lesions. Herpangina is an infectious disease that is caused by a coxsackievirus A that usually affects children in the late summer and early fall. The patients show fever, general malaise, and viral lesions of the soft palate and fauces. These viral lesions are multiple, vesicular, and distributed over a reddened soft palate. Like herpes they rupture quickly. Their localization to the soft palate usually distinguishes them from herpes, which seldom involves the soft palate except in patients who are receiving immunosuppressive drugs.

Hand-foot-mouth disease is also caused by a coxsackievirus A (various strains). As described by Germishuys (1980), children under 10 years of age are usually affected. Characteristic symptoms of a systemic viral disease occur, such as fever, malaise, nausea, and diarrhea. The feature that distinguishes hand-foot-mouth disease from primary intraoral herpes or recurrent intraoral herpes is that the vesiculoulcerative lesions occur simultaneously in the oral cavity (hard palate, gingiva, and tongue) and on the hands and feet.

A further discussion of the distinguishing features of similar-appearing intraoral ulcers is presented in the differential diagnosis section at the end of this chapter (pp. 215-219). For a discussion of generalized oral ulcerations or mucositides, see Chapter 6.

Management

Except for the major aphthae, RAU and IRHS resolve in 8 to 14 days without treatment. For the treatment of aphthous ulcers, Stanley (1973) recommends a tetracycline mouthwash (an oral suspension of uncoated Achromycin crystals, 250 mg/tsp, in 5 ml water) to be flushed over the affected region for at least 2 minutes. After debridement with the tetracycline mouthwash, the ulcer is coated by a thick layer of triamcinolone acetonide in emollient dental paste (Kenalog in Orabase) after meals and before bed. Systemic analgesics are administered if necessary. We have found this regimen to give very satisfactory results but usually reserve the use of tetracycline for multiple ulcers or major aphthae. Wray (1982) administered systemic zinc sulfate to 25 patients with RAU. He reported that no therapeutic effect was seen during a 3-month period. Hunter and Addy (1987) reported that ulcer duration was shortened when chlorhexidine mouthwash was used. Recently a new hydroxypropyl cellulose material (Zilactin) has been used effectively in the treatment of RAU (Rodu and Lakeman, 1988; Rodu and Russell, 1988; Rodu et al., 1988).

Major aphthous ulcers are difficult to treat. The patients often have had these painful nonhealing ulcers for months. The following modalities have been used with some success: excision with primary closure, cryosurgery, topical application of tetracycline followed by cortisone ointment, and injection of cortisol or cortisone directly into the lesion in combination with systemic administration of cortisone. Various procedures (for example, cryotherapy, photochemical activation) have been used to treat herpetic lesions, with varying results. Currently, photochemical activation is not recommended. Theoretically, Kenalog in Orabase should not be applied to IRHS, since the corticosteroid may contribute to the dissemination of the virus, but to date we have not observed any such sequelae, nor are we aware that any have been reported.

Various topical agents have been advocated, but benefits have not been consistent: ether and aqueous neutral red in conjunction with fluorescent light are two of the methods. Also large doses of lysine have been advocated to shorten the duration of the lesions and suppress recurrences. This approach has given equivocal results. Thein and Hurt (1984) suggested that prophylactic lysine may be useful in managing selected cases of recurrent herpes simplex labialis if serum lysine levels can be maintained at adequate concentrations.

The fraudulent nucleoside, idoxuridine (Stoxil), has proved beneficial when used topically as a 0.5% ophthalmic ointment in treatment of herpetic infections of the eye. Unfortunately, this drug has not been successful in treating herpes labialis or IRHS lesions.

Chemotherapeutic antiviral agents have been introduced that demonstrate success against HSV infections: vidarabine (Vira-A), acyclovir (Zovirax), foscarnet, and Ara-ADA (Food and Drug Administration, 1978-1979; Rowe et al., 1979; Pallasch et al., 1984). Vidarabine has been extremely successful, when given intravenously, in reducing the high mortality rate of patients with herpes simplex encephalitis. Rowe et al. (1979) used this drug to treat patients with herpes labialis. The drug was applied in ointment form, as a 3% vidarabine concentration in water-miscible gel. Beneficial results were minimal.

Acyclovir (Zovirax) has been shown to be effective against HSV-2 and is approved for use in the treatment of initial genital herpes (Pallasch et al., 1984). This agent is available for intravenous use and in ointment or capsule form. Results of the use of acyclovir ointment in the treatment of herpes labialis have been disappointing (Spruance and Crumpacker, 1982).

Forscarnet and Ara-ADA are two of several new experimental drugs that show effectiveness against herpes virus and are undergoing further testing (Pallasch et al., 1984). MacPhail et al. (1989) reported the effectiveness of foscarnet in a patient resistant to acyclovir. Results with acyclovir have been variable depending on dosage and mode of administration (topical 5% ointment, tablets, intravenous [IV] route). In immunosuppressed patients, IV administration is usually successful (Cawson, 1986; Cohen and Greenberg, 1985). Topical ointment has been ineffective in the treatment of herpes labialis (Raborn et al, 1989). Patients with herpes labialis who took 200 mg of acyclovir in tablet form 5 times a day showed some improvement (Raborn et al, 1987), but it was suggested that a higher dose may be more effective.

Partridge and Poswillo (1984) reported that the topical use of carbenoxolone in the management of herpetic gingivostomatitis and herpes labialis markedly reduced the healing time and pain associated with these lesions.

ULCERS FROM ODONTOGENIC INFECTIONS

Ulcers resulting from the drainage of pus from odontogenic infections are easily recognized. Two similar clinical situations can cause them: the ulcer may serve as the cloacal opening of a sinus draining a chronic alveolar abscess, or the ulcer may be the site of a superficial space abscess that has spontaneously ruptured.

Features

In most cases of chronic alveolar abscess, the ulcer is on the alveolar ridge on either the buccal or the lingual surface, usually near the mucobuccal fold, but occasionally it is on the palate (Figs. 11-6 and 13-6). The majority of chronic alveolar abscesses are seen in children of less than 14 years of age. Such draining sinuses and similar pathoses are discussed in detail in Chapter 13, so they are not considered here.

Other ulcers may represent the ruptured surface of an odontogenic space abscess situated on the palate or in the sublingual or vestibular areas (Fig. 11-6). Pressure on the adjacent soft tissue causing pus to exude from the ulcer identifies the condition. If odontogenic infection is suspected, a thorough clinical radiologic examination of the teeth and supporting structures almost always provides enough information to enable the examiner to either identify or rule out an odontogenic infection.

Should the results of the examination be equivocal, a gutta-percha point may be placed in the ulcer and passed into the tract as far as it will go without undue force. A radiograph may then be taken. If the ulcer is a cloaca of an alveolar abscess, the point frequently extends to the apex of an infected tooth.

Differential diagnosis

The odontogenic ulcer can be misdiagnosed only as the result of a cursory or careless examination. When a small ulcer (0.2 to 1 cm in diameter) is present on the mucosa of the palate, alveolus, or vestibule, an odontogenic ulcer must always be considered a likely possibility. Two other, less likely possibilities are sinus openings from osteomyelitis and infected malignant tumors. A more thorough discussion may be found in the differential diagnosis section at the end of this chapter (pp. 215-219).

Management

Endodontic therapy or extraction, which on occasion may have to be accompanied by the

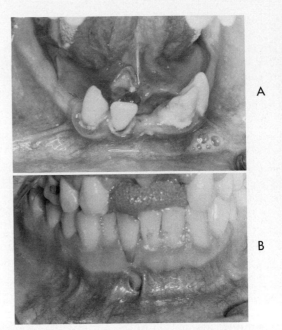

Fig. 11-6. Odontogenic ulcers. **A,** Sublingual abscess from the infected lateral incisor ruptured to produce this ulcer. **B,** The ulcer represents the oral opening of a draining chronic alveolar abscess from the pulpless lower incisor.

administration of antibiotics, usually results in the healing of the ulcer.

SLOUGHING, PSEUDOMEMBRANOUS ULCERS

Sloughing, pseudomembranous ulcers, described in detail in Chapter 8, are mentioned here because they are shown to have an ulcerated surface when the membrane is removed. Such lesions include crushing types of traumatic ulcers, acute necrotic ulcerative gingivitis (ANUG), candidiasis, and gangrenous stomatitis.

ANUG is the most common example of such lesions, and the fact that the necrotic and ulcerative process involves one or more of the tips of the interdental papillae is practically pathognomonic for the disease. However, similar lesions may be seen on the gingivae accompanying other oral lesions such as diffuse gangrenous stomatitis (Chapter 8).

GENERALIZED MUCOSITIDES AND VESICULOBULLOUS DISEASES

Generalized mucositides and vesiculobullous diseases have been included here, because even though singly the entities may be uncommon to rare, as a group they are relatively common. Although the diseases produce oral ulcerations, the ulcerations are secondary to primary mucositides and vesicular and bullous lesions. Thus in most cases the whole mucosal surface of the oral cavity is a mass of ulcers, blebs, and erosive erythematous areas. A list of such diseases includes the following:

Behçet's syndrome
Erosive lichen planus
Erythema multiforme
Primary herpetic gingivostomatitis
Gangrenous stomatitis
Stevens-Johnson syndrome
Vesiculobullous lesions (benign mucous membrane pemphigoid, bullous lichen planus, cat-scratch disease, epidermolysis bullosa, herpangina, herpes zoster, pemphigus and its variants, foot-and-mouth disease, hand-foot-mouth disease)

Some of these more common diseases are discussed in detail in Chapter 6. Their usually wide dissemination in the oral cavity precludes their being misdiagnosed as one of the discrete, frequently solitary ulcers discussed in this chapter, however. They are included here mainly because a solitary lesion may precede the more severe manifestations of the disease and thus be confused with the solitary ulcers that are the subject of this chapter.

SQUAMOUS CELL CARCINOMA

Squamous cell carcinoma is the most common oral malignancy and represents approximately 90% to 95% of all malignant tumors that occur in the mouth and jaws. It is discussed as a red lesion in Chapter 5, a white lesion in Chapter 8, a red and white lesion in Chapter 9, and an exophytic lesion in Chapter 10. In this chapter the ulcerative variety is stressed.

Although the cause of squamous cell carcinoma is unknown, chronic irritation from the use of tobacco products, alcohol, and other carcinogens either singly or in combination may trigger a malignant change in a genetically and systemically conditioned oral mucosa. The combination of heavy smoking and high consumption of alcohol is a particularly deadly combination of irritants involved in the development of oral carcinoma. Blot et al. (1988) reported a 35-fold increase in risk in heavy smokers and drinkers. Luce et al. (1988) reported different rates of risk for different oral sites in smokers, nondrinkers and drinkers, and nonsmokers. Actinic radiation and other ionizing agents also induce such malignant changes. Shillitoe and Silverman (1979), Scully (1983), and Kassim and Daley (1988) reviewed the current knowledge concerning the association of herpes simplex virus with oral cancer. They concluded that although there may be an association, a cause-and-effect relationship has yet to be established. Eskinazi (1987) discussed the potential of sexually transmitted viruses to cause oral cancer. Syrjanen et al. (1988) related the possible association of human papillomavirus with oral cancer. Whereas Weaver et al. (1979) offered evidence that pointed to the possible etiologic role of mouthwashes in the production of oral cancer, Blot et al. (1983a, 1982b), Wynder and Kabat (1983), and Wynder et al. (1983) obtained inconclusive results and recommended additional studies. Mashberg et al. (1985) were unable to find a correlation between the use of mouthwash and oral cancer.

Reif (1981) discussed the causes of cancer in general. Binnie et al. (1983) reviewed the current thoughts on the cause of oral squamous cell carcinoma. Silverman et al. (1983) discussed tobacco usage in patients with head and neck carcinomas, reporting that of 166 patients, 73% used tobacco (90% smoked cigarettes). These workers further reported that 30% of patients who did not change their tobacco habit showed second primary cancers. Reduction or discontinuation of smoking appeared to lower the risk of a secondary primary cancer.

Scully (1982) discussed the immunologic response to cancers of the head and neck, with particular reference to oral cancer.

At one time, implicating chronic mechanical trauma (sharp teeth or denture flanges) as a cause of intraoral squamous cell carcinoma was fashionable, but statistical studies have failed to confirm a relationship between chronic mechanical injury and this type of ulcer (Spouge, 1973, p. 394). We have not observed a squamous cell carcinoma in which mechanical trauma alone could be implicated. However, we have developed the clinical impression that squamous cell carcinoma does occur more frequently in septic mouths.

Features

Squamous cell carcinoma is the most common persistent ulcer to occur in the oral cavity or on the lips. Because it is almost always painless, the patient usually is not aware of its presence until it has become relatively advanced. Consequently the smaller ulcerative tumors are found during routine oral examinations.

In the United States, squamous cell carcinoma of the oral cavity and lips occurs approximately two times as frequently in men as in women, but this ratio is decreasing. Although it may affect any age-group, it is predominantly a disease of the middle aged and elderly populations. The classic ulcerative squamous cell carcinoma is described as a craterlike lesion having a velvety red base and a rolled indurated border (Figs. 11-7 and 11-8). If situated on the vermilion border, it may be covered with a crust because of the absence of saliva (Fig. 11-7, *A*). The intraoral ulcer is usually devoid of necrotic material.

When the tumor has infiltrated the surrounding connective tissue, the base and borders of the lesion are firm to palpation. When it is situated on a mucosal surface that is usually freely movable and it has infiltrated the deeper tissues, the mucosa is fixed to the deeper structures. When this occurs in specific locations, such as the undersurface of the tongue, the function of the organ may be im-

paired. In the case of an affected tongue, an alteration in speech is detectable.

The lower lip (95% of labial lesions are on the lower lip) and the tongue (especially the lateral borders and ventral surface) are the most frequent sites of occurrence of oral squamous cell carcinoma. (A large percentage of tongue carcinomas, however, are not ulcerative but are leukoplakial or erythroplakial.) The floor of the mouth, alveolar gingivae, retromolar area, buccal mucosa, and palate (soft palate or the region at the junction of the hard and soft palates) are also frequently involved. The anterior hard palate appears to be immune to squamous cell carcinoma.

A U-shaped section of the oval cavity identifies the mucosal sites at which most of the intraoral squamous cell carcinomas occur. These include the floor of mouth, ventral and lateral

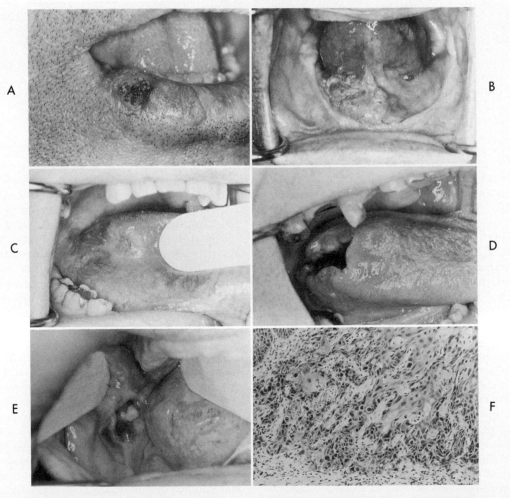

Fig. 11-7. Ulcerative squamous cell carcinomas. **F**, Photomicrograph of a poorly differentiated squamous cell carcinoma.   (**A** courtesy R. Oglesby, DDS, Chicago.)

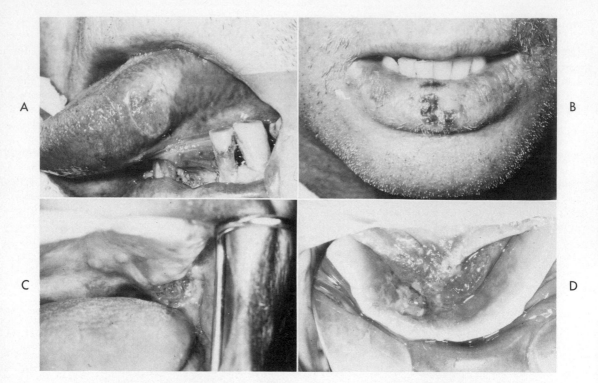

Fig. 11-8. Ulcerative squamous cell carcinomas. **A,** Lateral border of tongue associated with leukoplakia. **B,** Median region of vermilion border. **C,** Posterior to tuberosity in the left maxilla. **D,** Floor of the mouth and anterior ridge in the right incisor region. The ulcerated lesion is associated with a large erythroplakic patch on the floor of the mouth.   (**A, B,** and **D** courtesy J. Lehnert, DDS, Minneapolis.)

borders of the tongue, retromolar areas, tonsillar pillars, and lateral soft palate.

Lesions are usually solitary but in some cases have been multifocal. Eighteen percent of patients in the series of Silverman et al. (1983) showed the development of a second primary tumor. In the series of Ildstad et al. (1983) 23% of the patients showed the development of a second primary tumor. DeVries et al. (1986) reported that 17.6% of their patients had second primary tumors.

Intraoral carcinomas characteristically spread to the regional cervical lymph nodes, of which the submaxillary, superficial, and deep cervical nodes are the most commonly affected. In some cases contralateral nodes may be involved. In an extensive study of 898 cases of oral and oropharyngeal squamous cell carcinomas, Shear et al. (1976) reported statistics concerning lymph node metastasis. These investigators illustrated that poorly differentiated tumors have a markedly higher metastatic rate than well-differentiated or moderately differentiated tumors. (Crissman et al. [1980] reported, however, that depth of invasion appears to be

the only prognostic factor for lymph node metastases.) In addition, their study showed that lesions of the posterior third of the tongue or oropharynx have a higher tendency to metastasize than those that occur on the anterior two thirds of the tongue. In turn, this latter group show a higher tendency to metastasize than tumors that occur on the lips, oral floor, cheek mucosa, hard palate, and gingiva. Shingaki et al. (1988) concluded that depth of invasion is an important prognostic factor. Urist et al. (1987), reporting the same conclusion, added that tumor thickness is also an important factor.

Crissman et al. (1980), studying patients with squamous cell carcinoma of the floor of the mouth, reported that earlier lesions such as T1 and T2 lesions (for the staging of lesions, see p. 208) have little or no propensity for regional lymph node metastasis, whereas larger, deeper infiltrating tumors staged as T3 and T4 have a high frequency of regional lymph node metastasis. Crissman warned of inaccuracy of clinical findings of metastatic nodes when examining the neck. He found that 6 of 25 patients with no clinically detectable nodes had metastatic tumor on histologic examination. Conversely, 8 of 18 patients who showed lymph node metastasis on clinical examination were shown not to have metastatic tumor on histologic examination. These findings demonstrate that even experienced head and neck tumor surgeons are unable to tell, most of the time, whether enlarged nodes are inflammatory or metastatic. It is helpful to consider that almost all adults have at least one benign hyperplastic node, which is a smoothly contoured, firm, and freely movable mass. The clinician may incorrectly diagnose this common entity as metastatic carcinoma.

Distant metastasis from head and neck cancer occurs in a significant percentage of patients. Papac (1984) reported that 30.7% of 169 patients with *advanced* cancers of the head and neck had distant metastasis. Postmortem findings, as well as findings from extensive premortem workups, were used in the study. Floor of the mouth lesions and tongue lesions showed a distant metastasis rate of 11.8% and 13.5%, respectively. The most frequent organs involved with distant metastasis were ranked in decreasing order: lung, bone, liver, gastrointestinal tract, brain, skin, and kidney. In this study 74% of the metastases were found in patients who had lesions staged as T3 to T4; 26% were from patients with T2 lesions.

On microscopic examination the intraoral squamous cell carcinoma may vary in degree of malignancy from a low grade with excellent differentiation to an anaplastic, high grade with poor or no differentiation.

The low-grade malignancy demonstrates a high degree of normal maturation of the basal cells up through the stratum corneum. Projecting fingers and nests of epithelium are seen at the borders of the ulcer infiltrating the subepithelial connective tissue. The fingers of epithelial tissue show malignant changes that may include increased numbers of mitotic figures, hyperchromatism, prominent or multiple nucleoli, an increased ratio of nucleus size to cell size, pleomorphism of the cells in size and shape, individual cell keratinization, keratin pearls deep to the epithelial surface, and a diminution or loss of intercellular bridges (Fig. 11-7, *F*).

The anaplastic, high-grade malignancy, on the other hand, shows no maturation of the cells. Identifying the tissue of origin may be difficult or even impossible. The malignant characteristics just mentioned in connection with the well-differentiated type are more prominent and severe, except that intracellular

keratinization and keratin pearls may not be present.

Varying degrees of malignancy may be present in the same tumor. Oral pathologists usually identify the degree of malignancy by characterizing the tumor as well-differentiated, moderately differentiated, poorly differentiated, or anaplastic.

Differential diagnosis

Ulcerative squamous cell carcinoma is classified as a persistent ulcer; a discussion of its distinguishing features may be found under the differential diagnosis of persistent ulcers at the end of this chapter (pp. 215-219).

Management

Early detection and treatment of oral cancer are mandatory. Unfortunately, valuable time often is lost before these two processes are accomplished. Bruun's study (1976) of 34 patients with oral cancer indicated the magnitude of the problem. This investigator reported that the average time delay between the onset of symptoms and the patient's initial professional examination was 4.9 months. A second statistic was even more alarming: the average additional delay between detection and correct diagnosis (treatment) was 5.6 months.

When a suspect ulcer is discovered on the oral mucosa, it should be observed carefully to determine whether it is transient. If it does not show signs of regressing within 2 weeks, a biopsy should be performed. Of course, if the suspicion index is high during the initial visit, immediate arrangements should be made to perform a biopsy of the lesion or the patient should be referred to a specialist without delay.

Preferably, an excisional biopsy should be performed, including a generous border of normal tissue. If the size of the lesion precludes excisional biopsy and the clinician suspects that the lesion is cancerous, the patient should be referred to a board of tumor specialists or a surgeon who is competent to undertake the complete management of the case.

As a rule, an incisional biopsy of a highly suspect lesion should not be performed until the patient has been prepared for resection. A frozen section should then be taken and examined to determine whether the lesion is malignant and the extent of the resection that should immediately follow the biopsy, depending on the proved nature of the lesion. This approach helps to eliminate a prolonged waiting period between the incisional biopsy and the resection.

The tumor board may decide that the particular lesion should be treated by surgical excision (with possibly a complete or partial neck dissection), by presurgical or postsurgical radiation (Ampil et al., 1988; Nair et al., 1988), by chemotherapy, or by a combination of these procedures. The current status of radiation therapy in the treatment of oral cancer has been reviewed by Vermund et al. (1974). Cryosurgery has been used in the treatment of intraoral carcinoma. Chemotherapy is gaining acceptance as a useful modality in the treatment of advanced squamous cell carcinoma of the head and neck. This approach used to be considered palliative only. However, Pennacchio et al. (1982) found that more patients survived when two chemotherapeutic agents in combination with surgery or radiation therapy or both were used than when radiation therapy was used alone. The agents most frequently considered in treatment of head and neck carcinoma are methotrexate, cyclophosphamide, vinblastine, doxorubicin (Adriamycin), 5-fluorouracil, bleomycin, and cis-platinum (Gumprecht and Jafek, 1980). Olasz et al. (1988) reported encouraging results using combined chemotherapy, and Vikram and Farr (1983) reviewed the use of chemotherapy.

Patterson (1979) reported the use of electrocoagulation (disk electrode) in the treatment of intraoral cancer. Of 25 patients treated in this manner, 11 survived for more than 5 years, 8 died of other disease, and only 6 died of recurrent tumor. Laser surgery is being used more and more frequently in the management of oral cancer. Nagorsky and Sessions (1987) discussed the use of laser surgery in cases of early tumors.

A summary comment regarding treatment of squamous cell carcinoma is in order. It is generally agreed that complete surgical excision of T1 and most T2 lesions without metastasis is the treatment of choice if the patient is a good surgical risk. Larger T2, T3, and T4 lesions are generally managed with a combined approach. The 5-year survival rate for patients with T1 and T2 lesions that show no clinical evidence of metastasis is approximately 67%, whereas the 5-year survival rate of patients with carcinomas that have metastasized is approximately 37%. The overall 5-year survival rate for all oral cancer patients is approximately 40% (American Cancer Society, 1984).

Management of the posttreatment period is important. Spouge (1973, p. 401) recommended the removal of any local irritation, with specific attention to the five "S's": smoking, spirits, spices, sepsis, and syphilis. A complete examination is necessary every 4 to 6 months to detect the recurrence of the tumor at the earliest possible date.

Close cooperation among the physician, dentist, and patient is necessary so that radiation caries is minimized. The combination of meticulous oral hygiene, frequent dental examination, and daily self-application of topical fluoride has given gratifying results (Carl et al., 1972; Levin, 1984).

If extractions are necessary before radiation therapy is initiated, a generous alveolectomy should be completed in the extraction site so that a good mucosal coverage may be accomplished. This helps reduce the incidence of osteoradionecrosis (osteomyelitis) after radiation therapy. This aspect of treatment is covered in detail in Chapter 25.

A 5-year survival rate may be predicted statistically for patients with a carcinoma, and this average expectancy can be anticipated to be altered by specific therapeutic modes. The prognosis of an individual lesion of ulcerative squamous cell carcinoma, however, can be determined only on the basis of the distinctive features of that particular tumor.

The assessment of a particular lesion has been referred to as "clinical staging" (Shafer et al., 1983, p. 111). The staging of an individual lesion is determined by such considerations as the following:

1. Size and extent of the primary lesion
2. Degree of infiltration by the primary lesion
3. Presence or absence of metastases to regional lymph nodes
4. Presence or absence of distant metastases
5. Involvement of contralateral or ipsilateral nodes
6. Whether or not nodes are fixed

Tumors are classified by primary tumor (T), cervical lymph node (N), and distant metastasis (M) according to the TNM staging categories described by Shafer et al. (1983) (Baker, 1983).

The T (primary tumor) categories are as follows:

T1—Greatest diameter of primary tumor is 2 cm or less

T2—Greatest diameter of primary tumor is more than 2 cm but not more than 4 cm

T3—Greatest diameter of primary tumor is more than 4 cm

T4—Massive tumor of more than 4 cm involves adjacent structures

The N (cervical lymph node) categories are as follows:

N0—No clinically positive nodes

N1—Single clinically positive homolateral node 3 cm or less in diameter

N2—Single clinically positive homolateral node more than 3 cm but not more than 6 cm in diameter, or multiple clinically positive homolateral nodes, none more than 6 cm in diameter

N3—Massive homolateral node(s), bilateral nodes, or contralateral node(s)

The M (distant metastasis) categories are as follows:

M0—No (known) distant metastasis

M1—Distant metastasis present—specify site(s)

In addition to providing the clinician with information that contributes to a more accurate prognosis of an individual lesion, clinical staging provides the clinician with a systematic basis for selecting the most appropriate mode of treatment—whether surgery, radiation therapy, radium, or a combination of irradiation and surgery.

The anatomic site of the lesion modifies the prognosis (staging) markedly, as does the degree of histologic differentiation.* For instance, in regard to anatomic location, a lesion on the lower lip has the best prognosis, whereas a lesion on the posterior third of the tongue has the poorest. The degree of differentiation must be modified on the basis of the lesion's other features: a poorly differentiated carcinoma that is restricted to a primary site has a better prognosis than does a well-differentiated lesion that has already metastasized to a lymph node. Langdon et al. (1977) reported on a study of 131 cases of intraoral cancer, corroborating that site and histodifferentiation are indeed important factors in prognosis. They suggested a new classification for oral cancer, the STNMP system, in which "S" stands for site and "P" stands for histopathology.

Crissman et al. (1980) contended that degree of differentiation was not a significant factor in predicting lymph node metastasis. Platz et al. (1983) pointed out inadequacies of the TNM system as a prognosticator. Factors that have proved to be prognostically relevant are (1) tumor size, (2) degree of infiltration, (3) degree of histologic differentiation, (4) site, (5) combination of evidence + clinical appearance + degree of fixation of the regional lymph nodes, (6) age of the patient, and (7) evidence of distant metastasis (Platz et al., 1983).

SYPHILIS (CHANCRE AND GUMMA)

Syphilis is a venereal disease caused by the motile spirochete *Treponema pallidum;* it may be congenital or acquired. The untreated acquired form has three easily recognizable stages:

1. The primary lesion is the *chancre*, which is usually solitary.
2. The secondary lesions are numerous *macules, papules, mucous patches,* or *condylomas* or combinations of these.
3. The tertiary (oral) lesions are *gummas* and *interstitial glossitis.*

The mucous patch is a grayish white, sloughing lesion and has been included in the list of rarities under sloughing, pseudomembranous, nonkeratotic white lesions in Chapter 8. Both the chancre and the gumma are ulcerated lesions, so they are included here, but because they are completely different lesions from the standpoint of pathogenesis and clinical appearance, they are described separately.

Congenital syphilis may include findings of Hutchinson's incisors, mulberry molars, saddle nose, interstitial keratitis,* and deafness.

Hutchinson's incisors are bell-shaped or screwdriver-shaped central incisors with notches in the middle of their incisal edges. Mulberry molars are first permanent molars that are a little smaller than normal with hypoplasia so severe on the occlusal one third of the teeth that the cusps are dwarfed and the resultant biting surface has a mulberry appearance.

Chancre

Chancres are found on the genitalia in 90% of syphilis patients but may occur on the oral mucous membrane. They develop at the site of inoculation, usually where there is a defect in the surface continuity of the skin or mucosa. The *T. pallidum* organisms are transferred by direct contact with primary or secondary lesions of an infected individual. The chancres develop approximately 3 weeks after inoculation and persist for 3 weeks to 2 months.

---

*Histologic classification of a lesion is not one of the features involved in clinical staging.

*Interstitial keratitis is a diffuse chronic inflammation of the cornea involving the whole thickness of the cornea and is associated with superficial and deep vascularization.

FEATURES

Chancres on the genitalia are characteristically painless.

Oral lesions, on the other hand, almost invariably become painful soon after they ulcerate because of contamination by the oral fluids and flora. A cervical lymphadenitis is almost always present and is usually tender and painful because of the contamination.

The primary oral lesions occur most often on the lips, on the tip of the tongue, in the tonsillar region, or on the gingivae, commencing as small erythematous macules that become papules or small nodules and then ulcerate. Mature chancres measure from 0.5 to 2 cm in diameter and have narrow, copper-colored, slightly raised borders with a reddish brown base, or center (Figs. 11-9 and 11-10). The lesions are ulcerated over nearly their entire surface and have a base that is shiny and usually clear of necrotic material and debris. Occasionally chancres retain white, sloughy material (see Fig. 8-47, A) and have to be differentiated from the other white pseudomembranous ulcers. Chancres occurring on the vermilion border are usually crusted.

The chancres are extremely contagious. They are teeming with spirochetes, which may be detected by means of dark-field microscopy or phase microscopy—the usual methods for examining material from the lesions. These methods are not diagnostic for oral lesions, however, because of the probable contamination of the ulcers by nonpathogenic oral spirochetes; the *T. pallidum* can be positively identified if immobilized by syphilis antiserum.

Screening tests (Kahn, Wassermann, reactive plasma reagin) are used routinely, and although not specific, they are quite sensitive. Consequently, if one of these screening tests gives a positive result, another specific test for the diagnosis of syphilis should be performed, for example, the fluorescent treponemal antibody (FTA) test or the microhemagglutinin antibody (MHA) test, both of which are usually available from the state department of health. Results of serologic tests are usually negative until the chancre has been present for 2 or 3 weeks. If the disease is not treated, the antibody levels rise slowly and remain elevated for the life of the patient. If the patient receives successful treatment in an early stage, antibody levels soon return to normal.

Since the lesions are contaminated by the oral flora, the microscopic examination of a mature oral chancre seldom yields information specific enough to identify the chancre. Hence the microscopic diagnosis is usually "nonspecific" ulcer. Sometimes, however, the characteristic obliterative endarteritis and perivascular cuffing by lymphocytes are apparent deep in the tissue. Silver stain also reveals the presence of numerous spirochetes in the inflamed areas of the biopsy specimen.

DIFFERENTIAL DIAGNOSIS

Because chancres may be present for a period of 3 weeks to 2 months, they must be classified as both short-term and persistent ulcers.

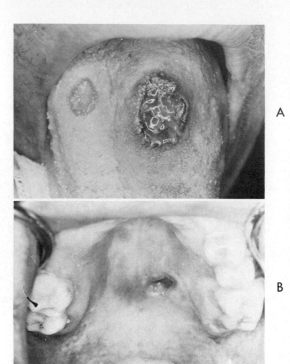

Fig. 11-9. Chancre. **A,** Two lesions on the dorsal surface of the tongue. **B,** Lesion at the junction of the hard and soft palates.

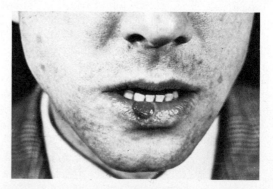

Fig. 11-10. Chancre of the lower lip.   (Courtesy R. Gorlin, DDS, Minneapolis.)

The distinguishing features are discussed in the differential diagnosis section at the end of this chapter (pp. 215-219).

MANAGEMENT

When systemic penicillin is initiated during the primary stage of the disease, in several days it successfully eliminates syphilis in the vast majority of cases.

The multiple secondary lesions of syphilis appear 5 to 6 weeks after the disappearance of the chancres and undergo spontaneous remission within a few weeks, but recurrences may be manifested periodically for months or several years.

Gumma

Although a variety of lesions may occur in different locations during the tertiary stage of untreated syphilis, gummas develop in 33% to 66% of such cases. They are the most common syphilitic lesion seen in the oral cavity (Meyer and Shklar, 1967) and appear to be the result of a type of sensitivity, since the severity of the lesion is vastly out of proportion to the few *Treponema* organisms present.

FEATURES

Intraoral gummas occur most often in the midline of either the palate or the tongue, starting as small, firm, painless, nodular masses and often growing to become several centimeters in diameter. Necrosis commences within the nodules and produces an ulceration of the surface epithelium. The lesions are sharply demarcated, and the necrotic tissue at the base of the ulcers may slough away, leaving a punched-out defect. The semifirm type of necrosis imparts a rubberlike consistency to the nodular, ulcerative masses. On occasion the necrosis is destructive, causing perforation of the palate and formation of a persistent oronasal fistula. The nodular ulcers heal after several months.

On microscopic examination a nonspecific ulcer with an extraordinary amount of necrosis is seen, and occasionally a few giant cells are present. The result of serologic examination at this stage is usually positive and often at a high titer.

DIFFERENTIAL DIAGNOSIS

Gummas may be confused easily with *tubercular lesions, sarcoidosis, granulomatous fungal (mycotic) infections, oral malignancies, necrotizing sialometaplasia,* and the *rare nonhealing midline granuloma.* The differential features are discussed in the differential diagnosis section at the end of this chapter (pp. 215-219).

MANAGEMENT

Patients with gummas should be managed by clinicians who have been trained in all aspects of syphilitic disease because (1) intraoral gummas imply the presence of additional gummas in other locations, which cause more serious complications and (2) treatment must be tailored to minimize the possibility and intensity of the Jarisch-Herxheimer reaction.

ULCERS SECONDARY TO SYSTEMIC DISEASE

The incidence of ulcers that occur secondary to a particular systemic disease is not high enough to warrant the assignment of separate categories to the individual ulcers. However, when all the ulcers that result from such systemic diseases are considered as a group, their combined incidence is high enough to preclude listing them among the rarities.

Such ulcers most often occur in patients with uncontrolled diabetes, uremia, and blood dyscrasias (such as pancytopenia, leukemia, cyclic neutropenia, and sickle cell anemia).

Except in the cases of sickle cell anemia and uremia, the pathogenesis of ulcer formation is similar. The resistance of the host tissue and the leukocytic defense is so diminished that a small break in the integrity of the mucosa becomes superficially infected by the oral flora and an ulcer results. Although a diffuse gangrenous stomatitis may also occur in these diseases (Chapter 8), the discrete ulcers are emphasized in this chapter.

Features

The ulcers are tender or painful, usually well demarcated, and shallow with a narrow erythematous halo; they may contain some yellowish or gray necrotic material. They may vary in size from 0.5 to 2 or 3 cm in diameter. A painful regional cervical lymphadenitis is almost invariably present.

In sickle cell anemia the ulcers form in regions of ischemic infarcts caused by the plugging of small blood vessels by sickle cell thrombi that occurs during the sickle cell crisis. Such ulcers are usually painless and frequently involve the marginal gingivae and interdental papillae (Fig. 11-11).

Ulcers that occur in patients with uremia may also involve the marginal gingivae (Fig. 11-11) or other regions of the oral mucosa.

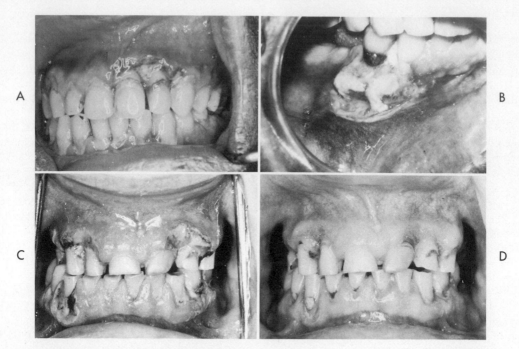

Fig. 11-11. Ulcers in systemic disease. **A,** Gingival ulcer in a patient with sickle cell anemia. **B,** Gingival ulcer in a patient with acute leukemia. **C** and **D,** Ragged, sloughing gingival ulcers in a uremic patient. (**D** was taken 2 weeks after **C.** The uremia had been corrected and a regimen of hydrogen peroxide mouthwashes instituted.) (**A** courtesy R. Dixon, DDS, Chicago. **B** courtesy G. MacDonald, DDS, Belleville, Ill.)

These ulcers are related to (1) the bacterial breakdown of urea (present in high concentrations in the saliva) to ammonia, (2) mouth breathing in acidosis, (3) dehydration, and (4) bacterial or fungal infection.

It has been recognized that oral candidiasis, usually of the pseudomembranous type, is a frequent complication of systemic diseases that decrease the resistance of the patient. However, Tyldesley et al. (1979) drew attention to superficial oral bacterial infections in patients who were taking immunosuppressive drugs after receiving renal transplants. These authors stressed that these superficial bacterial infections looked almost identical to pseudomembranous candidiasis and that only culturing the lesions revealed their true nature.

Differential diagnosis

The distinguishing features of these ulcers secondary to systemic disease are discussed in the differential diagnosis section at the end of this chapter (pp. 215-219).

Management

In the management of oral ulcers secondary to a systemic disease, it is most important that the dental clinician recognize the possibility of a predisposing condition and realize that the condition is basic to the oral problem.

When the patient's history indicates that the suspected systemic disease has not been detected by his or her physician, it is especially important that the dentist seek medical consultation. The dentist and the physician together are able to manage the problem as a team, whereas the oral condition is not likely to respond satisfactorily to local treatment alone. While the physician is treating the systemic disease, the dental clinician initiates procedures to ensure the establishment of the best possible oral hygiene. Toward this end, a regimen of hydrogen peroxide mouth rinses many times a day is recommended (Fig. 11-11). The hydrogen peroxide debrides the ulcerated tissues. In addition, the systemic administration of antibiotics (penicillin) compensates for the patient's diminished defenses and helps control the oral ulcers. It is critical at this juncture to determine whether the pseudomembranous ulcerative lesions are infected with either bacteria or *Candida albicans*.

TRAUMATIZED TUMORS (TYPES USUALLY NOT ULCERATED)

As described in Chapter 3, exophytic growths *originating in tissues separate from and beneath the surface epithelium* characteristically have smoothly contoured, nonulcerated surfaces. Such lesions include benign and malignant mesenchymal tumors, inflammatory hyperplasias, metastatic tumors (situated deep to the surface epithelium), most types of minor salivary gland tumors, and odontogenic tumors. These entities are discussed in detail in Chapter 10 as exophytic lesions. Some of them become ulcerated, so they are included as a group in this chapter. The cause of the ulceration is usually obvious but should always be identified, so the lesion is not confused with a primarily ulcerative lesion.

The ulceration is often the result of mechanical trauma from mastication with ill-fitting dentures. Fig. 11-12, *C*, illustrates a case in which a central ameloblastoma became ulcerated when an extruded upper third molar repeatedly traumatized the posterior mandibular swelling produced by the ameloblastoma. In our experience even malignant mesenchymal tumors almost always have a smooth surface until some traumatic episode causes a surface erosion or ulceration. Such a surface ulceration is frequently the result of an incisional biopsy. Fig. 11-12, *A* and *B*, shows a smooth-surfaced exophytic chondrosarcoma of the maxilla that became necrotic and ulcerated after an incisional biopsy.

In other instances masses of tumor cells interfere with the blood supply of the surface epithelium to such an extent that the epithelium becomes necrotic and ulcerative. Occasionally a tumor mass extrudes from a recent extraction wound, and since the growth does not have an epithelial covering, it soon becomes necrotic and ulcerated because of the irritating nature of the oral environment.

It is important to recognize that these ulcerated lesions are primarily exophytic; their classification as such facilitates their identification.

MINOR SALIVARY GLAND TUMORS

The majority of salivary gland tumors are firm exophytic lesions that seldom ulcerate ex-

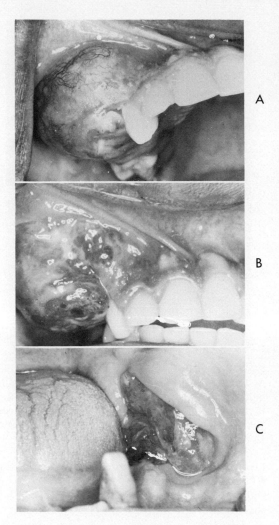

Fig. 11-12. Ulcerated tumors. **A** and **B**, Chondrosarcoma. (**B** was taken 2 weeks after an incisional biopsy of the lesion in **A**.) **C**, Ameloblastoma with an unusual surface ulceration inflicted by an upper molar.   (**A** courtesy R. Nolan, DDS, Waukegan, Ill.)

cept as a result of conditions described in the preceding discussion. Some types of salivary gland tumors, however, *contain quantities of pooled liquid and are relatively soft and fluctuant*. Such lesions include low-grade mucoepidermoid tumor, mucous adenocarcinoma, papillary cyst adenoma, and papillary cystadenoma lymphomatosum (Warthin's tumor). If the collection of fluid is near the surface, the pool eventually ruptures and causes the formation of an ulcerated surface. These tumors may ulcerate at a relatively early stage, even before they have attained sufficient mass to produce an exophytic lesion. They therefore appear as shallow persistent ulcers that can easily be mis-

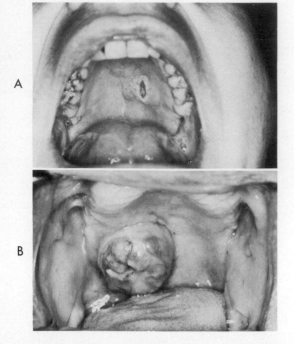

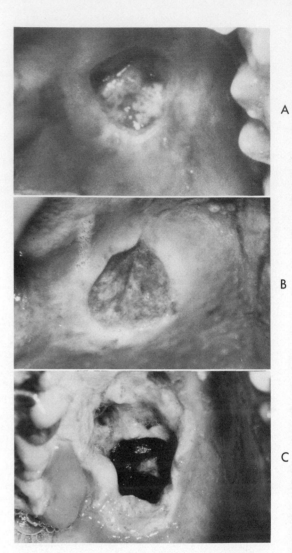

Fig. 11-13. Ulcerated minor salivary gland tumors. **A,** Low-grade mucoepidermoid tumor. **B,** Pleomorphic adenoma 1 week after incisional biopsy. Before the biopsy the surface was smooth and nonulcerated. (**A** courtesy D. Bonomo, DDS Flossmoor, Ill.)

taken for a squamous cell carcinoma (Fig. 11-13). A discussion of these tumors is included in the differential diagnosis section at the end of this chapter (pp. 215-219).

Differential diagnosis

Lesions that should be considered in the differential diagnosis with ulcerated minor salivary gland tumors of the posterior hard palate are squamous cell carcinoma, necrotizing sialometaplasia, midline nonhealing granuloma, chancre, gumma, leukemic ulcer, malignancy of the maxillary sinus, neurotrophic ulcer, traumatic ulcer, and major aphthous ulcer (Fig. 11-4, *D,* and 11-14).

RARITIES

A multitude of rare lesions may occur as oral ulcers. A partial list, arranged in alphabetical order, includes the following (Fig. 11-15):

Actinomycosis
Adenoid squamous cell carcinoma
Basal cell carcinoma
Basidiobolus haptosporus
Botryomycosis hominis
Cancrum oris

Fig. 11-14. **A** and **B,** Two cases of necrotizing sialometaplasia on the palate. **C,** Midline lethal granuloma. (**A** courtesy A. Abrams, DDS, Los Angeles. **B** courtesy C. Dunlap, DDS, and B. Barker, DDS, Kansas City, Mo. **C** courtesy S. Goldman, DDS, Maywood, Ill.)

Crohn's disease
Foot-and-mouth disease
Fungal infections (blastomycosis, coccidioidomycosis, cryptococcosis, histoplasmosis, sporotrichosis)
Gonococcal stomatitis
Granulomatous disease of the newborn
Hand-foot-mouth disease
Herpangina
Herpes zoster
Keratoacanthoma
Midline nonhealing granuloma (midline malignant reticulosis)

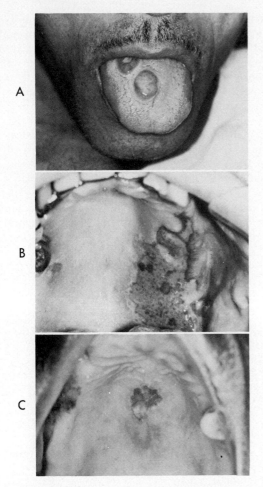

Fig. 11-15. Rare oral ulcers. **A,** Metastatic carcinoma from squamous cell carcinoma of the esophagus in a 46-year-old man. **B,** Benign mucous membrane pemphigoid. **C,** Palatal lesion of psoriasis. (**A** courtesy E. Robinson, DDS, Toledo, Ohio. **B,** courtesy P.D. Toto, DDS, Maywood, Ill. **C** courtesy D. Bonomo, DDS, Flossmoor, Ill.)

Leukemia
Lymphoma
Median rhomboid glossitis—ulcerative variety
Metastatic tumor
Mucormycosis
Mycosis fungoides
Necrotizing sialometaplasia
Neurotrophic ulcer
Phycomycosis
Sarcoidosis
Self-mutilation wounds
Sutton's disease
Syringomyelia
Tuberculosis
Waldenström's macroglobulinemia
Warty dyskeratoma

DIFFERENTIAL DIAGNOSIS OF ORAL ULCERS

Since oral ulcers may be conveniently divided into two groups, short-term (those that usually disappear within 3 weeks) and persistent (those that usually last longer than 3 weeks), it is also convenient to discuss the differential diagnosis of these two groups separately. Nonetheless, both groups have in common that (1) the complaint of *pain in an oral ulcer does not permit* a definite identification of the ulcer, since the majority of oral ulcers, regardless of their cause, soon become painful from contamination by the oral liquids and flora and (2) because of contamination by oral fluids, *a painful regional lymphadenitis almost always accompanies* oral ulcers.

Thus the presence or absence of pain in the ulcer or the associated enlarged nodes is not a conclusive diagnostic feature. Exceptions to this rule are squamous cell carcinoma and other peripheral malignancies, which are characteristically painless early in their course because most of the peripheral sensory nerve endings are destroyed or their surfaces are covered by tumor epithelium. These malignant lesions often do not become painful until they have attained a large size. When metastatic spread to regional lymph nodes has occurred, the enlarged nodes are likewise characteristically painless, as well as quite firm.

Again, it should be emphasized that these characteristics are not diagnostic because such entities as benign lymph node hyperplasias and enlarged fibrosed nodes are usually firm and painless.

Short-term ulcers are shallow lesions; they are not raised above the mucosal surface. In contrast, persistent ulcers are frequently exophytic; in other words, they are frequently situated over a slight nodular, dome-shaped, or plateaulike mass (see Fig. 11-7).

Short-term ulcers

The more common short-term ulcers, ranked according to their approximate frequency of occurrence in the general population, are as follows:

Traumatic ulcer
Recurrent aphthous ulcer and intraoral recurrent herpes simplex lesion
Ulcer occurring as a result of odontogenic infection
Ulcer occurring with generalized mucositis or vesiculobullous disease
Ulcer secondary to systemic disease

With *ulcers secondary to systemic disease* the clinician usually determines this circumstance from the patient's history, if the disease has been previously detected. If the patient is not aware of the predisposing disease, however, a careful history should reveal information that suggests the possibility of a specific disease or group of diseases. For instance, the patient may complain of fatigue, dizziness, and nausea with some of the anemias or of polydipsia and polyuria with diabetes. The patient may have a fever or a paleness of the mucosa, or both, which should alert the clinician to the possibility of one of the anemias, leukemias, or pancytopenias. Appropriate laboratory procedures are invaluable in helping to identify the specific disease. Since there is nothing specific in the appearance of these oral ulcers, the clinician must obtain a complete history and rely on it in every case.

The *single ulcer* that heralds the arrival of any of the *generalized mucositides or vesiculobullous diseases* appears perhaps a few days or weeks before the diffuse nature of the disease manifests itself. A discussion of the differential diagnosis of the oral mucositides is included in Chapter 7.

Ulcers resulting from odontogenic infection are easily diagnosed if the clinician remembers to include them in the differential diagnosis. Although there is no fluctuant painful swelling at this stage, a careful systematic approach identifies the involved tooth from which the infection is draining. The clinician should suspect any small ulcer on the alveolus or palate of being associated with an odontogenic infection. He or she should then attempt to demonstrate the presence of a sinus with a gutta-percha cone and if successful should take a radiograph of the area with the cone in place to determine whether the tract leads to the apex of a tooth. Sometimes digital pressure on the involved tooth or the alveolus causes a drop of pus to be expressed from the opening in the ulcer, and this helps the clinician determine the correct diagnosis.

The *recurrent aphthous ulcers* and *intraoral recurrent herpes simplex lesions* can be differentiated, in most cases, by the criteria listed in Table 11-1. As a general rule, a cluster of small punctate ulcers that is not more than 0.5 cm in diameter and occurs on mucosa that is fixed to periosteum is intraoral recurrent herpetic lesions (hand-foot-mouth disease shows these small ulcers in the three locations). On the other hand, a yellowish ulcer measuring between 0.5 and 2 cm in diameter with a narrow erythematous halo and occurring on a loose mucosal surface is a recurrent aphthous ulcer. This conclusion is made if trauma cannot be implicated and the patient does not have an underlying systemic disease associated with a stomatitis or if an odontogenic infection cannot be identified.

Traumatic ulcers are easily recognized if the clinician can establish the cause of the physical injury. In some cases the origin or nature of the trauma is obscure, and consequently the diagnosis is difficult to establish. Occasionally, traumatic lesions, especially those occurring on the tongue, may persist for weeks; these lesions are discussed with the differential diagnosis of persistent ulcers.

Persistent ulcers

The most common persistent ulcers, ranked according to their approximate incidence in the general population, include the following:

Traumatic ulcer
Ulcer from odontogenic infection
Major aphthous ulcer
Squamous cell carcinoma
Keratoacanthoma
Necrotizing sialometaplasia
Chancre
Gumma
Ulcer secondary to systemic disease
Traumatized tumor that does not usually ulcerate
Low-grade mucoepidermoid tumor
Metastatic tumor

Metastatic tumors to the oral soft tissues are quite uncommon and occur usually in the lower half of the oral cavity. In the absence of a primary tumor elsewhere or symptoms of such, secondary tumors are assigned a low rank on the differential list.

If a cystic area in a *low-grade mucoepidermoid tumor* ruptures, the resemblance to a squamous cell carcinoma may be striking, since both tumors may appear as deep ulcers with firm, raised, rolled borders (Fig. 11-13, *A*). Although the squamous cell carcinoma is a much more common oral malignancy, if the questionable lesion is situated in the posterolateral region of the hard palate, it is most likely to be a minor salivary gland tumor, such as a mucoepidermoid tumor, since the hard palate is an unlikely site for a squamous cell carcinoma. If a mucocele-like lesion was reported to be in the same location a few days earlier, mucoepidermoid tumor must be given a high priority in the differential diagnosis. If the lesion in question is painless, the possibility that it is a traumatic ulcer, a chancre, an ulcer secondary to systemic disease, or major aphthae is eliminated. If an odontogenic infection cannot be found, the probability that it is an odontogenic ulcer is lessened. Intraoral gummas occur most often in the midline of the palate or tongue and are not as common as the mucoepidermoid tumor.

Tumors and *growths* originating in tissues separate from and beneath the stratified squamous epithelial surface do not characteristically ulcerate, but they may do so because of a mechanical injury or as the result of an incisional biopsy. If such ulcers are the result of an incisional biopsy, they should be easily identified from the history; on the other hand, if they have resulted from mechanical trauma, a careful intraoral examination discloses the cause. The differential diagnosis of exophytic lesions is discussed in detail in Chapter 10.

Ulcers secondary to systemic disease are usually short term, but they may persist if the predisposing systemic disease is not detected and controlled. They may be confused with any of the shallow persistent ulcers—traumatic ulcer, early squamous cell carcinoma, chancre, early mucoepidermoid tumor. Usually the systemic problem becomes apparent through the history or clinical examination and prompts the proper diagnosis. These ulcers secondary to systemic disease are usually painful, in contrast to early squamous cell carcinoma or early mucoepidermoid tumors. A traumatic ulcer can generally be ruled out by establishing the absence of physical injury. Although serologic tests of a patient who appears to have an ulcer secondary to a systemic disease may have positive findings, a chancre can be ruled out if a smear of the lesion does not provide spirochetes that are immobilized by syphilitic antiserum.

Gummas are uncommon oral lesions that occur mostly in the midline of the palate or the midline of the dorsum of the tongue. Similar-appearing pathoses rarely develop at these sites. A traumatic ulcer on a palatal torus or a midline nonhealing granuloma might be considered, but the ulcerated torus should be recognized, and the latter entity is so rare as to be an unlikely diagnosis. Also the rubbery consistency of the gumma eliminates both the torus and the midline nonhealing granuloma from consideration. The serologic findings are usually strongly positive in the case of gummas but only incidentally so in the case of a torus or the rare midline lethal granuloma.

Tests for *chancres* usually result in positive serologic findings, especially after the lesion has been present for 2 or more weeks. If the patient states that he or she was recently in contact with a person who may have had syphilis, this establishes a high priority for chancre in the differential diagnosis. If the ulcer is reddish brown, has a copper-colored halo, and is shallow and if there is no history of mechanical trauma, the diagnosis is strengthened; the impression may be additionally strengthened if the patient is under 40 years of age, because then the lesion is less likely to be an early squamous cell carcinoma or mucoepidermoid tumor. If spirochetes immobilized by syphilitic antiserum are found in the ulcer, the diagnosis of chancre is firmly established.

Necrotizing sialometaplasia is an uncommon, benign, ulcerative, inflammatory process of the minor salivary glands, which is primarily found in the posterior hard palate (Grillon and Lally, 1981; Samit et al., 1979) (Fig. 11-14, *A* and *B*). The cause is unknown. Infarction has been suggested, although the underlying predisposing factors are not clear. The lesion is usually a nodule of slight elevation, and the surface may be ulcerated. These lesions, although uncommon, mimic minor salivary gland tumors in appearance and location and so must always be considered as a possible diagnosis when a soft tissue mass is observed in the posterior hard palate. Necrotizing sialometaplasia is basically a self-limiting disease that usually heals in 6 to 12 weeks. During its ulcerated stage (see Fig. 11-14) it very much resembles a squamous cell

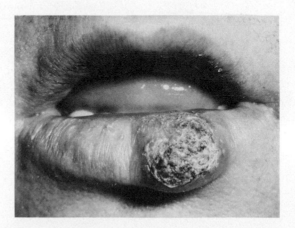

Fig. 11-16. Keratoacanthoma on the lower lip of a 20-year-old man. This was a slowly growing, intermittently tender lesion of 4 to 5 months' duration. This lesion is indistinguishable on clinical examination from squamous cell carcinoma. (From Bass KD: J Oral Surg 38:53-55, 1980, Copyright by the American Dental Association. Reprinted by permission.)

carcinoma and also an ulcerated mucoepidermoid carcinoma. As reported in Anneroth and Hansen's article (1982) it is found more in men than women and at an average patient age of 46 years. Biopsy is indicated to establish the diagnosis and to differentiate between necrotizing sialometaplasia and these other, similar lesions.

Keratoacanthoma is similar to ulcerative types of squamous cell carcinoma (Fig. 11-16). It rarely occurs in the oral mucosa but often is seen on the lower lip, where it may look identical to a squamous cell carcinoma (Bass, 1980). Its rapid growth may help differentiate it from carcinoma, but excision is necessary. Ellis (1983) reported that although there are some histopathologic (histochemical) differences between keratoacanthomas and squamous cell carcinomas, the differences are not significant and are not reliable for differentiation.

Major aphthous ulcer is a persistent ulcer that may closely resemble a squamous cell carcinoma on clinical examination (Fig. 11-4, *D*). However, two striking features help the clinician rule out the malignancy and make the identification of major aphthous ulcer: the severe pain and the inflammatory (nonvelvety red) border.

Squamous cell carcinoma is the most common malignant ulcer of the oral mucosa. The early lesion may be a painless shallow ulcer with a velvety red base. The healing traumatic ulcer, because its base may be filled with reddish pink granulation tissue, may resemble this early lesion. A lesion is most likely a squamous cell carcinoma, however, if (1) the patient is over 40 years of age, is a man, and smokes or drinks heavily; (2) there is no evidence that the lesion is related to trauma or systemic disease; (3) the serologic findings are negative, and the presence of spirochetes cannot be demonstrated; and (4) the lesion is not located on the posterolateral region of the hard palate.

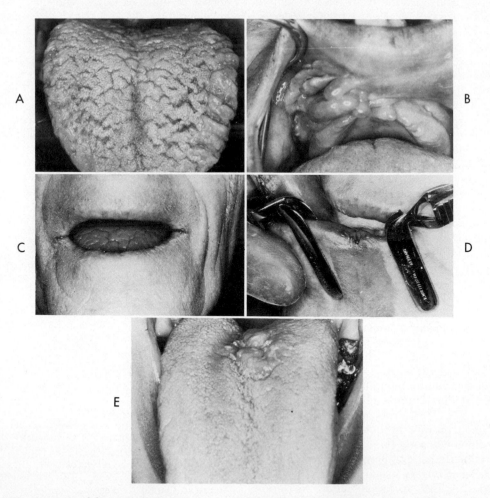

Fig. 11-17. Oral fissures. **A,** Fissured tongue. **B,** Large epulis fissuratum. **C,** Angular cheilosis. **D,** Squamous cell carcinoma. **E,** Fissured type of median rhomboid glossitis.

Ulcers from odontogenic infection are discussed with the differential diagnosis of short-term ulcers.

Traumatic ulcers, especially on the tongue, may in some cases persist for several weeks after the traumatic factor has been eliminated. Such ulcers cannot be differentiated from malignancies on a clinical basis alone and often require complete excision before they resolve. This procedure is recommended because it permits the microscopic examination of the ulcerated tissue.

Fissures

Fissures represent a clinical entity separate from the ulcers and should be grouped separately. The more common fissures that occur in the oral region, ranked according to approximate frequency, include the following (Fig. 11-17):

Angular cheilosis
Congenital cleft
Epulis fissuratum
Fissured tongue
Median rhomboid glossitis—fissured variety
Melkersson-Rosenthal syndrome
Squamous cell carcinoma—fissured variety
Syphilitic rhagades

The differential diagnosis for these entities is not included in this text.

REFERENCES

American Cancer Society: Cancer facts and figures, 1984, New York, The Society.

Ampil F, Datta R, and Shockley W: Adjuvant postoperative external beam radiotherapy in head and neck cancer, J Oral Maxillofac Surg 46:569-573, 1988.

Anneroth G and Hanson LS: Necrotizing sialometaplasia, Int J Oral Surg 11:283-291, 1982.

Antoon JW and Miller RL: Aphthous ulcers—a review of the literature on etiology, pathogenesis, diagnosis and treatment, J Am Dent Assoc 101:803-808, 1980.

Baker HW: Staging of cancer of the head and neck: oral cavity, pharynx, larynx and paranasal sinuses, CA 33(3):130-133, 1983.

Barrett AP: A long-term prospective clinical study of orofacial herpes simplex virus infection in acute leukemia, Oral Surg 61:149-152, 1986.

Barrett AP, Buckley DJ, Greenberg ML, and Earl MJ: The value of exfoliative cytology in the diagnosis of oral herpes simplex infection in immunosuppressed patients, Oral Surg 62:175-178, 1986.

Bass KD: Solitary keratoacanthoma of the lip, J Oral Surg 38:53-55, 1980.

Binnie WH, Rankin KV, and MacKenzie IC: Etiology of oral squamous cell carcinoma, J Oral Pathol 12:11-29, 1983.

Blot WJ, McLaughlin JK, Winn DM, et al: Smoking and drinking in relation to oral and pharyngeal cancer, Cancer Res 48:3282-3287, 1988.

Blot WJ, Winn DM, and Fraumeni JF: Oral cancer and mouthwash (letter to the editor), J Natl Cancer Inst 71:1104-1105, 1983a.

Blot WJ, Winn DM, and Fraumeni JF: Oral cancer and mouthwash, J Natl Cancer Inst 70:251-253, 1983b.

Brooks SL, Rowe NH, and Drach JC: Prevalence of herpes simplex virus disease in a professional population, J Am Dent Assoc 102:31-34, 1981.

Bruun JP: Time lapse by diagnosis of oral cancer, Oral Surg 42:139-149, 1976.

Budtz-Jorgensen E: Oral mucosal lesions associated with the wearing of removable dentures, J Oral Pathol 10:65-80, 1981.

Carl W, Schaat NG, and Chan TY: Oral care of patients irradiated for cancer of the head and neck, Cancer 30:448-453, 1972.

Cawson RA: Update on antiviral chemotherapy: the advent of acyclovir, Br Dent J 161:245-252, 1986.

Cohen SG and Greenberg MS: Chronic oral herpes simplex virus infection in immunocompromised patients, Oral Surg 59:465-471, 1985.

Crissman JD, Gluckman J, Whitley J, and Quenelle D: Squamous cell carcinoma of the floor of the mouth, Head Neck Surg 3:2-7, 1980.

Davis LE, Redman JC, Skipper BJ, and McLaren LC: Natural history of frequent recurrences of herpes simplex labialis, Oral Surg 66:558-561, 1988.

DeVries N, van der Waal I, and Snow GB: Multiple primary tumors in oral cancer, Int J Oral Maxillofac Surg 15:85-87, 1986.

Ellis GL: Differentiating keratoacanthoma from squamous cell carcinoma of the lower lip: an analysis of intraepithelial elastic fibers and intracytoplasmic glycogen, Oral Surg 56:527-531, 1983.

Eskinazi DP: Oncogenic potential of sexually transmitted viruses with special references to oral cancer, Oral Surg 64:35-40, 1987.

Eversole LR, Shopper TP, and Chambers DW: Effects of suspected food stuff challenging agents in the etiology of recurrent aphthous stomatitis, Oral Surg 54:33-38, 1982.

Ferguson MM, Carter J, and Boyle P: An epidemiological study of factors associated with recurrent aphthae in women, J Oral Med 39:212-217, 1984.

Flaitz CM and Hammond HL: The immunoperoxidase method for the rapid diagnosis of intraoral herpes simplex virus infection in patients receiving bone marrow transplants, Spec Care Dent 8:82-85, 1988.

Food and Drug Administration: FDA Drug Bulletin: Vidarabine approved for herpes simplex virus encephalitis, FDA Drug Bull 8:36, Dec 1978-Jan 1979.

Fox SF, Meiller TF, Lohr JT, and Sydiskis RJ: Evaluation of a monoclonal antibody typing system for herpes simplex virus, Oral Surg 64:165-170, 1987.

Germishuys PJ: Hand-foot-and mouth disease: a case report, J Oral Med 35:4-6, 1980.

Grillon GL and Lally E: Necrotizing sialometaplasia: literature review and presentation of five cases, J Oral Surg 39:747-753, 1981.

Gumprecht TF and Jafek BW: Chemotherapy of epidermoid head and neck carcinoma, Colo Oral Cancer Bull 3(11):1-5, 1980.

Hay KD and Reade PC: The use of an elimination diet in the treatment of recurrent aphthous ulceration of the oral cavity, Oral Surg 57:504-507, 1984.

Hunter L and Addy M: Chlorhexidine gluconate mouthwash in the management of minor aphthous ulceration, Br Dent J 162:106-110, 1987.

Ildstad ST, Bigelow ME, and Remensynder JP: Intraoral cancer at Massachusetts General Hospital: squamous cell carcinoma of the floor of the mouth, Ann Surg 197:34-41, 1983.

Kassim KH and Daley TD: Herpes simplex virus type 1 proteins in human oral squamous cell carcinoma, Oral Surg 65:445-448, 1988.

Langdon JD, Rapidis AD, Harvey PW, and Patel MF: ST-NMP—a new classification for oral cancer, Br J Oral Surg 15:49-54, 1977.

Levin AC: Dental management of the irradiated patient. In Million RR and Cassisi NJ: Management of head and neck cancer, Philadelphia, 1984, JB Lippincott Co, pp 133-136.

Lindemann RA, Riviere GR, and Sapp JP: Oral mucosal antigen reactivity during exacerbation and remission phases of recurrent aphthous ulceration, Oral Surg 60:281-284, 1985.

Luce D, Guenel P, Leclerc A, et al: Alcohol and tobacco consumption in cancer of the mouth, pharynx, and larynx: a study of 316 female patients, Laryngoscope 98:313-316, 1988.

MacPhail LA, Greenspan D, Schiødt M, et al: Acyclovir-resistant, foscarnet-sensitive oral herpes simplex type 2 lesion in a patient with AIDS, Oral Surg 67:427-432, 1989.

Mader CL: Lingual frenum ulcer resulting from orogenital sex, J Am Dent Assoc 103:888-890, 1981.

Main DMG: Acute herpetic stomatitis: referrals to Leeds Dental Hospital 1978-1987, Br Dent J 166:14-16, 1989.

Mashberg A, Barsa P, and Grossman ML: A study of the relationship between mouthwash use and oral and pharyngeal cancer, J Am Dent Assoc 110:731-734, 1985.

Merchant VA, Molinari JA, and Sabes WR: Herpetic whitlow: report of a case with multiple recurrences, Oral Surg 55:568-571, 1983.

Meyer I and Shklar G: The oral manifestations of acquired syphilis: a study of eighty-one cases, Oral Surg 23:45-57, 1967.

Miller MF, Garfunkel AA, Ram CA, et al: The inheritance of recurrent aphthous stomatitis: observations on susceptibility, Oral Surg 49:409-412, 1980.

Nagorsky MJ and Sessions DG: Laser resection for early oral cavity cancer: results and complications, Ann Otol Rhinol Laryngol 96:556-560, 1987.

Nair MK, Sankaranarayanan R, and Padmanabhan TK: Evaluation of the role of radiotherapy in the management of carcinoma of the buccal mucosa, Cancer 61:1326-1331, 1988.

Olasz L, Szabo I, and Horvath A: A combined treatment for advanced oral cavity cancers, Cancer 62:1267-1274, 1988.

Olson J, Feinberg I, Silverman S, et al: Serum vitamin B$_{12}$, folate, and iron levels in recurrent aphthous ulceration, Oral Surg 54:517-520, 1982.

Pallasch TJ, Joseph CE, and Gill CJ: Acyclovir and herpes virus infections: a review of the literature, Oral Surg 57:41-44, 1984.

Papac RJ: Distant metastasis from head and neck cancer, Cancer 53:342-345, 1984.

Partridge M and Poswillo DE: Topical carbenoxolone sodium in the management of herpes simplex infection, Br J Oral Maxillofac Surg 22:138-145, 1984.

Patterson WB: Treatment of intraoral cancer by electrocoagulation, Cancer 43(3):821-824, 1979.

Pattison GL: Self-inflicted gingival injuries: literature review and case report, J Periodontol 54:299, 1983.

Pennacchio JL, Hong WK, Shapshay S, et al: Combination of cis-platinum and bleomycin prior to surgery and/or radiotherapy compared with radiotherapy alone for the treatment of advanced squamous cell carcinoma of the head and neck, Cancer 50:2795-2801, 1982.

Peters TED, Blair AE, and Freeman RG: Prevention of self-inflicted trauma in comatose patients, Oral Surg 57:367-370, 1984.

Platz H, Fires R, Hudec M, et al: The prognostic relevance of various factors at the time of the first admission of the patient: retrospective DOSAK study on carcinoma of the oral cavity, J Maxillofac Surg 11:3-12, 1983.

Raborn GW, McGaw WT, and Grace M: Herpes labialis treatment with acyclovir 5 per cent ointment, Can Dent Assoc J 55:135-137, 1989.

Raborn GW, McGaw WT, Grace M, et al: Oral acyclovir and herpes labialis: a randomized double-blind, placebo-controlled study, J Am Dent Assoc 115:38-42, 1987.

Reif AE: The causes of cancer, Am Scient 69:437-447, 1981.

Rennie JS, Reade PC, and Scully C: Recurrent aphthous stomatitis, Br Dent J 159:361-367, 1985.

Rodu B and Lakeman F: In vitro virucidal activity by components of a topical film-forming medication, J Oral Pathol 17:324-326, 1988.

Rodu B and Russell CM: Performance of a hydroxypropyl cellulose film former in normal and ulcerated mucosa, Oral Pathol 65:699-703, 1988.

Rodu B, Russell CM, and Desmarais AJ: Clinical and chemical properties of a novel mucosal bioadhesive agent, J Oral Pathol 17:564-567, 1988.

Rowe NH, Brooks SL, Young SK, et al: A clinical trial of topically applied 3 percent vidarabine against recurrent herpes labialis, Oral Surg 47:142-147, 1979.

Rowe NH, Hëine CS, and Kowalski CJ: Herpetic whitlow: an occupational disease of practicing dentists, J Am Dent Assoc 105:471-473, 1982.

Samit AM, Mashberg A, and Greene GW: Necrotizing sialometaplasia, J Oral Surg 37:353-356, 1979.

Savage NW, Mahanonda R, Seymour GJ, et al: The proportion of suppressor-inducer T-lymphocytes is reduced in recurrent aphthous stomatitis, J Oral Pathol 17:293-297, 1988.

Savage NW, Seymour GJ, and Kruger BJ: T-lymphocyte subset changes in recurrent aphthous stomatitis, Oral Surg 60:175-181, 1985.

Savage NW, Seymour GJ, and Kruger BJ: Expression of class I and class II major histocompatibility complex antigens on epithelial cells in recurrent aphthous stomatitis, J Oral Pathol 15:191-195, 1986.

Schiødt M: Traumatic lesions of the gingiva provoked by tooth brushing (letter to the editor), Oral Surg 52:261, 1981.

Schroeder HE, Muller-Glauser W, and Sallay K: Pathomorphologic features of the ulcerative stages of oral aphthous ulcerations, Oral Surg 58:293-305, 1984.

Scully C: The immunology of cancers of the head and neck with particular reference to oral cancer, Oral Surg 53:157-169, 1982.

Scully C: Viruses and cancer: herpesviruses and tumors in the head and neck, Oral Surg 56:285-292, 1983.

Shafer WG, Hine MK, and Levy BM: A textbook of oral pathology, ed 4, Philadelphia, 1983, WB Saunders Co.

Shear M, Hawkins DM, and Farr HW: The prediction of lymph node metastasis from oral squamous cell carcinoma, Cancer 37(4):1901-1907, 1976.

Shillitoe EJ and Silverman S: Oral cancer and herpes simplex virus—a review, Oral Surg 48:216-223, 1979.

Shingaki S, Suzuki I, Nakajima T, and Kawasaki T: Evaluation of histopathologic parameters in predicting cervical lymph node metastasis of oral and oropharyngeal carcinomas, Oral Surg 66:683-688, 1988.

Ship II: Socioeconomic status and recurrent aphthous ulcers, J Am Dent Assoc 73:120-123, 1966.

Silverman S, Greenspan D, and Gorsky M: Tobacco usage in patients with head and neck carcinomas: a follow-up study on habit changes and second primary oral/oropharyngeal cancers, J Am Dent Assoc 106:33-35, 1983.

Spouge JD: Oral pathology, St. Louis, 1973, The CV Mosby Co.

Spruance SL and Crumpacker CS: Topical 5 percent acyclovir in polyethylene glycol for herpes simplex labialis: antiviral effect without clinical benefit, Am J Med (Acyclovir Symposium) 73:315-319, 1982.

Stanley HR: Management of patients with persistent recurrent aphthous stomatitis and Sutton's disease, Oral Surg 35:174-179, 1973.

Syrjanen SM, Syrjanen KJ, and Happonen RP: Human papilloma virus (HPV) DNA sequences in oral precancerous lesions and squamous cell carcinoma demonstrated by in situ hybridization, J Oral Pathol 17:273-278, 1988.

Thein DJ and Hurt WC: Lysine as a prophylactic agent in the treatment of recurrent herpes simplex labialis, Oral Surg 58:659-666, 1984.

Tyldesley WR: Stomatitis and recurrent oral ulceration: is a full blood screen necessary? Br J Oral Surg 21:27-30, 1983.

Urist MM, O'Brien, CJ, Soorg SJ, et al: Squamous cell carcinoma of the buccal mucosa: analysis of prognostic factors, Am J Surg 154:411-414, 1987.

Vermund H, Rappaport I, and Nethery WJ: Role of radiotherapy in the treatment of oral cancer, J Oral Surg 32:690-695, 1974.

Vikram B and Farr HW: Adjuvant radiation therapy in locally advanced head and neck cancer, CA 33(3):134-138, 1983.

Weathers DR and Griffin JW: Intraoral ulcerations of recurrent herpes simplex and recurrent aphthae: two distinct clinical entities, J Am Dent Assoc 81:81-87, 1970.

Weaver A, Fleming SA, and Smith DB: Mouthwash and oral cancer: carcinogenic or coincidence? J Oral Surg 37:250-253, 1979.

Wray D: A double blind trial of systemic zinc sulfate in recurrent aphthous stomatitis, Oral Surg 53:469-482, 1982.

Wray D, Graykowski EA, and Notkins AL: Role of mucosal injury in initiating recurrent aphthous stomatitis, Br Med J 283:1569-1570, 1981.

Wynder EL and Kabat GC: Oral cancer and mouthwash (letter to the editor), J Natl Cancer Inst 71:1105, 1983.

Wynder EL, Kabat GC, Rosenberg S, and Levenstein M: Oral cancer and mouthwash use, J Natl Cancer Inst 70:255-260, 1983.

12

Intraoral brownish, bluish, or black conditions

NORMAN K. WOOD
PAUL W. GOAZ
DANNY R. SAWYER

The intraoral conditions classified as brownish, bluish, or black may be categorized according to whether they produce distinct and discretely circumscribed lesions or a generalized and diffuse discoloration of the patient. (Features of these conditions are summarized in Tables 12-1 and 12-2 on pp. 251-253).

Distinct circumscribed types
Melanoplakia
Varicosity
Amalgam tattoo
Petechia and ecchymosis
Early hematoma
Late hematoma
Hemangioma
Oral melanotic macule
Mucocele
Ranula
Superficial cyst
Giant cell granuloma
Black hairy tongue
Lymphangioma
Pigmented fibroma
Melanoma
Nevus
Mucus-producing salivary
   gland tumors
von Recklinghausen's
   disease
Albright's syndrome
Heavy metal lines
Kaposi's sarcoma
Rarities
   Acanthosis nigricans
   Acromegaly
   Addison's disease
      (distinct circumscribed
      lesions)
   AIDS-related
      pigmentation
   Amyloidosis

Angioma bullosa
   haemorrhagica
Angiosarcoma
Blue nevus
Blue rubber-bleb nevus
   syndrome
Chlorpromazine therapy
Chronic obstructive
   pulmonary disease
   (COPD)
Cushing's syndrome
Fabry's disease
Gaucher's disease
Hemangioendothelioma
Henoch-Schönlein
   purpura
Hereditary hemorrhagic
   telangiectasia
Incontinentia pigmenti
Kaposi's sarcoma
   (non-AIDS)
Lentigo
Lichen planus
Lupus erythematosus
Lymphangiomas of
   neonates
Lymphoma (superficial)
Maffucci's syndrome
Melanoacanthoma
Melanotic
   neuroectodermal tumor
   of infancy
Minocycline pigmentation
Nelson's syndrome
Pernicious anemia

Peutz-Jeghers syndrome
Pheochromocytoma
Quinidine pigmentation
Rheumatic fever
Scleroderma
Smoker's mucosal
   melanosis
Submucous fibrosis
Superficial cartilaginous
   tumor in patient with
   ochronosis or
   alkaptonuria
Superficial Pseudomonas
   aeruginosa infection
Tattoo
Thyrotoxicosis
Uremia (petechiae)
Wegener's
   granulomatosis
Xeroderma pigmentosa

Generalized brownish, bluish, or black conditions
Cyanosis
Chloasma gravidarum
Addison's disease
Hemochromatosis
Argyria
Rarities
   Aniline intoxication
   Arsenic poisoning
   Carotenemia
   Chloroquine therapy
   Dermatomyositis
   Idiopathic familial
      juvenile
      hypoparathyroidism,
      Addison's disease,
      superficial candidiasis
   Pellagra
   Porphyria
   Sprue
   Wilson's disease

The brownish, bluish, or black color that serves as the basis for this category of disorders originates from one of two sources: (1) the accumulation of colored material in abnormal amounts or locations in the superficial tissues or (2) a pooled, clear fluid just beneath the epithelium. The amassed material that effects these color changes may be either exogenous or endogenous in origin.

The exogenous substances that produce the brownish, bluish, or black conditions usually include heavy metals not normally found in the body, commercial dyes, vegetable pigments, and various other stains that have been either ingested or introduced directly into the tissues. The point of introduction may be at the site of or remote from the lesion in question.

The endogenous chromatic materials that produce the brownish, bluish, or black conditions usually result from increased melanin states or are derived from blood pigments or abnormal aggregations of metals normally found in the body. It is interesting that the color imparted by such exogenous or endogenous materials is a function of not only the amount of pigment but also the depths at which the pigments have been deposited in the tissues. For example, the more superficial melanin deposits appear browner, whereas the deeper melanin deposits seem more bluish.

Refraction phenomena cause abnormal coloration in superficial, fluid-filled cavities such as some cysts, and retention phenomena cause abnormal coloration in the minor salivary glands. Although in these pathoses the distinctive bluish color might appear to be caused by pigment in the area, it is actually the result of altered reflection and absorption of light in the area.

Distinct circumscribed types

MELANOPLAKIA (BLACK PIGMENTATION)

All people except albinos* have a discernible degree of melanin pigmentation distributed throughout the epidermis of the skin.

Melanin is thought to be produced by the dendritic melanocytes in the basal layer of the

---

*Melanin formation is impaired by a congenital decrease in tyrosinase in albinism.

epidermis (Fig. 12-1). It is formed by the oxidation of tyrosine, a reaction that is catalyzed by the copper-containing enzyme tyrosinase and mediated by the melanocyte-stimulating hormone (MSH), from the anterior pituitary. The melanin is secreted by the melanocytes and then picked up by the adjacent basal cells of the epithelium.

Features

The clinical appearance of melanin varies from light brown through blue to black, depending on the amount present and its depth in the tissues. The deeper and heavier the deposit of melanin in the skin or mucosa, the darker it appears. There is great variation in the degree of pigmentation of the skin among the races and between individuals of the same race. Although much of this variation is genetically controlled, the remainder is caused by various degrees of tanning from exposure to sunlight.

Most light-skinned individuals have a relatively even coloration throughout the oral cavity; however, dark-complexioned people, especially blacks, frequently have macules of pigmentation (melanoplakia) of various configurations and sizes on their oral mucosae (Fig. 12-2). Gorsky et al. (1984) reported findings on differences in physiologic oral pigmentation in Israeli Jews of three different ethnic origins. The gingivae are frequent sites of this patchy pigmentation, but variation in physiologic pigmentation is not limited to the gingivae. Such areas of melanoplakia on the oral mucous membranes in blacks are not usually a cause for con-

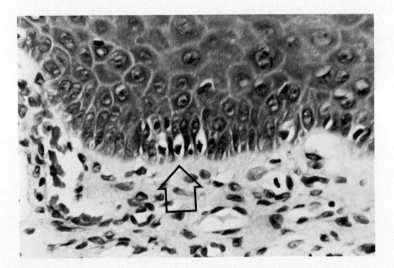

Fig. 12-1. The clear cells in the basal cell layer of the epithelium are melanocytes. The arrow indicates three melanocytes.

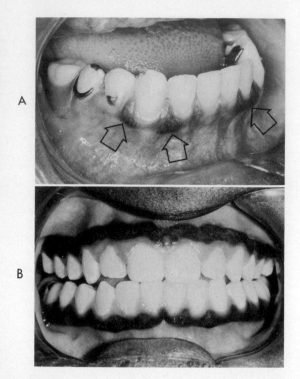

Fig. 12-2. Melanoplakia. **A,** Arrows indicate areas of involvement. **B,** Unusual, ribbonlike appearance of melanoplakia.

cern, but if they are known to be of recurrent origin, they may complicate the formulation of a differential diagnosis and prompt a biopsy.

Differential diagnosis

A solitary, small, circumscribed, darkly pigmented lesion in a black person cannot be clinically distinguished from an *amalgam tattoo, junctional nevus, melanoma,* or local area of *hemosiderin deposition* after trauma. Should such an area be observed in a white person, it is unlikely to be melanoplakia but more likely to be an oral melanotic macule or one of the entities just mentioned. Hertz et al. (1980) reported a condition similar to melanoplakia (melanosis) in female patients with light complexions. All of these patients were taking the combination (high-estrogen) type of oral contraceptives.

On microscopic examination the increased pigmentation in the basal layer is the only significant observation in melanoplakia.

Management

The diagnosis of melanoplakial patches in blacks is seldom a problem, and after correct identification this entity requires no further attention. However, it is not always possible to differentiate between a patch of melanoplakia

and a superficial spreading melanoma on a clinical basis. Hence the pigmented patch should be excised along with an adequate border of normal-appearing tissue and submitted for microscopic study if the pigmented patch has (1) appeared recently rather than at birth or during childhood, (2) decreased or increased in size, (3) become elevated in part or whole, (4) undergone color changes of any type, or (5) undergone surface ulceration or fissuring.

VARICOSITY

A varicosity is a distended vein and is a common occurrence in the oral cavity, especially in older individuals. It may also result from partial blockage of the vein proximal to the distension either by a structure causing external pressure or from a plaque that has formed on the lumen side of the wall as a result of an injury.

Features

The varicosities most frequently observed by the clinician are superficial, painless, and bluish; they appear somewhat congested and accentuate the shape and distribution of the vessel. The most frequent site is the ventral surface of the tongue (Fig. 12-3).

When many of the sublingual veins are involved, this condition is called "caviar tongue" (or phlebectasia linguae) (Fig. 12-3). The clinician should know that varicosities in the oral cavity, although occurring for the most part normally, may on rare occasions be caused by a tumor pressing on the superior vena cava at a proximal site, such as in the mediastinum. Congested veins in the head and neck region are also seen in apprehensive individuals and in children who are holding their breath.

Differential diagnosis

The clinical identification of a lesion as a varicosity usually does not present a problem, but occasionally one is found with a bulbous shape (Fig. 12-3, *C*) and then must be differentiated from all the other fluid-filled bluish lesions of the oral cavity: hemangioma, aneurysm, mucocele, ranula, and superficial nonkeratotic cyst.

In contrast to the *superficial nonkeratotic cyst, ranula,* and *mucocele,* which are fluctuant and cannot be emptied by digital pressure because they contain fluid in a closed chamber, the varicosity, the hemangioma (especially the cavernous variety), and the aneurysm do not demonstrate fluctuance and usually can be emptied by digital pressure.

An *aneurysm* is exceedingly rare in the oral cavity and demonstrates a pulse, as does an *ar-*

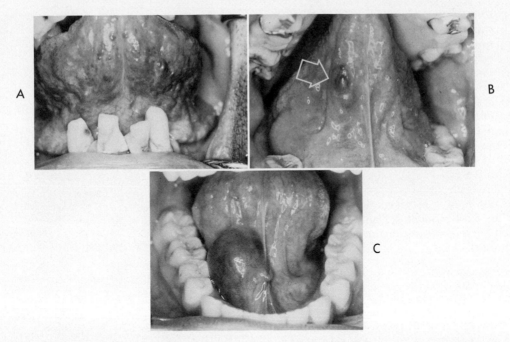

Fig. 12-3. A, Caviar tongue (phlebectasia linguae). **B,** Small varicosity. **C,** Large, bulbous varicosity that resembled a ranula.

teriovenous shunt. An angiogram may be an additional aid in the identification of an arteriovenous lesion.

Although the *cavernous hemangioma* can be readily emptied into the afferent and efferent vessels by digital pressure, the *capillary hemangioma* cannot be as readily emptied because the vascular spaces and the afferent and efferent vessels are so small that they may be immediately sealed when pressure is applied to the lesion. Also the capillary hemangioma is seldom a bluish domed mass like its cavernous counterpart but is more reddish.

The varicosity, on the other hand, collapses if the vein distal to it is occluded by digital pressure (provided the proximal end is not totally blocked by a process that may have caused the varicosity). A hemangioma, however, usually does not collapse when manipulated in this manner because the blood tends to pool in the many vascular spaces.

A more dependable test to identify a varicosity is to completely occlude the vessel proximally by digital pressure and try to evacuate the lesion by massaging in a distal direction. If the lesion is a varicosity, it cannot be easily evacuated in a distal direction because the valves in the normal segment of the vein distal to the varicosity do not readily permit the retrograde passage of blood.

Management

Usually all that is required is to positively diagnose the lesion as a varicosity. Except for the large bulbous types, which may be regularly irritated, oral varicosities seldom require treatment. It is extremely important, however, that they be differentiated from other pathoses. The clinician must develop a thorough differential diagnosis and a positive working diagnosis of varicosity and must completely rule out other vascular lesions.

If the lesion relates to a general cardiovascular condition, contemplated dental work should be deferred until the patient's physician indicates that it is safe to proceed.

AMALGAM TATTOO

The amalgam tattoo is a frequently occurring, asymptomatic, dark bluish lesion usually seen on the gingiva in mouths in which teeth have been restored with silver amalgam (Fig. 12-4). It usually is produced when the gingiva is abraded at the time a tooth is prepared for restoration. Subsequently, when the amalgam is placed, some of the silver or mercury contacts the abraded tissue and precipitates the protein of the immature collagen fibers, thus fixing them.

Buchner and Hansen (1980a) reported their findings on an unusually large series of amalgam tattoos (268 cases). They found that the most common locations were the gingiva, the alveolar mucosa, and the buccal mucosa, in order of decreasing frequency. Almost one half of the lesions were located on the gingiva and the alveolar mucosa, and the mandibular region was affected more than the maxillary. Sixty-one percent of the patients were between the ages of 20 and 49, and the mean age was 43.1 years. The lesions were prevalent in females with a ratio of 1.8:1. Ninety-six percent of the patients were white.

The amalgam tattoo is a permanent stain and can also be seen in histologic sections of the tissue (Fig. 12-4). Buchner and Hansen (1980a) detailed their histologic findings in the following manner:

> The amalgam was present in the tissues as discrete, fine, dark granules and as irregular solid fragments. The dark granules were arranged mainly along collagen bundles and around blood vessels. They were also associated with the walls of blood vessels, nerve sheaths, elastic fibers, and acini of minor salivary glands. Dark granules were also present intracellularly within macrophages, multinucleated giant cells, endothelial cells and fibroblasts.

These writers explained that in 45% of cases there was no tissue reaction to the amalgam, in 17% of cases there was a macrophagic reaction, and in 38% of cases there was a chronic inflammatory response usually in the form of a foreign body granuloma with foreign body and Langhans' giant cells. Unfortunately, on microscopic study amalgam may at times be difficult to differentiate from hemosiderin and melanin. Hartman et al. (1986) described "energy dispersive x-ray analysis," a technique that clearly identifies amalgam in the tissues.

Radiographs of the region are normal except when actual fragments of amalgam have been introduced into the tissue; the fragments are then detectable as dense radiopacities.

Differential diagnosis

On visual examination an amalgam tattoo often cannot be differentiated from a junctional nevus, an oral melanotic macule, a macular type of melanoma, or a hemangioma (see Figs. 12-11 and 12-17).

A *superficial hemangioma* blanches on pressure, and a *nevus* or *melanoma* seldom occurs in the oral cavity. From the Buchner and Hansen study (1980a) we obtained an estimate of the relative frequency of these lesions. From 9 years of biopsy service they reported 262 cases of amalgam tattoo, 105 melanotic macules, and 32 pigmented nevi.

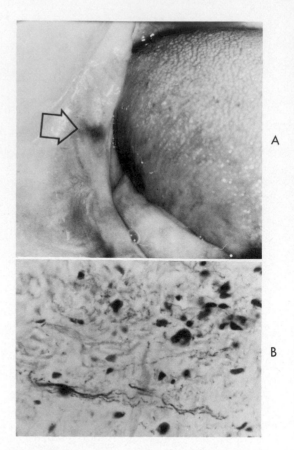

Fig. 12-4. Amalgam tattoo. **A,** Dark macule on the crest of the ridge in the mandibular molar area. **B,** The black granules forming the wavy lines are particles of silver that have stained reticulin fibers.

Furthermore, an increase in size or a change in color is expected with a melanoma, and if there is an amalgam restoration adjacent to such a quiescent lesion, this is almost conclusive evidence that the suspected area is an amalgam tattoo.

Management

Amalgam tattoos do not require treatment, but if there is a suspicion that the lesion could be a nevus or a melanoma, it should be excised and microscopically examined. A similar course should be followed if the patient is worried about the nature of the lesion.

PETECHIA AND ECCHYMOSIS (PURPURA)

Petechiae and ecchymoses are purpuric submucous or subcutaneous hemorrhages. They have the same basic mechanism: both appear as bluish macules differing only in size; petechiae are minute pinpoint hemorrhages, whereas ec-

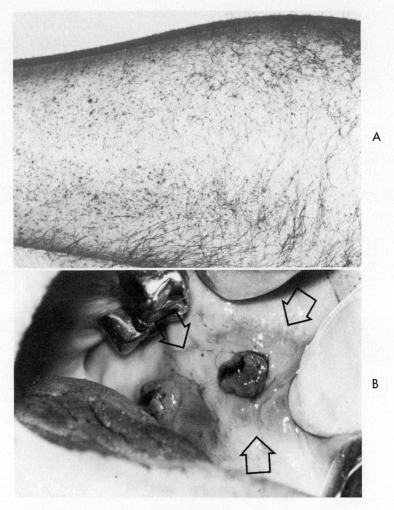

Fig. 12-5. A, Petechiae on the arm of a patient with thrombocytopenic purpura. **B,** Ecchymosis *(arrows)* surrounding an exophytic blood clot in the same patient.   (Courtesy S. Svalina, DDS, Maywood, Ill.)

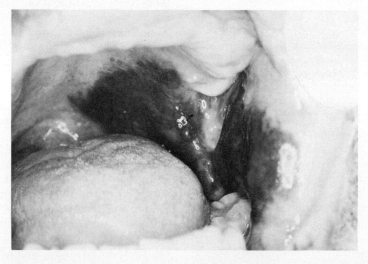

Fig. 12-6. Large, purpuric lesion in the buccal and palatal mucosa after a mandibular fracture.   (Courtesy D. Bonomo, DDS, Flossmoor, Ill.)

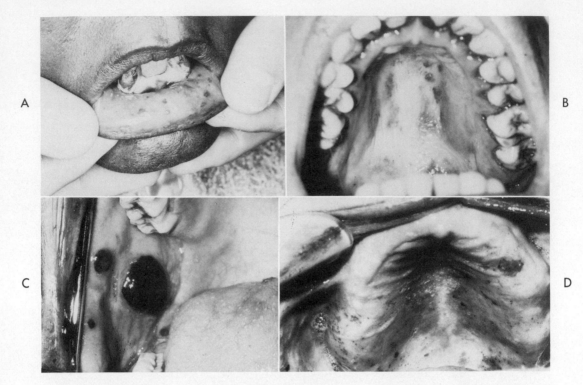

Fig. 12-7. Purpuric macules in hemostatic disease. **A,** Petechial purpuric macules that occurred during a sickle cell crisis. **B,** Petechiae and gingival bleeding occurring in a patient with acute myelogenous leukemia. **C,** Purpuric macules and blood clots in a patient with heroin-induced thrombocytopenic purpura. **D,** Purpuric macules in a patient with leukemia. (**A** courtesy S. Smith, DDS, Chicago. **B** courtesy J. Canzona, DDS, Chicago. **C** from Kraut RA and Buhler JE: Oral Surg 46[5]:637-640, 1978. **D** courtesy M. Lehnert, DDS, Minneapolis.)

chymoses are larger than 2 cm in diameter (Figs. 12-5 to 12-7). If these lesions are observed soon after their inception, they are red. Within a few hours they change to a bluish brown color.

Features

The hemorrhaging is slow in this spectrum of lesions; hence there is not sufficient blood to pool and develop the fluctuant swellings characteristic of the early hematomas. Trauma and perhaps more frequently disorders of the hemostatic mechanisms or other systemic disease may be the causative factors involved. It is important to obtain a complete history from a patient who is discovered to have these lesions. If the person has had several such episodes, he or she almost certainly has a systemic problem and must be examined for hemostatic defects such as thrombocytopenia, leukemia, and hemophilia or other diseases such as subacute bacterial endocarditis, Waterhouse-Friderichsen syndrome, infectious mononucleosis, sickle cell anemia, polycythemia, disseminated fat emboli, or vitamin C deficiency.

Differential diagnosis

On clinical examination petechiae and ecchymoses begin as reddish macules of varying shape and outline. On palpation their consistency is similar to that of normal mucosa. They do not blanch on pressure, but within a few days their color changes from red to blue to greenish blue to yellowish green to yellow and then disappears as the hemoglobin is degraded to hemosiderin and removed.

A single petechial macule resulting from local trauma takes on a bluish brown appearance within a day or two and must be differentiated from an *amalgam tattoo,* an *oral melanotic macule,* a *junctional nevus,* and a *melanoma.* A history of recent trauma, accompanied by the change from bluish brown to green to yellow and then finally the disappearance within 4 or 5 days, indicates its identity.

Early petechial lesions must be differentiated from *telangiectasis* in patients with Rendu-Osler-Weber syndrome (hereditary hemorrhagic telangiectasia). This syndrome manifests itself as small, reddish, macule-papule lesions that are dilated capillaries situated just under the epithelium; the lesions blanch on pressure. They can thus be differentiated from petechiae.

Palatal petechiae and ecchymotic patches require further differentiation when they occur as a solitary lesion at or near the junction of the hard and soft palate. The diagnoses to be considered are (1) trauma from fellatio, (2) trauma from severe coughing, (3) trauma from severe vomiting, (4) prodromal sign of infectious mononucleosis, and (5) prodromal sign of hemostatic disease.

There seems little doubt that *oral sexual practices* are on the increase. Thus the dentist must consider this possibility first when a reddish or bluish macule is detected on the posterior palate and has been produced by extravasated blood (see Fig. 5-4). If the lesion is indeed caused by fellatio, the bruise disappears in a few days after passing through changes from blue to green to yellow. Frequently it reappears in another week or so. A careful history taken in confidential surroundings confirms the diagnosis in almost all cases.

Bruising of the palate from severe attacks of *vomiting* and *coughing* appears as a broad linear red or bluish bruise that follows the junction of the hard and soft palate. Again the history is diagnostic in these cases.

Prodromal signs of *infectious mononucleosis* may occur a few days before the patient becomes ill as 6 to 20 petechiae in the soft palate. These petechiae may also occur between the fifth and twentieth days of illness. This feature, along with malaise, enlarged nodes in the neck, and a positive Monospot test followed by a positive Paul-Bennell heterophil test, establishes the diagnosis of the disease.

Because the soft palate sustains a considerable degree of stimulation and mild trauma during swallowing of food, this location is frequently the first to show the petechiae that may herald the onset of *hemostatic disease*. A complete series of blood tests usually identifies the specific diagnosis. However, the clinician must remember that some individuals bruise easily and so a few scattered petechiae may be present from time to time on the normal palates of these individuals.

Management

The associated hemostatic disorders may be conveniently divided into three groups according to the basic defect: disorders of the vessels, disorders of the platelets, and disorders affecting coagulation. A suitable study of the patient, including a thorough history and clinical examination and the appropriate laboratory tests,

identifies the specific underlying systemic defect. Surgery should not be performed until the defect has been identified and treated, or at least the surgical procedure has been modified on the basis of the defect's recognition and nature.

EARLY HEMATOMA

The hematoma is a pool of effused blood confined within the tissues. When it is superficial, it appears as an elevated bluish swelling in the mucosa (Fig. 12-8). The early hematoma is fluctuant, rubbery, and discrete in outline, and the overlying mucosa is readily movable. The temperature of the overlying mucosa may be elevated slightly. Digital pressure on the surface

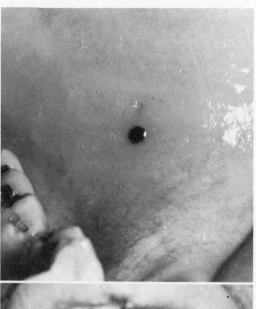

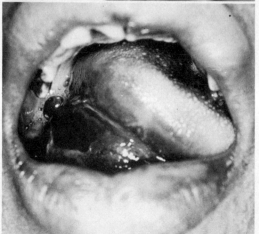

Fig. 12-8. Hematoma. **A,** Small lesion on the buccal mucosa. **B,** Large, dome-shaped hematoma in the right sublingual region caused by damage to the lingual artery during a surgical procedure.

may induce a stinging sensation as the pressure on the contained pool of blood causes further separation of the tissues.

Differential diagnosis

A history of a traumatic incident (such as accident, surgery, or administration of a local anesthetic) can almost always be elicited from the patient and is useful in establishing the diagnosis of early hematoma. Not to be overlooked is the possibility of spontaneous hemorrhage that accompanies the development of a hematoma in patients who have a blood dyscrasia or other bleeding diathesis; this may be the first indication of their systemic disease. Generally, however, petechia and ecchymosis are more often seen in these patients than is a hematoma, although a hematoma may be encountered after a surgical procedure in such patients if they have not been properly prepared for surgery.

Early hematoma must be differentiated from all the soft and rubbery bluish lesions that occur in the oral cavity: *mucocele, ranula, varicosity, hemangioma, lymphangioma,* and *superficial cyst.* The history of a sudden onset after a recent traumatic incident strongly favors a diagnosis of early hematoma. The lesion is tender and fluctuant and cannot be evacuated by digital pressure. Although an early hematoma is usually not painful, palpation generally induces a stinging sensation. There is no thrill or crepitus. The early hematoma is almost always a solitary lesion that yields dark blue blood on aspiration.

Management

The hematoma is usually self-limiting in size because the increasing pressure of the blood in the tissue equalizes with the hydrostatic pressure in the injured vessel and thus terminates the extravasation. If a large arteriole is damaged, however, a pressure bandage may be placed over accessible areas to control the hemorrhage and limit the expansion of the hematoma.

Occasionally it may be feasible to evacuate an expanding or painful hematoma with an aspirating syringe and then apply a pressure bandage to prevent its re-formation. If indicated, the patient may be hospitalized for observation and the offending vessel located surgically and ligated.

An enlarging hematoma in the neck or sublingual area may encroach on the airway, and its management must be evaluated in the light of this possibility. Goldstein (1981) reported three cases of acute dissecting hematomas and discussed the management of this life-threatening condition.

Since the hematoma presents an excellent medium for the growth of opportunistic bacteria, the clinician must be aware that the probability of infection is high if the patient is not immediately placed on a suitable regimen of antibiotic medication for several days.

LATE HEMATOMA

A hematoma is usually completely clotted within 24 hours and then becomes a hard, black, painless mass. It often requires this prolonged period to completely clot because blood continues to leak into the clotting pool from the injured vessels. If the hematoma is superficially located, changes from black to blue to green to yellow may be observed during the following days. It disappears finally when all the hemosiderin from the extravasated blood has been removed from the tissues.

If a hematoma becomes infected, it is painful. Although the clot initially is firm, if the infection is a pyogenic type, the firm clot softens and becomes fluctuant as pus accumulates.

Differential diagnosis

In postextraction patients, clinicians frequently see hematomas that have formed inferior to the extraction site. The submaxillary space is a frequent site for the development of such postextraction hematomas, which must be differentiated from an *early space infection.*

The late hematoma is firm and painless, whereas the infection is firm but acutely painful to palpation. In addition, the tissue over the infection has an increased temperature and may be inflamed. Later the infection may become fluctuant and yield pus on aspiration.

Management

If the patient with a large hematoma has not been protected with antibiotics, such prophylactic treatment should be initiated immediately and the patient observed carefully for the next few days. If the patient has or appears to be developing a problem with respiration, he or she should be hospitalized and appropriate measures instituted to establish and maintain a patent airway.

HEMANGIOMA

The hemangioma is a benign tumor of patent blood vessels that may be congenital or traumatic in origin. It may appear similar to a telangiectasia, which is a dilation of a previously existing vessel. The hemangioma, however, is a

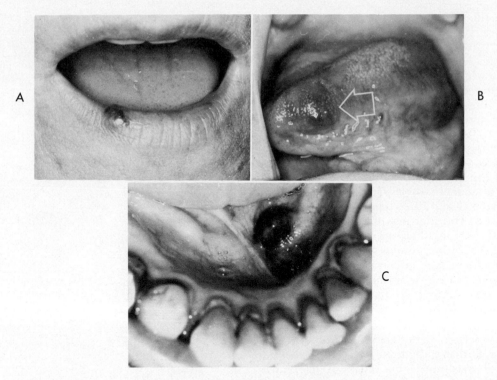

Fig. 12-9. Cavernous hemangioma. **A,** Of the lip. **B,** Of the anterolateral border of the tongue. **C,** Of the floor of the mouth, mimicking a ranula.   (Courtesy G. MacDonald, DDS, Belleville, Ill.)

new formation of blood vessels. Seventy-three percent of hemangiomas occur within the first year of life (Watson and McCarthy, 1940).

Only those hemangiomas that occur superficially are considered in this section. The deeper hemangiomas are rarely detected and do not appear blue, since the deeper tissue covering obscures the color imparted by the vascular mass; the capillary hemangiomas are not included in this discussion, since they are usually a reddish lesion.

The cavernous hemangioma is a soft, nonfluctuant, domelike, bluish nodule that may vary in size from a millimeter or less to several centimeters in diameter (Fig. 12-9). It frequently appears on the lips, buccal mucosa, palate, and other sites in the oral cavity.

Maffucci's syndrome features (1) multiple enchondromas, (2) multiple hemangiomas, and (3) phleboliths. Laskaris and Skouteris (1984) reported a case in which the intraoral hemangiomas were the only ones present.

Differential diagnosis

The hemangioma blanches and may be emptied by the application of digital pressure, which forces the blood from the vascular spaces. This feature accounts for the finding that the lesion is not fluctuant and, in turn, helps to differentiate the cavernous hemangioma from the *mucocele, ranula,* and *superficial cysts,* which though soft are, in contrast, fluctuant and nonemptiable. (Refer to Chapter 3 for a broader discussion of these differences.) A varicosity usually is seen as an elongated enlargement of a superficial vein rather than as a nodule or dome-shaped mass.

Furthermore, a pulse is not detectable within the cavernous hemangioma. This feature serves to distinguish the hemangioma from an *arteriovenous shunt* or an *aneurysm,* both of which may occur as rubbery, nonfluctuant, domelike, bluish nodules with a usually discernible throbbing.

In addition to the foregoing characteristics, the aspiration of bluish blood with a fine-gauge needle contributes convincing evidence for a working diagnosis of cavernous hemangioma.

Management

Surgery or sclerosing techniques or both are used for treatment of a hemangioma. Sclerosing solutions such as sodium psylliate or sodium morrhuate are injected into the lesion to induce the formation of fibrous tissue, which scleroses and shrinks the vascular spaces (Fig. 12-10). Chin (1983) indicated this technique to be useful particularly with slowly flowing lesions in which the sclerosing agent would have more time to act. This technique is often used before surgery to reduce the amount of surgery needed and to reduce the hemorrhage that attends the removal of these conditions. Angiograms are advised if the lesions appear to be extensive, to help determine the size and location of the lesion as well as the number and size of attendant vessels (Zhao-ju et al., 1983).

Minkow et al. (1979) reported on treating a series of 24 hemangiomas of the oral cavity and lips with sodium tetradecyl sulfate (Sotradecol). The smaller lesions disappeared after injection, whereas the larger lesions required up to 10 treatments with 2 weeks between treatments. These investigators reported that all lesions disappeared without scarring and no side effects occurred.

The injection of a sclerosing agent is frequently all that is required. A lesion so treated becomes firm and loses much of its bluish color. The exact size and extent of the tumor must be determined before any treatment, however, since the visible portion may represent just the tip of the iceberg. Angiograms are used to advantage for this purpose. The excision of a moderately large or large hemangioma should not be attempted in the dental office; rather, the patient should be hospitalized and the procedure performed in an operating room, where blood is available for transfusions and where extraoral ligation of cervical arteries may be accomplished more readily.

Cryotherapy has gained acceptance in the treatment of hemangiomas (Leopard, 1975; Murphy, 1978). Gongloff (1983) reported good to excellent results using nitrous oxide cryosurgery in nine cases of intraoral hemangioma.

ORAL MELANOTIC MACULE

The oral melanotic macule is a pigmented entity of the oral mucosa and lips (Buchner and Hansen, 1979a; Page et al., 1977; Weathers et al., 1976). This lesion is the most common pigmentation to occur in the oral cavity of light-skinned individuals. Concerning incidence Buchner and Hansen (1979a) studied 105 cases and reported that the oral melanotic macule accounted for 0.5% of cases accessioned in their laboratory. The cause of the oral melanotic macule is uncertain in the majority of cases but may represent posttraumatic (inflammatory) pigmentation in some cases. Buchner and

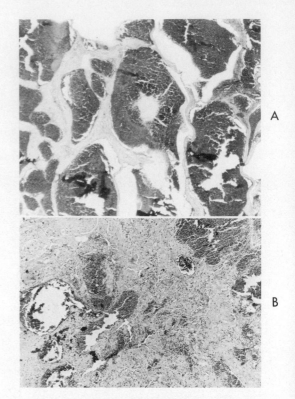

Fig. 12-10. A, Photomicrograph of a cavernous hemangioma showing the many vascular spaces separated by thin, connective tissue septa. B, Photomicrograph of a cavernous hemangioma that has been sclerosed by an injected agent shows a decreased number of vascular spaces and the increased fibrous tissue component.

Hansen suggested the possibility that it is an atypical manifestation of physiologic pigmentation, since the histologic appearance is identical to that of melanoplakia.

Features

The oral melanotic macule is usually a solitary lesion that occurs mostly in light-skinned individuals. The lesion is usually well circumscribed and gray, brownish, black, or bluish (Fig. 12-11). The majority were less than 1 cm in diameter; the largest reported lesion was 2 cm in diameter (Page et al., 1977). In Buchner and Hansen's study the most frequent site was the lower lip (28.7%), followed by the gingiva (22.8%), the buccal mucosa (16.2%), and the hard palate (6.7%). Page et al. and Weathers et al. reported the same site predilections, although they considered the lip lesions a separate entity from the oral lesions.

The mean patient ages were 41.0 years, 45.4 years, and 31.5 years, respectively, for the

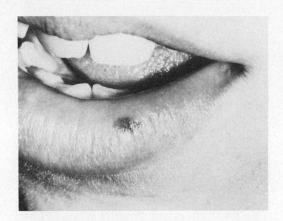

Fig. 12-11. Oral melanotic macule of the lower lip.

Buchner, Page, and Weathers (labial melanotic macule) studies. Buchner and Hansen reported that the ratio of women to men was 2.2:1. Page et al. reported an approximately equal sex ratio. The majority of the lesions remain constant in size and do not tend to become malignant. The only significant histologic observation is the increased pigment contained in the basal cell layer. Lesions also may show melanin in the lamina propria, some of which is contained in melanophages. In some instances an increase in the number of clear cells is seen. The microscopic appearance is identical to that of melanoplakia.

Differential diagnosis

Entities that should be included in the differential discussion of oral melanotic macule are melanoplakia, amalgam tattoo, ecchymotic patch, superficial spreading melanoma, nevi, lentigo, focal melanosis and oral melanoacanthomas.

Melanoplakia is not always distinguishable from the oral melanotic macule, but usually the latter entity is smaller and has a configuration different from that of the melanoplakic patches present in the rest of the mucosa of the patient. The condition commonly occurs in blacks.

The *amalgam tattoo* in most cases is in a location where it could be associated with a juxtaposed amalgam filling. However, that is not always the case; amalgam tattoos have been seen on mucosa far removed from the alveolar processes.

The *ecchymotic patch* can be easily differentiated from all the melanin-containing macules. The former entity usually has a browner color and disappears within a few days.

Superficial spreading melanoma is much less common, is seen in patients who are, on the average, 8 years older than those with an oral melanotic macule, and slowly spreads by circumferential growth. Oral melanoma occurs twice as frequently in men as does the oral melanotic macule, and the palate is the most commonly affected site.

Flat *nevi* and *lentigo* are rare lesions in the oral cavity but may look identical clinically to the oral melanotic macule.

Focal melanosis as described by Buchner and Hansen (1979a) shows a similar increase in pigmentation of the basal cell layer. However, focal melanosis, unlike the oral melanotic macule, is not seen as a pigmented lesion clinically. Hence focal melanosis must be considered in the histologic process of differential diagnosis.

Goode et al. (1983) reported 10 cases of *oral melanoacanthomas*, which mimic closely the clinical appearance of melanotic macules and also junctional nevi.

If multiple melanotic patches are present in the oral cavity of a patient, melanoplakia, multiple oral melanotic macules, melanoma, Addison's disease, Albright's syndrome, Peutz-Jeghers syndrome, and postinflammatory pigmentation should be considered.

Management

The oral melanotic macule should be excised as soon as possible along with an adequate border of normal tissue and submitted for microscopic study. This is necessary because these lesions cannot be differentiated from small, superficial, spreading melanomas on a clinical basis. Only one exception is permitted: if a melanin patch has been known to be present for at least 5 years and *no* changes have occurred, it is sufficient to observe the lesion every 6 months. If the patient's information is known to be unreliable, such a lesion should be excised without further surveillance.

MUCOCELE

The superficial mucocele is one of the most frequent bluish lesions to occur on the lower lip, but it can occur anywhere on the oral mucosa. It is unlikely to be found on the attached gingiva or the anterior hard palate, however, because of the usual absence of minor salivary glands in these regions. The upper lip is another uncommon location for a mucocele. The mucocele is also discussed in Chapter 10 with the exophytic lesions.

The mucocele is thought to occur when a duct of a minor salivary gland is severed by trauma and the secretion is spilled and pooled in the superficial tissues. It seldom possesses an epithelial lining and thus is classified as a false cyst.

A superficial mucocele appears as a bluish mass (Fig. 12-12) because the thin overlying mucosa permits the pool of mucous fluid to absorb most of the visible wavelengths of light except the blue, which is reflected. A deep mucocele, on the other hand, may be normal mucosal pink because of the thickness of the covering mucosa. If a mucocele is subjected to chronic irritation, its mucosal covering is inflamed.

Differential diagnosis

A mucocele is usually a fluctuant, bluish, soft, nodular or dome-shaped elevation that is freely movable on the underlying tissue but cannot be moved independent of the mucosal layer. It cannot be emptied by digital pressure, and on aspiration it yields a sticky, viscous, clear fluid. This result helps to rule out the *vascular lesions* and also the *superficial nonkeratotic cyst*, which usually contains a thin, straw-colored fluid.

The patient may report that the swelling is somewhat paroxysmal—suddenly recurring, rupturing, and draining periodically. In spite of these characteristic features, the differential diagnosis developed for a mucocele must include *early mucoepidermoid tumor* and *mucinous adenocarcinoma*. Both these neoplastic entities may mimic a mucocele in that superficial pools of mucus may be apparent in all three. Hence the clinician must inspect and palpate the tissue at the base and periphery of the mucocele for induration, which might indicate the presence of such tumors. A salivary tumor is rare in the lower lip but occurs with a higher frequency in the palate, buccal mucosa, and upper lip (Krolls and Hicks, 1973).

Management

Any mucocele should be completely removed and the excised tissue examined microscopically. This procedure is particularly important because some mucin-producing salivary tumors mimic a mucocele clinically. The lesion should be excised in such a way as to sever a minimum of the ducts of adjacent acini. A good practice is to remove all the glandular units that protrude into the incision because their ducts are likely to have been severed. This practice helps avoid the embarrassing occurrence of numerous iatrogenic satellite mucoceles.

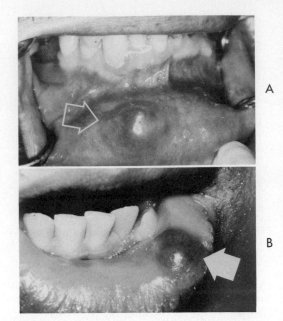

Fig. 12-12. Mucocele *(arrows)*. (**B** courtesy G. MacDonald, DDS, Belleville, Ill.)

Investigators (Wilcox and Hickory, 1978) have suggested steroid injection as an alternative to surgery in the treatment of mucoceles. Abrams (1978) pointed out the danger of overlooking early mucin-producing tumors when such a treatment approach is used.

RANULA

A ranula is, in effect, a mucocele that occurs in the floor of the mouth—a retention cyst in the sublingual salivary gland (Fig. 12-13). It derives its name from the diminutive form of the Latin word for frog, *rana;* it is said to resemble a frog's belly. Galloway et al. (1989) discussed the various theories regarding causes in detail. The ranula is also discussed in Chapter 10 with the exophytic lesions.

Features

A pertinent feature to be noted in the history of a ranula is fluctuation in size. The lesion is generally smallest early in the morning before the patient rises and largest just before meals. This fluctuation in size reflects both the increased secretory activity during periods of gustatory stimulation and water absorption from the pooled mucus during inactive periods of sleep.

When superficially located, a ranula is quite bluish (Fig. 12-13), but a deep ranula appears

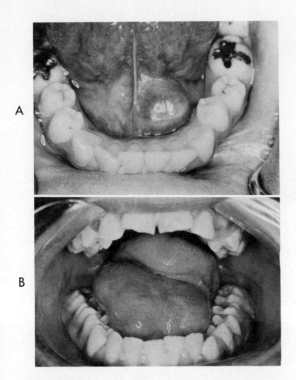

Fig. 12-13. Ranula. **A,** Small, unilateral, dome-shaped, bluish lesion. **B,** Large, bluish ranula occupying the floor of the mouth.

pinker, reflecting the thicker mucosal covering. It usually occurs unilaterally, is dome shaped, and may vary greatly in size. It is soft and fluctuant and cannot be emptied by digital pressure. It does not pulsate, and on aspiration it yields the sticky, clear fluid characteristic of salivary retention phenomena.

Differential diagnosis

The differential diagnosis for a ranula is identical to that described for a mucocele (p. 234). It is interesting how closely the vascular lesions depicted in Figs. 12-3, *C*, and 12-9, *C*, resemble a ranula in both location and appearance.

Management

Initially, conservative treatment by marsupialization is recommended—excising the entire roof of the ranula and permitting the area to heal without a dressing. Such an approach necessitates the careful examination of the lesion's base, in case the mucin-producing entity is really a salivary tumor. For the same reason, close postoperative surveillance is necessary. The lesion so treated may recur in a low percentage of cases. When the lesion does recur,

it is an indication that ducts from neighboring sublingual gland units have been severed during operation or occluded by scarring.

Recurrences of the condition may well signal the need to adopt a more radical form of treatment, such as the removal of sections of the involved gland or at times the entire gland. If the ranula is large and a considerable degree of postoperative swelling is anticipated, the patient must be hospitalized to care for airway problems that may develop.

SUPERFICIAL CYST

The odontogenic and some of the "fissural" cysts that occur just under the epithelial surface and contain straw-colored fluid appear on clinical examination as bluish, nodular swellings. Although they do occur in patients with a mixed dentition, the most common example is the eruption type of follicular cyst seen in infants.

Actually, several types of odontogenic cysts (radicular, dentigerous, or residual, and eruption) appear as nodular, bluish, fluctuant swellings if they are not confined in bone and are located near enough to the surface that the intervening soft tissues can transmit some light to the cyst's mass (Fig. 12-14).

Epidermoid cysts, however, are filled with keratin, so they appear white and are called "Epstein's pearls" when they are small and situated superficially. Superficial keratocysts also appear white for the same reason.

Differential diagnosis

The superficial cyst must be differentiated from all the other soft bluish lesions.

A *cavernous hemangioma* can be evacuated by digital pressure, whereas a superficial cyst cannot.

A radiograph helps differentiate a superficial cyst from a *mucocele*, since the bony superficial cyst causes demonstrable bone destruction, whereas the mucocele is not apparent on radiographic examination.

A *gingival cyst* generally does not involve bone, so a radiograph is not helpful in differentiating it from a mucocele. In addition, a mucocele, unlike a gingival cyst, rarely if ever occurs on the gingiva or the alveolar ridges, since minor salivary glands are not normally present in these locations.

Provided the cyst is not infected, a thin, straw-colored fluid is obtained on aspiration, whereas a clear, viscous, sticky fluid is found in the mucocele.

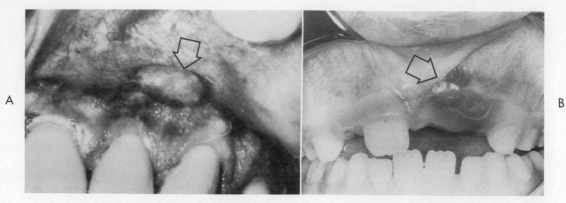

Fig. 12-14. Bluish cysts. **A,** Bluish, translucent, shallow, dome-shaped mass *(arrow)*, which proved to be a gingival cyst. **B,** Bluish eruption cyst *(arrow)* involving the left central incisor tooth. The cyst is similar in appearance to an eruption hematoma.   (**A** courtesy E. Seklecki, DDS, Tucson. **B** courtesy A.C.W. Hutchinson collection, Northwestern University Dental School Library, Chicago.)

Eruption cysts in infants and youngsters in the mixed-dentition-stage are rather common lesions. They characteristically occur in the incisor region, especially in infants (Clark, 1962). The dome-shaped, fluid-filled swelling is readily seen on the ridge, where the involved tooth is attempting to erupt (Fig. 12-14). The eruption cyst usually has a light bluish hue and is rubbery.

An *eruption hematoma*, caused by trauma to the tissue just superficial to the crown of the erupting tooth, closely resembles an eruption cyst. Usually the darker blue color of the eruption hematoma helps the clinician make this distinction.

Also the *lymphangiomas of the alveolar ridges in neonates* as reported by Levin et al. (1976) closely mimic eruption cysts in infants. These authors reported that this special type of lymphangioma occurred on the posterior crests of the maxillary ridges and on the posterior lingual surface of the mandibular ridges. They were dome shaped, blue, and fluid filled. Fifteen infants had single lesions, 32 had two lesions each, two had three lesions each, and nine infants had four lesions, one in each quadrant. The majority were 3 to 4 mm in diameter. In this study the lesions were only found in black infants; 3.7% of the black infants examined had a lesion or lesions. During biopsy the lesions collapsed and the fluid escaped. No teeth were observed deep in the lesion during excision. The fact that eruption cysts in infants almost always occur in the incisor region of the mouth aids in making the distinction between these two entities.

Management

The treatment of intrabony cysts is discussed in Chapters 17 and 19. Eruption cysts usually rupture spontaneously, but if the parents are concerned, simple incision or excision may be performed and followed by microscopic study.

GIANT CELL GRANULOMA

The giant cell granuloma may be either central or peripheral. The central variety is discussed in detail in Chapter 19, whereas the peripheral giant cell granuloma (PGCG) is described in Chapter 10 as an exophytic lesion. The exophytic giant cell granuloma, as well as some of the other inflammatory hyperplastic lesions, may be bluish, so it is also included in this chapter.

Apparently the exophytic giant cell granuloma tends to undergo intermittent episodes of internal hemorrhage because often a considerable amount of hemosiderin is observed in the tissue. If the hemosiderin is located near the surface, it often imparts a bluish brown appearance to the superficial (peripheral) lesion. The numerous vascular spaces filled with bluish blood also account for the bluish color. Katsikeris et al. (1988) reported on 224 new cases and reviewed 956 other cases reported in the literature.

Differential diagnosis

The lesions that should be considered in the differential diagnosis of the PGCG are other inflammatory hyperplastic lesions, hemangioma, lymphangioma, metastatic tumors of the gingiva, nevi, and nodular melanomas.

Other *inflammatory hyperplastic* lesions need not be differentiated because they represent the same basic pathosis as the PGCG.

The majority of *hemangiomas* have been present from birth, whereas the PGCG is of relatively recent onset. Also, congenital hemangiomas seldom occur on the gingiva, yet the gingiva and alveolar mucosa are the only locations of the PGCG.

Oral *lymphangiomas* are much less common than the PGCG and rarely occur on the gingiva. In addition, the lymphangioma has a much paler color.

Metastatic carcinoma to the gingiva must be considered also. However, in the absence of a history of a primary tumor elsewhere, this entity deserves a low ranking. Evidence of bone destruction under the exophytic lesions prompts the clinician to consider metastatic tumor more likely.

Oral nevi and nodular melanomas occur much less frequently than does the PGCG and in almost all cases are firmer to palpation, and they are usually darker in color except for the amelanotic varieties. Finally, a nodular melanoma produces a history of rapid growth.

Management

The cardinal rule is that radiographic examination is a necessary adjunct in the clinical evaluation of all exophytic lesions. Therefore adequate radiographs of the area in question must be available to determine whether underlying bone is involved. Also the giant cell lesion of hyperparathyroidism must be ruled out by examining the serum for the biochemical signs of this disease. Surgical excision is the treatment of choice.

Although less than 10% of these lesions recur after excision, patients who have had them removed should receive two or three yearly examinations so that any recurrence does not go undetected.

BLACK HAIRY TONGUE

Hairy tongue is a harmless entity that occurs on the dorsum of the tongue in approximately 0.15% of the general population (Farman, 1977). This condition is the result of an elongation of the filiform papillae, in some cases to such an extent that they resemble hair (Fig. 12-15). This alteration in the papillae results from an increased retention and accumulation of keratin (hyperkeratosis) (Fig. 12-15). The condition has been thought to be provoked by irritation from one or a combination of local factors: (1) food debris remaining on the tongue

and becoming impacted between the papillae as a result of inadequate oral hygiene, (2) habitual use of oxidizing or astringent agents in oral preparations, (3) local use of some antibiotics, (4) use of tobacco, and (5) *Candida albicans* infection. Systemic influences such as systemic antibiotic therapy, anemia, and general debilitation have been suspected to play an etiologic role (Farman, 1977). Mann et al. (1974) showed that zinc deficiency was associated with hairy tongue in sheep.

The hyperplastic, hyperkeratotic papillae are essentially light colored, but the color they assume is a consequence of local factors in and about them. Chromogenic bacteria, mineral and vitamin preparations, drugs, and dark-colored food may be responsible for changing a white hairy tongue from tan to brown and then to black. Pain is usually not a feature, but gagging may be a problem.

Farman (1977) reported in an extensive study of hairy tongue that patients with malignant neoplasia are prone to this condition (22.06% of his patients with a malignant neoplasm had hairy tongue). This investigator also found a slightly increased incidence in elderly patients (0.72%). Additional findings indicated that hairy tongue is generally associated with candidal organisms and that the pH of saliva on hairy tongues was 6 or less. The majority of Farman's patients with hairy tongue were not smoking at the time of the study, but most had smoked previously in their lives.

Management

Improved tongue-brushing techniques after shearing the elongated papillae with scissors are generally all that is necessary.

LYMPHANGIOMA
Features

A lymphangioma is similar to a cavernous hemangioma. Like the hemangioma it is congenital, but it is much less common. Its most frequent intraoral sites are the dorsal surface and lateral borders of the tongue (Fig. 12-16). (Zachariades and Koundouris [1984] described an interesting case of the buccal mucosa.) Its color is less blue than that of a hemangioma, ranging from normal mucosal pink to bluish, and may be quite translucent. Aspiration yields lymph fluid that is high in lipid content.

The dilated lymphatic channels of a lymphangioma characteristically reach high into the lamina propria and often contact epithelial basement membranes. This feature is often pronounced enough to impart a pebbly appear-

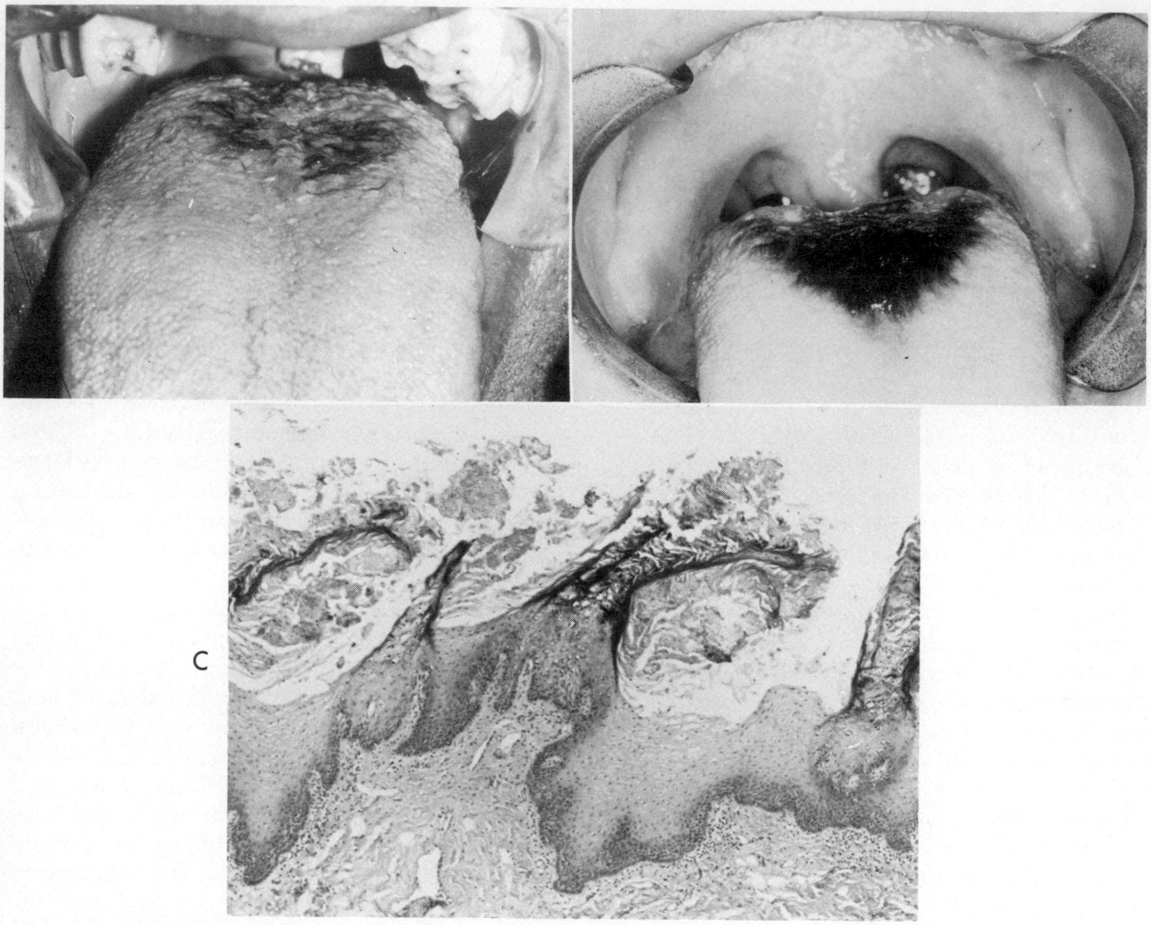

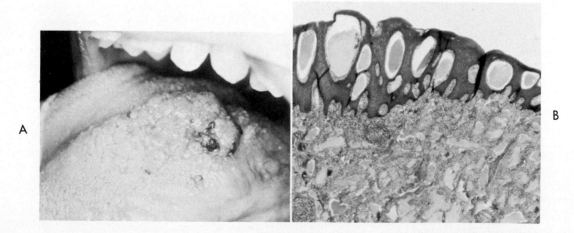

Fig. 12-15. Black hairy tongue. **A** and **B,** Clinical views of patients. **C,** High-magnification photomicrograph shows elongated filiform papillae with increased keratin retention. (**C** courtesy A.C.W. Hutchinson collection, Northwest University Dental School Library, Chicago.)

Fig. 12-16. Lymphangioma. **A,** Lesion with a pebbly surface on the dorsum of the tongue. **B,** The numerous lymphatic spaces appear to be in intimate contact with the surface epithelium. (**A** courtesy D. Bonomo, DDS, Flossmoor, Ill.)

ance to the surface of the lesion. In addition, this feature may hinder the evacuation of the lesion by digital pressure.

Differential diagnosis

The differential diagnosis of a lymphangioma is identical to that of a cavernous hemangioma. Aspiration with a fine-gauge needle may be used to differentiate these two lesions.

Management

Even small lesions on the dorsal surface and lateral borders of the tongue are often continually irritated and become a worry to the patient. It follows that surgical excision is the treatment of choice, but a hemangioma must be ruled out before the excisional procedure is undertaken. Excision of a lymphangioma is not as hazardous a procedure as is excision of a hemangioma; still, if the lesion is larger than 2 cm and is located on the tongue, the patient should be hospitalized because of the possibility of extensive postoperative edema and a related airway problem.

PIGMENTED FIBROMA (PIGMENTED EPULIS)

The pigmented fibroma occurs occasionally in the oral cavity. It is a small, moderately firm, nodular or polypoid mass light bluish or brownish in appearance. It is frequently mistaken for a nevus, and its true identity depends on microscopic examination, which demonstrates it to be a fibroma or a myxofibroma with increased melanin deposition in the basal layer of the epithelium (fibroma in melanoplakic patch). The entity, then, must be included in the differential diagnosis of "nevoidlike" lesions.

MELANOMA

Melanoma is a relatively uncommon malignant tumor of melanocytes; approximately 27,000 new cases for all body sites are diagnosed each year (American Cancer Society, 1989). Bale et al. (1989) reported finding two genetic markers linked to a gene that predisposes people to cutaneous melanoma–dysplastic nevus. Oral melanomas are rare, accounting for approximately 1% of all melanomas (Weathers et al., 1976). Incidence varies significantly with race. Oral melanomas are much more common in the Japanese and in Ugandan Africans than in whites (Batsakis et al., 1982).

In the past, melanomas of the skin had been more or less lumped together as a single entity with a uniformly poor prognosis, but this con-

cept has changed dramatically (Clark et al., 1969; McGovern, 1976). Most primary melanomas of the skin may now be classified as separate lesions on a clinical, histologic, and behavioral basis: (1) lentigo maligna melanoma, (2) superficial spreading melanoma, and (3) nodular melanoma (Regezi et al., 1978). These lesions are listed in ascending order of malignant behavior.

Lentigo maligna melanoma has a predilection for the exposed surfaces of older patients. On clinical examination it is seen as a pigmented macule with an ill-defined margin. During phase one it grows slowly in a radial (developing uniformly around a central axis) and a superficial manner. This slow-growth phase usually continues for many years, and then behavior becomes more aggressive as phase two begins. In this second stage invasion becomes advanced and metastasis frequent (Regezi et al., 1978). Prognosis for the lentigo maligna melanoma is considered to be good, particularly if it is completely excised during the radial-growth phase. McDonald et al. (1983) recommended the use of the term "acral lentiginous melanoma" of the oral cavity because it more closely reflects the usual behavior.

Superficial spreading melanoma is the most common form of melanoma and shows some behavioral characteristics similar to lentigo maligna melanoma. It begins as a pigmented macule that enlarges slowly for several years in a superficial radial growth pattern (Fig. 12-17). As the name implies, the superficial malignant melanocytes are restricted mostly to the epithelium and the junction. If the lesion is left untreated, it shifts into the more aggressive, vertical-growth phase and shows as a pigmented nodule or nodules within the larger pigmented patch. Metastasis usually does not occur while the lesion is in the superficial spreading (radial-growth) phase. Thus if the lesion is completely excised during the superficial phase, the prognosis is much better than for nodular melanoma.

Nodular melanoma, which arises by itself without a superficial spreading component, grows rapidly, may metastasize early, and carries the poorest prognosis.

Clark et al. (1969) reported the mortality rate for the three types of skin melanomas: lentigo maligna melanoma, 10.3%; superficial spreading melanoma, 31.5%; and nodular melanoma, 56.1%.

Oral melanomas and melanomas of the lips are rare tumors. Like their skin counterparts, over the years the oral tumors have been

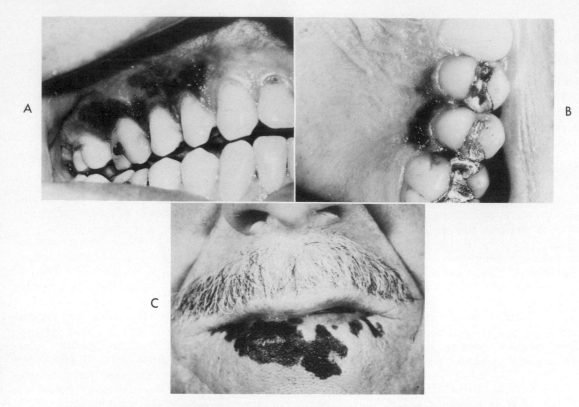

Fig. 12-17. Superficial spreading melanomas. A and B, Two views of a superficial spreading melanoma on the maxillary ridge of a 45-year-old man. The patient had watched it slowly grow for several months. B, Mirror shot showing spread of tumor from the labial gingiva through the interproximal area to involve the lingual gingiva. C, Superficial spreading melanoma of the lower lip in a 59-year-old man had been present for 8 years, spreading from two small, pigmented patches. Nodules were now present on the mucosal surface.   (A and B from Robertson GR, Defiebre BK, and Firtell DN: J Oral Surg 37:349-352, 1979. Copyright by the American Dental Association. Reprinted by permission. C from Regezi JA, Hayward JR, and Pickens TN: Oral Surg 45[5]:730-740, 1978.)

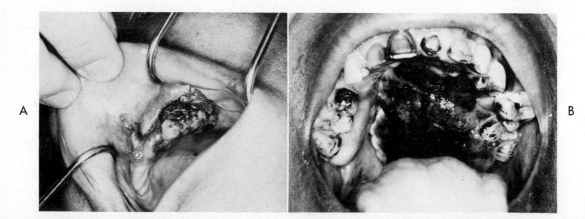

Fig. 12-18. Advanced melanomas of the maxillary ridge and palate. A, Nodular melanoma appeared to have a superficial spreading component at the periphery. B, Large, advanced nodular melanoma in a 56-year-old woman.   (A courtesy S. Smith, DDS, Chicago.)

grouped as one entity with a uniformly grave prognosis (Bina, 1979; Chaudry et al., 1960; Eneroth, 1975). It has been recognized, however, that there are behavioral differences among oral melanomas (Jackson and Simpson, 1975; Liversedge, 1975). Also a few superficial spreading melanomas of the oral cavity have been reported (Bennett et al., 1976; Regezi et al., 1978; Robertson et al., 1979). In addition to these developments, a history of a previously existing pigmented patch (melanosis) in a significant number of large nodular melanomas has been reported (Regezi et al., 1978). Thus it seems likely that many oral melanomas are of the superficial spreading type, are present for several years, and are not diagnosed until the lesion has changed to the more aggressive, vertical-growth phase.

Features

The oral melanoma may be encountered on clinical examination as one of four enlarging lesions: a pigmented macule, a pigmented nodule, a large pigmented exophytic lesion, or an amelanotic (unpigmented) variety of any of these three forms (Figs. 12-17 and 12-18). It may vary from a mucosal pink through brown and blue to black. It is usually firm to palpation but not as firm as a squamous cell carcinoma. The oral variety frequently ulcerates but does not possess a rolled, raised border. An erythematous border in the mucosa often surrounds the tumor and represents an inflammatory reaction of the surrounding tissue to the tumor.

The oral melanoma occurs most frequently in the maxillary alveolar mucosa and on the hard and soft palates (Figs. 12-17 and 12-18). The rate of growth in superficial spreading melanoma is slow until the vertical phase is reached. The growth rate for the nodular melanoma, although usually rapid, may be variable. The tumor is usually painless unless ulcerated or infected or both. Rapid infiltration of the adjacent deep tissues frequently occurs in the nodular type and fixes the superficial tissues to the deeper layers.

Differential diagnosis

The early melanoma, which appears clinically as a small brownish blue macule, may be readily confused with an *amalgam tattoo,* an *oral melanotic macule,* a *focal hemosiderin deposit* after trauma, or a localized area of *melanoplakia.*

The clinician who must choose from these entities with only the information available from the patient examination has difficulty arriving at a working diagnosis.

On clinical examination the early nodular melanoma is difficult or impossible to differentiate from an *intramucosal, compound,* or *blue nevus,* a *pigmented fibroma,* or a small pigmented *peripheral giant cell granuloma* that contains a large amount of hemosiderin. Occasionally the nodular melanoma has an irregular, fissured, or ulcerated and bleeding surface—features that strongly suggest malignancy. Rapid growth is a feature of melanoma.

Although the rapidly enlarging pigmented exophytic variety is not easily confused with other entities, the clinician may be confronted with a lesion in a patient being seen for the first time and the patient may not be able to tell how long the lesion has been present or whether it is enlarging.

If the melanin is deposited near the surface, the *melanotic neuroectodermal tumor of infancy* may be similar in appearance to the pigmented melanoma. Many of these appear on clinical examination with a nonpigmented, pink surface, however, because the melanin is deposited in the deeper tissue. The anterior maxilla is a common site for either of these tumors, but the average patient age at occurrence of an oral melanoma is in the 50s (the youngest occurrence reported was in a child 5 years old), whereas the melanotic tumor of infancy occurs in children of less than 1 year of age.

On clinical examination the amelanotic melanoma is sometimes mistaken for a *pyogenic granuloma,* or it may resemble many of the *benign* or *malignant tumors* that have nodular, polypoid, or exophytic shapes.

The macular bluish, brownish, or black lesions such as melanoplakia, oral melanotic macule, and ecchymotic patch must be considered in the differential diagnosis of superficial spreading melanoma. All are macules with similar coloring.

The *ecchymotic patch* disappears within a few days, passing through the various characteristic color changes. Frequently its occurrence is related to a traumatic episode.

Melanoplakia, the physiologic pigmentation found in the oral cavities of blacks, is present from infancy or puberty without change. Most designs are similar throughout the mouth, so if a patch of unusual design is present, the clinician suspects as a more likely possibility a superficial spreading melanoma. If the patch had appeared within the preceding 2 or 3 years in an adult between 40 and 70 years of age and had increased in size, the working diagnosis is superficial spreading melanoma.

The *oral melanotic macule* cannot be differentiated from an early lesion of superficial spreading melanoma. If the pigmented patch is more than 2 cm in size and has shown evidence of enlargement, it must be considered a superficial spreading melanoma until proved otherwise by microscopic study.

Management

If the suspicion index is low, a melanoma may be ruled out by just observing the small pigmented area for a period of 3 to 6 months. If the working diagnosis is amalgam tattoo, for example, the lesion should be reexamined in 6 months.

If the suspicion index is higher and the lesion is small, however, the lesion should be excised early with a wide margin of normal tissue and microscopically examined. Radical resection with removal of regional lymph nodes may be necessary in cases of larger lesions. The effectiveness of intralesional injections of interferon and polyvalent melanoma antigen vaccines is currently being evaluated (Bystryn et al., 1988; von Wussow et al., 1988).

The prognosis for oral melanomas is poor because characteristically they are discovered in advanced stages and they metastasize early to the regional nodes and via vascular routes to the lungs, liver, skin, brain, and bones. However, the prognosis is much improved if the tumor is of the superficial spreading type and is excised in the radial-growth phase, when the lesion is small. The possibility that the oral lesion is a secondary (metastatic) lesion should always be considered (see Fig. 10-30).

NEVUS

A nevus is a congenital or acquired benign tumor of the melanocytes or nevus cells that occurs on the skin but seldom intraorally. It is usually but not always pigmented, ranging from gray to light brown to blue to black. There are four types of oral nevi: intramucosal, junctional, compound, and blue.

The intramucosal (intradermal*) nevus is composed of a bulk of nevus cells in the lamina propria, which do not contact the basement membrane. Because this bulk of cells is packed within the usually dense, collagenous, connective tissue stroma, the nevus is firm to palpation and is usually raised in the form of a smooth nodule, but sometimes it appears as a polypoid mass (Fig. 12-19). The intramucosal

---

*The intradermal nevus or common mole is one of the most frequently occurring pigmented lesions of the skin.

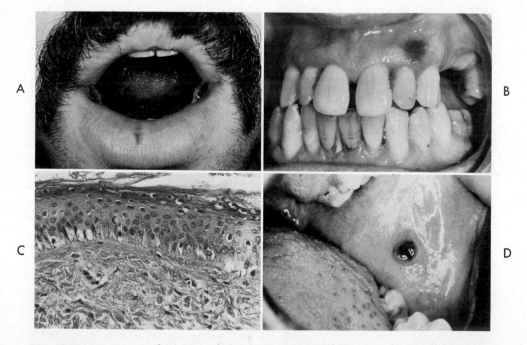

Fig. 12-19. Nevus. **A** and **B,** Junctional nevi. **C,** Junctional nevus on histopathologic examination. **D,** On histologic examination this exophytic lesion proved to be an intramucosal nevus.   (**D** courtesy N. Herrod, DDS, Provo, Utah.)

nevus must be differentiated from a *pigmented fibroma* and a *small nodular melanoma.*

The junctional nevus derives its name from the nevus cells that are in the basal layer just above the junction of the epidermis and dermis. It is usually not raised because there are only a few nevus cells present (Fig. 12-19). This lesion must be differentiated from *melanoplakia*, an *amalgam tattoo*, a *melanotic macule*, and a *melanoma.*

The compound nevus cells are in both locations—lamina propria and basal layer of the epithelium. This lesion therefore is a firm, raised, nodule or polypoid mass having a clinical appearance identical to that of the intramucosal nevus.

The blue nevus is also a raised nodule It is usually dark blue and has stellate and fusiform cells that usually contain melanin. These cells are commonly located deep in the lamina propria, which is why the lesion may appear more darkly pigmented than the other nevi. It can be moved over the submucosal structures but cannot be moved independent of the mucosa. It must be differentiated from a melanoma but cannot be differentiated on clinical examination.

Buchner and Hansen (1980b) reported on 32 new cases of intraoral nevi: 66% were the intramucosal type, 25% were common blue nevi, 6% were compound, and 3% were the junctional type. The locations of the lesions were as follows: 37.5% on the hard palate, 16% on the buccal mucosa, and 12.5% each on the labial mucosa, the vermilion border, and the gingiva. Ninety-one percent of the nevi exhibited pigmentation on clinical examination. The mean age of the patients was 29.6 years and the female-to-male ratio was 36:1.

In a series of 17 nevi reported by Watkins et al. (1984) 12 were intramucosal nevi, 2 were compound nevi, and 1 was a blue nevus. In 1987 Buchner and Hansen reported their findings on 36 new cases and reviewed findings of 155 cases from the literature.

Differential diagnosis

The firmness of a nevus to palpation distinguishes this lesion from a *cyst*, a *retention phenomenon* of the minor salivary glands, and a *hemangioma*. An exception might be a *sclerosing hemangioma*, but even it has vascular spaces that are reddish and blanch on digital pressure, a characteristic not shared by the nevi.

The occurrence of a dark bluish lesion in proximity to an amalgam restoration, or the probability of such a previous relationship in an edentulous area, lends support to the identification of the condition as an *amalgam tattoo.*

Small areas of hemorrhage may resemble a junctional nevus but the former lesion shows color changes and disappears within a week or two.

A nevus cannot be definitely differentiated from an early *melanoma* except by microscopic study, but a change in degree of pigmentation, bleeding, or surface appearance is an ominous sign.

The *oral melanotic macule* looks identical to a nonraised nevus or an early superficial spreading melanoma. The latter lesions are much less common, however, and so are ranked much lower in the differential process.

Management

A nevus should be excised along with a wide border of normal tissue and studied microscopically. The opinion persists today that some melanomas may arise from nevi. Hansen and Buchner (1980b) recommended that junctional nevi be completely excised because their malignant potential is uncertain.

MUCUS-PRODUCING SALIVARY GLAND TUMORS

The mucoepidermoid tumor is a malignancy of the salivary glands that originates in the oral cavity with some frequency. Three cell types are seen: a mucous cell, an epidermoid cell, and an intermediate–type cell. The greater the percentage of mucous cells present, the less malignant the tumor is thought to be. This low-grade variety is included with the blue lesions because pools of mucus are frequently present (Fig. 12-20). Thus the tumor may resemble a mucocele on clinical examination.

The mucous cell adenocarcinoma is another tumor of salivary glands that produces mucus and can mimic a mucocele in its early stages.

An advanced tumor of these two types might have a firm consistency overall, with discrete, soft, fluctuant areas intermixed.

Differential diagnosis

The lower lip is an uncommon site for a salivary gland tumor but a frequent site for a mucocele. Hence a bluish, fluctuant, dome-shaped, nonemptiable swelling on the lower lip is most likely a *mucocele.*

A lesion resembling a mucocele on the palate or even the buccal mucosa or upper lip, however, should be viewed with suspicion, since mucoceles are less common in these areas.

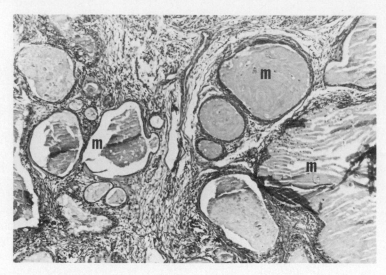

Fig. 12-20. Low-grade mucoepidermoid tumor showing pools of mucus (*m*), which on clinical examination may cause this lesion to mimic a mucocele.

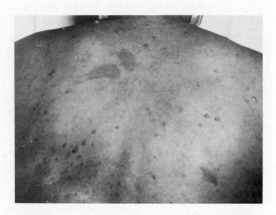

Fig. 12-21. Café-au-lait spots on a patient with von Recklinghausen's disease. Note the small, nodular, multiple neurofibromas.   (Courtesy P.D. Toto, DDS, Maywood, Ill.)

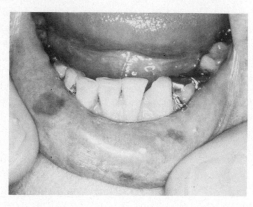

Fig. 12-22. Perioral macular pigmentation in patient with Addison's disease.   (Courtesy S. Smith, DDS, Chicago.)

Management

The base of any clinical mucocele should be examined closely for induration, which might indicate an infiltrating tumor. Of course, all excised tissue from a lesion of this type must be microscopically examined to establish the nature of the lesion. Wide resection is the treatment of choice for a mucoepidermoid tumor.

VON RECKLINGHAUSEN'S DISEASE (MULTIPLE NEUROFIBROMATOSIS)

Multiple neurofibromatosis is a hereditary disease that is thought to be transmitted as an autosomal dominant trait. The two most common features of this disorder are the multiple neurofibromas and the café-au-lait spots (Fig. 12-21). The tumors are frequently of the plexiform variety and thus are soft, smooth, fluctuant, usually flesh colored, and nodular or pedunculated; however, they occasionally assume large, pendulous, flabby proportions.

Multiple cutaneous neurofibromas are a characteristic sign. Axillary freckling is also characteristic. These spots, as their color suggests, are the result of increased pigment in the basal layer, and like the neurofibromas, are sometimes encountered in the oral cavity.

The café-au-lait spots are brownish macules that occur at any cutaneous site, including genitalia, soles, and palms. Larger than 1.5 cm in diameter, they are present in more than 90% of the cases and are diagnostic when more than five are present.

Differential diagnosis

The multiple cutaneous neurofibromas identify von Recklinghausen's disease.

The *basal cell nevus syndrome* (BCNS) has cutaneous tumors and is accompanied by cysts in the jaws. Unlike the neurofibromas of von Recklinghausen's disease, however, the tumors of the basal cell nevus syndrome are restricted to the skin of the face, neck, and chest. Furthermore, pigmentation is not a feature of BCNS.

Multiple mucosal plexiform neurofibromas are also seen as part of a syndrome with *nodular carcinoma of the thyroid gland* and *pheochromocytoma*, but cutaneous neurofibromas and pigmentation are not features.

Multiple desmoid tumors, fibromas, and epidermoid cysts occur on the skin of patients who have *Gardner's syndrome*, but no pigmented macules are present. In addition, patients with Gardner's syndrome have multiple osteomas of the cranial and facial bones, including the jaws, and multiple polyposis of the colon.

The differential diagnosis of diseases with café-au-lait spots is discussed in this chapter with Albright's syndrome.

Management

The café-au-lait spots do not require treatment, but surgical excision of individual neurofibromas may be necessary for various reasons. Approximately 7% of these patients develop a neurogenic sarcoma.

ALBRIGHT'S SYNDROME

Albright's syndrome is a developmental defect of unknown cause that features: (1) café-au-lait macules, (2) single or multiple involvement of bones with fibrous dysplasia leading to deformity and fractures, and (3) precocious puberty in girls. This entity is uncommon in its complete form and more frequently occurs with the first two features only, which combination is known as Jaffe's type. The café-au-lait spots are irregularly shaped, brownish tan macules seen in the skin and sometimes in the oral mucosa. They represent melanin deposition.

Differential diagnosis

When pigmented macules are found on the skin and oral mucosa, syndromes and diseases that must be considered are Albright's syndrome, von Recklinghausen's disease, Peutz-Jeghers syndrome, and Addison's disease.

Patients with *Addison's disease* in some instances have discrete macules instead of the diffuse tanning (Fig. 12-22). Chuong and Goldberg (1983) described a case of Addison's disease in which oral hyperpigmentation was the only finding at first. Usually the classic symptoms of adrenal insufficiency differentiate this disease from the others.

Peutz-Jeghers syndrome can be excluded from consideration, since the pigmented macules on the skin in this disorder are restricted to the area surrounding body orifices or the fingers or both. (Fig. 12-23). Then too the symptoms that result from the accompanying intestinal polyposis of Peutz-Jeghers syndrome prevent the clinician from confusing this condition with Albright's syndrome and von Recklinghausen's disease.

The café-au-lait spots occuring in *Albright's syndrome* are seen in young patients with fibrous dysplasia and precocious puberty. In contrast, the café-au-lait spots occurring in *von Recklinghausen's disease* are associated with concomitant cutaneous and mucosal multiple neurofibromas.

Management

The café-au-lait spots of Albright's syndrome do not require treatment. The jaws, however, may be affected with the lesions of fibrous dysplasia and thus may require recontouring for esthetic considerations.

HEAVY METAL LINES

Chronic poisoning with heavy metals (such as mercury, lead, and bismuth) may result in a dark brownish to blue-black discoloration in the oral cavity. Most frequently the heavy metals are deposited as a line or band on inflamed marginal gingiva. In 1975, ten Bruggenkate et al. reported a case of a painter who habitually used an electric grinder to remove old paint. Lockhart (1981) described a case of a patient who was mentally retarded and lived in a dormitory with much old paint peeling from the walls.

The line or band pattern of deposition is the result of increased capillary permeability in the free gingivae caused by inflammation, which permits perivascular infiltration of the tissues by the metal. The pigmentation does not disappear when the irritation is removed and the accompanying inflammation resolved. Information obtained from the history is the most useful in establishing a positive identification of the offending metal. Ten Bruggenkate et al.

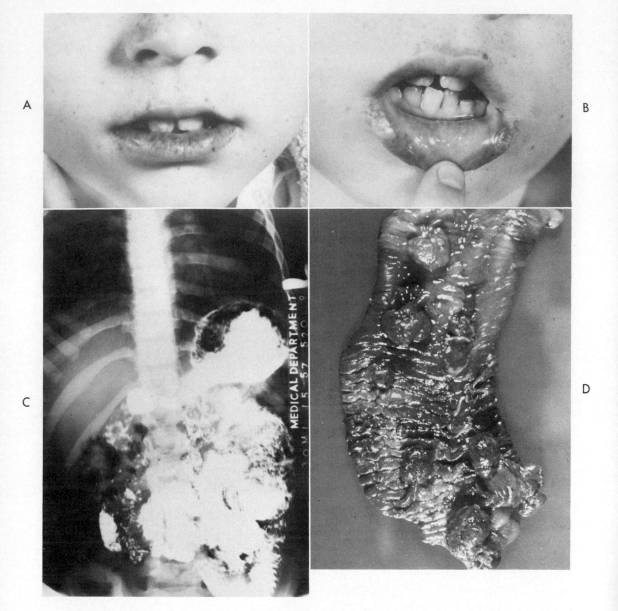

Fig. 12-23. Peutz-Jeghers syndrome. **A** and **B,** Perioral pigmentation. **C,** Radiograph showing intestinal polyposis. **D,** Specimen of intestine showing numerous polyps on the luminal surface.   (Courtesy D. Cooksey, DDS, Los Angeles.)

(1975) described the characteristic findings of the blood, urine, bone marrow, and radiographic tests of patients with lead poisoning.

More stringent regulation of working conditions in factories that use heavy metals, more careful inspection and elimination of chipping lead paint in the interior of old houses, and the elimination of these metals from medicines have greatly reduced the incidence of this type of lesion.

KAPOSI'S SARCOMA

Intraoral Kaposi's sarcoma is a common occurrence in patients with acquired immunodeficiency syndrome (AIDS). In a study by Lozada et al. (1983) 51% of their patients had these lesions. The lesions of Kaposi's sarcoma may appear as broad, reddish to reddish brown to bluish brown swellings with minimal elevation (Fig. 12-24). They may also present as discrete nodules that bleed easily and may measure

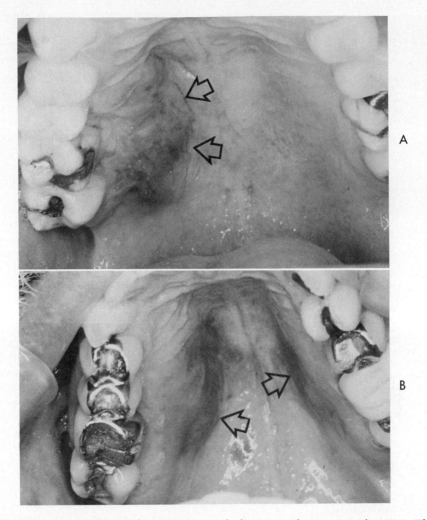

Fig. 12-24. Two cases of Kaposi's sarcoma in male homosexual patients with AIDS. These palatal lesions were bluish brown with minimal swelling. **A,** Single lesion on the right side of the palate *(arrows).* **B,** Bilateral lesions *(arrows).*   (**A** and **B** courtesy S. Silverman, DDS, San Francisco.)

from a few millimeters to a centimeter or more in diameter (see Figs. 10-10, *B,* and 5-22). In the nodular form they may closely resemble a pyogenic granuloma or other inflammatory hyperplastic lesions. They are frequently tender or painful. On histologic examination, Kaposi's sarcoma in patients with AIDS is similar to that which occurs in patients who do not have AIDS. The treatment of Kaposi's sarcoma consists of radiotherapy, chemotherapy, and interferon therapy, singly or in combination (Fauci et al., 1984). By and large, the treatment of Kaposi's sarcoma in patients with AIDS has not been as successful as its treatment in patients who do not have AIDS. Ficarra et al. (1988) reported on their study of Kaposi's sarcoma in

134 patients with AIDS. Kaposi's sarcoma and AIDS are further described and illustrated in Appendix D.

RARITIES

Although the disease conditions listed as rarities do have distinctly circumscribed, brownish, bluish, or black oral lesions, either they occur rarely or, if found more frequently, these entities seldom occur as oral lesions. No ranking according to frequency of occurrence has been attempted:

Acanthosis nigricans
Acromegaly
Addison's disease (distinct circumscribed lesions)
AIDS-related pigmentation

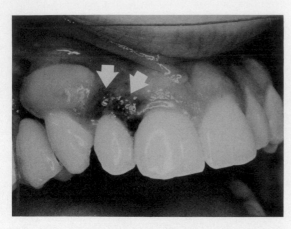

Fig. 12-25. Hemangioendothelioma of the gingiva (*arrows*). (Courtesy Victor Barresi, DDS, De-Kalb, Ill.)

Amyloidosis
Angina bullosa hemorrhagica
Angiosarcoma
Blue nevus
Blue rubber-bleb nevus syndrome
Chlorpromazine therapy
Chronic obstructive pulmonary disease (COPD)
Cushing's syndrome
Fabry's disease
Gaucher's disease
Hemangioendothelioma (Fig. 12-25)
Henoch-Schönlein purpura
Hereditary hemorrhagic telangiectasia
Incontinentia pigmenti
Kaposi's sarcoma (non-AIDS)
Lentigo
Lichen planus
Lupus erythematosus
Lymphangiomas of neonates
Lymphoma (superficial)
Maffucci's syndrome
Melanoacanthoma
Melanotic neuroectodermal tumor of infancy
Minocycline pigmentation
Nelson's syndrome
Pernicious anemia
Peutz-Jeghers syndrome
Pheochromocytoma
Quinidine pigmentation
Rheumatic fever
Scleroderma
Smoker's mucosal melanosis
Submucous fibrosis
Superficial cartilaginous tumor in patient with ochronosis or alkaptonuria
Superficial *Pseudomonas aeruginosa* infection
Tattoo
Thyrotoxicosis
Uremia (petechiae)
Wegener's granulomatosis
Xeroderma pigmentosa

Generalized brownish, bluish, or black conditions

CYANOSIS

Cyanosis is caused by a substantial rise in the proportion of reduced hemoglobin to oxygenated hemoglobin in the blood. The cyanosis may be local or generalized according to the cause. For instance, a tourniquet that has been applied to a patient's arm soon produces a local cyanosis of the arm, whereas a hysterical, crying child who is hypoventilating has a generalized cyanosis.

A rule of thumb holds that cyanosis becomes clinically apparent when the reduced hemoglobin reaches 5 g/100 ml. The generalized bluish cast to the skin is readily seen in light-skinned individuals but is easy to overlook in dark-skinned individuals. It can be detected readily in the oral mucous membranes of individuals of all races and complexions.

Coldness may cause a peripheral cyanosis on the lips and extremities but is readily apparent as the cause.

The three causes of generalized cyanosis are respiratory deficiency, cardiovascular pathology, and abnormal hemoglobin metabolism. Respiratory diseases that cause generalized cyanosis are advanced tuberculosis, emphysema, and pneumonia. Common cardiovascular diseases that cause generalized cyanosis are congenital heart defects, right ventricular failure, and ventricular fibrillation. Clubbing of the fingers often accompanies cyanosis, if the cyanosis has persisted as a chronic condition.

Differential diagnosis

The patient should be referred to a competent physician for the diagnosis of the general medical problem.

Management

Before composing a treatment plan or initiating any dental treatment for the patient, the clinician must be aware of the serious implications of cyanosis and the problems that may be encountered. Thus it is imperative that the physician's advice be sought, obtained, and followed. Of course, if the patient is having an acute attack, the dental clinician must initiate emergency measures that support the patient's circulation and respiration until the patient is in the care of a competent medical team.

CHLOASMA GRAVIDARUM

Chloasma gravidarum is the tanned mask seen on the cheeks, nose, and infraorbital areas of pregnant, light-skinned women during the latter half of pregnancy. It is occasionally accompanied by a diffuse browning of the oral mucosa. The pigmentation slowly disappears after delivery. The increased ACTH level during pregnancy is thought to account for the increased melanocyte activity.

ADDISON'S DISEASE

Addison's disease occurs in approximately one in 100,000 of the population and is extremely rare in children. Bilateral adrenocortical destruction after tuberculous or fungal infection and an idiopathic atrophy are the most frequent causes. Occasionally bilateral tumor metastasis, leukemic infiltration, and amyloidosis of the adrenal cortex have been found to be responsible. Whatever the cause, the loss of adrenal cortex results in a deficiency in both glucocorticoids and mineralocorticoids.

It has been shown that ACTH and melanocyte-stimulating hormone (MSH) are similar in structure, and ACTH is believed to have some degree of melanocyte-stimulating activity. Normally the pituitary gland produces ACTH, which causes the adrenal cortex to produce glucocorticoids (such as hydrocortisone), which in turn are secreted into the circulation. When the glucocorticoids reach a certain concentration in the blood, they cause the anterior pituitary to cease production of ACTH. In Addison's disease, however, the defective cortex is unable to produce much glucocorticoid, so this feedback mechanism is not activated and the pituitary continues to produce ACTH. As a result the increased production of melanin changes the color of the skin to a smoky tan or a chestnut brown.

Pigmentation usually appears early and is one of the most prominent signs of the disease. It may take one of two forms, the more usual being a deep tanning of the skin and mucous membranes with heavier deposits of melanin over pressure points. The cheek is the most common site for this pigmentation in the oral mucosa. More infrequently the increased melanocytic activity is expressed by the development of distinct brownish macules on the oral mucosa and skin (see Fig. 12-22).

Other clinical features that attend the disease are hypotension, lymphocytosis, hyperkalemia, hypoglycemia, hyponatremia, and a reduced basal metabolic rate.

Differential diagnosis

A thorough history and clinical appraisal should guide the practitioner to the correct working diagnosis. The type of pigmentation in Addison's disease that produces an overall, deep tanning of the skin and mucous membranes must be differentiated from hemochromatosis, argyria, and several rarer entities (such as hyperpituitarism).

Addison's disease may be distinguished from *hyperpituitarism* by the use of urine tests: levels of 17-ketosteroids in the urine are decreased in the former but elevated in the latter condition. Although *chronic adrenal insufficiency* is rare in children, it does occur to complete the occasional and little-understood genetic syndrome characterized by superficial candidiasis, idiopathic familial juvenile hypoparathyroidism, and Addison's disease.

A history of silver ingestion identifies *argyria*.

The accompanying hepatic fibrosis, diabetes, other endocrinopathies, and iron deposition in the affected organs and the skin that are seen in *hemochromatosis* differentiate this conditon from Addison's disease.

The macular type of discoloration that occasionally develops in place of the more generalized tanning might be mistaken for *Peutz-Jeghers syndrome*, *Albright's syndrome*, or *von Recklinghausen's disease;* however, the attending features of these individual syndromes should preclude any such confusion.

Management

The dentist should not begin treatment without first consulting the patient's physician. If the disease is well controlled, the patient is able to withstand dental procedures. Supplementation of the patient's corticosteroid medication is generally required before dental work is initiated.

HEMOCHROMATOSIS (BRONZE DIABETES)

Bronze diabetes is a disorder in which excess iron is deposited in the body and results in eventual sclerosis and dysfunction of the tissues and organs so involved. The iron is stored in the form of hemosiderin and ferritin. Three circumstances are generally believed to be contributing influences—idiopathy, diet, and excessive blood transfusions—and all three relate to increasing iron levels in the body.

No agreement has yet been reached as to the exact pathogenesis of the three types of hemochromatosis (or even whether they are different). The most frequently involved organs are the liver, the skin, and the endocrine glands, especially the pancreas and the adrenal glands.

In the idiopathic type there appears to be a defect in the iron-absorption mechanism permitting increased intestinal absorption. The gradual surplus of iron accumulates until enough is present to produce the symptoms, usually in the patient's fourth and fifth decades of life.

The cause of the tanning in hemochromatosis, like that in Addison's disease, is an increased melanin production and not the deposition of hemosiderin in the skin. This increased production, as in Addison's disease, results from the high levels of ACTH that accompany the destruction of the adrenal cortex by the heavy iron deposits. The effect is a blue gray color of the skin, especially over the genitalia, face, and arms.

The disease is primarily manifested in men; more than 80% of the cases occur in men. This prevalence is attributed to the greater intake of dietary iron in men, which they are unable to excrete. On the other hand, women apparently lose enough iron during menses and pregnancy to prevent the tissue deposits of iron from reaching toxic levels. In addition, the genetic defect in the iron absorption mechanism that has been proposed may have greater penetrance in males.

Differential diagnosis

Similar skin and oral pigmentation is seen in *Addison's disease*, *argyria*, and some of the rare diseases (for example, *Wilson's disease* [hepatolenticular degeneration] and *porphyria*); a careful history and clinical examination eliminate these from consideration. When the triad of hemochromatosis (skin pigmentation, liver disease, and diabetes) is present in a male patient, the diagnosis is not difficult.

Although a skin biopsy showing iron deposits is of value in confirming the diagnosis, determination of the iron content and iron-binding capacity of the serum and biopsies of the bone marrow and liver are considered more reliable than the skin biopsy.

Management

The dental clinician must work closely with the patient's physician when oral treatment is planned. The patient is particularly susceptible to infection, cardiovascular collapse, and hypoglycemic episodes—tendencies that are characteristic of adrenal insufficiency and diabetes.

ARGYRIA (SILVER PIGMENTATION)

Whites who have silver pigmentation develop a striking, bluish gray (slate-colored) skin, especially in the exposed areas. They in-

variably give a history of having used some type of self-medication, such as nose drops, containing silver salts, for a long period of time. Plack and Bellizzi (1980) described a case of argyria in which the patient had chewed photographic film as an aid to discontinue smoking. Silver deposition often causes accompanying neurologic and hearing damage, which in turn affects the equilibrium. It also stimulates melanocyte activity in the skin, hence the more intense color in exposed areas. The bluish gray discoloration has also been reported to occur in the oral mucosa.

Differential diagnosis

The bluish gray color is usually easily distinguished from the more brownish, *Addisonian color*. *Hemochromatosis* also produces a browner color. Exposed areas of the skin that are not more discolored than the covered areas differentiate *cyanotic states* from argyria. Histologic identification of silver particles fixed to protein complexes in the corium is diagnostic for the disease.

Management

The only special precaution to take during oral treatment is to consider the patient's disturbance in equilibrium. Hence the clinician should avoid rapid changes in the position of the dental chair while the patient is seated.

RARITIES

Although the disease conditions included in this section may show generalized brownish, bluish, or black conditions, the diseases either occur rarely or seldom show this feature. No ranking according to frequency of occurrence has been attempted:

Aniline intoxication
Arsenic poisoning
Carotenemia
Chloroquine therapy
Dermatomyositis
Idiopathic familial juvenile hypoparathyroidism, Addison's disease, superficial candidiasis
Pellagra
Porphyria
Sprue
Wilson's disease

Table 12-1. Distinct, circumscribed types of brownish, bluish, or black conditions

Condition	Appearance	Usual history	Usual age of occurrence (years)	Frequency
MACULES				
Melanoplakia	Macules of varying size, shape, and location on oral mucosa	No symptoms	Birth to 1	Common in dark-skinned races
Amalgam tattoo	Macule on gingiva or edentulous ridge	No symptoms Amalgam-filled tooth	5 and older	Common
Petechia and ecchymosis	Macule anywhere in oral cavity or skin	Recent trauma or bleeding diathesis	(young children and older adults)	Occasional
Melanotic macule	Small macule (less than 2 mm in diameter) on lower lip, gingiva, or buccal mucosa	No symptoms	Mean age 41 to 42	Occasional Male/female ratio 1:2.2
Superficial spreading melanoma	Enlarging macule on palate or maxillary gingiva	Present for several years Slowly enlarging	Mean age 50.5	Rare Male/female ratio 2:1
Junctional nevus	Macule anywhere on oral mucosa (palate, lips)	No symptoms	Mean age 38	Rare in oral cavity Equal frequency for men and women
Heavy metal lines	Macular ribbon following free gingivae	Malaise Anemia	(working age)	Rare
Peutz-Jeghers syndrome	Macules around lips, buccal mucosa, fingers, body orifices	Melena Intestinal colic	More distinct at puberty	Rare
Albright's syndrome	Macules (café-au-lait spots) anywhere on skin or mucous membranes	Skeletal problems Precocious puberty in girls	6 to 10	Rare
FIRM LESIONS				
Amalgam fragment	Macule on gingiva or edentulous alveolus	Present for some years Firm mass in tissue	5 and older	Common
Late hematoma	Mass or swelling	Previous trauma or bleeding diatheses with repeated bleeding episodes		Occasional
Giant cell granuloma	Moderately firm macule, nodule, or polypoid mass on gingiva or alveolus	Slowly expanding mass	30 and older	Occasional
Pigmented fibroma	Papule, nodule, or polypoid mass Usually on buccal mucosa	Present for some time		Occasional
Intramucosal nevus	Papule, nodule, or polypoid mass	Present from birth		Rare
Compound nevus	Papule, nodule, or polypoid mass	Present from birth		Rare
Melanoma	Pigmented or amelanotic; nodule, polypoid mass on palate or maxillary gingiva	Rapidly enlarging mass	Mean age 50.5	Rare Twice as common in men
Neuroectodermal tumor	Expansion of labial alveolus Pigment or pink	Slowly expanding mass in anterior maxilla	Birth to 1	Rare

Table 12-1. Distinct, circumscribed types of brownish, bluish, or black conditions—cont'd

Condition	Appearance	Fluctu-ance	May be emptied	Usual history	Usual age of occurrence (years)	Frequency
EXOPHYTIC LESIONS OF SOFT CONSISTENCY						
Black hairy tongue	Patch of hairy growth, varying in length, on dorsal surface of tongue	No	No	Feels like hairs on tongue Gagging sensation	Older than 30	Occasional
Mucocele	Nodular swelling	Yes	No	Variation in size Occasional rupture and drainage	Older than 40	Occasional Significantly more common in males
Ranula	Nodular swelling on floor of mouth	Yes	No	Slowly enlarging Smaller in early morning		Occasional Significantly more common in females
Cavernous hemangioma	Nodular swelling	Usually not	Yes	Present from birth or after trauma Occasional bleeding		Occasional
Early hematoma	Nodular swelling	Yes	No	Recent trauma or bleeding diatheses		Occasional
Superficial cyst	Nodular swelling	Yes	No	Displaced teeth Slowly enlarging swelling		Occasional
Lymphangioma	Nodular swelling Surface frequently has pebbly appearance	Usually not	Partially	Present from birth or after trauma		Rare
Mucoepidermoid tumor	Mucocele-like nodule	Some areas	No	Slowly expanding mass	40	Rare Mucocele-like epidermoid tumor is rare
Multiple neurofibromatosis	Macules (cafe-au-lait spots) present on skin and occasionally on oral mucosa	Macule—no Tumors—yes	Multiple skin tumors present from birth		Rare	
Hereditary hemorrhagic telangiectasia (Rendu-Osler-Weber)	Purple papules on skin and mucous membranes, which blanch on pressure	No	Yes	Bleeding from lesions and body orifices	12	Rare

Table 12-2. Generalized brownish, bluish, or black discolorations*

Condition	Distribution	Usual history	Usual age of occurrence (years)	Accompanying conditions	Special tests
Cyanosis	Total skin surface Oral mucosa (if systemic type)	Increased severity of symptoms on exertion	1 month to 2 years (infants); 60 to 90	Malaise Dyspnea Orthopnea	Color decreases when circulation and oxygenation of blood is increased
Chloasma gravidarum	Skin of face, most frequently over nose and cheek	Increased brownish color of skin as pregnancy progresses	Older than 13	Pregnancy	
Addison's disease	Skin, especially exposed areas Oral mucosa	Hypoglycemia Weakness Decreased resistance to stress	18 and older	Symptoms and signs of adrenocortical insufficiency	Negative ACTH test Improvement with cortisone and aldosterone administration
Hemochromatosis†	Skin, especially, exposed areas Oral mucosa	Slowly increasing pigmentation, recent increased iron intake, or multiple blood transfusions	Older than 35	Liver disease Diabetes Adrenocortical insufficiency	Tests of skin, liver, and bone marrow positive for iron Serum iron-binding capacity
Argyria	Skin, especially exposed areas Oral mucosa	Chronic self-administration of silver-containing medication	18 and older	Equilibrium and hearing problems Headaches	Skin biopsy positive for silver

*With the exception of argyria, which is rare, all these entities are of occasional frequency. Chloasma gravidarum, of course, is not seen in men.
†Eighty percent of the patients are men.

REFERENCES

Abrams AM: Danger of treating mucoceles by steroid injection, J Oral Surg 36:583, 1978.

American Cancer Society: Cancer facts and figures, New York, 1989, The Society.

Bale SJ, Dracopoli NC, Tucker MA, et al: Mapping the gene for hereditary cutaneous malignant melanoma–dysplastic nevus to chromosome I_p, N Engl J Med 320:1367-1372, 1989.

Batsakis JG, Regezi JA, Solomon AR, et al: The pathology of head and neck tumors: mucosal melanomas, Part B, Head Neck Surg 4:404-418, 1982.

Bennett AJ, Solomon MP, and Jarrett W: Superficial spreading melanoma of the buccal mucosa: report of case, J Oral Surg 34:1109-1111, 1976.

Bina S: Primary malignant melanoma of the oral cavity in Iranians (review of 18 cases), J Oral Med 34:51-52, 1979.

Buchner A and Hansen LS: Melanotic macule of the oral mucosa: a clinicopathologic study of 105 cases, Oral Surg 48:244-249, 1979a.

Buchner A and Hansen LS: Amalgam pigmentation (amalgam tattoo) of the oral mucosa, Oral Surg 49:139-147, 1980a.

Buchner A and Hansen LS: Pigmented nevi of the oral mucosa: a clinicopathologic study of 32 new cases and review of 75 cases from the literature. II. Analysis of 107 cases, Oral Surg 49:55-62, 1980b.

Buchner A and Hansen LS: Pigmented nevi of the oral mucosa: a clinicopathologic study of 36 new cases and review of 155 cases from the literature. I. A clinicopathologic study of 36 new cases, Oral Surg 63:566-572, 1987.

Bystryn JC, Oratz R, Harris MN, et al: Immunogenicity of a polyvalent melanoma antigen vaccine in humans, CA 61:1065-1070, 1988.

Chaudry AP, Burke RJ, and Gorlin RJ: Malignant melanoma of the oral cavity, Oral Surg 13:584-588, 1960.

Chin DC: Treatment of maxillary hemangioma with a sclerosing agent, Oral Surg 55:247-249, 1983.

Chuong R and Goldberg MH: Clinicopathologic conferences. Case 47, Part I. Oral hyperpigmentation, J Oral Maxillofac Surg 41:613-615, 1983.

Chuong R and Goldberg ML: Clinicopathologic conferences. Case 47, Part II. Oral hyperpigmentation associated with Addison's disease, J Oral Maxillofac Surg 41:680-682, 1983.

Clark CA: A survey of eruption cysts in the newborn, Oral Surg 15:917, 1962.

Clark W, From L, Bernardina E, and Mihm M: The histogenesis and biologic behavior of primary human malignant melanomas of the skin, Cancer Res 29:705-726, 1969.

Eneroth CM: Malignant melanoma of the oral cavity, Int J Oral Surg 4:191-197, 1975.

Farman AG: Hairy tongue (lingua villosa), J Oral Med 32:85-91, 1977.

Fauci AS, Macher AM, Longo DL, et al: NIH Conference: acquired immunodeficiency syndrome; epidemiologic, clinical immunologic and therapeutic considerations, Ann Intern Med 100:92-106, 1984.

Ficarra G, Gerson AM, Silverman S, et al: Kaposi's sarcoma of the oral cavity: a study of 134 patients with a review of the pathogenesis, epidemiology, clinical aspects, and treatment, Oral Surg 66:543-550, 1988.

Galloway RH, Gross PD, Thompson SH, and Patterson AL: Pathogenesis and treatment of ranula: report of three cases, J Oral Maxillofac Surg 47:299-302, 1989.

Goldstein BH: Acute dissection hematoma: a complication of oral and maxillofacial surgery, J Oral Surg 39:40-43, 1981.

Gongloff RK: Treatment of intraoral hemangiomas with nitrous oxide cryosurgery, Oral Surg 56:20-24, 1983.

Goode RK, Crawford BE, Callihan MD, et al: Oral melanoacanthoma, Oral Surg 56:622-628, 1983.

Gorsky M, Buchner A, Fundoianu-Dayan D, and Aviv I: Physiologic pigmentation of the oral mucosa in Israeli Jews of different ethnic origin, Oral Surg 58:506-509, 1984.

Hartman LC, Natiella JR, and Meenaghan MA: The use of elemental microanalysis in verification of the composition of presumptive amalgam tattoo, J Oral Maxillofac Surg 44:628-633, 1986.

Hertz RS, Beckstead PC, and Brown WJ: Epithelial melanosis of the gingiva possibly resulting from the use of oral contraceptives, J Am Dent Assoc 100:713-714, 1980.

Jackson D and Simpson HE: Primary malignant melanoma of the oral cavity, Oral Surg 39:553-559, 1975.

Katsikeris N, Kalarantza-Angelopoulou E, and Angelopoulos AP: Peripheral giant cell granuloma: clinicopathologic study of 224 new cases and review of 956 reported cases, Int J Oral Maxillofac Surg 17:94-99, 1988.

Krolls SO and Hicks JL: Mixed tumors of the lower lip, Oral Surg 35:212-217, 1973.

Laskaris G and Skouteris C: Maffucci's syndrome: report of case with oral hemangiomas, Oral Surg 57:263-266, 1984.

Leopard PJ: Cryosurgery and its application to oral surgery, Br J Oral Surg 13:128-152, 1975.

Levin LS, Jorgenson RJ, and Jarvey BA: Lymphangiomas of the alveolar ridges in neonates, Pediatrics 58:881-884, 1976.

Liversedge RL: Oral malignant melanoma, Br J Oral Surg 13(1):40-55, 1975.

Lockhart PB: Gingival pigmentation as the role presenting sign of chronic lead poisoning in a mentally retarded adult, Oral Surg 52:143-149, 1981.

Lozada F, Silverman S, Migliorati CA, et al: Oral manifestations of tumors and opportunistic infections in the acquired immunodeficiency syndrome (AIDS): findings in 53 homosexual men with Kaposi's sarcoma, Oral Surg 56:491-493, 1983.

Mann SO, Fell BF, and Dalgarno AC: Observations on the bacterial flora and pathology of the tongue of sheep deficient in zinc, Rev Vet Sci 17:91-101, 1974.

McDonald, JS, Miller RL, Wagner W, et al: Acral lentigenous melanoma of the oral cavity, Head Neck Surg 5:257-262, 1983.

McGovern VJ: Malignant melanoma: clinical and histological diagnosis, New York, 1976, John Wiley & Sons, Inc, pp 55-84.

Minkow B, Laufer D, and Gutman D: Treatment of oral hemangiomas with local sclerosing agents, Int J Oral Surg 8:18-21, 1979.

Murphy JB: The management of a large hemangioma of the oral cavity with cryotherapy, J Oral Med 33:104-106, 1978.

Page LR, Corio RL, Crawford BE, et al: The oral melanotic macule, Oral Surg 44:219-226, 1977.

Plack W and Bellizzi R: Generalized argyria secondary to chewing photographic film, Oral Surg 49:504-506, 1980.

Regezi JA, Hayward JR, and Pickens TN: Superficial melanomas of oral mucous membrane, Oral Surg 45:730-740, 1978.

Robertson GR, Defiebre BK, and Firtell DN: Primary malignant melanoma of the mouth, J Oral Surg 37:349-352, 1979.

ten Bruggenkate CM, Cardoza EL, Maaskant P, et al: Lead poisoning with pigmentation of the oral mucosa: review of the literature and report of a case, Oral Surg 39:747-753, 1975.

von Wussow P, Block B, Hartmann F, and Deicher H: Intralesional interferon-alpha therapy in advanced malignant melanoma, Cancer 61:1071-1074, 1988.

Watkins KV, Chaudhry AP, Yamane GM, et al: Benign focal melanotic lesions of the oral mucosa, J Oral Med 39:91-96, 1984.

Watson WL and McCarthy WD: Blood and lymph vessel tumors: a report of 1,056 cases, Surg Gynecol Obstet 71:569-588, 1940.

Weathers DR, Corio RL, Crawford BE, et al: The labial melanotic macule, Oral Surg 42:196-205, 1976.

Wilcox JW and Hickory JE: Nonsurgical resolution of mucoceles, J Oral Surg 36:478, 1978.

Zachariades N and Koundouris I: Lymphangioma of the oral cavity: report of a case, J Oral Med 39:33-34, 1984.

Zhao-ju Z, Yun-tang W, Xuan-peng Z, et al: Clinical application of angiography of oral and maxillofacial hemangiomas: clinical analysis of seventy cases, Oral Surg 55:437-447, 1983.

13

Pits, fistulas, and draining lesions

HENRY M. CHERRICK
NORMAN K. WOOD

Pits, fistulas, and draining lesions of the oral cavity include the following:

Pits
Fovea palatinae
Commissural lip pit
Postsurgical pit
Postinfection pit
Rarities
    Congenital lip pits

Intraoral fistulas and sinuses
Chronic draining alveolar abscess
*Suppurative infection of the parotid and
    submandibular glands*
Draining mucocele and ranula
Oroantral fistula
Oronasal fistula
Draining chronic osteomyelitis
Draining cyst
Patent nasopalatine duct

Cutaneous fistulas and sinuses
Pustule
*Sinus draining a chronic dentoalveolar abscess
    or chronic osteomyelitis*
Extraoral draining cyst
Specific sinuses
    Thyroglossal duct
    Second branchial sinus
    Congenital aural sinuses
Salivary gland fistula or sinus
Auriculotemporal syndrome
Orocutaneous fistula
Rarities
    First branchial arch sinus and fistula

Pits, fistulas, and draining lesions of the cervicofacial complex may present perplexing diagnostic problems, partially because numerous types may occur in the oral cavity and on the skin of the face and neck. The process of differential diagnosis may be facilitated, however, by dividing these lesions into three categories: pits, intraoral fistulas and sinuses, and cutaneous fistulas and sinuses.

The terms "fistula" and "sinus" are used in the present discussion as prescribed by their traditional definitions. A *fistula* (Latin, reed instrument or pipe) is an abnormal pathway between two anatomic cavities; it has two openings. A *sinus* (Latin, hollow, bay, or curve) represents the tract of a lesion; it has but one opening. The fistula and the sinus are designated according to the surface or surfaces on which they open (for example, oroantral fistula, cutaneous sinus). The clinician is undoubtedly aware that most writers do not strictly adhere to these definitions; there is, furthermore, an increasing tendency to use the terms interchangeably in the literature.

Pits

A "pit" is defined as a hollow fovea or indentation. Pits, generally being blind tracts lined with epithelium, are either normal, anatomic landmarks or congenital, postsurgical, or inflammatory defects.

FOVEA PALATINAE

The fovea palatinae are two indentations formed by a coalescence of several mucous gland ducts near the midline of the palate. These round to oval depressions are always located in soft tissue on the anterior part of the soft palate. They can usually be accentuated when the patient holds his or her nose and attempts to blow it. The depressions may be probed to a depth of 0.5 to 2 mm, and when manipulated, may secrete a clear, mucinous fluid. On occasion the foveae palatinae are abnormally large and may be confused with fistulas or sinuses (Fig. 13-1).

COMMISSURAL LIP PIT

The commissural lip pit is a relatively common developmental disorder, although there is no agreement concerning its incidence. Everett and Wescott (1961) reported that approximately 0.2% of the population showed this anomaly; however, Baker (1966) found that 12% of whites and 20% of blacks in his series demonstrated it.

The commissural lip pit may be bilateral or unilateral. Unilateral pits occur as often on the right as on the left side of the mouth. The pits are located at the angles of the mouth, with the tracts diverging dorsolaterally into the cheek (Fig. 13-2). They range in size from a shallow dimple to a tract measuring 4 mm in length, and the tissue is slightly raised about the opening.

On microscopic examination the tract is lined with stratified squamous epithelium that continues into the vermilion tissue of the lip. Mucous gland ducts may empty into the sinus, and as a result mucus frequently can be milked from the tract.

Differential diagnosis

The differential diagnosis of the commissural lip pit is discussed in the differential diagnosis section at the end of the chapter (p. 270). The commissural lip pit especially must be differentiated from the *congenital lip pit*, which is seen on the vermilion border of the lower lip but not at the commissures. The congenital lip pit, however, is extremely rare, occurring in approximately one of 2 billion births (Gorlin and Pindborg, 1964, p. 117).

Management

The commissural lip pit is asymptomatic and requires no treatment.

POSTSURGICAL PIT

The postsurgical pit is the result of wound breakdown secondary to infection or failure to obliterate dead space in wound closure (improper layer closure and inadequate eversion of the wound). The postsurgical pit appears on clinical examination as a dimple or puckering of either a portion or the entire surface of a wound with a comparatively shallow depression that can be probed easily (Fig. 13-3).

Differential diagnosis

The differential diagnosis of the postsurgical pit is discussed in the differential diagnosis section concerning the postinfection pit.

Management

The management of the postsurgical pit is discussed in the management section concerning the postinfection pit.

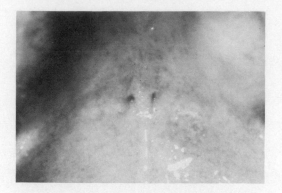

Fig. 13-1. Fovea palatinae on the anterior aspect of the soft palate.

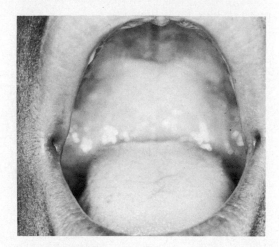

Fig. 13-2. Bilateral commissural lip pits.   (Courtesy D. Bonomo, DDS, Flossmoor, Ill.)

POSTINFECTION PIT

The postinfection pit usually results from loss of tissue, often because of necrosis. After the infection has been resolved, a subsequent inversion of the surface tissue into the resultant defect forms a postinfection pit, which clinically resembles the postsurgical pit (Fig. 13-4). Accurate diagnosis may be determined from facts obtained through the patient interview.

Differential diagnosis

The postsurgical pit and the postinfection pit may appear similar to a *stitch abscess, sinus, fistula,* or *congenital pit;* however, they may be distinguished from the latter entities by a careful history and physical examination, including depth exploration (with lacrimal probes), and by radiographic examination (performed with lacrimal probes or gutta-percha points inserted into the pits).

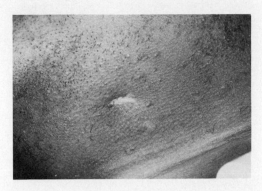

Fig. 13-3. Postsurgical pit after incision and drainage.

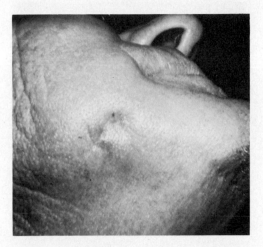

Fig. 13-4. Postinfection pit after successful treatment of actinomycosis with antibiotic therapy.

Management

Shallow postsurgical and postinfection pits within the oral cavity do not usually require treatment. If food debris tends to become deposited in them, however, they should be surgically eliminated. Esthetic consideration prompts the same excision and layer closure as for extraoral pits.

RARITIES

The congenital lip pit represents one of the rarest defects in the human body; thus it is not discussed further here.

Intraoral fistulas and sinuses

CHRONIC DRAINING ALVEOLAR ABSCESS

The dentoalveolar abscess is one of the most common lesions observed by dentists and fre-

quently occurs as a draining lesion. The pathogenesis and radiologic appearance of this lesion are discussed in Chapter 16.

The vast majority of dentoalveolar abscesses result from a direct extension of an acute pulpitis or an acute nonsuppurative periodontitis or from an acute exacerbation of a periapical granuloma, cyst, or chronic abscess. Less commonly the dentoalveolar abscess is of the postoperative type, arising from an infection of the alveolar socket after surgical removal of a tooth. The pulp tissue of the extracted tooth may have been infected before removal, or the infection may have been implanted during the extraction. In either case the process remains essentially the same: a pyogenic infection of the periodontal ligament and bone (Eisenbud and Klatell, 1951).

The surrounding tissue attempts to localize the pyogenic infection by forming an enclosure of granulation tissue, which in turn is surrounded by fibrous connective tissue. This results in a well-circumscribed lesion containing necrotic tissue, disintegrated and viable polymorphonuclear leukocytes, and other inflammatory cells in the periapical region of the tooth or alveolus.

This well-circumscribed, periapical abscess may penetrate the surrounding fibrotic capsule and form a sinus that opens on the mucosa or the skin of the face or neck, usually as a result of one or more of the following circumstances:

1. Inability of the body to completely contain or localize the causative organisms
2. Increase in the number of the causative organisms, or introduction of a more virulent organism through the carious tooth or by surgical intervention
3. Lowering of the patient's general resistance during the course of formation of the periapical abscess
4. Trauma or surgical intervention, mechanically producing an opening in the fibrous capsule

The enlarging dentoalveolar abscess contains purulent material that is under pressure. Because of this pressure, the pus proceeds through the bone along the path of least resistance until it reaches the surface, where because of the limiting fibrous periosteal layer, it temporarily forms a subperiosteal abscess. Eventually it erodes through the periosteum and penetrates the soft tissue, again following the path of least resistance.

The path of least resistance is determined by the location of the breakthrough in the bone and the anatomy of the muscles and fascial planes in the area. In the majority of cases the expanding abscess points and discharges onto the nearest external surface in the oral cavity; there are other, more complicated paths of infection, but their discussion is beyond the scope of this text.

Features

In the majority of cases the intraoral sinuses open on the labial and buccal aspects of the alveolus (Fig. 13-5) because usually the apices of both the maxillary and the mandibular teeth are located nearer to the buccal than to the lingual cortical plate. Thus this route offers the shorter distance for the burrowing pus.

In the maxilla, however, the roots of the lateral incisors and the palatal roots of the molars frequently lie closer to the palatal cortical plate than to the buccal plate; therefore an infection in these roots often produces a palatal abscess and perhaps a sinus (Fig. 13-6). Also the mandibular molar roots, particularly of the third molars, are located closer to the lingual plate. In addition, since most of the root tips of these teeth lie below the mylohyoid muscle, the pus drains into the submandibular space and the deeper planes of the neck instead of through an intraoral sinus.

On clinical examination the sinus opening has the appearance of a small ulcer. This opening is most commonly found on the buccal alveolus adjacent to the infected tooth. The palatal sinus, on the other hand, may burrow for a variable distance on the palate before it points and erodes the palatal mucosa. The mucosal sinus opening may be red and bleeds easily. It may be level with the mucosa or raised (a parulis). Occasionally, after temporary emptying of an abscess, the sinus heals and forms a slightly raised pale papule. After a period of time, pus accumulates and another sinus opening develops. Therefore in some cases the clinician may find multiple sinus scars or patent sinuses or both. Palpation of the surrounding mucosa may cause the expression of pus from the sinus(es).

The patient frequently gives a history of pain that started as a dull ache and progressed to an increasingly severe throbbing. A sudden decrease in the pain usually signals the formation of a sinus; the pain may disappear completely at this stage. Although the offending tooth is often tender to percussion, vitality tests are negative, since the pulp is nonvital.

Dentoalveolar abscesses and sinuses usually appear on radiographic examination as radiolucent areas of bone resorption around a root apex. The radiolucent area is frequently ragged

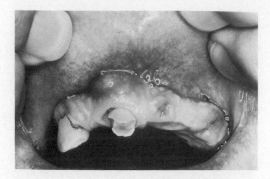

Fig. 13-5. Intraoral sinus from a chronic alveolar abscess of the central incisor. Parulis is evident on the labial aspect.

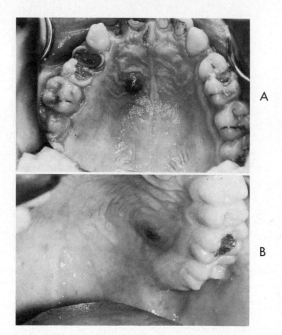

Fig. 13-6. Openings of palatal sinus draining chronically infected pulpless teeth. **A,** Lateral incisor. **B,** Maxillary first molar.

in outline and generally lacks a sclerotic margin, although such a margin may develop. This feature is discussed in detail in Chapter 16.

Differential diagnosis

The differential diagnosis of a chronic draining alveolar abscess is discussed in the differential diagnosis section at the end of the chapter (p. 270). Rossman et al. (1982) discussed the endodontic periodontic fistula.

Management

The management of pulpoperiapical sequelae is discussed at length in Chapter 16. Culture and sensitivity tests of the draining fluid usually identify the causative organism(s). Occasionally, unusual organisms such as *Actinomyces* are found (Craig et al., 1984).

SUPPURATIVE INFECTION OF THE PAROTID AND SUBMANDIBULAR GLANDS

Purulent discharge from Stensen's papillae and the sublingual caruncles indicates the presence of a suppurative infection of the parotid and submandibular salivary glands, respectively (Fig. 13-7). Thus pus-forming infections of these two major salivary glands are included in this discussion of intraoral draining lesions.

Suppurative infection of the parotid or submandibular salivary glands characteristically occurs in extremely ill or debilitated patients; most often these are patients of more than 65 years of age or within the first 4 weeks after birth (Gustafson, 1951; Krippachne et al., 1962; Shulman, 1950). In the delicate or debilitated newborn of low birth weight, inflammation of the glands usually develops from complicating diseases that produce dehydration (Gustafson, 1951). In the older individual there are many predisposing factors, among which are dehydration, malnutrition, and oral cancer. Surgery, especially abdominal and orthopedic procedures, is one of the most common predisposing factors for suppurative infection of the salivary glands (Krippachne et al., 1962).

The route taken by the microbes is thought to be either (1) retrograde, from the oral cavity to the affected gland via the secretory duct, or (2) antegrade, from the bloodstream to the gland (Shulman, 1950). *Staphylococcus aureus* is the most frequent infectious agent found, but infections of *Streptococcus viridans* and *Escherichia coli* are also common; in addition, many bacteria of the oral flora may induce this infection.

For an infection to be introduced via the secretory duct, a change in the person's wellbeing must have occurred, usually in one of four ways: (1) increase in the number of microorganisms in the oral cavity, or introduction of a more virulent type than is normally present at the duct opening, (2) lowering of the individual's general resistance, (3) decrease in salivary secretion, or (4) decrease in the bactericidal effect of the saliva (Gustafson, 1951).

The infection commences in the epithelial cells of the large secretory duct and spreads progressively to the smaller ducts and finally to the gland parenchyma. Once infection of the parenchyma has occurred, multiple abscesses

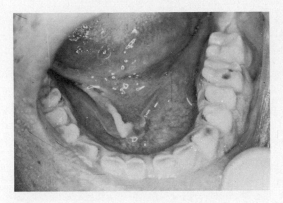

Fig. 13-7. Purulent discharge from Wharton's duct during an acute infection of the submandibular gland.

may form and then coalesce. If the infection is not eradicated, pus may penetrate the gland capsule and spread into the surrounding tissue, usually along one of three pathways: (1) downward into the deep fascial planes of the neck, (2) backward into the external auditory canal, or (3) outward onto the skin of the face (Gustafson, 1951; Krippachne et al., 1962).

Features

Often the first manifestation of a parotid infection is pain in the temporomandibular joint region; this is followed by swelling of the gland, which usually becomes hot, indurated, and tender to palpation. Redness may be found around the orifices of the infected gland's duct, and pus may be expressed by pressure on the gland (Fig. 13-7).

The patient may be febrile and quite ill, often out of proportion to what would be expected from such a localized infection. In the majority of cases, there is a concomitant rise in the number of leukocytes in the blood, especially in the neutrophil fraction.

Differential diagnosis

The differential diagnosis of suppurative infection of the parotid and submaxillary glands is discussed in the differential diagnosis section at the end of the chapter (p. 270).

Management

Treatment of choice is the immediate institution of antibiotic therapy. Since many of the infections are resistant to the most frequently used antibiotics, the most effective treatment is with type-specific antibiotics, indicated by determining the type of the causative organism from pus expressed from the duct. If there is

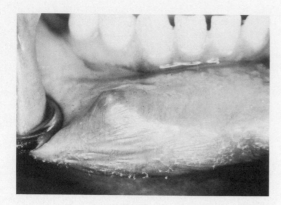

Fig. 13-8. Sinus opening from a chronic draining mucocele.

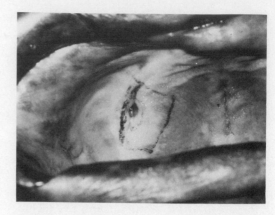

Fig. 13-9. Oroantral fistula in an edentulous patient. (Courtesy P. Akers, DDS, Chicago.)

no improvement within 3 to 4 days, incision and drainage should be undertaken.

DRAINING MUCOCELE AND RANULA

The mucocele and ranula are retention phenomena of the minor salivary glands and the sublingual salivary gland, respectively. These lesions are included in Chapter 10 as exophytic lesions and are discussed in Chapter 12 with the bluish lesions. They are included in this chapter because occasionally they occur as chronic draining lesions.

As a mucocele or a ranula increases in size, the overlying epithelium and mucous membrane become stretched. As it grows progressively larger, it may cause the mucous membrane to become extremely thin and undergo spontaneous rupture. Often a traumatic incident in the oral cavity promotes rupture. The exudate is usually clear, viscous, and sticky. When drainage occurs, the mucocele or ranula decreases in size; however, healing of the rupture occurs rapidly and the lesion gradually fills and expands again. Continual repetition of these events can produce a chronic sinus (Fig. 13-8).

Differential diagnosis

The differential diagnosis of the mucocele and ranula is discussed in Chapters 10 and 12 and at the end of this chapter (p. 270).

Management

Treatment consists of either total enucleation or marsupialization. During the surgical correction other salivary ducts or glands may be injured, so recurrences are fairly common.

OROANTRAL FISTULA

The oroantral fistula is a pathologic pathway connecting the oral cavity and the maxillary sinus (Fig. 13-9). In the majority of cases it is caused by the extraction of a tooth, but it may also be caused by other trauma, tuberculosis (Juniper, 1973), syphilis (Shafer et al., 1983), or leprosy (Lighterman et al., 1962). Occasionally it results from tooth-associated pathoses, such as periapical infection or cyst formation. The oroantral fistula is also discussed in Chapter 35.

Most oroantral fistulas are initiated by the extraction of a maxillary tooth, the primary reason being the proximity of the sinus floor to the apex of the tooth. Usually the apices of the posterior teeth are within 3 mm of the cortical floor of the maxillary sinus, or they may project into the maxillary sinus with only a small amount of bony covering. The roots of the second molar are closest to the maxillary sinus, followed by those of the first molar, third molar, second premolar, first premolar, and canine.

The palatal root apices of the molars are most frequently involved in the formation of a fistula. Extraction of the maxillary first molar accounts for 50% of the oroantral fistulas with the other 50% almost evenly accounted for by extraction of the second and third molars (Killey and Kay, 1967; Mustian, 1933; Wowern, 1971).

An oroantral fistula generally forms as a result of inadequate blood clot formation in the alveolus after violation of the maxillary sinus. This may be consequential to a sinusitis or secondary infection or the introduction of packs or other hemostatic agents in the socket.

Features

On clinical examination an oroantral fistula is frequently seen immediately after extraction of a tooth, especially if the root has been fractured and displaced into the antrum; however, it may not always be apparent or suspected, especially if the extraction was atraumatic.

A patient with a chronic oroantral fistula may experience one or more symptoms. The most frequent complaint is the passage of fluids from the oral cavity into the nose, or the patient may have a foul or salty taste in the mouth. Facial pain or an associated frontal headache may develop from an acute maxillary sinusitis. The headache is generally of a throbbing nature and is exacerbated by any movement of the head. A unilateral nasal discharge accompanied by a sensation of nasal obstruction or nocturnal coughing resulting from the draining of exudate into the pharynx may also occur. The swallowed exudate may produce a morning anorexia. The patient may also experience an epistaxis on the affected side.

Other, less common symptoms are the eversion of an antral polyp through the fistula, resulting in the sudden appearance of an exophytic mass on the alveolar crest, the aspiration of air into the mouth through the tooth socket, and the inability to blow out the cheeks or draw on a cigarette (Killey and Kay, 1967).

A patient with an oroantral fistula has a pathologic pathway by which microorganisms of the oral flora may enter the maxillary sinus and cause a sinusitis. The severity of the sinusitis depends on several factors, varying usually inversely with the diameter of the fistula. If the opening is large, pressure does not increase because the exudate escapes freely into the oral cavity; hence the patient complains of little if any pain. On the other hand, if the diameter of the fistula is quite small, an acute sinusitis is more likely to develop.

A patient with an acute maxillary sinusitis may experience swelling and redness overlying the sinus and the molar eminence, as well as pain beneath the eye. Palpation over the maxilla increases the pain, and the teeth with roots adjacent to the sinus are often painful or sensitive to percussion. The pain may also be referred to other teeth in the arch and to the ear.

In a chronic sinusitis from an oroantral fistula, nasal and postnasal discharges are ordinarily present along with a fetid breath and a vague pain or stuffiness in the affected side of the face (Burket, 1971, p. 233; Shafer et al., 1983).

On radiologic examination the maxillary sinus may appear cloudy because of an accumulation of blood, mucus, or purulent exudate. In some cases a distinct fluid level may be evident (Worth, 1963, p. 706).

Differential diagnosis

When the fistula is large and a definite communication between the oral cavity and the maxillary sinus can be demonstrated, the diagnosis is obvious. In other cases, when the inflammation of the sinus mucosa has sealed the fistula, the diagnosis may be more difficult because the clinician is unable to identify the tract on clinical examination. A radiograph, however, may reveal a break in the continuity of the sinus floor, which identifies the site of the previously patent defect. Ehrl (1980) details in excellent fashion a program of diagnostic steps for cases of suspected oroantral fistula.

Management

An oroantral fistula should be repaired as soon as possible after it has occurred. Ehrl (1980) stated that the longer the interval between genesis of the fistula and treatment, the greater the complications. In cases of sinusitis or an infection, however, the surgical repair of the fistula must wait until the infection has been eliminated. An intensive course of antibiotic therapy should be instituted for a minimum of 1 week, the duration depending on the extent of the infection. A decongestant should also be employed to encourage free drainage of the pus and mucus. Antral lavage is necessary in some cases and may be accomplished through the fistulous opening. Occasionally an antrostomy may be necessary to help in draining the sinus (Anderson, 1969; Killey and Kay, 1967).

Many elaborate surgical methods have been developed for closing oroantral fistulas. In all methods the fistula is excised and the surrounding necrotic tissue is curetted. The methods include bone grafts, the use of gold foil grids, and buccal and palatal flap techniques (Goldman et al., 1969; Ziemba, 1972). Once the antral infection has been eliminated, closure of the defect is usually successful regardless of the surgical technique employed; however, some surgeons prefer to augment the closure by packing the maxillary sinus with gauze and subsequently removing the gauze through a nasal antrostomy. This procedure helps to ensure that a sinusitis does not develop during the critical stage of closure of the fistula.

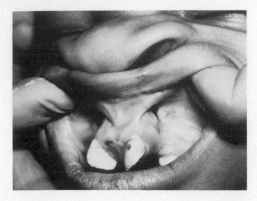

Fig. 13-10. Oronasal fistulas in a patient with congenital cleft palate. (Courtesy P. Akers, DDS, Chicago.)

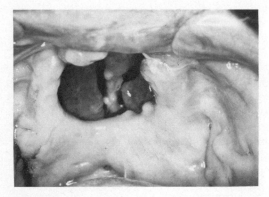

Fig. 13-11. Oronasal fistula as a result of a healed syphilitic gumma.

ORONASAL FISTULA

The oronasal fistula is a pathologic, epithelium-lined defect connecting the oral and nasal cavities. The most frequent causes of this type of fistula are congenital cleft palate, trauma, infection, neoplasm, and unsuccessful surgical procedures. The most common traumatic injuries are automobile accidents and gunshot wounds (Clarkson et al., 1946).

Although a complete midline cleft of the palate is not a diagnostic problem, occasionally a partial cleft, an unsuccessful repair of a complete cleft, or an anterior cleft resembles an oronasal fistula that results from some other cause (Fig. 13-10).

Occasionally an acute dentoalveolar abscess of a maxillary central incisor burrows through the maxilla into the floor of the nasal cavity. Infrequently the abscess may exit high on the nasolabial aspect of the maxilla and tunnel up beneath the periosteum into the floor of the nose, where it usually forms an opening in the anterior portion of the nasal cavity (Gorlin and Goldman, 1970, p. 346). Other less frequent infectious causes are leprosy, syphilitic gumma, and mycotic infections (Gorlin and Goldman, 1970, p. 346; Lighterman et al., 1962) (Fig. 13-11). The fistula may also be produced during the surgical removal of teeth, buried roots, odontomas, tori, cysts, or benign and malignant neoplasms.

Features

When there is an obvious defect in the maxilla, the patient complains of food passing into the nose and often demonstrates nasal speech. Probing of the defect during radiographic examination usually establishes a definitive diagnosis of an oronasal fistula.

Management

The indicated treatment is usually the surgical removal of the fistula with subsequent flap advancement. When the fistula is considered too large to close surgically, a prosthetic appliance can be used to cover the defect.

DRAINING CHRONIC OSTEOMYELITIS

Chronic osteomyelitis is discussed in Chapter 16 as a periapical radiolucency, in Chapter 21 as an ill-defined radiolucency, in Chapter 25 as a mixed radiolucent-radiopaque lesion, and in Chapter 28 as a radiopacity. In the present chapter its draining aspect is featured.

Features

On clinical examination a sinus extends from the medullary bone through the cortical plate to the mucous membrane or skin (Figs. 13-12 and 13-13). Should the infection exit the bone above a muscle attachment, the sinus opening may be a considerable distance from the offending infection. The mandible is much more frequently involved than the maxilla (Chapter 21). Cases that involve chronic draining are ordinarily painless unless there is an acute or subacute exacerbation. On radiographic examination the involved bone may be radiolucent, mixed radiolucent-radiopaque, or completely radiopaque, depending on the course of the infection. Formation of sequestra and involucra is often noted.

Differential diagnosis

The differential diagnosis of a draining chronic osteomyelitis is discussed in the differential diagnosis section at the end of the chapter (p. 270).

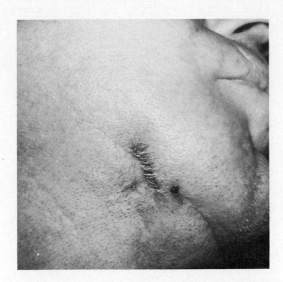

Fig. 13-12. Cutaneous sinus secondary to chronic osteomyelitis at a fracture site.

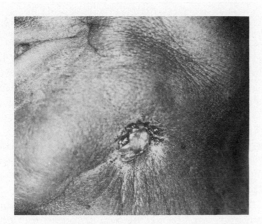

Fig. 13-13. Cutaneous sinus secondary to osteoradionecrosis.

Management

The management of a draining chronic osteomyelitis is discussed in detail in Chapter 21.

DRAINING CYST

Odontogenic and nonodontogenic cysts of intraosseous origin may perforate and produce sinuses that drain onto the oral mucosa. Secondary infections, or direct extensions by expansion of the cysts, generally produce these lesions. Cysts caused by inflammation and cysts that frequently become large (for example, periapical cysts, dentigerous keratocysts, odontogenic keratocysts) are the greatest offenders. Giunta et al. (1983) describe an intraoral dermoid cyst with a sinus tract.

Features

Before sinus formation, there is usually pain or swelling of the involved area. When the periosteum and mucosa are perforated, the pain ceases and a purulent discharge ensues. If the sinus is small, the drainage may continue as a chronic case. If the sinus is large, however, the infection regresses because of the excellent drainage established and the cyst may disappear completely because of its decompression. On clinical examination, when the cyst is large, there is expansion of the cortical plate. Palpation of the area commonly elicits pain, crepitus, and a purulent or cheesy discharge. On radiologic examination a well-delineated radiolucency is visible.

Differential diagnosis

The differential diagnosis of a draining cyst is discussed in the differential diagnosis section at the end of the chapter (p. 270).

Management

After the infection has been eliminated, the cyst must be treated by enucleation, marsupialization, or decompression. Associated teeth may require extraction or root canal therapy.

PATENT NASOPALATINE DUCT

A completely patent nasopalatine duct or canal is an extremely rare condition, especially in the adult. It arises when the embryologic nasopalatine ducts fail to become obliterated. In embryonic life the nasopalatine ducts are paired, epithelium-lined tubes extending from the nasal cavity to the oral cavity within the incisive canal. The nasal orifices of the ducts lie on each side of the nasal septum in the anterior nasal floor.

The nasopalatine duct is funnel shaped and continuous with the nasal epithelium. It extends downward in an anterior direction more or less parallel with the facial contour of the premaxilla to exit as two slits, one on each side of the palatine papilla, which overlies the incisive foramen (Hill and Darlow, 1945; Rosenberger, 1944).

The nasopalatine duct is lined with ciliated, pseudostratified, columnar epithelium to within 3 or 4 mm of the palatal opening. At this level there is a transition to cuboidal epithelium and then to stratified squamous epithelium (Abrams et al., 1963; Burket, 1937; MacGregor, 1964).

Under normal circumstances the nasopalatine ducts disintegrate during fetal life and this oronasal communication is eliminated. In un-

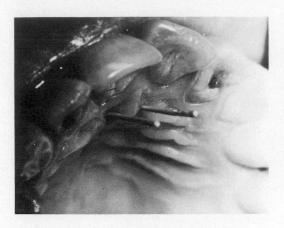

Fig. 13-14. Bilateral patent nasopalatine ducts with gutta-percha cones inserted into the defects. (Courtesy W. Goebel, DDS, Edwardsville, Ill.)

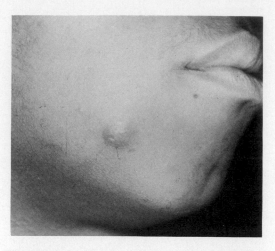

Fig. 13-15. Cutaneous sinus secondary to a periapical infection. This cutaneous lesion resembles a pustule.

usual cases all or part of the duct persists and remains patent in postnatal life. The completely patent nasopalatine duct is rare; however, circumstances in which only sections of the duct are patent at the nasal or oral end are more frequent. These sections exist as variable-length cul-de-sacs, with the nasal variety being more common. The oral variety of the patent nasopalatine duct may be identified by exposing a radiograph of the region with an orthodontic wire or gutta-percha point inserted into the defect (Fig. 13-14). Moskow (1982) and Allard et al. (1982) reported one case each of bilaterally patent nasopalatine ducts. Farman et al. (1982) also reported a case and reviewed the literature.

Features

The patent nasopalatine duct is usually asymptomatic except when small particles of food or liquid are aspirated into the nose via the duct. This happens most often after the patient has begun wearing dentures, which may force liquid up the canal and into the nose.

Differential diagnosis

The differential diagnosis of a patent nasopalatine duct is discussed in the differential diagnosis section at the end of the chapter (p. 270).

Management

Since the nasopalatine duct is usually asymptomatic, it seldom requires treatment.

Cutaneous fistulas and sinuses

PUSTULE

A pustule is a small, superficial elevation of the skin or mucous membrane filled with pus. Pustules are included in this chapter primarily because they become draining lesions for a short time after they rupture, and they are included secondarily because a solitary pustule on the skin overlying the jaws may easily be mistaken for a draining sinus from a chronic alveolar abscess or a chronic osteomyelitis (Fig. 13-15).

Pustules in the skin are common lesions and generally are the result of psoriasis, impetigo, acrodermatitis continua, or superficial bacterial diseases. Intraoral pustules are less common and are the result of superficial foreign bodies or specific diseases such as pustular psoriasis or subcorneal pustular stomatitis. Pustules are classified as primary or secondary (that is, preceded by a vesicle or papule).

Features

On clinical examination the pustule appears as a small, superficial elevation filled with pus and possibly surrounded by a small area of erythema. These lesions are generally asymptomatic but may be tender or painful.

Differential diagnosis

The differential diagnosis of a pustule is discussed in the differential diagnosis section at the end of the chapter (p. 270).

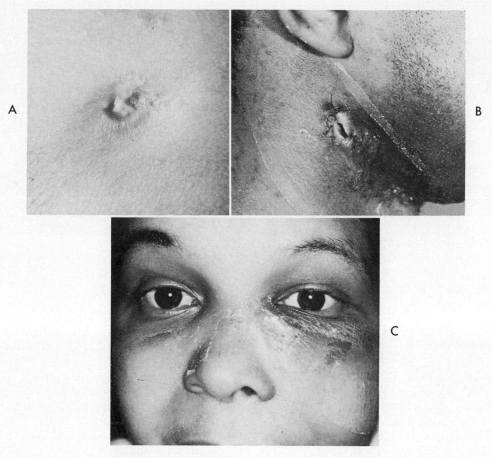

Fig. 13-16. Cutaneous sinuses. **A,** Secondary to a draining dentoalveolar abscess. **B,** Caused by a submandibular space infection. **C,** Secondary to a canine space infection. (**A** courtesy S. Rosen, DDS, Los Angeles.)

Management

A pustule seldom requires definitive treatment.

SINUS DRAINING A CHRONIC DENTOALVEOLAR ABSCESS OR CHRONIC OSTEOMYELITIS

As with intraoral draining lesions, pus from an enlarged dentoalveolar abscess or chronic osteomyelitic lesion burrows along the path of least resistance in both hard and soft tissues. This burrowing usually results in the formation of a sinus that empties into the vestibule adjacent to the offending tooth. In some instances, however, the path of least resistance leads to the skin and thus to the formation of cutaneous sinuses (Figs. 13-15 and 13-16).

If the pus exits from bone deep within soft tissue, its spread is governed by structures such as muscles and fascial sheets. Usually the infection spreads via fascial planes to the most available fascial space. A fascial space is a potential space that exists between two or more layers or planes of fasciae and is occupied by loose areolar tissue.

The infections of the head and neck are usually classified by their anatomic location. *Maxillary* dentoalveolar infections usually spread to the canine fossa, the buccal space, and the infratemporal space, whereas *mandibular* infections spread to the mandibular, submandibular (submaxillary), submental, pterygomandibular, masseteric, parapharyngeal, parotid, and carotid spaces. The infection may spread by direct continuation from the dentoalveolar abscess along the fascial planes or by the lymphatic and blood systems. A detailed discussion of the individual space abscesses is beyond the scope of this chapter; the space abscesses of the neck are discussed in Chapter 31. Calman et al. (1980) published eight cases of cutaneous sinus tracts on the face and anterior part of the neck that represented draining periapical infections. Braun and Lehman (1981) reported a similar case. McWalter et al. (1988) added two more cases to the literature. Salamat and Rezai (1986) described a successful method of nonsurgical treatment.

EXTRAORAL DRAINING CYSTS

The phenomenon of intraoral draining cysts is discussed earlier in the chapter (p. 257). Draining cysts can also occur on the skin of the face and neck (Fig. 13-17). The more common cysts to occur in these cutaneous regions are sebaceous, epidermoid, dermoid, thyroglossal, preauricular, and branchial and are discussed more completely in Chapter 15 with masses in the neck.

SPECIFIC SINUSES
Thyroglossal duct

The thyroglossal duct is a hollow tube of epithelial cells marking the embryonic descent of the thyroid anlage from the tongue to the normal position of the thyroid gland in the neck. The duct normally becomes a solid stalk and usually undergoes degeneration and disappears. The original opening of the thyroglossal duct persists as a vestigial pit, the foramen cecum of the tongue. Occasionally this communication fails to become obliterated and persists as a thyroglossal duct.

FEATURES

The thyroglossal duct is most commonly seen within the first two decades of life, although a duct may begin to drain later in life because of local irritation, with resultant proliferation of the duct tissue. The sexes are approximately equally affected (Marshal, 1949; Stahl and Lyall, 1954; Ward, 1949).

The sinus opening from the thyroglossal duct may be at any level in the midline of the neck from the foramen cecum to the suprasternal notch. Most frequently it is located in the area adjacent to the hyoid bone, being more often observed just below the hyoid than just above (see Fig. 31-13).

Rarely is the duct seen in the suprasternal area or in the foramen cecum region. Although mainly a midline phenomenon, it is found on either side of the midline in a small percentage of cases; on rare occasions it is far enough from the midline to be confused with a branchial

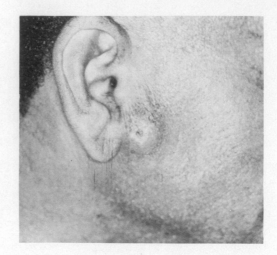

Fig. 13-17. Chronic draining sebaceous cyst.

cleft sinus (Pollock and Stevenson, 1966). The epithelial lining of the duct is usually squamous epithelium or ciliated, pseudostratified, columnar epithelium. Ducts in which inflammation has recurred may show little or no epithelial lining; chronic inflammation is usually present in the surrounding connective tissue. Rarely, thyroid tissue is entrapped in the duct lining and neoplastic transformation into papillary thyroid carcinoma occurs (Jacques, 1970).

The literature suggests that the duct opening is usually secondary to either infection of a thyroglossal duct cyst or incomplete removal in previous operations. The cutaneous openings are 1 to 3 mm in diameter with a reddish, inflamed margin. Mucoid (clear) or purulent exudate may be expressed from the opening. The tract may be palpable back to the cyst. Rarely, patent thyroglossal ducts empty into the oral cavity via the foramen cecum. The patient then usually complains of a bad taste in the mouth. A purulent exudate resulting from an infection with oral microorganisms may be seen emanating from the foramen cecum.

DIFFERENTIAL DIAGNOSIS

The differential diagnosis of a thyroglossal duct is discussed in the differential diagnosis section at the end of the chapter (p. 270).

MANAGEMENT

The indicated treatment is complete surgical excision of all thyroglossal duct epithelium. Because such excision is frequently difficult to complete, however, the recurrence rate is high (Brown, 1961).

Second branchial sinus (lateral cervical sinus)

A sinus or fistula of the second branchial cleft or pouch is fairly common; it constitutes the vast majority of sinuses and fistulas of the lateral neck. This anomaly is thought to occur when the second branchial cleft or the second pharyngeal pouch or both fail to become obliterated in the embryologic development of the fetus. The second branchial cleft separates the second and third branchial arches and, continuous with the second pharyngeal pouch internally, forms the second branchial membrane. The second branchial cleft and membrane usually become obliterated and disappear, whereas the endoderm of the pouch gives rise to the palatine tonsil and tonsillar fossa. The line of obliteration of the second branchial cleft extends from the lower anterior border of the sternocleidomastoid muscle, through the fork of the carotid artery bifurcation, and upward toward the tonsillar fossa (Gore and Masson, 1959). Thus there can be three distinct types of branchial tracts (Bailey, 1933): (1) a cutaneous sinus that results from failure of obliteration of the second branchial cleft, (2) a mucosal sinus that results from failure of obliteration of the second pharyngeal pouch, and (3) a fistula with both external and internal openings that results from failure of obliteration of both the cleft and the pouch.

FEATURES

A second branchial sinus occurs equally in males and females, and although there appears to be a strong familial tendency at times, the majority of sinuses lack any known hereditary influence (Carp and Stout, 1928; Hyndman and Light, 1929). The sinus or fistula may be unilateral, bilateral, or rarely, near the midline. The majority of anomalies are either external sinuses (50%) or complete fistulas (39%), and only occasionally is an internal sinus observed (Neel and Pemberton, 1945). The sinus or fistula is usually found at birth or within the first year of life. Adults with this anomaly commonly give a history of either intermittent drainage since childhood or a spontaneous discharge caused by infection and rupture of a cervical cyst.

These branchial sinuses or fistulas appear as small dimples or small openings in the lateral region of the neck. The openings are usually close to the anterior border of the sternocleidomastoid muscle, the majority being in the lower neck just above the sternoclavicular joint. They sometimes occur in the middle or upper third of the neck along the anterior border of the sternocleidomastoid, but in these cases there is the possibility that the sinus was acquired through the formation of a sinus tract after infection of a branchial cyst.

DIFFERENTIAL DIAGNOSIS

A second branchial sinus may be differentiated from any other fistulas or sinuses of the neck by its position.

A *thyroglossal duct sinus* or *fistula* is found high in the midline, and the *first branchial sinus* may be found high in the neck posterior and inferior to the angle of the mandible. Rarely is a second branchial sinus seen near the midline or high in the neck.

The only other common draining lateral sinus in the neck is *suppurative lymphadenitis*, most commonly *tuberculous adenitis*. This entity can usually be differentiated by the history or by appropriate clinical diagnostic tests. Sometimes radiographs taken after the injection of radiopaque dye into the sinus or fistula are of diagnostic help.

MANAGEMENT

Once the diagnosis is made, the sinus or fistula must be excised in its entirety or it recurs.

Congenital aural sinuses (auricular fistulas, preauricular fistulas, preauricular pits)

Congenital aural sinuses occur in approximately 1% of the population (Ewing, 1946). They are more common in blacks and Orientals than in whites (Selkirk, 1935) and are present equally in males and females, occurring bilaterally in approximately 25% of the cases. They are believed to be a non-sex-linked mendelian dominant trait with variable expressivity (Cowley and Calman, 1971). Occasionally they are associated with other ear and facial anomalies, but as a rule they occur alone.

Current opinion on the cause of aural sinuses maintains that they evolved during the embryologic development of the external ear from the six ectoderm-covered mesenchymal nodules (the auditory tubercles) of the first two branchial arches. By the third fetal month these six nodules have proliferated and merged around the primitive external auditory meatus to form the external ear. Abnormal development may have resulted in the formation of congenital sinuses between the auditory tubercles.

FEATURES

Although there are seven possible sites about the ear for these pits to occur, by far the most common is the marginal helix (90%); sinuses

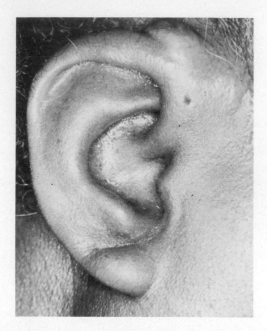

Fig. 13-18. Congenital aural sinus and cyst.

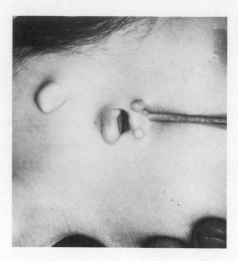

Fig. 13-19. Auricular tags (and clinical instrument) in a case of congenital aural sinus.

are rarely seen at the other possible sites. The majority of congenital aural sinuses open at the anterior margin of the ascending limbs of the helices where the skin of the face joins the skin of the external ear (Fig. 13-18).

The openings of the aural sinuses vary in size from pinpoint to 2 mm in diameter, and unless infected, are level with the surrounding skin.

The aural sinuses usually range in size from a slight fossa to a depression with a depth of 1 cm; they extend internally in an inferoposterior direction anterior to the cartilaginous external auditory meatus (Fig. 13-19). They may be attached to the meatus by a ribbon of fibrous tissue, but they never pierce or open into the meatus (Sykes, 1972).

The majority of aural sinuses are asymptomatic, but sometimes occlusion of the orifices results in formation of a cyst. Once the sinuses have been infected, they seldom become completely asymptomatic but usually undergo a chronic, low-grade inflammation with occasionally recurring, acute inflammatory exacerbations.

DIFFERENTIAL DIAGNOSIS

Most commonly these sinuses are confused with *first branchial cleft anomalies*. The two can be differentiated by remembering that the aural sinuses never open into the external auditory canal and are generally located on the anterosuperior aspect of the external ear, whereas the first branchial cleft anomalies commonly open into the external auditory canal and produce a purulent discharge with no evidence of middle ear infection. Also the first branchial anomalies usually have another opening on the inferoposterior side of the angle of the mandible, forming a fistula.

MANAGEMENT

Treatment is rendered only when the aural sinuses become cystic or infected: in such a case, complete removal of the tract is necessary to prevent recurrence of symptoms.

SALIVARY GLAND FISTULA OR SINUS

Parotid and submandibular gland fistulas are relatively rare lesions and are caused primarily by accidental trauma, surgery, or infection. For a fistula to be produced, there must usually be damage to the parotid or submandibular duct or one of its large branches. The saliva that escapes from the damaged duct either forms a pool within the soft tissue or drains through a fistula in the skin (Figs. 13-20 and 13-21).

The parotid duct lies in the middle third of an area determined by imagining a line drawn across the face from the tragus of the ear to a point midway between the vermilion border of the lip and the ala of the nose. It arises from the merger of numerous smaller branches at the anterior border of the gland. Occasionally there is an accessory parotid duct that joins the main duct somewhat distal to this border.

The main parotid duct then crosses superficially to the masseter muscle and turns inward at the anterior border of the muscle, passing

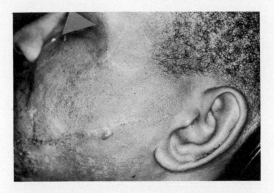

Fig. 13-20. Posttraumatic parotid fistula caused by laceration of the parotid duct.

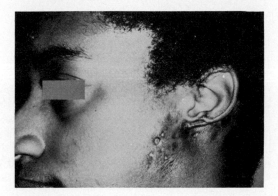

Fig. 13-21. Multiple fistulas resulting from a chronic parotitis.

through the fat pad of the cheek and forward in an oblique direction to open into the oral cavity opposite the maxillary second molar. When it crosses the outer surface of the masseter muscle, it lies close to the skin and is vulnerable to injury at this site (Baron, 1960).

Parotid gland fistula has been reported to occur as a result of infection caused by actinomycosis, tuberculosis, syphilis, cancrum oris, salivary calculi, and malignancies.

A fistula of the submandibular salivary gland complex is rare and is not discussed. Bronstein and Clark (1984) discussed the rare case of a salivary fistula developing in the mental region from a plunging ranula of a sublingual gland.

DIFFERENTIAL DIAGNOSIS

Differential diagnosis of salivary gland fistula includes the consideration of *fistulas and sinuses that occur as a result of specific and nonspecific infections and foreign bodies* in the area of the salivary glands. Definitive diagnosis is accomplished by the history, the probing of the involved duct, and the use of sialography.

MANAGEMENT

Once diagnosed, there are various surgical modes of treating salivary gland fistula. If the fistula is the result of trauma, the most common method is apposition of the severed duct ends. Another method is creation of a second mucosal opening by suturing the proximal intact portion of the duct to the buccal mucosa. Yet another method is formation of an artificial internal fistula, using various materials. If a chronic fistula does not respond to these conservative operations, the gland may be removed.

AURICULOTEMPORAL SYNDROME (FREY'S SYNDROME)

The auriculotemporal syndrome is included in this chapter because patients with this disorder have profuse sweating from a small, cutaneous area in the temporal region. Perspiration exuding from such a small area could be confused with an exudate from a draining lesion.

The disorder is caused by damage to the auriculotemporal nerve and reinnervation of the sweat glands by parasympathetic salivary fibers. Surgeries involving the parotid gland, ramus, or condyle are the most common cause. Tuinzing and Van Der Kwast (1982) described a case that followed sagittal splitting of the ramus. Olson et al. (1977) described a case caused by blunt trauma to the side of the face during a motorcycle accident. Accidental trauma and infections have also been implicated. Kryshtalskyj and Weinberg (1989) discussed the occurrence of this phenomenon following temporomandibular joint surgery.

Features

On clinical examination the auriculotemporal syndrome becomes evident approximately 5 weeks after damage to the auriculotemporal nerve. The first signs are sweating on the involved side of the face during and after gustatory stimuli. Eventually a feeling of warmth may precede flushing and sweating (Laage-Hellman, 1957).

Differential diagnosis

The definitive diagnosis of auriculotemporal syndrome is made by eliciting a history of trauma or infection in the involved area. The simplest way to identify the fluid as sweat is to use the Minor starch-iodine test (Laage-Hellman, 1957). Other aspects of the differential diagnosis are discussed in the differential diagnosis section at the end of the chapter (p. 270).

Management

The auriculotemporal syndrome is usually considered to be permanent, although an estimated 5% of these patients show regression or disappearance of the disorder.

OROCUTANEOUS FISTULA

Orocutaneous fistula is a troublesome defect because it permits the continual leaking of saliva onto the lower face or neck. It is a common sequela of trauma to the head and neck regions. The lesion is also seen with oral malignancies and inflammatory conditions. Cancrum oris, a lesion rarely seen in the United States, may produce an orocutaneous fistula.

Features

On clinical examination there is an abnormal communication of the oral cavity with the skin surface. A traumatic fistula primarily involves soft tissue, but in many neoplastic and infectious conditions the fistula may involve the osseous structures of the jaws.

Traumatic fistula is generally an epithelium-lined communication resulting from either an accident or an attempt at surgical repair. It usually does not exhibit the signs of inflammation commonly seen in neoplastic fistulas or fistulas induced by infection.

Neoplastic fistula may be the result of disease that has progressed through soft tissue or bone, beginning either in the oral cavity or on the skin surface (Fig. 13-22). Often the fistula is the result of surgical intervention for the neoplastic disease.

Inflammatory fistula is generally not lined with epithelium unless it is of long duration. The fistula may originate in either soft tissue or bone (for example, actinomycosis).

Differential diagnosis

Establishing a diagnosis of orocutaneous fistula is usually readily accomplished, and the cause plainly evident.

Management

Surgical repair may be successful in most cases of traumatic fistula, but treatment of a fistula caused by malignancy is usually hopeless because of the advanced stage of the tumor.

Small, infectious-type fistulas may heal spontaneously after elimination of the infection.

RARITIES

Rare defects such as the first branchial arch sinus and fistula are included in this category.

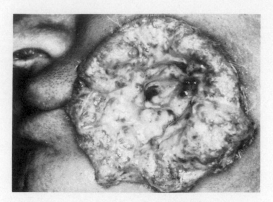

Fig. 13-22. Orocutaneous fistula resulting from a squamous cell carcinoma.

DIFFERENTIAL DIAGNOSIS OF PITS, FISTULAS, AND SINUSES

Pits, fistulas, and sinuses may be misdiagnosed easily, if the clinician fails to employ a systematic diagnostic approach. When encountering these lesions, the clinician should be certain to establish answers to the following questions during the patient interview: (1) Was the defect present at birth? If not, when did it become apparent? (2) Is fluid draining from it? (3) Does the patient complain of a bad taste in the mouth?

During the clinical examination pressure should be exerted on the surrounding or associated tissue to determine whether fluid can be expressed from the pit. If fluid is obtained, it should be carefully scrutinized to determine its nature—saliva, pus, blood, or cyst fluid.

In addition, the clinician should attempt to probe the depression to determine whether it is just a shallow diverticulum or indeed a tract. If the instrument or gutta-percha cone can be inserted to a considerable depth, a radiograph of the area should be obtained to aid in determining the depth, direction, and termination of the tract.

Routine radiographs of the adjacent bone helps to identify lesions of bone as origins of such tracts.

In some cases shallow pits represent all that remains of quiescent or eradicated tracts.

Intraoral pits, fistulas, and sinuses

The following entities must be considered, in this approximate order of frequency:

Fovea palatinae
Chronic draining dentoalveolar abscess
Commissural lip pits
Postsurgical and postinfection pit or depression

Oroantral fistula
Oronasal fistula
Draining cyst
Draining chronic osteomyelitis
Draining mucocele or ranula
Suppurative infection of the parotid and submaxillary salivary glands
Patent nasopalatine duct

The *patent nasopalatine duct* is a rare entity. When it is present, the patient may complain of a bad taste. The diagnosis is established by determining the duct's course through the incisive canal, which can be illustrated by exposing a radiograph after a gutta-percha cone has been inserted into the tract.

Suppurative infection of the parotid and submaxillary salivary glands is also quite uncommon. It should be suspected especially when there is a predisposing dehydration. Expressing pus from the respective duct openings by application of pressure on the glands establishes the diagnosis and differentiates this disorder from infections involving other tissues.

Draining mucocele or ranula is slightly more common. The mucocele is most often located on the lower lip, and the ranula occurs in the floor of the oral cavity. A history of repeated episodes of swelling and draining with regression in these locations prompts the clinician to assign a high rank to mucocele and ranula, especially when the fluid is clear, viscous, and sticky.

A *chronic osteomyelitis* more frequently drains through an extraoral sinus opening than through an intraoral opening. Findings of suggestive changes in the basal bone and pus that can be expressed by exerting pressure on a tender or painful expansion of the mandible suggest the assignment of a high rank to osteomyelitis. The probability that chronic osteomyelitis is the likely diagnosis is enhanced if (1) the patient has an uncontrolled systemic disease, such as diabetes, (2) the jawbone has been previously irradiated, or (3) the patient has Paget's disease.

Drainage from a cyst is almost always caused by infection. If the cyst is in bone, a radiograph reveals the defect but may not help differentiate between an abscess and a cyst. Such a distinction is academic anyway because an infected cyst may be considered an abscess. Soft tissue cysts within the oral cavity are uncommon.

A large *oronasal fistula* is easily recognized, so a discussion of its differential features is not necessary. Small fistulas in the anterior midline could be confused with a patent nasopalatine duct, but these two entities can be distinguished by observing the position of an inserted gutta-percha point on an occlusal radiograph.

Since the majority of *oroantral fistulas* occur on the ridge in the premolar-molar area, a defect in this region that permits passage of food or drink into the nose is almost certainly an oroantral fistula. Small tracts from *infected cysts* or *abscesses* in this region could be confused with purulent drainage of an infected sinus through an oroantral fistula; however, a radiograph made after the insertion of a gutta-percha cone reveals the image of the cone terminating inferior to the antrum when the case is an infected cyst or abscess.

A *postsurgical or postinfection defect* is seen most often on the alveolus and is diagnosed by learning of the causative experience.

Commissural lip pits always occur in the characteristic location; the probability that other pits or sinus openings could occur in this location is remote.

Chronic draining dentoalveolar abscesses constitute the majority of intraoral draining lesions. If pus can be expressed from the opening by pressing on a tender tooth, the diagnosis is almost certainly chronic abscess. This impression is confirmed if a radiograph exposed after the insertion of a gutta-percha cone shows the image of the cone leading to the tooth.

The *fovea palatinae* are normal anatomic landmarks; however, in some patients these depressions are so prominent that they may resemble fistulas or sinus openings. Their characteristic location on each side of the midline of the anterior soft palate and the presence of mucus that can be expressed from them by pressing on the surrounding soft tissue should permit identification.

Fistulas and sinuses of the face and neck

The following entities must be considered in the differential diagnosis when a draining lesion is encountered on the skin of the face and neck:

Pustule
Draining cyst
Chronic alveolar abscess or osteomyelitis
Salivary gland fistula
Orocutaneous fistula
Congenital aural sinus
Auriculotemporal syndrome
Thyroglossal sinus
Lateral cervical sinus

Determination of the location, depth, and course of tracts in the neck and face often permits the differentiation of these lesions. Thus injecting radiopaque dye into the defects, along with the use of radiographs, is frequently beneficial as a diagnostic indicator.

Identifying the fluid draining from these lesions may provide a valuable clue for diagnosis. In various cases the fluid may prove to be saliva, cyst fluid, pus, or sweat.

Saliva is found emanating from orocutaneous and salivary gland fistulas and through the second branchial arch sinus:

1. The *second branchial arch sinus* can be differentiated from the orocutaneous fistula by the fact that the former is a developmental lesion and so is usually observed early in life. Also in most cases the former defect is more posterior, extending downward through the hyoid bone to the lateral tonsillar fossa.
2. The *orocutaneous fistula* may be differentiated from the salivary fistula in that the defect does not extend from skin surface to mucosal surface in the latter. Also the characteristic location of the salivary gland fistula aids in the differentiation.

When the drainage is *clear, thin cyst fluid,* a tract from a *branchial* or *thyroglossal cyst* must be suspected. If the sinus is in the lateral neck, it is most likely draining from a branchial cyst. If it is in or near the midline in the region of the hyoid bone, however, and if it is stressed when the tongue protrudes, the lesion is most likely thyroglossal in origin.

If *purulent material* is emanating from a cutaneous sinus, the entities that must be considered are pustule, infected cyst, chronic alveolar abscess or chronic osteomyelitis, and infected congenital aural sinus:

1. If the lesion is an infected *aural sinus,* swelling and tenderness are present, as is a small sinus opening in or just anterior to the external ear. This entity may be confused with a *first branchial arch sinus,* but the latter is extremely rare (only 24 cases have been reported in the literature).
2. A *draining alveolar abscess* or *chronic osteomyelitis* of the mandible may empty onto the skin of the lower face or upper neck. On radiographic examination bony changes are evident with both entities. If the cause is *Actinomyces,* fine yellow granules frequently are present in the purulent material (which usually emanates from multiple sinuses).

3. *Infected draining cysts* most often encountered in these regions are the thyroglossal, branchial, sebaceous, and dermoid.
   a. The *sebaceous* and *dermoid* varieties can usually be differentiated from the other two by their more superficial location. The dermoid cyst occurs most often in the midline and is firm, whereas the sebaceous variety may occur anywhere and is not so firm.
   b. The deeper, *thyroglossal* and *branchial* types usually can be differentiated by observing that the former are near or in the midline, whereas the latter are situated more laterally.
4. *Purulent infections in lymph nodes* and *draining space infections* must also be considered.

A *pustule* is the most common of all purulent draining lesions and is readily recognized by its short course and superficial location and by the presence of multiple skin lesions.

The *auriculotemporal syndrome* need not be confused with any of the other entities included in this chapter. A history of trauma to the parotid region followed by sweating on gustatory stimulation is practically pathognomonic.

REFERENCES

Abrams AM, Howell FV, and Bullock WK: Nasopalatine cysts, Oral Surg 16:306-332, 1963.

Allard RHB, de Vries K, and van der Kwast WAM: Persisting bilateral nasopalatine ducts: a developmental anomaly, Oral Surg 53:24-26, 1982.

Anderson MF: Surgical closure of oroantral fistula: report of a series, J Oral Surg 27:862-863, 1969.

Bailey H: The clinical aspects of branchial fistulas, Br J Surg 21:12-21, 1933.

Baker BR: Pits of the lip commissures in Caucasoid males, Oral Surg 21:56-60, 1966.

Baron HD: Surgical correction of salivary fistula, Gen Pract 21:89-98, 1960.

Braun RJ and Lehman J: A dermatologic lesion resulting from a mandibular molar with periradicular pathosis, Oral Surg 52:210-212, 1981.

Bronstein SL and Clark MS: Sublingual gland salivary fistula and sialocele, Oral Surg 57:357-361, 1984.

Brown PM and Judd ES: Thyroglossal duct cysts and sinuses, Am J Surg 102:494-501, 1961.

Burket LW: Nasopalatine duct structures and a peculiar bony pattern observed in the anterior maxillary region, Arch Pathol 23:793-800, 1937.

Burket LW: Oral medicine: diagnosis and treatment, ed 6, Philadelphia, 1971, JB Lippincott Co.

Calman HI, Gradjesk JE, Eisenberg M, et al: The external fistula: its diagnostic importance, Dent Radiogr Photogr 53(2):26-30, 1980.

Carp L and Stout AP: Branchial anomalies and neoplasms: a report of thirty-two cases with follow-up results, Ann Surg 87:186-209, 1928.

Clarkson P, Wilson THH, and Lawrie RS: Treatment of 1,000 jaw fractures, Br Dent J 80:69-75, 1946.

Cowley DJ and Calman JS: Pre-auricular fistulae in four generations: a study in heredity, Br J Plast Surg 24:388-390, 1971.

Craig RW, Andrews JD, and Wescott WB: Draining fistulas associated with an endodontically treated tooth, J Am Dent Assoc 108:851-852, 1984.

Ehrl RA: Oroantral communication: epicritical study of 175 patients with special concern to secondary operative closure, Int J Oral Surg 9:351-358, 1980.

Eisenbud L and Klatell J: Acute alveolar abscess, Oral Surg 4:208-224, 1951.

Everett FG and Wescott WB: Commissural lip pits, Oral Surg 14:202-209, 1961.

Ewing MR: Congenital sinuses of the external ear, J Laryngol Otolaryngol 61:18-23, 1946.

Farman AG, Gould AR, and Schuler ST: Patent nasopalatine ducts: a developmental anomaly, J Am Dent Assoc 105:473-475, 1982.

Giunta JL, Friedman AL, and Karp R: Dermoid cyst of the tongue with sinus tract, Oral Surg 53:450-453, 1983.

Goldman EH, Stratigos GT, and Arthur AL: Treatment of oroantral fistula by gold foil closure: report of a case, J Oral Surg 27:875-877, 1969.

Gore D and Masson A: Anomaly of the first branchial cleft, Ann Surg 150:309-312, 1959.

Gorlin RJ and Goldman HM: Thoma's oral pathology, ed 6, St. Louis, 1970, The CV Mosby Co.

Gorlin RJ and Pindborg JJ: Syndromes of the head and neck, New York, 1964, McGraw-Hill, Inc.

Gustafson JR: Acute parotitis, Surgery 29:786-801, 1951.

Hill WC and Darlow HM: Bilateral perforate nasopalatine communication in the human adult, J Laryngol Otolaryngol 60:160-165, 1945.

Hyndman OR and Light A: The branchial apparatus: its embryologic origin and the pathologic changes to which it gives rise, with presentation of a familial group of fistulas, Arch Surg 19:410-452, 1929.

Jacques DA, Chambers RG, and Oertel JE: Thyroglossal tract carcinoma: a review of the literature and additions of eighteen cases, Am J Surg 120:439-446, 1970.

Juniper RP: Tuberculosis causing bilateral oroantral fistulae, Br J Oral Surg 10:352-356, 1973.

Killey HC and Kay LW: An analysis of 250 cases of oroantral fistula treated by the buccal flap operation, Oral Surg 24:726-739, 1967.

Krippachne W, Hunt TK, and Dunphy J: Acute suppurative parotitis: study of 161 cases, Ann Surg 156:251-257, 1962.

Kryshtalskyj B and Weinberg S: An assessment for auriculotemporal syndrome following temporomandibular joint surgery through the preauricular approach, J Oral Maxillofac Surg 47:3-6, 1989.

Laage-Hellman JE: Gustatory sweating and flushing after conservative parotidectomy, Acta Otolaryngol 48:234-252, 1957.

Lighterman I, Watanabe Y, and Hidaku T: Leprosy of the oral cavity and adnexa, Oral Surg 15:1178-1194, 1962.

MacGregor AJ: Patent nasopalatine canal, Oral Surg 18:285-292, 1964.

Marshall SF: Thyroglossal cysts and sinuses, Ann Surg 129:642-651, 1949.

McWalter GM, Alexander JB, del Rio CE, and Knot JW: Cutaneous sinus tracts of dental etiology, Oral Surg 16:608-14, 1988.

Moskow BS: Bilateral congenital nasopalatine communication, Oral Surg 53:458-460, 1982.

Mustian WF: The floor of the maxillary sinus and its dental, oral and nasal relations, J Am Dent Assoc 20:2175-2187, 1933.

Neel HB and Pemberton J: Lateral cervical (branchial) cysts and fistulas, Surgery 18:267-286, 1945.

Olson RE, Walters CL, and Powell WJ: Gustatory sweating caused by blunt trauma, J Oral Surg 35:306-308, 1977.

Pollock WF and Stevenson EO: Cysts and sinuses of the thyroglossal duct, Am J Surg 112:225-232, 1966.

Rosenberger HC: Fissural cysts, Arch Otolaryngol 40:288-290, 1944.

Rossman LE, Rossman SR, and Graber DA: The endodontic-periodontic fistula: report of a case, Oral Surg 53:78-81, 1982.

Salamat K, and Rezai RF: Nonsurgical treatment of extraoral lesions caused by necrotic nonvital tooth, Oral Surg 61:618-623, 1986.

Selkirk TK: Fistula auris congenita, Am J Dis Child 49:431-447, 1935.

Shafer WA, Hine MK, and Levy BM: A textbook of oral pathology, ed 4, Philadelphia, 1983, WB Saunders Co.

Shulman BH: Acute suppurative infections of the salivary glands in the newborn, Am J Dis Child 80.413-416, 1950.

Stahl WM and Lyall D: Cervical cysts and fistulae of thyroglossal tract origin, Ann Surg 139:123-128, 1954.

Sykes PJ: Pre-auricular sinus: clinical features and the problems of recurrence, Br J Plast Surg 25:175-179, 1972.

Tuinzing DB and Van Der Kwast WAM: Frey's syndrome: a complication of sagittal splitting of the mandibular ramus, Int J Oral Surg 11:197-200, 1982.

Ward GE: Thyroglossal tract abnormalities: cysts and fistulas, Surg Gynecol Obstet 89:727-734, 1949.

Worth HM: Principles and practice of oral radiologic interpretation, Chicago, 1963, Year Book Medical Publishers.

Wowern NV: Oroantral communications and displacements of roots into the maxillary sinus: a follow-up of 231 cases, J Oral Surg 29.622-627, 1971.

Ziemba RB: Combined buccal and reverse palatal flap for closure of oral-antral fistula, J Oral Surg 30:727-729, 1972.

14

Yellow conditions of the oral mucosa

RONALD E. GIER

Yellow lesions, with the exception of Fordyce's granules, rarely occur in the oral cavity. The variety of yellow lesions is also limited:

Fordyce's granules
Superficial abscess
Superficial nodules of tonsillar tissue
Yellow hairy tongue
Acute lymphonodular pharyngitis
Lipoma
Lymphoepithelial cyst
Epidermoid and dermoid cysts
Pyostomatitis vegetans
Jaundice or icterus
Lipoid proteinosis
Carotenemia
Rarity
   Pseudoxanthoma elasticum

Many potentially yellow lesions may not appear yellow because the covering mucosa masks their color.

Normal fat covered by a thin layer of mucosa appears yellow. Salivary gland tissue infiltrated with fat appears yellow. This condition occurs most often in the soft palate. Bone and salivary stones covered by a thin mucosa may impart a yellowish tinge to the mucosa.

The thrombin clot over some ulcers and the pseudomembranes of several conditions may become stained by food or microorganisms or both and have a yellowish color.

FORDYCE'S GRANULES

Fordyce's granules occur in the oral mucosa as multiple, small, slightly raised granules that vary from a whitish yellow to a distinct yellow. They may occur in clusters or may form plaquelike areas. They are considered a normal variation made up of collections of sebaceous glands covered with intact mucosa. The lobules of these glands may be quite distinct.

The patient is usually unaware of the presence of Fordyce's granules; when he or she does become aware of their presence, the patient may be worried that they are early cancer. This is frequently the reaction of a patient with cancerophobia.

Features

Fordyce's granules have been reported by Miles (1958) to increase rapidly in number at puberty and to continue to increase during adult life. There is no established hereditary pattern to their occurrence. Halprin et al. (1953) found that approximately 80% of the individuals in a series they studied had Fordyce's granules and there was no difference in the distribution according to sex. They found in the population they examined that the granules were present in approximately 60% of patients under the age of 10 years and in 88% of those over the age of 10. Gorsky et al. (1986) reported an incidence of 94.9% in nearly 2500 Israeli Jews.

Fordyce's granules occur most often in the buccal mucosa and are usually bilaterally symmetric. They are also found in the retromolar pad area and in the labial mucosa; occasionally they occur on the gingiva, frenum, and palate. They are sharply delineated, with surfaces that are smooth and not ulcerated, and the solid nodules give the involved area a slightly cheesy feeling.

The histologic features are the same as those of normal sebaceous glands in the skin. The glands have ducts that may be plugged with keratin, and frequently extrusions of sebum into the oral cavity are found.

Differential diagnosis

The differential diagnosis of Fordyce's granules should include the possibility that the granules might be focal collections of Candida and that the plaquelike areas could possibly be a hyperkeratotic leukoplakia.

There is no special laboratory test for the diagnosis of Fordyce's granules; however, the appearance and distribution of the condition are so distinctive that, once recognized, there is little probability that the granules could be confused with another entity.

Management

Since this entity is innocuous, the importance of the condition is exclusively in the differential diagnosis. The involved glands are normal, and, unless malignant changes occur, as on rare occasion they may in sebaceous glands, no treatment is indicated for this condition.

SUPERFICIAL ABSCESS

A superficial bacterial or mycotic abscess may appear as a yellow lesion. The yellow color is imparted by the pus pooling below the thinned mucosa stretched over the enlarging abscess. If a fistula forms and allows the pus to discharge, however, the lesion may no longer be yellow. The superficial swelling of odontogenic abscesses is the visual part of an infection that has its deeper origin at the periapex or the periodontal ligament or subgingivally. Over the years, the term "gum boil" has been applied to some of these superficial lesions.

Features

Pain is usually the chief complaint in superficial abscesses, and the history and oral examination frequently reveal its origin.

Superficial abscesses may be single or multiple; they may occur at all ages in either sex and primarily in the tooth-bearing areas. A single abscess is a raised, sessile swelling with a smooth, frequently reddened mucosa over the yellow pus. On palpation the abscess is fluctuant and, when aspirated, yields pus. The surface may ulcerate and complete the sinus from the initiating infection, resulting in a draining lesion.

Teeth most often are the precipitating cause of this condition and can usually be identified as such, because they are either badly broken down by caries or involved with large restorations that have produced pulpal disease. At times the offending tooth or teeth are associated with a deep periodontal pocket in which a lateral periodontal abscess has developed.

Differential diagnosis

When a painful, fluctuant swelling is present and pus is close enough to the surface to give the swelling a yellow color, there is little question that the diagnosis is an abscess. The diagnosis is especially certain if the swelling is opposite the apex of an elevated tooth that is sensitive to percussion.

Management

The management of these lesions involves treating the underlying cause of infection.

SUPERFICIAL NODULES OF TONSILLAR TISSUE

It is not uncommon to find discrete, yellowish pink nodules distributed over the posterior wall of the oropharynx and occasionally on the oral mucosa. These are nodes of lymphatic tissue that supplement the major tonsils composing Waldeyer's ring, and they are discussed in detail in Chapter 10.

Features

When the nodes of tonsillar tissue are present and situated in areas that are visible during a routine examination of the oropharynx, from one to ten may be apparent. They vary in size but are usually 3 to 5 mm in diameter, and have a yellowish pink sheen.

Differential diagnosis

The appearance and distribution of superficial tonsillar nodules are so characteristic that these structures are readily identified as a variation in the normal distribution of lymphatic tissue surrounding the entrance to the digestive and pulmonary systems.

Management

Since the nodules do not represent a pathologic reaction, their importance relates only to the differential diagnosis.

YELLOW HAIRY TONGUE

The conditions contributing to the development and discoloration of a hairy tongue are described in Chapters 8 and 12. It suffices to say here that the hypertrophied filiform papillae of a hairy tongue may be stained yellow by food, tobacco, medicines, or chromogenic microorganisms.

ACUTE LYMPHONODULAR PHARYNGITIS

Acute lymphonodular pharyngitis is manifested by whitish to yellowish papular lesions on the soft palate and oropharynx. The causative factor is the coxsackie virus A10, and the occurrence of this disease today is probably widespread.

Features

The incubation period for the virus is approximately 5 days after exposure. The patients, who are primarily children and young adults, complain of a sore throat. There is an elevation of temperature from 38° to 41° C (100° to 105° F) along with headache and loss of appetite. The oral lesions appear on about the third day. The course of the disease runs from 4 to 14 days, and the oral lesions resolve in 6 to 10 days after the onset of the symptoms. No sexual predilection has been reported for the disease (Steigman et al., 1963).

The lesions are raised, discrete papules 3 to 6 mm in diameter. The whitish to yellowish papules are surrounded by a narrow, well-defined zone of erythema. Their surfaces are not vesicular and do not ulcerate. The nodules are extremely tender, completely superficial, and bilateral; they generally occur as multiple lesions on the uvula, soft palate, anterior tonsillar pillars, and posterior oropharynx.

The histopathology of these lesions consists of densely packed nodules of lymphocytes. There may be some inclusion bodies in the overlying epithelium.

Differential diagnosis

The differential diagnosis must include *herpangina*, although the lesions of lymphonodular pharyngitis are not vesicular and do not ulcerate.

Management

Since acute lymphonodular pharyngitis is self-limiting and causes few if any complications, no treatment other than supportive therapy is recommended.

LIPOMA

The lipoma is one of the most common benign neoplasms, but it seldom occurs in the oral cavity. It is a tumor of mature fat cells that is found in the subcutaneous tissue. No significant mechanical, dental, familial, or social history is consistent with the occurrence of lipomas.

The lipoma is classified as an exophytic lesion in Chapter 10.

Features

The lipoma has been reported to occur in individuals from 6 weeks of age to 21 years; most lipomas, however, are found after the age of 40, with the peak incidence at 50 years (Burzynski et al., 1971; Yoshimura et al., 1972). The patient is usually aware of a slow-growing mass that may have been present from 1 month to 30 years before treatment is initiated (Hatziotis, 1971; Pisanty, 1976). There does not appear to be a racial distribution of these lesions, and the sexual distribution seems to be approximately equal. Burzynski et al. (1971) reported 55 in men and 41 in women; Seldin et al. (1967) found 14 in women and 10 in men.

The review by Burzynski et al. (1971) indicated that the buccal mucosa and mucobuccal fold are the most common areas of occurrence of lipoma, followed by the tongue, floor of the mouth, and lip; lipomas in the palate, gingiva, and other oral locations are rare.

In deVisscher's series (1982) of 19 lipomas and fibrolipomas, the age of patients at time of excision ranged from 11 to 75 years and had a mean of 53 years. Fifty-eight percent of the patients were between 39 and 63 years of age. There were 10 men and 9 women. Areas of occurrence were similar to those indicated by Burzynski except that the lip was the second most common site.

Lekkas and van Hoof (1979) and Coghlan (1983) reported lipomas of the tongue, whereas Miles et al. (1984) described a lipoma in the soft palate.

The lipoma usually occurs as a solitary lesion that may be sessile, pedunculated, or submerged. It ranges in size from a small lesion approximately 1 cm in diameter to a massive tumor 5 × 3 × 2 cm (Seldin et al., 1967). The lesion varies in contour and shape, ranging from a well-contoured, well-defined, round swelling to a large, ill-defined, lobulated mass. The color, which often is yellow, depends on the thickness of the overlying mucosa. The surface is smooth and nonulcerated except when the tumor occurs in an area that causes it to be subjected to trauma.

On palpation the lesion is nontender, soft, and almost cheesy in consistency, but it may be fluctuant. It is usually relatively superficial, but it may infiltrate muscle and become fixed to the surrounding tissue and therefore not be freely movable. The more deeply occurring lesions may produce only a slight surface elevation and may be well encapsulated, more diffuse, and less delineated than the superficial variety. This more diffuse form gives the clinical impression of fluctuance. Most reported lesions have been solitary, but multiple lesions have been described. There is no tooth involvement with these lesions.

On microscopic examination, the lipoma is mature fat enclosed within a connective tissue capsule. A fibrous stroma divides the fat into lobules, and these septa contain small blood vessels. Cartilage formation has been reported in a lipoma of the lip (McAndrew and Greenspan, 1976). Various combinations of histologic features have been reported. Brahney et al. (1981) described a case of an angiolipoma. A myxoid lipoma was detailed by Chen et al. (1984). Fibrolipomas have been reported by de Visscher (1982), Gallagher et al. (1982), and Kiehl (1980). McDaniel et al. (1984) reported an interesting case of a spindle cell lipoma. Such combinations are not of prognostic significance, although the clinical appearance of color and tissue consistency may vary with the combination of histologic features.

Differential diagnosis

Differential diagnosis of this lesion must include an *epidermoid* or *dermoid cyst* and a *lymphoepithelial cyst.*

Management

If the lesion is not imposing an inconvenience on the patient, it may be ignored. Otherwise the treatment should be surgical excision, making certain to remove the tumor completely. There is a reported 20% recurrence.

LYMPHOEPITHELIAL CYST

The lymphoepithelial cyst is relatively uncommon in the oral cavity. It is apparently the result of cystic degeneration of epithelial inclusions in lymphoid aggregates in the oral cavity. In this respect it is not unlike a branchial cyst in the cervical area, which also results from cystic degeneration of epithelial inclusions. Knapp (1970) described this entity as a pseudocyst of oral tonsil tissue. Chaudhry et al. (1984) proposed that lymphoepithelial cysts arise in excretory ducts of the sublingual glands or occasionally from the ducts of the minor salivary glands and that the lymphoid components are a localized inflammatory response, perhaps of an autoimmune type.

Features

Lymphoepithelial cysts are asymptomatic and nontender, so the patient is frequently not aware of how long they have been present. Lesions reported by Acevedo and Nelson (1971) were present for 1 to 10 years before treatment. There is no related social or familial history.

The studies by Acevedo and Nelson (1971), Bhaskar (1966), and Buchner and Hansen (1980) showed that lymphoepithelial cysts occur predominantly in men; all of Acevedo and Nelson's cases were in men, Bhaskar and Buchner and Hansen reported a 2:1 incidence in men. The age range of the patients included in these two studies was 14 to 81 years, and the most common area of occurrence was the floor of the mouth. In the series of 24 cases of Chaudry et al. (1984) 75% of the patients were in the second to fifth decades. The lesions occurred in 15 women and 9 men and were almost exclusively limited to the floor of the mouth or the lateral border of the tongue.

On clinical examination the lesion is solitary and appears as a raised, yellowish white or white nodule with a smooth surface. It is usually small, with a diameter of only a few millimeters, but it may be as large as 2 cm in diameter. It is fairly mobile, usually superficial, soft in consistency, variably fluctuant, and sharply delineated.

Since these lesions occur predominantly in the floor of the mouth, no teeth are involved.

On aspiration the cyst produces an amorphous coagulum composed predominantly of keratin.

Microscopic examination illustrates that the nodule is a cyst lined with a thin, stratified squamous epithelium containing nucleated, partially keratinized cells and keratin. Circumscribed lymphoid follicles are embedded in the walls.

Differential diagnosis

The differential diagnosis of this lesion should include *lymph node, mucocele, sialolith, dermoid cyst, neuroma, lipoma,* and *other benign tumors of the floor of the mouth.*

Management

Lymphoepithelial cysts are treated by conservative excision; recurrence is improbable.

EPIDERMOID AND DERMOID CYSTS

Epidermoid and dermoid cysts are developmental anomalies. They are basically cystic teratomas, resulting primarily from trapped germinal epithelium. They occur in all areas of the body but are rare in the oral cavity. Usually the patient with an oral epidermoid or dermoid cyst complains of a swelling in the floor of the mouth.

Features

The floor of the mouth is the most common area in the head and neck for the epidermoid or dermoid cyst to occur, followed by the submaxillary and submental areas. These cysts may lie above or below the mylohyoid muscle:

if above, the tongue is displaced superiorly; if below, the soft tissue in the submental region is distended. The cysts may be in the midline or located laterally. Although they have been reported to occur at any age from birth to 72 years, they usually become apparent in patients between the ages of 15 and 35 (Meyer, 1955). They may be slow growing, as reported by Meyer, or of sudden onset.

Epidermoid and dermoid cysts are nontender and range in size from a relatively small lesion to a 10 × 5 × 5 cm mass (Chakravorty and Schatzki, 1975; New and Erich, 1937). There is no pertinent medical or dental history that is unique to patients with these lesions and no recognizable familial pattern of occurrence or sexual predilection.

The cyst is usually not fixed to the surrounding tissue. Its color varies, depending on the position of the cyst and the thickness of the overlying tissue. If the cyst is relatively superficial, it is yellow to white, and its surface is smooth and nonulcerated unless traumatized.

The cyst varies in consistency from soft to firm; it may be fluctuant and frequently is rubbery or cheesy, depending on the elements within it.* The lesion is usually sharply delineated, and aspiration produces a variety of materials other than the typical, straw-colored cyst fluid.

Since this is usually a midline structure, the teeth are not involved unless some dental structures are included in the cyst.

The histopathology of this entity ranges from a simple cyst, usually lined with stratified squamous epithelium and showing some keratinization, to a cyst composed of other germ layers and various types of epithelium:

1. The lumen of the simple cyst is filled with cyst fluid or keratin and no other specialized structure; such a cyst is defined as an *epidermoid cyst.*
2. On the other hand, the lumen may contain other elements, depending on the germinal potential of the originating epithelium; consequently, in the case of these more complex cysts, the lumen may be filled with sebum, hair, and even teeth.

a. If the lumen contains sebaceous material as well as keratin, the lesion is called a *dermoid cyst.*
b. If the lumen contains elements such as bone, muscle, or teeth from various germinal layers, the entity is called a *teratoma.*

Differential diagnosis

The differential diagnosis should include *ranula, thyroglossal duct cyst, cystic hygroma, branchial cleft cyst, cellulitis, tumors,* and *fat masses.*

Management

The treatment for epidermoid and dermoid cysts is surgical removal; the cyst usually does not recur.

PYOSTOMATITIS VEGETANS

The oral lesions of pyostomatitis vegetans are composed of large numbers of small, closely set papillary projections with a broad base and usually on an intensely erythematous mucosa. Although the small projections are red to reddish pink, they may show tiny yellow pustules beneath the epithelium. These lesions were first described by McCarthy (1949) as a rare inflammatory disease of the oral mucosa. The cause of the disease is unknown, but McCarthy and Shklar (1963) suggested that psychosomatic factors may be involved. The chief complaint is usually "eruptions in the mouth."

The lesions may be present for months before the patient seeks professional attention, and occasionally they may be found on routine examination. McCarthy and Shklar (1963) suggested that pyostomatitis vegetans is part of a syndrome that includes ulcerative colitis. Hansen et al. (1983) expanded on this concept in an excellent paper on the differential diagnosis of pyostomatitis vegetans.

Features

The lesions of pyostomatitis vegetans are painless, and there is little if any lymphadenitis. They occur in any area of the mouth and are usually multiple; however, few appear on the tongue. When the condition is present, the buccal and labial mucosal lesions have many folds and the papillary projections develop on these folds. The erythema surrounding the lesions on the buccal mucosa is generally not as intense as in the rest of the mouth.

The yellow vesicles that develop on the papillary projections resemble pustules and, if

---

*The cyst may contain (1) only keratin, (2) sebaceous material and keratin, (3) sweat glands and hair follicles, or (4) in the case of a lesion that represents a complex teratoma, keratin, sebum, bone, muscle, and gastrointestinal tissue (Shafer et al., 1983, p. 379).

opened, these vesicles discharge small amounts of purulent material. This is the only disease known to produce an oral pustular eruption (Cataldo, 1981).

No sexual predilection has been reported for this disease, and the patients who were described by McCarthy (1949) and McCarthy and Shklar (1963) ranged in age from 15 to 47 years.

On histologic examination the involved mucosal tissue is characterized by a chronic inflammatory infiltration, with occasional localized accumulations of polymorphonuclear leukocytes. The lymphocytic infiltration is arranged in patterns of small abscesses or is spread diffusely throughout the tissue. Basophils are predominant in the early lesions.

Bacterial studies have not demonstrated consistent findings in cases of pyostomatitis vegetans. Only microorganisms of the normal oral flora are isolated from the lesions, so the disease is not believed to be infectious.

Differential diagnosis

A diagnosis is possible only if the following can be ruled out: *generalized papillomatosis* of the oral mucosa, Crohn's disease, the group of vesicular eruptions that includes *pemphigus vegetans, viral* and *fungal infections, systemic drug reactions*, and allergic reactions such as *erythema multiforme*.

Management

In most cases the lesions are completely resistant to any kind of therapy, including antibiotics. Those lesions that are concomitant with ulcerative colitis frequently improve when the colitis is controlled, and an exacerbation of the colitis is followed by a similar change in the oral lesions. Topical and systemic steroids have proved to be of some benefit for the oral lesions.

JAUNDICE OR ICTERUS

Jaundice or icterus is a condition that is recognized by the yellowish discoloration of the skin, mucous membranes, and sclerae of the eyes. The discoloration is produced by an increase in the blood level of bilirubin and the deposition of this bile pigment in the tissues. The jaundice appears when the serum concentration exceeds 2 to 3 mg/dl (Jeffries, 1971, p. 1389). The hyperbilirubinemia is caused by (1) excessive pigment production, (2) reduced hepatic uptake, or (3) decreased transport, conjugation, and biliary excretion of bilirubin.

Hemolysis is the most common cause of excessive production of bilirubin. It is a feature of a number of diseases, such as thalassemia, sickle cell anemia (discussed in Chapter 21), pernicious anemia, polycythemia, and neonatal jaundice. A reduced conjugation of bilirubin in the liver in neonatal jaundice and in some other rare syndromes is caused by the immaturity of the hepatoexcretory system.

Reduced uptake of bilirubin in the liver is usually the result of a defect in the transport of plasma bilirubin to the liver cells. Such a defect occurs in Gilbert's syndrome, acute viral hepatitis, and congestive heart failure and follows portacaval shunt surgery. Some drugs interfere with bilirubin uptake. Viral hepatitis is discussed in Appendix C.

The reduced excretion of the conjugated bilirubin is found in cases of hepatocellular injuries such as in viral hepatitis or in inflammatory granulomatous or neoplastic infiltration of the liver, resulting in an obstruction of the biliary tree or bile ducts.

Features

The physical manifestation of jaundice includes a yellow tinge of the eyes, skin, and oral mucous membranes. Icterus is frequently the first and sometimes the only manifestation of liver disease. The appearance of bilirubin in the urine, however, may precede for some time the development of clinical jaundice. The discoloration of the oral mucosa is most often seen first at the junction of the hard and soft palates. This may be caused by the accentuation of the yellow color by the fat in this area.

Depending on the cause of the jaundice, there may be pruritus, pain, and an enlarged liver. If there is partial, intermittent, or total biliary obstruction, the feces is light in color and the urine is dark.

Differential diagnosis

Jaundice must be distinguished from other causes of yellow pigmentation of the skin such as *carotenemia* and *quinacrine therapy*.*

Management

A patient with icterus who is suspected of having liver disease or one of the hemolytic diseases should be referred to a physician for consultation and treatment.

---

*An anthelmintic used for the treatment of tapeworms.

LIPOID PROTEINOSIS

Lipoid proteinosis is a rare disease that severely affects the oral cavity, with the formation of characteristic yellowish white papular plaques on the oral mucosa. The same type of plaques also develops on the skin. The disease, thought to be a disturbance of the mucopolysaccharide metabolism or an alteration in the formation of lipoprotein, is transmitted as an autosomal recessive trait (Gorlin, 1969).

The chief complaints with lipoid proteinosis are an inability to cry as a baby, a husky voice from birth, and scarring maculopapular eruptions on the skin. Calcification of the hippocampal gyri may occur; when it does, it is pathognomonic of this disease (Bearn, 1971, p. 1703).

Features

Lipoid proteinosis is present from birth, and lesions occur on the lips, oral mucosa, face, neck, hands, axillae, scrotum, perineal areas and intergluteal cleft, eyelids, knees, and elbows. Lesions also occur on the epiglottis, the aryepiglottic folds, and the interarytenoid region. The patient may have a recurrent painful parotitis.

The yellowish white lesions are multiple and appear to occur in all races; no sexual predilection has been reported for this disease. The lesions are characteristically raised, waxy nodules that are whitish to yellow and have smooth, nonulcerated surfaces. They may be of varying size, from 2 mm to 0.5 cm in diameter, and they are solid in consistency and firmly fixed to the underlying tissue. They increase in number and prominence from childhood into adult life. Congenital absence of teeth and enamel hypoplasia have been reported to accompany this disease. Hofer and Bergenholtz (1975) were unable to substantiate these associated tooth anomalies.

Histologic study shows hyalinosis of the connective tissue of the upper layer of the corium in the plaques. Small blood vessels are affected much like those in diabetes mellitus. The hyalin material stains intensely with the periodic acid–Schiff stain.

Differential diagnosis

The lesion may be mistaken for an unusual scar formation, but the nature of the plaques can be determined from a biopsy specimen.

Management

The treatment of this disease is symptomatic. Corticosteroids have been employed, but there is no convincing evidence that they are effective.

CAROTENEMIA

Carotenemia is an extremely rare condition in which there is a generalized yellowness of the skin and mucosa. It is produced by an excessive deposition of carotenoid (lipochrome), which is the result of a high intake of foods containing carotene pigments (Blankenhorn, 1960; Jeghers, 1943; Josephs, 1944). There is usually no other systemic problem, but increased yellowness is seen in hyperlipemia, diabetes, nephritis, and hypothyroidism and in conditions in which the conversion of carotene to vitamin A is impaired by an inborn metabolic error or hepatic disease (Ebling and Rook, 1968, p. 1111).

Features

Carotenemia is a generalized yellowness of the skin and mucous membrane. No unusual statistical relationship exists between the occurrence of this phenomenon and the sex or age of the individual. The history usually discloses that the patient has an extremely high intake of food containing relatively large amounts of carotene (for example, carrot juice, oranges, halibut liver oil).

Differential diagnosis

The differential diagnosis must include *jaundice*, which can be ruled out by clinical laboratory tests showing a high serum level of the carotenoid pigments. (If equal parts of serum, alcohol, and petroleum ether are shaken together, the carotenoids are absorbed by the ether.) Also most of the laboratory tests that give elevated values in jaundice are within the range of normal values in carotenemia. In addition, since the carotenoids have a great affinity for fat and bilirubin has a great affinity for elastic tissue, there is an early involvement of the sclera in jaundice, whereas the eye is not discolored in carotenemia.

Management

The treatment involves restricting the dietary intake of food containing carotenoids.

REFERENCES

Acevedo AE and Nelson JF: Lymphoepithelial cysts of the oral cavity: report of nine cases, Oral Surg 31:632-636, 1971.

Bearn AG: Lipoid proteinosis. In Beeson PB and McDermott W, editors: Cecil-Leob textbook of medicine, ed 13, Philadelphia, 1971, WB Saunders Co.

Bhaskar SN: Lymphoepithelial cysts of the oral cavity: report of twenty-four cases, Oral Surg 21:120-126, 1966.

Blankenhorn DH: The infiltration of carotenoids into human atheromas and xanthomas, Ann Intern Med 53:944-954, 1960.

Brahney CP, Aria AA, Koval MH, et al: Angiolipoma of the tongue: report of case and review of literature, J Oral Surg 39:451-453, 1981.

Buchner A and Hansen L: Lymphoepithelial cysts of the oral cavity, J Oral Surg 50:441-449, 1980.

Burzynski NJ, Sigman MD, and Martin TH: Lipoma of the oral cavity: literature review and case report, J Oral Med 26:37-39, 1971.

Cataldo E, Covino MC, and Tesone PE: Pyostomatitis vegetans, Oral Surg 52:172-177, 1981.

Chakravorty RC and Schatzki PF: Lateral sublingual dermoid, Oral Surg 39:862-866, 1975.

Chaudhry AP, Yamane GM, Scharlock SE, et al: A clinicopathological study of intraoral lymphoepithelial cysts, J Oral Med 39:79-84, 1984.

Chen SY, Fantasia JE, and Miller AS: Myxoid lipoma of oral soft tissue: a clinical and ultrastructural study, Oral Surg 57:300-307, 1984.

Coghlan KM: Lipoma of the tongue, Oral Surg 56:29-30, 1983.

de Visscher JG: Lipomas and fibrolipomas of the oral cavity, J Maxillofac Surg 10:177-181, 1982.

Ebling FJ and Rook A: Disorders of skin color. In Rook A, Wilkinson DS, and Ebling FJ, editors: Textbook of dermatology, Philadelphia, 1968, FA Davis Co.

Gallagher DM, Goldman E, and Schaffer SD: Fibrolipoma of the cheek in a child, J Oral Maxillofac Surg 40:824-827, 1982.

Gorlin RJ: Genetic disorders affecting mucous membrane, Oral Surg 28:512-525, 1969.

Gorsky M, Buchner A, Fundoianu-Dayan D, and Cohen C: Fordyce's granules in the oral mucosa of adult Israeli Jews, Community Dent Oral Epidemiol 14:231-232, 1986.

Halprin B, Kolas S, Jefferis KR, et al: The occurrence of Fordyce spots, benign migratory glossitis, median rhomboid glossitis and fissured tongue in 2,487 dental patients, Oral Surg 6:1072-1077, 1953.

Hansen LS, Silverman S, and Daniels TE: The differential diagnosis of pyostomatitis vegetans and its relation to bowel disease, Oral Surg 55:363-373, 1983.

Hatziotis JCH: Lipoma of the oral cavity, Oral Surg 31:511-524, 1971.

Hofer P and Bergenholtz A: Oral manifestations in Urbach-Wiethe disease (lipoglycoproteinosis; lipoidproteinosis; hyalinosis cutis et mucosae), Odont Revy 26:39-58, 1975.

Jeffries GH: Diseases of the liver. In Beeson PB and McDermott W, editors: Cecil-Loeb textbook of medicine, ed 13, Philadelphia, 1971, WB Saunders Co.

Jeghers H: Medical progress: skin changes of nutritional origin, N Engl J Med 228:678-686, 1943.

Josephs HW: Hypervitaminosis A and carotenemia, Am J Dis Child 67:33-43, 1944.

Kiehl RL: Oral fibrolipoma beneath complete mandibular denture, J Am Dent Assoc 100:561-562, 1980.

Knapp MJ: Pathology of oral tonsils, Oral Surg 29:295-304, 1970.

Lekkas C and van Hoof R: Lipoma of the tongue, Oral Surg 48:214-215, 1979.

McAndrew PG and Greenspan JS: Lipoma of the lip with cartilage formation, Br Dent J 140:239-240, 1976.

McCarthy FP: Pyostomatitis vegetans: report of 3 cases, Arch Dermatol Syph 60:750-764, 1949.

McCarthy P and Shklar GA: A syndrome of pyostomatitis vegetans and ulcerative colitis, Arch Dermatol 88:913-919, 1963.

McDaniel RK, Newland JR, and Chiles DG: Intraoral spindle cell lipoma: case report with correlated light and electron microscopy, Oral Surg 57:52-57, 1984.

Meyer I: Dermoid cysts (dermoids) of the floor of the mouth, Oral Surg 8:1149-1164, 1955.

Miles AEW: Sebaceous glands in the lip and cheek mucosa of man, Br Dent J 105:235-248, 1958.

Miles DA, Langlais RP, Aufdemorte TB, et al: Lipoma of the soft palate, Oral Surg 57:77-80, 1984.

New EB and Erich JB: Dermoid cysts of the head and neck, Surg Gynecol Obstet 65:48-55, 1937.

Pisanty S: Bilateral lipomas of the tongue, Oral Surg 42:451-453, 1976.

Seldin HM, Seldin SD, Rakower W, and Jarrett WJ: Lipoma of the oral cavity: report of 26 cases, J Oral Surg 25:270-274, 1967.

Shafer WG, Hine MK, and Levy BM: A textbook of oral pathology, ed 4, Philadelphia, 1983, WB Saunders Co.

Steigman AJ, Lipton MM, and Braspennickx H: Acute lymphonodular pharyngitis: a newly described condition due to Coxsackie A virus, J Pediatr 61:331-336, 1963.

Yoshimura Y, Miyagi K, Shoju M, et al: Lipoma in the infant and child: report of cases, J Oral Surg 30:690-693, 1972.

BIBLIOGRAPHY

Brooke RI: Traumatic herniation of buccal pad of fat (traumatic pseudolipoma), Oral Surg 45:689-691, 1978.

Leung AKC: Carotenemia, Adv Pediatr 34:223-248, 1987.

Messenger KL and Cloyd W: Traumatic herniation of the buccal fat pad: report of case, Oral Surg 43:41-43, 1977.

Vindenes H: Lipomas of the oral cavity, Int J Oral Surg 7:162-166, 1978.

Part III

Bony lesions

The risks versus the benefits of the screening type of radiographic surveys, as well as the changes observed on subsequent radiographs, has been the subject of considerable research (Burgess, 1985; Garcia et al., 1987; Keur, 1986; Langland et al., 1980; Valachovic et al., 1986; Weems et al., 1985).

Adherence to the following general guidelines is essential for accurate radiographic interpretation and the development of a differential diagnosis:

1. Radiographs must be of good quality.
2. The radiograph represents only a portion of the available clinical data relative to a particular pathologic process or change.
3. The proper evaluation of radiographic information necessitates an intimate working knowledge of osseous and soft tissue anatomy, radiographic anatomy, and the basic nature and varieties of the pathologic processes that affect the tissues in the areas of concern.
4. A differential diagnosis leading to a working diagnosis is as necessary in evaluating bony lesions as it is in evaluating soft tissue lesions.

Good-quality radiographs

Even at the risk of a wearing effect, it must be stressed that good-quality radiographs are essential. There is little doubt that quality is frequently disregarded, apparently on the grounds of inconvenience; in other words, to determine the proper radiographic techniques and then apply them just does not seem to be convenient.

Corroborative data

The radiographic evaluation must in every case be qualified on the basis of information obtained from the complete examination of the patient. Basing an opinion on radiographic findings alone is risky and often leads to error. Thus, when a radiolucency is discovered on a radiograph, the patient must be questioned in

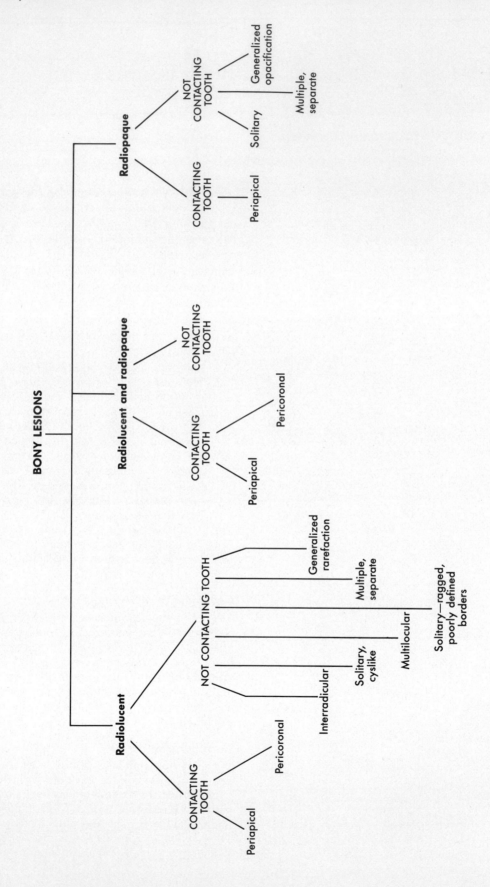

an attempt to outline the onset and course of the suspected lesion and to obtain other pertinent historical facts. Furthermore, the adjacent soft tissue, the cortical plates of the bone, and any teeth in the region must be examined. This examination should include a thorough inspection and a systematic tissue-knowledgeable palpation.* The clinician thereby is able to determine much about the lesion, such as whether the process in the bone has enlarged sufficiently to expand or erode the cortical plates and possibly invade the adjacent soft tissue.

Basic knowledge necessary for diagnosis

A further explanation of the third guideline mentioned relates to the clinician's basic preparation for the evaluation of radiologically detectable changes in the bone. To become accomplished in this area of diagnosis, he or she must acquire and use a general knowledge of anatomy, pathology, and radiology. The pertinence of such a contention is well illustrated by the wide variability that anatomic structures can manifest and yet be considered to fulfill the requirements of the normal order. Consequently the clinician must be not only aware of the potential for deviation from the usual morphology but also familiar with the altered radiographic appearances these irregularities can assume. The true nature of many normal anatomic variations has often been recognized only during the surgery for their intended removal.

After the student has become quite familiar with the normal radiographic appearances and variations that anatomic structures can assume, he or she is ready to study the radiographic changes produced by disease states. The breadth of this information may appear awesome at first encounter because of the multitudinous lesions that may occur in bone. Fortunately, however, a comprehension of these diseases is facilitated by considering that practically all bony lesions can be categorized into three groups, depending on whether their radiographic appearances are completely radiolucent, mixed radiolucent-radiopaque, or totally radiopaque.

To emphasize this concept, Part III is divided into three sections. In addition, each section is divided into chapters that represent a subclassification of the lesions based on more subtle radiographic differences, for example, periapical radiolucencies and cystlike radiolucencies.

A factor complicating this simplified scheme is that frequently a lesion occurs with two or even three different images, which usually represent different stages of maturation. Thus it has been necessary to include some entities in more than one chapter. Appendix A lists the more common bony lesions that are appropriately placed in two or more of the basic categories (radiolucent, mixed, radiopaque).

Differential diagnosis

In most cases the microscopic examination of biopsy tissue provides the final diagnosis. Yet before biopsy the clinician is without such explicit information but nevertheless must formulate his or her own list of possibilities supported by the results from physical, radiologic, and laboratory examinations. To emphasize the need for carefully formulated working diagnoses, imagine the chagrin and the problems encountered by credulous clinicians who find themselves well into surgical procedures on unsuspected vascular tumors. In summary, when osseous lesions are being studied, the formulation of a differential diagnosis—with the disease entities arranged in decreasing order of probability, as indicated by the strength of their supporting clinical evidence—is just as necessary as it is for the study of soft tissue lesions.

Furthermore, when studying a radiolucent lesion, the clinician must be cognizant of the possibility that such a lesion may not have originated in the bone but rather may have developed in the overlying mucosa and subsequently extended into the bone. A careful clinical examination of the patient in conjunction with the radiographic findings usually indicates the correct inference. This distinction is, of course, important when a list of pertinent pathoses is being considered, since the soft tissue entities can usually be deemphasized if the evidence suggests an origin in bone. A rare exception would be concomitant lesions—one originating in bone and another in the adjacent soft tissue.

Careful adherence to these principles ensures that the clinician approaches lesions of the bone in a logical manner. Valuable information on this process has been presented by Chomenko (1980), Frommer (1982), Mourshead (1980), and Reiskin and Valachovic (1980).

---

*In Chapter 3 the manner in which careful palpation of a pathologic area, swelling, or mass can provide considerable definitive information is described. Therefore, when a lesion is suspected or discovered in a bone, all the physical characteristics of the region must be considered.

REFERENCES

Burgess JO: A panoramic radiographic analysis of Air Force basic trainees, Oral Surg 60:113-117, 1985.

Chomenko AG: Removing "shades of gray" in radiographic interpretation of jaw lesions, Dent Surv 56:32-38, 1980.

Frommer HH: Differential diagnosis from pantomograms, Dent Radiogr Photogr 55:25-36, 1982.

Garcia RI, Valachovic RW, and Chauncey HH: Longitudinal study of the diagnostic yield of panoramic radiographs in aging edentulous men, Oral Surg 63:464-497, 1987.

Keur, JJ: Radiographic screening of edentutous patients: sense or nonsense? a risk-benefit analysis, Oral Surg 62:463-467, 1986.

Langland OE, Langlais RP, Morris CR, and Preece JW: Panoramic radiographic survey of dentists participating in ADA health screening programs: 1976, 1977, 1978, J Am Dent Assoc 101:279-282, 1980.

Mourshead F: An approach to the teaching of radiographic interpretation of bony lesions, Oral Surg 50:92-93, 1980.

Reiskin AB and Valachovic RW: Radiologic considerations in evaluation of radiolucent lesions of the mandible, J Am Dent Assoc 101:771-776, 1980.

Valachovic RW, Douglass CW, Reiskin AB, et al: The use of panoramic radiography in the evaluation of asymptomatic adult dental patients, Oral Surg 61:289-296, 1986.

Weems RA, Manson-Hing LR, Jamison HC, and Greer DF: Diagnostic yield and selection criteria in complete intraoral radiography, J Am Dent Assoc 110:333-338, 1985.

15

Anatomic radiolucencies

NORMAN K. WOOD
PAUL W. GOAZ

The following structures produce anatomic radiolucencies:

Structures peculiar to the mandible
Mandibular foramen
Mandibular canal
Mental foramen
Lingual foramen
Airway shadow
Submandibular fossa
Mental fossa
Midline symphysis
Medial sigmoid depression

Structures peculiar to the maxilla
Intermaxillary suture
Incisive foramen, incisive canal, and superior
  foramina of incisive canal
Nasal cavity
Naris
Nasolacrimal duct or canal
Maxillary sinus
Greater palatine foramen

Structures common to both jaws
Pulp chamber and root canal
Periodontal ligament space
Marrow space
Nutrient canal
Developing tooth crypt

In view of the foregoing comments relative to the diagnosis of radiographically apparent lesions, any consideration of the differential diagnosis of pathologic radiolucencies of bones should be prefaced by a discussion of the normal anatomic radiolucencies and their variations.

Discussing entities in the order of their decreasing frequency of occurrence, the procedure followed in the other chapters of this book, is not appropriate for these entities, since they are normal and are to be expected in most adequate radiographs of the anatomic regions considered.

Some circumstances may seem to contradict the above comment, however; those that require mention relate to the mitigating factors that alter the nature and radiographic reproduction of the usual normal landmarks. For ex-

ample, the presence or absence of certain normal radiolucencies is related to age. The developing tooth crypts in persons under 16 years of age are usually not present in older individuals. Likewise pulp chambers, root canals, and periodontal ligament spaces decrease in size with age and are, of course, not present at all in edentulous persons. There is also considerable variation in the frequency of occurrence and radiographic representation of the lingual foramen, but this variability does not appear to be related to age. Nutrient canals are another example of radiolucencies that may be prominent in the radiographs of some patients but difficult to identify or even find in others. Consequently only an arbitrary decision accounts for the order of the following discussion: first, the radiolucencies of the mandible; second, those of the maxilla; and finally, those that are common to both jaws.

Structures peculiar to the mandible

MANDIBULAR FORAMEN

The mandibular foramen is usually situated just above the midpoint in the medial surface of the ramus and just posterior to the midpoint between the anterior and posterior borders (Hayward et al., 1977). It receives the inferior dental nerve and artery after they traverse the pterygomandibular space. Because of its position in the ramus, this foramen is seldom seen on periapical films, but it may often be identified on panographic and lateral oblique films, in which its outline varies from triangular to oval to funnel shaped and its definition varies from faint to prominent (Fig. 15-1).

The radiographic image of the mandibular foramen is seldom larger than 1 cm in diameter, and the foramen can be positively identified by its bilateral occurrence and its association with the relatively radiolucent mandibular canal, which passes from it in an anteroinferior direc-

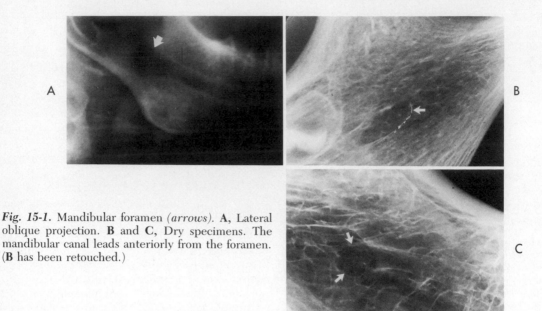

Fig. 15-1. Mandibular foramen *(arrows)*. **A,** Lateral oblique projection. **B** and **C,** Dry specimens. The mandibular canal leads anteriorly from the foramen. (**B** has been retouched.)

tion. Frequently the lingula can be detected as a triangular radiopacity of variable density at the foramen's anterior border. These associated structures, the mandibular canal and the lingula, can be mistaken for pathologic entities.

MANDIBULAR CANAL (INFERIOR DENTAL CANAL)

The outline of the mandibular canal, the largest of the nutrient canals in the jaws, may be seen on a panographic or periapical view of the molar region. The canal appears as a relatively radiolucent channel, bounded by definite, thin radiopaque lines (cortical bone) throughout its length (Fig. 15-2). Its course can be followed from the mandibular foramen anteroinferiorly to a point where it frequently appears to sweep upward to meet the mental foramen (now called the mental canal). Occasionally it is seen to extend some distance anteriorly and inferiorly from the mental foramen (Fig. 15-3) where it is called the incisive canal.

There is great variation in the width and prominence of the mandibular canal, but in most individuals the bilateral appearance is similar. There is some variation also in the position of the canal within the body of the mandible; some canals are near the inferior border, whereas others lie just below the apices of the molars. The curvilinear course is normally rather gentle; abrupt changes in outline,

whether it narrows, broadens, becomes discontinuous, or alters in direction, are suggestive of pathosis (Fig. 15-4). Farman et al. (1977) described alterations in the radiographic appearance of the mandibular canal induced by disease of the mandible.

MENTAL FORAMEN

The mental foramen permits the exit of the mental branches of the mandibular artery and nerve to the soft tissue in the area of the chin, lower lip, and labial gingiva. It can usually be located on a radiograph of the area, generally in the vicinity of the premolar apices (Fig. 15-5).

The relative definition of the foramen may vary, however, because the mental canal does not often meet the buccal cortical plate at a right angle. When the angle approaches 90 degrees, the resultant radiographic image is the most conspicuous because the beam is directed parallel to the canal (Fig. 15-6).

Since this foramen frequently occurs at the apices of the premolars, there is a tendency for the unwary clinician to confuse it with periapical pathosis (Fig. 15-7).

Green (1987) observed that the position of the mental foramen varies somewhat from race to race. Goodday and Precious (1988) described a case in which two mental nerves and two mental foramina occurred on the right side.

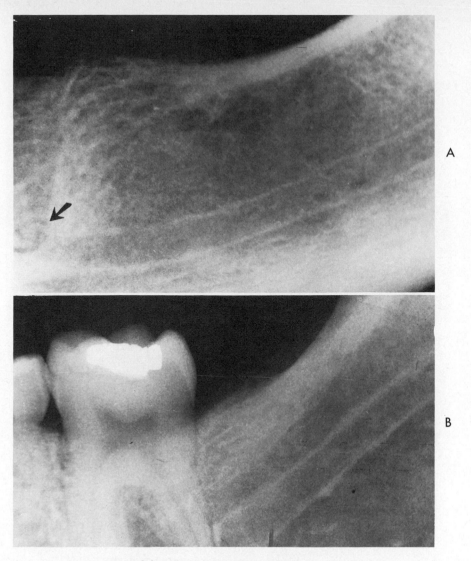

Fig. 15-2. Mandibular canal delineated by two thin radiopaque lines. **A**, In an edentulous jaw. The mental foramen *(arrow)* appears at the anterior terminal of the canal. **B**, In a dentulous jaw.

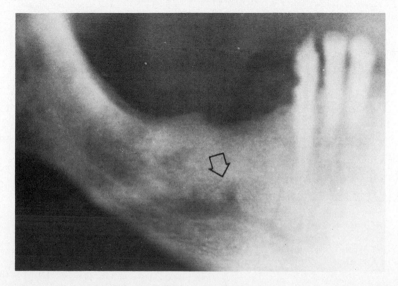

Fig. 15-3. The continuation of the mandibular canal anterior to the mental foramen *(arrow)*.

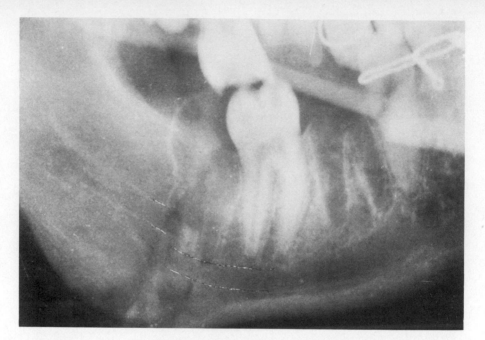

Fig. 15-4. Lateral oblique view of a mandible fractured at the angle. The interrupted course of the canal is caused by displacement of the fragments. (Photograph has been retouched.)

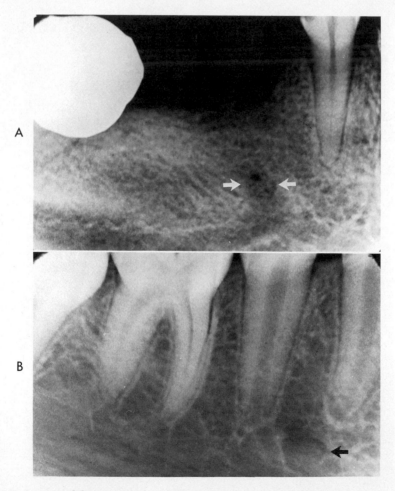

Fig. 15-5. A, Mental foramen *(arrows)*. **B,** Occasionally the mental foramen is confused with an adjacent foramen-like marrow space *(arrow)*, as illustrated in this radiograph.

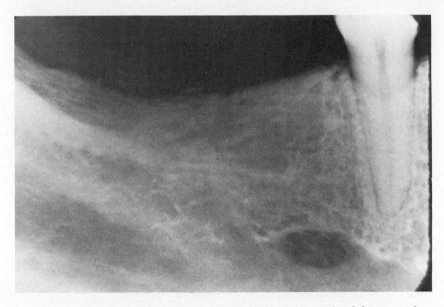

Fig. 15-6. This prominent image of the mental foramen is a result of directing the x rays parallel to the mental canal.

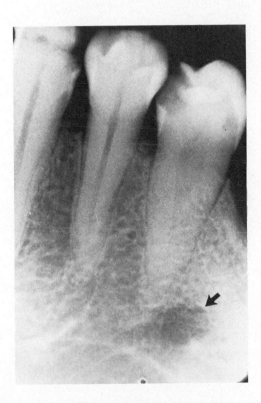

Fig. 15-7. Mental foramen *(arrows).* Occasionally the foramen is projected near or over the roots of adjacent teeth and may be misinterpreted as periapical pathosis. This happens especially when the pulps of the teeth are suspect.

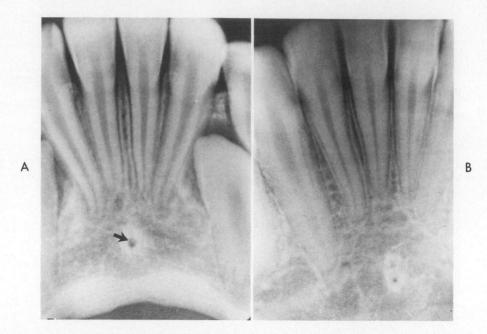

Fig. 15-8. Lingual foramen. **A,** A single foramen *(arrow)* is accentuated by the radiopaque projections of the geniotubercles that usually encircle it. **B,** This radiographic view shows a double foramen.

LINGUAL FORAMEN

The lingual foramen can often be seen on periapical views of the lower central incisors. It is located well below the apices of these teeth in the midline, is generally surrounded by a prominent radiopaque ring of cortical bone, and is variable in frequency, size, and appearance (Fig. 15-8, *A*). It seldom is more than 1 or 2 mm in diameter. Occasionally two or more foramina are present (Fig. 15-8, *B*). Terminal branches of the inferior dental artery (incisive branches) exit at this point to supply the lingual incisive gingiva.

AIRWAY SHADOW

An airway shadow is bilateral, relatively radiolucent, and especially well recorded on panographs and cephalometric and lateral oblique radiographs.

This image, which runs in an inferoposterior direction across the angle of the mandible just posterior to the molar region, is frequently troublesome to the inexperienced clinician (Fig. 15-9). It results from the lack of soft tissue between the posterodorsal surface of the tongue and the region of the soft palate and posterior pharynx.

SUBMANDIBULAR FOSSA

The submandibular fossa is a concave area on the lingual side of the mandible below the molar area. It accommodates the submandibular salivary gland and usually appears as a poorly defined, relatively radiolucent area (Fig. 15-10, *A*). Often its contrast is enhanced by a prominent radiopaque mylohyoid ridge that runs across the top of the depression, thus making its radiolucency more pronounced (Fig. 15-10, *B*).

MENTAL FOSSA

The image of the mental fossa is similar to the image produced by the submandibular fossa. The mental fossa is situated on the labial aspect of the midline of the mandible just above the mental tubercle. Radiographs of the area often show such a relative radiolucency over the incisor roots that this fossa may be mistaken for periapical pathosis (Fig. 15-11).

MIDLINE SYMPHYSIS

The mandibular midline symphysis is present on radiographs at the midline of the mandibles of infants and is represented by a radiolucent line that may be misinterpreted as a

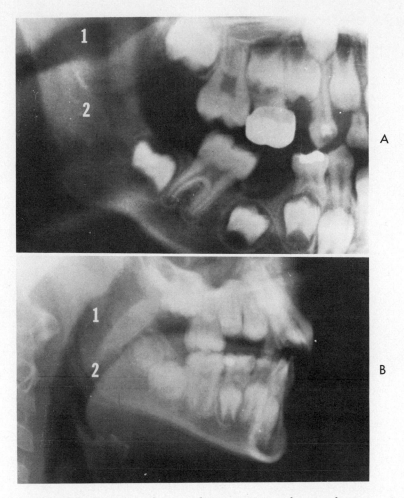

Fig. 15-9. Airway shadow. *1*, Nasopharyngeal airway; *2*, oropharyngeal airway. **A**, Panograph. **B**, Cephalometric view.

fracture (Fig. 15-12). The symphysis usually fuses and ossifies by the age of 1 year and is then no longer apparent. It is not frequently encountered by the dental clinician on radiographs, since few patients have cause to be radiographically examined at this young age.

MEDIAL SIGMOID DEPRESSION

Langlais et al. (1983) described a radiolucency that appeared below and just anterior to the greatest depth of the sigmoid notch of the mandibular ramus. It may be observed occasionally on a panoramic radiograph (Fig. 15-13). The authors referred to the bony depression that caused this image as the medial sig-

moid depression. This depression is defined by the temporal crest and the crest of the mandibular neck; its degree of expression, which is quite variable, depends on the robustness (prominence) of these two crests. According to the authors the medial sigmoid depression is encountered radiographically on approximately 10% of the films examined. However, they point out that the image of the depression, regardless of the depression's size, depends on the geometry of the machine used and a particular positioning of the patient. This normal feature of the mandible is important only in that its recognition precludes its misinterpretation as pathosis.

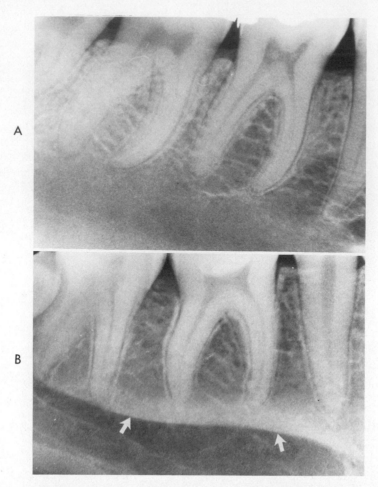

Fig. 15-10. Submandibular fossa. **A,** The fossa appears as a poorly defined radiolucency below the apices of the molars. **B,** The prominent mylohyoid ridge *(arrows)* in this view accentuates the fossa.

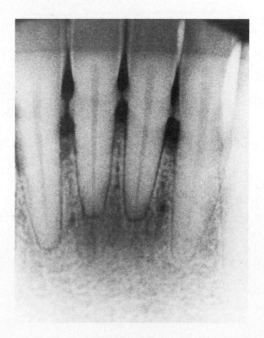

Fig. 15-11. Mental fossa. This radiograph showing a generalized radiolucency in the periapical incisor region illustrates the thinning of the bone resulting from the mental fossa.

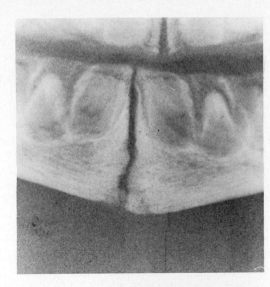

Fig. 15-12. This radiograph of a stillborn child shows the mandibular symphysis at birth. The structure has been erroneously identified as a fracture.

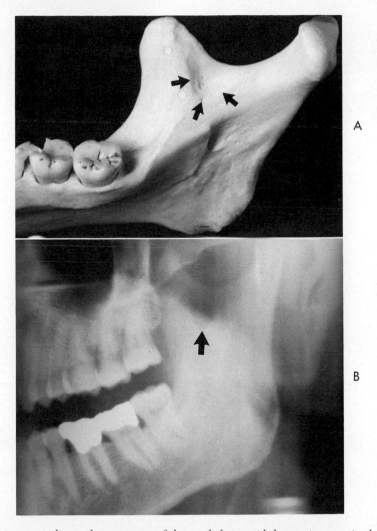

Fig. 15-13. Arrows indicate the presence of the medial sigmoid depression on, **A,** the medial aspect of the bone and, **B,** the panoramic projection.

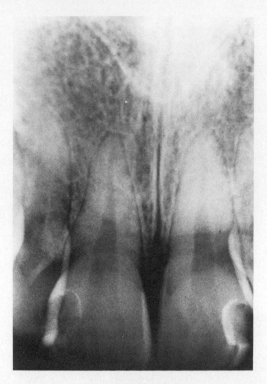

Fig. 15-14. The intermaxillary suture can be identified as a vertical radiolucent line in the central incisor region. It becomes less distinct with age.

Structures peculiar to the maxilla

INTERMAXILLARY SUTURE

The intermaxillary suture, between the right and left maxillary bones, can be identified as a thin vertical radiolucency in the midline between the central incisors (Fig. 15-14). It is usually delineated by two thin vertical radiopaque lines (cortical bone). It generally fuses later in life and is then no longer represented on the radiograph.

INCISIVE FORAMEN, INCISIVE CANAL, AND SUPERIOR FORAMINA OF INCISIVE CANAL

The incisive foramen (incisive fossa, anterior palatine foramen) frequently shows as a well-defined round, oval, diamond-shaped, or heart-shaped radiolucency on occlusal films; less often, on periapical films, especially of the central incisors, it appears as a rounded to ribbon-shaped, poorly defined radiolucency. The variation in size of this foramen also parallels its nonuniformity in shape. The position of the foramen on the radiograph ranges from between the roots of the central incisors, close to the alveolar ridge, to the level of the apices (Fig. 15-15).

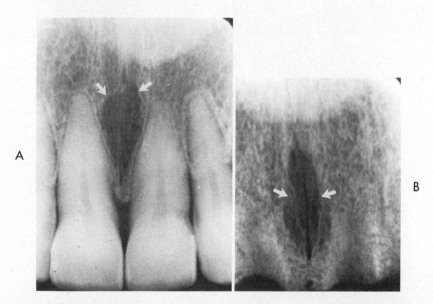

Fig. 15-15. The incisive foramen (*arrows*) represents the oral terminal of the incisive canal. **A,** It is frequently projected onto the central incisor region near the crest of the alveolar process. **B,** The foramen of a nutrient canal is immediately inferior to the incisive foramen.

This variability in the position of the foramen on radiographs relates to both the angulation of the rays used to expose the film and the position of the foramen itself. The location of the foramen, which is in the midline, may range from the crest of the alveolar ridge to some distance posteriorly.

The incisive canals (nasopalatine or anterior palatine canal) that end at the incisive foramen are occasionally seen on periapical films of the central incisors. Their radiolucency on the film, more apparent than real, is emphasized by the contrast with their relatively sharp opaque lateral walls, which actually delineate the canals (Fig. 15-16). The images vary greatly in width and length and may be seen to converge from the nasal fossa toward the foramen, but they usually become indistinct before reaching this terminal (Fig. 15-18).

The images of the superior foramina of the incisive canals are found on periapical films of the maxillary central and lateral incisors and canines, especially if the vertical angle of the radiographic beam is increased sharply (Fig. 15-17). These foramina are seen on the floor of the nasal fossa bordering the septum. On the periapical films their radiolucent images may be projected over the apices of any of the incisor teeth, prompting an impression of periapical pathosis.

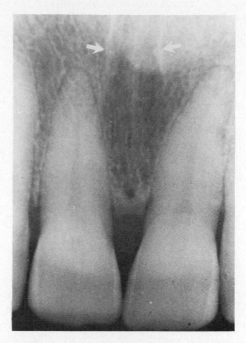

Fig. 15-16. Incisive canals *(arrows)*.

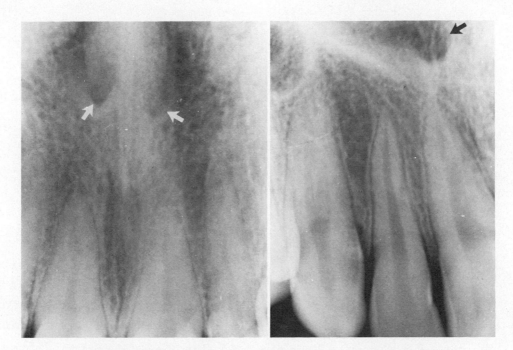

Fig. 15-17. Arrows indicate the nasal terminals of the incisive canals.

NASAL CAVITY (NASAL FOSSA)

The inferior aspect of the nasal cavities is often seen on periapical radiographs of the incisor and canine regions, especially if the vertical angulation is increased. These cavities appear as twin radiolucencies separated by the radiopaque septum and are delimited by radiopaque cortical bone (Fig. 15-18). The inferior border of the cavities is often projected above the apices of the incisors and canines.

NARIS

The image of the nose is sometimes projected over the image of the alveolar bone on anterior periapical films. The density of this soft tissue added to the density of the bone results in a radiographic impression of increased bone density in the area of the superimposition.

Contrariwise, the images of the nares project onto this area of increased density as relative radiolucencies that frequently appear over or on the maxillary incisor region (Fig. 15-19). The nares may then be misinterpreted by the uninitiated diagnostician as evidence of periapical pathosis.

NASOLACRIMAL DUCT OR CANAL

The nasolacrimal duct on each side is usually enclosed in such a thin tube of cortical bone that it is seldom discernible on the usual periapical radiograph (Fig. 15-20, A). The orbital extreme of the structure, however, does appear on the maxillary occlusal radiograph, projected onto the posterior hard palate near the first or second molar area as a relatively large bilateral radiolucency that is well defined by sharp radiopaque borders (Fig. 15-20, B).

On the well-centered radiograph the image of each duct is usually at the junction of the radiopaque lines representing the maxillary sinuses and the nasal fossa. These radiopaque lines are situated lateral to and roughly parallel with the midsagittal plane, where the median suture may still be radiographically apparent before fusion.

MAXILLARY SINUS

The maxillary sinus on each side appears as a well-defined radiolucency with thin, sharp, radiopaque borders (Fig. 15-21). The radiolucency may be crisscrossed by one or more thin radiopaque lines that represent bony septa ap-

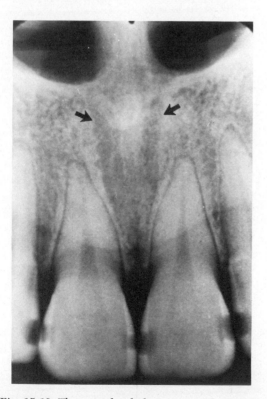

Fig. 15-18. The paired radiolucencies at the superior border represent the nasal cavities. Arrows indicate the divergent branching of the incisive canals toward their nasal terminals.

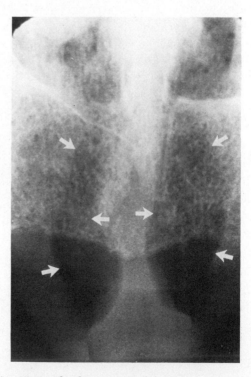

Fig. 15-19. The faint image of the nose and outlines of the nares (*arrows*) are seen in this periapical view of the maxillary incisor region.

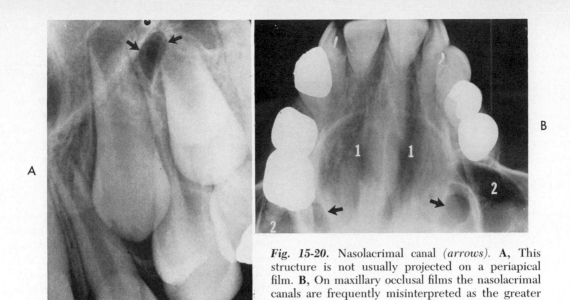

Fig. 15-20. Nasolacrimal canal *(arrows).* **A,** This structure is not usually projected on a periapical film. **B,** On maxillary occlusal films the nasolacrimal canals are frequently misinterpreted as the greater palatine foramina. Note the nasal cavities, *1,* and the maxillary sinuses, *2.*

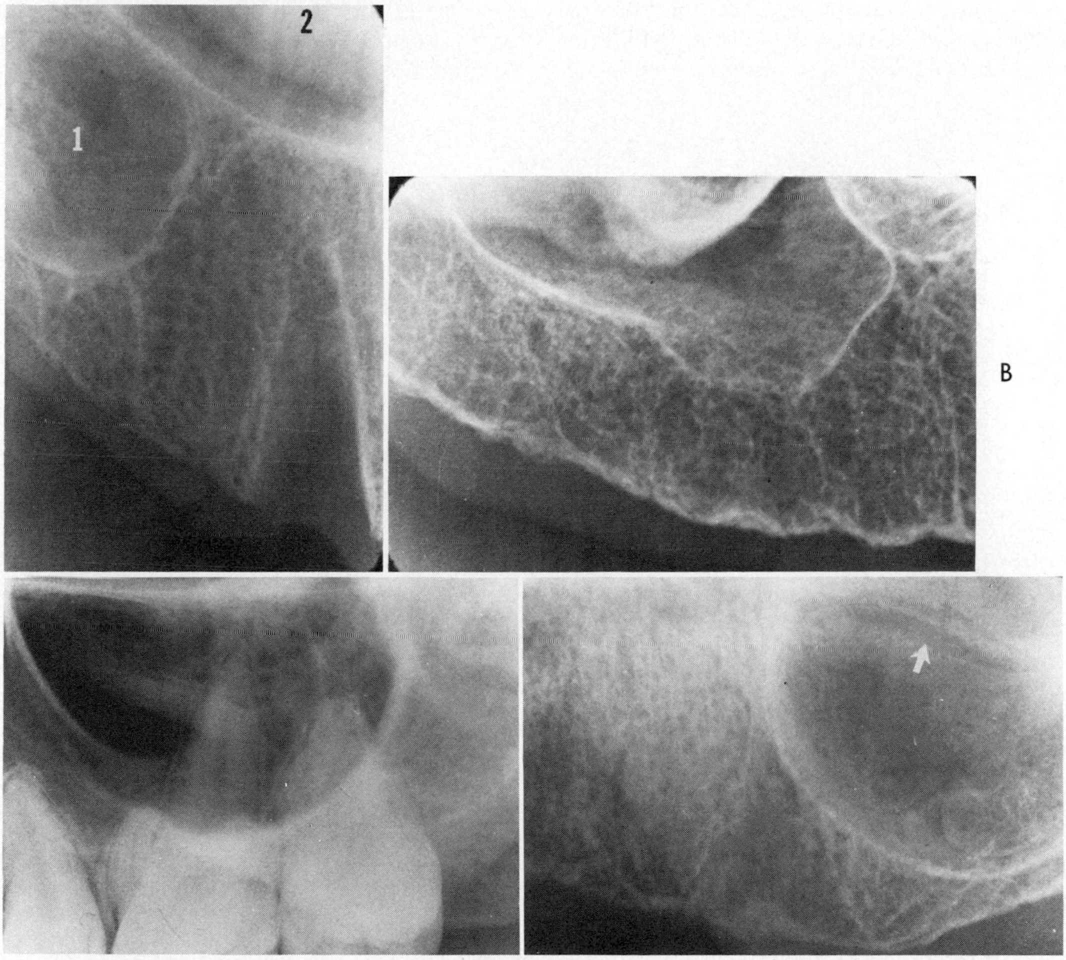

Fig. 15-21. Maxillary sinus. **A,** This periapical view of the canine region shows the maxillary sinus, *1,* the nasal cavity, *2,* and the antral Y. **B,** Maxillary sinus in an edentulous molar region. **C,** Maxillary sinus, showing complex contours and unusual extensions. **D,** Maxillary sinus with a cystlike configuration. A nutrient canal *(arrow)* in the sinus wall aids in differentiating the sinus from a cyst.

pearing to subdivide the sinus. The sinus occurs bilaterally over the molars and premolars and may vary in anteroposterior extent from tuberosity to canine root, or even to the lateral incisor root.

Each maxillary sinus may appear to border or overlap the nasal fossa, depending on the angle of exposure. In the adult the inferior aspect of each sinus lies below the level of the floor of the nasal fossa; frequently nutrient canals are seen in the sinus wall and, when present, help to distinguish this anatomic structure from a cyst or other pathosis. Poyton (1972) discussed the radiographic appearance of the maxillary sinus in detail. The maxillary sinus is also discussed in Chapter 35.

GREATER (MAJOR) PALATINE FORAMEN

Occasionally the greater palatine foramen can be identified on each side as a round to oval ill-defined radiolucency over or between the apices of the maxillary second and third molars (Grier, 1970).

Structures common to both jaws

PULP CHAMBER AND ROOT CANAL

The shadows of pulp chambers and root canals, along with the variations in these anatomic structures, are of great importance in restorative dentistry and in root canal therapy, but a discussion of these features is beyond the scope of this text.

PERIODONTAL LIGAMENT SPACE

Clinicians are well oriented to the radiographic appearance of the smooth radiolucent outline of the periodontal ligament spaces, and dental students are equally well instructed in its appearance. When the spaces are superimposed over anatomic radiolucencies, however, the resultant radiographic images can simulate a broadening of the spaces and occasionally be mistaken for disease.

MARROW SPACE

The marrow spaces between the trabeculae of spongy bone appear as radiolucent areas that

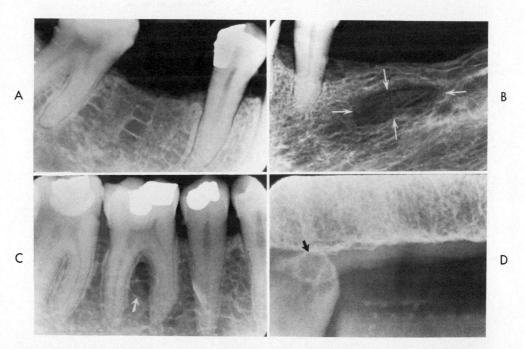

Fig. 15-22. Marrow space. **A,** This pattern occurs with some frequency adjacent to the mandibular molar roots. **B,** Large marrow space *(arrows)* that was mistaken for a lesion. **C,** Large marrow spaces *(arrow)* frequently occur in the bifurcation of the mandibular molars. These variations must be differentiated from periodontal involvement in the bifurcation. **D,** A large marrow space *(arrow)* in the coronoid process was mistaken for a lesion. Note the relatively small marrow spaces in the maxilla as compared with those usually occurring in the posterior region of the mandible.

vary greatly in size, shape, and distribution from person to person as well as throughout the jaws of the same individual (Fig. 15-22). In general, however, the radiographic representations of these structures throughout the maxilla are relatively uniform in size, whereas throughout the mandible the marrow spaces are smaller and more numerous in the anterior portion and tend to be larger in the posterior areas.

In some persons the trabecular spaces above and below the roots of the molars are so large and the trabeculae so sparse that the combined appearance may resemble and be misinter-preted as cysts, traumatic bone spaces, rarefying osteitis, or other such pathoses. In areas where trabeculae are few and marrow spaces are large, the thinly scattered trabeculae are often relatively dense. It is pertinent to emphasize that the size of the marrow spaces is not a particularly reliable criterion for evaluating the status of the jawbone.

NUTRIENT CANAL

The nutrient canals appear as linear ribbon-like radiolucencies of fairly uniform width that are most often found between the roots of teeth (Figs. 15-15, *B*, and 15-23). These inter-

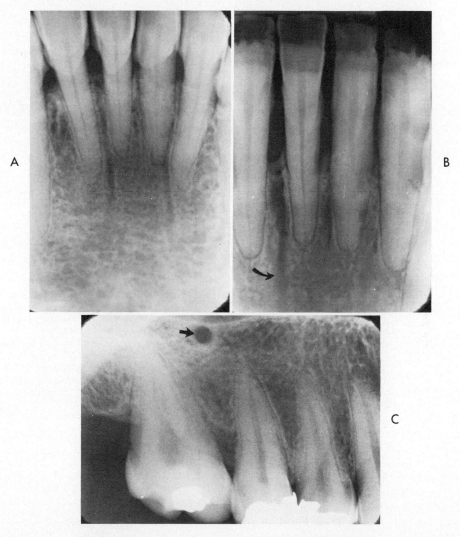

Fig. 15-23. Nutrient canal. **A,** These canals are frequently prominent between the roots of the mandibular incisors and they terminate as small foramina on the crest of the interseptal bone. **B,** The prominent nutrient canal *(arrow)* in this view could be mistaken for a fracture. **C,** The prominence of this unusually large nutrient canal or accessory foramen *(arrow)* is produced by directing the x rays parallel to the canal.

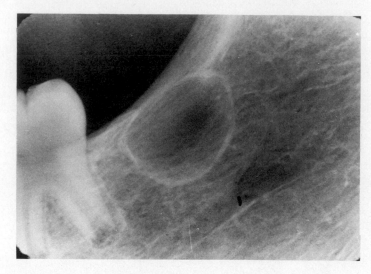

Fig. 15-24. Developing tooth crypt of a third molar. This cystlike radiolucency may be correctly identified by its position in the jaw, its bilateral occurrence, the age of the patient, and serial radiographs.

dental canals, which are most frequently observed on radiographs of the mandibular incisor region, become less numerous in the mandibular premolar area, and the bone supporting the maxillary premolars is the third most likely area in which they are found.

Occasionally a relatively large nutrient canal, carrying the posterior superior alveolar artery and tranversing the lateral wall of the maxillary sinus, is apparent on a maxillary posterior radiograph (Fig. 15-21, *D*). Although nutrient canals are rarely seen in the anterior region of the maxilla and are seldom recognized below or between the mandibular molars, infrequently one is found in the mandibular posterior region, where the trabeculae are few in number and the marrow spaces large. In this region a canal or two accentuated by fine radiopaque walls may be apparent.

In all the regions of both jaws, the canals become much more marked when the teeth are missing. If the beam of the radiograph is directed parallel to a canal and through its foramen in the cortical bone, the canal appears as a small round radiolucency (Fig. 15-23, *C*). These radiolucencies technically are accessory canals and foramina. Occasionally, however, they are confused with pathologic radiolucencies. Patel and Wuehrmann (1976) and Kishi et al. (1982) studied the radiographic appearance of nutrient canals in the jaws.

DEVELOPING TOOTH CRYPT

Tooth crypts are seen on radiographs of developing dentitions, so they are seldom present in patients over 15 years of age. If the developing tooth is uncalcified, the crypt appears as a roundish homogeneous radiolucency and is mistaken for a cyst by the uninitiated diagnostician (Fig. 15-24). If just the tips of the cusps have calcified, the radiographic appearance is of a well-defined radiolucency containing radiopaque foci.

REFERENCES

Farman AG, Nortje CJ, and Grotepas FW: Pathological conditions of the mandible: their effect on the radiographic appearance of the inferior dental (mandibular) canal, Br J Oral Surg 15:64-74, 1977.

Green RM: The position of the mental foramen: a comparison between southern (Hong Kong) Chinese and other ethnic and racial groups, Oral Surg 63:287-290, 1987.

Goodday RHB and Precious DS: Duplication of mental nerve in a patient with cleft lip-palate and rubella syndrome, Oral Surg 65:157-160, 1988.

Grier DC: Radiographic appearance of the greater palatine foramen, Dent Radiogr Photogr 43:34-38, 1970.

Hayward BS, Richardson ER, and Malhotra SK: The mandibular foramen: its anteroposterior position, Oral Surg 44:837-843, 1977.

Kishi K, Nagaoka T, Gotoh T, et al: Radiographic study of mandibular nutrient canals, Oral Surg 54:118-122, 1982.

Langlais RP, Glass BJ, Bricker SL, and Miles DA: Medial sigmoid depression: a panoramic pseudoforamen in the upper ramus, Oral Surg 55:635-638, 1983.

Patel JR and Wuehrmann AH: A radiographic survey of nutrient canals, Oral Surg 42:693-701, 1976.

Poyton HG: Maxillary sinuses and the oral radiologist, Dent Radiogr Photogr 45:43-59, 1972.

16

Periapical radiolucencies

NORMAN K. WOOD
PAUL W. GOAZ
MARIE C. JACOBS

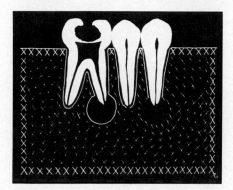

Periapical radiolucencies include the following:

Anatomic periapical radiolucencies (false)
Marrow spaces and hematopoietic defect of the
  jaws
Dental papillae
Maxillary sinus
Incisive foramen and canals
Nasolacrimal duct
Naris
Greater palatine foramen
Mental foramen
Submandibular fossa
Mandibular canal

True periapical radiolucencies
Periapical radiolucencies
  Sequelae of pulpitis
    Granuloma
    Radicular cyst
    Scar
    Chronic and acute dentoalveolar abscesses
    Surgical defect
    Osteomyelitis
  Dentigerous cyst
  Periapical cementomas
  Periodontal disease
  Traumatic bone cyst
  Nonradicular cysts
  Malignant tumors
Rarities
  Ameloblastic variants
  Ameloblastoma
  Aneurysmal bone cyst
  Benign nonodontogenic tumors
  Buccal cyst
  Cementifying and ossifying fibromas
  Cementoblastoma—early stage
  Gaucher's disease
  Giant cell granuloma
  Giant cell lesion of hyperparathyroidism
  Histiocytosis X
  Leukemia
  Lingual salivary gland depression (anterior)
  Mandibular infected buccal cyst
  Odontoma—early stage
  Osteoblastoma—early stage
  Paradental cyst
  Solitary and multiple myeloma

Radiolucent shadows are cast over the periapical regions of teeth in practically all oral radiographic surveys of dentulous patients. Some of these periapical radiolucencies represent innocent anatomic variations, whereas others are caused by benign conditions and require treatment to preserve the associated teeth; still others represent systemic disease conditions that many times become the responsibility and obligation of the dental clinician to recognize and bring to the attention of the patient's physician. The dental clinician should in every case afford whatever cooperation facilitates the most effective treatment.

Malignancies represent a small group of these periapical shadows, and early detection, recognition, and treatment currently represent the only hope the patient has of being cured.

Marmary and Kutiner (1986) reported that in their survey of periapical jawbone lesions, 51% showed radiographic evidence of an inflammatory process in the jawbone. The high incidence and broad spectrum of conditions causing periapical radiolucencies combine to make it imperative that all dental clinicians acquire a broad and comprehensive working knowledge of the conditions listed or discussed in this chapter.

TRUE OR FALSE PERIAPICAL RADIOLUCENCIES

All periapical radiolucent shadows may be readily divided into two categories: true or false. *True* periapical radiolucencies represent lesions that truly are located in contact with the apex of a tooth: their shadow cannot be shifted from the periapex by taking additional radiographs at different angles. In contradistinction, *false* periapical radiolucencies are produced by anatomic cavities or lytic bony lesions that do not contact the apex of a tooth: these radiolucent shadows may be shifted from the periapex by taking additional radiographs at different angles.

Classifying a periapical radiolucency as *true* or *false* is useful in the differential diagnosis process because if it can be clearly demonstrated that the radiolucency in question is truly periapical in location, it is most likely that the lesion has resulted from a pulpitis. On the other hand, if the radiolucency can be shifted from the apex, it most likely is produced by an anatomic cavity or space.

ANATOMIC PERIAPICAL RADIOLUCENCIES

Anatomic radiolucencies are projected over the periapical regions in almost every radio

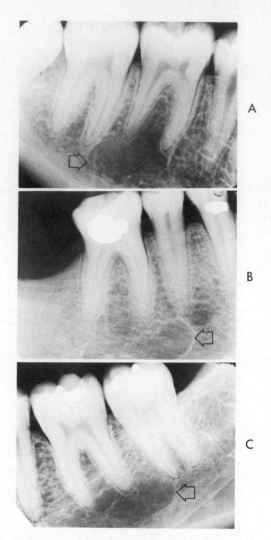

Fig. 16-1. Periapical marrow spaces and hematopoietic marrow defects *(arrows).* **A,** Poorly defined borders. **B** and **C,** Well-defined, smoothly contoured borders.

graph of jawbone-bearing teeth. Different views of the area in question (for example, a panoramic, occlusal, or Waters' projection) frequently aid in differentiating the normal anatomic shadows from periapical radiolucencies that result from disease processes. Also radiographs of suspect periapical regions made with the central beam directed from at least two different angles cause structures not in the periapical region to be displaced in succeeding films. Richards (1980) described this technique in detail.

Thus the shadow of a distant anatomic structure may be demonstrated to overlie the image of the apex and thereby create a radiolucent area. Furthermore, a complete examination, including the patient history and clinical, labo

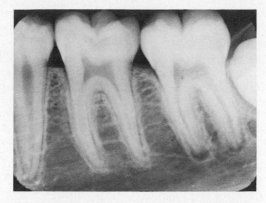

Fig. 16-2. Dental papillae (radiolucencies) at the apices of the second molar.

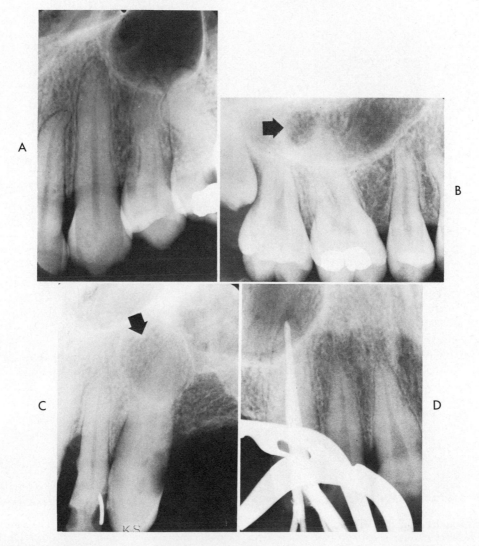

Fig. 16-3. Maxillary sinus projected as a periapical radiolucency *(arrows).*   (**D** courtesy M. Smulson, DDS, Maywood, Ill.)

ratory, and pulp tests, aids in this differentiation. If the radiolucencies are anatomic in origin, a comparison with the radiographs of the opposite side frequently reveals an identical situation. Clinicians should be not only aware of the normal location and appearance of the anatomic cavities, canals, and foramen that produce innocent periapical radiolucencies but also familiar with the normal ranges and variations of these structures.

The normal structures that may be responsible for radiolucencies that could be confused with those caused by disease processes are discussed in some detail in Chapter 14. Therefore anatomic radiolucencies that may appear on periapical films are only listed here with their illustrations for convenience:

Marrow spaces (Fig. 16-1)
Dental papillae (Fig. 16-2)
Maxillary sinus (Fig. 16-3)

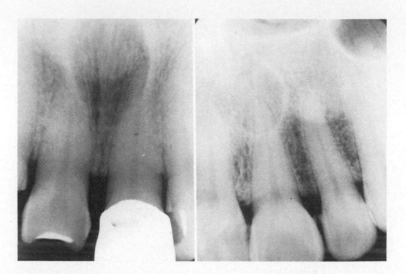

Fig. 16-4. Incisive foramina projected as periapical radiolucencies.

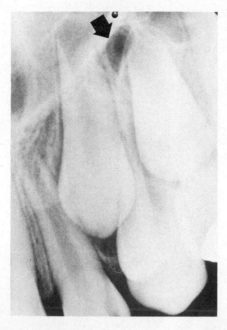

Fig. 16-5. Nasolacrimal duct as a radiolucency at the apex of the first premolar *(arrow)*. Not observed in most periapical films unless the vertical angle is exaggerated.

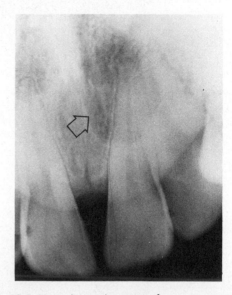

Fig. 16-6. Naris *(arrow)* projected as a periapical radiolucency over the apex of the central incisor.

Incisive foramen and canals (Fig. 16-4)
Nasolacrimal duct (Fig. 16-5)
Naris (Fig. 16-6)
Greater palatine foramen (Fig. 16-7)
Mental foramen (Fig. 16-8)
Submandibular fossa (Fig. 16-9)
Mandibular canal (Fig. 16-10)

Bone marrow patterns are seen scattered throughout jaws in radiographs and vary greatly in size and shape. Occasionally, larger examples are observed that are usually solitary and frequently cystlike (Fig. 16-1, *B* and *C*), or may have ragged, well-defined borders (Fig. 16-1, *A*). These larger examples are referred to as *osteoporotic bone marrow defects*. Makek and Lello (1986) reported their findings on 20 cases. When these defects occur in the periapex, the unwary clinician may assume them to be pulpoperiapical lesions. This entity is described in more detail in Chapter 19.

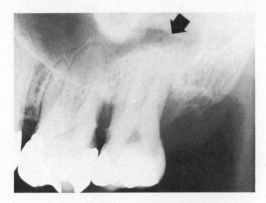

Fig. 16-7. Greater palatine foramen *(arrow).*

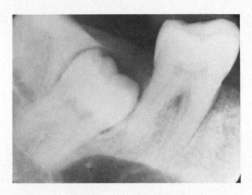

Fig. 16-9. A radiolucency near the apices of the second molar proved to be the submandibular fossa. (Courtesy L. Schwartz, DDS, Maywood, Ill.)

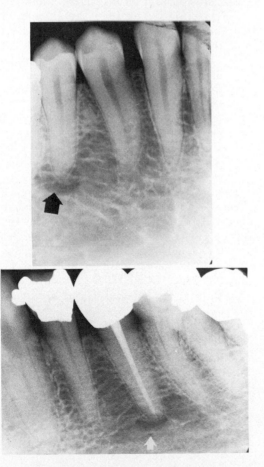

Fig. 16-8. Mental foramen *(arrows).*

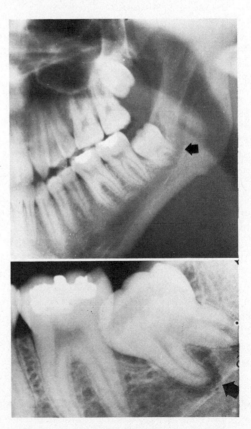

Fig. 16-10. Mandibular canal superimposed over apices of the third molars *(arrows).*

PERIAPICAL RADIOLUCENCIES

Sequelae of pulpitis (pulpoperiapical pathoses)

The seven pathologic entities included in the group of pulpoperiapical pathoses initially share a common cause: irritating inflammatory products from a pulpitis. These products escape from the pulp canal and initiate a local inflammatory response in the periapical area. It is thought that antigen-antibody reactions may play an important initiating role (Torabinejad and Kettering, 1979). Various factors (for example, host resistance, presence, number, and virulence of bacteria, amount of antigenic material and other toxins emanating from the canal, degree of tooth function, extent of other trauma, presence of epithelial rests of Malassez, thickness of adjacent cortical plates, and nature of previous treatment) determine the type of sequelae.

Interventional treatment might include any of the following:

1. Pulp capping (Jordan et al., 1978)
2. Preparation and obliteration of the canal with or without a root resection or apical curettage or both
3. Establishment of drainage either via the pulp canal or through the soft tissues
4. Administration of drugs through the pulp canal or systemically
5. Extraction

Such measures frequently modify the sequelae of pulpal infection, in contrast to what might result from an uninterrupted sequence of pathologic events.

Thus the information provided by the history of the circumstances attending a periapical radiolucency, including the response to previous treatment, as well as the information gained from clinical and radiographic examinations, is needed for the development of a working diagnosis. The final diagnosis of an asymptomatic radiolucency, however, can be determined only by microscopic examination of the periapical tissue.

It has been believed that without exception periapically involved teeth included in this group have nonvital pulps. It has been recognized for years that occasionally one root of a multirooted tooth contains a gangrenous pulp and has a periapical radiolucency, whereas the other root(s) may remain vital. Such a tooth frequently gives a vital reaction with the electrical pulp tester.

However, it has been suggested and partially substantiated that periapical lesions discernible on radiographic examination may occur at the apex of those teeth that have a localized area of pulpitis in the coronal portion of the pulp. Such a pulp is vital and gives positive responses to electrical pulp testing. Block et al. (1976) explain the process in this manner: "One could assume that the accumulated disintegration products and bacterial toxins travel from their place of origin through the lymph vessels of the remaining vital pulp and gather in the periapical tissue. This would explain the seemingly illogical appearances of a remaining nearly unaltered pulp tissue between two areas of severe inflammation." The study by Jordan et al. (1978) lends credence to this general concept. These investigators treated, by indirect pulp capping, 24 vital posterior teeth that had deep carious lesions and periapical lesions demonstrable on radiographic examination. Eleven of the teeth showed apparent resolution of periapical pathology, absence of pain, and continued vitality in the posttreatment follow-up.

The periapical lesions in this group share several clinical characteristics, as well as a similar cause:

1. The periapical lesion is radiolucent.
2. The roots associated with the lesion usually contain nonvital pulps that are clinically apparent on instrumentation.
3. The crown may often be discolored or show deep caries or have a restoration that is close to the pulp.
4. The crown may be partially or completely missing because of a traumatic incident; this is more frequently seen in anterior teeth.
5. A history of painful pulpitis, which heralded the death of the pulp some time before the radiolucency formed, may be reported by or can be elicited from the patient.

Teeth with a dens in dente have a higher incidence of pulp death and also a higher incidence of pulpoperiapical lesions (Fig. 16-11). Burton et al. (1980) described various characteristics of dens in dente, which explains its frequent association with pulpoperiapical lesions. Stewart et al. (1978) described dens evaginatus, which may also lead to pulpoperiapical lesions.

In the discussion of the differential diagnosis of lesions that follows, it must be understood that frequently the clinician is unable to differentiate clearly between a granuloma, a radicular cyst, a scar, a surgical defect, and a cholesteatoma on the basis of the history or by the clinical and radiographic findings alone. The final diagnosis can be decided by the microscopic examination of the periapical tissue.

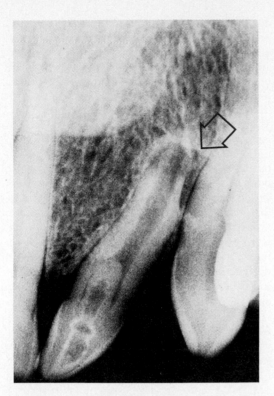

Fig. 16-11. Lateral incisor tooth in a 22-year-old patient with a nonvital pulp, an extensive dens in dente, and a pulpoperiapical radiolucent lesion. Arrow indicates the arrested development of the pulp canal.

The foregoing statement notwithstanding, in most cases of periapical radiolucencies the astute diagnostician can develop a working diagnosis or impression from a well-conceived differential diagnosis. Approximately 90% of the pathologic periapical lesions are either granulomas or cysts; this consideration greatly aids the clinician in the development of a valid differential diagnosis.

SEQUENCE OF EVENTS AFTER PULP DEATH

As a consequence of pulpitis with or without pulp death, from whatever cause, one or a combination of sequelae can be expected at the periapex.

First, none (or at most a very limited amount) of the irritating products of pulp necrosis may reach the periapical tissues. As a result no periapical pathosis is induced and no change is suggested by the patient's history or detectable on clinical or radiographic examination.

Second, irritating products may arrive at the periapex but in such moderate amounts that the host's defenses are able to effectively com-

bat and localize their effects. The resultant inflammation in the circumscribed area is of a chronic nature, and a "primary-type"* periapical granuloma develops.

Third, in teeth with contaminated gangrenous pulp(s), the number and virulence of the bacteria passing from the root canal(s) may be sufficient to overwhelm the defenses of the periapical tissue; consequently an acute periapical abscess develops.

Fourth, the resultant infection may be partially controlled by the body's defenses, by surgically induced drainage, or by antibiotic therapy. The most probable result, however, is the development of a chronic periapical periodontitis or chronic alveolar abscess.

The dental granuloma may in turn evolve into one of several entities, depending on the presence and interaction of certain factors.

If the odontogenic epithelial rests of Malassez (present in the periodontal ligament and frequently identified in periapical granulomas) proliferate and become cystic, a *radicular cyst* results. If bacteria of sufficient virulence and in sufficient numbers to counteract the host resistance are introduced into the granuloma or cyst, an *acute periapical abscess* develops.

If, in the course of the infection of a cyst or granuloma, the correct antibiotics are administered in adequate amounts or the abscess is drained, the infection is aborted and the periapical lesion may regress into a "secondary-type"† *dental granuloma* or *cyst*. If a sinus develops from the abscess to the surface, the lesion becomes a *chronic alveolar abscess*.

Another possible sequence of events that may influence the course of a dental granuloma is the effective treatment of the associated tooth's root canal(s), resulting in the ultimate disappearance of the granuloma and the complete resolution of the radiolucency to normal bone. If the granuloma has been subjected to repeated exacerbations of inflammation as a result of periodic contact with irritants from the root canal, however, areas of it may become fibrosed during the quiescent interludes. Then, if the tooth is successfully treated by conserva-

---

*In the present discussion the term "primary-type" or "virgin-type" granuloma refers to the lesion that is the first pathologic entity developing at the apex. This is in contrast to the granuloma that replaces another periapical entity, such as a cyst converted by infection or mechanical disruption ("secondary type").

†In contrast to the primary-type granuloma, the secondary type replaces another periapical entity such as a cyst or a primary granuloma that has been converted by acute infection or mechanical disruption or both.

tive endodontic techniques, the remaining inflammation and granulomatous tissue resolves, leaving only the fibrosed area. Such entities are referred to as periapical scars and frequently remain for many years, during which time they may be repeatedly observed unchanged as a periapical radiolucency.

RADIOGRAPHIC CONSIDERATIONS

Lamina dura. Clinicians have found through evaluating many sets of full mouth radiographs that the shadow of the lamina dura normally varies greatly from person to person. A wide range in degree of prominence is also seen from region to region in the full mouth radiographs of the same person. The lamina dura at the periapex of the maxillary canines often is impossible to discern even in good radiographs. The thin bone over the apex, as well as the pointed shape of the canine root, is responsible for this phenomenon. The lamina dura at the apices of the other teeth, in contrast, may be quite distinct in the same patient. Furthermore, the lamina dura may be prominent in some patients and faint in others. This information must be kept in mind when evaluating radiographs for early bony change at the apex of a suspicious tooth. If the lamina dura is consistently faint, the apparent diminution of lamina dura at the apex of the suspect tooth may be within normal limits. In such a case radiographs taken a year or two earlier might be helpful because the present appearance could be checked with that on the former radiograph to see if the shadow of the lamina dura has changed (Wood, 1984).

Apropos to the above discussion is the importance of the angle of projection when evaluating images of the lamina dura. If the beam is not tangential to the lamina dura, its image is either inapparent or faint. Thus the lamina dura may be well apparent in one projection and burned out in another of the same region.

Amount of bone destruction. It has generally been considered that 30% to 60% of regional bone destruction must have occurred for a radiolucency to be detected on radiographs. Thus an actively growing lesion might actually be slightly larger than it appears on radiographs. For many years when radiolucent lesions at the apex have been discussed, controversy has existed as to how much bone or what region of the periapical bone needs to be resorbed before the lesion shows on periapical radiographs. Earlier reports of research indicated that the lesion needed to expand to the point at which the bony spicules were destroyed all the way

out to their broad junctions with the inner aspect of the cortical plate. Thus, even though all of the cancellous bone was resorbed, the periapical radiograph would not show any change unless at least the junctional portion of the trabecula on the cortical plate was destroyed (Bender, 1961; Ramadan and Mitchell, 1961). Shoha et al. (1974) reported that in the premolar region (more often than in the molar region) radiographic change cannot be detected without involvement of the junctional or cortical bone. These researchers reported that periapical lesions on anterior teeth would show when just the lamina dura and a small amount of medullary bone were destroyed. Valasek and Emmering (1983), using wet cadaver specimens, demonstrated that very small areas of destruction of the apices of mandibular molar teeth could be detected as radiographic change. Van der Stelt (1985), using long bones, reported that removal of cancellous bone only did not change the radiographic image visibly.

Root resorption. Slight to moderate root resorption cannot be observed on radiographs but must be demonstrated by histologic examination. A considerable amount of resorption must have occurred for it to be obvious on radiographs, and even then its appearance is unpredictable (Ford, 1984). External root resorption may be caused by (1) orthodontic movement of teeth, (2) inflammation or infection or both, and (3) benign and malignant tumors. Thus root end resorption is a common finding in pulpoperiapical lesions. In the senior author's experience (N.K.W.) resorption caused by inflammation or infection is characteristically more ragged in outline, whereas resorption resulting from tumor is usually more linear or curvilinear.

GRANULOMA

The periapical granuloma represents the most common type of pathologic radiolucency. Block et al. (1976) reported that microscopic evaluation of 230 cases of pulpoperiapical radiolucent lesions treated by apicoectomy revealed that approximately 94% were granulomas and 6% were cysts. Stockdale and Chandler (1988) reported that approximately 83% of the lesions were granulomas and 17% were cysts.

Basically the periapical granuloma is the result of a successful attempt by the periapical tissues to neutralize and confine the irritating toxic products that are escaping from the root canal. The continual discharge of chronic irritating products from the canal into the periapical tissue is, however, sufficient to maintain a low-grade inflammation in these tissues; this inflammatory reaction continues to induce a vascular inflammatory response, which makes up the entity. McKinney (1981) explained the difference between the terms "granulomatous" and "granulation tissue." This author pointed out that "granulomatous" refers to a *specific type of inflammation*, the outstanding feature of which is the presence of mononuclear phagocytic cells—monocytes, macrophages, and sometimes epithelioid cells. McKinney further explained that this entity generally has a distinctive pattern and arrangement of cells with a central area of necrosis or fibrinoid material surrounded by a cellular reaction consisting mainly of mononuclear phagocytes and some lymphocytes. New collagen fibers and ground substance predominate toward the periphery. From this description dental granuloma would best be considered an example of "granulomatous tissue." McKinney explained that, in contrast, "granulation tissue" is the tissue of *healing* and *repair*. It usually occurs after the injury and on microscopic examination is characterized by proliferating capillaries, many fibroblasts, new collagen fibers, ground substance, and macrophages. It may be found as a component of granulomatous inflammation. As granulation tissue matures, it becomes less vascular and more fibrous.

In addition, the granuloma represents a stage in the repair process, which is altering the defect that has resulted from the lysis of bone in the immediate vicinity of the root end. Consequently the clinician should consider the presence of a periapical granuloma an indication that the natural defenses have contained the insult from the related diseased root canal. The *insult* from the diseased pulp may represent a broad spectrum of inflammatory mediators. It is assumed that the many irritating products of inflammation, such as prostaglandins, kinins, and also lysosomes from the disintegrating cells, play an important role. Likewise, bacterial products and toxins are present in infected cases. Shonfeld et al. (1982) demonstrated that the presence of endotoxin correlated well with the presence of inflammation in pulpoperiapical lesions. Immunologic reactions also appear to enjoy a prominent part in the process of inflammation and lysis at the periapex. Morse (1977) summarized pertinent information in this regard. Greening and Schonfeld (1980) demonstrated elevated levels of immunoglobulin G in pulpoperiapical lesions. In 1980 Yanagisawa reported the presence of cells containing IgE and also IgG and C3 in the connective tissue of periapical granulomas. Skauq et al. (1984) produced more evidence that cellular immune reactions were involved by demonstrating infiltrates of T lymphocytes in periapical granulomas. Torabinejad et al. (1983) suggested that chronic periapical lesions do not act as a focus to cause systemic disease via immune complexes.

The microstructure of the granuloma consists of proliferating endothelial cells, capillaries, young fibroblasts, a minimal amount of collagen, and chronic inflammatory cells (lymphocytes, plasma cells, macrophages) (Fig. 16-12). Occasionally nests of odontogenic epithelium, Russell bodies, foam cells, and cholesterol clefts are present. On the basis of histopathology Yanagisawa (1980) classified the periapical granuloma into (1) exudative, (2) granulomatous, (3) granulofibrous, and (4) fibrous types. We assume that the fibrous type would be identical to the lesion that we describe as "periapical scar" in this chapter.

Classically, more inflammation is seen in the center of the lesion, where the apex of the tooth is usually located, because at this point the irritating substances from the pulp canal are most concentrated. At the periphery of the lesion, fibrosis (healing) may already have begun, since the irritants are diluted and neutralized some distance from the apex. Practically, though, the orderly picture just described may not often be found. Occasionally cholesterol clefts may form a major portion of the lesion. Hirschberg et al. (1988) termed these examples "cholesterol granuloma of the jaws."

Features. On radiographic examination the lesion is a well-circumscribed radiolucency somewhat rounded and surrounding the apex of the tooth (Fig. 16-12). This periapical radiolucency may or may not have a thin radiopaque (hyperostotic) border. Radiographs of the involved tooth may reveal the presence of deep restorations, extensive caries, fractures, or a narrower pulp canal than in the contralateral tooth. All these features would lead the clinician to suspect the presence of pulp pathosis. A periapical granuloma cannot be differentiated from a radicular cyst by radiographic appearance alone; however, when a periapical radiolucent lesion has attained a diameter of 1.6 cm or larger, the likelihood of its being a radicular cyst is much greater (Lalonde, 1970). Few granulomas ever become larger than 2.5 cm in diameter. In our opinion any granuloma with a diameter of more than 2.5 cm probably represents a resolving chronic alveolar abscess rather than a primary-type granuloma.

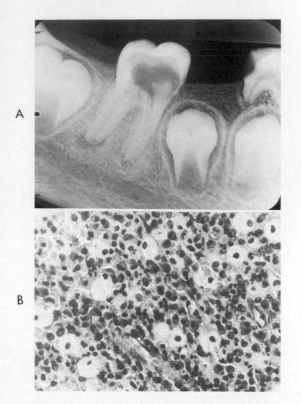

Fig. 16-12. Periapical granuloma. **A,** The pulp of the first molar was nonvital. **B,** Photomicrograph.

When the offending tooth is subjected to electrical and thermal pulp testing, the response of the patient usually indicates that the pulp is nonvital. The tooth is completely asymptomatic, including usually an absence of sensitivity to percussion. The crown may have a darker color than that of its neighbors because of blood pigments that have diffused into the empty dentinal tubules. Swelling or expansion of the cortical plates over the area of the apex is most unusual, since periapical granulomas rarely reach a size to produce such an effect.

Differential diagnosis. A differential diagnosis for a periapical granuloma is included in the corresponding section in the discussion of the radicular cyst (p. 315).

Management. The management of a periapical granuloma is included in the management section of the discussion of the radicular cyst.

RADICULAR CYST

The radicular (periapical) cyst is the second most common pathologic periapical radiolucency. Only 6% of a series of periapical radiolucent lesions reported by Block et al. (1976) were radicular cysts, and approximately 17% of

lesions in a study by Stockdale and Chandler (1988) were periapical cysts. The radicular cyst may be classified as an inflammatory cyst because this process is thought to initiate the growth of the epithelial component. It may also be classified as an odontogenic cyst because of its origin in the cell rests of Malassez, which are remnants of Hertwig's root sheath; the latter, in turn, is a product of the odontogenic epithelial layers (the inner and outer enamel epithelia).

Practically all radicular cysts originate in preexisting periapical granulomas, and their pathogenesis depends on an inflammatory reaction. Hence they are also classified as inflammatory cysts. A significant number of granulomas contain epithelial remnants (Block et al. [1976] reported that 20% do), which may start to proliferate because of the irritation* that induced the proliferation of the granuloma. As the masses of proliferating epithelial nests increase in size, the central cells start to degenerate and liquefy because they are blocked from an adequate blood supply in the surrounding connective tissue and because the capillaries in the tissue surrounding the developing cyst are being compressed. This sequence of events leads to the formation of a liquid-filled cavity lined with epithelium (that is, a cyst). The cyst continues to grow because of a combination of factors. The products from cell lysis are probably irritating and may provide a growth stimulus. In addition, epithelial cells (their products, as well as the contents of the degenerating cells) are discharged into the cyst lumen and thus increase the protein content and the osmotic pressure of the cyst fluid. The result is that more water diffuses into the lumen, further expanding the cyst. Wilk et al. (1983) suggested that soluble proteins, their levels elevated as a result of local immunoglobulin production, encourage protein diffusion into the lumen. The pressure exerted by the enlarging cyst on the alveolar bone induces osteoclastic action and resorption of the peripheral bone.

Features. The vast majority of radicular cysts involve the apices of the permanent teeth. Stockdale and Chandler (1988) reported that 58% involved the lateral incisors. Lustmann and Shear (1985) reported 23 cases that involved deciduous teeth, most commonly the

---

*The inflammatory products are suspected of causing a shift in the oxidative metabolism of the rests of Malassez, which permits them to proliferate in the milieu of the granulation tissue, whereas apparently the quiescent cells are maintained by the aerobic pathway (Grupe et al., 1967).

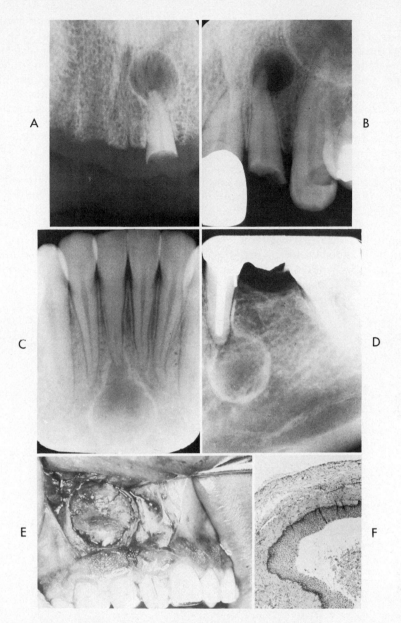

Fig. 16-13. Radicular cyst. **A** to **D**, Smoothly contoured, well-defined margins are evident in periapical radiographs. Hyperostotic borders can be seen in **A, C,** and **D. E,** Erosion of the labial cortex can be seen under the mucoperiosteal flap. **F,** Photomicrograph of a cyst wall shows the epithelial layer that surrounds the lumen.

molars. The patient's history and the clinical and radiographic findings associated with a pulpless asymptomatic tooth that has a small, well-defined periapical radiolucency at its apex are identical whether the lesion is a periapical granuloma or a radicular cyst.

The preceding statement notwithstanding, the more pronounced the hyperostotic border of the lesion is, the more likely the lesion is to be a cyst (Fig. 16-13). Studies by Lalonde (1970) showed that such a lesion is more likely to be a radicular cyst if the periapical radiolucency is at least 1.6 cm in diameter. Root resorption can occur: 18% of radicular cysts showed this effect in a study reported by Struthers and Shear (1976). An untreated cyst may slowly enlarge and cause expansion of the cortical plates. In these instances the expansion can be observed on clinical examination as a domelike swelling on the alveolus over the periapical region of the involved tooth.

The swelling may develop on either the buccal or the lingual side of the alveolar process and is covered with normal-appearing mucosa. Initially it is bony hard to palpation, but later it may demonstrate a crackling sound (crepitus) as the cortical plate becomes thinned. Usually the cortical plates remain intact, although numerous cases have been encountered in which a radicular cyst completely resorbed the overlying cortical bone (Fig. 16-13). In these cases the clinical swelling is rubbery and fluctuant because of the cyst fluid within. Large cysts may involve a complete quadrant with some of the teeth occasionally mobile and some of the pulps nonvital. Root resorption is also seen.

Neither the causative tooth nor the alveolar swelling produced by an expanding cyst is painful in sterile cysts. If such a cyst becomes infected, however, the tooth and swelling develop all the painful symptoms of an abscess.

On microscopical examination the radicular cyst is classically described with a connective tissue wall that may vary in thickness from region to region and from cyst to cyst. This wall may also vary in character throughout its width. Peripherally it is fibrous, although its inner regions may be composed of granulomatous tissue. Within the wall, and especially within its granulomatous portions, foci of chronic inflammatory cells, foam cells, Russell bodies, and cholesterol slits may be found. The wall surrounds the fluid-filled lumen; its lumen side is usually covered with various types of ep-

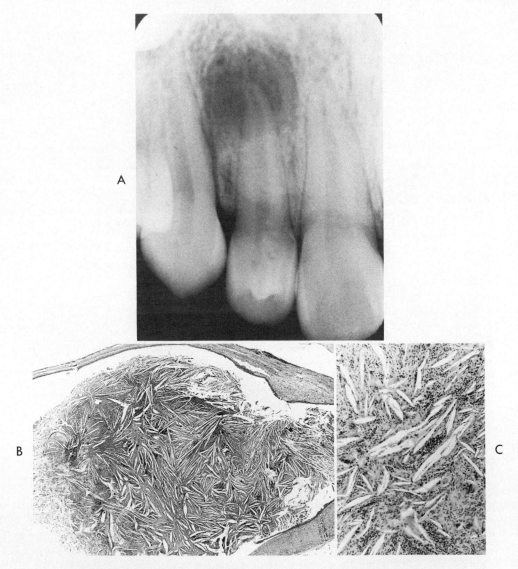

Fig. 16-14. Periapical cholesteatoma. **B** and **C**, Histopathologic appearance.

ithelium, which may also vary greatly in form, thickness, and continuity.

Although the lumen lining is usually stratified squamous epithelium, occasionally ciliated pseudostratified columnar and even keratinizing epithelium is found, whether the cyst is in the mandible or the maxilla (Fig. 16-13). Practically, however, these layers of tissue do not often occur so uniformly; inflammation may be present in some areas, resulting in the destruction of the epithelial lining in that region. Frequently the radicular cyst is, in fact, a combination of dental granuloma and radicular cyst. Aspiration of a noninfected radicular cyst produces a light straw-colored fluid, usually containing an abundance of shiny granules (cholesterol crystals). Occasionally so much cholesterol is formed that the whole lumen is filled with this material and the accompanying foreign body reaction (Fig. 16-14).

Differential diagnosis. When the clinician encounters a periapical radiolucency, he or she must consider that it could represent any of the entities discussed or listed in this chapter.

If a well-defined radiolucency is at the apex of an untreated asymptomatic tooth with a nonvital or diseased pulp and if anatomic structures can be ruled out, in approximately 90% of the cases the radiolucency is either a *dental granuloma* or a *radicular cyst*. Although these two entities cannot be distinguished by radiographic features alone, if the radiolucency is 1.6 cm or more in diameter, as stated earlier, it is more likely to be a cyst.

Occasionally, however, tissue obtained from large periapical lesions are diagnosed by the pathologist as a *periapical granuloma*. Our experience with these cases has led us to expect such a report, especially when the tooth in question has precipitated repeated episodes of pain and alveolar swelling, has spontaneously developed intermittent drainage, or has been incised and drained a number of times. By way of explanation of this apparent contradiction, the history of the involved tooth is reasonably good evidence that the larger granuloma is not the primary type but is the secondary type, which has perhaps proliferated in an infected cyst whose epithelium was destroyed by acute inflammation and necrosis and has just resolved to the healing granulomatous stage.

Many attempts have been made to develop a technique that consistently differentiates between a periapical granuloma and a radicular cyst without resorting to biopsy.

The radiographic examination of periapical radiolucencies after the injection of a radiopaque contrast medium, either directly into the area or through the root canals, has been proposed but has not proved to be dependable.

Electrophoretic studies of fluid from root canals of pulpless teeth with periapical radiolucencies have proved interesting. The fluid from teeth that were subsequently found to have radicular cysts gave a segment characteristic of serum globulin, but this segment was not given by fluid from teeth that had periapical granulomas.

Aspiration of straw-colored fluid via the extracanalicular approach has long been recognized as indicating the presence of a cyst rather than a granuloma. In practice, however, it is not necessary to differentiate between small periapical granulomas and cysts, since both respond well to conservative root canal therapy.*

Periapical scars and *surgical defects* are frequently confused with a periapical granuloma or cyst. In teeth that have received nonsurgical endodontic treatment for granulomas and cysts and are assumed to be well sealed, a persistent, asymptomatic, nonenlarging radiolucency is most likely a periapical scar. Similarly an asymptomatic radiolucency that persists after root resection can be either a scar or a surgical defect, but it is unlikely to be any type of residual pathosis if the tooth remains asymptomatic and the radiolucency does not increase in size.

The *periapical cementoma* in its early lytic fibroblastic stage cannot be distinguished from a periapical granuloma or cyst by radiographic examination. In the tooth with a cementoma, however, the pulp is vital and healthy, whereas the tooth with a granuloma or cyst has a nonvital pulp. On rare occasions a pulpless tooth may have a concomitant early cementoma at the apex, so the criterion of pulp vitality would be confusing; however, periapical cementomas most frequently involve the lower teeth (in a ratio of about 9:1), especially the incisors.

Although a *traumatic bone cyst* in a periapical area may be mistaken for a dental granuloma or cyst, as with a cementoma, the pulps of the associated teeth are usually vital. Also a traumatic bone cyst differs from a periapical cyst and a granuloma, since approximately 90% of traumatic bone cysts occur in the mandible, where they are most frequently seen in the molar, premolar, and incisor regions (in that order), whereas periapical cysts and granulomas have no predilection for the lower jaw.

---

*The term "conservative root canal therapy" encompasses all the procedures required to properly obliterate the root canal(s) but does not include any direct surgical intervention in the periapex.

When a patient's history indicates a *systemic disorder* (for example, hyperparathyroidism, primary malignant tumor, multiple myeloma), obviously the working diagnosis of periapical granuloma or cyst must be broadened to include these more serious entities.

The periapical lesion associated with periodontal disease usually shows moderate to severe crestal bone loss. According to Brynolf (1978) this is coupled with a pattern of periapical bone loss morphologically distinct from that usually produced by pulpitis in that the radiolucency associated with marginal bone loss is of greatest width around the apex but extends laterally tapering along the root for a short distance.

The mandibular infected buccal cyst (molar area) is an interesting lesion recognized by Stoneman and Worth (1983) and further discussed by Camarda et al. (1989). This cyst is located on the buccal aspect of a lower molar tooth, which is usually but not invariably erupted. On periapical radiographs the inferior aspect of the shadow of the cyst can be seen crossing the root at variable levels and sometimes includes the periapex. The size varies from 1 cm in diameter to considerably larger. The patient is usually young, the first molar is the most frequently involved, the pulp is usually vital, and the lamina dura around the apices is intact. These last two characteristics permit differentiation from a periapical granuloma or cyst.

Management. A small periapical cyst or granuloma may be treated in either of two ways. The clinician may decide the offending tooth interferes with plans for restoring the dentition, and the tooth may be extracted. The periapical soft tissue in this case should be removed and examined microscopically. On the other hand, the clinician may decide the tooth should be retained. In this case most clinicians prefer to resort to conservative root canal therapy alone and observe the lesion radiographically every 6 months to ensure that it is not enlarging or is regressing. Shah (1988) reported a 84.4% success rate for 132 teeth with periapical radiolucencies that were treated in this manner.

Reported clinical experience has shown that routine root canal obliteration is the indicated treatment for most small lesions whether granulomas or cysts. Jordan et al. (1978) used indirect pulp capping on teeth with endodontic periapical lesions and reported disappearance of the periapical lesions in a significant number of cases.

Why do cysts respond so well to nonsurgical endodontic treatment? Several theories have been proposed.

One suggests that instrumentation beyond the apex in these nonvital cases permits the cyst to drain into the canal and produces an inflammatory reaction that results in the lysis of the epithelial cells lining the lumen. The overinstrumentation theory has few adherents (Block et al., 1976).

Another theory holds that when the root canal is sealed, the irritating products from the gangrenous pulp are no longer present and the inflammation subsides. Healing then commences at the periphery, where such dense collagen is laid down that the blood supply to the epithelial lining becomes impaired and the epithelial cells necrose. The products from these degenerating epithelial cells are responsible for inflammatory reaction that stimulates the proliferation of granulation tissue, and the tissue, in turn, fills the cystic space. The resulting granuloma then regresses, since the inflammation-inducing material is no longer draining into the area from the root canal or being produced in the area by degenerating cystic epithelia.

In general, then, a radicular cyst is initiated in a granuloma and may be subsequently replaced by the granuloma in a sequence of events that attend its healing. Regardless of the mechanism responsible, apparently many small cysts are successfully treated by nonsurgical root canal therapy. When a conservative type of endodontic therapy has been employed, it is imperative that the clinician observe the patient radiographically at regular intervals to be certain that the radiolucency is resolving or at least is not enlarging.

This close supervision of the area is of utmost importance because a final definite diagnosis has not been verified by such a nonsurgical approach; the clinician must be cognizant that the radiolucency could represent a more serious entity (for example, a malignant tumor). If there did prove to be an enlarging radiolucency, the clinician would then know that a biopsy via a buccal window must be performed to determine the nature of the lesion. Schlagel et al. (1973) discussed apicoectomy in conjunction with microscopic study as an important adjunct to diagnosis when the suspicion index warrants it. Weisman (1975) stresses the importance of submitting for microscopic study all tissues removed during endodontic surgical procedures. Frequently an enlarging lesion is demonstrated to be an expanding granuloma or cyst caused by an inadequate root canal seal and the continued irritation of the periapex by degradation products. Barbakow et al. (1981) reported that of 192 teeth with periapical areas treated with root canal therapy, in 1 year or more after therapy 59% of the lesions disappeared completely and 29% decreased in size. Natkin et al. (1984) cites a success rate of 80% or less for the nonsurgical treatment of periapical lesions.

Although management varies somewhat with the clinician, some believe that apical curettage or a more extensive root resection procedure is indicated for periapical radiolucencies measuring 2 cm in diameter or larger, since most of these are radicular cysts. Conditions also arise that dictate the surgical approach for smaller lesions. For example, when a patient cannot be available for three or four appointments, a direct root canal filling with surgical curettage and periapical retrograde sealing might be the best way to manage the case; or if the root canal was found to be nonnegotiable, a surgical approach to facilitate a retrograde filling of the canal and periapical curettage might be indicated.

On occasion large radicular cysts that have destroyed a considerable amount of bone are encountered. Currently six approaches may be used for the management of such lesions. These approaches, described in detail in Chapter 17, are surgical enucleation; surgical enucleation and restoration of the defect with a graft, preferably autogenous bone; marsupialization; decompression; decompression with delayed enucleation; and creation of a common chamber with the maxillary sinus or the nasal cavity (used occasionally for large maxillary cysts).

Liposky (1980) described a technique of decortication and bone replacement for large cysts.

Sequential postsurgical radiographs are essential to ensure that the defect is regressing, no matter which method is employed. The average healing time for cysts of more than 10 mm in diameter is approximately 2½ years. Incomplete removal of the cyst lining may result in the formation of a residual cyst or in rare instances a more aggressive type of pathosis.

SCAR

Scar tissue represents one of the possible end points of healing, whether it occurs on the surface of the body or in the deeper tissues (for example, at the periapex). The periapical scar is composed of dense fibrous tissue and is situated at the periapex of a pulpless tooth in which usually the root canals have been successfully filled. This entity is represented by a periapical granuloma, cyst, abscess, or cholesteatoma whose healing has terminated in the formation of dense scar tissue (cicatrix) rather than bone in the defect (Fig. 16-15). From 2% to 5% of all periapical radiolucent lesions are estimated to be periapical scars, although there is a little information in the literature concerning this entity.

This paragraph explains how a periapical scar is formed. If the introduction of the irritant into the inflamed area is continued, as might be possible from the apex of an untreated pulpless tooth, chronic inflammatory cells accumulate, young fibroblasts, endothelial cells, and capillaries proliferate, and subsequently a granuloma is formed. Grossly the granulomatous tissue is soft, compressible, and reddish. Fluctuations in the severity of the irritant are paralleled by cyclic changes in the associated inflammation. In periods of minimal irritation and inflammation, the young fibroblasts present in the granulomatous tissue mature and are transformed into a more dense connective tissue (scar) instead of being replaced by bone (if that is the normal tissue of the area, as it is in the case of a periapical scar).

When the tooth is successfully treated by nonsurgical endodontic techniques, the irritants from the root canal are eliminated and the periapical granuloma or cyst frequently resolves, being replaced by bone, and is no longer apparent on the radiograph. In some instances, however, the granulation tissue slowly organizes, with the production of more and more collagen fibers, and eventually a dense contracted connective tissue scar results, which is quite permanent and radiolucent.

On microscopic examination a mature periapical scar shows a few spindle-shaped fibroblasts scattered throughout dense collagen bundles, and the collagen bundles often show an advanced degree of hyalinization. Inflammatory cells are not a feature, and vascularity is meager (Fig. 16-15, C).

In our experience a significant percentage of lesions diagnosed microscopically as periapical granulomas have contained isolated areas of scar tissue, as well as regions of granulation tissue. Such lesions are in reality mixed lesions and probably should be thought of as scarring periapical granulomas or perhaps as relatively

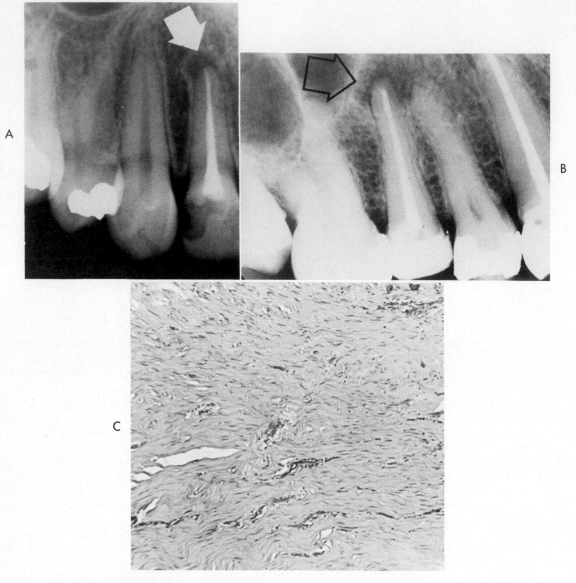

Fig. 16-15. Periapical scars. **A** and **B,** The periapical lesions had become markedly smaller in these two asymptomatic teeth following conservative root canal therapy. **C,** Photomicrograph showing dense fibrous tissue that makes up the periapical scar.

young, less dense scar that is experiencing intermittent inflammation. Since a substantial portion of periapical granulomas microscopically examined are found to be such mixed lesions, the contention would seem to be substantiated that if the lesions are properly treated by nonsurgical (conservative) procedures, their granulomatous portion readily resolves and their reduced area may persist as periapical scar tissue.

Serial radiographs of such lesions would be expected to show a decrease in the size of the periapical radiolucency proportional to the amount of granulomatous tissue present at the time the endodontic treatment was initiated.

It would seem, then, that the majority of persisting radiolucencies at the apex of asymptomatic teeth whose canals have apparently been successfully sealed by nonsurgical endodontic procedures are periapical scars. Of course, since there is little justification, few of these apparent periapical areas are surgically explored or their contents microscopically examined. Consequently evidence bearing on this question is extremely limited. Periapical scars also frequently occur in patients initially treated by periapical curettage or root resection (Arwill et al., 1974).

Features. The periapical scar causes a well-circumscribed radiolucency that is more or less round and on radiographic examination resembles the periapical granuloma and cyst (Fig. 16-15). It is frequently smaller than either of these entities. The tooth and associated radiolucency are asymptomatic, and the scar, if observed radiographically over the years as it should be, is seen to remain constant in size or perhaps diminish slightly. Such a history, of course, depends on the establishment and maintenance of a good apical seal.

The periapical scar occurs most often in the anterior region of the maxilla. Most of the involved teeth have been treated endodontically. Occasionally such a scar occurs at the periapex of a pulpless tooth that has not been endodontically treated, however; in these cases the body's natural defenses are assumed to have completely neutralized the irritants emanating from the root canal after an initial successful inflammatory response to the irritants. In other cases the root canal may have sealed itself off, thus restricting the irritants within the canal.

Differential diagnosis. The differential diagnosis of these lesions is included in the corresponding section in the discussion of periapical surgical defects (p. 324).

Management. When the periapical scar is associated with an asymptomatic root canal–filled tooth, it requires no treatment. Such a tooth presents a problem to the clinician who is contemplating extensive restorative procedures, however, since he or she cannot differentiate by clinical or radiographic examination between a dental granuloma or cyst and the scar. The tooth in question may appear to have an adequate root canal filling but in fact not have a good apical seal, which would cause the cyst or granuloma to persist.

The asymptomatic root canal–filled tooth, of course, imposes the potential of an acute inflammatory reaction that may not be evident until after extensive restorative work has been completed; at that time the inflammatory reaction can be successfully treated only by procedures that adversely alter the restoration. If the tooth has remained asymptomatic since the root canal filling and the perapical area has not increased in size, the radiolucency can be safely assumed to be a periapical scar.

As a general rule a tooth that is to be used as an abutment but has a periapical radiolucency should be observed radiographically for about 6 months after endodontic treatment.

CHRONIC AND ACUTE DENTOALVEOLAR ABSCESSES

Abscesses make up about 2% of all pathologic periapical radiolucencies. In the context of this chapter, the periapical or dentoalveolar abscesses are subdivided as follows, according to whether they are radiolucent or not:

1. *Primary or neoteric abscesses* are pulpoperiapical inflammatory conditions associated with teeth that have not developed apparent periapical radiolucent lesions; they are usually described as an acute apical periodontitis or an acute periapical abscess (Fig. 16-16).
2. *Secondary or recrudescent abscesses* develop in a previously existing asymptomatic periapical radiolucent lesion (for example, granuloma, cyst, scar, cholesteatoma) (Fig. 16-16).

The primary (neoteric) abscess develops in a periapical region that is normal on radiographic examination. The infection is almost always acute and exudative, involving the periodontal tissues at the apex of the tooth with a necrotic pulp. The canal contains large numbers of virulent bacteria that rapidly spread to the periapical tissues and cause an acute periodontitis, a

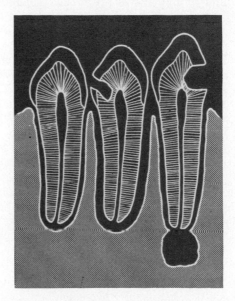

Fig. 16-16. Diagram illustrating radiographic changes in pulpoperiapical infection. The middle tooth, illustrating primary acute abscess displays (1) the absence of a preexisting pulpoperiapical lesion and (2) the widened periodontal ligament space caused by the fluid exudate at the apex, which has shifted the tooth in a coronal direction. The tooth on the right represents a pulpoperiapical, secondary abscess where a radiolucent lesion has been present before this acute onset.

very sensitive tooth, and perhaps alveolar swelling. The onset and course of the infection are so sudden that resorption of bone has not yet occurred; hence a periapical radiolucency is not a feature. Frequently the infection and inflammation in the apical area cause a swelling of the periodontal ligament and force the tooth slightly from its socket, thus creating an increased periodontal ligament space around the entire root (Fig. 16-16). The increased space is usually apparent on the radiograph, but because a periapical radiolucency is not a feature of the neoteric abscess, a detailed discussion is not presented in this chapter.

The secondary (recrudescent) abscess may be either of the chronic or the acute type, depending on various factors—the number and virulence of the invading organisms, the resistance of the host, and the type and timing of the treatment instituted. Although various strains of staphylococci and streptococci are frequent causative microorganisms, a wide variety of other microorganisms have been found to be offenders in certain instances. Studies by Kannangara et al. (1980) and Labriola et al. (1983) demonstrated that a much higher percentage of anaerobic organisms were present in odontogenic infections than was previously thought. In Kannangara's series, 74% of patients had anaerobic infections, whereas in the Labriola study 86% of the specimens contained anaerobes. (It should be pointed out that both of these studies included all cases of infections of the jaws and space abscess; thus the cases were not limited to pulpoperiapical infections. Nevertheless much of the information is apropos to the subject here.) The anaerobes most frequently encountered were *Bacteroides*, *Peptococcus*, *Peptostreptococcus*, *Actinomyces*, *Eubacterium*, and *Fusobacterium*. Most of the cases represented mixed infections or polyinfections. Many bacterial isolates were resistant to penicillin (Kannangara et al., 1980; Labriola et al., 1983).

Features. The primary lesion in which the infection occurs may be a granuloma, cyst, scar, or cholesteatoma; thus a periapical radiolucency is a feature of the secondary abscess. The radiolucency may vary from small to quite large and may involve much of the jaw. The initial periapical lesion may even have caused an expansion of the cortical plate.

If the acute infection is discovered soon after its onset, and depending on its duration, acuteness, or chronicity, the margins of the radiolucency may vary from well defined with possibly a hyperostotic border to poorly defined in chronic cases (Fig. 16-17). Sometimes the radiolucency is represented as a blurred area of somewhat lessened density than the surrounding bone. Radiographs of the related tooth frequently show such features as deep restorations, caries, narrowed pulp chambers, or canals, which suggest that the pulp is nonvital. The roots of these teeth may also show resorption at the apex.

The microscopic picture varies somewhat, depending on the stage of the infection, but basically it consists of a central region of necrosis containing a dense accumulation of polymorphonuclear leukocytes surrounded by an inflamed connective tissue wall of varying thickness. A chronic resolving abscess may have fewer polymorphonuclear leukocytes, less necrosis, and more lymphocytes, plasma cells, macrophages, and granulation tissue (Fig. 16-17). On the contrary, an acute abscess may contain only necrotic and unidentifiable soft tissue.

On clinical examination the tooth with an acute abscess is painful to percussion, and if it is in occlusion, the patient complains that it seems "high" when it occludes with the opposing tooth. As a rule it does not respond to electrical pulp tests. The application of ice, however, relieves the pain somewhat, in contrast to heat, which intensifies the pain. The tooth may demonstrate increased mobility.

If permitted to progress without treatment, the abscess may penetrate the cortical plate at the thinnest and closest point to the apex and form a space infection in the adjacent soft tissues. The space abscess is painful, and the surface of the skin or mucosa over the abscess feels warm and rubbery to palpation and demonstrates fluctuance. The systemic temperature may be elevated. Aspiration usually produces yellowish pus. Regional lymph nodes may become enlarged and painful.

Serial, total, and differential leukocyte counts are valuable in determining the course and nature of the infection. If circumstances are unfavorable, such as lowered host resistance combined with virulent multiplying organisms and inadequate early treatment, serious complications may ensue—osteomyelitis, septicemia, septic emboli, asphyxia from a Ludwig's angina or other space infection that compromises the airway, cavernous sinus thrombosis—any of which could be fatal.

A chronic infection ensues when the virulence and number of the organisms are low and the host resistance is high. If untreated, the chronic abscess frequently forms a sinus tract,

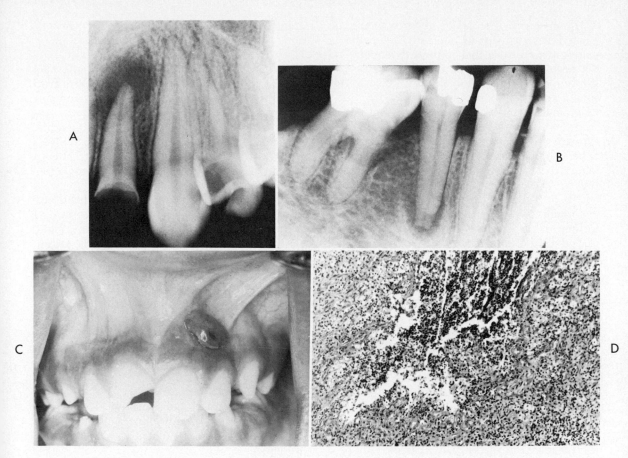

Fig. 16-17. Chronic periapical abscess. **A** and **B**, Ill-defined ragged borders. **C**, Parulis resulting from a chronic draining abscess at the apex of the pulpless left central incisor. **D**, Microscopy of a chronic abscess surrounded by granulation tissue.

permitting the pus to drain to the surface. A small proliferation of granulomatous tissue often forms on the surface and is referred to as a parulis (Fig. 16-17, *C*).

When drainage is established, the tooth and associated swelling are no longer painful, since the pain-producing pressure of the abscess is reduced.

Differential diagnosis. When a painful fluctuant swelling is present, there is little question that the diagnosis is *abscess*. When the abscess is determined to be of the secondary type, however, the original periapical lesion may not be easy to identify. Actually such an identification is often impossible because the histomorphology has been destroyed by the infection.

If the abscess is a sequela of pulpitis, whether it was a cyst, granuloma, scar, or cholesteatoma is not of practical concern, but the clinician must always be alert to the possibility that the apical radiolucency might be either a *secondarily infected primary tumor* or a *secondary malignant tumor*.

In addition, any of the nonodontogenic cysts (for example, incisive canal, globulomaxillary, median) may become infected and on radiographic examination be projected over the apices of teeth with vital pulps, simulating an infected *radicular cyst*. Thus if the clinician fails to recognize this possibility and establish the exact location of the radiolucency in question, teeth could be unnecessarily compromised.

It is also necessary to consider that not all abscesses involving teeth are of pulpal origin. The *periodontal abscess*, originating in a deep periodontal pocket, is a common lesion and can be distinguished from the incited periapical abscess by proper radiographic procedures showing the absence of a periapical radiolucency and usually the presence of a periodontal pocket. In addition, the pulps of teeth with such periodontal abscesses are almost always vital.

Management. The acute abscess should be treated aggressively to alleviate the patient's pain and to ensure that untoward sequelae do not occur. In our opinion it is better to establish drainage immediately if possible, since this speeds the resolution of the abscess.

Drainage may be established in some cases by opening the pulp chamber and passing a file through the canal into the periapical region. When drainage cannot be established in this manner, a trephination procedure is indicated; that is, an opening is made through the mucosa and bone to the abscess at the apex. When a vestibular palatal or lingual space abscess has formed, a through-and-through drain* may be placed in the abscess and frequently irrigated with a 1:1 mixture of 3% hydrogen peroxide and normal saline solution.

A sample of pus should be obtained for culture and sensitivity tests. In more severe cases penicillin therapy should be instituted immediately (not less than 500 mg 4 times a day for at least 5 days), since many of the microorganisms responsible for odontogenic infections are sensitive to penicillin (if the infection is not by one of the resistant strains indigenous to many hospitals). Nevertheless, before the antibiotic therapy is initiated, the patient must be questioned to determine whether he or she is allergic to penicillin; if the patient is or if there is some question that he or she might be, erythromycin should be substituted. Later the type and dosage of antibiotic may be tailored as indicated by the results of the culture and sensitivity tests.

It is generally deemed unwise to extract a severely abscessed tooth (especially if much surgical manipulation is required) unless the patient has been adequately treated with antibiotics to ensure an effective blood level that protects against the bacterial shower in the circulation produced by surgical manipulation in an abscessed area. Pellegrino (1980) advised that the correct time to extract must be determined by personal judgment, but in most cases aggressive treatment and early extraction shorten the course of the disease and the patient returns to health sooner.

Patients with severe abscesses are frequently discovered to have a decreased resistance caused by a debilitating systemic disease such as diabetes. Thus it is mandatory to effect a good medical evaluation, including the history and a physical and laboratory examination of the patient. If an underlying systemic disease is found, the patient's physician can undertake treatment of the concomitant medical problem, thus increasing the patient's resistance and aiding in the management of the abscess.

If it is advantageous to retain the offending tooth once the acute phase of the infection has been controlled, routine endodontic treatment may be performed with or without a root resection.

When there is a chronic abscess with a draining sinus, the exact origin of the abscess must be located. This can usually be accomplished by inserting a gutta-percha cone to the extent of the sinus and making a radiograph of the area. On the radiograph, the image of the cone points to the abscess. The procedure may not only direct attention to the offending tooth but also demonstrate whether the abscess is of pulpal or periodontal origin. Sinus defects usually close when the infection has been eradicated and the root canals have properly obliterated. These treated teeth must be radiographically reexamined at 6-month intervals to ascertain that the periapical radiolucency is regressing because treatment with apparent healing does not provide a definite diagnosis of the original periapical lesion.

SURGICAL DEFECT

A surgical defect in bone is an area that fails to fill in with osseous tissue after surgery. It is frequently seen periapically after root resection procedures, especially when both labial and lingual plates have been destroyed. Approximately 45% of all periapical radiolucencies treated surgically require from 1 to 10 years for complete resolution, and another 30% take longer than 10 years. In the remaining 25% the surgical defects resulting from root resection procedures do not heal completely. The post–root resection defect represents an area where the cortical plate is entirely lacking. In addition to the defect in the cortical plate, a periapical scar may be present.

Features. The periapical radiolucency produced by a surgical defect is rounded in appearance and smoothly contoured, and it has well-defined borders. It accounts for approximately 3% of all the periapical radiolucencies. It usually does not measure more than 1 cm in diameter and is frequently smaller. The radiolucent shadow may be projected directly over the apex or a few millimeters beyond the apex of the resected root of the endodontically treated tooth (Fig. 16-18). If a time-sequence

---

*An appliance of nonabsorbent material, such as a perforated tube or strip of rubber dam material, is passed through the abscess to maintain a passage for irrigation by injecting fluid into one opening and letting it escape through another.

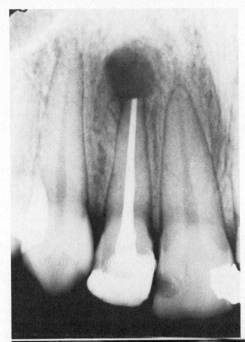

Fig. 16-18. Periapical surgical defects.

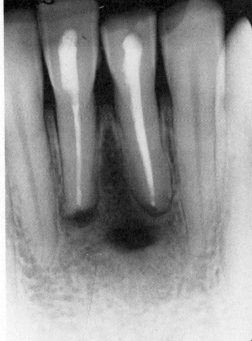

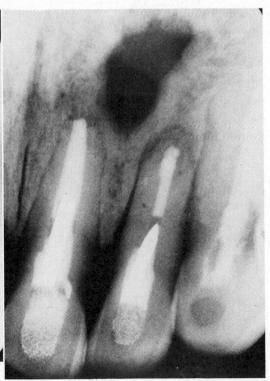

series of radiographs is available, from the time of the resection, the radiolucency usually shows a decrease in size. Frequently it resolves to a certain size and then remains constant.

The tooth and periapical area are completely asymptomatic. A careful clinical examination may reveal the mucosal scar from the previous surgery. If the defect is large enough, it may be detected by palpation.

Differential diagnosis. The periapical radiolucency produced by a surgical defect may be confused with any of the periapical lesions included in this chapter, especially the granuloma, radicular cyst, secondary abscess, and periapical scar.

The entity most likely to be confused with the surgical defect is the *periapical scar*. The periapical scar, however, is not displaced from the apex by radiographic localization techniques, whereas the surgical scar usually is.

A history of root resection, combined with the radiographic appearance of a resected, asymptomatic, endodontically treated tooth associated with a well-defined periapical radiolucency not larger than 1 cm and a small depression in the mucosa over the apical area, alerts the clinician to the probability that the lesion is not an *abscess, cyst,* or *granuloma.*

If changing the angle of the beam shifts the radiolucent shadow about in the periapical area, this can be taken as additional evidence that the entity is not at the periapex but in the cortical plate. If the shadow is caused by a surgical defect, it should show a reduction in size as it is periodically reexamined, especially during the first 6 months after surgery.

Management. Correct identification and periodic surveillance with radiographs are required for the management of periapical surgical defects.

OSTEOMYELITIS

Occasionally a periapical abscess develops into an acute or chronic osteomyelitis, especially in patients who have an underlying systemic disease that has depressed their systemic resistance or who have received large doses of radiation therapy to the jaws. Osteomyelitis is defined as an infection of bone that involves all three components: periosteum, cortex, and marrow. On this basis the periapical abscess can be considered a localized type of osteomyelitis (Chapter 21).

Although the terms "osteomyelitis" and "osteitis" are often used interchangeably, the latter actually describes the more localized condition and the former describes the more active diffuse conditions. We believe this distinction of nomenclature should be made, because although the pathologic processes may be fundamentally similar, there are clinical and radiographic differences between the entities and a difference in the regions of the jaw involved. Furthermore, the differences in the architecture, circulation, and character of the marrow between the alveolus and the body of the jawbone are apparently responsible for the usual localized restricted nature of the osteitis—in contrast to the diffuse, almost unrestricted spread of the infection through the medullary spaces of the jawbone in an osteomyelitis. Differing responses to treatment also aid in the delineation of the two entities: an osteitis may be readily managed, whereas an osteomyelitis often proves difficult to eradicate. Inasmuch as osteomyelitis is discussed in detail in Chapter 21, only a brief description in relation to periapical radiolucencies is presented here.

Acute osteomyelitis is similar to an acute primary alveolar abscess, since the onset and course may be so rapid that bone resorption does not occur and thus a radiolucency may not be present. Chronic osteomyelitis, on the other hand, represents a low-grade infection of bone, which if untreated follows a protracted course of bone destruction and produces a radiolucent lesion. Chronic osteomyelitis may demonstrate four distinct radiographic pictures: completely radiolucent, mixed radiolucent and radiopaque, completely radiopaque, and Garré's osteomyelitis. This last can be recognized as a somewhat opaque layering of the periosteum, with bone proliferating peripherally. In this discussion only the chronic destructive type, causing a periapical radiolucency, is considered.

Features. Osteomyelitis is seldom observed in the maxilla, probably because of the comparatively rich blood supply; when it does occur, however, it may be a much more fulminating infection than in the mandible, where it prevalently occurs.

The exciting tooth usually contains a nonvital pulp, may be sensitive to percussion, and may have been previously associated with an acute or chronic periapical abscess. There is a periapical radiolucency—somewhat rounded in shape—resembling the image seen in a periapical cyst, granuloma, or abscess. Frequently, however, the borders of the radiolucency are poorly defined and ragged (Fig. 16-19). Such an appearance is characteristic of infections in bone and results from the irregular extensions of the inflammation through marrow spaces and channels in the bone.

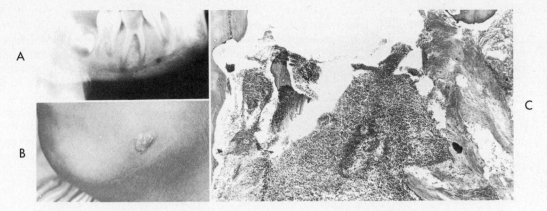

Fig. 16-19. Chronic osteomyelitis. **A,** Radiolucencies around the roots of the first molar. **B,** Sinus draining extraorally. **C,** Nonvital bony trabeculae (empty lacunae), inflammatory infiltrate, and necrotic material.   (**A** courtesy R. Moncada, MD, Maywood, Ill.)

The bony course of a draining tract traversing the body of the jawbone may be seen as a radiolucent band from the periapical radiolucency through the cortical plate beneath the sinus opening on the mucosa or skin (Fig. 16-19). The course of this tract is deeper or longer than that seen with a pointed chronic alveolar abscess, since it is traversing the body of the jaw, in contrast to the shorter course characteristic of the draining restricted to the alveolar process.

If a sequestrum (segment of dead bone) is present and large enough, it shows as a radiopacity within a radiolucency. The patient complains of malaise and may have a fever, and there is a concomitant swelling on the bone and mucosa around the osteomyelitis that may vary from slight to moderate. The swelling is firm, painful, and hot to palpation; pressure on the swelling or tooth may cause pus to be discharged from the sinus opening. Cultures of the purulent drainage usually demonstrate varieties of streptococci or staphylococci.

The microscopic picture is identical to that produced by a chronic alveolar abscess: necrotic tissue containing polymorphonuclear leukocytes and also regions of granulation tissue. More dead bone (spicules with empty lacunae) are seen in osteomyelitis than in a chronic alveolar abscess (Fig. 16-19). Although such spicules may be found in the radiolucent lesions, they are not large enough to show on the radiographs.

Differential diagnosis. The entities that should be included in the differential diagnosis are osteomyelitis, chronic alveolar abscess, an infected malignant tumor, Paget's disease complicated with osteomyelitis, and eosinophilic granuloma. If the draining sinus involves the body of the jawbone and courses through the marrow, the prognosis for the lesion is less favorable than for a chronic alveolar abscess.

If the area of bone destruction is large and the region not painful, *eosinophilic granuloma* must be considered. A biopsy establishes the final diagnosis.

An *osteomyelitis superimposed on a malignant tumor* of bone may completely disguise the more serious lesion, which becomes apparent again only after successful treatment of the osteomyelitis. Thus valuable time may be lost in the treatment of the malignancy. Since the concomitant occurrence of an osteomyelitis and a malignancy of bone is not common, such an entity is assigned a low ranking in the differential diagnosis.

The suspicion that a lesion may be an osteomyelitis can be qualified in light of the following circumstances:

1. If only the alveolar portion of the jawbone is infected, the diagnosis is *alveolar abscess.*

2. On the other hand, if the tooth suspected of precipitating the condition is in a fracture line, the diagnosis of *chronic osteomyelitis* is strengthened.* This diagnosis is also supported if an accompanying uncontrolled systemic disease such as diabetes is present.

---

*The occurrence of teeth in the fracture line and the failure to remove them in patients with poor oral hygiene may cause complications in the management of jaw fractures.

3. Also an attending bone disease, such as *Paget's disease*, or previous radiation therapy, along with some pathognomonic symptoms of infection, tends to strengthen the impression of osteomyelitis. Paget's disease is evident when several bones are found to have the classic cotton-wool appearance.

When considering Paget's disease, the clinician must remember that there is an increased incidence of osteosarcoma in this disease and the radiographic appearance of the disease and osteogenic sarcoma can be confused with that of chronic sclerosing osteomyelitis.

Management. The management of osteomyelitis is discussed in detail in Chapter 21. The clinician must predicate any treatment he or she may be inclined to administer on the premise that the patient has an uncontrolled systemic disease. As a rule the osteomyelitis is difficult to eliminate. Usually the best treatment is to extract the offending tooth rather than attempt to conserve it by endodontic procedures.

Dentigerous cyst

Although a dentigerous cyst forms adjacent to the crown of an unerupted tooth, sometimes the position of the crown of the involved tooth and the extension of the cyst is such that the pericoronal radiolucency is projected over the apex of a neighboring tooth (Fig. 16-20, A). In 55% of such instances root resorption of the neighboring tooth occurs (Struthers and Shear, 1976). On rare occasion the radiolucency is projected over the apex of the same tooth, especially in cases of a circumferential or lateral dentigerous cyst (Fig. 16-20, B). In such situations, whether the radiolucency is pericoronal or periapical may not be immediately apparent; the confusion is compounded if the tooth over whose apex the image of the follicular cyst is cast has a nonvital pulp. Dentigerous cysts are discussed in detail in Chapter 17.

Periapical cementomas

The periapical cementomas, cementifying or ossifying fibromas, and benign cementoblastomas arise from elements in the periodontal ligament. Thus an increasing number of oral pathologists currently consider these lesions related (Waldron and Giansanti, 1973; Waldron, 1985). Within the versatile periodontal ligament are mature osteoblasts and cementoblasts, as well as precursor cells, with the capacity to form cementum, alveolar bone, or fibrous tissue.

Periapical cementomas are by far the most common of this group of lesions and have been called many names: periapical cemental dysplasia, periapical osteofibroma, and periapical osteofibrosis. Periapical cementomas are thought to arise on a reactive basis rather than on a neoplastic basis like their "cousins," the cementifying and ossifying fibromas.

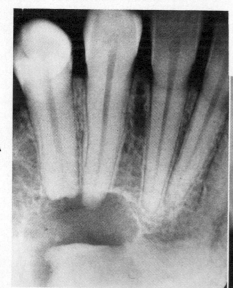
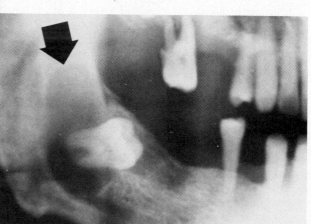

Fig. 16-20. Dentigerous cysts seen as periapical radiolucencies. **A,** The pulps of the canine and first premolar tooth tested vital. **B,** Unusual radiographic shadow of a circumferential dentigerous cyst *(arrow)*, which gives the illusion that the cyst is associated with the root rather than the crown. **(B** courtesy R. Latronica, DDS, Albany, N.Y.)

These periapical lesions have three stages of development, which are apparent on radiographic examination:

1. The early (osteolytic or fibroblastic) stage is radiolucent; the microstructure consists chiefly of a cellular fibroblastic stroma that may contain a few small foci of calcified material (Fig. 16-21).
2. As these lesions mature, they pass through an intermediate stage, which is indicated by a radiolucent area containing radiopaque foci.
3. The final stage is referred to as the mature lesion; the cementoma has become almost completely calcified and appears as a well-defined, solid, homogeneous radiopacity surrounded in most cases by a thin radiolucent border.

The calcified material in periapical lesions may seem to be entirely cementum, both cementum and bone, or all bone; however, to differentiate between cementum and bone by routine microscopic techniques is usually difficult if not impossible. It has been suggested

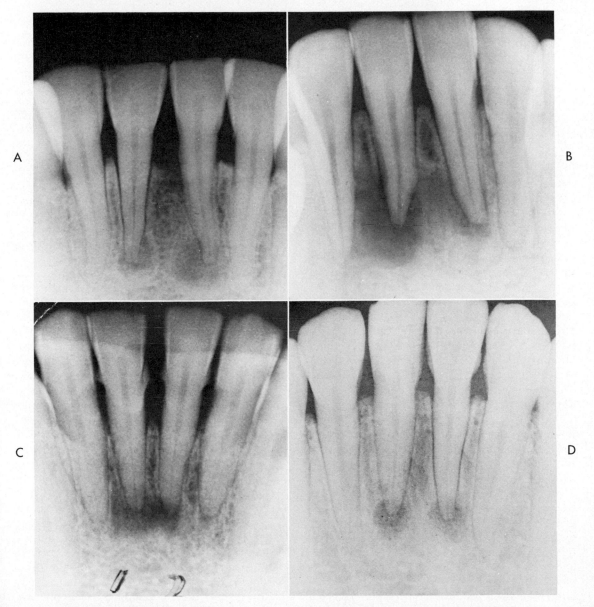

Fig. 16-21. Periapical cementomas (early stage). **A** to **D,** All incisors were vital and all patients were over 30 years of age.   *Continued.*

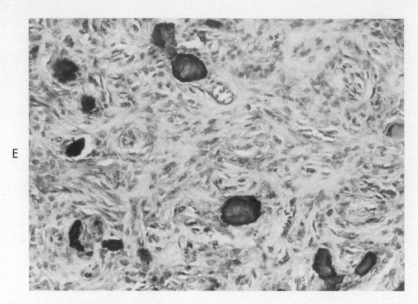

Fig. 16-21, cont'd. E, Photomicrograph of an early cementoma showing a few small droplets of cementum in a fibroblastic field.

that polarizing microscopy can distinguish the patterns of cemental fibers from those of bone (Waldron and Giansanti, 1973).

In this chapter, which deals with the periapical radiolucencies, only the osteolytic (fibroblastic) or radiolucent stage of the lesion is discussed.

Features. In the early stage of the development, the periapical cementomas occur as radiolucencies that are usually somewhat rounded, have well-defined borders, and are associated with teeth having vital pulps (Fig. 16-21). Blacks are more commonly affected than whites; 80% of the lesions occur in women. Neville and Albenesius (1986) reported that this lesion occurred in 5.9% of black women. The lesions are seldom seen before the fourth decade of life.

Although any tooth may be affected, approximately 90% of periapical cementomas occur in the mandible, where the periapical region of the incisors is the most frequently involved site. Tanaka et al. (1987), reporting on their own cases and reviewing the Japanese literature, found that the premolar and molar regions were the most commonly involved sites in Japanese patients. The lesions may be solitary or multiple, are completely asymptomatic, and seldom exceed 1 cm in diameter. It is unusual for a periapical cementoma to become large enough to produce a detectable expansion of the cortical plate.

Differential diagnosis. The osteolytic or early stage of the periapical cementoma could be confused with the periapical radiolucencies that are related to pulpal disease, and the inattentive clinician might needlessly extract or institute endodontic treatment on a tooth with a normal pulp. There is little excuse for this type of error, however, because the lesions can usually be readily recognized.

The cementoma is totally asymptomatic, the pulp of the involved tooth is usually vital, and the lesion most frequently affects the mandibular incisors. These features are in contrast to those of a *pulpoperiapical lesion*, which is associated with pulp disease or pulp death in a tooth that is frequently (or has been) sensitive to pressure or percussion or both. The two lesions cannot be differentiated on radiographic examination while the cementoma is at the radiolucent stage. In some instances, however, although not always, the apex of a tooth with a cementoma gives the appearance of having been sharpened in a pencil sharpener (Fig. 15-16, *C*).

A *traumatic bone cyst* may be projected over the apex of a tooth with a vital pulp and may be confused with a periapical cementoma, but it is usually much larger and is characteristically found in a younger age-group. If its identity is in doubt, however, radiographs taken at a later date reveal the developing calcifying foci within the radiolucency if the lesion is a cementoma. In the intermediate stage, differentiating the cementoma from pulpoperiapical pathosis is also easier because of the radiopaque areas present at this time within the radiolucent area. The *cementifying* or *ossifying fibroma* occurs at the apices of vital teeth, is more commonly seen in the mandible, goes through maturation stages similar to the periapical cementoma, and so could be confused with this latter entity. It differs in this regard: (1) it occurs in younger people; (2) it does not have a predilection to the lower incisors but occurs most often in the premolar region; (3) it has the potential to be a large lesion; and (4) it requires prompt enucleation.

The *cementoblastoma* in its early stage may also be confused with an early cementoma, but the former is a rare lesion that occurs almost exclusively at the periapices of the mandibular molars (see Fig. 16-29, *C*). Furthermore, it characteristically extends higher on the root.

Management. Once the clinician has established a working diagnosis of periapical cementoma, it is sufficient to observe the lesion radiographically. In the rare instance in which a cementoma reaches a sufficient size to expand the cortical plate and become infected because of ulceration of the mucosa, the lesion must be enucleated surgically and the material examined microscopically. Hall et al. (1987) described a particularly aggressive lesion that required block resection. The final diagnosis was aggressive cemento-ossifying fibroma.

The development of a cementoma apparently is not related to the condition of the pulp, and although the entity classically occurs at the apex of a vital tooth, this does not preclude the subsequent or concomitant development of a gangrenous pulp and an inflammatory reaction attending a cementoma. Such a case could present a confusing diagnostic problem, but the significance of such an episode is only academic, since treatment is necessarily directed at the inflammatory process. Conservative endodontic intervention is the initial choice of treatment in such a case.

Periodontal disease

As stated in the preface, a discussion of periodontal disease is not within the purview of this text. Nevertheless, periodontal disease must be considered here because it occasions a relatively common periapical radiolucency. Such a radiolucency is usually caused by advanced periodontal bone loss involving one tooth much more severely than teeth immediately adjacent. The entire bony support of the

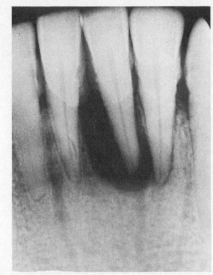

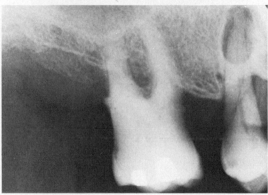

Fig. 16-22. Periodontal disease. Periapical radiolucencies caused by periodontal disease. The teeth tested vital.

involved tooth may be completely destroyed and the tooth may appear to be floating in a radiolucency (Fig. 16-22). Sometimes a narrow vertical pocket extends to the apex and appears to be a fairly well-defined periapical radiolucency, which in one projection seems to be completely surrounded by bone (Fig. 16-22). Brynolf (1978) described specific characteristics that she considered useful in differentiating between periodontal disease–produced periapical radiolucencies and pulpoperiapical radiolucencies. However, these findings remain to be substantiated by other investigators.

This presentation may lead the unwary clinician to a false conclusion of pulpoperiapical pathosis if the diagnosis is not based on clinical as well as radiographic evidence. A misdiagnosis of the condition can usually be obviated by a clinical examination of the supporting structures through identifying and probing all periodontal pockets. Pocket depth relative to the root length of associated teeth can be demonstrated by placing gutta-percha points in the pockets to their full depths and then taking a radiograph of the area with the points in place.

Teeth with advanced periodontal destruction are usually quite mobile and sensitive to percussion; surprisingly many remain vital, however, and the demonstration of such vitality aids the clinician in determining the correct diagnosis. Nevertheless, endodontic and periodontal problems may be concomitant. Feldman et al. (1981) discussed this aspect in an excellent paper. DiFranco and Gargiulo (1983) reported a case giving an example of an advanced periodontally involved tooth, which had a nonvital pulp that almost certainly occurred as a result of the periodontal condition.

Extraction of the tooth may be the indicated treatment. The soft tissue must be curetted from the region of the apex and sent for microscopic examination to establish the final diagnosis and rule out the more serious diseases that can cause a similar pattern of bone loss.

Traumatic bone cyst

Although the traumatic bone cyst (hemorrhagic bone cyst, extravasation cyst, simple bone cyst, solitary bone cyst, progressive bony cyst, blood cyst) is discussed in detail in Chapter 17, it should also be included in this series, since it may present a difficult diagnostic problem when it occurs as a periapical radiolucency. The traumatic bone cyst is classified as a false cyst of bone because it does not have an epithelial lining. Its cause has not been definitely established, although some authors favor trauma as the provoking factor.

Features. A history of trauma may or may not be elicited. The lesion is usually discovered on routine radiographs and is asymptomatic except when it occasionally reaches a size sufficient to cause expansion of the jaw. In such instances cortical plates are expanded rather than eroded and this produces a bony hard bulge on the jaw. Sometimes the lesion involves half the mandible. The mandible is involved much more frequently than the maxilla. The premolar and molar region is the most common location, but the symphysis is also involved with some frequency (Fig. 16-23). Bilateral cases have been reported (Patrikiou et al., 1981).

Teeth involved with this type of periapical radiolucency are vital, and the lamina dura is intact. Tipping, migration of teeth, and root re-

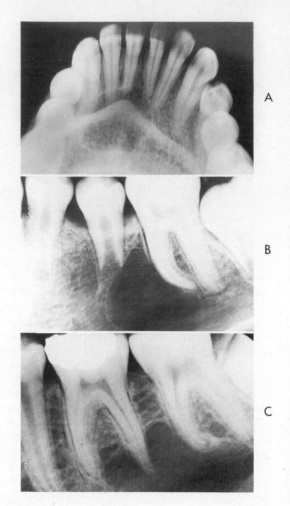

Fig. 16-23. Traumatic bone cyst. All teeth tested vital.   (**B** courtesy the late M. Kaminski, DDS.)

sorption are not features. Traumatic bone cysts usually occur in patients under 25 years of age.

On radiographic examination a traumatic bone cyst is a well-defined (cystlike) radiolucency above the mandibular canal either predominantly round and positioned somewhat symmetrically about the periapex of a root (Fig. 16-23) or more elongated and oriented in a mesiodistal direction extending superiorly between the premolar and molar roots and producing a scalloped appearance. The lateral and inferior borders of the elongated variety have smooth, regular contours (Fig. 16-23).

Aspiration usually is fruitless, but in some cases serosanguineous fluid or even a small quantity of blood may be obtained. At surgery scanty tissue may be found, which on microscopic examination proves to be loose or dense fibrous connective tissue containing some hemosiderin.

Differential diagnosis. The traumatic bone cyst that is projected around and between the roots of teeth is most frequently mistaken for a *radicular cyst.* The pulps of the associated teeth are vital in traumatic bone cysts, however, which makes the distinction between the two entities clear in most cases.

Differentiating between a periapical traumatic bone cyst and a relatively large, early-stage *periapical cementoma* may pose a diagnostic problem, since the pulps of the associated teeth in both cases should be vital (barring a concomitant nonrelated pulpal problem). In distinguishing between these two, the clinician can take a clue from the size of the lesion; the periapical cementoma is seldom more than 0.7 cm in diameter, whereas the traumatic bone cyst is usually larger than 1 cm. Also the traumatic bone cyst usually occurs in individuals under 25 years of age, whereas the cementoma is seen in patients over 30 years of age. Periodic radiographs show the maturation changes of the radiolucent cementoma—through the mixed radiopaque-radiolucent stage to the mature radiopaque stage—and thus permit the identification of the lesion as a cementoma.

A traumatic bone cyst may also be confused with the rare *median mandibular cyst.* Both entities have similar features. The surrounding teeth have vital pulps. Both can occur in the midline of the lower jaw and both may project between the teeth, although the median mandibular cyst frequently causes a separation of the teeth, whereas the traumatic bone cyst does not. Both are usually asymptomatic. Even though expansion of the cortical plates is an unusual finding in either case, such a deformity is even less common in the traumatic bone cyst. Aspiration may produce similar and confusing results.

When the characteristics of a lesion in the symphysis of the mandible do not tend to delineate one lesion or the other and establishing a priority between the entities is difficult, the traumatic bone cyst should be given a higher ranking, since the mandibular developmental cyst is quite rare. The microscopic examination of surgical specimens from a median mandibular cyst reveals a substantial cyst wall lined with epithelium, whereas the tissue from a traumatic bone cyst consists of only a few strands of connective tissue.

Management. In our opinion the traumatic bone cyst cannot be positively identified on the basis of the patient's history and the clinical and radiographic features alone. Thus we do not think that a lesion suspected of being a traumatic bone cyst should be managed by periodic radiographic examination. This contention is based on the possibility that such a cyst-like radiolucency could represent many types of serious pathosis, so a final definite diagnosis must be established. In addition, if the radiolucency has reached a fair size, it predisposes the jaw to pathologic fracture.

The treatment of choice is to open the area surgically, establish a diagnosis of traumatic bone cyst, remove the tissue debris present, curette the walls of the bony cavity to induce bleeding, and close the soft tissue flap securely. The patient should be protected with antibiotics, since the clinician has in effect produced an intrabony hematoma. This mode of treatment has proved to be quite successful, with bone filling the defect after the clot has organized. A careful follow-up to confirm healing is advised (Forssell et al., 1988).

An alternative method of treatment has been suggested for the clinician who is confident of his or her diagnosis; it involves injecting venous blood into the bony defect. Although good results have been obtained, a serious objection to this injection technique is that it precludes establishing a firm diagnosis. Consequently the clinician may discover in periodic radiographic follow-up examinations that the radiolucency is not resolving after the injections but rather is expanding. In such instances the clinician may have lost valuable time for the treatment of a more serious lesion.

Nonradicular cysts

On occasion nonradicular cysts may be projected over the apices of teeth. Thus, their description is appropriate in this chapter.

The most common offenders are the incisive canal cyst, midpalatal cyst, median mandibular cyst (refer to foregoing discussion of traumatic bone cyst), and primordial cyst (Fig. 16-24). With the exception of primordial cysts, these occur in specific regions of the jawbones. In general, they must be differentiated from anatomic shadows, radicular cysts, periapical granulomas, traumatic bone cysts, early cementomas, and other less common entities.

Changing the angle at which the radiograph is taken frequently projects the radiolucent image of the nonodontogenic cyst away from the apices that may be superimposed over it, and this differentiates the nonodontogenic from the radicular cyst and from the dental granuloma or other pulpoperiapical lesions. Also the teeth seemingly associated with these nonradicular cysts are usually vital.

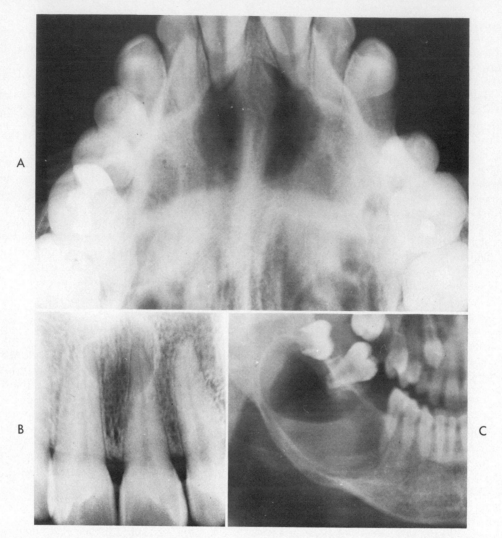

Fig. 16-24. Nonradicular cyst. **A** and **B,** Incisive canal cysts. **C,** Primordial cyst.   (Courtesy N. Barakat, DDS, Beirut, Lebanon.)

Differential diagnosis. If a cystlike radiolucency larger than 2 cm in diameter is present over the apex of a vital maxillary incisor and can be projected away from the apex by changing the horizontal angle at which a second radiograph is taken, the most likely diagnosis for the lesion is *incisive canal cyst.*

If a cystic area at the periapex of a maxillary first molar on a periapical film is shown on an occlusal film to involve the whole palate and if all the maxillary teeth are vital, the most appropriate diagnosis is *midpalatal cyst.*

Malignant tumors

Malignant tumors may be found as a single periapical radiolucency mimicking a more common benign lesion. Unfortunately, the clinician sometimes ignores this fact. Schlagel et al.

(1973) and Weisman (1975) discussed the importance of biopsy of periapical lesions that do not respond to endodontic therapy, are surgical cases, or are otherwise suspect. Burkes (1975) and Gingell et al. (1984) both reported cases of malignant salivary gland tumors occurring as periapical radiolucencies that were mistaken for pulpoperiapical lesions. Malignant tumors may be either primary or secondary. Primary malignancies that cause radiolucent lesions are discussed in detail in Chapter 19. Metastatic tumors of the jaws often produce a variable radiographic appearance, and those that resemble benign conditions escape early diagnosis most often.

The discussion of malignant tumors is limited to their appearance as periapical radiolucencies. The most commonly occurring malignan-

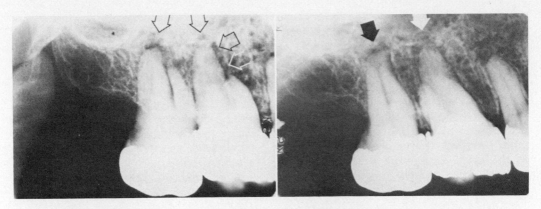

Fig. 16-25. Periapical radiographs. Arrows indicate bony destruction and periapical radiolucencies at the apices of the premolar and molar teeth, all caused by squamous cell carcinoma of the maxillary sinus.   (Courtesy R. Copeland, DDS, Libertyville, Ill.)

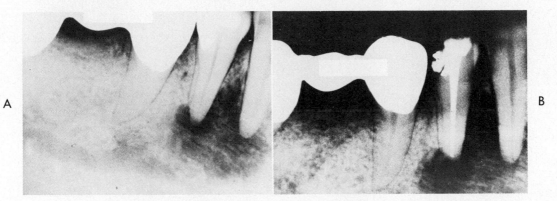

Fig. 16-26. Adenoid cystic carcinoma. **A,** Periapical radiograph showing the existing periapical radiolucency before endodontic treatment. **B,** Periapical radiograph taken 4 months later showing enlargement of the radiolucency. Surgery and microscopic study established the diagnosis.   (From Burkes J: J Endodont 1:76-78, 1975. Copyright by the American Dental Association. Reprinted by permission.)

cies producing this image are the squamous cell carcinoma, malignant tumor of the minor salivary glands (Figs. 16-25 and 16-26), metastatic tumors, osteolytic sarcoma, chondrosarcoma, melanoma, fibrosarcoma, reticulum cell sarcoma, and multiple myeloma.

Secondary tumors metastasizing to the jaws include malignant tumors of the lungs, the gastrointestinal tract, the breasts, the prostate and thyroid glands, and the kidneys. Milobsky et al. (1975) reported a case of renal adenocarcinoma that presented as a periapical radiolucency of the central incisor tooth.

Malignant tumors (for example, the squamous cell carcinoma, the malignant salivary gland tumor originating on or in the surface mucosa) usually erode much alveolar crest bone before they arrive at the apex, so they generally do not produce an isolated periapical radiolucency. Rather, the apical area of the tooth is included in a large radiolucency with ragged borders, representing a large area of bone destruction (Fig. 16-27). On the other hand, a low-grade, slow-growing, malignant salivary gland tumor that has destroyed some cortical bone may project over the periapex as

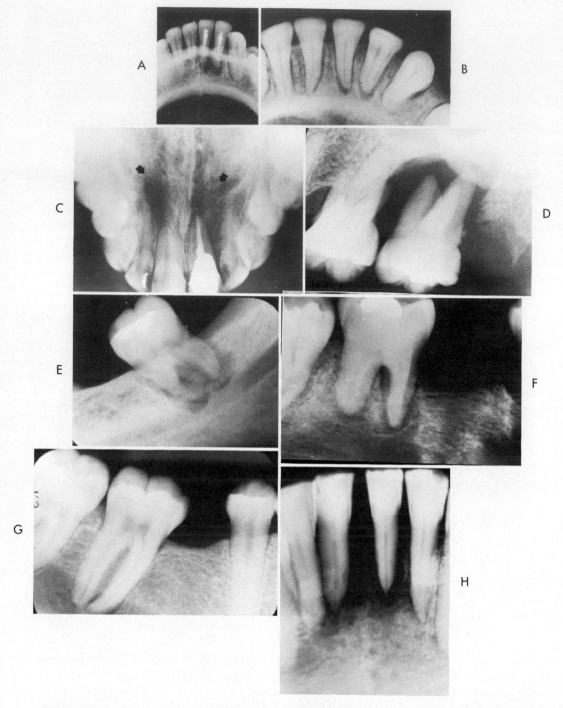

Fig. 16-27. Malignant periapical radiolucencies. **A,** Chondrosarcoma. **B** and **C,** Osteogenic sarcoma. (The bandlike widening of the periodontal ligament spaces around the incisor roots is evident in **B.**) **D,** Adenoid cystic carcinoma on the posterolateral hard palate. **E,** Metastatic carcinoma from the pancreas. **F,** Hemangiosarcoma. The radiolucencies at the apices of the molar and the bandlike widening of the periodontal ligament spaces are evident on all teeth shown. **G,** Metastatic rhabdomyosarcoma at the periapex of a molar. **H,** Metastatic carcinoma at the apices of the central incisors.   (**A** courtesy O.H. Stuteville, DDS, MD, St. Joe, Ark. **B** and **G** courtesy R. Goepp, DDS, Zoller Clinic, University of Chicago. **C** from Curtis M: J Oral Surg 32:125-130, 1974. Copyright by the American Dental Association. Reprinted by permission. **F** courtesy D. Skuble, DDS, Maywood, Ill. **H** courtesy R. Oglesby, DDS, Chicago.)

a rather discrete, well-defined radiolucency. Mesenchymal malignant tumors and metastatic tumors originating within bone are more apt to produce a more localized periapical radiolucency than a peripheral squamous cell carcinoma, which almost always originates in the surface and erodes through the alveolar bone to arrive at the apex. However, a squamous cell carcinoma originating within a cyst could be seen as a localized periapical radiolucency.

In summary, malignant periapical radiolucencies may be indicated by (1) a well-defined periapical radiolucency, (2) a poorly defined periapical radiolucency, or (3) a large, ragged, well-defined radiolucent tumor that has destroyed a large segment of the surface bone and has involved the apex of a tooth. The feature of root resorption may accompany any of the three images.

Features. The signs and symptoms of most malignancies of the oral cavity and jaws have much in common. Although these tumors occur in patients of all ages, they are much more common in patients of middle and old age. Pain may or may not be a feature. The involved teeth may retain their vitality. If the tumor is advanced, there may be migration, loosening, tipping, and spreading of teeth. There may also be gingival bleeding. Paresthesia or anesthesia of the soft tissues is sometimes present.

Expansion of the jaw is a feature in advanced lesions. With the exception of squamous cell carcinoma, at first this expansion has a smooth surface covered with normal-appearing mucosa. Later in the course of the tumor's growth, the mucosa breaks down because of chronic trauma, ulcerates, and then develops into a fulminating necrotic growth of tissue because the surface is continually traumatized.

Differential diagnosis. The advanced lesions are readily recognized as malignancies, so a differential diagnosis is not so important in these cases, except as it may help to arrive at a definitive diagnosis. The earlier lesions, however, do present a problem because they may mimic the benign conditions just discussed, and unless other subtle symptoms of malignancy are recognized, the clinician is not alerted to the seriousness of the case.

A well-defined rounded radiolucency produced by a malignant tumor may resemble a *radicular cyst, granuloma, scar, cholesteatoma, cementoma,* or *traumatic bone cyst,* whereas an ill-defined periapical radiolucency resembles a *chronic alveolar abscess* or an *osteomyelitis* (radiolucent type). The diagnostic problem blends with the philosophy of treatment of all periapical radiolucencies.

Management. Fortunately, two basic principles are employed by clinicians who manage periapical radiolucencies.

First, if the lesion and tooth are treated with conservative endodontics only, the tooth and the area in question are observed with periodic clinical and radiographic examination. Thus if a small malignant periapical radiolucency has been misdiagnosed and treated as a pulpal sequela, this error soon becomes apparent as a result of the clinician's continued surveillance.

Second, if the clinician chooses to perform a root resection in addition to the root canal filling, the tissue recovered from the periapex is routinely sent for microscopic study. Thus the malignancy is diagnosed immediately and the more extensive procedures, such as surgical resection, radiation, or antitumor medication, may be instituted at the discretion of the local tumor board.

RARITIES

The following list, although not complete, includes pathologic entities that at times occur as periapical radiolucencies. Thus the clinician must be aware that even though these lesions are either rare or rarely present primarily as periapical radiolucencies, a specific lesion under study could indeed be one of them:

Ameloblastic variants
Ameloblastoma
Aneurysmal bone cyst
Benign nonodontogenic tumor
Buccal cyst
Cementifying and ossifying fibroma
Cementoblastoma—early stage
Gaucher's disease
Giant cell granuloma
Giant cell lesion of hyperparathyroidism
Histiocytosis X
Leukemia
Lingual salivary gland depression (anterior)
Mandibular infected buccal cyst
Odontoma—early stage
Osteoblastoma—early stage
Paradental cyst
Solitary and multiple myeloma

Specific points obtained from the patient's history or by clinical, radiographic, or laboratory examination would presumably direct the examiner to the lesion most likely responsible for the patient's periapical radiolucency (Figs. 16-28 to 16-30).

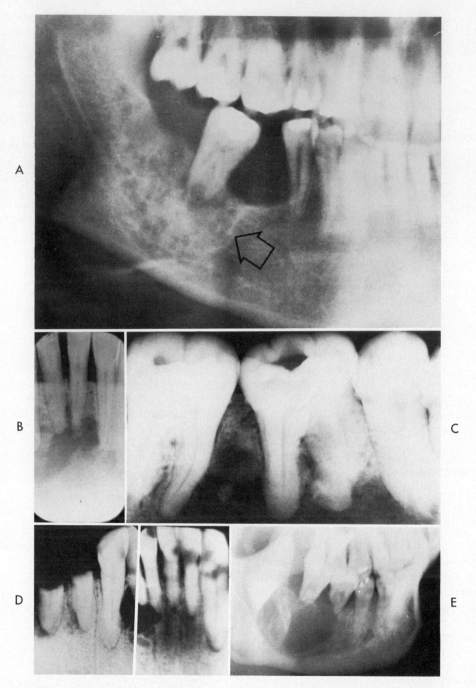

Fig. 16-28. Rare periapical radiolucencies. **A** to **C**, Giant cell granuloma involving teeth that were vital. The arrow in **A** indicates the lesion. **D** and **E**, Ameloblastoma. **F** and **G**, Histiocytosis X. (**F**, Radiolucency at the apex of the lateral incisor and canine in an adult patient; **G**, three periapical radiolucent lesions *[arrows]* in a 14-year-old boy.) **H**, Periapical lesion in a 62-year-old woman with multiple myeloma. The lesions in myeloma usually have smoother contours than shown.   (**A** courtesy N. Barakat, DDS, Beirut, Lebanon. **B** and **F** courtesy R. Goepp. DDS, Zoller Clinic, University of Chicago. **C** courtesy J. Ireland, DDS, and J. Dolci, DDS, Mundelein, Ill. **D** courtesy P. Akers, DDS, Chicago. **E** courtesy O.H. Stuteville, DDS, MD, St. Joe, Ark.)

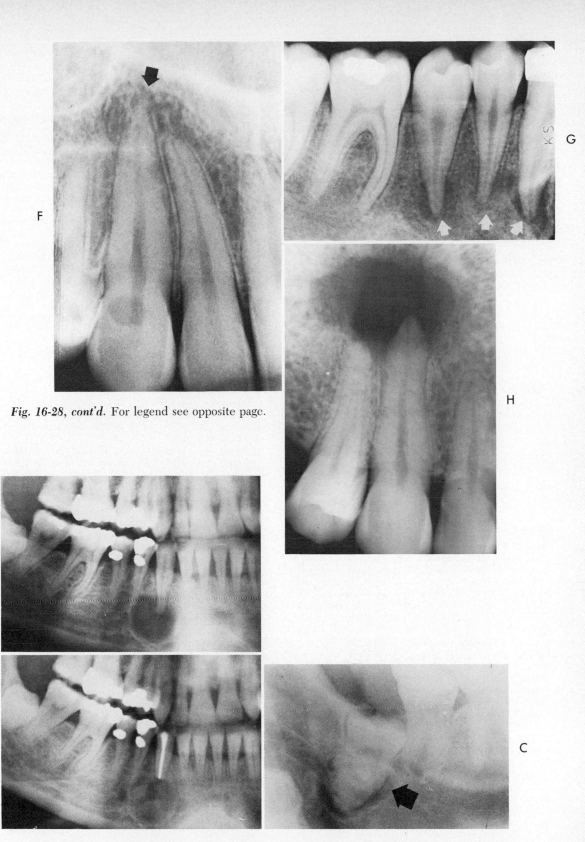

Fig. 16-28, cont'd. For legend see opposite page.

Fig. 16-29. Uncommon or rare benign fibro-osseous lesions of periodontal origin. **A,** Ossifying fibroma at apex of a vital mandibular canine tooth. **B,** Radiograph taken 9 months after root canal therapy, root resection, and enucleation of the lesion. **C,** Cementoblastoma in the early radiolucent stage associated with the root of an unerupted third molar tooth. The lesion is in contact with a considerable length of the root. Periapical cementomas seldom extend to this extent in a cervical direction. (**A** and **B** courtesy N. Barakat, DDS, Beirut, Lebanon. **C** courtesy P. Pullen, DDS, St. Louis.)

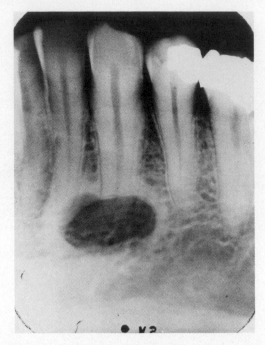

Fig. 16-30. Periapical radiograph showing well-defined radiolucency projected over the apex of the mandibular canine tooth. This radiolucency was produced by an anterior lingual mandibular bone concavity. (From Connor MS: Oral Surg 48:413-414, 1979.)

REFERENCES

Arwill R, Persson G, and Thilander H: The microscopic appearance of the periapical tissue in cases classified as "uncertain" or "unsuccessful" after apiectomy, Odont Revy 25:27-42, 1974.

Barbakow FH, Cleaton-Jones PE, and Friedman D: Endodontic treatment of teeth with periapical radiolucent areas in a general dental practice, Oral Surg 51:552-559, 1981.

Bender IB: Roentgenographic and direct observation of experimental lesions in bone. I, J Am Dent Assoc 62:152-160, 709-716, 1961.

Block RM, Bushell A, Rodridgues H, and Langeland K: A histopathologic, histobacteriologic, and radiographic study of periapical endodontic surgical specimens, Oral Surg 42:656-678, 1976.

Brynolf I: Radiography of the periapical region as a diagnostic aid. I. Diagnosis of marginal changes, Dent Radiogr Photogr 51:21-39, 1978.

Burkes JE: Adenoid cystic carcinoma of the mandible masquerading as periapical inflammation, J Endodont 1:76-78, 1975.

Burton DJ, Saffos RO, and Scheffer RB: Multiple bilateral dens in dente as a factor in the etiology of multiple periapical lesions, Oral Surg 49:496-499, 1980.

Camarda AJ and Forest D: Mandibular infected buccal cyst: report of two cases, J Oral Maxillofac Surg 47:528-534, 1989.

DiFranco CF and Gargiulo AV: Isolated advanced periodontal defects with pulpal involvement, Perio Case Rep 5:1-4, 1983.

Feldman G, Moskowitz E, Solomon C, et al: Endodontic treatment of periodontal problems, Dent Radiogr Photogr 54(1):1-15, 1981.

Ford TRP: The radiographic detection of periapical lesions in dogs, Oral Surg 57:662-667, 1984.

Forssell K, Forssell H, Happonen R-P, and Neva M: Simple bone cyst: review of the literature and analysis of 23 cases, Int J Oral Maxillofac Surg 17:21-24, 1988.

Gingell JC, Beckerman T, Levy BA, et al: Central mucoepidermoid carcinoma: review of the literature and report of case associated with an apical periodontal cyst, Oral Surg 57:436-440, 1984.

Greening AB and Schonfeld SE: Apical lesions contain elevated immunoglobulin G levels, J Endodont 6:867-869, 1980.

Grupe HE Jr, Ten Cate AR, and Zander HA: A histochemical and radiobiological study of in vitro and in vivo human epithelial cell rest proliferation, Arch Oral Biol 12:1321-1329, 1967.

Hall EH, Naylor GD, Mohr RW, and Warnock GR: Early aggressive cemento-ossifying fibroma: a diagnostic and treatment dilemma, Oral Surg 63:132-136, 1987.

Hirschberg A, Dayan D, Buchner A, and Freedman A: Cholesterol granuloma of the jaws: report of a case, Int J Oral Maxillofac Surg 17:230-231, 1988.

Jordan RE, Suzuki M, and Skinner DH: Indirect pulp-capping of carious teeth with periapical lesions, J Am Dent Assoc 97:37-43, 1978.

Kannangara DW, Thadepalli H, and McQuirter JL: Bacteriology and treatment of dental infections, Oral Surg 50:103-109, 1980.

Labriola JD, Mascaro J, and Albert B: The microbiologic flora of orofacial abscesses, J Oral Maxillofac Surg 41:711-714, 1983.

Lalonde ER: A new rationale for the management of periapical granulomas and cysts: an evaluation of histopathological and radiographic findings, J Am Dent Assoc 80:1056-1059, 1970.

Liposky RB: Decortication and bone replacement technique for the treatment of a large mandibular cyst, J Oral Surg 38:42-45, 1980.

Lustmann J and Shear M: Radicular cysts arising from deciduous teeth: review of the literature and report of 23 cases, Int J Oral Surg 14:153-161, 1985.

Makek M and Lello GE: Focal osteoporotic bone marrow defects of the jaws, J Oral Maxillofac Surg 44:268-273, 1986.

Marmary Y and Kutiner G: A radiographic survey of periapical jawbone lesions, Oral Surg 61:405-408, 1986.

McKinney RV: Letter to the editor: clarification of the terms granulomatous and granulation tissue, J Oral Pathol 10:307-310, 1981.

Milobsky SA, Milobsky L, and Epstein LI: Metastatic renal adenocarcinoma presenting as periapical pathosis in the maxilla, Oral Surg 39:30-33, 1975.

Morse DR: Immunologic aspects of pulpal-periapical diseases: a review, Oral Surg 43:436-451, 1977.

Natkin E, Oswald RS, and Carnes LI: The relationship of lesion size to diagnosis, incidence, and treatment of periapical cysts and granulomas, Oral Surg 57:82-94, 1984.

Neville BW and Albenesius RJ: The prevalence of benign fibroosseous lesions of periodontal ligament origin in black women: a radiographic survey, Oral Surg 62:340-344, 1986.

Patrikiou A, Sepheriadou-Marropoulou T, and Zambelis G: Bilateral traumatic bone cyst of the mandible: a case report, Oral Surg 51:131-133, 1981.

Pellegrino SV: Extension of dental abscess to the orbit, J Am Dent Assoc 100:873-875, 1980.

Ramadan AE and Mitchell DF: Roentgenographic study of experimental bone destruction, Oral Surg 15:934-943, 1961.

Richards AG: The buccal object rule, Dent Radiogr Photogr 53:37-56, 1980.

Schlagel E, Seltzer RJ, and Newman JI: Apicoectomy as an adjunct to diagnosis, NY State Dent J 39:156-158, 1973.

Schonfeld SE, Greening AB, Glick DH, et al: Endotoxic activity in periapical lesions, Oral Surg 53:82-87, 1982.

Shah N: Nonsurgical management of periapical lesions, Oral Surg 66:365-371, 1988.

Shoha RR, Dowson J, and Richards AG: Radiographic interpretation of experimentally produced bony lesions, Oral Surg 38:294-303, 1974.

Skauq N, Johannessen AC, Niles R, et al: *In situ* characterization of cell infiltrates in human dental periapical granulomas. 3. Demonstration of T lymphocytes, J Oral Pathol 13:120-127, 1984.

Stewart RE, Dixon GH, and Graber RB: Dens evaginatus (tuberculated cusps): genetic and treatment considerations, Oral Surg 46:831-836, 1978.

Stockdale CR and Chandler NP: The nature of the periapical lesion: a review of 1108 cases, J Dent 16:123-129, 1988.

Stoneman DW and Worth HM: The mandibular infected buccal cyst—molar area, Dent Radiogr Photogr 56:1-14, 1983.

Struthers R and Shear M: Root resorption by ameloblastoma and cysts of the jaws, Int J Oral Surg 5:128-132, 1976.

Tanaka H, Yoshimoto A, Toyama Y, et al: Periapical cemental dysplasia with multiple lesions, J Oral Maxillofac Surg 16:757-763, 1987.

Torabinejad M and Kettering JD: Detection of immune complexes in human dental periapical lesions by anticomplement immunofluorescence techniques, Oral Surg 48:256-261, 1979.

Torabinejad M, Theofilopoulos AN, Ketering JD, et al: Quantitation of circulating immune complexes, immunoglobulins G and M, and C_3 complement component in patients with large periapical lesions, Oral Surg 55:168-190, 1983.

Valasek P and Emmering TE: Unpublished data, 1983.

Van der Stelt PF: Experimentally produced bone lesions, Oral Surg 59:306-312, 1985.

Waldron CA: Fibro-osseous lesions of the jaws, J Oral Maxillofac Surg 43:249-262, 1985.

Waldron CA and Giansanti JS: Benign fibro-osseous lesions of jaws: a clinical-radiologic-histologic review of sixty-five cases. II. Benign fibro-osseous lesions of periodontal ligament origin, Oral Surg 35:340-350, 1973.

Weisman MI: The importance of biopsy in endodontics, Oral Surg 40:153-154, 1975.

Wilk AE, Milobsky S, Reynolds D, et al: The demonstration of alpha 1 antitrypsin in periapical lesions, Oral Surg 55:86-90, 1983.

Wood NK: Periapical lesions. In Taylor G: Endodontics, Dent Clin North Am 28(4):725-766, 1984.

Yanagisawa S: Pathologic study of periapical lesions. I. Periapical granulomas: clinical, histopathologic and immunohistopathologic studies, J Oral Pathol 9:288-300, 1980.

17

Pericoronal radiolucencies

NORMAN K. WOOD
PAUL W. GOAZ

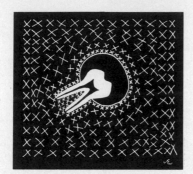

The entities producing pericoronal radiolucencies include the following:

Pericoronal or follicular space
Dentigerous cyst
Unicystic (mural) ameloblastoma
Ameloblastoma
Calcifying odontogenic cyst
Adenomatoid odontogenic tumor
Ameloblastic fibroma
Rarities
  Ameloblastic variants
  Calcifying epithelial odontogenic tumor
  Envelopmental primordial cyst
  Ewing's sarcoma
  Extrafollicular dentigerous cyst
  Follicular primordial cyst
  Histiocytosis X
  Malignant teratoma
  Odontogenic carcinoma
  Odontogenic fibroma
  Odontogenic keratocyst
  Odontogenic myxoma
  Odontoma in pericoronal location
    (premineralized stage)
  Ossifying fibroma
  Other radiolucencies projected onto images of
    impacted tooth crowns
  Paradental cyst
  Pseudotumor of hemophilia
  Salivary gland tumors (central)
  Squamous cell carcinoma
  Squamous odontogenic tumor

Characteristic features of the entities that most commonly produce periocoronal radiolucencies are shown in Table 17-1 (p. 359).

PERICORONAL OR FOLLICULAR SPACE

The crowns of unerupted teeth are normally surrounded by a follicle—a soft tissue remnant of the enamel organ that is frequently referred to as the reduced enamel epithelium.

On microscopic examination the follicle is shown to be composed of soft myxomatous to dense collagenous fibrous tissue containing nests or cords of odontogenic epithelium (Fig. 17-1).

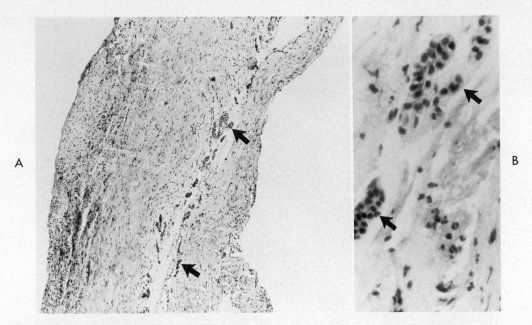

Fig. 17-1. Photomicrographs of a pericoronal follicle. **A,** Low magnification and, **B,** high magnification. Nests and cords of odontogenic epithelium *(arrows)* are found throughout the fibrous and myxomatous stroma.

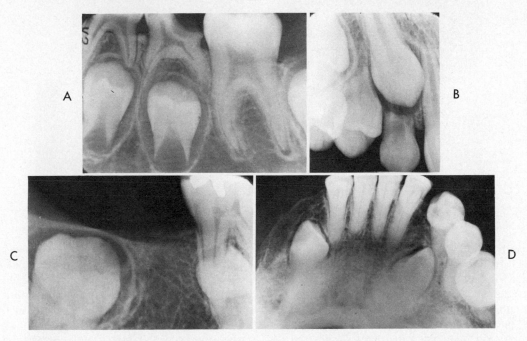

Fig. 17-2. Normal follicular space. **A,** Mandibular premolars. **B,** Maxillary canine. **C,** Mandibular second molar. **D,** Impacted mandibular canines.

The follicle appears on radiographic examination as a homogeneous radiolucent halo. The halo has thin outer radiopaque border (Fig. 17-2) representing compact bone that is continuous with lamina dura in the area of the cementoenamel junction. This halo, which appears as a space, merges with the periodontal ligament space; the halo varies in breadth because of the varying thicknesses of the follicles and the accumulation of fluid between the capsule of the reduced epithelium and the crown of the tooth.

Fig. 17-3. Meager follicular space associated with an impacted premolar. Diminished follicular spaces are frequently seen with impacted teeth of long standing.

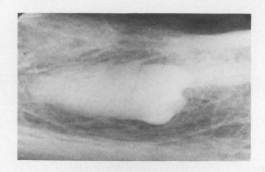

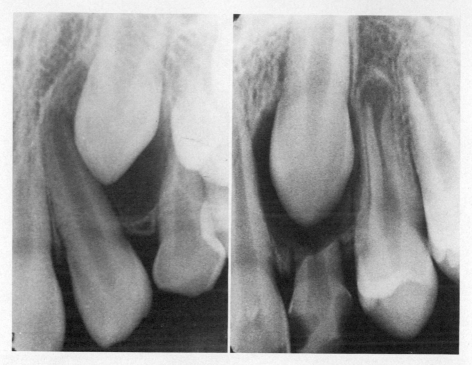

Fig. 17-4. Pericoronal spaces surrounding maxillary canines frequently achieve these proportions and are often misdiagnosed as follicular cysts.

Teeth that have been impacted for some years frequently show a meager pericoronal space (Fig. 17-3). By contrast, the unerupted maxillary canines frequently have an enlarged follicular space, especially when their eruption has been delayed (Fig. 17-4). Because cystic change can take place in such follicles and effect delayed eruption or displacement of unerupted teeth, it is important to identify any developing pathosis. Unfortunately, these entities are usually painless and there is no specific criterion that enables the dentist to distinguish between a normal and an abnormal (enlarging) follicle.

Some children have generalized enlargement of their follicular spaces. Fig. 17-5 illustrates

such a case. Almost all the follicular spaces surrounding the unerupted teeth were abnormally large, but only the largest one, which surrounded the crown of the mandibular left first premolar tooth, represented a lesion (a dentigerous cyst). The clinicians in charge of this case observed the boy closely to ensure that tooth eruption was not delayed.

Two guidelines have been used to distinguish between a normal and an abnormal follicle. Worth (1963) proposed that when an asymptomatic follicular radiolucency becomes approximately 2.5 cm in diameter and the surrounding cortical plate is poorly defined, disease is strongly suggested. Stafne (1969) contended that if the pericoronal space reaches 2.5

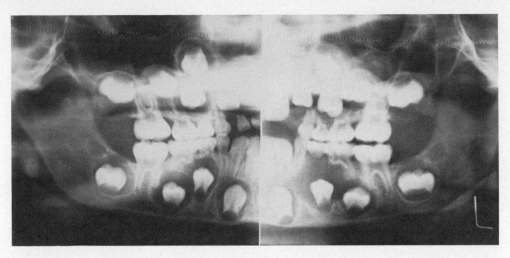

Fig. 17-5. Enlarged follicular spaces within normal limits. Panorex radiograph of an 8-year-old child showing multiple enlarged follicular spaces around unerupted permanent teeth. Surgery and microscopic study demonstrated a dentigerous cyst associated with the crown of the lower left first premolar tooth. Follow-up examinations showed the eruption of the remainder of the teeth without surgical intervention.   (Courtesy J. Dolce, DDS, and the late J. Ireland, DDS.)

mm in width on the radiograph, the size is presumptive evidence that fluid is collecting within the follicle and pathosis is present in 80% of the cases.

In our experience the contention of Stafne (1969) has not proved useful for evaluating the pericoronal spaces of upper canines, which are consistently larger than those surrounding other erupting teeth.

Differential diagnosis

For a discussion of the differential diagnosis of a pericoronal or follicular space, refer to the differential diagnosis section at the end of this chapter.

Management

In the absence of clinical symptoms, it is advisable to radiographically examine equivocally enlarged or enlarging follicles at least every 6 months or until it becomes apparent that eruption is being delayed, the tooth is being displaced, or the tooth actually erupts. If eruption is being delayed, a dentigerous cyst or other pericoronal pathologic condition must be considered and surgical intervention is indicated.

DENTIGEROUS (FOLLICULAR) CYST

After the radicular cyst, the dentigerous cyst is the most common odontogenic cyst. Dentigerous cysts are associated with the crowns of unerupted or developing teeth.

Features

The dentigerous cyst is the most common pathologic pericoronal radiolucency. It has a lumen lined with epithelium derived from the enamel organ or from other remnants of the dental lamina (Fig. 17-6). Various types of epithelial linings may be seen; occasionally, keratinizing epithelial linings occur. In these cases the lesion may be either an odontogenic keratocyst or a keratinizing odontogenic cyst.

The teeth most frequently affected are the mandibular third molars, the maxillary canines, the mandibular premolars, and the maxillary third molars (in that order). The highest incidence occurs during the second and third decades of life.

If multiple dentigerous cysts are found, the patient should be examined for either multiple basal cell nevus syndrome or cleidocranial dysplasia. In the latter condition there are many supernumerary teeth, and thus multiple impactions with increased possibilities of dentigerous cyst formation. Lustmann and Bodner (1988) reviewed the literature on the association of this type of dentigerous cyst with supernumerary teeth and presented six cases of their own. They reported that this type constituted 5% to 6% of all dentigerous cysts. Approximately 90% of this type of dentigerous cyst were associated with a maxillary mesiodens. They did not comment on syndromes with supernumerary teeth.

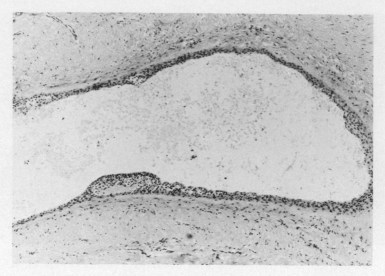

Fig. 17-6. This follicular cyst wall is lined with stratified epithelium. The thick wall consists mostly of dense fibrous connective tissue.

It has been reported that 2.6% of patients with one or more unerupted teeth have dentigerous cysts (Mourshed, 1964). Stanley et al. (1988) estimated that dentigerous cystic changes occur in 81% of impacted third molars. The cysts vary greatly in size, from less than 2 cm in diameter to massive expansions of the jaws (Fig. 17-7). The expansion may in turn produce gross deformity of the region involved.

Although a slowly expanding cyst may markedly thin the cortical plates, it seldom erodes them. This, however, is by no means a hard and fast rule. When the cortical plates are eroded, palpation reveals a rubbery, fluctuant, nonemptiable mass (in contrast to the crepitus or crackling quality of the sensation revealed on palpation of the expanded, thin walls of the bony cyst). Struthers and Shear (1976) reported that dentigerous cysts cause resorption of adjacent tooth roots in 55% of cases. Ackermann et al. (1987) prefer the term "paradental cyst" for cysts that occur at the distal or buccal surfaces of the crown of the impacted tooth.

Aspiration is often useful in the examination of cystic or cystlike lesions. Odontogenic cysts frequently yield a straw-colored thin liquid and usually yield cholesterol crystals, which may be seen in the aspirate when the syringe is slowly rotated in front of a strong light. The introduction of contrast medium into the evacuated cyst lumen occasionally provides additional diagnostic information, since the outline and extent of the cystic defect are sometimes made more distinct.

Because a cyst is usually painless, delayed eruption of a tooth may be the only clinical sign suggesting pericoronal pathosis. A painful cyst usually indicates the presence of infection. Rarely does a dentigerous cyst expand so rapidly that it presses on a sensory nerve and causes pain. When this does occur, however, the pain may be referred to any part of the face and is frequently described as headache. Paresthesia, anesthesia, or mobile teeth are almost never produced.

One exception to the foregoing comments on pain is the occurrence of a particular type of eruption cyst, usually involving a premolar below a deciduous molar. This circumstance has been observed to precipitate a severely painful condition, possibly resulting from the pressure of the cyst on the unprotected pulp of the resorbing deciduous tooth. The situation may be relieved by removing the deciduous tooth, whose loss is usually not considered premature in view of the position of the permanent tooth when the condition develops.

The eruption cyst is a dentigerous cyst that has developed, or is discovered, when the associated tooth is near the surface. It may be found immediately below the gingiva, producing a domelike swelling on the ridge. The eruption cyst should not be considered a separate entity. It is described in greater detail in Chapter 12.

Pathologic fracture is an inherent danger associated with a large cyst that has destroyed an

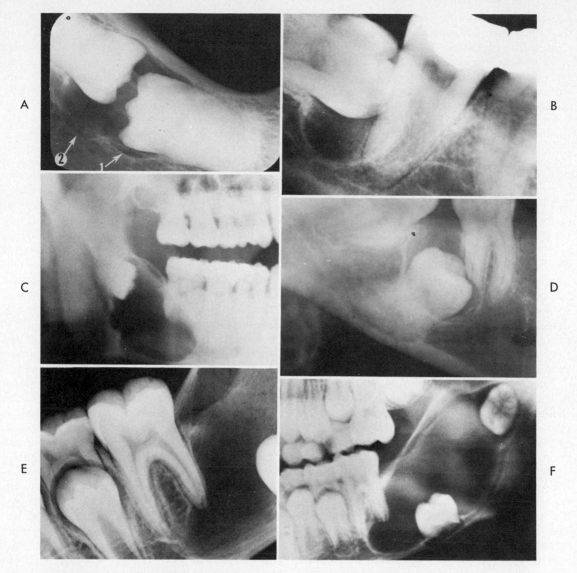

Fig. 17-7. Dentigerous cyst. **A,** Molar impactions showing, *1,* a follicular space and, *2,* a dentigerous cyst. Microscopic examination confirmed this impression. **B,** and **C,** Dentigerous cysts associated with impacted mandibular third molars. **D,** Dentigerous cyst surrounding an impacted second molar. **E,** and **F,** Two views of the same cyst surrounding the crowns of impacted second and third molars. This case illustrates the importance of obtaining adequate radiographs to grossly determine the extent of the lesion. (**C** courtesy D. Skuble, DDS, Hinsdale, Ill.)

extensive segment of the jaw. The jaw may become so weakened that it must be splinted before surgery to prevent fracturing during the enucleation. The splint is placed on the teeth.

Differential diagnosis

For a discussion of the differential diagnosis of a dentigerous cyst, refer to the differential diagnosis section at the end of this chapter.

Management

The position of a cyst should be confirmed before surgery by the Clark technique (studying several radiographs of the area taken from various angles) and by careful clinical examination. Since ameloblastic change may happen in islands of odontogenic epithelium that occur in the cyst lining or that extend from the epithelial lining itself, complete enucleation must be accomplished. Such a precaution reduces the possibility that potentially dangerous cells remain in the region after surgery.

To ensure that these latently dangerous foci are specifically noticed by the pathologist, the surgeon should carefully examined the lumen of any cyst removed and identify suspect areas before the specimen is sent for evaluation of the frozen section. Most follicular cysts have smooth uniformly thin walls, but some have smooth thick walls. If, on examination of a cyst lining, a local thickening or elevation projecting into the lumen is observed, the clinician can direct the attention of the pathologist to the area by placing a suture in the specimen to identify the region of special interest (Fig. 19-9, *B*). Should microscopic examination of the frozen section show that the elevation is a tumor (most likely an ameloblastoma) and that it has penetrated the cyst wall, the surgeon must recognize the corresponding area in the bony defect. This recognition enables the surgeon to return to the appropriate place and excise more tissue from the area to ensure all traces of tumor are removed.

Enucleation and primary closure are successful in the treatment of smaller cysts, and the defect resulting from the removal of a larger cyst can be repaired with a graft, preferably using autogenous cancellous bone. Some surgeons prefer to use surgical dressings, which are changed and reduced as the bony cavity decreases in size by secondary intention healing. The treated area must be periodically examined radiographically, since there is no way the surgeon can be certain that all the epithelium was removed at operation.

Marsupialization (or the Partsch procedure) is a conservative approach to the treatment of especially large cysts. It is accomplished by removing just the roof of the cyst, making the defect saucer shaped (the overhanging bony edges are cut away until the cavity is shallow with gradually sloping walls), and then suturing the membrane of the cyst to the oral mucosa around the periphery of the opening.

Decompression is another procedure used in treating bony cysts. A small acrylic button or short section of rubber tubing is placed in a preformed surgical opening in the cyst; this button keeps the opening patent and permits drainage. Ramsey et al. (1982) described clasp-retained drainage tubes as a drainage device. The procedure effects a slow diminution in size of the cyst defect, which slowly fills with bone.

The main disadvantage of both marsupialization and decompression is that the surgeon does not have an opportunity to grossly or microscopically examine the epithelial lining in the deeper extremes of the cyst. Hence ameloblastic change or worse, if present in the lining, can go unnoticed. Such procedures then impose the liability of leaving the potentially dangerous cystic epithelial lining in situ.

The serious drawback of these approaches is that approximately one half the cyst lining is left in place and so has not been examined microscopically. However, close examination of the retained lining by the surgeon reveals any *clinically* suspect rough spot, nodule, or ulcer, which would prompt the excision of such an area. Schultz et al. (1981) advised performing routine exfoliative cytology on the residual cyst lining. At any rate careful periodic postsurgical monitoring is mandatory with marsupialization and decompression cases to ensure that the surgical depression is filling in normally and that a previously unrecognized tumor is not present and enlarging.

When there is no clinical evidence of mural tumors, however, and a cyst is of such proportions that enucleation may result in pathologic or iatrogenic fracture, and if the condition of the patient precludes extensive enucleation and grafting procedures, marsupialization or decompression may be the treatment of choice.

Marsupialization or decompression may also be applied to advantage in the treatment of large dentigerous cysts that occur in tooth-bearing areas of children. Enucleation in children may result in the unnecessary loss of permanent teeth. This technique is used most frequently when a dentigerous cyst is preventing the eruption of a tooth and the tooth appears not to be impacted but to be ready to erupt once it is relieved of the cyst. Jacobi (1981) described a case in which the displaced permanent teeth erupted into normal position without orthodontic intervention. The operation can also be used for the patient who appears to be a poor surgical risk and not likely to tolerate the more traumatic procedure of total enucleation and bone grafting.

Occasionally a cyst bordering on the maxillary sinus has been treated by anastomosing the cyst with the sinus, which thus enlarges the sinus. This approach has proved successful, but it positions the sinus so near the crest of the ridge that a worrisome situation may be created.

Liposky (1980) described an interesting technique for treatment of large cysts of the jaws. Basically the buccal cortical bone is removed carefully in several sections over the cyst. The cyst is enucleated surgically and the sections of cortical plate are placed back in their original position and secured by wires. Such an approach helps to ensure a nicely contoured alveolar process.

UNICYSTIC (MURAL) AMELOBLASTOMA

This ameloblastoma that possibly forms in the wall of a dentigerous cyst ranks next to the dentigerous cyst as the most frequently occurring pathologic pericoronal radiolucency. The terms "mural" and "unicystic" are used to identify this type.

Shteyer et al. (1978) reviewed nearly 80 cases of mural ameloblastoma and reported that this entity represents approximately 5% of all ameloblastomas. The ameloblastoma and mural ameloblastoma were similar in predilections for sex (occurring approximately equally in men and women) and site (mandibular third molar region). However, they differed markedly in average age of patient affected: 21.8 years for the mural ameloblastoma versus 38.9 years for the ameloblastoma. Of unicystic ameloblastomas 85% were associated with dentigerous cysts, all of which were found in patients under 30 years of age. Other cyst types associated with mural ameloblastoma are residual, radicular, globulomaxillary, and primordial cysts. In 1988, Ackermann et al. reported on their study of 57 unicystic ameloblastomas. The vast majority occurred in the mandible, and the mean patient age at diagnosis was approximately 24 years. The authors divided histopathologic fea-

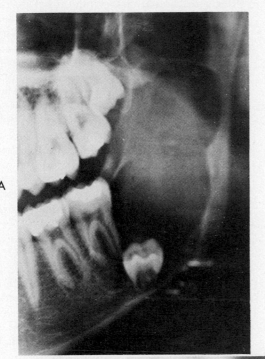
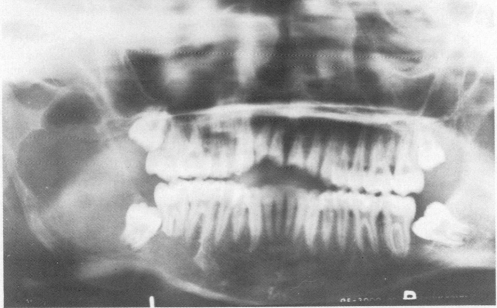

Fig. 17-8. **A,** Unicystic ameloblastoma in a young adult, seen as a pericoronal radiolucency associated with the impacted mandibular third molar tooth. **B,** Orthopantomograph showing another case of a unicystic ameloblastoma seen as a pericoronal radiolucency. (**A** courtesy D.E. Cooksey, DDS, Los Angeles. **B** courtesy E. Casper, DDS, Chicago.)

tures into (1) lining of variable nondescript epithelium, (2) intraluminal plexiform proliferation of epithelium, and (3) invasion of epithelium into cyst wall. Leider et al. (1985) reported on 33 new cases and concluded that these lesions occur as mural and luminal ameloblastomatous changes in preexisting cysts.

Various studies have shown that between 15% and 30% of all ameloblastomas form in the wall of a dentigerous cyst (Kane, 1951; Mehlisch et al., 1972). Stanley and Diehl (1965) found the ameloblastomatous potential of dentigerous cysts to decline markedly in patients over 30 years of age.

Gorlin (1970) stated that only rarely does an ameloblastoma arise from a nonneoplastic cyst. From the clinician's viewpoint, however, the identification of a radiolucent cystlike area as a nonneoplastic entity must await surgery and microscopic examination, since the clinical and radiographic appearances of the early mural ameloblastoma are identical to those of the dentigerous cyst (Fig. 17-8). Nevertheless, if the latter entity enlarges and remains untreated, it develops all the locally invasive characteristics of the ameloblastoma. The clinical characteristics of the larger ameloblastoma are detailed in Chapters 19 and 20.

Features

Sufficient to the present discussion is the recognition that a localized thinning and haziness of the hyperostotic radiopaque rim of the pericoronal radiolucency should prompt the clinician to suspect that a mural ameloblastoma may have penetrated the fibrous capsule of a follicular cyst and is initiating the invasion of bone between trabeculae.

The unicystic (mural) ameloblastoma, which occurs with greatest frequency in patients under 30 years of age (average age at discovery is 21 years), is asymptomatic and unsuspected and remains undetected until the pericoronal radiolucency is seen on the routine radiograph. Rapidis et al. (1982) recommended aspiration of the cyst fluid and injection of a radiopaque solution into the cyst cavity to help demonstrate the presence of a mural nodule, as well as its position and size. As the lesion slowly enlarges, however, a slight nontender swelling becomes apparent on clinical examination. This swelling is the result of an expansion of the cortical plates of the jaw and can be identified by palpation as hard and bony. With enlargement of the tumor, the overlying cortical plates are thinned to the point of destruction and palpation discloses softer areas, some of which may be fluctuant cystic spaces. Other softer areas are firm but not bony hard and represent solid masses of tumor or fibrous tissue that has extended through the eroded bone.

Differential diagnosis

For a discussion of the differential diagnosis of a mural ameloblastoma, refer to the differential diagnosis section at the end of this chapter.

Management

Before a surgeon undertakes the treatment of a pericoronal radiolucency, he or she should develop a differential diagnosis that includes the unicystic (mural) ameloblastoma. Subsequently, at surgery, if a distinct mass is discovered in the cyst wall projecting into the lumen, the surgeon should mark it with sutures to enable the pathologist to concentrate on this mass as the area of greatest concern. Such a discrepancy on the surface of the lining may prove to be any of the following:

1. Heavy localized deposits of cholesterol (Fig. 17-9, A)
2. Fibrous tissue nodule (Fig. 17-9, B)
3. Granulation tissue nodule (Fig. 17-9, C)
4. An area showing ameloblastic change (Fig. 17-9, D)
5. A mural ameloblastoma (Fig. 17-9, E)
6. Another type of odontogenic tumor (see Figs. 17-11, B and C, and 17-12)
7. Salivary tumor (Breitenecker and Wepner, 1973)
8. Central squamous cell carcinoma

Should the pathologist's examination establish the mass to be a tumor that has penetrated the capsule, the surgeon moderately excises more bone or soft tissue from the area of the bony defect that corresponded to the irregularity in the cyst lining.

In view of the foregoing information, the surgeon must develop a technique that enables him or her to identify the point on the wall of the cyst defect that corresponds to the suspect thickening in the cyst lining. If a cyst lining proves to be unusually adherent at a certain point, this site should be closely examined for the presence of a mural ameloblastoma. Some mural ameloblastomas do not show as elevations but are situated in the periphery of the wall, and the adherent lining may be the only clue the clinician has that another pathosis is present. Not all adhesions necessarily prove to be ameloblastomas, however, since inflammatory areas are often adherent too.

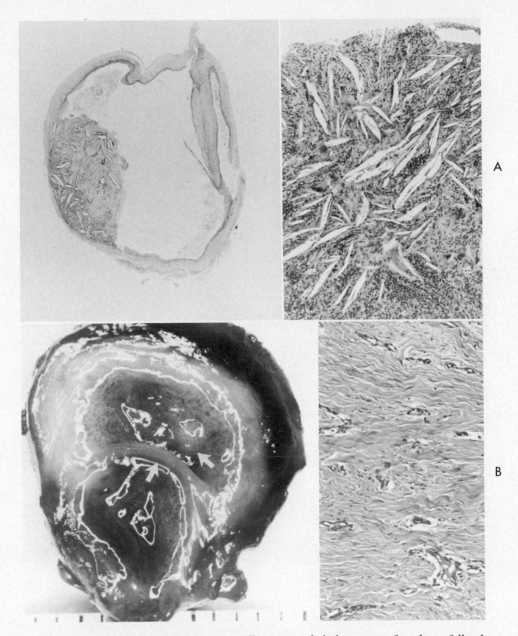

Fig. *17-9*. Mural nodules on follicular cyst walls. **A,** Mural cholesteatoma found in a follicular cyst wall (low and high magnification). **B,** Mural nodules *(arrows)* are composed of fibrous tissue.   *Continued.*

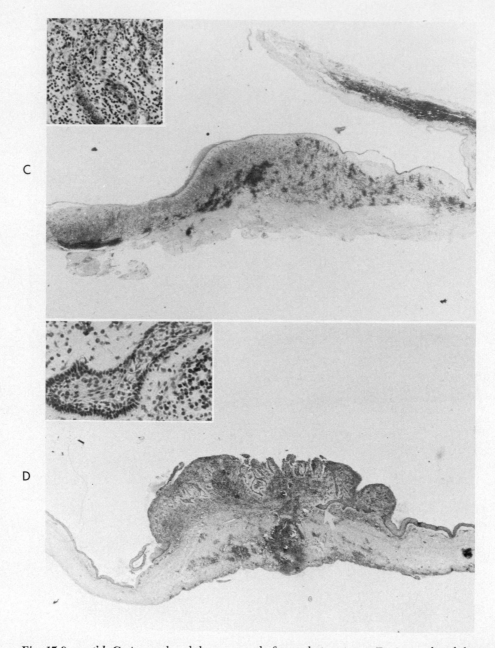

Fig. 17-9, cont'd. C, A mural nodule composed of granulation tissue. **D,** A mural nodule containing odontogenic epithelial nests, which are undergoing ameloblastic change.

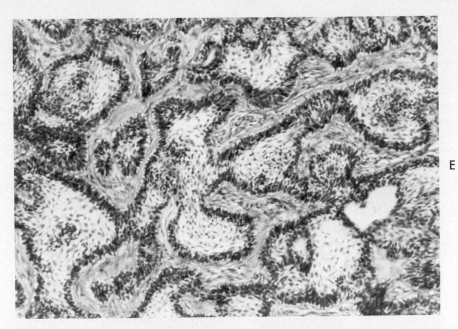

Fig. 17-9, cont'd. **E,** This mural nodule proved to be a follicular ameloblastoma.

The study of Shteyer et al. (1978) revealed that the frequency of recurrence after simple enucleation of cysts containing mural ameloblastomas is considerably lower than that of ameloblastomas that have been treated in a similar manner. Robinson and Martinez (1977) similarly reported a much lower recurrence rate for the unicystic (mural) ameloblastoma than for the ameloblastoma in general, which has a recurrence rate of 50% to 95%. These investigators, and Rapidis et al. (1982), Gardner and Corio (1983, 1984), and Marks et al. (1983) recommended that further and more extensive surgery for unicystic (mural) ameloblastoma be done only in event of recurrence. In cases of proven capsular infiltration of tumor into bone, more bone removal should be done in that region. The clinician should consider all findings in an individual case before deciding a treatment approach. In all cases careful periodic follow-up is mandatory.

Gardner (1981) and Gardner and Corio (1983, 1984) discussed in detail the plexiform histologic variant of unicystic (mural) ameloblastoma. Their findings indicated that this variant (microscopic features aside) was similar in every way to the "garden-variety" unicystic (mural) ameloblastoma and should not be considered a separate entity. Gardner and Corio (1984) described the microscopic features of the plexiform type as an anastomosing network of stratified squamous epithelium within a delicate stroma of connective tissue. The basal cells are not remarkable and do not meet the criteria proposed by Vickers and Gorlin (1970) for ameloblastoma. The pathologist must recognize this epithelial proliferation as a type of ameloblastoma rather than consider it hyperplastic epithelium.

AMELOBLASTOMA

It is important to consider that the pericoronal radiolucency under investigation may prove to be a "garden-variety" ameloblastoma at surgery and microscopic study. In other words the radiolucent cavity may be completely filled by ameloblastoma that has infiltrated peripherally into the bony margins. Presumably such examples may represent mural (unicystic) ameloblastomas that have had time to develop into full-blown ameloblastomas. At any rate, these should be recognized as locally aggressive lesions that require more extensive surgery. The ameloblastoma is discussed in detail in Chapter 19 as a solitary cystlike radiolucency and in Chapter 20 as a multilocular radiolucency.

CALCIFYING ODONTOGENIC CYST

On first thought the calcifying odontogenic cyst should be included with the mixed radio-lucent-radiopaque lesions in Chapters 24 and 25 but not here. However, we have observed a wide variation in the amount of calcified material in these lesions; this variation ranges from extremely small foci that can only be seen at the microscopic level to moderate-sized foci that can readily be seen as white flecks in the cystic radiolucency (see Fig. 24-11) to a calci-fied component so large that it almost com-pletely obliterates the radiolucency. Hence it is apparent that in the early stage the calcifying odontogenic cyst appears as a completely ra-diolucent cystlike lesion. Many of these occur as pericoronal radiolucencies and so are in-cluded here (Fig. 17-10). We are unaware of any difference in site, age predilection, or behavior between this lesion and the "garden-variety" dentigerous cyst. The calcifying odon-togenic cyst is discussed in greater detail in Chapter 24 as a mixed radiolucent-radiopaque lesion.

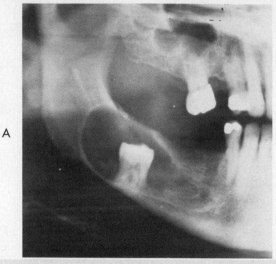

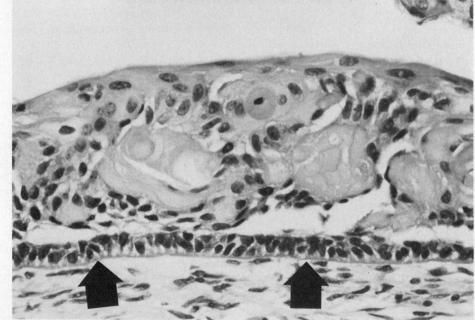

Fig. 17-10. Calcifying and keratinizing odontogenic cyst. **A,** Panorex radiograph shows a pe-ricoronal radiolucency in association with an impacted mandibular molar tooth. The calcified areas in this case were so small that they could not be seen in the radiograph as radiopaque flecks. **B,** Photomicrograph of an early lesion before calcification showing the ghost cells with keratinization. Arrows indicate the basal cell layer of the cyst wall.

ADENOMATOID ODONTOGENIC TUMOR (ADENOAMELOBLASTOMA)

The adenomatoid odontogenic tumor (AOT) is uncommon and benign and makes up approximately 3% of all odontogenic tumors, according to the study reported by Regezi et al. (1978). The origin of the AOT is still in dispute, but it seems certain that it arises from residual odontogenic epithelium. Some authorities suggest that instead of classifying the AOT as a benign tumor it might be better to consider it a hamartoma of residual odontogenic epithelium (Courtney and Kerr, 1975). At any rate it is important to distinguish the AOT from the amelo-

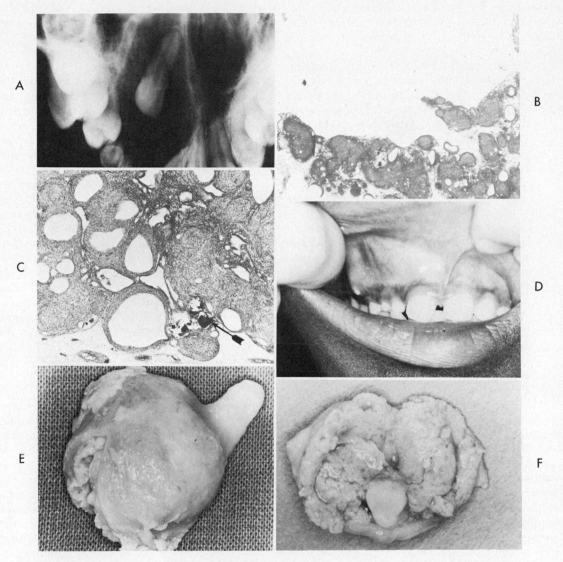

Fig. 17-11. Adenomatoid odontogenic tumor. **A,** Maxillary occlusal radiograph showing a large radiolucency involving and displacing the maxillary right canine. **B,** Low-power photomicrograph of an adenomatoid odontogenic tumor showing fingers of tumor tissue projecting into the lumen. **C,** Higher-power photomicrograph of an adenomatoid odontogenic tumor showing the typical picture of pseudoducts and pseudoacini. The small areas of calcification *(arrow)* were not large enough to show as radiopaque foci on the radiograph of this lesion. **D,** Expansion of the alveolar process and vestibule in the upper right canine region in a 14-year-old patient with an adenomatoid odontogenic tumor. This tumor had destroyed the labial plate. **E,** Surgical specimen from this patient. The smooth regular periphery permitted ready separation from the surrounding bone. The root tip of the permanent canine is protruding from the mass. **F,** Bisected specimen from the same patient. Papillomatous projections are evident from the wall into the lumen of this cystic tumor.   (**A, D, E,** and **F** courtesy W. Smith, DDS, MD, San Diego.)

blastoma. Actually these two lesions differ radically in clinical, radiographic, and microscopic features and behavior, so the AOT must not be considered a type of ameloblastoma.

Some pathologists have described the AOT as passing through definite stages of maturation (early, middle, and mature). Although this concept is still unproved, two distinct radiographic appearances are known to exist, depending on whether sufficient calcification is present in the tumor to be evident on radiographic examination.

1. In one stage, perhaps representing an early period, the tumor is completely radiolucent (Fig. 17-11, A). On macroscopic examination it may be solid or may contain large, cystlike areas (Fig. 17-11, B). On histologic examination it has an acinar pattern and in many areas shows nodules, cords, and swirls in addition to ductlike structures lined with cuboidal or columnar epithelial cells (Fig. 17-11, C). Minute calcifications are also apparent in the microscopic picture of this stage, although the degree and extent of the calcification are not sufficient to produce radiopacities. Hatakeyama and Suzuki (1978), Poulson and Greer (1983), Schlosnagle and Someren (1981), Smith et al. (1979), and Takagi (1967), describe the ultrastructure of the AOT.

2. In the more advanced stage sufficient calcification has occurred to produce clusters of radiopaque foci within the radiolucency.

Although the clinician may not observe any apparent difference in the clinical behavior of the tumors that could be related to their histologic or radiographic picture or both, the clinician nevertheless might suspect that the more radiopaque the tumors are, the less active they would be.

The AOT is twice as common in women and usually occurs in the second decade of life; the average age at occurrence is 16 years. At least 75% of these tumors occur in association with unerupted teeth or in the walls of dentigerous cysts. Several of the tumors have been reported in areas where teeth failed to develop, suggesting that they could have arisen from primordial cysts or directly from the enamel organ before the development of the hard dental structures. Approximately 90% have occurred in the anterior portions of the jaws; they are about one and one-half times more frequent in the maxilla than in the mandible.

Unerupted teeth that are most frequently associated with this tumor (in order of frequency) are the maxillary canine, lateral incisor, and mandibular premolar. The lesions are slow growing, and the radiolucent type previously described is similar to a dentigerous cyst in both growth pattern and appearance (Fig. 17-11, A). Thus the tumor may be small and show no clinical signs or symptoms. Conversely, continued slow growth may expand the cortical plates and produce a clinical swelling and asymmetry but invasion of the soft tissue does not occur (Fig. 17-11, D).

Management

The AOT is best treated by conservative surgical removal, since it separates easily and cleanly from its bony defect, has an extremely low recurrence rate, and shows no evidence of metastatic tendency (Fig. 17-11, E). Its behavior is much more benign than that of the simple ameloblastoma.

The surgical specimen may be solid or cystic, and on gross inspection, elevations of varying size and shape may be found projecting from the lining into the fluid-filled lumen (Fig. 17-11, F). Some areas of the cystic wall are thinner and smooth, however, and are in essence segments of typical dentigerous cyst wall. An examination of frozen sections should be undertaken at the time of surgery to establish a definite diagnosis. This diagnosis also permits the surgeon to remove more tissue if the biopsy report so indicates.

AMELOBLASTIC FIBROMA

The ameloblastic fibroma is a true mixed odontogenic tumor, containing nests and strands of odontogenic and ameloblastic epithelium in a primitive dental papilla-like connective tissue (Fig. 17-12, B). Calcified dental structures are not present. Slootweg (1981) recommended that the ameloblastic fibroma be considered a separate entity that does not develop into an odontoma. The ameloblastic fibroma is usually found as a unilocular radiolucency that is well defined, although occasionally multilocular lesions occur in areas surrounding the crowns of unerupted teeth or in tooth-bearing regions where teeth have failed to develop (Fig. 17-12, A).

Features

The ameloblastic fibroma is not as frequently associated with an unerupted tooth as the AOT is, although both are usually found in the same age-group (under 20 years of age).

The ameloblastic fibroma does not demonstrate a predilection for either sex. More than 70% of these fibromas occur in patients under

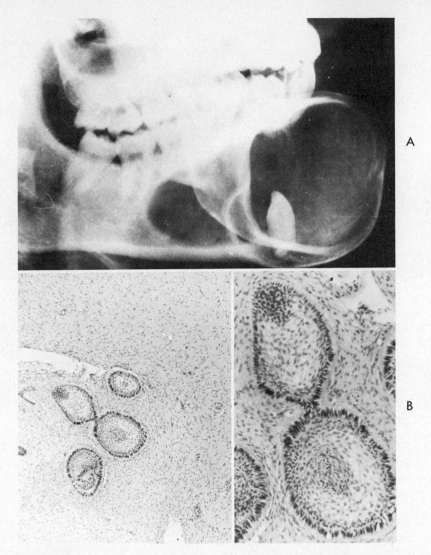

Fig. 17-12. Ameloblastic fibroma. **A,** This large, well-defined radiolucency displacing the mandibular canine and expanding the cortical plates proved to be an ameloblastic fibroma. **B,** Low and high magnification of the histologic features of an ameloblastic fibroma showing ameloblastic nests in a pulplike stroma.   (**A** courtesy O.H. Stuteville, DDS, MD, St. Joe, Ark.)

20 years of age; the average age has been reported as 14 years (Gorlin et al., 1961) and 15½ years (Trodahl, 1972). Although this tumor may arise in either jaw, the vast majority occur in the mandible and the highest incidence is in the premolar and molar region. This mixed odontogenic tumor grows slowly by expansion of the cortex and usually does not invade bone.

On radiographic examination the ameloblastic fibroma may appear as a unilocular or multilocular radiolucency that may or may not show cortical expansion (Fig. 17-12). The tumor is often associated with unerupted teeth and may spread to roots of adjacent teeth (Hager et al., 1978).

Management

The treatment suggested for the ameloblastic fibroma by most surgeons is conservative enucleation. The tumor readily separates from the bone, and since the ameloblastic cells generally do not invade the connective tissue capsule, a high number of recurrences are not observed. Zallen et al. (1982) reported from a survey of the literature that 14 of 74 recurred. The recurrence rate is higher for this tumor than for the AOT, however, and in rare instances there have been several recurrences. Consequently, periodic radiographic reexamination of the treated area is a necessary precaution. Ameloblastic fibrosarcomas have been reported.

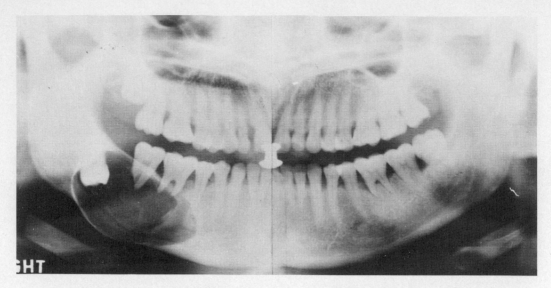

Fig. 17-13. Calcifying epithelial odontogenic tumor (Pindborg tumor) seen as a well-defined pericoronal radiolucency involving the impacted third molar in a 30-year-old woman. (From Smith RA, Roman RS, Hansen LS, et al: J Oral Surg 35:160-166, 1977. Copyright by the American Dental Association. Reprinted by permission.)

RARITIES

Almost any pathologic process may occur around the crowns of unerupted teeth, including primary and metastatic malignant tumors. These processes are rare and do not generally produce well-defined radiolucent lesions; nevertheless, in this discussion of rarities, it is appropriate to mention the odontogenic fibroma and the odontogenic myxoma, which do occur (infrequently) around unerupted teeth and indeed can displace associated teeth from their normal position. Both tumors may enlarge and produce expansion and thinning of the cortical plates, but rarely do they destroy the plates. An unusual case of a malignant teratoma (Hudson et al., 1983) and an unusual manifestation of histiocytosis X (Jensen et al., 1982) occurred as pericoronal radiolucencies.

An incomplete list of lesions that rarely produce a pericoronal radiolucent lesion is as follows:

Ameloblastic variants
Calcifying epithelial odontogenic tumor (Fig. 17-13)
Envelopmental primordial cyst
Ewing's sarcoma (Fig. 17-14)
Extrafollicular dentigerous cyst
Follicular primordial cyst
Histiocytosis X
Malignant teratoma
Odontogenic carcinoma
Odontogenic fibroma
Odontogenic keratocyst
Odontogenic myxoma (Fig. 17-15)
Odontoma in pericoronal location (premineralized stage)
Ossifying fibroma (Fig. 17-16)
Other radiolucencies projected onto images of impacted tooth crowns
Paradental cyst
Pseudotumor of hemophilia (Fig. 17-17)
Salivary gland tumors (central)
Squamous cell carcinoma
Squamous odontogenic tumor

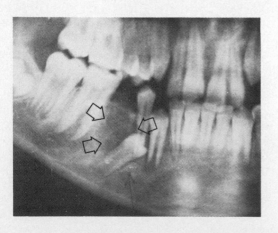

Fig. 17-14. Arrows indicate ragged ill-defined pericoronal radiolucency involving the impacted mandibular right second premolar tooth. Biopsy specimen in this 15-year-old adolescent revealed Ewing's sarcoma. (Courtesy N. Barakat, DDS, Beirut, Lebanon.)

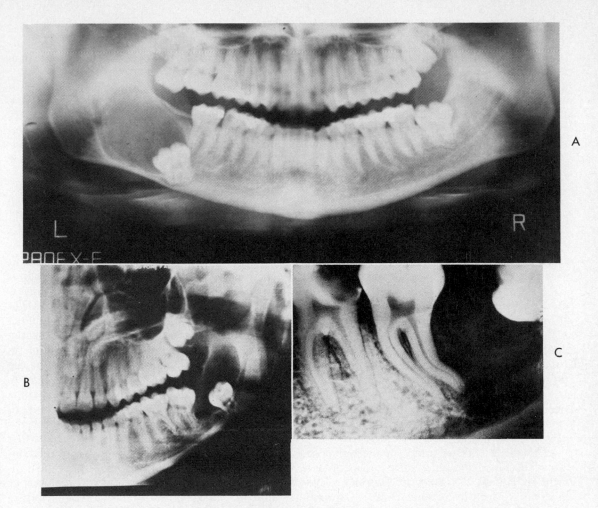

A

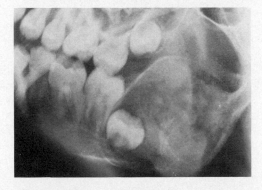

B

C

Fig. 17-15. **A,** Odontogenic fibromyxoma seen as a pericoronal radiolucency associated with the impacted left mandibular third molar. **B** and **C,** Another case of fibromyxoma seen as a pericoronal radiolucency. **B,** Panoramic film. **C,** Periapical film.   (Courtesy D.E. Cooksey, DDS, Los Angeles.)

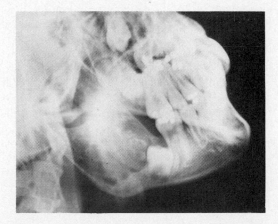

Fig. 17-16. Ossifying fibroma. The large radiolucent area appears to contact the crown of the displaced mandibular third molar. The thin radiopaque borders of the lesion are evident. The increased buccolingual thickness of the ramus composed of dense fibrous tissue imparts a hazy semiradiopaque appearance to this lesion that contained minimal foci of calcification.

Fig. 17-17. Pseudotumor of hemophilia seen as a pericoronal radiolucency in this lateral oblique radiograph of a young man with a hereditary deficiency of factor VIII.   (Courtesy G. Blozis, DDS, Columbus, Ohio.)

DIFFERENTIAL DIAGNOSIS OF PERICORONAL RADIOLUCENCIES

When the clinician is confronted by a pericoronal radiolucency, he or she must prepare the surgical team for the anticipated procedure. This is best accomplished by the formulation of a list of possible diagnoses arranged in order of probability, with the most probable lesion heading the list, as the basis of a working diagnosis. Thus, if all the discernible features of the pathosis under study give ameloblastoma a low level of probability, the need to prepare the surgical team for an extensive procedure (for example, a block resection with bone graft) is obviated.

To illustrate the usefulness of formally developing a differential diagnosis, we close this chapter with an analysis of the circumstances attending a 50-year-old woman with a well-defined pericoronal radiolucency associated with an impacted lower right third molar.

The lesion was discovered on a routine radiographic survey. It was asymptomatic and measured 2 cm in diameter with an intrafollicular space measuring 1 cm. Because normal follicular spaces usually decrease in size with age, it was initially recognized, on the basis of its proportions, as not a simple, enlarged, uncomplicated follicle but rather a pathologic process.

Although the lesion under investigation occurred in the mandibular third molar area, a frequent site of the *unicystic (mural) ameloblastoma*, this entity was not assigned a prominent rank, since it seldom occurs in persons over 30 years of age (Stanley and Diehl, 1965).

The *odontoma* and its *ameloblastic variants* commonly occur in a supracoronal position in close approximation to the occlusal surface of an unerupted tooth. Thus in radiographs these lesions in their unmineralized stages could be seen as pericoronal radiolucencies. However, the chances of the lesion in question representing an odontoma or one of its ameloblastic variants is remote because these lesions develop at the same time as the dentition and so would have already passed into the completely radiopaque stage in a patient who is 50 years old.

The *calcifying odontogenic cyst* may occur as a pericoronal radiolucency and be unsuspected until small radiopaque foci appear. Inasmuch as its management is identical to that of the uncomplicated dentigerous cyst, extensive attempts at ranking are academic rather than practical.

Although the *ameloblastic fibroma* is four times more common in the mandible, the choice of this entity as the working diagnosis was inappropriate, since this mixed odontogenic tumor occurs most frequently in the mandibular premolar–first molar area and seldom is seen in patients over 20 years of age.

Further, none of the lesion's characteristics (for example, location, age of patient) suggested an *adenomatoid odontogenic tumor (AOT)*, since these entities show a predilection for the anterior region of the jaws of young persons.

Envelopmental primordial cysts and *follicular primordial cysts* are interesting possibilities to consider here. These lesions have been discussed by Altini and Cohen (1982). As described by these authors the envelopmental primordial cyst is a true primordial cyst that occurs in close proximity to the crown of an unerupted tooth, and superimposition of the image may cause the cystlike radiolucency to appear as a dentigerous cyst on radiographic examination. The follicular primordial cyst, in counterdistinction, actually surrounds the crown, and the cyst lining is attached to the neck of the tooth in a true dentigerous relationship. To enhance the process of differential diagnosis, different angulations of radiographs shift the image into a different relationship in the case of envelopmental primordial cysts, thus showing that they are not true dentigerous cysts. The follicular primordial cyst image could not be differentiated from that of the dentigerous cyst. The important point is that a high percentage of the primordial cysts are odontogenic keratocysts (high recurrence rate), whereas only a small percentage of true dentigerous cysts are odontogenic keratocysts.

Thus the working diagnosis—or the condition assigned the highest rank in the differential diagnosis for this radiolucent lesion—was dentigerous cyst. The possibility that any of the other pericoronal radiolucencies might be found at operation was remote; nevertheless, the unicystic (mural) ameloblastoma was a distant second on the formulated list.

Table 17-1. Pericoronal radiolucencies*

	Predominant sex	Peak age (year)	Most frequent jaw involved	Most frequent area of jaw involved	Most frequent tooth involved	Signs or symptoms	Recurrence
Follicular spaces Developing teeth		4-12				None	
Impacted teeth	M ~ F	Over 18	Mandible	Posterior	Mandibular third molar	Delayed eruption of tooth	Recurs as cyst or ameloblastoma
Dentigerous cysts	?	Over 18	Mandible	Posterior	Mandibular third molar	Delayed eruption of tooth Swelling; asymmetry	Recurs as cyst or ameloblastoma
Unicystic (mural) ameloblastomas	M ~ F	85% under 30 (average 21)	Mandible	Posterior	Mandibular third molar	Delayed eruption of tooth Swelling; asymmetry	Occasional
Ameloblastoma	M ~ F	Average 38.9	Mandible	Posterior	Mandibular third molar	Delayed eruption of tooth Swelling	Significant
Adenomatoid odontogenic tumors	$\frac{F}{M} = \frac{2}{1}$	10-21 (average 16.5)	Maxilla	Anterior (90%)	Maxillary canine (60%)	Delayed eruption of tooth Swelling; asymmetry	Unusual
Ameloblastic fibromas	M ~ F	70% under 20 (average 14 to 15.5)	Mandible	Posterior	Mandibular molar and premolar	Delayed eruption of tooth Advanced swelling; asymmetry	Unusual

*Entities listed according to frequency of occurrence.

~, Approximately equal.

REFERENCES

Ackermann GL, Altini M, and Shear M: The unicystic ameloblastoma: a clinicopathological study of 57 cases, J Oral Pathol 17:541-546, 1988.

Ackermann G, Cohen MA, and Altini M: The paradental cyst: a clinicopathologic study of 50 cases, Oral Surg 64:308-313, 1987.

Altini M and Cohen M: The follicular primordial cyst – odontogenic keratocyst, Int J Oral Surg 11:175-182, 1982.

Breitenecker G and Wepner F: A pleomorphic adenoma (so-called mixed tumor) in the wall of a dentigerous cyst, Oral Surg 36:63-71, 1973.

Courtney RM and Kerr DA: The odontogenic adenomatoid tumor, Oral Surg 39:424-435, 1975.

Gardner DG: Plexiform unicystic ameloblastoma: a diagnostic problem in dentigerous cysts, Cancer 47:1358-1363, 1981.

Gardner DG and Corio RL: The relationship of plexiform unicystic ameloblastoma to conventional ameloblastoma, Oral Surg 56:54-60, 1983.

Gardner DG and Corio RL: Plexiform unicystic ameloblastoma: a variant of ameloblastoma with a low-recurrence rate after enucleation, Cancer 53:1730-1735, 1984.

Gorlin RJ: Odontogenic tumors. In Gorlin RJ and Goldman HM, editors: Thoma's oral pathology, ed 6, St. Louis, 1970, The CV Mosby Co, vol 1, p 484.

Gorlin RJ, Chaudhry AP, and Pindborg JJ: Odontogenic tumors, classification, histopathology and clinical behavior in man and domestic animals, Cancer 14:73-101, 1961.

Hager RC, Taylor CG, and Allen PM: Ameloblastic fibroma: report of case, J Oral Surg 36:66-69, 1978.

Hatakeyama S and Suzuki A: Ultrastructure study of adenomatoid odontogenic tumor, J Oral Pathol 7:295, 1978.

Hudson JW, Jaffrey B, Chase DC, et al: Malignant teratoma of the mandible, J Oral Maxillofac Surg 41:540-543, 1983.

Jacobi R: Spontaneous repositioning of displaced molars after marsupialization of a dentigerous cyst, J Am Dent Assoc 102:655-656, 1981.

Jensen JL, Correll RW, and Bloom CY: Painful mandibular and maxillary bone lesions in a young adult, J Am Dent Assoc 105:673-674, 1982.

Kane JP: Odontogenic tumors: a statistical and morphological study of 88 cases, thesis, Washington, DC, 1951, Georgetown University.

Leider AS, Eversole LR, and Barkin ME: Cystic ameloblastoma, Oral Surg 60:624-630, 1985.

Liposky RB: Decortication and bone replacement technique for the treatment of a large mandible cyst, J Oral Surg 38:42-45, 1980.

Lustmann J and Bodner L: Dentigerous cysts associated with supernumerary teeth, J Oral Maxillofac Surg 17:100-102, 1988.

Marks R, Block M, Sanusi DI, et al: Unicystic ameloblastoma, Int J Oral Surg 12:186-189, 1983.

Mehlisch DR, Dahlin DC, and Masson JK: Ameloblastoma: a clinicopathologic report, J Oral Surg 30:9-22, 1972.

Mourshed F: A roentgenographic study of dentigerous cysts. I. Incidence in a population sample, Oral Surg 18:47-53, 1964.

Poulson TC and Greer RO: Adenomatoid odontogenic tumor: clinicopathologic and ultrastructural concepts, J Oral Maxillofac Surg 41:818-824, 1983.

Ramsey WO, Denegri RF, and King WF: Clasp retained devices for drainage of marsupialized cysts, J Oral Maxillofac Surg 40:759-761, 1982.

Rapidis AD, Angelopoulos AP, Skouteris, CA, et al.: Mural (intracystic) ameloblastoma, Int J Oral Surg 11:166-174, 1982.

Regezi JA, Kerr DA, and Courtney RM: Odontogenic tumors: an analysis of 706 cases, J Oral Surg 36:771-778, 1978.

Robinson L and Martinez MG: Unicystic ameloblastoma: a prognostically distinct entity, Cancer 40:2278-2285, 1977.

Schlosnagle DC and Someren A: The ultrastructure of the adenomatoid odontogenic tumor, Oral Surg 52:154, 1981.

Schultz P, von Skerst H, Rummel HH, et al: Cytological findings in cases of marsupialized odontogenic cysts: a contribution to early diagnosis of malignant changes, J Maxillofac Surg 9:35-41, 1981.

Shteyer A, Lustmann J, and Lewin-Epstein J: The mural ameloblastoma: review of the literature, J Oral Surg 36:866-872, 1978.

Slootweg PJ: An analysis of the interrelationship of the mixed odontogenic tumors—ameloblastic fibroma, ameloblastic fibro-odontoma, and the odontomas, Oral Surg 51:266-276, 1981.

Smith RRL, Olson JL, Hutchins GM, et al: Adenomatoid odontogenic tumor: ultrastructural demonstration of two cell types and amyloid, Cancer 43:505, 1979.

Stafne EC: Oral roentgenographic diagnosis, ed 3, Philadelphia, 1969, WB Saunders Co., p 149.

Stanley HR, Alattar M, Collett WK, et al: Pathological sequelae of "neglected" impacted third molars, J Oral Pathol 17:113-117, 1988.

Stanley HR and Diehl DL: Ameloblastoma potential of follicular cysts, Oral Surg 20:260-268, 1965.

Struthers P and Shear M: Root resorption by ameloblastomas and cysts of the jaws, Int J Oral Surg 5:128-132, 1976.

Takagi M: Adenomatoid ameloblastoma: an analysis of nine cases by histopathological and electron microscopic study, Bull Tokyo Med Dent Univ 14:487, 1967.

Trodahl JN: Ameloblastic fibroma, a survey of cases from the Armed Forces Institute of Pathology, Oral Surg 33:547-558, 1972.

Vickers RA and Gorlin RJ: Ameloblastoma: delineation of early histologic features of neoplasia, Cancer 26:699-710, 1970.

Worth HM: Principles and practice of oral radiologic interpretation, Chicago, 1963, Year Book Medical Publishers, Inc., p 76.

Zallen RD, Preskar MH, and McClary SA: Ameloblastic fibroma, J Oral Maxillofac Surg 40:513-517, 1982.

18

Interradicular radiolucencies

NORMAN K. WOOD
CHARLES G. BAKER

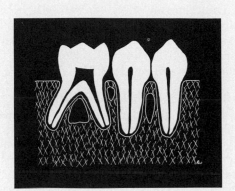

In this chapter the following interradicular radiolucencies are presented:

Anatomic radiolucencies
Primary tooth crypt
Mental foramen and mental canal
Maxillary sinus
Incisive foramen
Lateral fossa
Bone marrow pattern
Nutrient canal

Pathologic radiolucencies
Periodontal pocket (bony)
Furcation involvement
Lateral radicular cyst
Traumatic bone cyst
Primordial cyst
Other odontogenic cysts
Odontogenic tumors
Globulomaxillary radiolucencies
Incisive canal cyst
Malignancies
Lateral (inflammatory) periodontal cyst
Lateral (developmental) periodontal cyst
Benign nonodontogenic tumors and tumorlike
  conditions
Median mandibular cyst

Rarities
Buccal cyst
Histiocytosis X
Osteoradionecrosis
Paradental cyst

Interradicular radiolucencies, as the name and introductory drawing imply, are radiolucencies that occur between the roots of teeth. The most common are the harmless anatomic radiolucent shadows that may occur in this location and are usually readily recognizable. Logic dictates that the majority of actual lesions in this location be related to teeth or odontogenesis or are tumors of odontogenic tissue; in practice this proves to be true. A third group comprises lesions that could develop anywhere in the skeleton but by chance occur occasionally in the alveolar bone between the roots of teeth; neurofibroma is an example of this type of lesion.

ANATOMIC RADIOLUCENCIES

Some of the anatomic radiolucencies seen in films of the jawbone, described in detail in Chapter 15, may occur between the roots of teeth (Fig. 18-1).

Radiolucent *primary tooth crypts* are normal structures seen as radiolucencies of young children. The interradicular ones represent the developing premolars and are located between or among the roots of the deciduous molar teeth at approximately 2 years of age (Fig. 18-1).

The *mental foramen* is seen as a small roundish radiolucency in the periapices of the mandibular premolar teeth. Occasionally it occurs between the roots of these teeth, and occasionally the bandlike radiolucency of the mental canal is also observed.

The shadow of the *maxillary sinus* has many variations. In some individuals it dips down between the molar roots (Fig. 18-1). Its configuration usually is bilaterally similar. In unusual circumstances a small buccal outpouching of the sinus wall shows as a cystlike radiolucency between the tooth roots.

The shadow of the *incisive foramen* is prominent in some individuals and faint in others. When present it usually projects as a well-defined contoured radiolucency between the roots of the central incisors in the midline (Fig. 18-1). Its superior or inferior position is influenced by the degree of vertical angulation at which the radiograph was taken.

The *lateral fossa* is the vertical depression often present in the labial alveolar plate between the lateral incisor and canine teeth. This narrowing of the alveolus, which produces a definite radiolucency in this region (see Fig. 18-9), is discussed in this chapter with the globulomaxillary shadows. Such a normal narrowing of the alveolus may occur in other interradicular sites also.

Bone marrow patterns in the mandible are prominent in some individuals and nondescript in others. In the former instance variously shaped radiolucent patterns are dispersed throughout the alveolar and basal bone; some occur interradicularly and are recognizable by the characteristic patterns seen throughout the mandibular films (see Fig. 18-3).

Nutrient canals are obvious in the mandibular periapical radiographs of some individuals. In radiographs of dentate persons these are seen as vertical, narrow, bandlike radiolucencies running between the teeth (Fig. 18-1) and sometimes to the apices of the teeth. Occasionally, when the x-ray beam is directed to the long axis of the particular canal (Fig. 18-1), a nutrient canal is seen as a small "worm hole."

PERIODONTAL POCKETS

Periodontal bone loss of the horizontal variety produces familiar changes on periapical films. In cases of intrabony pockets or vertical bone loss that occurs locally on the mesial or distal aspect of a tooth, the resultant radiolucency is interradicular but closer to the involved tooth contacting its surface (Fig. 18-2, A). The relatively straightforward diagnosis in such cases is established by placing a periodontal probe into the defect. In cases of severe bone loss the radiolucency completely surrounds the root (Fig. 18-2, B).

FURCATION INVOLVEMENT

Advanced periodontal disease frequently produces furcation involvement. The defect is easily detected, particularly in films of mandibular molars, since the bifurcation is devoid of bone and shows as a radiolucency (Fig. 18-3). Usually a periodontal probe can be maneuvered into bifurcation defects from either the buccal or the lingual aspect. Two entities may mimic this condition: (1) a bone marrow space in the bifurcation (Fig. 18-3) and (2) *endodontic involvement* with rarefying osteitis in the bifurcation area as a result of an accessory canal connecting the floor of the pulp chamber to the bifurcation. (Vertucci and Anthony [1986] showed that a significant number of molar teeth have this particular accessory canal.) In these two cases the clinician is usually unable to enter the bifurcation with a probe. In the case of the bone marrow pattern the lamina dura remains unchanged over the bone in the bifurcation area but is absent in periodontal disease and in the pulp-related rarefying osteitis. In the case of the rarefying osteitis of endodontic origin, the pulp gives abnormal readings to pulp testing. Occasionally, tooth fractures also produce rarefying osteitis in the furcation region (Fig. 18-3).

LATERAL RADICULAR CYST

The radicular cyst is discussed in detail as a periapical radiolucency in Chapter 16. Associated teeth have nonvital pulps, and lateral radicular cysts may occur when a sizable accessory canal opens to the lateral root surface (Fig.

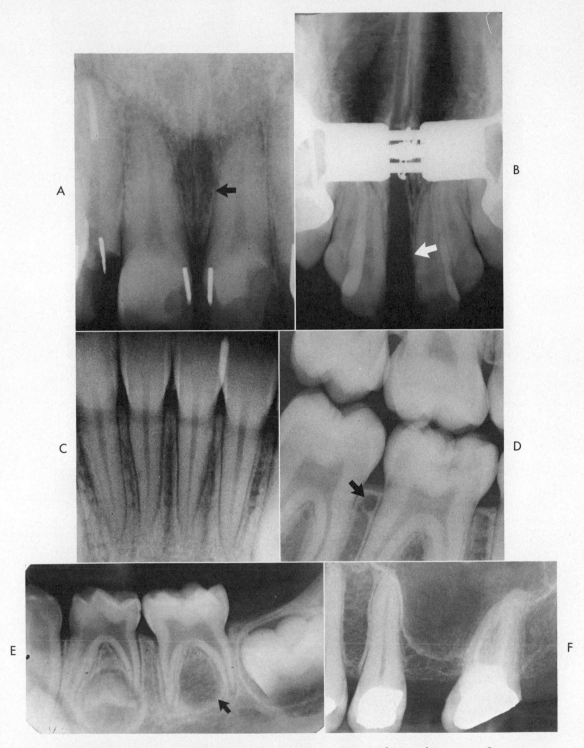

Fig. 18-1. Anatomic interradicular radiolucencies. **A,** Arrow indicates the incisive foramen. Vertical radiolucent line is the midline suture. **B,** Marked widening of the midline suture (*arrow*) is a result of an orthodontic appliance. **C,** Vertical radiolucent lines in several interradicular areas represent nutrient canals. **D,** Near the alveolar crest the arrow shows a "worm hole" radiolucency that is a nutrient canal running parallel to the direction of the x rays. **E,** Radiolucent tooth crypt of a second premolar tooth (*arrow*) between the roots of the primary deciduous molar tooth. **F,** Radiolucent shadow of a maxillary sinus extending down between the molar and premolar teeth.

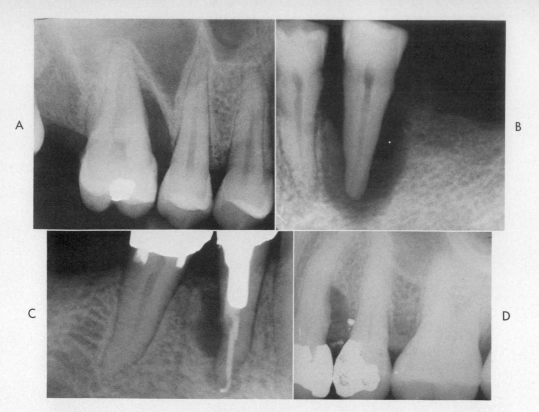

Fig. 18-2. Periodontal bone loss. **A,** Deep intrabony pocket on the mesial side of the first molar. **B,** Extensive periodontal bone loss associated with a premolar tooth. **C,** Root fracture with distal bone destruction. **D,** Periodontal bone destruction distal to the root of the first premolar tooth is a reaction to amalgam.

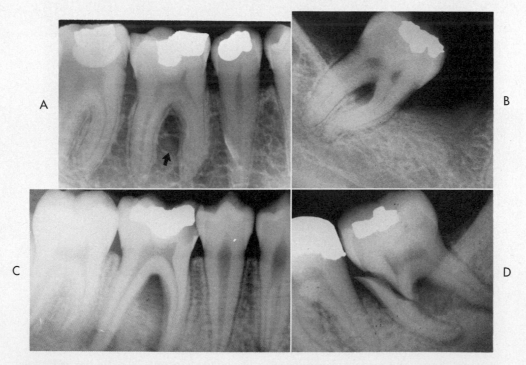

Fig. 18-3. Furcation involvement. **A,** Prominent bone marrow pattern *(arrow)*. **B,** Periodontal involvement of a molar bifurcation. **C,** Bone destruction in bifurcation associated with the first molar caused by pulp disease. **D,** Bone destruction in bifurcation of the second molar caused by tooth fracture.

18-4). An early small cyst is seen to be restricted to a small area of the interradicular bone adjacent to the root surface. In larger cysts the thickness of interseptal bone is destroyed and it may be more difficult to make the diagnosis or to identify which is the offending tooth. When the cyst becomes infected, pain and swelling occur and the offending tooth or both teeth may become sensitive to percussion.

TRAUMATIC BONE CYST

The traumatic bone cyst (TBC) is discussed in detail as a cystlike radiolucency not contacting teeth in Chapter 19. Characteristically the TBC primarily involves the bone inferior to the apices of the mandibular premolars and first molar and may extend superiorly into the area between the roots of these teeth. In unusual cases, when the primary involvement is in the interradicular bone (Fig. 18-5), there may be very little classic destruction of the bone just inferior to the apices. These interradicular radiolucencies are more oval or slitlike and are not as round as the lateral radicular cyst or the lateral periodontal cyst. The traumatic bone cyst occurs primarily in the tooth-bearing region of mandibles in people under 30 years of age.

PRIMORDIAL CYST

Discussed in Chapter 19 as cystlike radiolucencies not contacting teeth, primordial cysts may occur interradicularly in a region where a tooth may have failed to develop.

OTHER ODONTOGENIC CYSTS

Almost any of the other odontogenic cysts can involve the interradicular region occasionally. The dentigerous cyst is an example, but its pericoronal location usually aids in its recognition (Fig. 18-6).

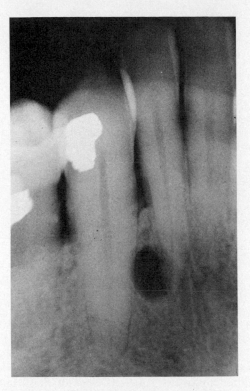

Fig. 18-4. Lateral radicular cyst involved with a nonvital canine tooth with a lateral canal.

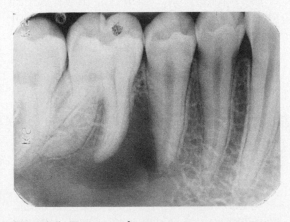

Fig. 18-5. Traumatic bone cyst in a young patient with extensive interradicular involvement between the molar and second premolar roots.

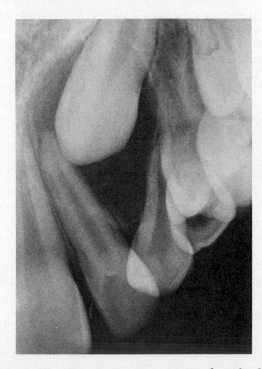

Fig. 18-6. Dentigerous cyst associated with the crown of a permanent canine tooth, which appears as an interradicular radiolucency.

ODONTOGENIC TUMORS

Odontomas, by far the most common odontogenic tumors, in almost all cases involve at least a portion of the alveolar bone. Thus they frequently occur as interradicular lesions (Fig. 18-7). They are seldom seen in their completely radiolucent stage; small odontomas in the radiolucent stage are cystlike with a well-defined border, and foci of mineralization soon begin to appear within the radiolucency in subsequent radiographs.

Ameloblastomas have been discussed in Chapter 19 as cystlike radiolucencies and in Chapter 20 as multilocular radiolucencies. They can originate in the interradicular bone and so in the early stage mimic many of the other lesions discussed in this chapter (Fig. 18-8).

GLOBULOMAXILLARY RADIOLUCENCIES
Globulomaxillary cyst

The origin of the epithelial nests that form the globulomaxillary cyst is a matter of dispute (Christ, 1970; Little and Jakobsen, 1973). Some pathologists favor the theory that epithelial nests are left in the fusion line between the embryonic maxillary processes. Others believe that these primitive processes merge rather than fuse, and since there is no fusion line, there cannot be nests of epithelium entrapped.

Most recent embryonic studies have illustrated, however, that both mechanisms (fusion and merging) are involved and that epithelial nests could easily be trapped in the bottom of the grooves during obliteration of the nests by the merging processes. Another reasonable school of thought holds that globulomaxillary cysts are really primordial cysts that have occurred in supernumerary tooth buds in the area.

To further complicate the issue, many radicular cysts positioned between the lateral incisor and the canine have been misdiagnosed as globulomaxillary cysts. It is therefore important that the vitality of adjacent teeth be ensured before the diagnosis of globulomaxillary cyst is made. This rules out the possibility that the cyst is pulpal in origin. Wysocki (1981) stated that if true globulomaxillary cysts occur at all, they must be very rare. Hollingshead and Schneider (1980) went even further, advising that the use of the term be discontinued.

The classic radiographic picture is of a more or less inverted pear-shaped or tear-shaped, well-defined radiolucency between the roots of the lateral incisor and canine (see Fig. 18-10).

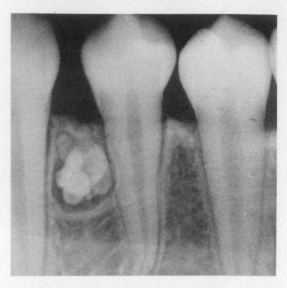

Fig. 18-7. Complex odontoma in an interradicular position. In its premineralization stages this would have appeared as a radiolucency.

Furthermore, a careful examination of the radiograph discloses that the lamina dura around the roots of both teeth is intact.

FEATURES

The globulomaxillary cyst (if it occurs at all) is asymptomatic and discovered on routine radiographic examination. As it becomes larger and expands the cortical plate buccally, the patient may complain of swelling or of pain, especially if it becomes secondarily infected. The astute examiner notices that the contact point between the lateral incisor and canine has shifted toward the incisal edges of these teeth because of rotation of the crowns by the spreading roots. The mucosa over the buccal swelling is normal in appearance, and palpation of the surface produces crepitus if the cortical plate is still intact but fluctuance if not. Aspiration often yields typical amber-colored cyst fluid. The microscopic picture is similar to that of other cysts. Hollingshead and Schneider (1980) did a thorough histologic and embryologic analysis of so-called globulomaxillary cysts.

DIFFERENTIAL DIAGNOSIS

When an inverted tear-shaped radiolucency is found on the radiographs of a patient, the clinician must be especially careful not to make an impulsive diagnosis.

An *odontogenic cyst,* a *giant cell granuloma,* an *adenomatoid odontogenic tumor, surgical*

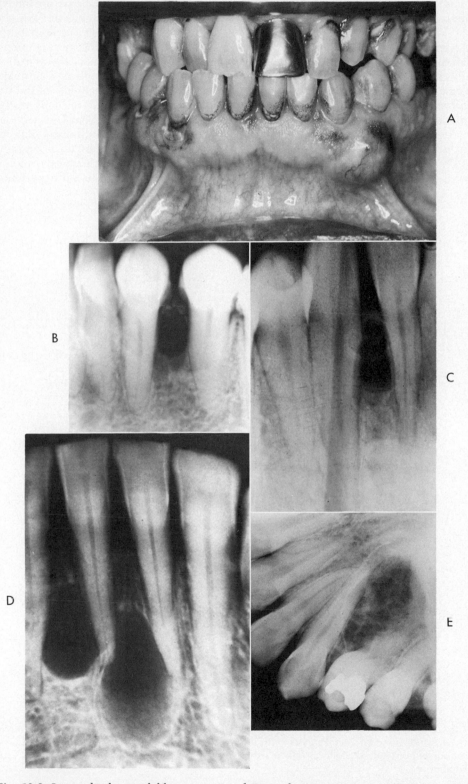

Fig. 18-8. Interradicular ameloblastomas. **A** and **B** are the same patient.   (**C** courtesy M. Wolfe, DDS, Chicago. **D** courtesy of K. Tsiklakis, DDS, Athens, Greece.)

defects, *myxomas, anterior bony clefts,* and especially *anatomic variations* have masqueraded as a globulomaxillary cyst (Figs. 18-9 and 18-10).

If the clinician finds an amber-colored fluid on aspiration, he or she can be reasonably sure that the lesion is a *cyst,* although there is a remote chance that the lesion is a *mural* or *cystic ameloblastoma.*

Having determined a working diagnosis of cyst, the clinician must establish whether it is a *radicular lateral periodontal* or a *globulomaxillary cyst.* This distinction must be made before treatment is initiated because the root canals of the involved teeth have to be treated and filled before surgery if the pulps are nonvital. Pulp vitality tests aid in establishing whether the radiolucency is a sequela of a nonvital pulp.

In our experience the most common cause of a radiolucency between the maxillary canine and lateral incisor tooth is a normal anatomic depression in the labial plate of the lateral fossa in this region (Fig. 18-9). This trough can be readily identified by visual inspection and also by palpation. In contradistinction almost all pathologic bony lesions do not produce a depression but expand the jaws as soon as growth is sufficient to do so. In our experience the sec-

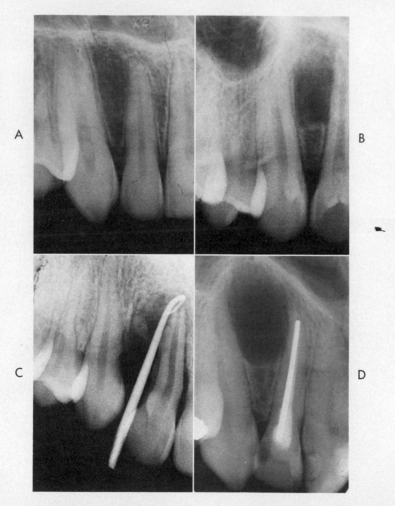

Fig. 18-9. Globulomaxillary radiolucencies. **A,** Shadow of a lateral fossa. **B,** Lateral rarefying osteitis in a nonvital lateral incisor with dens in dente. **C,** Chronic alveolar abscess. Lateral incisor is nonvital. **D,** Lateral radicular cyst from the lateral canal of a lateral incisor, after treatment.

ond most common cause of radiolucencies is pulpopcriapical lesions perhaps positioned laterally because of the presence of lateral canals. Zegarelli and Zegarelli (1973) have published a worthwhile paper on radiolucent lesions in the globulomaxillary region as have Taicher and Azaz (1977). In 1981 Wysocki published an excellent paper on "differential diagnosis of globulomaxillary radiolucencies." Dunlop and Barker (1980) described an interesting case of myospherulosis in this region.

MANAGEMENT

The management of this cyst is identical to that described for other bony cysts in Chapters 16 and 17. Special care must be taken during surgery to avoid devitalizing the adjacent teeth. As with other cysts, the lining must be carefully investigated to ascertain that no mural tumors are present. The surgical site must be observed radiographically until the defect has completely resolved or until time has lessened concern for recurrence.

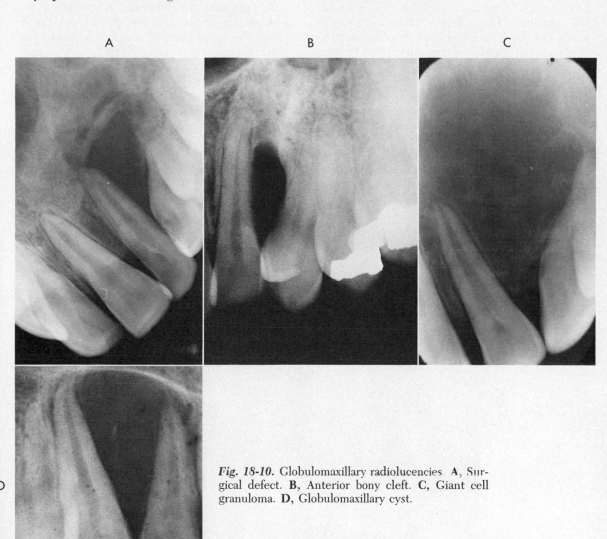

Fig. 18-10. Globulomaxillary radiolucencies **A,** Surgical defect. **B,** Anterior bony cleft. **C,** Giant cell granuloma. **D,** Globulomaxillary cyst.

INCISIVE CANAL CYST

Cysts of the incisive canal and of the palatine papilla are subclassifications of nasopalatine cysts originating in nests of epithelium that remain after the disintegration of the nasopalatine duct, an early epithelial fetal structure that is present in the area of the incisive canal (Fig. 18-11).

This bilateral epithelium-lined duct structure runs superiorly through the incisive canal area to become Jacobson's organ, which is bilaterally positioned on the lateral aspects of the nasal septum. These lateral structures disintegrate in later fetal life, but nests of epithelium remain and are sometimes stimulated to produce cysts of the incisive canal and palatine papilla. Bodin et al. (1986) reported their findings of nasopalatine duct cysts in seven patients.

The incisive canal cyst is situated within bone and thus shows as a cystlike radiolucent enlargement of the canal (Fig. 18-11). It is the most common nonodontogenic cyst of the maxilla and is reported to occur in one of every 100 persons. A cyst of the palatine papilla is located in soft tissue, so it usually does not produce a radiolucency.

Features

The incisive canal cyst is evident as a cystlike radiolucency on occlusal and periapical radiographs of the maxillary central incisor area (Fig. 18-11). Frequently its image is projected over the apices of the central incisors and must be differentiated from a radicular cyst. Often the anterior nasal spine is seen over the superior portion of the cyst as a radiopaque shadow, thus producing a heart-shaped radiolucency (Fig. 18-11).

On occasion, the cyst forms in a superior aspect of one of the incisive canals at a point where the canals are discernibly separate, in which case it is positioned slightly to one side of the midline and the displacement is perceptible on radiographs. Sometimes two separate cysts develop simultaneously in the left and right branches of the canal and cause paired cystlike radiolucencies. The appearance of separate cysts, however, may be an illusion resulting from a cyst at the juncture of canals extending superiorly into the separate branches of the incisive canal.

A cyst of the palatine papilla may be evident on clinical examination as a nodular fluctuant

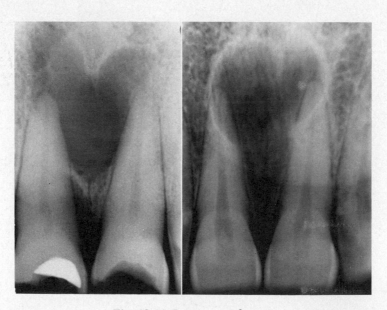

Fig. 18-11. Incisive canal cysts.

mass involving the area of the papilla, but it is not demonstrable on radiographs, since it is primarily of soft tissue and extends into the soft tissue more readily than into bone; bony destruction in the incisive foramen therefore does not usually result. On occasion, however, an incisive canal cyst at the oral limits of the bony canal bulges out of the canal into the soft tissue papilla and produces a nodular swelling that appears on clinical examination to be a cyst of the palatine papilla but can be correctly recognized from the obvious bony destruction that is apparent on the radiograph. A cyst in the canal may also erode the bone posterior to the canal, bulge into the mucosa posterior to the papilla, and create the clinical impression of a midpalatal cyst.

The majority of incisive canal cysts are small, asymptomatic, and found on routine radiographic surveys. Frequently the patient complains of a salty taste in the mouth, produced by a small sinus or a remnant of the nasopalatine duct that permits cystic fluid to drain into the oral cavity. Besides drainage, a feeling of fullness and a burning and numbness of the palatal mucosa over the papilla are frequent complaints.

When a sinus is not present and the cyst slowly enlarges, the patient usually observes a palatal swelling just posterior to the maxillary central incisors. This swelling becomes painful if it is in a position that permits it to be traumatized during mastication or if it becomes secondarily infected. The swelling becomes fluctuant as soon as it projects through the bone. Aspiration may yield the typical amber-colored fluid. On occasion, a very large cyst is seen to produce an obvious facial swelling in the region of the philtrum-lip junction.

Other cysts may bulge into the nasal cavity and extend so far posteriorly as to appear to be midline cysts of the palate.

The microscopic structure of the incisive canal cyst is similar to that of other cysts, although the epithelium lining the lumen is occasionally of the respiratory type and mucous glands are frequently present in the cyst wall.

Differential diagnosis

Several types of cysts may occur in the anterior maxillary region and be projected over the apices of the incisors. Also it is important to be aware that the incisive canal and foramen may normally vary greatly in size. Consequently the clinician may have some difficulty distinguishing between a large incisive foramen and a small asymptomatic incisive canal cyst on the basis of radiographic evidence alone. Some clinicians follow the rule of thumb that radiolucencies of the incisive canal measuring less than 0.6 cm in diameter should not be considered cystic in the absence of other symptoms.

A diagnostic problem frequently arises when a cystlike radiolucency is projected over the apex of a maxillary central incisor. The clinician must distinguish whether this is an incisive canal cyst or a radicular cyst (Fig. 18-11).

If the lesion is an *incisive canal cyst*, the radiolucency in many instances may be projected away from the apex of the tooth in question by changing the horizontal angulation of the x-ray tube. Also if the pulps prove to be vital, the possibility of a *radicular cyst* is eliminated.

When an *incisive canal cyst* has reached large proportions and extended posteriorly, destroying most of the hard palate, or has contacted and perhaps resorbed the roots of the incisors, the correct diagnosis often proves difficult. In such situations the lesion may be confused with a *midline palatal cyst* or a *radicular cyst*, respectively.

Occasionally a *primordial cyst*, arising in a supernumerary tooth bud, occurs in the midline and must be differentiated from a radicular and an incisive canal cyst. Radiographs taken at different angles and vitality tests of the adjacent teeth aid in making the distinction.

Some older texts describe a *midalveolar cyst* that was thought to occur in the anterior midline and to arise from epithelial remnants left in the midfusion line of the median nasal process. Clearly, however, the median nasal process is not a paired structure, so it does not have a fusion line. These cysts were most likely examples of primordial cysts.

Management

Surgical excision is the treatment of choice for small incisive canal cysts; if possible, the defect should be entered from the palate to avoid devitalization of the adjacent incisor teeth. The nasopalatine nerve is frequently severed during surgery, and as a result the small patch of mucosa surrounding the incisive papilla and including the lingual incisive gingivae is numb for some time. Because the nasopalatine nerve innervates such a small area of palatal mucosa, numbness in the area is readily accepted by the patient, especially if he or she is informed of this possibility before surgery.

Occasionally large cysts have been treated by marsupialization.

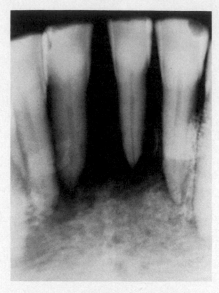

Fig. 18-12. Metastatic carcinoma.

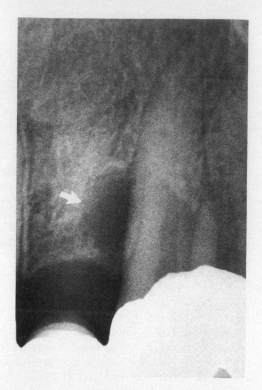

Fig. 18-13. Lateral (inflammatory) periodontal cyst (*arrow*).

MALIGNANCIES

Malignancies can begin in the interseptal bone and usually present as radiolucencies with poorly marginated borders (Fig. 18-12). Further, malignancies that involve the periodontal ligament early in their development characteristically produce a bandlike widening of the periodontal ligament image. These features are described in detail in Chapter 21.

LATERAL (INFLAMMATORY) PERIODONTAL CYST

Lateral (inflammatory) periodontal cysts are cysts that occur in the periodontal ligament, usually near the alveolar crest. They are thought to arise as the result of periodontal disease and can affect any tooth. Pocket contents may be the irritant that stimulates adjacent rests of Malassez in the periodontal ligament. Fig. 18-13 illustrates a case in a periapical film. These cysts must be distinguished from lateral (developmental) periodontal cysts (Killey et al., 1977), which are next described.

LATERAL (DEVELOPMENTAL) PERIODONTAL CYST

The lateral (developmental) periodontal cyst is an unusual odontogenic cyst whose cause is unclear. These cysts occur in an interradicular position and have a high predilection for the mandibular premolar region (Fig. 18-14). The adjacent teeth have vital pulps. On radiographic examination these small to medium-sized cysts are round to oval and usually have a well-marginated, often hyperostotic border. Some authors include the botryoid odontogenic cyst as an example of the lateral periodontal cyst (Phelan et al., 1988).

Theories of the formation and development of the cyst hold that it results from (1) an early dentigerous cyst left in place after eruption of the tooth, (2) a primordial cyst, (3) the rests of Malassez in the periodontal ligament, and (4) remnants of the dental lamina (Wysocki et al., 1980). These authors discussed the microscopic characteristics of this cyst and its many similarities to the gingival cyst of the adult.

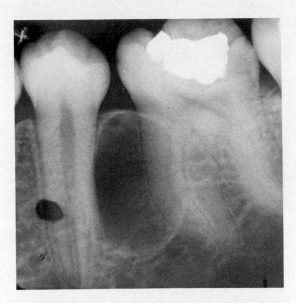

Fig. 18-14. Lateral (developmental) periodontal cyst.

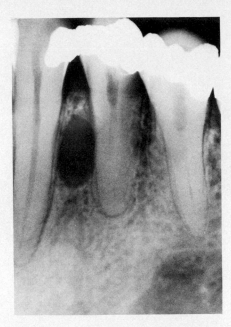

Fig. 18-15. Neurilemoma. (From Morgan G and Morgan P: Oral Surg 25:182-189, 1968).

Entities among those to be considered in the differential diagnosis are the lateral radicular cyst, lateral (inflammatory) periodontal cyst, radiolucent odontogenic tumors, and benign mesenchymal tumors.

Management

Management involves surgical enucleation and microscopic study of the specimen. Care should be taken to preserve teeth if possible.

BENIGN NONODONTOGENIC TUMORS AND TUMORLIKE CONDITIONS

Any benign tumor of the tissues found within bone may occur and characteristically appear as a smoothly contoured, well-defined radiolucency much like a cyst (Fig. 18-15). These tumors or tumorlike conditions occur uncommonly in the jaw bone and less commonly in the interradicular region.

MEDIAN MANDIBULAR CYST

The median mandibular cyst occurs in the symphyseal region of the lower jaw. It is uncommon, and its origin is in dispute. Some authorities contend that it is a true fissural cyst originating from epithelium trapped in the fusion or merging of the paired mandibular processes during the fourth week of embryonic life; others suggest that it probably represents a primordial cyst that formed in a supernumerary tooth bud; others favor a theory of developmental origin with nests of odontogenic epithelium from the dental lamina (Tenaca et al., 1985); still others raise the possibility that it may be a lateral periodontal cyst developing on the medial aspect of the central incisors (DiFiore and Hartwell, 1987). Soskolne and Shteyer (1977) discussed these possibilities in detail. Nanavati and Gandhi (1979) detailed five criteria that they thought should be fulfilled before identifying a lesion as a median mandibular cyst. Rapidis and Langdon (1982) were of the opinion that this is not a true clinical entity.

Research techniques have not yet been sufficiently refined to demonstrate the genesis of this cyst in all cases. Certainly, though, if the central incisors adjacent to a median mandibular cyst are nonvital, it is reasonable to conclude that the particular example is a radicular cyst; conversely, if the teeth are vital, a radicular cyst can reasonably be eliminated from consideration.

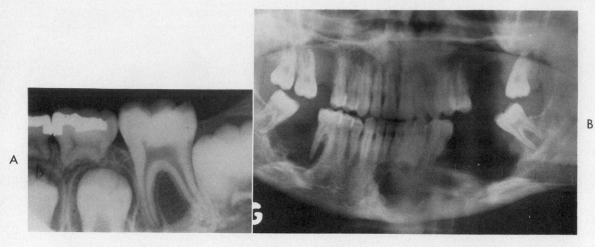

Fig. 18-16. A, Buccal cyst. **B,** Eosinophilic granulomas in all four quadrants.

RARITIES

Rare entities that can occur interradicularly are the adenomatoid odontogenic tumor, buccal cyst, histiocytosis X, osteoradionecrosis, and paradental cyst (Fig. 18-16). Other, more common entities such as giant cell granulomas may rarely appear primarily as interradicular radiolucencies (Fig. 18-17).

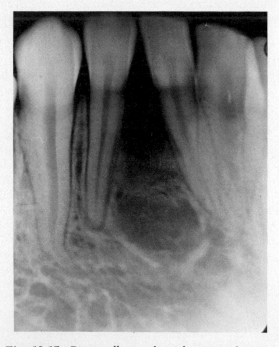

Fig. 18-17. Giant cell granuloma between the central incisors.

REFERENCES

Bodin I, Isacsson G, and Julin P: Cysts of the nasopalatine duct, Int J Oral Maxillofac Surg 15:696-706, 1986.

Christ TF: The globulomaxillary cyst: an embryonic misconception, Oral Surg 30:515-526, 1970.

DiFiore PM and Hartwell GR: Median mandibular lateral periodontal cyst, Oral Surg 63:545-550, 1987.

Dunlap CL and Barker BF: Myospherulosis of the jaws, Oral Surg 50:238-243, 1980.

Hollingshead MB and Schneider LC: A histologic and embryologic analysis of so-called globulomaxillary cysts, Int J Oral Surg 9:281-286, 1980.

Killey HC, Kay LW, and Seward GR: Benign cystic lesions of the jaws: their diagnosis and treatment, Edinburgh, 1977, Churchill Livingstone, Inc.

Little JW and Jakobsen J: Origin of the globulomaxillary cyst, J Oral Surg 31:188-195, 1973.

Nanavati SD and Gandhi PP: Median mandibular cyst, J Oral Surg 37:422-425, 1979.

Phelan JA, Kritchman D, Fusco-Ramer M, et al: Recurrent botryoid odontogenic cyst (lateral periodontal cyst), Oral Surg 66:345-348, 1988.

Rapidis AD and Langdon JD: Median cysts of the jaws—not a true clinical entity, Int J Oral Surg 11:360-363, 1982.

Soskolne WA and Shteyer A: Median mandibular cyst, Oral Surg 44:84-88, 1977.

Taicher S and Azaz B: Lesions resembling globulomaxillary cysts, Oral Surg 44:25-29, 1977.

Tenaca JI, Giunta JL, and Norris LH: The median mandibular cyst and its endodontic significance, Oral Surg 60:316-321, 1985.

Vertucci FJ and Anthony RL: A scanning electron microscopic investigation of accessory foramina in the furcation and pulp chamber floor of molar teeth, Oral Surg 62:319-326, 1986.

Wysocki GP: The differential diagnosis of globulomaxillary radiolucencies, Oral Surg 51:281-286, 1981.

Wysocki GP, Brannon RB, Gardner DG, et al: Histogenesis of the lateral periodontal cyst and the gingival cyst of the adult, Oral Surg 50:327-334, 1980.

Zegarelli DJ and Zegarelli EV: Radiolucent lesions in the globulomaxillary region, J Oral Surg 31:767-771, 1973.

19

Solitary cystlike radiolucencies not necessarily contacting teeth

NORMAN K. WOOD
PAUL W. GOAZ

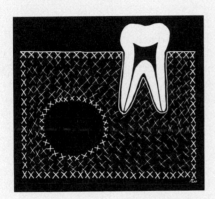

In this chapter the cystlike radiolucencies that usually do not involve the teeth are presented:

Anatomic patterns
  Marrow spaces
  Maxillary sinus
  Early stage of tooth
   crypts
  Mandibular foramen
  Median sigmoid
   depression
Postextraction socket
Residual cyst
Traumatic bone cyst
Primordial cyst
Lingual mandibular bone
 defect
Odontogenic keratocyst
Ameloblastoma
Hematopoietic defect of the
 jaws
Surgical defect
Giant cell granuloma
Giant cell lesion
 (hyperparathyroidism)
Incisive canal cyst
 Midpalatal cyst
Cementifying and ossifying
 fibromas (early stage)
Benign nonodontogenic
 tumors
Rarities
 Adenomatoid odontogenic
  tumors
 Ameloblastic variants
 Aneurysmal bone cyst
 Aneurysms in bone

Arteriovenous
 malformation in bone
Artifact
Calcifying epithelial
 odontogenic tumor
Calcifying odontogenic cyst
Cementoma
Central fibroma
Central hemangioma of
 bone
Central squamous cell
 carcinoma in cyst lining
Desmoplastic fibroma
Hemangioma of bone
Histiocytosis X
Lipoma (intraosseous)
Low-grade metastatic
 carcinoma
Metastatic carcinoma
Minor salivary gland
 tumor in bone
Myospherulosis
 (paraffinoma)
Myxoma
Odontogenic fibroma
Odontoma (early stage)
Oral pulse granuloma
Osteoblastoma (early stage)
Postoperative maxillary
 cyst
Plasmacytoma
Squamous odontogenic
 tumor
Unicystic ameloblastoma

The term "cystlike radiolucency" describes a dark radiographic image that is approximately circular in outline and usually smoothly contoured with well-defined borders. On occasion

375

the radiolucency may be somewhat elongated, especially in the horizontal plane, and thus appear more elliptic in shape. The radiolucency is sometimes accentuated by a narrow radiopaque rim that is cast by a thin hyperostotic layer of bone.

When confronted by such radiographic evidence, the unwary, less perceptive clinician is inclined to conclude immediately that he or she has encountered a cyst, thus disregarding the myriad possibilities of the cystlike appearance. This lack of discernment may well precipitate an unpleasant experience if the clinician surgically enters the cystlike radiolucency without conducting a careful examination or developing an adequate differential diagnosis. Such preliminary procedures not only ensure the appropriate therapeutic approach but also help obviate the possibility of an unexpected encounter with any of the potentially dangerous cystlike lesions. This group includes the imposing spectrum of entities from normal anatomic spaces to cysts of various types, benign tumors, ameloblastomas, dangerous intrabony hemangiomas, and malignancies (for example, slow-growing metastatic tumors, squamous cell carcinomas within cysts).

Consequently it cannot be overemphasized that all cystlike radiolucencies in the jaws must be given careful consideration before they are treated.

The radicular, lateral, and follicular cysts are not discussed here but are taken up in other chapters. Some lesions included in this chapter (for example, traumatic bone cysts, early cementomas) also occur as periapical radiolucencies and so are included in Chapter 16, but since these entities also occur with some frequency independent of the roots of teeth, they satisfy the criterion for inclusion in the present chapter.

Cysts, giant cell granulomas, giant cell lesions of hyperparathyroidism, ameloblastomas, aneurysmal bone cysts, myxomas, metastatic carcinomas, and hemangiomas may all have more than one radiographic appearance, so these lesions are also included in other chapters.

Finally, lesions such as metastatic carcinoma are not discussed here but are merely listed in the rarities section because they do not commonly cause a cystlike radiolucency. They are dealt with in other chapters, however, in which their more common appearances are discussed. The characteristic features of the more common solitary cystlike radiolucencies are shown in Table 19-1 (p. 400).

ANATOMIC PATTERNS

The anatomic radiolucencies found in radiographs of the jawbones are discussed in Chapter 15. Consequently consideration of them is restricted here to a brief comment on the four entities: marrow spaces, maxillary sinus, early tooth crypts, and the inferior dental (mandibular) foramen.

Marrow spaces

There is great variation among the patterns of marrow spaces from person to person and also from one jaw to the other in the same person. When marrow spaces occur as larger than normal, somewhat rounded radiolucencies with borders that appear to be hyperostotic and not contacting teeth, they may be mistaken for any of the cystlike radiolucencies included in this chapter (Fig. 19-1). Larger examples may be termed hematopoietic bone marrow defects.

Such unusual marrow space patterns occur more frequently in the mandible; they are seldom seen on radiographs of the maxilla. When the clinician encounters what he or she interprets as an uncommon marrow space pattern, a comparison with the spaces in the same area on the opposite side of the jaw usually shows a similar picture if indeed the clinician is dealing with an anomalous condition. This finding, coupled with an absence of local or systemic symptoms, is usually sufficient to permit the correct diagnosis.

It should be borne in mind, however, that if the contralateral areas being compared are subject to different magnitudes of stress, as might be the case when the occlusion on one side has been altered by the loss of teeth, such a comparison is not valid without some qualification in light of these extenuating circumstances. Furthermore, some abnormal changes in size

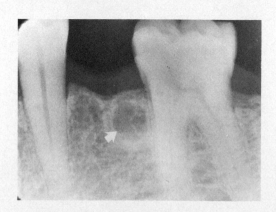

Fig. 19-1. Cystlike marrow space (*arrow*).

of the marrow spaces occur with certain systemic disorders, and these changes are usually bilateral. Thus comparison of contralateral patterns might be misleading.

Nevertheless, if the clinician is in doubt as to the diagnosis, he or she should reexamine the area radiographically at regular intervals to ascertain that it is not enlarging. On the contrary, if symptoms that can be related to the region in question are present, a careful examination and complete differential diagnosis must be formulated and a biopsy of the area performed.

Maxillary sinus

Frequently a cystlike outpouching of the maxillary sinus occurs on a radiograph of an edentulous upper jaw, and this normal variation presents a difficulty in differentiation from a pathologic process (Fig. 19-2). Radiographs of the area taken from different angles (Clark technique), however, often show a connection between such an outpouching and the larger maxillary sinus cavity and resolve the question of identity. Large nutrient canals in the walls of the sinus also contribute to a tentative identification.

Although the maxillary sinuses are frequently asymmetric, comparing their configurations may be helpful in the correct interpretation of a cystlike projection. Again, however, as is true of the changes in marrow space patterns in response to altered function, the sinus may expand and its shape may be altered when stresses are reduced as a result of the loss of maxillary posterior teeth on the corresponding side.

Finally, if the clinician cannot satisfy his or her doubts as to the nature of the structure in question, periodic radiographs demonstrate whether the radiolucency is changing. As a last resort, aspiration of air from the cavity identifies it as the maxillary sinus.

Early stage of tooth crypts

The radiographic picture of a tooth crypt in the early stages of development before calcification is round, smooth, and well defined and has a radiopaque rim identical to that of a cyst (Fig. 19-3).

Since periapical radiographs of younger dentitions are not often made when the developing crypts of the permanent canines and premolars are in the radiolucent stage, these teeth do not usually cause a diagnostic problem. Furthermore, the clinician who is familiar with the chronologic development and calcification of the permanent dentition readily identifies such

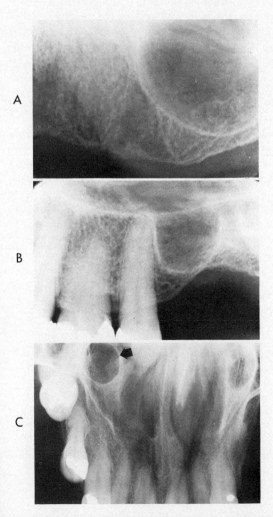

Fig. 19-2. A, Cystlike maxillary sinus. **B,** Cystlike outpouching of the maxillary sinus. **C,** Large nasolacrimal duct *(arrow)*.

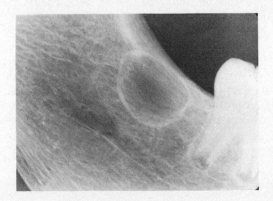

Fig. 19-3. Early molar crypt.

areas as developing tooth crypts and verifies their identity by relating to the contralateral sites in the jaw. Nevertheless, a single tooth may be delayed in its development as compared with the corresponding tooth in the opposite quadrant and may present a diagnostic problem. The diagnosis of primordial cyst is then assigned a high rank in the order of possible entities.

The clinician can differentiate between the two entities (delayed calcification or primordial cyst) by periodically examining the region radiographically for approximately 6 months.* If the radiolucent area is a retarded developing tooth, radiopaque foci representing the initiation of mineralization at the cusp tips are soon found. If no calcification is detected within 6 months to 1 year, the discontinuity in the bone is most likely a primordial cyst that began within the odontogenic epithelium of the tooth bud before calcification was initiated.

Mandibular foramen

The mandibular foramen, which provides the entrance for the inferior dental vessels and nerve into the mandibular canal, is usually apparent on lateral oblique and panoramic views of the jaws. It is located on the medial surface of the ramus at the approximate center and can be readily identified by its position and by the presence of the mandibular canal, which runs anteroinferiorly from it. The mandibular canal, however, may not be radiographically diagnostic; in such instances the round to oval to funnel-shaped radiolucency of the inferior dental foramen may be mistaken for a lesion in the ramus.

As is usual with anatomic structures, however, a comparison with the opposite side aids in making the correct diagnosis. Occasionally the triangular lingula is projected over the shadow of the foramen in such a manner as to give the illusion of a mixed radiolucent-radiopaque lesion.

Median sigmoid depression

The median sigmoid depression is an anatomic radiolucent shadow recognized and described by Langlais et al. (1983). The radiolucent foramen-like shadow is produced by an osseous depression in some mandibles in the me-

dial portion of the ramus just below the sigmoid notch area. The radiolucency may be unilateral or bilateral. Langlais reported that this radiolucency was seen in 10% of panoramic radiographs of patients with 6% occurring unilaterally and 4% bilaterally.

POSTEXTRACTION SOCKET

Sometimes after an extraction the socket resembles a cystlike radiolucency and presents a difficult problem in developing a working diagnosis. This situation usually occurs in edentulous molar areas of the mandible but is also seen in the mandibular incisor region (Fig. 19-4).

Questioning the patient frequently yields the information that there has been a recent extraction in the region, which may be verified by a clinical examination revealing a depressed area on the ridge. Sockets at extraction sites sometimes remain uncalcified for years as unchanging cystlike radiolucencies, but a check of other edentulous areas usually reveals similar-appearing sockets.

In some cases the history of an extraction is of little value to the differential diagnosis, since the patient with a *residual cyst* gives the same history of an extraction from the area.

If the examiner is reasonably certain that a cystlike radiolucency is indeed an old extraction wound, periodic radiographic examination of the area is indicated to confirm this impression. If the clinician has serious doubts as to the true nature of the radiolucency, however, he or she should surgically explore the area and remove tissue for examination, regardless of whether a typical cyst aspirate is obtained.

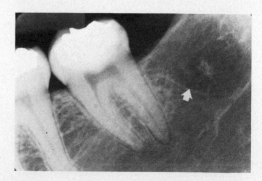

Fig. 19-4. Extraction site *(arrow)* 3 years after tooth's removal.

---

*The alert clinician should consider, however, that occasionally teeth are unusually slow in developing. Cunat and Collard (1973) described premolars that developed 5 to 8 years later than normal.

RESIDUAL CYST

A residual cyst, as the name implies, is a radicular, lateral, or dentigerous cyst that has remained after its associated tooth has been lost. In practice, to determine whether it was present at the time of extraction or developed later in the residual rests of Malassez (residual odontogenic epithelial nests from Hertwig's root sheath) is not possible unless a radiograph showing that it was present before the extraction can be obtained. High and Hirschmann (1988) postulated that low-grade inflammation of the parent cyst (or nest of epithelium) might predispose it to the formation of residual cysts. The residual cyst appears as a rounded radiolucency with well-defined borders (Figs. 19-5 and 19-6).

Sometimes, because of the resistance of the cortical plates, the cyst enlarges in a more elliptic shape. Its borders frequently are accentuated by a thin radiopaque line that is produced by hyperostosis resulting from the minimal pressure of the expanding cyst. There are no radiographic features that permit differentiation between this type of cyst and any of the other lesions included in this chapter.

Features

The residual cyst occurs in the alveolar process and body of the jawbones in edentulous areas, but it may also be found in the lower ra-

mus area. Patients over 20 years of age show the highest incidence of residual cysts, the average age being 52 years. The ratio of men to women is 3:2, and the maxilla is more commonly involved than the mandible (Cabrini et al., 1970). The cyst seldom reaches more than 0.5 cm in diameter but may at certain times be large enough to cause jaw expansion and asymmetry. Its symptoms, clinical characteristics, and histopathologic features are identical to those of the other odontogenic cysts discussed in Chapters 16 and 17. High and Hirschmann (1988) found in their series that nearly half were symptomatic. In an earlier paper (1986) these authors discussed age changes in radicular residual cysts.

Differential diagnosis

All the entities included in this chapter must be considered when a residual cystlike radiolucency is found; however, the *cystlike anatomic patterns, primordial cyst, keratocyst,* and *traumatic bone cyst* are the entities most likely to cause confusion. Kaneshiro et al. (1981) described a maxillary cyst that occurs with significant frequency 10 to 30 years after surgical intervention in the maxillary sinus. Such an entity must be differentiated from residual radicular cysts of the posterior maxilla. Differential diagnoses for these entities are given in detail in the discussion of keratocysts (p. 388).

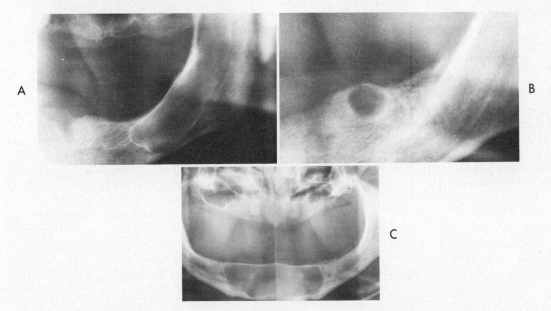

Fig. 19-5. **A** and **B,** Residual cysts. **C,** Midline cyst of the mandible; type not identified (could be a residual, primordial, or true midline cyst).   (Courtesy F. Prock, DDS, Joliet, Ill.)

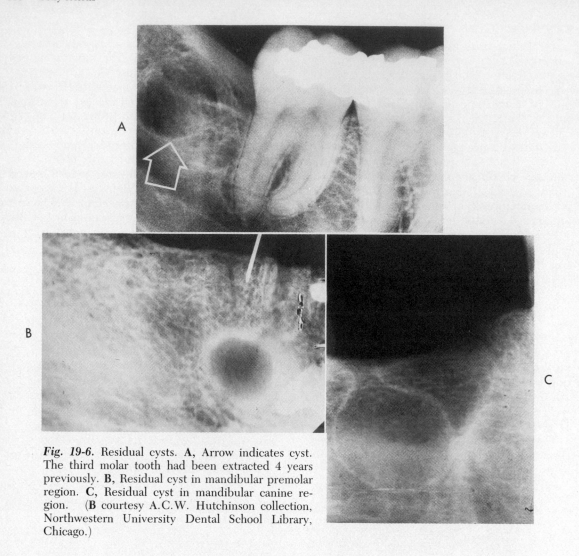

Fig. 19-6. Residual cysts. **A,** Arrow indicates cyst. The third molar tooth had been extracted 4 years previously. **B,** Residual cyst in mandibular premolar region. **C,** Residual cyst in mandibular canine region.   (**B** courtesy A.C.W. Hutchinson collection, Northwestern University Dental School Library, Chicago.)

Management

The treatment of a residual cyst is identical to that of any other intrabony odontogenic cyst except that in these cases the offending teeth have already been lost. Such circumstances as the patient's age and systemic condition and the size of the cyst may prompt the use of one of the following methods in preference to the others:

1. Complete enucleation of the cyst wall with its epithelium and primary closure of the mucoperiosteal flap
2. Complete enucleation of the cyst tissue with the placement of a surgical pack, which is slowly withdrawn as the defect fills in
3. Complete excision and replacement with autogenous particulate bone or a single segment of bone fixed in place

4. Marsupialization
5. Decompression
6. Decompression combined with delayed enucleation

Just before surgical intervention, aspiration of the area with at least an 18-gauge needle is a wise precautionary measure and circumvents the unpleasant surprise of encountering a more serious lesion than the surgeon anticipated (for example, solid tumor, intrabony hemangioma, or aneurysmal bone cyst). High and Hirschmann (1988) postulated that if inflammation is not a feature, these cysts tend to undergo slow resolution.

The management of cysts is discussed more thoroughly in Chapter 16 with the radicular cysts.

TRAUMATIC BONE CYST

The traumatic bone cyst (hemorrhagic bone cyst, extravasation cyst, simple bone cyst, solitary bone cyst, progressive bony cyst, blood cyst) occurs in other bones as well as the jaws and is classified as a false cyst because it does not have an epithelial lining.

A substantial percentage of traumatic bone cysts are found in the inferior portion of the alveolar process adjacent to the apices of teeth, although not actually contacting the apices (as evidenced by an intact lamina dura and the persistence of pulp vitality). Such examples are not discussed further here because they are included in Chapter 16 with the periapical radiolucencies. This ordering was necessary to compare and differentiate them from the periapical radiolucencies, which are sequelae of pulpal involvement. However, occasional examples are associated with retained roots (Cohen, 1984; Shiratsuchi et al., 1987).

On the other hand, the traumatic bone cyst occurs with some frequency in the basal bone of the jaws and may then be clearly seen on radiographs as separate from the apex of the tooth (Figs. 19-7 and 19-8). Thus it is included in this chapter, since it satisfies the criteria for cystlike radiolucencies dissociated from teeth. It is frequently round to oval and, in contrast to cysts in the alveolar bone, has a scalloped superior margin produced by its molding around the roots of the mandibular premolars or molars or both (Figs. 19-7 and 19-8).

The cause of the traumatic bone cyst has not been conclusively established. Some pathologists favor the theory that the lesion is a sequela of a trauma-induced intrabony hematoma. Others believe that it represents a dissipated cyst. Still others contend that it is a cyst whose lining is so membrane thin that the surgeon does not detect it but, nevertheless, the inflammation induced by surgery is sufficient to destroy this epithelial lining and account for the resolution of the lesion. Finally, a theory of tumor degeneration has been proposed.

Features

The traumatic bone cyst is frequently found unexpectedly on routine radiographs. When questioned about the lesion, half the patients give a history of trauma to the region. The cyst is usually totally asymptomatic, pain being experienced by only a few of the patients, and only occasionally does the jaw show regional expansion.

The mandible is involved in the majority of reported cases, with the premolar and molar area, the inferior region of the ramus, and the incisor region being affected in this order of frequency. Paresthesia is not a feature of the entity. The lesion seldom occurs in the maxilla (Winer and Doku, 1978) and seldom in a person over 25 years of age, although Kaugers and Cale (1987) reported that 27% of their 161 patients were over 30 years of age. It is found slightly more frequently in men. Multiple lesions have been reported in the same person (Patrikios et al., 1981). Furthermore, although jaw expansion has been observed in some patients, pathologic fractures have not been reported when expansion has been described. The surface has been smoothly contoured, and the covering mucosa has been normal in appearance.

Kuroi (1980), in an extensive review of the literature, reported the following findings: (1) 63% of the lesions were discovered in patients between 11 and 20 years of age; (2) 59% of patients were male; (3) 61% were asymptomatic; (4) 18% had pain and swelling; (5) a history of trauma was elicited in 54%; (6) frequency of mandibular to maxillary lesions was 6.5 to 1; (7) 94% of the lesions were empty or contained fluid; and (8) 96% had no epithelial lining.

Generally the lesion does not measure more than 3 cm in diameter, but examples have been reported in which there was involvement and expansion of almost the entire ramus and body (Fig. 19-7, C). Narang and Jarrett (1980) described a lesion that extended from the mandibular left molar to the second molar on the right side. Aspiration may yield a little straw-colored or even serosanguineous fluid, although on occasion copious amounts have been reported. Chapman and Romaniuk (1985) reported complete remission of a case following aspiration. Microscopic examination of the lesion usually reveals sparse shreds of fibrous tissue along with small deposits of hemosiderin.

Differential diagnosis

For a discussion of the differential diagnosis of a traumatic bone cyst, refer to the section on the differential diagnosis of keratocysts (p. 388). Fig. 19-8, D, shows an intrabony hemangioma that resembles a traumatic bone cyst.

Management

It is important not to rely on the radiographic image or the usual clinical features to establish a final diagnosis of traumatic bone

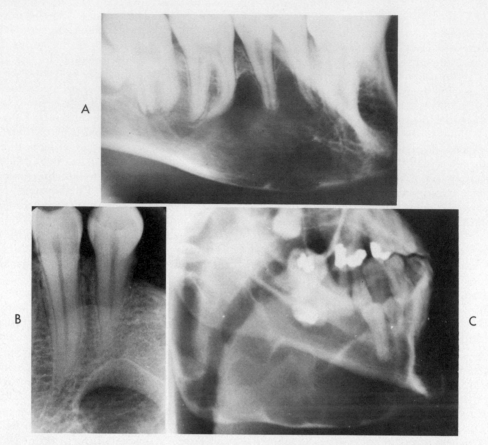

Fig. 19-7. Traumatic bone cyst. **C,** The pseudomultilocular appearance and cortical expansion of this large lesion are evident.   (**A** and **C** courtesy M. Kaminski, DDS, and S. Atsaves, DDS, Chicago. **B** courtesy R. Goepp, DDS, Zoller Clinic, University of Chicago.)

cyst. These radiolucencies of the jaws should be positively identified.

Even after carefully evaluating all the radiographic and clinical evidence obtained from a complete examination, including the results from any indicated laboratory test, the clinician should not conclude that a particular cystlike radiolucency is unquestionably a traumatic bone cyst or another kind of cyst. Before surgically entering any such defect, he or she must rule out by aspirating the area the remote possibility that the lesion could be a dangerous vascular tumor. When the clinician opens the region of a traumatic bone cyst, he or she discovers either an empty bone cavity or, on occasion, a cavity containing some friable loose

brownish material. A thin lining of the bony walls is sometimes observed.

Since this lesion must be surgically explored to ensure the correct diagnosis, the subsequent enucleation and curettement, which produces hemorrhage into the cavity, usually ensures a successful regression of the defect as it is slowly obliterated by bone. The healing period should be closely observed radiographically (Forssell et al., 1988a).

Biewald (1967) reported a different approach that involved injecting the patient's venous blood into the cavity through a small opening. Precious and McFadden (1984) reported using the same technique successfully with a large lesion.

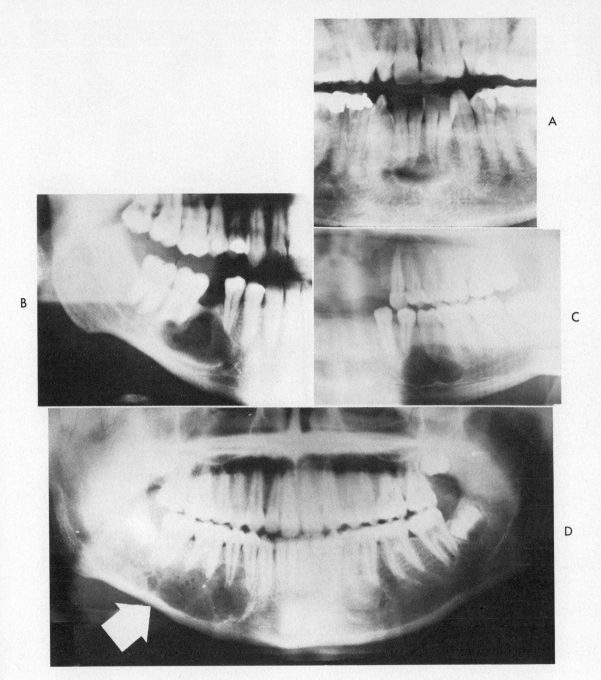

Fig. 19-8. **A** to **C**, Traumatic bone cysts. **A**, Lesion is in the symphysis region, where it has projected over the apices of the incisor teeth. **B**, Lesion is in the first molar region. **C**, Lesion is in the premolar region. **D**, Central cavernous hemangioma of bone, which resembles a traumatic bone cyst (arrow). Note the "worm hole" appearance sometimes seen in bony hemangiomas.   (**A** courtesy P. Akers, DDS, Evanston, Ill. **B** courtesy J. Lehnert, DDS, Minneapolis. **C** courtesy W. Heaton, DDS, Chicago. **D** from Zalesin HM, Rotskoff K, and Silverman H: J Oral Surg 33:877-884, 1975. Copyright by the American Dental Association. Reprinted by permission.)

PRIMORDIAL CYST

A primordial cyst is thought to develop as the result of some influence causing cystic degeneration in the odontogenic epithelium of the tooth germ before mineralization has been initiated. The involved tooth bud may be of either the regular permanent dentition or a supernumerary tooth. The radiographic picture is nonspecific, showing only a cystlike radiolucency.

The patient with a primordial cyst usually has a missing permanent tooth because of failure of the tooth to develop. When a permanent tooth is not missing but the patient shows a tendency to the development of supernumerary teeth, the clinician must consider that a cystlike radiolucency is possibly a primordial cyst developing in the germ of a supernumerary tooth. In practice, however, it is often difficult to establish with certainty whether a particular missing tooth has been extracted, because frequently the tooth (for example, 6-year molar) may have been removed at an early age and the patient failed to realize that a permanent tooth had been lost. Consequently the examiner often must determine the true nature of the situation through an intuitive process involving such considerations as the state of the patient's oral health, the particular permanent teeth missing, and the frequency with which the teeth in question are congenitally absent in the appropriate population.

Features

The primordial cyst shows no sexual predilection and occurs most frequently in patients between the ages of 10 and 30 years. The mandibular molar region, especially the third molar and the area just distal to it, represents the most frequent site of development (Fig. 19-9). These cysts demonstrate all the usual features of cysts and seldom cause cortical expansion. On microscopic examination they are usually keratocysts, which are next discussed. Thus on aspiration the clinician frequently obtains a thick yellowish granular fluid composed primarily of exfoliated cells and keratin.

Differential diagnosis

The differential diagnosis of this lesion is discussed in the section dealing with keratocysts (p. 388).

Management

Because a significant percentage of primordial cysts appear on microscopic examination as odontogenic keratocysts, which have a high re-

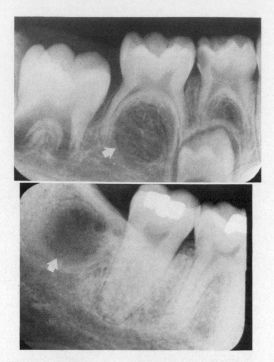

Fig. 19-9. Arrows indicate primordial cysts. The permanent tooth failed to develop in each case.

currence rate, they require more vigorous curettement and vigilant postsurgical attention than do other types of bony cysts. Partridge and Towers (1987) made the point that primordial cysts frequently mimic the behavior of benign tumors.

LINGUAL MANDIBULAR BONE DEFECT (STAFNE'S CYST)

The developmental bone defect of the mandible (known also as static bone cyst or defect, latent bone cyst or defect, idiopathic bone cavity, developmental submandibular gland defect of the mandible, aberrant salivary gland defect in the mandible, and lingual mandibular bone concavity) is a depression in the medial surface of the mandible usually in the third molar–angle area. Azaz and Lustmann (1973), examining dry mandibles, reported that 8% of their specimens had either anterior or posterior lingual depressions (Figs. 19-10 and 19-11).

Because a lobe of the submandibular salivary gland has been found to extend into this bony depression in several cases, the defect is generally believed to be caused by the mandible's developing around the lobe of the gland during embryonic life. Rarely the sublingual gland may produce a similar invagination in the canine and premolar region. Pogrel et al. (1986)

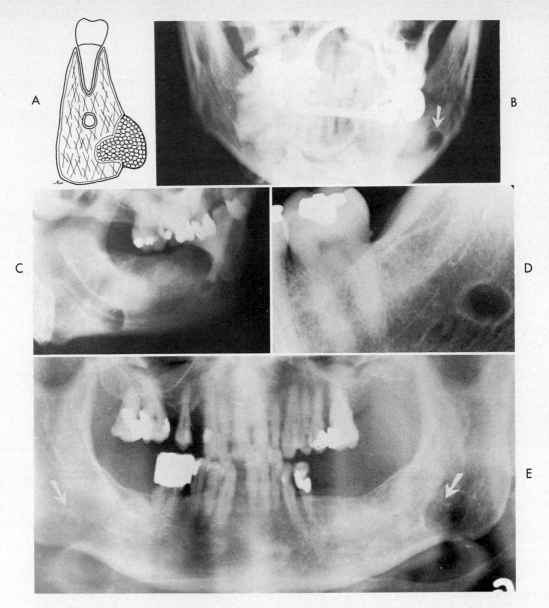

Fig. 19-10. Lingual mandibular bone defects. **A,** Diagram of a cross section of the mandible showing part of the submandibular gland within the defect. **B** to **D,** Radiographs of several different cases. **E,** Bilateral defects. Arrows in *B* and *E* indicate the defects.   (**B** and **C** courtesy O.H. Stuteville, DDS, MD, St. Joe, Ark. **E** courtesy N. Barakat, DDS, Beirut, Lebanon.)

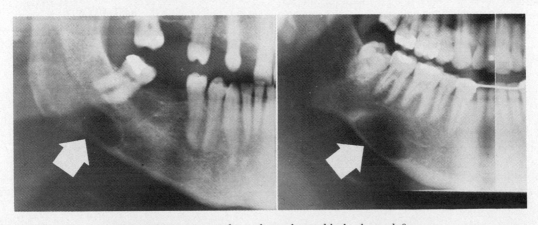

Fig. 19-11. Arrows indicate lingual mandibular bone defects.

reported a case of a defect that contained a lymph node rather than salivary tissue.

In a report of an interesting case, Hansson (1980) described a lingual mandibular bone cavity in an 11-year-old boy. Serial radiographs revealed that the radiolucency appeared in the patient between 11 and 12½ years of age, expanded, and became more prominent during the next 5 years. Wolf et al. (1986) described a lesion in a 36-year-old man that became much more prominent and developed a prominent radiopaque border within the next 8 years.

Features

The pouch extending through the medial plate of the mandible produces a well-circumscribed radiolucency surrounded by a heavy radiopaque border (Fig. 19-10). This border is the result of x rays passing parallel through the relatively greater thickness of cortical bone that makes up the walls of the defect.

The radiolucency may vary from 1 to 2 cm in diameter and be oval, elliptic, round, or semicircular. On occasion the defect is completely enclosed by bone. Bilateral defects have been described (Fig. 19-10).

The developmental bone defect of the mandible is completely asymptomatic and usually found on routine radiographic surveys. It is generally located near the angle of the mandible between the mandibular canal and the inferior border. It does not contact the apices of molars whose pulps are vital unless concomitant caries has produced gangrenous pulps. Statistical reports indicate that it is observed radiographically more frequently in males and occurs in approximately one of every 250 patients. Karmoil and Walsh (1968) and Oikarinen and Julku (1974) reported that all their cases were in males.

Correll et al. (1980) reviewed many lingual mandibular bone defects presented in the literature and reported on their series. They found that the average incidence of this defect in various series of living patients was 0.3%, or one defect for every 312 radiographs. The incidence in their own series was somewhat higher: 0.48%, or one defect for every 208 patients. All of their lesions were found in males. Most of their patients were from a V.A. Medical Center where 96% of the patients were males. Scott et al. (1981) described a defect that was so large that the complete inferior border of the mandible was missing.

Occasionally these defects are located in the anterior portion of the mandible. These are referred to as anterior lingual mandibular bone concavities and are, at least in some cases, associated with the sublingual gland. Connor (1979), Layne et al. (1981), and Hayashi et al. (1984) all reported cases in the anterior region of the mandible in which the radiographic radiolucent shadows were cast over the roots of anterior teeth.

Differential diagnosis

The position and appearance of this radiolucency are all but diagnostic. Occasionally when the defect is small and situated in a more superior position in a region where teeth are present or have only recently been extracted, it may be mistaken for a *radicular* or *residual cyst*. Confusion more frequently occurs with the anterior variety because the entity is often cast over the apices of the teeth (see Fig. 16-30).

Some clinicians use the following procedure to strengthen their impression of developmental bone defect: a curved needle, of approximately 16 gauge for rigidity, is advanced into the tissue either intraorally or extraorally until the medial surface of the mandible is encountered; thus the lingual surface of the mandible can be explored by walking the needle along the surface of the bone; if a recess is found on the medial wall, the diagnosis of developmental bone defect is certain provided all the other findings concur. Also sialography may show the distribution of dye in the radiolucency, since a portion of the submandibular salivary gland usually lies within this bony pocket.

Management

Recognition of this entity is all that is necessary. In our opinion these defects should no longer be surgically explored unless the clinician has reason to suspect a more serious diagnosis. It must not be forgotten, however, that *salivary gland tumors* have been reported to occur within these defects.

ODONTOGENIC KERATOCYST

The odontogenic keratocyst (OKC) has been recognized and classified as distinct from other types of bony cysts on the basis of its somewhat different clinical behavior and its distinct and unique microscopic structure.

The OKC cuts across the usual classification of cysts because its diagnosis depends entirely on its microscopic features and is independent of its location. For example, a primordial cyst, a follicular cyst, or a radicular cyst may prove to be a keratocyst on microscopic examination of the specimen. Interestingly the primordial cyst, the lateral periodontal cyst, and the multiple jaw cysts of the basal cell nevus syndrome are predominantly OKCs. Also a reported 7.8% of all jaw cysts, 8.5% of all dentigerous cysts, and 0.9% of all radicular cysts are OKCs (Payne, 1972). In Shafer's series (1978) 45% of primordial cysts were OKCs.

On radiographic examination the OKC cannot be distinguished from other intrabony cysts. On occasion its lumen, densely filled with keratin, causes the usual radiolucent cystlike image to have a hazy appearance (Fig. 19-12, A). Sometimes it has scalloped borders (Fig. 19-12, B), and it often occurs with a multilocular appearance. Frame and Wake (1982) recommended computerized axial tomography (CAT) to determine the complete extension of the larger cysts.

In this chapter the discussion of OKCs is limited to those that do not contact teeth, representing about 28% of these cysts.

Features

The symptoms produced by the OKC are identical to those of the other bony cysts. The cyst may occur in all age-groups, but its peak incidence falls in the second and third decades and shows a gradual decline through the later years; 56.9% occur in males; 65% are found in the mandible (Brannon, 1976).

Although multiple OKCs of the jaws have been reported, only some of these were accompanied by the basal cell nevus syndrome. Occasionally the cyst expands the cortical plates and perforates; when palpated, it demonstrates a firmer fluctuance than the usual bony cyst that has perforated the bony plates because the lumen of the OKC is filled with keratin having a somewhat doughy consistency.

For this reason the clinician should use a large-bore needle when attempting to aspirate these cysts to recover the thick, cheesy yellow substance that fills the lumen. The OKC differs from other bony cysts in showing a relatively high recurrence rate, reported to vary between 12% and 51% (Brannon, 1976; Vedtofte and Praetorius, 1979). Some of these lesions recurred as long as 15 years after their initial removal. It has also been observed by some that the recurrence is higher in males and in the young and that this rate can be reduced by removing the cyst in one piece (Chuong et al., 1982; Forssell et al., 1974a).

On microscopic examination the keratocyst also presents a characteristic picture and must be distinguished from a keratinizing odontogenic cyst, which seldom recurs. The lumen of

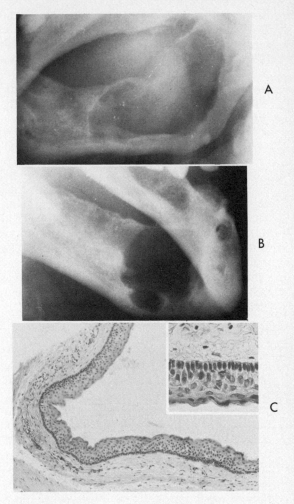

Fig. 19-12. Odontogenic keratocyst. **A,** The hazy appearance is evident. **B,** The scalloped margins are apparent. **C,** Characteristic histopathologic study.

the keratocyst is frequently filled with keratin produced by an epithelial lining whose appearance is distinct from that of the usual stratified squamous keratinizing epithelium and is peculiar to this type of cyst (Fig. 19-12). The wall is frequently thin and has a similarly thin epithelial lining deficient in rete ridges. The basal cells are either columnar or cuboidal and are arranged in a well-defined palisading row. The prickle cells are often vacuolated, usually sparse, and sometimes absent altogether in certain regions. The stratum corneum may be atypical in appearance, with the keratinized cells generally retaining their nuclei; hence the keratinization is predominantly of the parakeratotic type. A buddinglike proliferation from the basal layer is frequently seen in OKCs. Brannon (1977) published an extensive paper on the histologic features of the OKC. Wilson and Ross (1978) discussed the ultrastructure of the OKC. In a study of 272 OKCs, Woolgar et al. (1987) were unable to identify differences in microscopic features between cysts that later recurred and those that did not recur; they did report a greater incidence of inflammation in the nonrecurrent cysts.

Wright (1981) described the *orthokeratinized varient* of the *odontogenic keratocyst:* on microscopic examination this distinct clinicopathologic entity has a thin uniform epithelial lining with orthokeratinization and a granular cell layer just beneath the keratinized layer. The basal cells are usually cuboidal or flattened. Wright described the clinical features as follows: (1) a single cyst; (2) a predilection for males; (3) most common in second to fifth decade; (4) appears most often as a dentigerous cyst in the posterior mandible; and (5) shows little aggressiveness on clinical examination.

Differential diagnosis

Because of its unusually high recurrence rate, the OKC must be distinguished from all other cystlike radiolucencies listed in this chapter.

For example, a cystlike radiolucency measuring 1 cm in diameter is found on a radiograph of an edentulous third molar region of the mandible in a 21-year-old white man. The entity is completely asymptomatic, and there are no related clinical signs. On the radiograph the mandibular canal appears to be displaced inferiorly by the lesion. The differential diagnosis for this radiolucency is discussed in the two sections that follow.

LESS LIKELY

An assessment of the circumstances surrounding the discovery of a cystlike radiolucency undoubtedly lessens the probability that any of the entities in this group warrant further consideration in the differential diagnosis. Nevertheless, since they do have some features in common with the lesion under investigation the clinician is compelled to include them in the list of possibilities albeit they represent unlikely choices.

Benign nonodontogenic tumors of the mandible are uncommon and hence would be assigned a low ranking in the list of possibilities.

The *cementifying* or *ossifying fibroma* is not a common lesion.

Although a *developmental bone defect* might occur in the third molar region, it would almost never be found superior to the mandibular canal and would not cause displacement of the canal—except (rarely) when an expanding soft tissue tumor in the submaxillary space protruded into it, causing it to enlarge.

Fissural cysts do not occur in the third molar region.

The *giant cell granuloma* is usually found in the anterior regions of the jaws.

The *giant cell lesion of hyperparathyroidism* can often be ruled out by studies of the serum chemistry.

Although the third molar region is a likely location for an *ameloblastoma*, the young age of the patient and the less frequent occurrence of this odontogenic tumor characterize this possibility as less likely.

The possibility that the radiolucency is a *third molar tooth crypt* is not likely because the calcification of this tooth is usually initiated in the eighth year and the tooth is fully formed by age 21. Also the contralateral third molar area can be used for a comparison if delayed calcification is suspected. Radiographs taken 6 months later confirm the presence of the calcifying crown, but taking radiographs again in 6 months' time is not a suitable practice if the clinician strongly suspects that the lesion represents a serious pathologic condition.

Comparing the bone trabeculation in the remainder of the jaws aids in determining whether the entity is a *cystlike marrow space,* since a single marrow space of this size and shape without similar areas elsewhere in the jawbone would be quite unusual.

MORE LIKELY

The clinician's attention is now directed to the following more likely entities, which are similar in several respects and are appropriate for inclusion in the working diagnosis (ranked in descending order of frequency):

Residual cyst
Traumatic bone cyst
Primordial cyst
Odontogenic keratocyst—primordial type
Ameloblastoma

All these entities show a predilection for the third molar area, and, except for the ameloblastoma (which usually occurs in an older age-group), for patients in their early to middle twenties. The patient's medical history may produce some clues that aid in arranging the entities in a differential diagnosis, but more often than not it adds to the confusion.

Although the mandibular third molar region is a characteristic site for the *ameloblastoma,* this tumor should not be given a high ranking in this 21-year-old patient unless paresthesia is present.

Aspiration may be helpful in developing a working diagnosis. If the procedure produces an amber-colored fluid, a *primordial cyst,* a *residual cyst,* or a *cystic ameloblastoma* would be suggested. Conversely, if a thick, yellow cheesy material is collected, a *primordial type of keratocyst* would be inferred. If aspiration proved to be nonproductive, the area could then be a *tooth crypt,* a *traumatic bone cyst,* or one of the *solid* entities listed at the beginning of the chapter.

If the cystlike radiolucency shows a haziness within a hyperostotic border, the increased opacity could be caused by keratin packed in the lumen and suggestive of a diagnosis of *keratocyst.*

If the clinician can determine that the third molar failed to develop in the affected quadrant, the *developing tooth crypt* or the *primordial cyst* should be considered as the most likely diagnosis. A patient who has had several posterior teeth extracted during a period of years can seldom be relied on to give sufficiently accurate information regarding whether a third molar ever developed, especially if the other molars are present. Also, if the first permanent molar was extracted relatively soon after its eruption, the patient often becomes confused and reports that a deciduous tooth was lost. Furthermore, the second molar frequently erupts into the position of the first molar and the third molar drifts into the position of the second molar.

The rarer *myxoma* also must be considered in such a circumstance because this lesion is compatible with the history of a tooth that failed to develop and may be seen as a cystlike radiolucency.

If the patient informs the clinician that a tooth was extracted from the area and a cyst was associated with the tooth, the impression that the radiolucent area is a *residual cyst* is reinforced—unless there is otherwise conflicting evidence.

A previous radiograph showing a tooth present and associated with a cyst, whether radicular, lateral, or follicular, adds credence to the choice of *residual cyst.*

Forssell et al. (1974b) indicated that the following findings are highly suggestive of the diagnosis of OKCs: (1) a cystlike radiolucency in

the third molar region or mandibular ramus, (2) a diameter of more than 3 cm, (3) a unilocular cystlike radiolucency with scalloped margins, (4) a multilocular cyst, and (5) odorless creamy or caseous contents.

Management

The OKC should be approached in the same manner as that recommended for other bony cysts (Chapters 16 and 17) with the following exceptions:
1. When the clinician encounters a cystic lumen filled with yellow, cheesy, granular keratin, he or she must curette the bony walls in a more vigorous and thorough manner than usual, since the recurrence rate of the keratocyst is approximately 40% to 60%.
2. After the microscopic examination confirms the working diagnosis of OKC, a more careful than usual postsurgical radiographic follow-up is indicated.

Both Forssell et al. (1988b) and Zachariades et al. (1985) found a higher recurrence rate in multilocular OKCs. In addition, Forssell et al. (1988) found a 43% recurrence rate with few recurrences after the 3-year postoperative period. These authors reported a higher recurrence rate in cases of (1) multilocular cysts, (2) syndrome cysts, (3) infection, fistula, and perforated bony wall and (4) cysts enucleated in several pieces.

Voorsmit et al. (1981) presented a useful discussion of the management of keratocysts.

AMELOBLASTOMA

The ameloblastoma is an odontogenic tumor usually described as a locally malignant lesion and thought to arise from ameloblasts. It represents approximately 11% of odontogenic tumors (Regezi et al., 1978). It may cast a unilocular cystlike radiolucency or a multilocular image. When it occurs in the maxilla, it is mostly unilocular; when it occurs in the mandible, it is more evenly divided between unilocular and multilocular. Either way the radiographic appearance is not diagnostic. The multilocular appearance of this tumor is emphasized in Chapter 20.

Features

The ameloblastoma is painless and slow growing; it can cause migration and loosening of teeth, as well as root resorption and paresthesia of the lip. Struthers and Shear (1976) reported that in their series 81% of ameloblastomas contacting roots showed root resorption on radiographic examination (dentigerous cysts showed resorption in 55% of cases). The ameloblastoma may expand the cortical plates, but frequently it erodes them and then invades the adjacent soft tissue. True metastasis is rare and, of course, indicates that the particular lesion is malignant. The cystlike appearance on the radiograph is identical to that of the other entities discussed in this chapter (Fig. 19-13).

Ameloblastomas are found to be slightly more common in men (Kameyama et al, 1987). The incidence peaks between 20 and 50 years of age and approximately average incidence occurs at 40 years (Minderjahn, 1979). Keszler and Dominguez (1986) discussed eight cases that occurred in patients younger than 16 years of age.

The tumors make up approximately 1% of all tumors of the jaws, occurring five times more frequently in the mandible than the maxilla (Regezi et al., 1978) and most commonly in the posterior part of both jaws. Waldron and El-Mofty (1987) reported from their study of 116 cases that 88% occurred in the mandible. This last feature is propitious, since the thick, compact bone of the mandible tends to restrict their extension. In contrast the maxilla lacks

this limiting barrier that confines the tumor to the mandible. Tumors in this area are close to the nasal cavity, paranasal sinuses, orbital contents, pharyngeal tissues, and vital structures at the base of the skull, which contributes to the unfavorable prognosis of any expanding tumors occurring in the maxilla.

Tsaknis and Nelson (1980) reported on 24 cases of ameloblastoma of the maxilla, explaining that (1) 85% of the tumors occurred distal to the canine tooth; (2) the antrum was involved in 50% of the cases; (3) 33% of the tumors recurred; and (4) 75% of those that recurred showed sinus involvement. These authors advised complete surgical resection for ameloblastoma of the maxilla. Batsakis and McClatchey (1983) called the ameloblastoma of the maxilla the most dangerous of the ameloblastomas. Cherrick (1983) reported that whereas 33.6% of mandibular ameloblastomas recurred in his large series, 53.3% of the maxillary ameloblastomas recurred and when conservative treatment was employed, the latter figure was raised to 82.5%. More than half of Waldron and El-Mofty's maxillary cases (1987) were of the desmoplastic variety.

The early ameloblastoma is asymptomatic, but later, as it expands and may perforate the

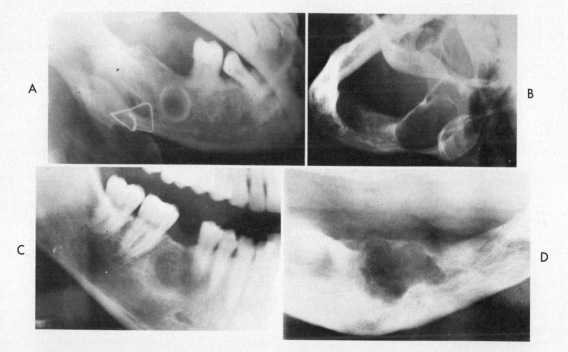

Fig. 19-13. Ameloblastoma. **A** to **D,** Four cystlike ameloblastomas. **E** to **I,** Histologic types of ameloblastoma: **E,** alveolar; **F,** plexiform; **G,** acanthomatous; **H,** granular cell; **I,** spindle cell. (**A** courtesy O.H. Stuteville, DDS, MD, St. Joe, Ark. **B** and **C** courtesy D. Skuble, DDS, Hinsdale, Ill. **D** courtesy J. Lehnert, DDS, Minneapolis.)

cortical plates, it becomes discernible and palpable on clinical examination. A particular ameloblastoma feels firm if it is of the solid type. If it is a cystic type, it is soft and fluctuant and straw-colored fluid can be aspirated, thus prompting the incorrect impression of a cyst. To distinguish between solid and cystic types on radiographic examination is not possible.

On microscopic examination there are at least six histologic types of true ameloblastoma: simple (alveolar) plexiform, acanthomatous, spindle cell, desmoplastic, and granular cell (Fig. 19-13). To date, a difference in invasive properties or recurrence rates among these types has not been shown. The very cellular ameloblastoma, however, may prove to be more aggressive than the less cellular types, which are composed of more fibrous tissue or large cystic spaces. Vickers and Gorlin (1970) delineated the histopathologic criteria for the ameloblastoma. Slootweg and Müller (1984) described in detail the malignant variants of the ameloblastoma and discussed efficacy of the two terms "malignant ameloblastoma" and "ameloblastic carcinoma."

Differential diagnosis

To avoid surprise at surgery, the surgeon must consider that every cystlike radiolucency of the jawbones could be an ameloblastoma. The differential diagnosis of the lesion is discussed with that of the odontogenic keratocyst (p. 388).

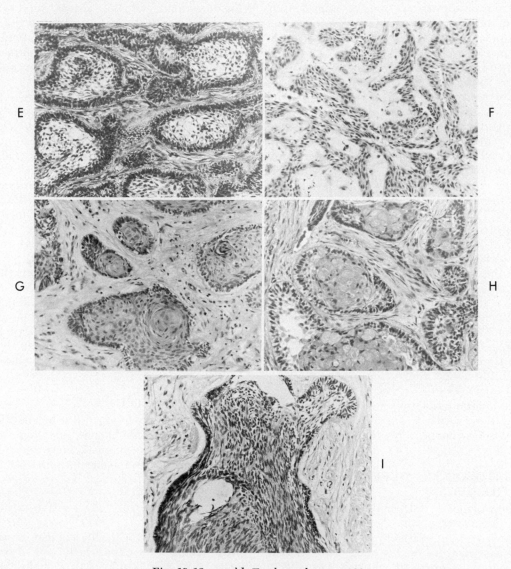

Fig. 19-13, cont'd. For legend see p. 390.

Management

The relatively radical surgical treatment of ameloblastomas is predicated on their high frequency of recurrence, which results from their tendency to develop small projections that extend beyond their apparent margins. Hence, careful follow-up is mandatory.

Mehlisch et al. (1972) aptly described the successful treatment of an ameloblastoma as that which achieves an acceptable prognosis and causes minimal disfigurement. Their criteria are based on a compromise between such variables as the age and general health of the patient and the size, location, and duration of the tumor. In light of these guidelines, judging whether treatment of an ameloblastoma is successful or not depends on the distinctive features of the tumor in question. The complete spectrum of approaches, ranging from conservative incision to wide block resection, has been practiced over the years. Wide block resection, with placement of a bone graft, has produced the lowest recurrence rate.

Less radical treatment appears to be effective for tumors located in the anterior part of the jaw and measuring less than 5 cm in diameter. Also, small lesions in older patients whose poor general health precludes resection have been well managed by vigorous curettement in conjunction with cautery. Ameloblastomas occurring in the anterior region of either jaw have the lowest recurrence rates. Marciani et al. (1977) recommended the use of cryotherapy in selected cases in the mandibular molar area. Veno et al. (1989), in a study of 91 patients with ameloblastoma of the mandible, developed the prognostic characteristic of a higher recurrence rate in older patients, multilocular lesions, and the follicular microscopic type.

Although radiation has been used from time to time as a modality of treatment for the ameloblastoma, recently increased interest has been shown in this approach (Atkinson et al., 1984; Gardner, 1982; Gould and Farman, 1984).

The unique unicystic ameloblastoma is a different entity with a much lower recurrence rate. Its management is discussed in Chapter 17.

HEMATOPOIETIC DEFECT OF THE JAWS

Hematopoietic defects of the jaws, also called *focal osteoporotic bone marrow defects* of the jaws, are relatively common and have been described by Barker et al. (1974), Crawford and Weathers (1970), Lipani et al. (1982),

and Standish and Shafer (1982). The cause is unknown in the vast majority of cases, but altered healing reactions or marrow hyperplasia may be the cause in a few cases (Barker et al., 1974).

Features

These radiolucent entities are usually asymptomatic, although Lipani et al. (1982) reported that pain and swelling are not uncommon. From a clinical point of view, the vast majority are detected on routine radiographs. Lipani et al. (1982) reviewed reports of four large series including their own and found that the average patient ages in the series ranged from 42 to 45 years, that there was a strong predilection for females, and that from 72% to 91% of lesions occurred in the premolar and molar region of the mandible. Of the lesions reported by Barker et al. (1974), 91% occurred in the mandible and less than 15% of the patients reported pain. Some lesions are bilateral, and 23% of the Barker series occurred in areas of previous extraction.

Radiographic appearance varied from radiolucencies with well-defined borders to the more common radiolucencies with ragged, poorly marginated borders. Occasionally trabeculations or spotty radiopaque flecks were seen within the radiolucency (Barker et al., 1974). Many of these defects are cast over or near the apices of teeth (see Fig. 16-1, *C*), but the teeth test vital and apical lamina duras are intact unless concomitant pulpal disease is present. Makek and Lello (1986) proposed five categories based on radiographic appearance.

The microscopic appearance is primarily that of bone marrow with hematopoietic components showing a variable fatty component. Twenty-five percent of the lesions reported by Barker et al. (1974) were primarily fatty. Some examples were composed of hypercellular marrow and possessed small lymphoid aggregates (Barker et al., 1974).

Differential diagnosis

A wide range of lesions must be considered, including dental granulomas, rarefying osteitis, odontogenic cysts, traumatic bone cysts, osteomyelitis, benign and malignant tumors of bone, manifestations of leukemia, histiocytosis X, and advanced anemias.

Management

Barker et al. (1974) advised that a radiolucent shadow with either distinct or ill-defined margins in the posterior aspect of the body of the mandible of a middle-aged woman should suggest an osteoporotic bone marrow defect. In our opinion, if conflicting evidence is not present in the form of worrisome signs or symptoms, such an area should be radiographed at intervals to ensure that change is not occurring. Special concern mandates biopsy.

SURGICAL DEFECT

Defects of a transitory or permanent nature result from the enucleation or resection of lesions occurring within bone. The majority of these defects possess well-defined borders; when they are round or ovoid, they have a cystlike appearance on radiographs (Fig. 19-14).

Usually a radiolucency may be recognized as a surgical defect when the patient informs the clinician of the prior surgery. Occasionally a surgical defect is permanent, usually because relatively large areas of cortical bone, along with the periosteum and marrow, have been lost; hence there is a deficiency of the bone forming elements. When a patient with such a deformity is seen by a different clinician some

years after the surgery, the cystlike radiolucency may present a dilemma. Is it a surgical defect or a recurrence of the original condition, or is it a new lesion? If a series of postsurgical radiographs have been taken during the intervening years and are available to the new clinician, he or she is readily able to tell whether the area is decreasing, remaining constant, or enlarging in size.

If the area has remained constant or is decreasing slightly in size or increasing in radiodensity, it is most likely a surgical defect. If it is increasing in size, however, it must be considered a recurrence of the original pathologic process or possibly a new lesion. For example, if a dentigerous cyst was removed some years before, an ameloblastoma may have developed from remnants of the epithelial lining.

If the clinician encounters an asymptomatic radiolucency in an area of the jaw that according to the patient's history was the site of previous surgery, and if the original diagnosis can be obtained, the clinician has enough information to consider whether the image is more likely to be a quiescent defect or a recurrence of disease.

If postsurgical radiographs of the area are not available, the size and shape of the asymptomatic radiolucency should be monitored every 6 months. Even though the original diagnosis was of a benign condition (that is, a cyst), this does not relieve the clinician of the obligation to periodically reexamine the presumed surgical defect until its innocent status has been convincingly demonstrated. Such a demonstration is established by the appearance of a constant or diminishing size in subsequent radiographs. If an increase in size is evident on successive radiographs, the area must be investigated to determine the cause of the change.

Palpation of the jawbone may reveal a depression on the medial or lateral surface in a position corresponding to the location of the radiolucency. Such a finding contributes to the description of the defect's identity.

CENTRAL GIANT CELL GRANULOMA

The central giant cell granuloma (GCG) of the jaws has often been compared with the giant cell tumor of long bones. In a recent study of a large number of both entities, Auclair et al. (1988) proposed that they represent a spectrum of a single disease process that is modified by the age of the patient and the site of occurrence.

The central GCG may occur initially as a solitary cystlike radiolucency (Fig. 19-15); as it

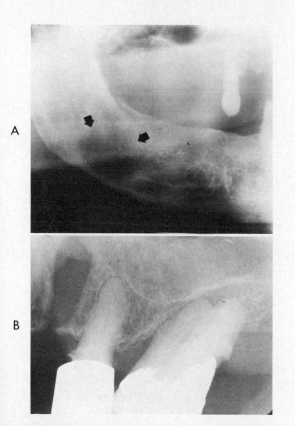

Fig. 19-14. Surgical defect. **A,** Defect *(arrows)* 20 years after cystectomy. **B,** One year after a traumatic extraction.

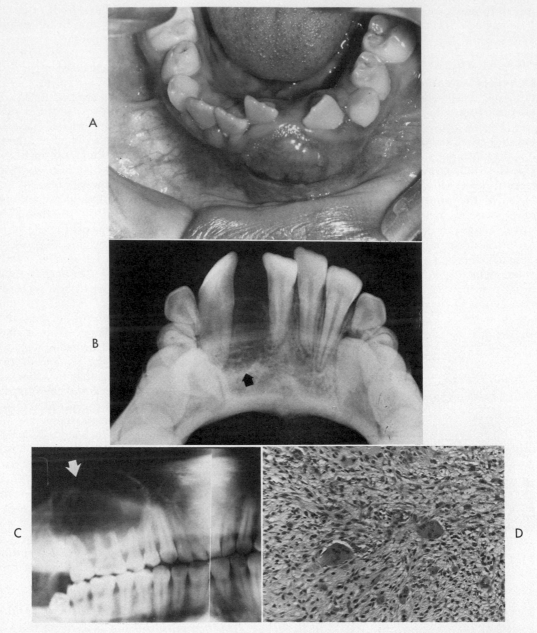

Fig. 19-15. Central giant cell granuloma. **A,** Clinical appearance of an anterior alveolar swelling in a 9-year-old boy. **B,** Radiograph of the lesion. **C,** Another cystlike central giant cell granuloma. **D,** Photomicrograph showing giant cells in the fibrovasular stroma.   (**C** courtesy the late J. Ireland, DDS, and J. Dolci, DDS, Mundelein, Ill.).

grows larger, it frequently develops an architecture that causes a soap-bubble type of multilocular radiolucency. Cohen and Hertzanu (1988) described in detail the radiographic appearances of the GCG, including those seen with computed tomography. Although trauma was thought to be the causative factor, many pathologists now believe that this is not the case; the factors that cause GCG are in doubt.

Features

The central giant cell granuloma occurs most frequently in women and girls under 30 years of age, and two of three lesions are found in the mandible. The portion of the jaws anterior to the molars is the usual site of involvement. Paresthesia is not a feature. In Raibley and Shafer's series (1979) of 90 central GCGs the mean patient age was 26.3 years, 65.5% of cases occurred in patients under 30 years of age, and 32% occurred in the second decade of life. The sex ratio was 2.4:1 in favor of women and girls. Predilection for women in their twenties was 8:1. Of the lesions 70.4% occurred in the mandible and 95.6% were situated anterior to the second molar teeth. Concerning appearance on radiographs, 71% were reported as being unilocular and 17.5% as multilocular.

The lesion is painless and grows slowly by expanding and thinning the cortical plates, but it seldom perforates the soft tissue. Thus the clinician usually finds a hard expansion demonstrating some flexibility. If the cortical plates are perforated, however, the swelling is moderately soft to palpation (Fig. 19-15). This is to be expected because on microscopic examination the lesion consists of multinucleated giant cells scattered throughout a vascular granulomatous tissue stroma that contains a minimum of collagen (Fig. 19-15).

Hemosiderin is often scattered throughout the tissue and, with the high vascularity, may impart a bluish cast to a lesion that has extended peripherally through the cortical plates and lies just beneath a thin mucosal surface. The covering mucosa appears normal unless traumatized. An expanding lesion may cause some migration of teeth, but root resorption is not the rule.

Differential diagnosis

All the cystlike lesions discussed in this chapter must be considered in the differential diagnosis of GCG. The clinical characteristics of the lesion in question should be compared with those listed for each entity at the end of the chapter.

Whenever a diagnosis of GCG is reported by the pathologist, the serum chemistry must be studied to exclude the possibility of a *giant cell lesion of hyperparathyroidism.*

Management

Surgical enucleation of the lesion with curettement is the treatment of choice. Recurrences are not common, but when they do happen, the possibility that the lesion is a giant cell lesion of hyperparathyroidism must be considered. Such a suspicion can be rejected or confirmed only by a study of the patient with emphasis on chemical study of the serum.

The serum should be analyzed particularly for calcium, phosphorus, and alkaline phosphatase levels to rule out hyperparathyroidism. Such analysis is imperative, since the GCG cannot be differentiated from this giant cell lesion on the basis of a clinical, radiographic, or microscopic examination.

Cherrick (1983), in a study of 292 central GCGs, reported a significantly higher recurrence rate than had been thought. He reported a 12% recurrence rate for lesions less than 2 cm in diameter and a 37% recurrence rate for lesions more than 2 cm in diameter. Eisenbud et al. (1988) reported a recurrence rate of approximately 16% when curettement with peripheral ostectomy was performed. Chuong et al. (1986) set parameters for differentiating between aggressive and nonaggressive types.

GIANT CELL LESION (HYPERPARATHYROIDISM)

The clinical, radiographic, and microscopic characteristics of the giant cell lesion of hyperparathyroidism are identical to those of the giant cell granuloma just discussed. The giant cell lesion occurs as a unilocular or a multilocular radiolucency and is found in patients with primary, secondary, or tertiary hyperparathyroidism. If the jaws show rarefaction (a possible finding in advanced hyperparathyroidism), the giant cell lesion appears to have poorly demarcated borders because of the osteoporosis of the surrounding bone (Fig. 19-16). Establishing its identity depends on demonstrating the concomitant parathyroid, kidney, or other systemic disorder.

Secondary hyperparathyroidism

Secondary hyperparathyroidism is discussed before the primary type because it is detected more frequently. One causative pathologic condition is impaired kidney function from disease (for example, an ascending infection), which induces a shift in the ionic balance of the blood that ultimately causes a lowered level of serum calcium. The mechanism of this shift is not yet a subject of complete agreement.

The reduced serum calcium level then leads to parathyroid hyperplasia and an increased production of parathyroid hormone, which in turn causes bone to resorb and return calcium to the blood to maintain serum calcium at normal levels. In moderate to severe cases, enough mineral is removed from the bones that the bones become rarefied and this rarefaction is discernible on radiographic examination (that is, osteitis fibrosa cystica generalisata, discussed in Chapter 23). The same phenomenon is observed in patients who are receiving prolonged dialysis.

In severe cases of hyperparathyroidism, the cortical plates are especially thinned and the lamina dura around the roots of the teeth may not be apparent on radiographs. Central giant cell lesions (brown tumors) are prone to occur in these patients with hyperparathyroidism and are found frequently in the jaws (Fig. 19-16). They are identical to the central giant cell granuloma in clinical, radiographic, and histologic features, but they differ insofar as the giant cell lesion of hyperparathyroidism may demonstrate a high recurrence rate if the systemic problem is not alleviated. Rao et al. (1978) reported on several cases of brown tumors associated with chronic renal failure. Kelly et al. (1980) detailed the radiographic changes of the jawbones in end-stage renal disease.

Primary hyperparathyroidism

Primary hyperparathyroidism that is detectable on clinical examination is less common than the secondary type and is caused by a functioning adenoma (less often by a carcinoma) of one of the parathyroid glands. The increased parathyroid hormone stimulates bone resorption and thus increases the level of serum calcium, concomitantly inducing an increased excretion of phosphate by the kidney. The skeletal changes and giant cell lesions are identical to those of the secondary type.

DIFFERENTIAL DIAGNOSIS

Primary and secondary hyperparathyroidism may be differentiated on the basis of history and laboratory findings.

Patients with *primary hyperparathyroidism* are usually in a younger age-group, between 30

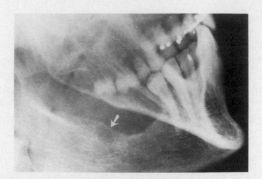

Fig. 19-16. Giant cell lesion of hyperparathyroidism *(arrow)*. The poorly defined borders of the tumor were caused by the generalized rarefaction of the jawbone.   (Courtesy O.H. Stuteville, DDS, MD, St. Joe, Ark.)

and 60 years, and may report polydipsia and polyuria because of the increased diuresis. Women are seven times more frequently involved than men. Serum values in advanced primary hyperparathyroidism are increased calcium levels, decreased phosphorus levels, and increased levels of alkaline phosphatase (which is characteristically elevated during increased bony resorption or apposition).

A patient with *secondary hyperparathyroidism* has the same symptoms and usually a history of kidney disease and is likely to have a decreased renal output. An older age-group (50 to 80 years) is involved, and women are only twice as often afflicted as men. Laboratory tests reveal an inverted relationship of the serum calcium and phosphorus levels as compared with those found in the primary disease (that is, the serum calcium levels are normal or decreased, whereas the serum phosphate and alkaline phosphate levels are increased).

MANAGEMENT

If the primary medical problem is corrected, the giant cell lesions often regress without surgery and the rarefaction disappears. Surgical excision of the parathyroid gland with its adenoma is the treatment for the primary type and is successful. The treatment of the kidney defect in the secondary type is usually more complicated.

INCISIVE CANAL CYST

The incisive canal cyst is discussed in detail in Chapter 18 as an interradicular radiolucency. In edentulous anterior maxillas it can occur as a cystlike radiolucency that does not contact the shadows of teeth (Fig. 19-17).

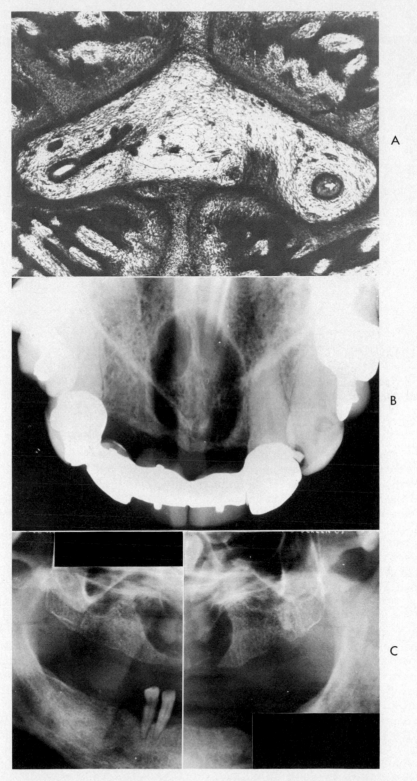

Fig. 19-17. **A,** Transverse section of a 15-week-old human embryo showing the incisive canal (inverted V-shaped structure). **B,** Occlusal radiograph of incisive canal cyst where some anterior teeth are missing. **C,** Large incisive canal cyst in a Panorex radiograph of an edentulous maxilla.

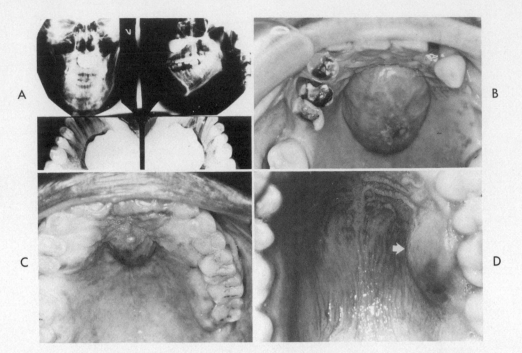

Fig. 19-18. **A,** Radiographs of a midpalatal cyst injected with radiopaque dye. **B,** Clinical appearance of a midpalatal cyst. **C,** Palatal swelling from an incisive canal cyst that destroyed the posterior bony boundary of the canal and simulated a midpalatal cyst. **D,** Palatal space abscess *(arrow)* from a pulpless premolar.   (**A** courtesy D. Skuble, DDS, Hinsdale, Ill.)

Midpalatal cyst

The midpalatal cyst is an uncommon bony cyst that develops in the midline of the palate posterior to the palatal papilla. It originates in residual embryonic epithelial nests in the fusion line of the lateral palatal shelves. On radiographic examination a unilocular radiolucency is seen in the midline of the palate (Fig. 19-18). Large cysts may completely destroy the bony palate.

FEATURES

The patient with a midpalatal cyst may complain of a painless bulging that is increasing in size in the roof of the mouth. If the cyst is not traumatized or secondarily infected, the dome-shaped mass is nontender and covered with normal mucosa, which perhaps appears more glossy than usual. The mass is situated over the midline of the palate posterior to the incisive papilla (Fig. 19-18).

Because the bone inferior to the cyst is so thin, the cortical plate is rapidly perforated as the cyst grows; consequently the swelling is soft and fluctuant but nonemptiable by digital pressure unless a sinus is present. If, as sometimes happens, the bony floor of the nose is completely eroded, the cyst may be slightly displaced superiorly by digital pressure. Aspiration produces an amber-colored fluid.

The microscopic picture is identical to that of other cysts. The epithelial lining may be of the respiratory type (with goblet cells).

DIFFERENTIAL DIAGNOSIS

Although many lesions occur on the palate with some frequency, it seems reasonable to limit the differential diagnosis to soft lesions: midpalatal cyst, incisive canal cyst, radicular cyst, palatal space abscess, lipoma, plexiform neurofibroma, mucocele, papillary cyst adenoma, and mucoepidermoid tumor (low grade).

Occasionally an early *low-grade mucoepidermoid tumor* appears on clinical examination as a mucocele when much mucus is produced by the mucous cells, which are the predominant cell type in the low-grade variety. However, minor salivary gland tumors and retention phenomena are seldom seen in the midline of the hard palate, since there is a paucity of minor salivary glands in this region. These tumors may be seen most frequently in the lateral aspect of the posterior palate in the region of the anterior palatine foramen. The clinician therefore assigns a low rank to mucoepidermoid carcinoma, *papillary cyst adenoma*, and *mucocele* in the differential diagnosis for a soft midpalatal swelling.

Furthermore, although both the low-grade mucoepidermoid tumor and the mucocele might demonstrate fluctuance and not be emptiable by digital pressure—characteristics similar to those of cysts—unlike cysts, on aspiration they do not yield a typical amber-colored fluid but a viscous, clear, sticky liquid (concentrated mucus).

The *plexiform neurofibroma* is the only peripheral nerve tumor that is soft and fluctuant. It is the usual type that occurs in von Recklinghausen's disease, so it is a likely choice if the patient has this disease. Also it can be readily differentiated from a cyst, since aspiration of a plexiform neurofibroma does not produce an aspirate.

A *lipoma* is not common in the oral cavity, and like the neurofibroma it can be readily distinguished from cysts by aspiration.

A *palatal space abscess* can be somewhat soft and fluctuant and yields pus on aspiration. It is generally associated with the palatal roots of nonvital posterior teeth or a vital or nonvital tooth with a lateral periodontal abscess on the lingual aspect of a palatal root. Consequently a palatal space abscess seldom is located in the posterior midline but is found adjacent to the tooth that gave rise to the infection (Fig. 19-18)—in contrast to an abscess resulting from a secondarily infected midpalatal cyst, which is more symmetrically situated in the midline.

A *radicular cyst* involving a canine or a premolar only rarely perforates the denser cortical bone of the lingual plate; rather this type of cyst extends through the thinner buccal plate into the buccal vestibule. Further vitality tests and periapical radiographs aid in the differentiation of the midpalatal cyst from the odontogenic palatal space abscess.

The *incisive canal cyst* is easily differentiated from the midpalatal cyst in most cases because it occurs in the canal above the palatine papilla, whereas the midpalatal cyst occurs in the midline of the palate posterior to the papilla. When either an incisive canal cyst or a midpalatal cyst expands and destroys the posterior limits of the incisive canal, however, distinguishing with certainty between the two is usually impossible (Fig. 19-18).

MANAGEMENT

After the working diagnosis of midpalatal cyst has been established and the possibility of more serious entities ruled out by all appropriate diagnostic techniques, including aspiration, an acrylic stent should be fabricated on a revised cast to cover the entire hard palate. A mucoperiosteal flap should then be raised from the anterior, including the entire palatal mucosa, by incising along the gingival sulci around the lingual necks of all the teeth from the first molar on the right to the first molar on the left. This ensures good access and permits complete removal of the cyst. If the full thickness of the bony palate has been destroyed, care should be taken to avoid perforating the nasal mucosa because such a perforation may well result in an oronasal fistula. The flap should be closed with sutures and the prefabricated stent placed securely in position. Clinical and radiographic follow-up is mandatory.

EARLY STAGE OF CEMENTIFYING AND OSSIFYING FIBROMAS (BENIGN FIBRO-OSSEOUS LESIONS OF PERIODONTAL LIGAMENT ORIGIN)

Cementifying and ossifying fibromas, as well as cemento-ossifying fibromas, are considered by most pathologists to be variants of the same basic entity.

These lesions are classified as neoplastic fibro-osseous lesions that arise from elements of the periodontal ligament (Hamner et al., 1968; Waldron and Giansanti, 1973a, 1973b). They differ from the much more common periapical cementomas in that they are seen in younger patients, occur most often in the premolar and molar region of the mandible instead of the incisor region, and if left untreated, attain a much larger size, frequently causing expansion of the jaws. The lesion may be labeled as ossifying or cementifying depending on which tissue is present. A mixture of bone and cementum may be seen in some lesions, which are identified as a "cemento-ossifying fibroma." Despite the foregoing, many oral pathologists believe it is not often possible to differentiate between cementum and bone. Hence such pathologists prefer to use the term "fibrocalcific lesions of periodontal ligament origin" (Cornyn, 1975). The majority of cementifying and ossifying fibromas occur in the periapex because they originate from elements in the periodontal ligament. Occasionally, however, they are not in contact with the roots of teeth but occur in the body of the maxilla or mandible in edentulous areas or, when teeth are present, are not associated with the teeth.

The early stage is osteolytic, in which the surrounding bone is resorbed and replaced by

Table 19-1. Solitary cystlike radiolucencies

Entity	Predominant sex	Usual age (years)	Predominant jaw	Predominant region	Other radiographic appearances	Additional features
Marrow spaces	M = F	All	Mandible	Molar	Routine Multilocular Multiple cystlike Osteosclerosis	Asymptomatic; similar patterns contralaterally
Postextraction sockets	M = F	Over 20	Mandible	Molar		Radiolucency does not enlarge; history of extraction; asymptomatic
Residual cysts	$\frac{M}{F} = \frac{3}{2}$	Over 20 (average 52)	Maxilla 57%		Multilocular	Asymptomatic; preextraction radiograph showing tooth with associated cyst
Traumatic bone cysts	M > F Slight	Under 30	Uncommon in maxilla	Premolar and molar Incisor	Periapical radiolucency	Teeth vital; asymptomatic; possible history of trauma; usually no aspirate
Primordial cysts	M ~ F	10-30	Mandible	Third molar	Multilocular	Permanent tooth fails to develop
Odontogenic keratocysts	M = 56.9%	Peak—10-30 (average 28)	Mandible 65%	Third molar	Scalloped borders Multilocular	Occasionally radiolucency appears hazy; high recurrence rate
Ameloblastomas	M ~ F	20-50 (average 40)	Mandible 80%	Posterior 70%	Ill-defined ragged borders Multilocular	Erode cortical plates; may cause paresthesia
Surgical defects	M = F	Over 10	Equal	Anterior	Ragged irregularly shaped borders	History of previous surgery; radiolucency does not enlarge
Central giant cell granulomas	$\frac{F}{M} = \frac{2.4}{1}$	Under 30 (average 26)	Mandible 70%	Anterior to second molars	Multilocular	History of previous trauma; serum chemistries normal
Giant cell lesions (secondary hyperparathyroidism)	$\frac{F}{M} = \frac{2}{1}$	50-80	Mandible	None	Multilocular Indistinct borders	History of kidney disease; serum calcium normal to ↓; serum phosphate ↑; serum alkaline phosphatase ↑
Giant cell lesions (primary hyperparathyroidism)	$\frac{F}{M} = \frac{7}{1}$	30-60	Mandible	None	Multilocular Indistinct borders	Polydipsia; polyuria; serum calcium ↑; serum phosphate ↓; serum alkaline phosphatase ↑

	Sex	Age	Jaw	Location	Shape	Features
Incisive canal cysts	$\frac{M}{F} = \frac{3}{1}$		Maxilla only	Incisive canal	Heart shaped	Teeth vital; salty taste
Midpalatal cysts			Maxilla only	Palatal midline; Posterior to papilla	None	Uncommon
Lingual mandibular bone defects	F > M	All ages	Mandible only	Third molar	Semicircular; oval	Teeth vital
Early cementifying and ossifying fibromas	M ~ F	26.4 (average)	Mandible 70%	Premolar and molar	Radiolucent-radiopaque	Teeth vital
Benign nonodontogenic tumors			Mandible	Molar Ramus	Radiopaque Elongated	Teeth vital

~, Approximately equal.

a fibrovascular type of soft tissue containing osteoblasts or cementoblasts or both. Cementifying cementomas and ossifying fibromas at this stage may appear as solitary cystlike radiolucencies that are not in contact with teeth (Fig. 19-19).

Features

Cementifying and ossifying fibromas, when small, are asymptomatic but frequently may grow sufficiently large to expand the jawbone; 70% occur in the mandible and are primarily found in the premolar and molar region. The average age of patients with ossifying fibroma is 26.4 years, and the sexes are approximately equally affected. The age range of patients in the study by Hamner et al. (1968) was 7 to 58 years. In contrast to the periapical cemento-

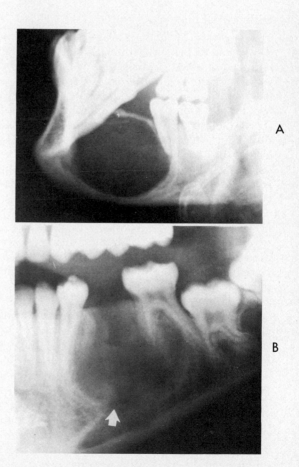

Fig. 19-19. Immature fibro-osseous lesions of periodontal ligament origin (PDLO). The biopsy report indicated ossifying fibroma in both cases. **B**, The arrow indicates the lesion. (**A** courtesy S. Atsaves, DDS, Chicago. **B**, courtesy R. Goepp, DDS, Zoller Clinic, University of Chicago.)

mas, these lesions classically occur as solitary entities.

During the initial radiolucent stage, the lesion usually changes progressively from a predominantly fibroblastic lesion to an increasingly calcified structure. During maturation, microscopic examination discloses a number of small droplets of cementum, spicules of bone, cementoblasts, and osteoblasts in a fibrous vascular stroma (see Fig. 19-18,C). As these entities continue to mature, the calcified components become larger, coalesce, and are then apparent on radiographs as radiopaque foci within a well-described radiolucency. Still later, in the mature stage, most of the lesion consists of calcified tissue and appears on radiographs as a well-defined radiopacity usually surrounded by a uniform radiolucent zone that represents a noncalcified area of fibrous tissue at the periphery.

Differential diagnosis

A period of at least 6 years is required for the lesion to pass from the radiolucent to the radiopaque stage. Usually this pathosis shows varying degrees of soft tissue density with a few small radiopaque foci present; accordingly it is usually included in the differential diagnosis of radiolucent areas with radiopaque foci, discussed in Chapter 24. When the lesion (infrequently) is found to be completely radiolucent and not in contact with teeth, however, it is assigned a low ranking in the differential discussion of such cystlike radiolucencies.

Management

To make the correct diagnosis, a surgical approach is necessary to obtain biopsy material. Excision and curettement of the lesion are all that is required, since this lesion does not have a tendency to recur. Only one of 16 lesions recurred in the series reported by Zachariades et al. (1984).

BENIGN NONODONTOGENIC TUMORS

Specific benign nonodontogenic tumors are rarely observed within the jawbones. If they are considered as a group, however, their composite incidence is high enough to warrant their exemption from the category of rarities. Tumors that have occurred with some frequency within the jaws as cystlike radiolucencies not necessarily in contact with teeth are lipoma, salivary gland adenoma, amputation neuroma, neurofibroma, schwannoma, fibroma, and myxoma. Because their growth is slow, they demonstrate well-defined radiolu-

cencies of varying shape (Fig. 19-20). Polak et al. (1989) reported a case of a solitary neurofibroma of the mandible and reviewed 29 other cases of neurofibromas in the literature.

Features

Most benign nonodontogenic tumors are asymptomatic, except for the peripheral nerve tumors that develop in conjunction with major sensory nerves. The patient then usually reports pain, paresthesia, or anesthesia in a region. The patient with an amputation neuroma almost invariably describes a previous traumatic incident: a tooth extraction, a jaw fracture, or major jaw surgery.

If benign tumors of the jaw go untreated, they slowly grow and expand the cortical plates, which because of the slow growth of the tumor frequently remain intact. Aspiration is nonproductive for the benign nonodontogenic tumors just discussed.

Differential diagnosis

Benign nonodontgenic tumors of the jawbone should be assigned a low ranking in the differential diagnosis of solitary cystlike radiolucencies.

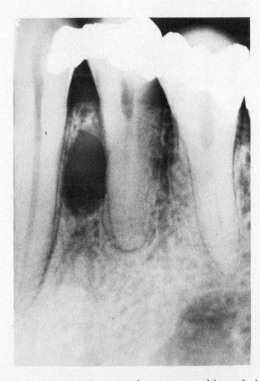

Fig. 19-20. Neurilemoma showing a cystlike radiolucency between the mandibular canine and premolar. (From Morgan G and Morgan P: Oral Surg 25:182-189, 1968.)

A *neurofibroma* involving the mandibular canal is sometimes found as an elongated broadening of the canal. When this picture is observed, therefore, the possibility that it represents a peripheral nervous tissue tumor should be considered. *Arteriovenous pathosis*, however, also must be considered in such a case.

When the patient gives a history of major surgery or fracture in a region that has a painful cystlike radiolucency, an *amputation neuroma* must be considered as a possibility.

If the patient has neurofibromatosis, the likelihood that a cystlike radiolucency of the jawbones is a peripheral nerve tumor is much greater than for the general population.

Management

Conservative excision—after a presurgical aspiration test has proved to be nonproductive—is the treatment of choice for these lesions. If the tumor involves the mandibular canal and its contents, the patient should be forewarned of the likelihood of a postoperative paresthesia or anesthesia of the lip and, if the radiolucency is large, of the possibility of jaw fracture during surgery.

RARITIES

The following entities, which may appear as cystlike radiolucencies not necessarily in contact with teeth, either represent rare pathoses or are more common lesions that rarely occur in the jaws (Fig. 19-21):

Adenomatoid odontogenic tumor
Ameloblastic variants
Aneurysmal bone cyst (Fig. 19-21, *D*)
Aneurysms in bone
Arteriovenous malformation in bone
Artifact
Calcifying epithelial odontogenic tumor
Calcifying odontogenic cyst
Cementoma
Central fibroma
Central hemangioma of bone
Central squamous cell carcinoma
    in cyst lining
Desmoplastic fibroma
Hemangioma of bone
Histiocytosis X (Fig. 19-21, *E*)
Lipoma (intraosseous)
Low-grade metastatic carcinoma
Metastatic carcinoma
Minor salivary gland tumor in bone
Myospherulosis (paraffinoma)
Myxoma (Fig. 19-21, *B* and *C*)
Odontogenic fibroma
Odontoma (early stage)
Osteoblastoma (early stage)
Plasmacytoma
Postoperative maxillary cyst
Squamous odontogenic tumor
Unicystic ameloblastoma

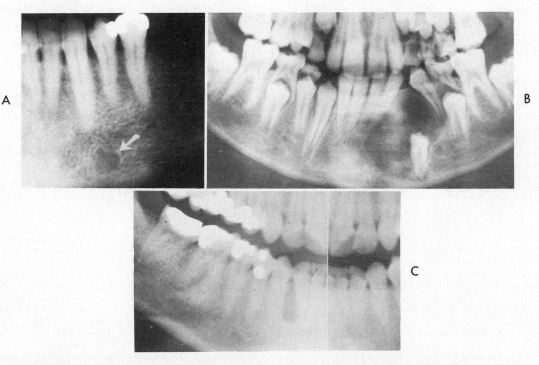

Fig. 19-21. Rarities. **A,** Cystlike metastatic bronchogenic carcinoma *(arrow).* **B,** Pericoronal radiolucency involving an impacted canine proved to be a myxoma. **C,** Myxoma between the canine and lateral incisor.   (**B** and **E** courtesy N. Barakat, DDS, Beirut, Lebanon. **C** and **D** courtesy R. Kallal, DDS, Chicago.)   *Continued.*

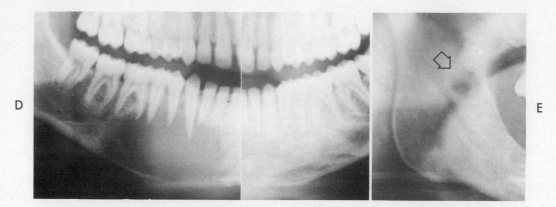

Fig. 19-21, cont'd. Rarities. **D,** Cystlike aneurysmal bone cyst. **E,** Eosinophilic granuloma *(arrow)*.

REFERENCES

Atkinson CH, Harwood AR, and Cummings BJ: Ameloblastoma of the jaw: a reappraisal of the role of megavoltage irradiation, Cancer 53:869-873, 1984.

Auclair PL, Cuenin P, Kratochuil FJ, et al: A clinical and histomorphologic comparison of the central giant cell granuloma and the giant cell tumor, Oral Surg 66:197-208, 1988.

Azaz B and Lustmann J: Anatomic configurations in dry mandibles, Br J Oral Surg 11:1-9, 1973.

Barker BF, Jensen JL, and Howell FV: Focal osteoporotic bone marrow defects of the jaws: an analysis of 197 new cases, Oral Surg 38:404-413, 1974.

Batsakis JG and McClatchey KD: Ameloblastoma of the mandibular bone concavity: report of case, Oral Surg 57:139-143, 1984.maxilla and peripheral ameloblastoma, Ann Otol Rhinol Laryngol 92:532-533, 1983.

Biewald HF: A variation in the management of hemorrhagic, traumatic or simple bone cyst, J Oral Surg 25:627-638, 1967.

Brannon RB: The odontogenic keratocyst: a clinicopathologic study of 312 cases. I. Clinical features, Oral Surg 42:54-72, 1976.

Brannon RB: The odontogenic keratocyst: a clinicopathologic study of 312 cases. II. Histologic features, Oral Surg 43:233-255, 1977.

Cabrini RL, Barros RE, and Albano H: Cysts of the jaws: a statistical analysis, J Oral Surg 28:485-489, 1970.

Chapman PJ and Romaniuk K: Traumatic bone cyst of the mandible: regression following aspiration, Int J Oral Surg 14:290-294, 1985.

Cherrick HM: Presentation to American Association of Oral and Maxillofacial Surgeons, Las Vegas, Sept. 1983.

Chuong R, Donoff RB, Guralnick W: The odontogenic keratocyst, J Oral Maxillofac Surg 40:797-802, 1982.

Chuong R, Kaban LB, Kozakewich H, and Perez-Atayde A: Central giant cell lesions of the jaws: a clinicopathologic study, J Oral Maxillofac Surg 44:708-713, 1986.

Cohen MA: Hemorrhagic (traumatic) cyst of the mandible associated with a retained root apex, Oral Surg 57:26-27, 1984.

Cohen MA and Hertzanu Y: Radiologic features including those seen with computed tomography of central giant cell granuloma of the jaws, Oral Surg 65:255-261, 1988.

Connor MS: Anterior lingual mandibular bone concavity: report of a case, Oral Surg 48:413-414, 1979.

Cornyn J: Fibro-calcific lesions to the jaws. Presentation to American Academy of Dental Radiology, Chicago, Oct 24, 1975.

Correll RW, Jensen JL, and Rhyne RR: Lingual cortical mandibular defects, Oral Surg 50:287-291, 1980.

Crawford B and Weathers D: Osteoporotic marrow defects of the jaws, J Oral Surg 28:600-603, 1970.

Cunat JJ and Collard J: Late developing premolars: report of two cases, J Am Dent Assoc 87:183-185, 1973.

Eisenbud L, Stern M, Rothberg M, and Sachs SA: Central giant cell granuloma of the jaws: experiences in the management of thirty-seven cases, J Oral Maxillofac Surg 46:376-384, 1988.

Forssell K, Forssell H, Happonen P, and Neva M: Simple bone cyst: review of the literature and analysis of 23 cases, Int J Oral Maxillofac Surg 17:21-24, 1988a.

Forssell K, Forssell H, and Kahnberg KE: Recurrences of keratocysts: a long-term follow-up study, Int J Oral Maxillofac Surg 17:25-28, 1988b.

Forssell K, Sorvari TE, and Oksala E: An analysis of the recurrence of odontogenic keratocysts, Proc Finn Dent Soc 70:135-140, 1974a.

Forssell K, Sorvari TE, and Oksala E: A clinical and radiographic study of odontogenic keratocysts in jaws, Proc Finn Dent Soc 70:121-134, 1974b.

Frame JW and Wake MJC: Computerized axial tomography in the assessment of the mandibular keratocyst, Br Dent J 153:93-96, 1982.

Gardner DG: The alleged radioresistance of ameloblastoma, J Oral Pathol 11:451, 1982.

Gould AR and Farman AG: Letter to the editor, J Oral Pathol 13:188, 1984.

Hamner JE, Scofield HH, and Cornyn J: Benign fibro-osseous jaw lesions of periodontal membrane origin, Cancer 22:861-878, 1968.

Hansson L: Development of a lingual mandibular bone cavity in an 11-year-old boy, Oral Surg 49:376-378, 1980.

Hayashi Y, Kimura Y, and Nagumo M: Anterior lingual

High AS and Hirschmann PN: Age changes in residual radicular cysts, J Oral Pathol 15:524-528, 1986.

High AS and Hirschmann PN: Symptomatic residual radicular cysts, J Oral Pathol 17:70-72, 1988.

Kameyama Y, Takehana S, Mizohata M, et al: A clinicopathological study of ameloblastomas, Int J Oral Maxillofac Surg 16:706-712, 1987.

Kaneshiro S, Nakajima T, Yoshikawa Y, et al: The postoperative maxillary cyst: report of 71 cases, J Oral Surg 39:191-198, 1981.

Karmoil M and Walsh RF: Incidence of static bone defect of the mandible, Oral Surg 26:225-228, 1968.

Kaugers GE and Cale AE: Traumatic bone cyst, Oral Surg 63:318-324, 1987.

Kelly WH, Mirahmadi MK, Simon JHS, et al: Radiographic changes of the jawbones in end stage renal disease, Oral Surg 50:372-381, 1980.

Keszler A and Dominguez FV: Ameloblastoma in childhood, J Oral Maxillofac Surg 44:609-613, 1986.

Kuroi M: Simple bone cyst of the jaw: review of the literature and report of case, J Oral Surg 38:456-459, 1980.

Langlais RP, Glass BJ, Bricker SL, et al: Medial sigmoid depression: a panoramic pseudoforamen in the upper ramus, Oral Surg 55:635-638, 1983.

Layne EL, Morgan AF, and Morton TH: Anterior lingual mandibular bone concavity: report of case, J Oral Surg 39:599-600, 1981.

Lipani CS, Natiella JR, and Greene GW Jr: The hematopoietic defect of the jaws: a report of 16 cases, J Oral Pathol 11:411-416, 1982.

Makek M and Lello GE: Focal osteoporotic bone marrow defects of the jaws, J Oral Maxillofac Surg 44:268-273, 1986.

Marciani RD, Trodahl JN, Suckiel MJ, and Dubick MN: Cryotherapy in the treatment of ameloblastoma of the mandible: report of cases, J Oral Surg 35:289-295, 1977.

Mehlisch RD, Dahlin DC, and Masson JK: Ameloblastoma: a clinicopathologic report, J Oral Surg 30:9-22, 1972.

Minderjahn A: Incidence and clinical differentiation of odontogenic tumors, J Maxillofac Surg 7:142-150, 1979.

Narang R and Jarrett JH: Large traumatic bone cyst of the mandible, J Oral Surg 38:617-618, 1980.

Oikarinen VJ and Julku M: An orthopantographic study of developmental bone defects, Int J Oral Surg 3:71-76, 1974.

Partridge M and Towers JF: The primordial cyst (odontogenic keratocyst): Its tumour-like characteristics and behaviour, Br J Oral Maxillofac Surg 25:271-279, 1987.

Patrickios A, Sepheriadou-Mavrapoulou Th, and Zambelis G: Bilateral traumatic bone cyst of the mandible: a case report, Oral Surg 51:131-133, 1981.

Payne TF: An analysis of the clinical and histopathologic parameters of the odontogenic keratocyst, Oral Surg 33:538-546, 1972.

Pogrel MA, Sanders K, and Hansen LS: Idiopathic lingual mandibular bone depression, Int J Oral Maxillofac Surg 15:93-97, 1986.

Polak M, Polak G, Brocheriou C, and Vigneul J: Solitary neurofibroma of the mandible: case report and review of the literature, J Oral Maxillofac Surg 47:65-68, 1989.

Precious DS and McFadden LR: Treatment of traumatic bone cyst of mandible by injection of autogenic blood, Oral Surg 58:137-140, 1984.

Raibley SO and Shafer WG: Unpublished data, 1979.

Rao P, Solomon M, Auramides A, et al: Brown giant cell tumors associated with second hyperparathyroidism of chronic renal failure, J Oral Surg 36:154-159, 1978.

Regezi JA, Kerr DA, and Courtney RM: Odontogenic tumors: analysis of 706 cases, J Oral Surg 36:771-778, 1978.

Scott R, Zech R, and Hayward JR: Large idiopathic bone defect of the mandible, J Oral Surg 39:709-712, 1981.

Slootweg PJ and Müller H: Malignant ameloblastoma or ameloblastic carcinoma, Oral Surg 57:168-176, 1984.

Shafer WG: Presentation to American College of Stomatologic Surgeons, Maywood, Ill, 1978.

Shiratsuchi Y, Tashiro H, and Kurihara K: Hemorrhagic cyst of the mandible associated with a retained root apex of the lower third molar, Oral Surg 63:661-663, 1987.

Standish S and Shafer W: Focal osteoporotic bone marrow defects of the jaws, J Oral Surg 20:123-128, 1962.

Struthers P and Shear M: Root resorption by ameloblastomas and cysts of the jaws, Int J Oral Surg 5:128-132, 1976.

Tsaknis PJ and Nelson JF: The maxillary ameloblastoma: an analysis of 24 cases, J Oral Surg 38:336-342, 1980.

Vedtofte P and Praetorius F: Recurrence of OKC in relation to clinical and histological features: a 20 year follow-up of 72 patients, Int J Oral Surg 8:412-420, 1979.

Veno S, Mushimoto K, and Shirasu R: Prognostic evaluation of ameloblastoma based on histologic and radiographic typing, J Oral Maxillofac Surg 47:11-15, 1989.

Vickers RA and Gorlin RJ: Ameloblastoma, delineation of early histopathologic features of neoplasia, Cancer 26:699-710, 1970.

Voorsmit RA, Stoelinga P, and van Haelst GJ: The management of keratocysts, J Maxillofac Surg 9:228-236, 1981.

Waldron CA and El-Mofty SK: A histopathologic study of 116 ameloblastomas with special reference to the desmoplastic variant, Oral Surg 63:441-451, 1987.

Waldron CA and Giansanti JS: Benign fibro-osseous lesions of the jaws: a clinical-radiologic-histologic review of sixty-five cases. I. Fibrous dysplasia of the jaws, Oral Surg 35:190-201, 1973a.

Waldron CA and Giansanti JS: Benign fibro-osseous lesions of the jaws: a clinical-radiologic-histologic review of sixty-five cases. II. Benign fibro-osseous lesions of periodontal ligament origin, Oral Surg 35:340-350, 1973b.

Wilson DF and Ross AS: Ultrastructure of odontogenic keratocysts, Oral Surg 45:887-893, 1978.

Winer RA and Doku HC: Traumatic bone cyst in the maxilla, Oral Surg 46:367-370, 1978.

Wolf J, Mattila K, and Ankkuriniemi O: Development of a Stafne mandibular bone cavity: report of a case, Oral Surg 61:519-521, 1986.

Woolgar JA, Rippin JW, and Browne RM: A comparative study of the clinical and histological features of recurrent and nonrecurrent odontogenic keratocysts, J Oral Pathol 16:124-128, 1987.

Wright JM: The odontogenic keratocyst. orthokeratinized variant, Oral Surg 51:609-618, 1981.

Zachariades N, Papanicolaou S, and Triantafyllou D: Odontogenic keratocysts: review of the literature and report of sixteen cases, J Oral Maxillofac Surg 43:177-182, 1985.

Zachariades N, Vairaktaris E, Papanicolaou S, et al: Ossifying fibroma of the jaws: review of the literature and report of 16 cases, Int J Oral Surg 13:1-6, 1984.

20

Multilocular radiolucencies

NORMAN K. WOOD
PAUL W. GOAZ
ROGER H. KALLAL

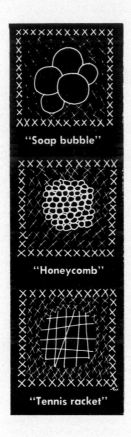

"Soap bubble"

"Honeycomb"

"Tennis racket"

Multilocular radiolucencies of the oral cavity include the following:

Anatomic patterns
Multilocular cyst
Ameloblastoma
Central giant cell granuloma
Giant cell lesion of hyperparathyroidism
Cherubism
Odontogenic myxoma
Odontogenic keratocyst
Aneurysmal bone cyst
Metastatic tumors to the jaws
*Vascular malformations and central
   hemangioma of bone*
Rarities
  Ameloblastic variants
  Arteriovenous malformations
  Burkitt's lymphoma
  Calcifying epithelial odontogenic tumor
  Cementifying and ossifying fibroma
  Central adenoid cystic carcinoma
  Central giant cell tumor
  Central mucoepidermoid tumor
  *Central odontogenic and nonodontogenic
   fibromas*
  Chondroma
  Chondrosarcoma
  Eosinophilic granuloma
  Fibromatosis
  Fibrous dysplasia
  Immature odontoma
  Leiomyoma
  Lingual mandibular bone defect
  Neurilemoma
  Neuroectodermal tumor of infancy
  Osteomyelitis
  Pseudotumor of hemophilia
  Squamous odontogenic tumor

Multilocular radiolucencies are produced by multiple, adjacent, frequently coalescing, and overlapping pathologic compartments in bone. They may occur in the maxilla but are found much more commonly in the mandible.

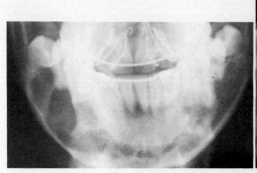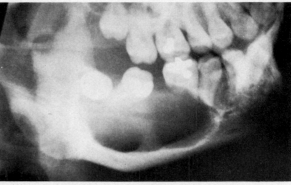

Fig. 20-1. Pseudomultilocular radiolucencies. Both lesions proved at surgery to be unilocular. **A,** Traumatic bone cyst. **B,** Ameloblastoma.   (Courtesy the late M. Kaminski, DDS, and S. Atsaves, DDS, Chicago.)

Whereas all the entities included in this chapter appear as multilocular lesions, they may also occur as a single, sharp, cystlike radiolucency or even as a poorly defined radiolucency. The presentation of these lesions in the outline at the beginning of this chapter and in Chapter 19 is according to incidence (to whatever extent such order is known or ordering is possible).

Unilocular lesions that have perforated the cortical plate in one or more areas may cause radiographic images that resemble those from multilocular entities (Fig. 20-1). The true multilocular lesion contains two or more pathologic chambers partially separated by septa of bone, which are usually discernible on radiographic examination. On occasion, the septa may be so thin and their images so indistinct as to cause the multilocular lesion to appear unilocular on radiographic examination.

The terms "soap bubble," "honeycomb," and "tennis racket" are frequently used to describe the various radiographic images of multilocular lesions. "Soap bubble" is reserved for lesions consisting of several *circular* compartments that vary in size and usually appear to overlap somewhat. "Honeycomb" applies to lesions whose compartments are *small* and tend to be *uniform* in size. The "tennis racket" designation is descriptive of lesions composed of *angular* rather than rounded compartments that result from the development of more or less straight septa. Thus these compartments tend to be triangular, rectangular, or square. (Refer to the introductory figure for this chapter.)

To amplify the connotation of the term "multilocular lesion" as used in this chapter, we merely remind the reader that multilocular is used only as a *radiographic*, not a microscopic, description. Many lesions demonstrate microscopic projections, but these tiny bosses are usually not large enough to be evident on radiographic examination. When studying radiographs of the lesions described in this chapter, the clinician should know that the radiolucent areas making up the images are not empty spaces, as they appear, but rather are compartments filled usually with neoplastic tissue or at least with cystic fluid or blood.

The following presentation includes descriptions of the primary and distinctive features of each lesion, illustrations of the development of a differential diagnosis, and discussion of the contributing circumstances and considerations that support a suggested course of treatment.

ANATOMIC PATTERNS

To preclude their being mistaken for multilocular lesions, two normal radiolucent structures of the perioral regions and their radiographic variations are described in this section: the maxillary sinus and bone marrow spaces.

The *maxillary sinus* usually has several compartments that project into the surrounding maxilla and zygoma and give the radiographic appearance of septa dividing the sinus into lobes.

When many such lobes or compartments are present, the soap bubble image may result (Fig. 20-2). The anatomic location of the variable extensions of the sinus and the relative location of adjacent structures on radiographs taken from different angles, coupled with the absence of symptoms, are usually sufficient to identify these areas as pouches from the maxillary sinus.

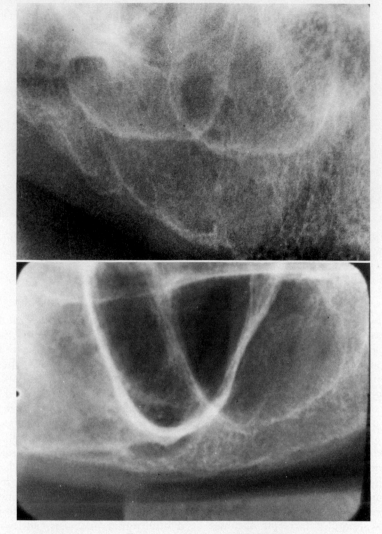

Fig. 20-2. Maxillary sinus showing multilocular patterns.

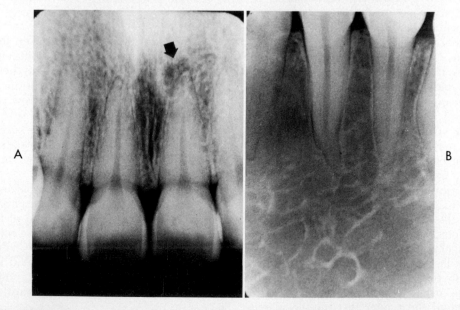

Fig. 20-3. Marrow spaces showing soap bubble patterns. **A,** The arrow identifies a multiloc-ular bone marrow space at the apices of the central incisor root.

Bone marrow spaces and trabecular patterns appear frequently as multilocular radiolucencies, especially in the mandible (Fig. 20-3). Usually when these spaces and patterns resemble pathologic multilocular radiolucencies, a comparison with the pattern of trabeculation in the remainder of the jawbone shows a similar image so the examiner can conclude with reasonable certainty that the suspect region is a normal variation.

When a trabecular pattern appears only as an isolated area, the correct diagnosis is more difficult to make. In the absence of additional manifestations of disease, however, a satisfactory technique is to observe the area semiannually with radiographs to be certain that no growth occurs and that it is an innocent variation of the normal trabecular pattern.

MULTILOCULAR CYST

The multilocular cyst is the most frequently encountered pathologic multilocular radiolucency in the jaws. It is always of the soap bubble variety, occurs most frequently in the mandible (usually in the premolar and molar region), and varies greatly in size (Fig. 20-4).

Theoretically any cyst that occurs in the jaws could develop multiple compartments, but the radicular and fissural cysts are almost always unilocular lesions, whereas in particular the odontogenic keratocyst, the primordial cyst, the follicular cyst, and the residual cyst occur with some frequency as multilocular cysts.

Features

The multilocular cyst is a true cyst of the jaws and may be found in any age-group but is

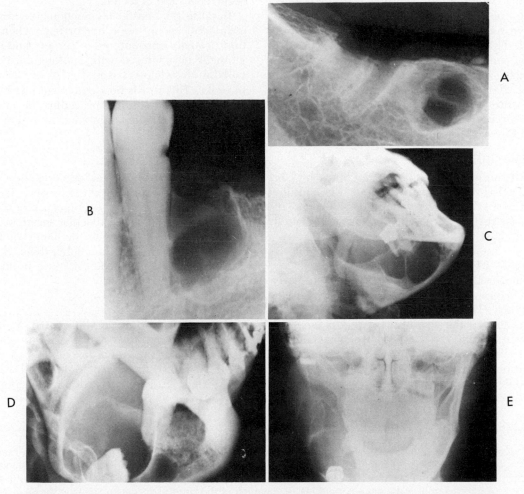

Fig. 20-4. Multilocular cysts **A,** Residual cyst. **B,** Botryoid cyst. **C,** Radicular cyst. **D** and **E,** Follicular cysts.   (**A** courtesy M. Smulson, DDS, Maywood, Ill. **C** courtesy R. Kallal, DDS, Flossmoor, Ill. **D** and **E** courtesy O.H. Stuteville, DDS, MD, St. Joe, Ark.)

more frequent in persons over 15 years of age. The small cyst is usually asymptomatic and generally noticed on routine radiographic examination (Fig. 20-4). It increases in size slowly and may cause displacement of adjacent teeth and occasionally root resorption, but it rarely gives rise to a paresthesia unless secondarily infected. If undetected, the cyst may expand the cortical plates as it enlarges and may become apparent on clinical examination as a smooth bony-hard swelling. If the overlying bone becomes quite thin, a crackling sound (crepitus) may be produced by palpation. Later, if the covering plate is destroyed, the cyst appears as a soft to rubbery fluctuant mass with perhaps a bluish color.

Aspiration usually yields a thin, straw-colored fluid unless the mass is a keratocyst, which yields a thick, granular, yellow fluid that requires a large-bore needle for successful aspiration. Microscopic study reveals lumina lined with epithelium and surrounded by a cyst wall varying in thickness and in fibrous tissue content. The botryoid odontogenic cyst is a particular multilocular cyst that gives a "grape bunch" multilocular radiolucent appearance (Fig. 20-4, B). It was first described by Weathers and Waldron (1973). Other authors have since reported on it, including Kaugers (1986) and Greer and Johnson (1988).

Differential diagnosis

All the lesions in this chapter must be considered in the differential diagnosis of multilocular cyst. These are given in the differential diagnosis section at the end of this chapter and in Table 20-1 (p. 426).

Management

The treatment of cysts is discussed in detail in Chapters 16 and 17. The alternative methods are (1) total surgical enucleation plus a bone graft if the size of the defect is large, (2) marsupialization, (3) decompression, and (4) partial decompression followed by surgical enucleation at a later date.

Many factors must be considered before a method of treatment is selected. Total removal is the treatment of choice for multilocular cysts because ensuring that all compartments have been eradicated is especially difficult if the more conservative methods are employed. A conservative approach may be preferable in some cases, however.

The final diagnosis must await results of surgery and microscopic examination. If the suspect lesion is a cyst, the surgeon usually encounters a thin lining of soft tissue and a lumen filled with fluid. Encountering any solid areas of soft tissue should alert the surgeon to the probability that he or she is dealing with a more serious lesion, such as one of those listed at the beginning of this chapter. In addition, the surgeon should be alert to the possibility of a mural ameloblastoma. Regardless of the method of treatment chosen, the surgical site must be observed radiographically for several years to ensure that healing is complete or that recurrences are detected.

Because the central hemangioma represents a threat of uncontrolled hemorrhage when it is unexpectedly encountered at surgery and since it might be confused with another entity detailed in this chapter, aspiration of any lesion is in order. This test is best employed just before initiation of the surgical procedure because of the possibility of contaminating the lesion during aspiration.

AMELOBLASTOMA

The ameloblastoma is an odontogenic tumor usually described as locally invasive. It may cast a unilocular cystlike radiolucency or a multilocular image. The multilocular image may be of either the soap bubble or the honeycomb variety (Fig. 20-5). The ameloblastoma is discussed in detail in Chapter 19 as a unilocular radiolucency.

Differential diagnosis

For a discussion of the differential diagnosis of ameloblastoma, refer to the differential diagnosis section at the end of this chapter (p. 427), Table 20-1 (p. 426), and the differential diagnosis section for ameloblastoma in Chapter 19 (pp. 391 and 388).

Fig. 20-5. Ameloblastoma. **A,** Facial asymmetry caused by the expansion of the left ramus in a 68-year-old man. **B,** Intraoral swelling in the third molar region of the same patient. The ulcerated surface was caused by trauma from a maxillary molar. **C,** Left lateral oblique radiograph in the same patient. **D,** Radiograph of the surgical specimen showing the soap bubble pattern. **E** to **J,** Radiographs of other ameloblastomas. (Honeycomb patterns are apparent in **E** and **G,** soap bubble patterns are evident in **H** and **I,** and the angular multilocular pattern is shown in **J.**)　(**E** courtesy P. Akers, DDS, Chicago. **F** to **J** courtesy O.H. Stuteville, DDS, MD, St. Joe, Ark.)

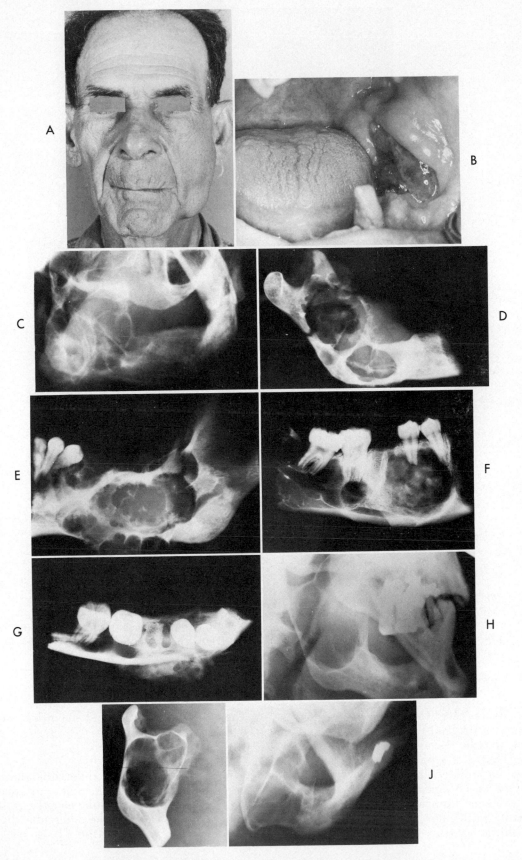

Fig. 20-5. For legend see opposite page.

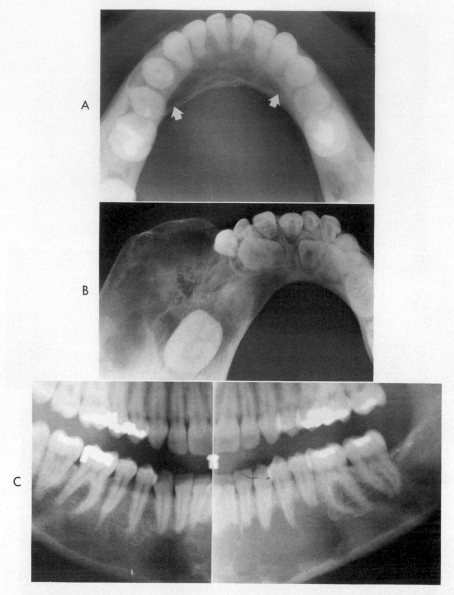

Fig. 20-6. Giant cell granuloma. **A,** Arrows indicate the lateral limits of the soap bubble lesion. **B,** Large soap bubble lesion producing marked expansion in the mandible of a 5-year-old boy. See Fig. 19-15, *D,* for the histopathologic features of the lesion. **C,** Lesion in a middle-aged woman.   (**A** and **B** courtesy R. Goepp, DDS, Zoller Clinic, University of Chicago. **C** courtesy V. Barresi, DDS, DeKalb, Ill.).

CENTRAL GIANT CELL GRANULOMA

The central giant cell granuloma (GCG) may occur initially as a solitary cystlike radiolucency, but as it grows larger, it frequently develops an architecture that causes a soap bubble type of multilocular radiolucency (Fig. 20-6). Although trauma was thought to be the causative factor, now many pathologists believe that this is not true; the cause is still in doubt.

The central giant cell granuloma is discussed in detail in Chapter 19.

Differential diagnosis

For a discussion of the differential diagnosis of central GCG, refer to the differential diagnosis section at the end of this chapter (p. 427), Table 20-1 (p. 426), and the differential diagnosis section for GCG in Chapter 19 (p. 395).

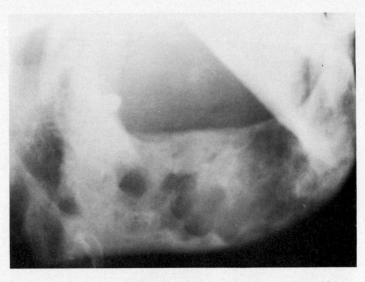

Fig. 20-7. Brown giant cell lesion of hyperparathyroidism. The soap bubble pattern is evident.   (From Rotblat S and Laskin D: J Oral Surg 27:820-825, 1969. Copyright by the American Dental Association. Reprinted by permission.)

GIANT CELL LESION OF HYPERPARATHYROIDISM

The clinical, radiographic, and histologic characteristics of the giant cell lesion of hyperparathyroidism are identical to those of the giant cell granuloma. It occurs as a unilocular or a multilocular radiolucency (Fig. 20-7) and is found in patients with primary, secondary, or tertiary hyperparathyroidism. Establishing its identity depends on demonstrating the concomitant parathyroid hormone or kidney disorder. This giant cell lesion is discussed in detail in Chapter 19.

Differential diagnosis

For a discussion of the differential diagnosis of the giant cell lesion of hyperparathyroidism, refer to the differential diagnosis section at the end of the chapter (p. 427), Table 20-1 (p. 426), and the differential diagnosis section of this giant cell lesion in Chapter 19 (p. 396).

CHERUBISM (FAMILIAL INTRAOSSEOUS SWELLING OF THE JAWS)

Although cases without familial involvement have been reported (DeTomasi et al., 1985), cherubism is usually inherited as an autosomal dominant trait. Expressivity and penetrance are more pronounced in males. The disease occurs with two or more separate multilocular-appearing lesions (Fig. 20-8). Sometimes the interlocular bone becomes so indistinct that the multilocular appearance is lost.

Features

Cherubism occurs in patients between the ages of 2 and 20 years. It usually commences bilaterally in the rami of the mandible and becomes apparent as painless swellings of the face in these areas. Occasionally the whole mandible is involved. Other bones (for example, the walls of the maxillary sinus, orbital floor, and tuberosity regions) may also be affected, and the resultant enlargement in these areas produces the cherublike expression by tilting the eyeballs superiorly (Fig. 20-8). The lesion grows slowly, expanding but not perforating the cortex. Paresthesia is not a feature.

At approximately 8 or 9 years of age, growth of the pathologic region may plateau—until puberty, when the lesion may begin to regress. Usually the bony architecture returns to normal by age 30, except for a few instances in which the involved bone of the ramus retains an appearance that resembles ground glass on radiographic examination. Some patients may demonstrate a persistent swelling for years.

A few posterior teeth may be missing in this disease because of the early-developing expanding masses; these expansions destroy the buds and the incipient follicles.

On posteroanterior views the teeth associated with the lesion often seem to be hanging in air. On microscopic examination the lesion is composed of mature fibroblasts in a surprisingly pale edematous background that contains little collagen. Multinucleated giant cells are

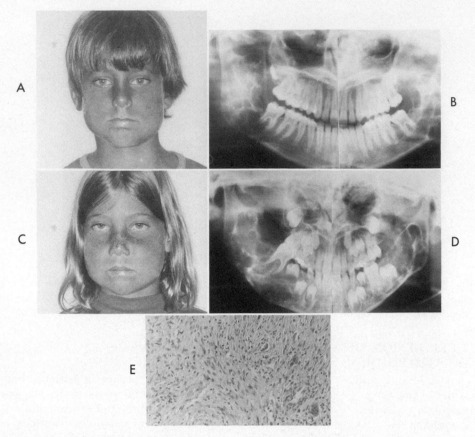

Fig. 20-8. Cherubism. **A,** Clinical appearance of bilateral expansion of the rami in a 12-year-old boy. **B,** Panograph reveals the bilateral soap bubble expansions of the rami. The maxilla was not involved in this case. **C** and **D,** Seven-year-old sister of this patient. Both the maxilla and the mandible are involved. The superior tilt of the eyeballs gives the cherubic appearance. **E,** Microscopy of cherubism.   (**A** to **D** courtesy J. Hebert, DDS, Houston.)

few and occur in clusters (Fig. 20-8). Coope et al. (1983) described a case of cherubism in which they constructed a serial stereophotogrametric assessment of the patient between the ages of 5 years 2 months and 10 years 3 months.

Differential diagnosis

The multiple lesions occurring bilaterally in the ramus—coupled with the cherubic appearance, the specific age-group, and a history of kindred involvement—should readily guide the clinician to the correct impression. This disease is the only entity in this chapter with characteristics specific enough to enable the clinician to feel confident of his or her working diagnosis. Nevertheless, because nonfamilial cases and unilateral lesions have been reported, the clinician should also consider a list of possible diagnoses. For more differential in-

formation concerning the differential diagnosis of cherubism the reader is referred to Table 20-1 and to the differential diagnosis section at the end of the chapter (p. 427).

Management

The correct identification of the condition and periodic clinical and radiographic examinations are required. If the clinical picture is confusing, an incisional biopsy provides the correct diagnosis.

Orthodontic care may be necessary to ensure proper alignment of the teeth, and occasionally surgical contouring of the lesion is necessary to improve esthetics, as well as in cases of rapid growth (Kuepper and Harrigan, 1978). Usually by the patient's fourth decade, most evidence of the disease has disappeared, although unusual cases show activity through age 60 (Waldron, 1976).

ODONTOGENIC MYXOMA

The odontogenic myxoma is a benign tumor of bone that apparently occurs exclusively in the jaws and is usually classified as an odontogenic tumor. The myxomatous tissue, of which this tumor is composed, is thought to originate (1) as a direct outgrowth of the dental papilla of a tooth, (2) as an inductive effect of nests of odontogenic epithelium on mesenchymal tissue, or (3) as a direct myxomatous change in fibrous tissue.

The myxoma is rarely seen in other bones of the skeleton; thus the theory of odontogenic origin is strengthened. Although it has been previously believed that the odontogenic myxoma frequently occurs in the region of a missing tooth, an extensive review of the literature failed to substantiate this opinion (Farman et al., 1977). There is also a malignant variant of this tumor.

On radiographic examination the odontogenic myxoma may be found as a unilocular cystlike radiolucency, a pericoronal radiolucency, or a mixed radiolucent-radiopaque image. More frequently it occurs as a multilocular radiolucency, however (Fig. 20-9).

The tennis racket appearance is the most common. The individual compartments may appear on radiographic examination in the form of triangles, rectangles, or squares, depending on the random arrangement of the bony septa. Fine trabeculation is often seen distributed within the individual compartments. The radiographic margins of the tumor may be well defined or poorly defined. Myxomas may also occur with soap bubble and honeycomb patterns.

Features

The myxoma accounts for 3% to 6% of all odontogenic tumors (Minderjahn, 1979; Regezi et al., 1978). Farman et al. (1977) reviewed the literature and found that the approximate ratio of maxillary to mandibular lesions is 3:4. Many of the maxillary lesions involved the maxillary sinus, and few cases crossed the midline. Farman et al. reported that most of the mandibular lesions occurred in the premolar and molar region. Only a few lesions involved the non–tooth-bearing areas of the jaw. A slight predilection for females was found. The average patient age for various categories ranged between 25 and 35 years. These reviewers found that root resorption was very rare. Harder (1978) reported that myxomas rarely occur before age 10 or after age 50.

The chief complaint of a patient with an odontogenic myxoma may be a slowly enlarging, painless expansion of the jaw with possible spreading, loosening, and migration of teeth in the involved area. Rarely there may be numbness of the lip and, occasionally, pain. The earlier asymptomatic stage, before cortical expansion occurs, may be detected only by a routine radiographic survey.

If the tumor is not detected and treated in the early stage, it causes facial asymmetry as it expands the cortical plates and effects a smooth enlargement of the alveolus of the jaw (Fig. 20-9). Sometimes it perforates the cortical plates in several places, thus producing a bosselated surface (several small nodules on the surface). The mucosa or skin over the tumor appears normal unless continually traumatized.

On histologic examination the tumor consists of tissue resembling that of the dental papillae. Thin, triangular cells with fibers streaming from the corners are seen scattered throughout a pale myxomatous background (Fig. 20-9). Small cords or nests of odontogenic epithelium may be present. Mature collagen fibers are scarce. The loosely arranged, fibrillar, pale-staining microscopic picture of this lesion confirms that if the cortical plates are perforated, the expanding mass is soft to palpation and gives the impression of fluctuance because of the high water content of the tissue. Aspiration, however, is nonproductive.

Differential diagnosis

Again, even though a lesion of this type may be suspected when the clinician encounters a typical multilocular radiolucency, all the lesions discussed in this chapter should be included in the differential diagnosis.

If there is a honeycomb or tennis racket picture, however, the myxoma must be considered along with the *ameloblastoma* and the *intrabony hemangioma*. The honeycomb variant of the myxoma usually shows fine trabeculations within the small lobules, which are not present in the ameloblastoma.

Since the myxoma occurs as a solitary lesion, usually in a slightly older age-group, confusing this lesion with the multiple lesions of *cherubism* should be obviated.

The *giant cell granuloma* occurs most commonly in the anterior regions of the jaws, whereas the myxoma is seen most frequently in the ramus and premolar and molar area of the mandible.

Management

Recurrences of the odontogenic myxoma are quite common and have been reported in 25%

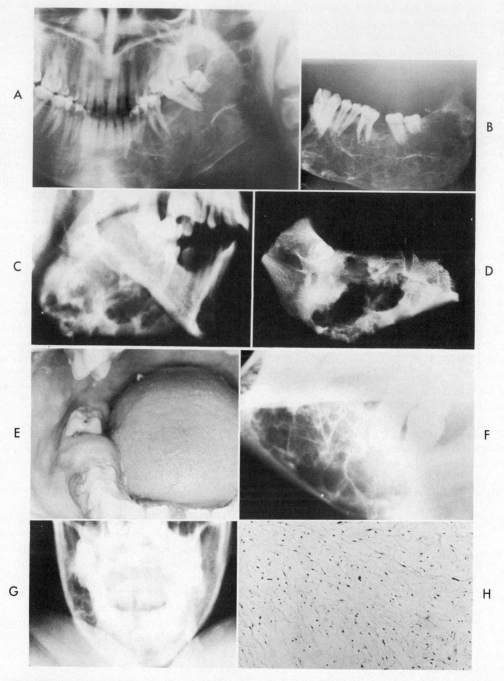

Fig. 20-9. Odontogenic myxoma. **A,** Orthopantomograph and, **B,** radiograph of a surgical specimen. **C,** Lateral oblique radiograph of another patient and, **D,** radiograph of the surgical specimen. **E,** Myxoma producing a smoothly contoured oral swelling. **F** and **G,** Radiographs of the lesion shown in **E. H,** Photomicrograph of a myxoma.   (**A** and **B** courtesy N. Barakat, DDS, Beirut, Lebanon. **C** and **D** courtesy O.H. Stuteville, DDS, MD, St. Joe, Ark. **F** courtesy R. Kallal, DDS, Flossmoor, Ill. **G** courtesy D. Bonomo, DDS, Flossmoor, Ill.)

of the treated patients. Apparently this behavior is a consequence of the tumor's tendency to spill into the surrounding marrow spaces. To minimize recurrences, normal resection of the tumor with a generous amount of surrounding bone is necessary in extensive lesions. Teeth in the region often must be included in the section. Many cases are successfully managed, however, with enucleation and cautery. The tumor does not respond to radiation.

Occasionally an odontogenic myxoma extends into the mandibular canal; in these cases the neurovascular bundle is usually sacrificed. Recurrences may on occasion be observed years after treatment, when the involved regions of the jaws have appeared on radiographic examination to be completely healed. A more extensive resection is then required, but the inferior border of the mandible should be retained if possible.

Adamo et al. (1980) reported a case of myxoma of the mandible in which the lingual plate and tumor were removed and the defect immediately grafted with autogenous iliac crest bone chips.

ODONTOGENIC KERATOCYST

The odontogenic keratocyst is discussed in detail as a cystlike radiolucency in Chapter 19. It is included in this chapter because it occurs with considerable frequency as a multilocular radiolucency and so must be considered in the differential diagnosis of the lesions included in this chapter. As high as the significant recurrence rate is for the odontogenic keratocyst, it will be of even greater concern to the surgeon when he or she plans a treatment approach for the multilocular variety.

ANEURYSMAL BONE CYST

The aneurysmal bone cyst (ABC) is characterized as a false cyst because it does not have an epithelial lining. It occurs as a unilocular or multilocular radiolucency (Fig. 20-10) that fre-

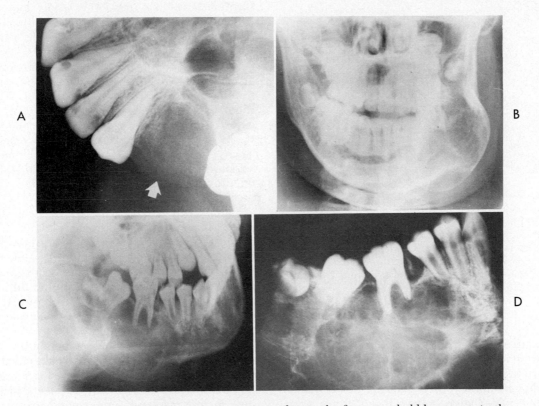

Fig. 20-10. Aneurysmal bone cyst. **A,** Arrow indicates the faint soap bubble pattern in the premolar region. **B** and **C,** Posteroanterior and lateral oblique radiographs and, **D,** radiograph of the surgical specimen from the 12-year-old girl shown in **B** and **C.** (**A** courtesy R. Goepp, DDS, Zoller Clinic, University of Chicago. **B** to **D** from Hoppe W: Oral Surg 25:1-5, 1968.).

Continued.

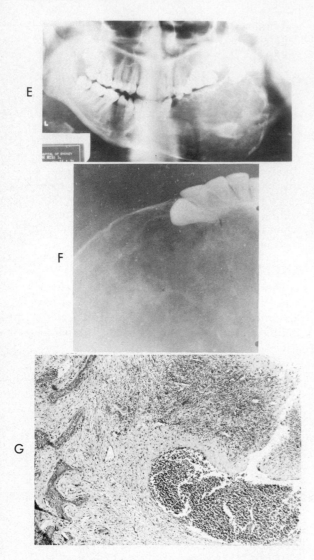

that the ABC is a secondary phenomenon that occurs in a primary lesion of bone. They studied histologic material from 303 lesions of bone to see if areas with histologic features similar to those of the ABC were present. They found areas similar to ABC in 28% of the giant cell granulomas, 10% of fibrous dysplasias, 1 of 7 cases of Paget's disease, 14% of fibrosarcomas, and 11% of osteosarcomas. These investigators postulated that the initiating process of the ABC is the microcyst that forms as a result of intercellular edema in a primary lesion with loose, unsupported stroma.

Features

The aneurysmal bone cyst is a slow-growing lesion that affects the mandible much more often than the maxilla (3:1) but is seldom encountered in the perioral regions. It most frequently involves persons under 20 years of age. Because it grows slowly, it may expand and thin the cortical plates, but it usually does not destroy them. It may be slightly tender and teeth may be missing or displaced, but root resorption is seldom seen. The lesion does not appear to show a predilection for either sex (Reyneke, 1978; Steidler et al., 1979). Paresthesia is not a feature.

Struthers and Shear (1984a, 1984b) reviewed 46 cases of ABC (42 well-documented cases from the literature and four of their own). They reported the following findings: (1) 93% occurred in the first three decades of life and two thirds of the patients were under 20 years of age; (2) 62% were women or girls; (3) the molar regions were the predominant sites; and (4) frequently there was a history of a period of rapid growth of the ABC.

Salmo et al. (1981) reported an interesting case of bilateral ABCs of the maxilla.

Grossly the lesion is soft and reddish brown; because of its rich blood supply it resembles a sponge filled with blood. On microscopic examination it contains giant cells scattered through a fibrous stroma that contains cavernous, thin-walled blood spaces (Fig. 20-10). Bone spicules and osteoid may be present.

Some pathologists are of the opinion that the ABC is actually a response to an alteration in the vasculature of the area involved (for example, trauma and subsequent intrabony bleeding). Such a response, an exaggerated proliferative reaction, is thought to be similar to that of the central and peripheral giant cell reparative granulomas, which it resembles in many respects; however, the developing ABC appar-

Fig. 20-10, cont'd. Aneurysmal bone cysts. **E,** Panograph and, **F,** occlusal radiograph of a large lesion found in a 20-year-old woman. The soap bubble pattern and retention of a thin cortex are characteristic of this benign condition. **G,** Photomicrograph showing a large vascular space. Multinucleated giant cells are frequently present. (**E** and **F** from Oliver LP: Oral Surg 35:67-76, 1973.)

quently balloons out the cortex. It has been reported most frequently in the long bones, the vertebrae, and occasionally the jaws. Its cause, although unproved, is thought to be trauma. Some pathologists believe that it forms a continuum with the traumatic bone cyst and the central giant cell granuloma.

Struthers and Shear (1984a, 1984b) undertook an extensive study to test the hypothesis

ently is continually effused with circulating blood from the injured vessels, whereas the granulomas are not.

In light of the suggested similarity in pathogenesis between the ABC and the two giant cell lesions, it is of interest that all three of these entities usually develop in younger patients (that is, patients under 30 years of age), at which time the repair response is more vigorous.

Differential diagnosis

The differential diagnosis of aneurysmal bone cyst is discussed in the differential diagnosis section at the end of this chapter (p. 427) and included in Table 20-1 (p. 426).

Management

As with the other lesions detailed in this chapter, the surgeon should organize a differential diagnosis, since the clinical and radiographic pictures of the ABC are similar to those of several other entities included in the group. Aspiration of the involved area of the bone is recommended to obviate a dangerous, unexpected entrance into an intrabony hemangioma or arteriovenous shunt.

Usually a copious amount of blood can be aspirated from an ABC—but not the syringefuls of blood that are readily obtained from hemangiomas or shunts. Surgical curettement is the treatment of choice. Hemorrhage is usually moderate, and its arrest is not difficult. ABCs do recur. El Deeb et al. (1980), in a review of the literature, found a recurrence rate of 26%. The treatment recommended by these investigators is surgical curettage with cryosurgery and immediate packing with bone chips. Struthers and Shear (1984) recommended thorough curettage using an extraoral approach if necessary to thoroughly accomplish the task. Ueno et al. (1982) performed a block resection for a large ABC of the mandible, and an immediate graft of the iliac crest was placed.

METASTATIC TUMORS TO THE JAWS

The malignant tumors that most commonly metastasize to the jaws are carcinomas of the lung, breast, gastrointestinal tract, kidney, prostate gland, testis, and thyroid gland. Metastatic jaw tumors have been reported to arise from parent tumors in other organs and sites, but these are rare.

Malignant cells from distant sites usually are carried via arterial blood. Some pathologists, believe, however, that malignant cells travel

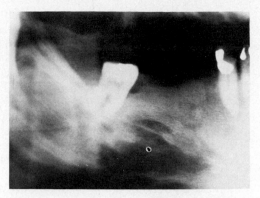

Fig. 20-11. Metastatic renal adenocarcinoma.

from their primary site to the jaws via the prevertebral veins of Batson.

The mandible is much more frequently the site of secondary tumors than is the maxilla, and the premolar and molar area is the most commonly affected region.

Although metastatic jaw tumors are included in this chapter, which is devoted to multilocular lesions, a multilocular pattern is not the only one produced by a secondary tumor.

Intrabony metastatic jaw tumors may cause several other radiographic appearances:

1. A *solitary, well-defined cystlike radiolucency.* Tumors giving this picture are usually of the slow-growing, well-differentiated type, or else the patient is being successfully treated with cytotoxic drugs.

2. A *solitary, poorly defined radiolucency.* This picture is usually caused by a localized, rapidly growing tumor.

3. *Multiple, separate, poorly defined radiolucencies.* This appearance usually occurs where several foci of malignant nests are present and growing separately from each other.

4. *Multiple punched-out radiolucencies (multiple myeloma–like radiolucencies).* This appearance is characteristic when several nests of slow-growing tumor cells are located close to each other in the bone.

5. *Radiopaque patterns with any of the foregoing radiolucent appearances.* The tumors in these cases have either induced osteoblastic activity or produced osteosclerosis in the bone.

6. *An irregular salt-and-pepper appearance.* This image usually involves a large segment of the jaws and indicates that the

tumor is widely disseminated in multiple nests in the bone. These nests appear as small radiolucencies (pepper). They induce sclerotic areas about themselves and thus sprinkle the overall image with small radiopaque foci (salt).

7. *A relatively dense, solitary radiopaque area.* Sometimes a prostatic or a mammary tumor demonstrates osteoblastic activity; the bone thus produced shows as a rather radiopaque area and may resemble condensing osteitis.

When a metastatic tumor of bone produces a multilocular radiographic lesion, it is almost always of the honeycomb or tennis racket structure (Fig. 20-11).

Features

The patient with a secondary tumor of the jaw may seek treatment for pain resulting from a local jaw metastasis or from the parent tumor itself (if it has not been successfully treated). Symptoms induced by the parent tumor usually reflect the altered physiology of the affected organ.

For example, a large bronchogenic carcinoma in the lung may produce symptoms that include chronic cough, hemoptysis, dyspnea, orthopnea, tachycardia, and an overall cachectic appearance. Thus, if a bony lesion is found in the jaws of such a patient, the clinician should consider the increased possibility that it is a metastatic tumor. The clinician must be aware, however, that in certain cases the metastatic lesion is the first discovered. In such cases the primary tumor is said to be occult and if the secondary tumor is poorly differentiated on histologic examination, the primary tumor may be difficult to locate.

The local symptoms produced by a metastatic tumor of the jaws are similar to those produced by a primary malignant jaw tumor. Thus a spectrum of manifestations may be expected, ranging from nonexistent in an early lesion to marked in an advanced lesion that has caused substantial bone destruction. Advanced tumors often involve the inferior dental canal and cause a paresthesia or anesthesia of the lower lip on the affected side. As the lesion becomes more extensive, pathologic fractures are possible.

An enlarging lesion may erode rapidly through the cortical plates, usually without expanding them, and then invade the surrounding soft tissues, which thus become fixed to the jawbone. The phenomenon of normally movable soft tissue fixed to bone is an ominous sign

and indicates either a sclerosing fibrosis or a malignant invasion. If fibrosis or invasion or both occur in a region where muscles are present, function is impaired. For example, a tumor that has perforated the bone and invaded one of the muscles of mastication causes restriction of mandibular opening or perhaps deviation to the affected side. Similarly, if the tongue is fixed in one region by the tumor, its movements may be curtailed and speech may also be affected.

Pain is not a frequent complaint, but occasionally it is present later in the course of growth of the tumor, when sensory nerves within the bone are encroached on. It is usually of short duration, however, because the tumor rapidly destroys the affected nerve.

The tumor usually erodes rather than expands the adjacent cortical plates. Thus detectable expansion is not bony hard to palpation but firm. This firmness is caused by the nests, cords, and sheets of closely packed tumor cells that are surrounded by a relatively broad and dense boundary of fibrous tissue. The exophytic mass is frequently nodular and smoothly contoured with a normal-appearing mucosal surface.

The microscopic structure of a metastatic tumor may vary greatly from that of the parent tumor, or both tumors may have an identical microstructure. In addition, a secondary tumor may appear to be more or less malignant than the primary tumor. When a tumor of the jaws is anaplastic (poorly differentiated) and aggressive and when a primary lesion has not been detected, a positive diagnosis may be difficult if not impossible to make. Such a nondescript lesion could actually be a primary anaplastic tumor of the jaws.

Differential diagnosis

Although the clinician must consider all the multilocular lesions, if the patient has a history of a primary malignancy elsewhere in the body, the possibility of metastatic tumor must be assigned a high rank in the differential diagnosis. For additional features, refer to Table 20-1.

Management

Once the diagnosis of a metastatic tumor has been made and the primary tumor identified, the case should be managed by a tumor board. The course of action of the tumor board is dictated by several factors:

1. If the primary tumor was successfully treated some time previously and the present jaw lesion is the only detectable

metastatic tumor after a complete examination (including a radiographic skeletal survey) and if the patient's general medical condition permits, the metastatic lesion should be *treated aggressively.*

2. Depending on the type and location of the jaw lesion and how the primary tumor responded to treatment, *surgery, radiation, antitumor medication,* or combinations of these techniques might be used. Despite this statement, however, the clinician must realize that the secondary tumor may react differently to similar treatment from the way the primary tumor reacted.

3. If the primary tumor has shown gross recurrence and there is wide metastasis, the jaw lesion should be *managed conservatively. Palliative measures* may be instituted to provide as much comfort as possible (for example, a nerve block of alcohol to arrest pain).

VASCULAR MALFORMATIONS AND CENTRAL HEMANGIOMA OF BONE

Vascular malformations in bone occur much more frequently than the central hemangioma of bone. Kaban and Mulliken (1986) reported that 35% of vascular malformations occur in bone, whereas central hemangiomas of bone are rare. The central hemangioma of bone is a benign tumor that rarely occurs in the jaws; it occurs more frequently in the skull and the vertebrae. It may be congenital or traumatic in origin.

The central hemangioma of bone has been referred to as "the great imitator" because it can produce so many different radiographic images. Worth and Stoneman (1979) have prepared an excellent and unusually thorough review of the various radiographic appearances of this tumor. In about 50% of cases a multilocular appearance can be detected (Fig. 20-12).

Another form this lesion can take reveals coarse, linear trabeculae that appear to radiate from an approximate center of the lesion. Small, angular locules of varying shape are seen; however, the general outline is round.

A third appearance that may be observed is a cystlike radiolucency with an empty cavity and sometimes a hyperostotic border.

The radiographic margins of these images may be either well defined or poorly defined. Resorption of roots of the involved teeth occurs with some frequency, and calcifications (phleboliths) appearing as radiopaque rings are occasionally seen.

Features

The usual complaint of a patient with an intrabony hemangioma is of a slow-growing asymmetry of the jaw or localized gingival bleeding. Numbness and tenderness or pain may also be described. This solitary tumor is found approximately twice as often in females, and about 65% occur in the mandible. Although the tumors affect patients of all ages, the majority have been discovered in patients between the ages of 10 and 20 years. Some tumors demonstrate pulsation and bruits. Paresthesia is occasionally a feature.

As the slow-growing tumor expands the cortical plates, the examiner may observe that the swelling has become bony hard and possesses a smooth or bosselated surface covered with a normal-appearing mucosa. Microscopic study reveals that the tumor comprises many thin-walled vascular spaces, some quite cavernous, separated by bony septa (Fig. 20-12).

Local hemorrhage may be evident about the cervices of the teeth encountered by the enlarging lesion. These teeth may also demonstrate a pumping action; that is, if the examiner depresses the crown of the tooth in an apical direction, the tooth rapidly assumes its former position when the pressure is removed.

Aspiration of an intrabony hemangioma readily yields a copious amount of blood, and caution is necessary. A recommended approach is to introduce the needle through the mucosa some distance from the point where the bone is to be perforated rather than to introduce the needle directly over the hemangioma. The bleeding that results from the former method usually is more easily arrested, since the mucosa over the point where the bone was penetrated is still intact and the channel through the mucosa can be more effectively compressed.

Differential diagnosis

Vascular malformations, including the intrabony hemangioma, are dangerous lesions of the jaw because rapid exsanguination often follows both tooth extraction and jaw fracture.

Because of this lethal potential, when a bony radiolucent lesion is encountered in the jaws, a central hemangioma or arteriovenous aneurysm must always be considered, especially since such a tumor often demonstrates a variety of radiographic appearances. Because the multilocular appearance is not pathognomonic for an intrabony hemangioma, however, the features listed in Table 20-1 must also be considered in the development of a differential diagnosis.

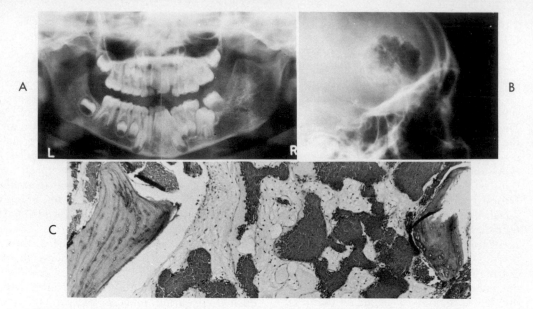

Fig. 20-12. Intrabony hemangioma. **A,** Panograph showing multilocular expansion of the right ramus and the malposition of the developing right mandibular molars. **B,** Multilocular lesion in the frontal bone. **C,** Histologic study showing many vascular spaces between the radiating spicules of bone. (**A** from Gamez-Araujo JJ et al: Oral Surg 37:230-238, 1974. **B** courtesy E. Palacios, MD, Maywood, Ill.)

Specifically the clinician should form a strong impression of intrabony hemangioma when encountering a pumping tooth (a tooth that can be pushed apically and then rebounds to its original position) or localized gingival bleeding around a loose tooth coupled with radiographic evidence of bony change in the region. This impression may be further strengthened when large quantities of blood are easily aspirated from the area.

Management

Once the surgeon has reached a working diagnosis of vascular malformation or intrabony hemangioma, it is incumbent on him or her to urge a complete examination of the patient and the institution of immediate treatment because death may accompany a traumatic incident to the jaws. Angiograms aid greatly in identifying a hemangioma or arteriovenous aneurysm.

Courses of radiation have successfully eliminated manifestations of the tumor and have even induced regression of the bony defects. If the treatment is to be surgery, a block resection of the lesion (including a safe margin of uninvolved bone) must be performed. Before surgery the external carotid artery must be ligated, but even this may not control the bleeding during surgery, since unusual vessel aberrations sometimes accompany these tumors.

A promising surgical approach involves ligating the external carotid artery and using muscle fragments, Gelfoam, and metallic pellets (which lodge in the hemangioma) to reduce the size of the vascular channels. Frame et al. (1987) reviewed these arterial embolization techniques in detail. The various treatment modalities have been reviewed by Sadowski et al. (1981).

RARITIES

Several other lesions in bone can cause multilocular radiolucencies. Although less than complete, a list of these entities includes the following (Figs. 20-13 to 20-18):

Ameloblastic variants
Arteriovenous malformation (Fig. 20-16)
Burkitt's lymphoma (Fig. 20-17)
Calcifying epithelial odontogenic tumor
Cementifying and ossifying fibroma (Fig. 20-18)
Central adenoid cystic carcinoma
Central giant cell tumor
Central mucoepidermoid tumor
Central odontogenic and nonodontogenic fibromas
Chondroma
Chondrosarcoma
Eosinophilic granuloma
Fibromatosis
Fibrous dysplasia (see Fig. 21-6, *B*)
Immature odontoma
Leiomyoma
Lingual mandibular bone defect
Neurilemoma (Fig. 20-16)
Neuroectodermal tumor of infancy
Osteomyelitis
Pseudotumor of hemophilia (Fig. 20-15)
Squamous odontogenic tumor

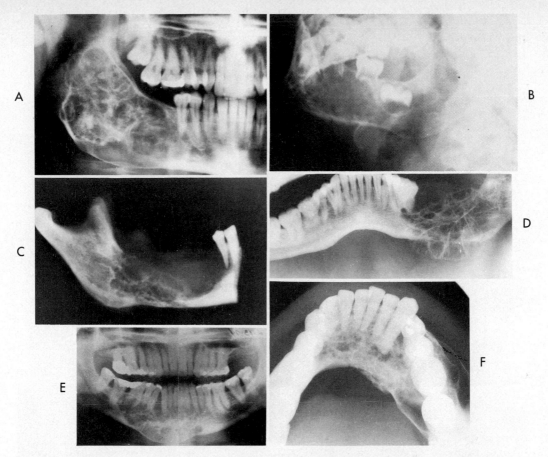

Fig. 20-13. Rare multilocular radiolucencies. **A,** Ameloblastic odontoma. **B,** Intrabony fibroma. **C,** Malignant ameloblastoma. **D,** Intrabony fibroma. **E** and **F,** Panographic and occlusal views, respectively, of intrabony central mucoepidermoid carcinoma of the mandible. (**A** and **C** courtesy O.H. Stuteville, DDS, MD, St. Joe, Ark. **B** courtesy N. Barakat, DDS, Beirut, Lebanon. **D** from Martis C and Karakasis D: J Oral Surg 30:758-759, 1972. Copyright by the American Dental Association. Reprinted by permission. **E** and **F** courtesy A. Morof, DDS, and W. Schoenheider, DDS, Maywood, Ill.)

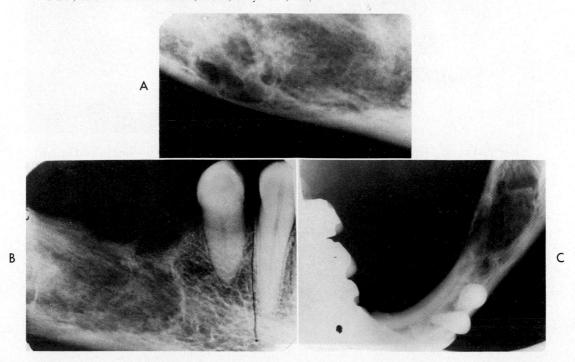

Fig. 20-14. Calcifying epithelial odontogenic tumor of the left mandible. Various views of the same case showing a multilocular pattern. **A** and **B,** Periapical radiographs. **C,** Occlusal radiograph. (Courtesy D. Waite, DDS, Minneapolis.)

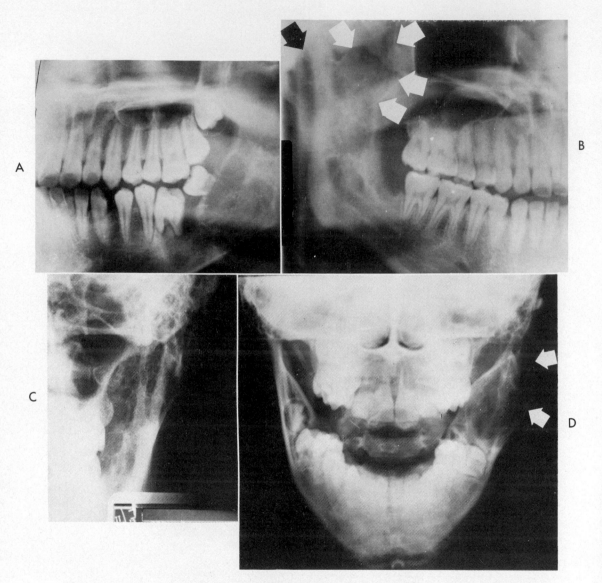

Fig. 20-15. Pseudotumor of hemophilia (three cases). **A,** Right side of a Panorex radiograph showing the multilocular lesion in a 16-year-old boy with severe hemophilia. **B** and **C,** Another case of pseudotumor in the left ramus of a 23-year-old patient with hemophilia. **B,** Panorex radiograph showing the multilocular expansion of the ramus, coronoid process, and condyle. **C,** Cropped posteroanterior radiograph of the affected ramus showing the mediolateral dimension of the multilocular expansion. **D,** Another case in an 11-year-old boy with severe hemophilia. Arrows in **B** and **D** identify the lesions.   (**A** from Mulkey TF: J Oral Surg 35:561-568, 1977. Copyright by the American Dental Association. Reprinted by permission. **B** and **C** courtesy T. Mulkey, DDS, Inglewood, Calif. **D** courtesy G. Blozis, DDS, Columbus, Ohio.)

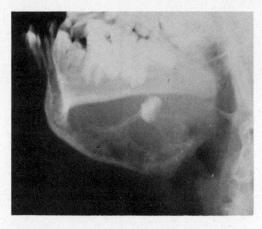

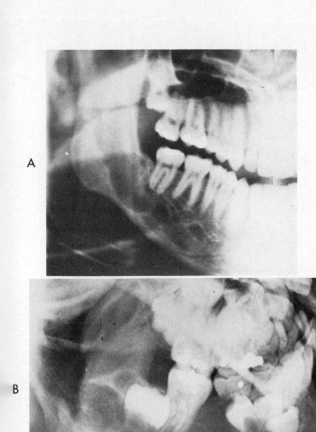

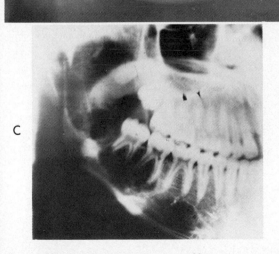

Fig. 20-17. Unilateral case of Burkitt's lymphoma in a young girl. Lateral oblique radiographs showing a rarefied and multilocular pattern of bone loss. (Courtesy D.R. Sawyer, DDS, and A.L. Nwoku, MD, DMD, Lagos, Nigeria.)

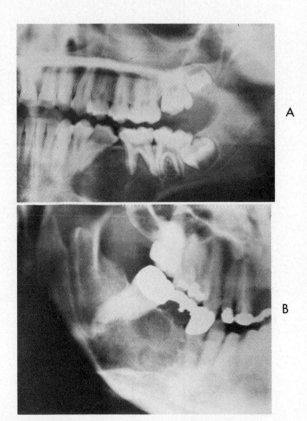

Fig. 20-16. A, Arteriovenous malformation in a 25-year-old man. **B,** Arteriovenous malformation in a 10-year-old patient. **C,** Intrabony neurilemoma. (**A** from Kelly DE, Terry BC, and Small EW: J Oral Surg 35:387-393, 1977. Copyright by the American Dental Association. Reprinted by permission. **B** and **C** courtesy J. Lehnert, DDS, Minneapolis.)

Fig. 20-18. Ossifying and cementifying fibroma. **A,** Multilocular-appearing lesion in premolar and first molar region of the mandible in a 13-year-old boy. **B,** Another multilocular-appearing lesion in the premolar and molar region of a 28-year-old woman. (**A** courtesy W. Heaton, DDS, Chicago.)

Table 20-1. Features of lesions producing multilocular radiolucencies

Lesion	Predominant sex	Usual age (years)	Predominant jaw	Predominant region	Predominant multilocular type	Other radiographic appearances	Additional features
Multilocular cysts	M = F	Over 16	Mandible Maxilla—rare	Posterior	Soap bubble	Unilocular cystlike	
Ameloblastomas	M ~ F	20-50 (average 40)	Mandible 80%	Posterior 70%	Soap bubble or honeycomb (Maxilla—unilocular)	Unilocular a. Ragged b. Ill defined	Paresthesia in some cases
Central giant cell granulomas	$\frac{F}{M} = \frac{2.4}{1}$	Under 30 (average 26)	Mandible 70%	Anterior to second molars	Soap bubble	Unilocular a. Cystlike b. Borders indistinct	Serum chemistries normal; 20% cross midline
Giant cell lesions of hyperparathyroidism (secondary)	$\frac{F}{M} = \frac{2}{1}$	50-80	Mandible	None	Soap bubble	Unilocular a. Cystlike b. Borders indistinct	Occasionally multiple; kidney disease; serum calcium ↓; serum phosphorus ↑; serum alkaline phosphatase ↑
Giant cell lesions of hyperparathyroidism (primary)	$\frac{F}{M} = \frac{7}{1}$	30-60	Mandible	None	Soap bubble	Unilocular a. Cystlike b. Borders indistinct	Occasionally multiple; polydipsia; polyuria; serum calcium ↑; serum phosphorus ↓; serum alkaline phosphatase ↑
Cherubism	M > F	2-20	Mandible Maxilla and zygoma	Ramus and molar Sinus and orbital floor	Soap bubble	Unilocular	Multiple; familial history of lesion
Odontogenic myxomas	M = F	10-50 (average 25-35)	Maxilla/ mandible =¾	Ramus, premolar and molar	Soap bubble Honeycomb Tennis racket	Unilocular a. Cystlike b. Borders indistinct	Congenitally missing tooth; pain and paresthesia occasionally

Lesion	Age	M:F	Location (%)	Region	Radiographic	Locularity	Other
Aneurysmal bone cysts	Under 20 70%	M ~ F	Maxilla/mandible = 1/3	Ramus and molar	Soap bubble	Unilocular	Tender
Metastatic tumors to jaws	50-80	M = F	Mandible 95%	Premolar and molar	Honeycomb	Many (see discussion in chapter)	History and symptoms of primary tumor ii. addition to local lesion
Central hemangiomas of bone	10-20	$\frac{F}{M}=\frac{2}{1}$	Mandible 65%	Body and ramus	Honeycomb	Tennis racket Unilocular a. Cystlike b. Borders indistinct	Local gingival bleeding; pumping action of tooth

~, Approximately equal.

DIFFERENTIAL DIAGNOSIS OF MULTILOCULAR RADIOLUCENCIES

As determined from the previous discussions of multilocular radiolucencies, it is fruitless to attempt to diagnose these lesions using radiographs alone. The clinician can, however, develop a sound differential diagnosis when confronted by a multilocular radiolucency.

If the suspect region is in the maxillary molar segment of the jaw, a *multilobed maxillary sinus* must be considered as the most likely diagnosis, especially if the pattern is bilateral and the region asymptomatic.

If the multilocular region is in the mandible, the diagnosis most likely is a soap bubble type of *marrow pattern*, especially if such a pattern is prominent throughout the mandible.

If the multilocular lesion is situated anteriorly in the jaws of a patient under 30 years of age, it is much more likely to be a *giant cell granuloma* than an ameloblastoma.

If the lesion is situated in the posterior of the mandible in a patient over 30 years of age, it is more likely to be an *ameloblastoma*, especially if there is an accompanying paresthesia of the lip. If no paresthesia is present, the lesion is more likely to be a *multilocular cyst*.

If the patient complains of polydipsia and polyuria or has a history of kidney disease along with abnormal serum calcium, phosphorus, and alkaline phosphatase levels, the lesion is most likely a *giant cell lesion of hyperparathyroidism*.

If the lesions occur in a child and are multiple and if there is a family history of such lesions, the diagnosis is almost certainly *cherubism*.

A history of primary malignant tumor elsewhere gives *metastatic carcinoma* a high rank.

Myxoma and *intrabony hemangioma* show several common features: both frequently have either a honeycomb or a tennis racket appearance; both are usually found in patients between 10 and 30 years of age; and both are usually found in the ramus and premolar and molar regions. A history of a developmentally missing tooth might prompt the clinician to favor a diagnosis of myxoma, whereas copious amounts of blood obtained by aspiration, the syndrome of the pumping tooth, or cervical hemorrhage are highly suggestive of intrabony hemangioma.

Finally, the clinician must know the various rarities and be ready to elevate one of these within his or her list of possibilities when the particular circumstances so dictate.

REFERENCES

Adamo AK, Locricchio RC, and Freedman P: Myxoma of the mandible treated by peripheral ostectomy and immediate reconstruction: report of case, J Oral Surg 38:530-532, 1980.

Coope JW, Ireland SL, and Burke PH: Cherubism with serial stereophotogrametric assessment, Br Dent J 155:127-130, 1983.

DeTomasi DC, Hann JR, and Stewart HM: Cherubism: report of a nonfamilial case, J Am Dent Assoc 111:455-457, 1985.

El Deeb M, Sedano HO, and Waite DE: Aneurysmal bone cyst of the jaws: report of a case associated with fibrous dysplasia and review of the literature, Int J Oral Surg 9:301-311, 1980.

Farman AG, Nortje CJ, Grotepass FW, et al: Myxofibroma of the jaws, Br J Oral Surg 15:3-18, 1977.

Frame JW, Putnam G, Wake MJC, and Rolfe EB: Therapeutic arterial embolisation of vascular lesions in the maxillofacial region, Br J Oral Maxillofac Surg 25:181-194, 1989.

Greer RO and Johnson M: Botryoid odontogenic cyst: clinicopathologic analysis of ten cases with three recurrences, J Oral Maxillofac Surg 46:574-579, 1988.

Harder F: Myxomas of the jaws, Int J Oral Surg 7:148-155, 1978.

Kaban LB and Mulliken JB: Vascular anomalies of the maxillofacial region, J Oral Maxillofac Surg 44:203-213, 1986.

Kaugers GE: Botryoid odontogenic cyst, Oral Surg 62:555-559, 1986.

Kuepper RC and Harrigan WF: Treatment of mandibular cherubism, J Oral Surg 36:638-642, 1978.

Minderjahn A: Incidence and clinical differentiation of odontogenic tumors, J Maxillofac Surg 7:142-150, 1979.

Mulkey TF: Hemophilic pseudotumors of the mandible, J Oral Surg 35:561-568, 1977.

Regezi JA, Kerr DA, and Courtney RM: Odontogenic tumors: analysis of 706 cases, J Oral Surg 36:771-778, 1978.

Reyneke J: Aneurysmal bone cyst of the maxilla, Oral Surg 45:441-447, 1978.

Sadowsky D, Rosenberg RD, Kaufman J, et al: Central hemangioma of the mandible: literature review, case report, and discussion, Oral Surg 52:471-477, 1981.

Salmo NAM, Shukur ST, and Abulkhail A: Bilateral bone cysts of the maxilla, J Oral Surg 39:137-139, 1981.

Steidler NE, Cook RM, and Reade PC: Aneurysmal bone cysts of the jaws: a case report and review of the literature, Br J Oral Surg 16:254-261, 1979.

Struthers PJ and Shear M: Aneurysmal bone cyst of the jaws. I. Clinicopathologic features, Int J Oral Surg 13:85-91, 1984a.

Struthers PJ and Shear M: Aneurysmal bone cyst of the jaws. II. Pathogenesis, Int J Oral Surg 13:92-100, 1984b.

Ueno S, Mushimoto K, Kurozumi T, et al: Aneurysmal bone cyst of the mandible, J Oral Maxillofac Surg 40:680-683, 1982.

Waldron CA: Personal communication, 1976.

Weathers DR and Waldron CA: Unusual multilocular cysts of the jaws (botryoid cysts), Oral Surg 36:235-241, 1973.

Worth HM and Stoneman DW: Radiology of vascular abnormalities in and about the jaws, Dent Radiogr Photogr 52:1-23, 1979.

21

Solitary radiolucencies with ragged and poorly defined borders

NORMAN K. WOOD
PAUL W. GOAZ
ORION H. STUTEVILLE

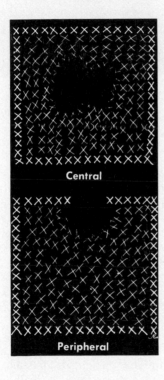

Central

Peripheral

Solitary radiolucencies of the jaws with ragged and poorly defined borders include the following:

Chronic osteitis
Chronic osteomyelitis
Hematopoietic bone marrow defect
Squamous cell carcinoma
Fibrous dysplasia—early lesion
Metastatic tumors to the jaws
Malignant minor salivary gland tumors
Osteogenic sarcoma—osteolytic type
Chondrosarcoma
Rarities
  Ameloblastic carcinoma
  Ameloblastoma
  Aneurysmal bone cyst
  Angiosarcoma
  Benign tumor in the rarefied jaw
  Burkitt's tumor
  Central hemangioma
  Desmoplastic fibroma
  Eosinophilic granuloma
  Ewing's sarcoma
  Fibromatosis
  Fibrosarcoma
  Histiocytosis
  Idiopathic histiocytosis (Langerhans' cell disease)
  Intrabony hemangioma
  Liposarcoma
  Lymphosarcoma
  Malignant ameloblastoma
  Malignant lymphoma of bone
  Medulloblastoma
  Melanoma
  Myeloma (solitary; plasmacytoma)
  Myosarcoma
  Myospherulosis (paraffinoma)
  Neuroblastoma
  Neuroectodermal tumor of infancy
  Neurosarcoma
  Odontogenic fibroma
  Odontogenic sarcoma
  Osteoblastoma

Phosphorus necrosis
Reticulum cell sarcoma
Sarcoidosis
Scleroderma
Spindle cell carcinoma
Surgical defect
Tuberculosis
Vascular malformations
Wilms' tumor

Most solitary radiolucencies with ragged and indistinct borders* are produced by three basic types of pathologic processes: inflammation or infection of bone, fibrous dysplasia (early stage), and osteolytic malignancy of bone. Because of the potentially serious nature of the lesion, every ill-defined radiolucency should be considered possibly malignant until proved otherwise.

Some clinicians depend too heavily on blood chemistry values (such as concentration of plasma calcium, phosphorus, and alkaline phosphatase) for the differentiation of osteolytic lesions. These lesions would have to induce a substantial amount of bony activity, either mineral absorption or mineral deposition, before significant changes in the blood chemistry values could occur. In addition, since pathologic bony activity does not progress at a constant rate, the biochemical values would fluctuate with shifts in activity of the pathologic processes. Thus specific altered values of blood chemistry would be pathognomonic only periodically and in only a few diseases.

Such instances are identified here when they complement the discussion of a particular entity.

CHRONIC OSTEITIS (CHRONIC ALVEOLAR ABSCESS)

Chronic osteitis is a local mild inflammation or infection in bone† that usually occurs around the roots of a tooth. It is commonly a sequela of pulpitis and is perhaps identical to the chronic alveolar abscess discussed as a periapical radiolucency in Chapter 16. It is included in this chapter because it often has ragged, poorly defined borders (Fig. 21-1). As described in Chapter 16, where the features of the chronic

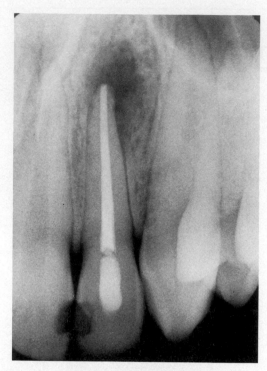

Fig. 21-1. Chronic alveolar abscess at the apex of a lateral incisor preceded the root canal filling, which had been recently completed.

alveolar abscess are discussed, the inciting tooth is pulpless and usually tender to percussion. A sinus may be present and may pass through the alveolar bone to open onto the mucosa generally near the level of the apex.

Differential diagnosis

The presence of an intra-alveolar draining sinus is not conclusive evidence that a radiolucent area is a *chronic osteitis, abscess,* or *osteomyelitis.*

Such a lesion could represent an *infected malignant tumor* in the periapical area. Because of the low incidence of such tumors, however, and also because a small malignant lesion is unlikely to become infected, this entity is assigned a low rank in the differential diagnosis of a draining periapical radiolucent lesion.

Management

Although the management of the chronic alveolar abscess is detailed in Chapter 16, it is important to reiterate at least three precepts pertaining to the treatment of radiolucent lesions of the jaws. Compliance with these rules enables the clinician to establish a valid initial

---

*The terms "ragged" and "moth-eaten" are also used to connote destructive lesions without smoothly contoured borders. The descriptive phrase "poorly defined" conveys the notion that the borders are fuzzy, indistinct, or difficult to delineate.
†The dry socket is a type of chronic or acute osteitis, but it is excluded from this discussion because it seldom if ever is a diagnostic problem.

diagnosis or at least provides the opportunity to reevaluate the initial impression and treatment. Such confirmation may obviate the disastrous delay that could result if a small periapical malignancy were misdiagnosed as a periapical sequela of pulpitis, treated as such, and then neglected. The three circumstances and the attending considerations are as follows:

1. If the clinician chooses to treat a periapical radiolucency nonsurgically by only obliterating the root canal(s) of the associated tooth, he or she must obtain *follow-up radiographs* to substantiate the initial impression that the bony lesion was the result of inflammation.
2. If the clinician believes that curettage with or without root resection is needed to complement the canal obliteration, the periapical tissue must be subjected to *microscopic examination*.
3. If the clinician chooses to extract the tooth, *the periapical lesion should also be removed and studied microscopically*. Since small malignancies in the area of the roots are uncommon, however, surgical removal and biopsy of every periapical radiolucency are not justified *except* in extraction cases.

The foregoing philosophy appears to be the best regarding the management of benign-appearing periapical radiolucencies, which include chronic osteitis (chronic alveolar abscess).

CHRONIC OSTEOMYELITIS

In its usual context the term "osteomyelitis" conveys the notion of an inflammatory reaction of bone marrow that produces clinically apparent pus. An effort to classify the inflammatory diseases of bone, however, according to whether the process is completely confined to the periosteum (periostitis), cortical bone, or marrow is more an academic exercise than a useful diagnostic procedure. In reality, there is seldom if ever such a sharp demarcation among these entities. For our purposes here, if the infection is restricted to the alveolar process, we refer to it as an alveolar abscess. If the basal bone is involved, this is considered an osteomyelitis.

The inflammation may involve any of the soft parts of the bone, the marrow, the haversian canals, and the periosteum—separately or in combination—depending on the initiating circumstances and the duration of the process. For example, an infection of local or hematogenous origin may be initiated in any area of the interstitial connective tissues of the bone and be confined to the area where the infectious agents were deposited, or the infection may subsequently spread to involve the other layers of the bone.

Another consideration that helps keep the concept of a bone infection in the proper perspective is that the calcified portion of the bone does not play an active role in the disease. The calcified portion is affected secondarily by the loss of blood supply, and a greater or lesser portion may die and be resorbed or sequestered. In contrast, however, some areas may become sclerotic as the result of a mild inflammation or infectious process that stimulates adjacent bone production.

Osteomyelitis of the jaws is a rare disease in healthy persons. The practitioner can readily appreciate this fact by noting the high incidence of odontogenic infections and the vast number of successful intraoral surgeries performed in contaminated fields without the development of an osteomyelitis.

A predisposing condition must be present for an osteomyelitis to develop. Uncontrolled or undiagnosed debilitating systemic diseases (such as diabetes, leukemia, alcoholic states, various anemias and neutropenias, uremias, trauma, and complications after jaw fracture) are common predisposing conditions. Daramola (1981) reported a case of massive osteomyelitis of the mandible in a patient with sickle cell disease. Furthermore, certain diseases (for example, Paget's, osteopetrosis, and sclerosing cemental masses) produce a dense, avascular type of bone, which is prone to the development of osteomyelitis.

Staphylococci and streptococci are the most frequent causative microorganisms in osteomyelitis of the jaws, but not the only ones (Gallo et al., 1976; Igo et al., 1978; Rosenquist and Beskow, 1977). For example, *Actinomyces israelii*, one of the etiologic organisms in cervicofacial actinomycosis (considered to be primarily a soft tissue infection, often situated at the angle of the mandible) may also cause an osteomyelitis of the bone (Fig. 21-2, *F*) (Musser et al., 1977; Walker et al., 1981; Yakata et al., 1978).

The acute type of osteomyelitis of the jaws is not discussed in this chapter because owing to its rapid onset, especially in an initial infection, this form does not produce radiolucent lesions. Furthermore, because of the widespread use of antibiotics for the treatment of odontogenic infections and traumatic injuries to the jaws, acute osteomyelitis of the jaws is not common today in the United States.

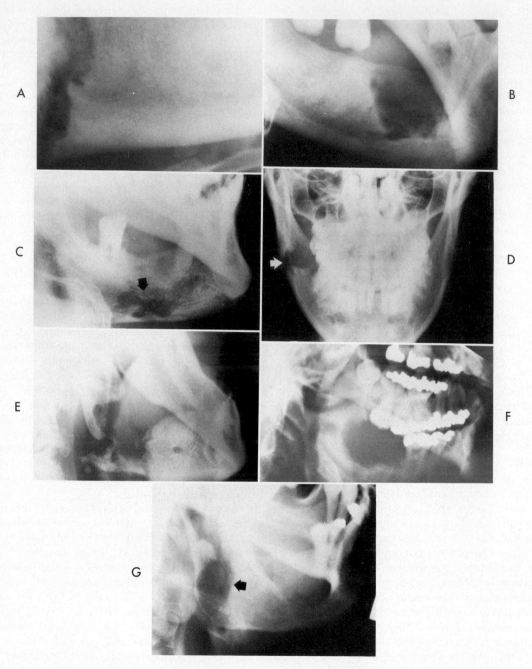

Fig. 21-2. Chronic osteomyelitis. **A,** In a fracture line. **B,** In an extraction site in a patient with diabetes. (Refer to Fig. 16-19, *B,* for an illustration of a draining sinus, and to Fig. 16-19, *C,* for the histopathologic appearance of chronic osteomyelitis.) **C** to **E,** Additional examples of osteomyelitis. The arrow in **D** indicates the lesion. **F,** Actinomycotic osteomyelitis. **G,** Airway shadow *(arrow)* simulating a radiolucent pathosis with ragged borders.   (**C, D,** and **E** courtesy O.H. Stuteville, DDS, MD, St. Joe, Ark. **F,** courtesy E. Palacios, MD, Maywood, Ill.)

Chronic osteomyelitis may produce at least four different radiographic images: a radiolucency with ragged borders, a radiolucency containing one or more radiopaque foci, a dense radiopacity, and a salt-and-pepper appearance. The patient history, clinical and laboratory features, and processes fundamental to the development of all four types of bony change are the same.

Examples of osteomyelitis that may appear as radiolucencies containing radiopaque foci are discussed in Chapter 25, as are the salt-and-pepper lesions. The completely radiopaque lesions are discussed in Chapter 28. The discussion in this chapter focuses on the conditions that attend the radiolucent type of lesion.

The completely radiolucent type of bony lesion that results from a chronic osteomyelitis usually has irregular shapes with ragged and poorly defined borders (Fig. 21-2).

The infection may originate in a recent extraction site or in a fracture line. When a fracture line is the site, the infection often appears as a more or less linear radiolucency having ragged, poorly defined borders and possibly varying in width as it follows the fracture line through the bone (Fig. 21-2).

Often the surrounding bony borders are denser than the adjacent normal bone, reflecting a degree of sclerosis induced by the chronic infection.

Osteoradionecrosis is a condition of bone that has some similarities to osteomyelitis. This disease, which is covered in detail in Chapter 25, seldom occurs as a completely radiolucent lesion. Usually there is a radiolucency with large radiopaque foci (sequestra) or perhaps a salt-and-pepper appearance.

Microscopic examination of the radiolucent lesions of chronic osteomyelitis shows small spicules of dead bone with empty lacunae scattered throughout necrotic tissue. The radiolucent areas contain varying numbers of lymphocytes, plasma cells, macrophages, and polymorphonuclear leukocytes (see Fig. 16-19). The small sequestra of bone that are microscopically apparent are not large enough to be seen on the radiographs.

Features

In an interview with a patient who has a confirmed or suspected chronic osteomyelitis of the jaws, the questioning should be especially directed to disclose symptoms that may be related to a contributing systemic disease.

For example, the patient may describe polydipsia or polyuria or both, symptoms suggesting diabetes. A disclosure that the patient is taking antitumor drugs* immediately suggests the possibility that the leukocyte count had been reduced to a level that would predispose the patient to infection. The patient may indicate having received radiation therapy directed to or near the oral cavity. He or she may report a history of facial trauma or a difficult extraction, followed by a suspected or confirmed jaw fracture.

If the examiner is aware of the spectrum of conditions that may contribute to the initiation of an osteomyelitis, appropriate questioning often leads to the discovery of such pertinent states as Paget's disease or osteopetrosis. In addition, the clinician should always be alert to the possibility that the patient may have a primary infection elsewhere (particularly in the skin or urinary tract).

Usually the patient's first complaint related to the local problem is tenderness or pain and swelling over the affected region of the bone. If a muscle of mastication is involved, trismus occurs during mandibular excursions. Regional lymph nodes may be inflamed and painful. A sinus from the abscess sometimes develops and discharges a purulent material onto the overlying skin or mucosa (see Fig. 16-19), but the drainage in chronic osteomyelitis is characteristically intermittent and of small volume.

Unlike a sinus that opens onto the face and is a frequent source of complaint, an osteomyelitic sinus that communicates with the oral cavity often goes unnoticed. The patient may complain of fetid breath, however, and if teeth are involved in an area of osteomyelitis, he or she may complain that they are loose and painful. A nonunited jaw fracture may lead to complaints of crepitus or abnormal jaw mobility. Intermittent fever may occur as the chronic condition flares into an acute phase because of occlusion of the sinus, a decrease in the patient's resistance, the introduction of a more virulent type of organism, or the interruption of therapy.

Osteomyelitis may occur at any age. In the absence of predisposing systemic disease, however, it is uncommon in the first three decades of life—except for the proliferative periostitis type, which is discussed in Chapter 28.

---

*The cytotoxic drugs commercially available for prescription by the medical profession are listed in the *Physicians' Desk Reference* (Medical Economics Co.) under the classification of antineoplastics. In general, they produce a marked depression of the bone marrow and may produce anemia, leukopenia, and thrombocytopenia.

The incidence of osteomyelitis slowly increases from the third decade on, which parallels the increase in systemic disease and the decreased resistance of bone to infection in later life. The latter is thought to result from the increased density of bone combined with a decreased vascularity.

Osteomyelitis is found more frequently in men, probably because they more commonly have traumatic incidents and their bones are usually denser.

The mandible is involved more often than the maxilla, which is rarely the site of an osteomyelitis, since the mandibular bone is much less vascular than the maxilla. Also, spontaneous drainage is more readily initiated from an alveolar abscess within the spongiosa of the maxilla because the cortical plates are thinner in this jaw. Such drainage often prevents the development of an osteomyelitis. Conversely, spontaneous drainage is not so readily established in the body of the mandible because the thicker and denser mandibular cortical plates tend to contain the purulent process within the bone and thus promote the development of a more serious lesion.

This difference in the incidence of osteomyelitis between the two jaws parallels the nature and frequency of fractures of these bones:

1. Fractures of the mandible are more common than fractures of the maxilla.
2. Fractures of the mandible anterior to the last tooth are the most common; these fractures, in turn, involve the largest bulk of the more easily infected dense cortical bone.
3. Fractures of the maxilla usually follow lines of low mechanical resistance that do not involve areas of dense cortical bone.

Osteomyelitis of the mandible most frequently occurs in the body because compound fractures occur more often in this segment.

Intraoral contamination of the fracture site, as often occurs in compound fractures, greatly increases the likelihood of the development of an osteomyelitis. Fractures of the ramus, condyle, and coronoid process seldom become infected, since they are rarely compounded intraorally because of the thick coverage of these segments of the lower jaw by muscles and other tissues. Furthermore, odontogenic infection does not commonly reach these areas because such abscesses occur primarily in the tooth-bearing areas of the jaws.

In a chronic osteomyelitis a sinus frequently opens onto the skin or the mucosal surface.

There is usually a firm swelling of the bone* and of the soft tissue covering the infected region. This swelling often has a reddish surface and is tender or painful on palpation. Pressure on the swelling may cause the expression of some purulent material from a sinus opening. Teeth in the radiolucent region may be somewhat sensitive when percussed. They may be loose and malposed and may show root resorption.

If the osteomyelitis has occurred in a fracture line, there may be a nonunion, which can be demonstrated by grasping both segments of the fractured bone in two hands and causing mobility about the fracture line.

When the mandible is involved at the angle or in the premolar-molar region, paresthesia of the lip may be a feature if the mandibular canal and its contents are compromised.

Occasionally before the sinus becomes patent or when it is later obliterated, a space abscess develops in the soft tissue over the segment of involved bone. This mass is fluctuant, nonemptiable, hot, and painful and yields pus on aspiration.

Laboratory tests are helpful in establishing a diagnosis of osteomyelitis. Not only may the picture of chronic bacterial infection be reflected by the blood cell counts (total leukocyte count increased with a lymphocytosis), but abnormal values consistent with a predisposing underlying systemic disease may also be evident.

Differential diagnosis

The differential diagnosis of osteomyelitis is discussed in the differential diagnosis section at the end of this chapter (p. 454).

Management

Because of the availability of many effective antibiotic preparations, osteomyelitis is not so serious today as it was a few decades ago, but it is still a difficult disease to eradicate. There are several reasons for this:

1. The blood supply to the involved bone was probably initially poor, and the decreased supply after the loss of tissue viability adds to the bone's susceptibility.

---

*This swelling is produced by the formation of pus (or edema fluid) under considerable tension beneath the periosteum. The pus lifts the membrane from the bone, causing a firm enlargement. Inflammation of the adjacent soft tissues, as well as fibrosis, increases the firmness.

2. The greatly diminished blood supply terminates at the periphery of the infected bony segment; thus the body's defenses and any systemically administered medication (such as antibiotics) can advance only to the perimeters of the disease process.

3. Frequently an open wound is communicating with the oral cavity, which permits the continual contamination of the osteomyelitic area by the oral flora and juices and indeed constitutes a serious problem to manage.

The clinician must first determine whether an underlying debilitating systemic disease is present. If so and if it is not being effectively treated, it must be brought under control as soon as possible with the cooperation of the patient's physician. Specimens must be obtained from the purulent drainage for culture and sensitivity tests. As soon as these results are available, the proper antibiotic therapy with adequate doses should be initiated and should continue for a suitable length of time. Even after the lesion becomes asymptomatic following treatment, small foci of bacteria within the affected bone remain to produce renewed flareups and recurrences of symptoms (Wannfors and Hammarstrom, 1985).

Any space abscesses must be incised and drained by a through-and-through rubber drain technique. The drains should be irrigated copiously several times a day with a solution of 3% hydrogen peroxide and normal saline (1:1).

If oral wounds are present, they must also be frequently and adequately irrigated. Excellent oral hygiene must be maintained. The use of hyperbaric oxygen has been reported to speed recovery from osteomyelitis (Goupil et al., 1978; Hart and Mainous, 1976; Kerley et al., 1981; Mainous et al., 1973; Mansfield et al., 1981; Marx and Ames, 1982).

Infected teeth in the area of osteomyelitis must usually be extracted. Attempting to conserve some of them through endodontic treatment at the risk of losing a large section of the jaw is unwarranted. Nevertheless, an attempt should be made to close any oral wound that may be present if the lesion is draining extraorally and especially after the initiation of antibiotic therapy. If bone is protruding through the wound, it should be adequately contoured to permit mucosal closure. If the osteomyelitis is complicating a nonunited fracture, the fragments should be reduced and immobilized as soon as possible.

If drainage continues through the sinus tract, surgical saucerization may be necessary (Nakajima et al., 1977). Such a procedure requires removing all dead bone along with the granulation and necrotic tissue and recontouring the remaining bone to eliminate sharp edges. If too much bone is lost, a bone graft may be needed to approximate the two ends.

In view of the difficult management problem posed by osteomyelitis, prevention is important. Detailing complete histories before surgery helps to reveal systemic disease, which can then be regulated before the surgical procedure is undertaken.

Patients undergoing surgical mandibular extractions may be given 500 mg of penicillin or erythromycin 1 hour before surgery and four times per day for 5 days thereafter, or until all the postoperative symptoms have subsided. When a tooth lies in the fracture line of a mandibular fracture and the oral hygiene is poor, some clinicians recommend that the tooth be removed before or at the time of reduction and fixation of the fracture.

HEMATOPOIETIC BONE MARROW DEFECT

The hematopoietic bone marrow defect has been described as a periapical radiolucency in Chapter 16 and as a cystlike radiolucency in Chapter 19. On occasion it can appear as a radiolucent lesion with ragged, poorly defined borders (see Fig. 16-1, A) and as such requires differentiation from the other lesions in this chapter. Usually the suspicion index is so low with these lesions that the clinician chooses to radiograph the lesion in 3 to 6 months' time to ensure that it is not enlarging. Nevertheless, in cases of suspected metastatic disease, such a lesion can be worrisome.

SQUAMOUS CELL CARCINOMA (EPIDERMOID CARCINOMA)

Squamous cell carcinoma is described as a red lesion in Chapter 5, as a white lesion in Chapter 8, as a red and white lesion in Chapter 9, as an exophytic lesion in Chapter 10, and as an ulcer in Chapter 11. This discussion primarily concerns its bone-destroying image.

Since squamous cell carcinoma is the most common malignant lesion to appear in the oral cavity, it is also the most common malignancy to produce radiolucent lesions in the jawbones. Not all intraoral squamous cell carcinomas invade and destroy bone, however. Squamous cell carcinomas of the tongue, floor of the mouth, buccal mucosa, lips, soft palate, and oropharynx do not invade bone unless they are permitted to reach a large size and develop unusual extensions. This is true because the mucosa in these sites is not close to bone. The carcinomas that originate on or near the crest of the mandibular ridge, the maxillary molar ridges, or the posterior hard palate are the tumors most likely to cause bony destruction. Not all types of squamous cell carcinoma seem to possess the same ability to invade bone. For example, the ulcerative variety seems to be more apt than the exophytic and verrucous types to invade and destroy bone.

Squamous cell carcinomas that destroy bone can be divided into two basic types according to origin: the peripheral or mucosal type, which is the more common, and the central type (within bone), which is rare. Since clinicians and pathologists have become increas-

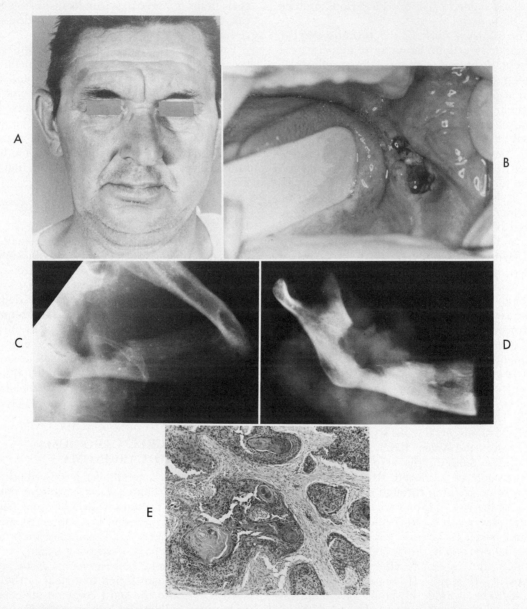

Fig. 21-3. Squamous cell carcinoma. **A,** Expansion of the face over the left molar region in a 58-year-old man. **B,** Intraoral ulcer in the same patient. **C,** Lateral oblique radiograph showing a craterlike radiolucency with ragged ill-defined borders. **D,** Radiograph of the surgical specimen. **E,** Histopathologic appearance of the tumor showing features of a moderately well-differentiated squamous cell carcinoma.

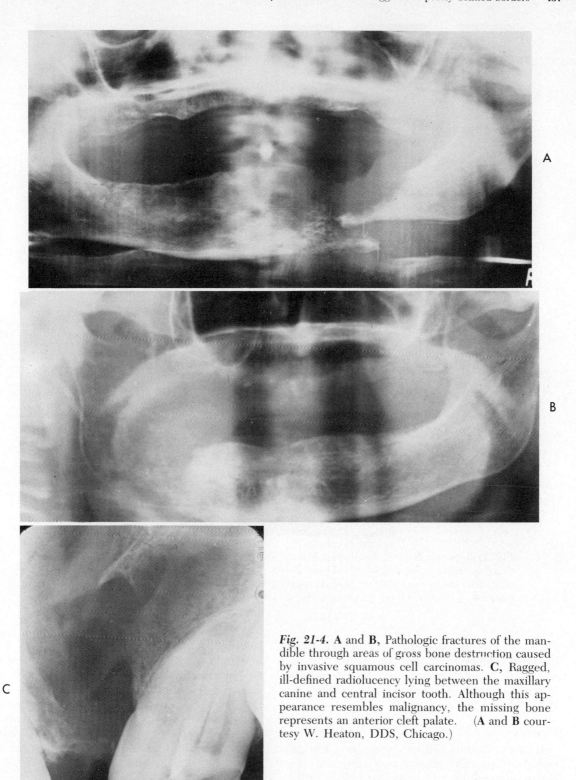

Fig. 21-4. **A** and **B,** Pathologic fractures of the mandible through areas of gross bone destruction caused by invasive squamous cell carcinomas. **C,** Ragged, ill-defined radiolucency lying between the maxillary canine and central incisor tooth. Although this appearance resembles malignancy, the missing bone represents an anterior cleft palate.   (**A** and **B** courtesy W. Heaton, DDS, Chicago.)

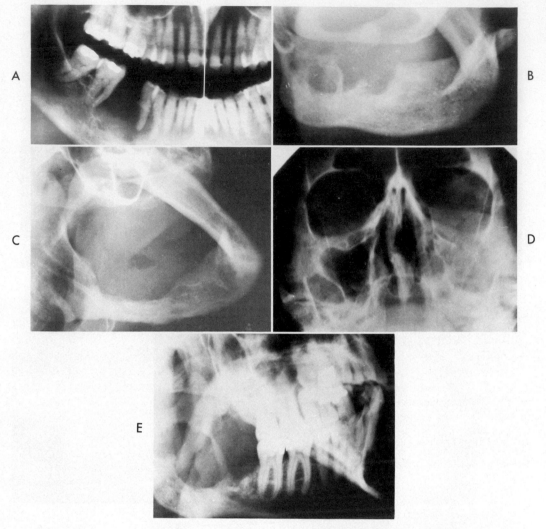

Fig. 21-5. Squamous cell carcinoma. **A** to **C,** Peripheral lesions in the mandible. **D,** In the maxillary sinus. Clouding of the left sinus with partial destruction of its walls is evident. **E,** central lesion in the ramus.   (**A** to **C** courtesy O.H. Stuteville, DDS, MD, St. Joe, Ark. **E** courtesy R. Nolan, DDS, Waukegan, Ill.)

ingly aware of the central type, however, more of these tumors are being recognized and reported; they are thought to originate in nests of epithelium either within the jawbone or within the epithelial lining of cysts.

Features

If the squamous cell carcinoma is of the peripheral type, the patient may complain of a worsening oral ulcer or mass that bleeds easily, may be somewhat tender, and is situated over bone of the alveolus or jaw or on the hard palate (Fig. 21-3). The patient usually has poor oral hygiene and admits to the heavy use of to-

bacco or alcohol or both. The question has been raised concerning the carcinogenic potential of mouthwashes (Weaver et al., 1979). Other frequent complaints are foul odor and taste, paresthesia or anesthesia of the lip, and if a pathologic jaw fracture is present, crepitus and pain on moving the jaw. Surprisingly, overt symptoms are frequently not present with pathologic fracture (Ciola, 1978). Fig. 21-4 illustrates advanced bone loss and fracture.

If the lesion is of the central type, the patient commonly complains of pain, paresthesia, and swelling of the jaw—the last in the more advanced stages of the disease (Fig. 21-5, *E*).

Radiographs of bone invaded by the peripheral type of squamous cell carcinoma show lytic defects with either of two forms:

1. A roughly semicircular or saucer-shaped erosion into the bony surface with ragged ill-defined borders that illustrate the varying, uneven osteolytic invasion (Fig. 21-3).

2. A mandibular lesion with advanced horizontal resorption of the ridge and basal bone in the involved area and only a thin, fairly well-defined inferior border of the mandible remaining (Fig. 21-5).

Small sequestra of bone may be present as ragged radiopacities in either type of radiolucent lesion (see Fig. 25-2).

Teeth involved with either type of lesion become loose, migrate, or have some root resorption.

If the advancing tumor has originated in the maxillary sinus, destroyed the sinus floor, and infiltrated the posterior maxillary ridge, its ragged and poorly defined borders will be toward the ridge away from the sinus. This is a useful feature for differentiating between a tumor that has originated in the maxillary sinus and one that has developed on the ridge.

The bony destruction usually delineates the path of the advancing lesion. If the maxillary sinus has been involved with a malignant tumor, the sinus walls are less well defined and perhaps one or more are destroyed. The sinus itself shows increased density (clouding) where it is filled with tumor (Fig. 21-5).

Enlarged regional lymph nodes are a frequent finding in oral squamous cell carcinoma and may represent either a benign lymphadenitis (caused by infection of the lesion by the oral flora) or metastatic spread. Inflamed nodes can usually be differentiated from nodes involved with metastatic tumor because the former tend to be enlarged, painful, firm, freely movable, and discrete whereas the latter are enlarged, painless, very firm, immovable, and frequently matted together. In advanced cases the lymph nodes are bound to adjacent structures by the infiltrating tumor and are not freely movable.

Central squamous cell carcinoma is rare and frequently appears radiographically as a more or less rounded radiolucency completely surrounded by bone (Fig. 21-5) (Coonar, 1979; Martinelli et al., 1977). When its early appearance suggests that it originated in the wall of a cyst, the radiographic borders are evenly contoured and well defined. Later, when the malignancy has infiltrated the cyst wall and destroyed the bone, its borders become ragged and lose their sharp definition (Nolan and Wood, 1976; Sirsat et al., 1973).

Central squamous cell carcinoma predominantly is seen in patients in the fourth through seventh decades of life. Males are affected two to three times as frequently as females. The mandible is involved almost four times as often as the maxilla (Shear, 1969). Conversely, peripheral squamous cell carcinoma affects an older age-group and shows a steady increase in incidence from the fourth decade on. No age-group is completely immune to either type, however. Elzay (1982) discussed primary intraosseous carcinoma of the jaws and recommended a new classification of these tumors.

The histologic picture of either the central or the peripheral type may be quite variable, ranging from a well-differentiated to a very anaplastic squamous cell carcinoma (Fig. 21-3).

Differential diagnosis

The problems attending a differential diagnosis of squamous cell carcinoma are discussed in the differential diagnosis section at the end of this chapter (p. 454).

Management

The management of patients with squamous cell carcinoma is discussed in Chapter 11.

FIBROUS DYSPLASIA—EARLY LESION

Fibrous dysplasia (benign fibro-osseous lesion not of periodontal ligament origin) is a lesion of bone that arises as a result of an abnormal proliferation of fibrous tissue. As the lesion matures and enlarges, destroying trabeculae and expanding cortices, peculiar trabecular shapes resembling Chinese characters are formed in the fibrous stroma (Fig. 21-6).

The proportion of fibrous to osseous tissue varies considerably among lesions, depending on the stage of development of the lesion. The radiographic features of fibrous dysplasia therefore vary depending on its stage of maturity. In an early fibrous (osteolytic) stage the lesion appears radiolucent, whereas an intermediate stage may be recognized by a smoky, mottled, or hazy pattern produced by the poorly defined intense aggregations of small spicules randomly distributed throughout the radiolucent area (see Chapter 25). Finally, a mature stage may be variously described as having a salt-and-pepper, ground-glass, or orange peel appearance, which varies in radiopacity depending on

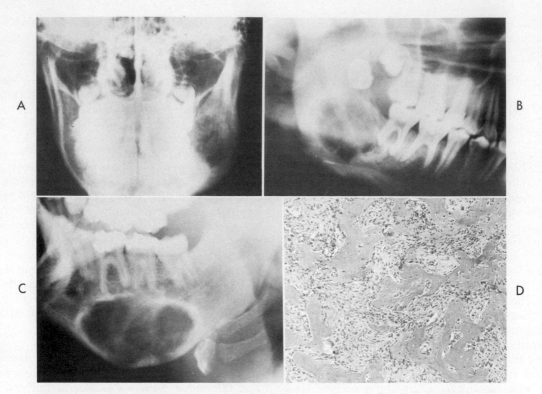

Fig. 21-6. Fibrous dysplasia. **A** and **B,** In a 16-year-old boy. The ill-defined margins of the radiolucency are evident. **C,** Advanced ossification at the periphery in this patient. The dense radiopaque appearance gives the illusion of well-defined borders. Periapical films of this peripheral region showed a ground-glass pattern. **D,** Chinese-character spicules of woven osteoid tissue among the active fibrous stroma. Osteoblastic rimming was not a feature.

the number, size, and degree of calcification of trabeculae. (Fibrous dysplasia is discussed as a solitary radiopacity in Chapter 28.)

When a lesion is discovered in the early osteolytic stage, its border is usually diffuse and appears to blend with the adjacent normal bony pattern without distinct demarcation (Fig. 21-6). Thus the early stage of fibrous dysplasia is included in this chapter, which encompasses the lesions having ill-defined borders.

Features

Although the cause of fibrous dysplasia is unknown, it primarily affects adolescents and young adults, showing no predilection for either sex. It may produce asymmetry of the jaws but usually no pain. If teeth are situated in an involved section of jawbone, malocclusion, spreading, or migration may be noted but not mobility. Growth is slow and usually ceases in the early twenties or before. The molar, premolar, and canine areas, the ramus and symphysis of the mandible, the premolar-molar regions of the maxilla, the zygoma, and the max-

illary sinus are the maxillofacial sites most frequently involved.

On radiographs the early lesion of fibrous dysplasia is radiolucent with poorly defined borders (Fig. 21-6). It is usually situated deep within the bone rather than superficially in the alveolus. The maturing changes that produce the ground-glass appearance frequently commence at the periphery of the lesion and are a clue to its correct identity (Fig. 21-6). Goldberg and Sperling (1981) noted that gross displacement of the mandibular canal is frequently associated with a lesion of fibrous dysplasia. Other features are discussed in detail in Chapter 25.

Differential diagnosis

The differential diagnosis of fibrous dysplasia is discussed in the differential diagnosis section at the end of this chapter (p. 454).

Management

The management of fibrous dysplasia is discussed in Chapter 25.

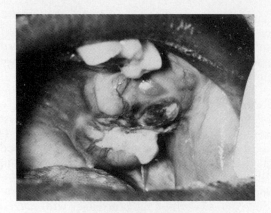

Fig. 21-7. Metastatic bronchogenic carcinoma to the maxillary molar and premolar region. Note the smoothly contoured expanded alveolar process in this region. The surface ulceration recently occurred as a result of masticatory trauma.   (Courtesy W. Heaton, DDS, Chicago.)

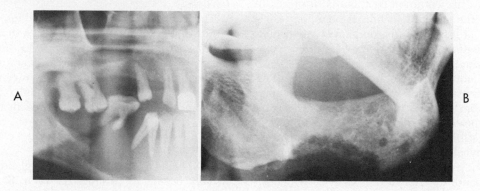

Fig. 21-8. Metastatic tumors. **A,** Metastatic bronchogenic carcinoma. **B,** Metastatic squamous cell carcinoma from the lower lip.   (**A** courtesy R. Latronica, DDS, Albany, N.Y. **B** courtesy O.H. Stuteville, DDS, MD, St. Joe, Ark.)

METASTATIC TUMORS TO THE JAWS

Metastatic tumors to the jaws are second only to primary squamous cell carcinoma as the most common group of malignant tumors in the jawbones. This group is discussed in Chapter 20, where it is stated that the secondary jaw tumor may produce some six different radiographic images. One possible image is a solitary radiolucency with ragged, poorly defined borders, which is the feature of metastatic tumors that explains their inclusion in this chapter.

Features

The more common primary tumors that metastasize to the jaws are from the breast, lung, gastrointestinal tract, prostate gland, kidney, and thyroid gland. Although the majority of secondary jaw tumors are found in the fifth decade and later, a few (such as neuroblastoma and retinoblastoma) have a high incidence in children and metastasize to bone in some cases; thus the possibility of metastatic tumors to the jaws in the lower age-groups must not be excluded.

Metastatic breast carcinomas to the jaws have been reported recently by Mizukawa et al. (1980), Yagan et al. (1984), and Zachariades and Papanicolaou (1982). Authors reporting cases of metastatic carcinoma from the kidney to the oral cavity include Fay and Weir (1983), Milobsky et al. (1975), and Quinn et al. (1981).

In 1982 Nishimura and coauthors in a review of the Japanese literature identified 41 metastatic tumors of the mouth and jaws. The incidence was 1.5 times higher in females, and 76% were in the fourth to seventh decades of life. It is interesting that the uterus was the most common site of origin, followed by the lung, kidney, and stomach. Carcinomas of glandular origin showed the highest rate of metastasis. Bony involvement was noted in 16 cases, and the gingiva was the location of the metastatic tumor in 16 cases.

Although a secondary jaw tumor may occur at the periphery and expand into the oral cavity, it is usually situated deep in the bone. When it produces an expansion, the exophytic lesion is usually dome shaped and covered with normal-appearing mucosa. Later, because it increases in size and there is concomitant masticatory trauma, a mucositis commonly develops on its surface; if the trauma continues, the surface ulcerates and becomes necrotic (Fig. 21-7).

Although metastatic tumors have been reported in different regions of the jaws, most occur in the premolar-molar area of the mandible; the incidence of secondary tumors in the maxilla is low.

A radiolucent area that may vary greatly in size with ragged poorly defined borders is one of the radiographic pictures produced by metastatic tumors in the jaws (Fig. 21-8). Pain and numbness are common complaints. If there are teeth in the affected section of bone, any combination of loss of lamina dura, root resorption, and loosening and spreading of teeth is a common finding.

Hashimoto et al. (1987) reported the findings of an extensive autopsy study of sectioned mandibles from patients with carcinoma. These authors reported on sites of metastatic tumors in the mandible and indicated that 16% of their cases revealed metastatic involvement of this bone. They concluded that hematopoietic areas in the mandible appeared to favor early deposition of tumor cells.

Differential diagnosis

A discussion of the differential diagnosis of metastatic tumors to the jaws is presented in the differential diagnosis section at the end of this chapter (p. 454).

Management

The management of metastatic tumors is discussed in Chapter 22.

MALIGNANT MINOR SALIVARY GLAND TUMORS

Malignant salivary gland tumors are discussed in Chapter 11 as mucosal ulcers and in Chapter 10 as exophytic lesions. In this chapter the features produced by these tumors when they infiltrate and destroy jawbone are emphasized. The more commonly occurring varieties are the pleomorphic and monomorphic adenocarcinoma, adenoid cystic carcinoma, mucoepidermoid tumor, and unclassified adenocarcinoma.

Although the incidence of malignant salivary gland tumors is much lower than that of the squamous cell carcinoma, they may occur as peripheral or central lesions, and like the squamous cell carcinoma, those originating within the jawbones are rare. Peripheral malignant salivary gland tumors may occur anywhere in the soft tissue lining of the oral cavity but seldom in the gingiva or on the anterior hard palate because the minor salivary glands are not usually found in these sites.

The posterior hard palate, upper lip and anterior vestibule, retromolar regions, and base of the tongue are the peripheral sites most commonly affected. The glandular tissue is most proximal to bone on the hard palate and in the retromolar areas, so these are the main sites where malignant minor salivary gland tumors invade the bone relatively early and produce poorly defined radiolucencies with ragged borders.

The central variety occurs so seldom that it is not discussed further here, other than to indicate that its features are similar to those produced by a central squamous cell carcinoma or any malignancy originating in the jawbones. An example that produced a multilocular radiolucency of the mandible is illustrated in Fig. 20-13.

Features

The malignant minor salivary gland tumor usually occurs in patients between 40 and 70 years of age and is more common in women. It usually grows slowly but may demonstrate alternate rates of growth. It frequently is found on routine examination, or sometimes the patient complains of a painful swelling. Because it develops as an increasing mass of tumor cells beneath and separate from the epithelial surface, it is most frequently somewhat dome shaped with a smooth surface and firm to palpation.

A mucus-producing adenocarcinoma and a mucoepidermoid tumor may have fluctuant areas because of pooling of the mucus produced by these special types of tumors. Aspiration yields clear, viscous, sticky mucus. When mucus pools near the surface of a mucus-producing tumor, the tumor may resemble a mucocele on clinical examination. Furthermore, if it has cystic areas of mucus retention, the areas may rupture and produce a persistent ulcerated surface.

Early in its development the malignant salivary tumor is usually covered with a smooth, normal-appearing mucosa. Later, if it is chronically traumatized, its surface demonstrates mucositis. If the trauma is severe or if a biopsy of the mass is performed, the surface ulcerates and remains ulcerated, this occurrence frequently leads to the production of a necrotic surface.

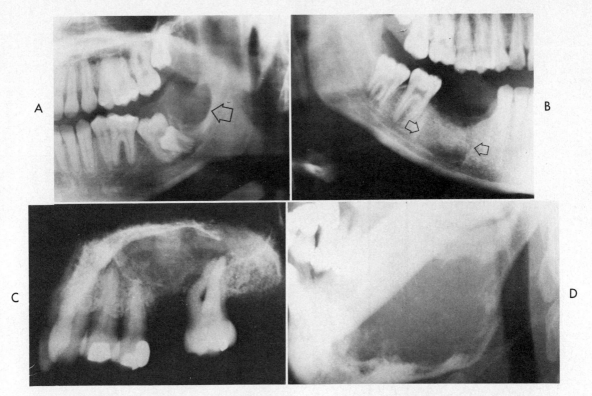

Fig. 21-9. Peripheral malignant salivary gland tumors. **A,** Mucoepidermoid tumor in the retromolar region destroying the alveolar bone *(arrow)*. **B,** Mucoepidermoid tumor *(arrows)*, which originated in the floor of the mouth and infiltrated the lingual alveolar plate in the premolar and molar region. **C,** Radiograph of a surgical specimen of an adenocystic carcinoma. **D,** Adenocarcinoma of minor salivary gland origin.   (**A** and **B** courtesy R. Kallal, DDS, Chicago. **C** courtesy O.H. Stuteville, DDS, MD, St. Joe, Ark. **D** courtesy R. Goepp, DDS, Zoller Clinic, University of Chicago.)

When a malignant salivary gland tumor infiltrates bone, it produces a radiolucency identical to that produced by a peripheral squamous cell carcinoma (that is, a semicircular radiolucency with poorly defined ragged advancing borders eroding from the surface into the bone Fig. 21-9). An undetected lesion on the posterolateral hard palate is apt to destroy the floor of the maxillary sinus and invade the air-filled cavity. Although the radiographic appearances of both tumors may be similar, the malignant salivary gland tumor seldom originates on the crest of the alveolar ridge, a fact that is useful in distinguishing this lesion from squamous cell carcinoma.

Differential diagnosis

Management of malignant minor salivary gland tumors is discussed in the section on differential diagnosis at the end of this chapter (p. 454).

Management

The management of malignant minor salivary gland tumors is discussed with peripheral oral exophytic lesions in Chapter 10.

OSTEOGENIC SARCOMA— OSTEOLYTIC TYPE

Osteogenic sarcoma is second only to multiple myeloma as the most frequently encountered *primary* tumor of the jawbones. It is thought to arise from primitive undifferentiated cells and from malignant transformation of osteoblasts. It has three basic radiographic appearances: completely radiolucent, radiolucent with radiopaque areas, and predominantly radiopaque. The classic sunburst effect may be seen in the latter two types. The various radiographic appearances of osteosarcoma are described in Table 21-1. Discussion in this chapter stresses the radiolucent variety of osteogenic sarcoma.

Table 21-1. Solitary ill-defined radiolucencies

Lesion	Predominant sex	Usual age (years)	Predominant jaw	Predominant region	Additional features	Other radiographic appearances
Chronic osteitis	M > F	50-80 and 5-15			Usually associated with root of pulpless tooth Slow course	Cystlike radiolucency Radiopacity
Chronic osteomyelitis	$\dfrac{M}{F} = \dfrac{5}{1}$	30-80	Mandible/maxilla = 7/1	Premolar-molar Angle Symphysis	History of debilitating systemic disease and/or fracture Slow course	Radiolucency with radiopaque foci Radiopacity
Peripheral squamous cell carcinomas	$\dfrac{M}{F} = \dfrac{2\text{-}4}{1}$	40-80 (peak 65)	Mandible/maxilla = 3/1	Mandibular molar	Tobacco, alcohol, poor hygiene Metastasizes—frequently early to regional lymph nodes Rapid growth	Radiolucency with radiopaque foci (sequestra)
Fibrous dysplasia (early stage)*	M ~ F	10-20 (peak 17)	Maxilla/mandible = 4/3	Rare in anterior maxilla and symphysis	No pain No paresthesia No root resorption Slow expansion	Mottled or smoky Ground-glass
Metastatic tumors to jaws						
Adults	$\dfrac{F}{M} = \dfrac{3}{2}$	40-60	Mandible/maxilla = 7/1	Premolar-molar	Signs and symptoms from primary tumor Unpredictable course	Solitary cystlike radiolucency Multiple cystlike radiolucencies
Children	M ~ F	0-10	Mandible > maxilla	Premolar-molar	Signs and symptoms from primary tumor Usually rapid course	Generalized rarefaction Salt and pepper Radiopacity Radiolucency with smooth, well-defined borders

Lesion	Sex	Age	Jaw	Site	Behavior	Radiographic features
Malignant minor salivary gland tumors	$\frac{F}{M} = \frac{2}{1}$	40-70	Mandible ~ maxilla	Posterior hard palate, Retromolar	Metastasizes to regional lymph nodes, Local extension by perineural space, Moderately slow but unpredictable course	
Osteogenic sarcomas	M > F	10-40 (peak 27)	Mandible/maxilla = 2/1	Mandibular body	Metastasizes by vascular route to lungs and other organs, Variable course	Radiolucency with radiopaque foci, Sunburst, Radiopacity
Chondrosarcomas	M > F	20-60 (avg. 40)	Maxilla > mandible		Metastasizes late by vascular route to lungs and other organs, Usually slow course	Asymmetric broadening of periodontal ligament, Widening of mandibular canal
Mesenchymal type	M > F	30-60 (peak 50s)			Metastasizes early by vascular route to lungs and other organs, Unpredictable course	Onionskin growth of periosteal bone, Codman's triangle, Cumulus cloud formation
Reticulum cell sarcomas	$\frac{M}{F} = \frac{2}{1}$	10-60 (avg. 37)	Rare in maxilla	Molar, Angle, Ramus	Metastasizes to bone or lymph nodes, Moderately slow course	Radiolucent and radiopaque
Ewing's sarcomas	$\frac{M}{F} = \frac{2}{1}$	5-24 (peak 14-18)	Rare in maxilla		Metastasizes to lymph nodes, lungs, and other bones, Rapid course	Onionskin growth of periosteal bone, Sunburst
Central squamous cell carcinomas	$\frac{M}{F} = \frac{2}{1}$	30-70 (peak 57)	Mandible/maxilla = 4.2/1	No predilection	Metastasizes to regional lymph nodes, Perhaps slow growth initially, then rapid growth	Cystlike radiolucency

*Pain, paresthesia, and root resorption are common features of all these lesions except fibrous dysplasia, although pain is not characteristically present in early lesions of peripheral squamous cell carcinoma and minor salivary gland tumors.
~, Approximately equal.

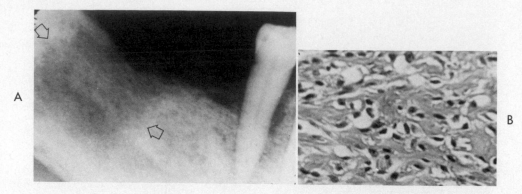

Fig. 21-10. A, Osteogenic sarcoma (osteolytic variety) *(arrows).* **B,** Microscopy of the lesion showing scanty osteoid and malignant osteoblasts.   (**A** courtesy R. Goepp, DDS, Zoller Clinic, University of Chicago.)

Like other malignant tumors the osteogenic sarcoma is of unknown cause. Bones that have been previously irradiated and bones affected with Paget's disease, however, show an increased incidence. Osteogenic sarcoma of the jaws differs from that found in other bones as follows:

1. The peak age of incidence is about 27 years, an average 10 years above the incidence observed in other bones.
2. The jaw lesions have less tendency to metastasize.
3. The prognosis is better for jaw lesions.

Osteogenic sarcoma metastasizes almost exclusively by hematogenous spread. Pulmonary metastasis, the most common, is frequently found at autopsy. Lymph node involvement is rare.

Features

A patient with an osteogenic sarcoma may complain of intermittent local pain, swelling, paresthesia or anesthesia, tooth mobility, intraoral bleeding, asymmetry of the jaws, and in some cases a mass on the ridge or gingivae. Garrington et al. (1967) reported that of their series, 40% had pain, 14% had paresthesia, and 25% had dental symptoms. There may be a history of recent tooth extraction with a nodular or polypoid, somewhat reddish, granulomatous-appearing mass growing from the tooth socket.

Approximately 60% of osteogenic sarcomas occur in men. The majority of patients affected are in the second to fifth decades, and incidence peaks at about 27 years of age. Investigators differ as to which jaw is more frequently involved, but most favor the mandible. In the series reported by Garrington et al. (1967) the mandible was affected twice as often as the maxilla.

Clark et al. (1983) reported on a series of 66 patients with osteosarcoma of the jaw at Mayo Clinic. The findings were as follows: (1) mean age was 34.2 years; (2) maxilla and mandible were approximately equally involved (51%/49%); (3) the most common sites were the body of the mandible and the alveolar ridge of the maxilla; (4) 50% of the maxillary lesions were osteoblastic whereas most mandibular lesions were osteolytic; and (5) chondroblastic osteosarcoma was the most frequent histologic type and was associated with the best survival rate (47%). Treatment included radical and local surgery with radiotherapy, chemotherapy, or various combinations. The overall recurrence rate was 70%. Patients treated with radical surgery initially had the best survival rate (80%). Those treated by local surgery had a survival rate of 27%. Most of the deaths resulted from uncontrolled local disease, and distant metastasis was documented in only four cases.

Rosen et al. (1982) reported receiving very promising results using preoperative and postoperative chemotherapy for osteosarcoma of the bones.

As the tumor grows, eroding the cortical plates, the expansion is very firm because of the dense fibrous tumor tissue produced. Initially the swelling is smoothly contoured and covered with normal-appearing mucosa. Later, when the expansion becomes chronically traumatized, mucosites develops on the surface; still later the surface ulcerates and a whitish gray necrotic surface results. This surface can be removed with a tongue blade.

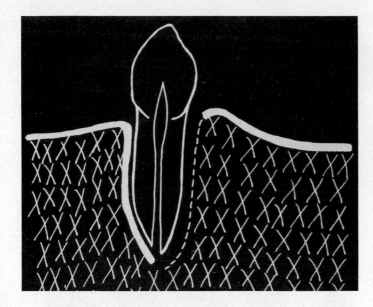

Fig. 21-11. Diagram of a periapical radiograph illustrating unilateral bandlike widening along right side of root. Such a bandlike widening of the periodontal ligament, either unilateral or bilateral, is suggestive of an intraosseous malignant tumor.

The bony lesion is radiolucent with poorly defined, ragged borders. Early in the course of the disease it is usually located centrally in the jaws (Fig. 21-10). Sometimes it is discovered as a radiolucency in the periapex or more toward the periphery of the ridge or cortical plates. It may originate adjacent to or seemingly in the periodontal ligament space, and in such cases it appears radiographically as a bandlike widening involving the complete length of the periodontal ligament space on one side of the root (Figs. 21-11 and 21-12, *B*) (Gardner and Mills, 1976). This particular picture is not pathognomonic for osteogenic sarcoma, however, but may also be seen with other types of mesenchymal malignancies, in patients undergoing orthodontic therapy, and with unusual unilateral bone resorption in periodontal disease (Fig. 21-12, *C* and *D*). In addition, Shafer (1980) described a case of osteoblastoma that produced a unilateral bandlike widening of the periodontal ligament. Lindquist et al. (1986) described a frequent involvement of the mandibular canal in their patients; this was accompanied by widening of the canal evident on radiographic examination and by paresthesia.

On microscopic examination the radiolucent type of osteogenic sarcoma is basically fibroblastic, showing malignant changes, good vascularity, and a few areas of osteoid tissue. It may also form some cartilage. A tumor composed primarily of osteoid or cartilage may rapidly calcify in these areas and become evident as a mixed radiolucent-radiopaque area or as a predominantly radiopaque lesion. The latter two types are discussed in Chapter 25.

Differential diagnosis

The differentiation of radiolucent lesions such as osteogenic sarcoma is discussed in the differential diagnosis section at the end of this chapter (p. 454).

Management

Although a diagnosis of osteogenic sarcoma of the jaws is grave (approximately 25% of the patients survive 5 years), the prognosis is better than for osteogenic sarcoma of other bones of the skeleton (Garrington et al., 1967). Lesions in the symphyseal region of the mandible have the best outlook, and those in the maxillary sinus have the poorest.

As with all malignant tumors, the management of a case of osteogenic sarcoma should be determined by the tumor board. Once the pathologist has made a positive diagnosis of osteogenic sarcoma, the patient must be thoroughly examined in an attempt to determine whether secondary lesions are present. If extensive secondary lesions are found, palliative radiation is usually decided on. If no secondary lesions are discovered, the tumor board usually decides on radical resection if possible. Regional lymph node dissection is rarely indicated or necessary, since spread to such nodes is infrequent. Some authors have advised presurgical radiation to reduce the threat of metastasis imposed by the surgical procedure. Recent studies have indicated that radiation or chemotherapy may yield as good results as radical surgery. High et al. (1978) reported achieving a complete remission in a recurrent case of osteosarcoma of the mandible. Jaffe et al. (1983) reported good re-

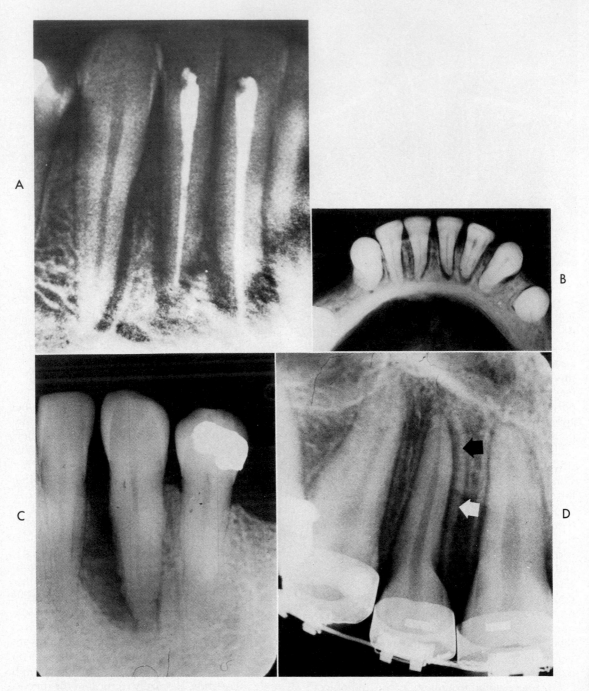

Fig. 21-12. Bandlike widening of the periodontal ligament. **A,** Chondrosarcoma of the anterior of the mandible in a young woman. **B,** Osteosarcoma of the anterior of the mandible Both symmetric and asymmetric bandlike widening of the periodontal ligament is evident in **A** and **B. C,** Asymmetric widening of the periodontal ligament on the mesial aspect of the canine tooth, which is caused by the presence of calculus. **D,** Asymmetric widening of the periodontal ligament on the mesial aspect of the upper lateral incisor tooth, which has been produced by recent orthodontic movement.   (**B** courtesy R. Goepp, DDS, Zoller Dental Clinic, University of Chicago. **C** courtesy O.H. Stuteville, DDS, MD, St. Joe, Ark.)

sults with intra-arterial infusion of a chemotherapeutic agent. The French Bone Tumor Group reported encouraging results with chemotherapy and prophylactic lung irradiation after treatment of the primary tumor (Trifaud et al., 1988). Burgers et al. (1988) also reported encouraging results with follow-up chemotherapy and prophylactic lung irradiation. Gebhart and Lane (1988) reported improved results with perioperative chemotherapy in sarcoma of the limbs.

The osteolytic type is the least differentiated and carries the poorest prognosis.

CHONDROSARCOMA

Chondrosarcoma follows multiple myeloma and osteogenic sarcoma as the third most common primary malignant tumor of the jawbones. It is, however, an uncommon jaw tumor; osteogenic sarcoma is at least three times more common. Although the exact origin of the chondrosarcoma is obscure, it may be found developing in normal cartilage, chondromas, or osteochondromas. It may originate centrally or on the periphery of the bone.

Chondrosarcomas show two quite different radiographic images: a frank radiolucency (usually in an early stage) or a radiolucency containing various shapes and sizes of radiopaque shadows. These radiopaque shadows are the result of calcification or ossification in areas of cartilage formation and are a feature of relatively long-standing tumors; they are found in the older parts of the tumors. Chondrosarcoma may mimic the appearance of osteosarcoma or radiographs (Table 21-1). Specifically, it may produce bandlike widening of the periodontal ligament (Garrington and Collett, 1988a, 1988b).

A comparatively rare, primitive type of chondrosarcoma, the mesenchymal chondrosarcoma, is apparently derived from cartilage-forming mesenchyme. Some authors believe this lesion is more aptly described as a mesenchymal sarcoma showing some chondroid differentiation.

In keeping with the subject of this chapter, only the completely radiolucent type is discussed.

Features

The chondrosarcoma is a tumor primarily of adulthood and old age; the majority of jaw tumors occur in patients between the ages of 20 and 60 years, with an average age of approximately 40 years (Sato et al., 1977). More than 60% of chondrosarcomas are found in men, and the maxilla is involved more often than the mandible. Some of the maxillary tumors represent lesions that originated in the cartilages of the nasal cavity and invaded the maxillary bone. The premolar and molar regions, symphysis, and coronoid and condyloid processes are the most frequent mandibular sites (Martis, 1978).

Unlike the osteogenic sarcoma, the chondrosarcoma metastasizes relatively rarely, especially in its early stages. As with osteogenic sarcoma, however, metastatic spread is almost entirely by vascular channels. Malignant cells may erode through the walls of a venule and extend along inside the venule without adhering to the vessel walls but still attached at their site of entry. When metastasis does occur, the lung is the organ most frequently involved.

Chondrosarcoma may recur when resection has been inadequate, usually only after many years. A patient whose tumor has not been adequately excised may have several recurrences and finally die because the tumor has invaded or metastasized to a surgically inaccessible site.

Although in the body as a whole the common type of chondrosarcoma occurs more frequently than the mesenchymal type, the mesenchymal type occurs more frequently in the jaws. The mesenchymal chondrosarcoma is a more malignant variety that grows faster and metastasizes earlier and more frequently; as a result it carries a much poorer prognosis.

Except for the mesenchymal variety, the chondrosarcoma behaves in a much less aggressive fashion than does the osteosarcoma. The patient frequently complains of a painful, slowly enlarging swelling in the affected region of the bone, often of several years' duration. The pain is strongly suggestive of an actively growing central type of bony tumor. Paresthesia is experienced in many cases. Occasionally when malignant transformation occurs in a previously benign cartilaginous tumor, an existing mass of long standing begins to grow rapidly.

Before the chondrosarcoma has caused expansion of the bone, pain may be the only clinical indication of the developing tumor. If it has eroded through the cortical plates, a tender or painful smoothly contoured mass can be palpated over the bone. The mass is firm if the tumor or region contains substantial amounts of cartilage or fibrous tissue. If much myxomatous-type tissue is present near its periphery, however, the tumor feels soft. The mucosal covering appears normal in the early stage but later may ulcerate and develop a necrotic surface if chronically traumatized. Teeth in the affected region may demonstrate spreading, migration, increased mobility, and root resorption. Sato et al. (1977) found that in maxillary tumors the most common symptoms were nasal.

The earlier lesion in bone is usually radiolucent because the neoplastic cartilage has not yet become calcified (Figs. 21-12, *A*, and 21-13).

On microscopic examination the lesion shows varying degrees of myxomatous-type tissue, atypical cartilage, endochondral bone, and nests of malignant chondrocytes (Fig. 21-13, *B*). A low-grade chondrosarcoma is difficult to differentiate by microscopic study from an aggressive chondroma.

Radiographs show a central tumor bordered by a ragged, poorly defined perimeter of bone. Conversely, the peripheral type may show only one border in bone and the rest of the tumor may be a vague hazy mass peripheral to the uneven area of bony erosion. The peripheral lesion generally tends to be more circumscribed. A lesion involving the teeth may appear as a periapical radiolucency or as an asymmetric broadening of the periodontal ligament space (Fig. 21-12, *A*).

Garrington and Collett (1988a) reported on a comprehensive survey of the chondrosarcoma literature. In that same year the same researchers reported on their analysis of 37 cases of chondrosarcoma of the jaws (Garrington and Collett, 1988b).

Differential diagnosis

The discussion of the differential diagnosis of the chondrosarcoma is included in the differential diagnosis section that begins on p. 454.

Management

Early extensive resection is mandatory for a good cure rate. The surgeon should be prepared for a radical procedure if the clinical appearance of the lesion suggests that it is malignant. If this precaution is observed, resection can be performed as soon as a frozen section is evaluated. Such preparedness reduces the time between the initial biopsy and the resection, when the potential for vascular dissemination of tumor cells is high because of the surgical manipulation.

The chondrosarcoma is quite radioinsensitive, and radiation therapy is used only as a palliative procedure with large inoperable tumors. Chemotherapy is also used as adjunctive therapy. More conservative local block resection, not including the full thickness of the bone, may be the treatment of choice in some early peripheral chondrosarcomas.

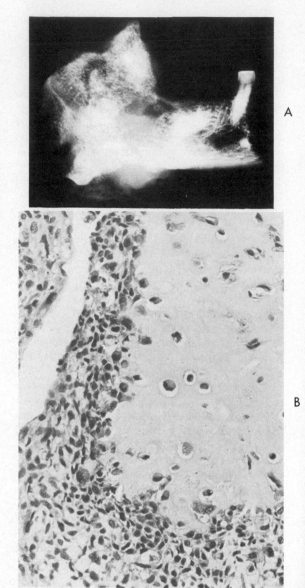

Fig. 21-13. Chondrosarcoma. **A,** Radiograph of surgical specimen of a mandibular lesion. **B,** Photomicrograph of a chondrosarcoma. (**A** courtesy O.H. Stuteville, DDS, MD, St. Joe, Ark.)

The long-term survival rate is good in 50% of the patients who have received early surgical treatment if wide margins of adjacent normal bone have also been excised. The prognosis for a jaw chondrosarcoma is not generally considered to be as good as for a chondrosarcoma of another bone, since jaw chondrosarcomas are more likely to be of the more aggressive mesenchymal variety. Well-differentiated tumors involving the symphyseal region have the most favorable prognosis (Garrington and Collett, 1988b).

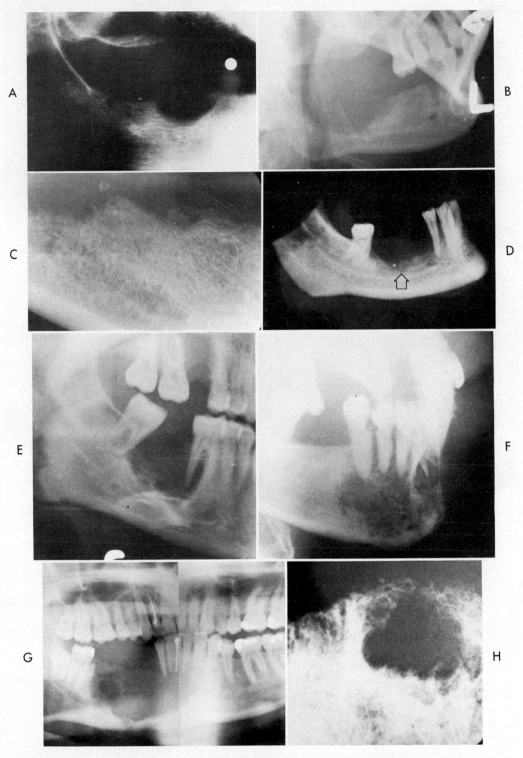

Fig. 21-14. Rare, ill-defined ragged radiolucencies. **A,** Ameloblastoma. **B,** Lateral oblique radiograph and, **C,** periapical radiograph of a reticulum cell sarcoma. **D,** Surgical specimen of a fibrosarcoma (*arrow*) of the mandible. **E,** Eosinophilic granuloma in the mandibular molar region. **F,** Central squamous cell carcinoma. **G,** Ameloblastic carcinoma. **H,** Simple ameloblastoma.   (**A** courtesy D. Skuble, DDS, Hinsdale, Ill. **B** and **C** courtesy R. Goepp, DDS, Zoller Clinic, University of Chicago. **D** courtesy R. Oglesby, DDS, Chicago. **E** courtesy N. Barakat, DDS, Beirut, Lebanon. **F** courtesy O.H. Stuteville, DDS, MD, St. Joe, Ark. **G** courtesy R. Latronica, DDS, Albany, N.Y. **H** courtesy R. Newman, DDS, Chicago.)

452

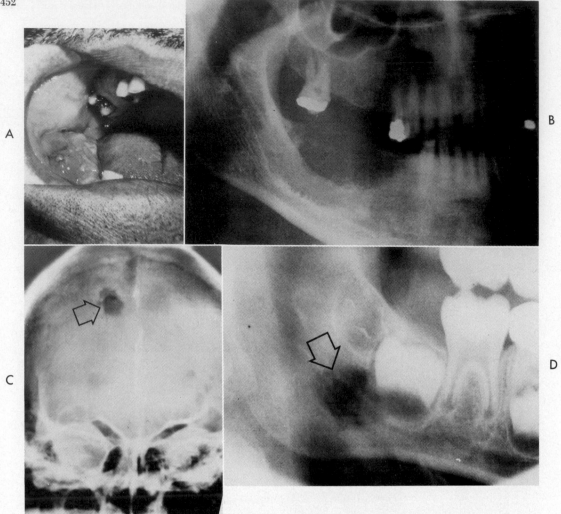

Fig. 21-15. **A** and **B,** Clinical and radiographic picture of a solitary myeloma in a 55-year-old man. **C,** Radiograph of a solitary myeloma *(arrow)* in the frontal bone. **D,** Eosinophilic granuloma *(arrow)* in a 9-year-old child. (**A** and **B** courtesy N. Barakat, DDS, Beirut, Lebanon. **C** courtesy W. Heaton, Chicago. **D** courtesy R. Warpeha, DDS, MD, Maywood, Ill.)

RARITIES

A considerable number and variety of rare lesions of the jaws may appear as solitary radiolucencies with ragged, poorly defined borders. Following is a partial list of such lesions. They are considered rarities because they seldom occur in the United States or do not usually cause a solitary radiolucent lesion with poorly defined borders characteristic of this group (Figs. 21-14 to 21-16):

Ameloblastic carcinoma (Fig. 21-14, *G*)
Ameloblastoma (Fig. 21-14, *A* and *H*)
Aneurysmal bone cyst
Angiosarcoma
Benign tumor in the rarefied jaw
Burkitt's tumor
Central hemangioma
Desmoplastic fibroma

Eosinophilic granuloma (Figs. 21-14, *E,* and 21-15, *D*)
Ewing's sarcoma (Fig. 21-16)
Fibromatosis
Fibrosarcoma (Fig. 21-14, *D*)
Histiocytosis X
Idiopathic histiocytosis (Langerhans' cell disease)
Intrabony hemangioma
Liposarcoma
Lymphosarcoma
Malignant ameloblastoma
Malignant lymphoma of bone
Medulloblastoma
Melanoma
Myeloma (solitary; plasmacytoma) (Fig. 21-15)
Myosarcoma
Myospherulosis (paraffinoma)
Neuroblastoma
Neuroectodermal tumor of infancy
Neurosarcoma

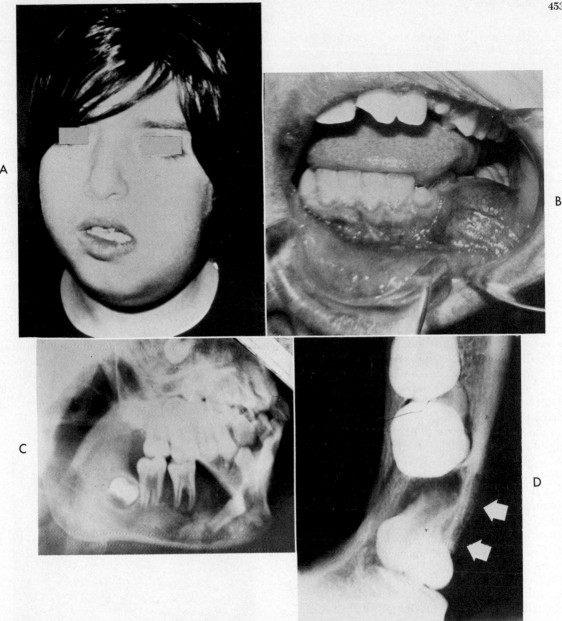

Fig. 21-16. Ewing's sarcoma in a 13-year-old girl. **A,** Full-face view showing asymmetry caused by a swelling in left mandible. **B,** Intraoral view showing smoothly contoured bony expansion in the premolar and first molar region. **C,** Lateral oblique radiograph showing ill-defined radiolucency and malposition of the premolar tooth. **D,** Occlusal view showing some central bone loss and also some destruction of the buccal plate *(arrows)*. Some bony spicules could be seen radiating out from the bone at this location in the original radiograph. The posteroanterior view of the mandible (see Fig. 28-12, *A*) showed periosteal bone growth at the inferior border of the mandible with an onionskin appearance. (Courtesy N. Barakat, DDS, Beirut, Lebanon.)

Odontogenic fibroma	Scleroderma
Odontogenic sarcoma	Spindle cell carcinoma
Osteoblastoma	Surgical defect
Phosphorus necrosis	Tuberculosis
Reticulum cell sarcoma (Fig. 21-14, *B* and *C*)	Vascular malformations
Sarcoidosis	Wilms' tumor

Furthermore, benign lesions in rarefied jaws may appear to have ill-defined borders. For example, a giant cell lesion in a jaw that is rarefied by osteitis generalisata of hyperparathyroidism appears as an ill-defined lesion because of the overall radiolucent appearance of the bone (see Fig. 19-16).

DIFFERENTIAL DIAGNOSIS OF SOLITARY RADIOLUCENCIES WITH RAGGED, POORLY DEFINED BORDERS

The finding of a radiolucency with ill-defined, ragged borders must be regarded as an ominous sign. When such a picture is observed on good diagnostic films, additional radiographs of the suspected area from various angles should be obtained to determine (1) whether the radiolucency actually has ill-defined borders or by happenstance the angle at which the original film was exposed combined with an unusual variation in anatomic structure to produce the misleading impression and (2) the exact size, extent, and location of the lesion. The differential diagnosis of lesions included in this chapter is relatively difficult, since the clinical characteristics of most of the entities are so similar—an enlarging tender or painful swelling of the jawbone accompanied by paresthesia or numbness. The radiographic appearances of these lesions are not uniquely characteristic during the radiolucent stage. Because of this similarity, the diagnostician must be alert to the more subtle features of each lesion: the relative frequency of occurrence, sexual predilection, age range of patients affected, incidence peaks, jaw regions usually involved, and accompanying systemic signs or symptoms.

An inflamed surface of an expanding jaw lesion, or even the presence of purulent drainage from a sinus, does not positively establish whether the pathosis is a chronic infection, however, since any of the tumors listed in this chapter may be complicated by the superimposition of an osteomyelitis.

Because the differential diagnosis of solitary, poorly defined, ragged radiolucencies in children is quite different from that of lesions having the same appearance in adults, this aspect is discussed separately for the two age-groups.

Solitary lesion in an adult
PERIPHERALLY LOCATED

A 59-year-old man complained of a tender swelling on the right side of the lower jaw in the molar area (Fig. 21-17). He also described a paresthesia of the lower lip on that side. He

had first noticed the swelling about 1 month previously. He smoked and drank excessively and had poor oral hygiene. On examination the clinician found an ulcer on the mucosa over the edentulous mandibular alveolar ridge in the right molar region (Fig. 21-17). The opposing posterior maxillary arch was also edentulous.

The ulcer had firm borders and was 2 cm in diameter. A firm, nontender expansion of soft tissue was present on the buccal and lingual surfaces of the ridge in the area of the ulcer. This soft tissue mass was tightly bound to the alveolar bone beneath. Several firm, nontender, enlarged, matted nodes were present in the right submandibular space. The hematologic examination revealed that although the patient was anemic, the total leukocyte count and differential count were within normal limits.

A broad, roughly semicircular, destructive lesion on the alveolar crest of the right mandibular molar region was apparent on a lateral oblique radiograph. The margin of this saucer-shaped erosion was ragged and poorly defined (Fig. 21-17).

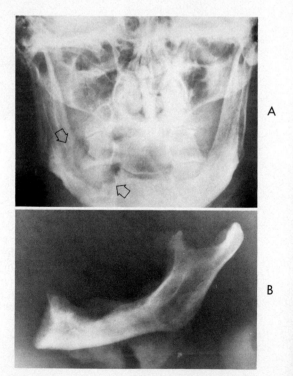

Fig. 21-17. Peripheral squamous cell carcinoma. **A,** Bony destruction *(arrows).* **B,** Radiograph of the surgical specimen. (Courtesy E. Palacios, MD, Maywood, Ill.)

In evaluating this lesion the clinician can initially rule out *fibrous dysplasia* because its early (radiolucent) stage would seldom if ever be seen at 59 years of age. Also, fibrous dysplasia almost never causes pain or paresthesia, and enlarged lymph nodes are not a feature of the disease.

The more common metastatic tumors of childhood, *neuroblastoma* and *retinoblastoma*, may be assigned a low rank on the basis of the patient's age. Also, *osteogenic sarcoma* usually occurs in a younger age-group. Other metastatic tumors more common to the patient's age would be assigned a low priority because of the absence of symptoms suggestive of a distant primary tumor.

Chronic osteomyelitis and *chronic osteitis* are not prime suspects for consideration because there are no manifestations of infection, such as local pain, cervical lymphadenitis, or leukocytosis.

The patient's age would not exclude *chondrosarcoma*, but a chondrosarcoma that had reached this size would usually show some calcified foci within the radiolucency. Furthermore, chondrosarcomas seldom involve the regional lymph nodes and are more common in the maxilla.

Squamous cell carcinoma, malignant minor salivary gland tumor, and *reticulum cell carcinoma* (see Table 21-1) must be considered possible diagnoses on the basis of the patient's age and the fact that they may involve lymph nodes. On the basis of incidence, these entities would be ranked in the following order in the working diagnosis: (1) squamous cell carcinoma, (2) malignant minor salivary gland tumor, and (3) reticulum cell sarcoma.

Peripheral squamous cell carcinoma is the most likely diagnosis for this lesion, since minor salivary gland tissue is unlikely to be found on the crest of the alveolar ridge. Also, the radiographic appearance of the tumor suggests that it originated in the soft tissue and was invading the bone from the periphery, which would be atypical of the usual initial manifestation of a localized reticulum cell sarcoma (a rare lesion). Finally, the diagnosis of peripheral squamous cell carcinoma is strongly supported by the fact that this oral lesion is frequently associated with poor oral hygiene, excessive smoking, and heavy alcohol consumption.

CENTRALLY LOCATED

A 30-year-old man described appreciable pain of about 1 month's duration in the right body of his lower jaw. Shortly before this time he had noticed a tingling in his lower lip on the right side. There was no history of trauma to the area.

During the examination the clinician noticed a slight swelling on the buccal aspect of the alveolus between and beneath the first molar and second premolar. These two teeth were found to be abnormally mobile, but they were not sensitive to percussion and they tested vital. The examination of the remainder of the oral cavity did not disclose additional significant abnormal conditions, and no cervical masses were found. A medical examination failed to disclose any systemic problems, and a skeletal radiographic survey revealed no other bony lesions. The results from all the appropriate laboratory tests* were within normal ranges.

Periapical radiographs of the right mandible revealed a solitary radiolucency at the junction of the molar and premolar areas. It was approximately round with irregular, poorly defined borders. The first molar and second premolar were found to have advanced and uneven root resorption, although the crowns of both appeared to be free of caries and there were no restorations. The lower borders of the radiolucency appeared to be encroaching on the mandibular canal.

Chronic osteitis and *osteomyelitis* can be excluded as likely causes of this man's discomfort, since there were no local signs of infection and no apparent evidence of predisposing conditions, fractures, or teeth with probable pulpitis.

Fibrous dysplasia can be eliminated from further consideration on the basis of the patient's pain, lip paresthesia, tooth mobility, and root resorption, which point to the probability of a malignancy.

Peripheral squamous cell carcinoma may be dismissed as an unlikely choice, since there is no mucosal involvement. The possibility that the lesion is a *central squamous cell carcinoma* can be assigned a low rank, since this tumor is rare. Also, the peripheral and central squamous cell carcinomas are usually seen in an older age-group.

Because of the patient's age, *Ewing's sarcoma*, which occurs most commonly at a younger age, *lymphosarcoma*, which is seldom seen between the ages of 20 and 30 years, and

---

*Erythrocyte and leukocyte counts (complete and differential) and levels of serum calcium, alkaline and acid phosphatase, urine calcium, and Bence Jones protein are usually determined.

metastatic lesions of childhood should be assigned a low ranking in the differential diagnosis.

Chondrosarcoma is more commonly seen in an older age-group, and it affects the maxilla more frequently than the lower jaw.

The patient is too young for *adult metastatic disease* to be strongly suspected, and there were no systemic symptoms to suggest a primary tumor elsewhere (although there could have been an occult primary lesion).

Central malignant minor salivary gland tumors are rare and are usually found in older individuals.

Reticulum cell sarcoma of bone is a possibility, but it is also usually found in older people and occurs much less frequently than osteogenic sarcoma.

Finally, the location, signs and symptoms, age of the patient, and incidence prompt the clinician to assign a top ranking to *osteogenic sarcoma (osteolytic type)*.

Solitary lesion in a child

A mother described the complaint of her 5-year-old daughter as a rapidly growing painful swelling in the molar region of the right mandible. The mother reported that she had first noticed the swelling approximately 1 month before and that pain had initially been intermittent but soon became constant. The child had recently had a tingling sensation on the right side of the lower lip. A history of recent trauma could not be established. Vital signs, including temperature, were normal. Examination of the child's neck failed to reveal any abnormalities such as lymph node involvement or tender areas.

The intraoral swelling, which was clinically apparent to the examiner, was tender and firm to palpation, and the jaw was somewhat expanded both buccally and lingually. The smoothly contoured swelling was covered with normal-appearing mucosa, and no draining sinus was present. The two deciduous molars in the area of the swelling were mobile, and there was some bleeding from their gingival sulci.

A complete radiographic survey of the skeleton disclosed only a solitary radiolucent lesion in the right mandible. It was completely surrounded by bone measuring approximately 2 cm in diameter, and its ragged borders were poorly defined. An occlusal radiograph showed that, although there was minimal evidence of destruction of both lingual and buccal cortical plates, multiple layers of subperiosteal new bone were faintly evident. The first and second right deciduous molars were not carious and had not been restored, but their roots were almost entirely resorbed. The lamina dura surrounding the root and crypt of the developing first permanent molar was missing.

A detailed medical examination, including complete blood and urine tests, failed to provide any pathognomonic results.

An early (osteolytic) lesion of *fibrous dysplasia* can immediately be eliminated as a possible diagnosis for this child's condition, since pain is not a feature of fibrous dysplasia and the lesion does not enlarge rapidly, does not cause root resorption, tooth mobility, or paresthesia, and infrequently develops in children as young as 5 years of age.

Chronic osteitis or *osteomyelitis*, with the exception of Garré's type, may be assigned a low rank because there was no obvious precipitating injury or predisposing systemic disease and the occurrence of osteomyelitis would be rare under such circumstances. Also, the local and systemic pictures did not show an infection. Since local inflammation was absent, there were no tender regional lymph nodes, and the patient's temperature, leukocyte count, and differential count were within normal limits.

The *neuroectodermal tumor* of infancy can be rejected as a possible diagnosis not only because this entity is rare but also because it almost always occurs in the anterior maxilla and is seldom if ever seen in children who have reached 5 years of age.

The patient's lesion is not likely to be an *intrabony hemangioma*, since pain is seldom a feature of the central hemangioma and such rapid expansion is not characteristic. Also, its superior border is usually contoured around the roots of the adjacent teeth. Furthermore, once the cortical plates were eroded, this vascular tumor would be relatively soft to palpation. If doubt still remained, judicious aspiration of the mass would provide convicing evidence of its vascular nature.

The foregoing considerations point to a conclusion of *malignant tumor* in bone. On the basis of age alone, however, this 5-year-old girl would not be likely to have a *squamous cell carcinoma, malignant minor salivary gland tumor,* or *chondrosarcoma.* Furthermore, a diagnosis of *peripheral squamous cell carcinoma* or *peripheral malignant minor salivary gland tumor* would be precluded by the radiographic appearance of the lesion—which indicated an origin in bone (central lesion)—and by the fact that there was no peripheral soft tissue mass or ulceration of the mucosa. Then, too, the *cen-*

tral varieties of squamous cell carcinoma and *minor salivary gland tumor* would be rare.

Although the foregoing speculations do not permit specific identification of the lesion, they do emphasize the important fact that the malignant tumors prone to involve this age-group are quite different from those that usually occur in adults. Also, malignant tumors in children are far less common than in adults and must be considered rare. Consequently, in identifying this child's pathosis, the clinician would be compelled to consider the entities listed as rarities.

The history, physical examination, and laboratory tests in this case provide presumptive evidence of a bone tumor, but there are no definite features that would permit the conclusion of either a primary or a metastatic lesion. To establish a working diagnosis, the clinician must consider a catalogue of the most frequent childhood tumors of bone.

The primary tumors are fortunately few and include osteogenic sarcoma, Ewing's sarcoma, lymphosarcoma, and chondrosarcoma. The most common metastatic bone tumors in children are Ewing's sarcoma (a primary osseous tumor that regularly metastasizes to other bones), neuroblastoma, and retinoblastoma. (Wilms' tumor might also be placed in this working diagnosis, since it occurs with some frequency in children, but it rarely metastasizes to bone.)

Two of the metastatic tumors, *retinoblastoma* and *neuroblastoma*, should be assigned a low ranking. Retinoblastoma seems unlikely, since the tumor is the most uncommon in this group of possibilities and since the physical examination failed to reveal any ocular symptoms. Neuroblastoma almost always produces multiple metastases, and the clinical examination of the patient did not suggest either the presence of a primary tumor of this type or that such a primary tumor had spread. Neither did the laboratory examination of the urine disclose high levels of catecholamines, which are almost always raised in neuroblastoma.

A diagnosis of *lymphosarcoma* seems less probable than one of osteogenic sarcoma or Ewing's sarcoma, since a lymphosarcoma is less common than either an osteogenic or a Ewing's sarcoma and, in contrast, does not form bone. Furthermore, its peak incidence occurs at a considerably older age.

Although *osteogenic sarcoma* is more common than *Ewing's sarcoma*, the age distribution of the latter is more skewed toward the younger ages. Osteogenic sarcoma also pro-

duces a more extensive erosion of the cortex than does Ewing's sarcoma (not a feature of this case). The concentric layers of laminated subperiosteal new bone (onionskin) observed in the patient may be produced by both tumors but are a more frequent characteristic of Ewing's sarcoma. (Such a pattern of laminated subperiosteal bone is also seen in proliferative periostitis, but this diagnosis is unlikely because there are no signs or symptoms of infection present.)

In view of this correlation of the patient's symptoms with the features of those bone tumors under suspicion, the order of working diagnosis that seems to provide the best compromise is (1) Ewing's sarcoma, (2) osteogenic sarcoma, (3) lymphosarcoma, and (4) metastatic tumor.

Although a working diagnosis of malignant tumor may be appropriate for this case, only the microscopic examination of representative excised tissue can identify the specific type of tumor and prove whether the lesion is really malignant.

REFERENCES

Burgers JMV, vanGlabbeke, M, Busson, A, et al: Osteosarcoma of the limbs: report of the EORTC-SIOP 03 trial 20781 investigating the value of adjuvant treatment with chemotherapy and or prophylactic lung irradiation, Cancer 61:1024-1031, 1988.

Ciola B: Pathologic fractures of the mandible following invasive oral carcinomas, Oral Surg 46:725-731, 1978.

Clark JL, Unni KK, Dahlin DC, et al: Osteosarcoma of the jaw, Cancer 51:2311-2316, 1983.

Coonar H: Primary intraosseous carcinoma of maxilla, Br Dent J 147:47-48, 1979.

Daramola JO: Massive osteomyelitis of the mandible complicating sickle cell disease: report of case, J Oral Surg 39:144-146, 1981.

Elzay RP: Primary intraosseous carcinoma of the jaws: review and update of odontogenic carcinomas, Oral Surg 54:299-303, 1982.

Fay JT and Weir GT: Metastatic renal cell carcinoma from a primary tumor removed 14 years previously, J Oral Maxillofac Surg 41:129-132, 1983.

Gallo WJ, Shapiro DN, and Moss M: Suppurative candidiasis: review of the literature and report of case, J Am Dent Assoc 92:936-939, 1976.

Gardner DG and Mills DM: The widened periodontal ligament of osteosarcoma of the jaws, Oral Surg 41:652-656, 1976.

Garrington GE and Collett WK: Chondrosarcoma I: a selected literature review, J Oral Pathol 17:1-11, 1988a.

Garrington GE and Collett WK: Chondrosarcoma II: chondrosarcoma of the jaws; analysis of 37 cases, J Oral Pathol 17:12-20, 1988b.

Garrington GE, Scofield HH, Cornyn J, and Hooker SP: Osteosarcoma of the jaws, Cancer 20:377-391, 1967.

Gebhart MJ and Lane JM: Management of bone sarcomas at Memorial Sloan-Kettering cancer center, World J Surg 12:299-306, 1988.

Goldberg MH and Sperling A: Gross displacement of the mandibular canal: a radiographic sign of benign fibro-osseous bone disease, Oral Surg 51:225-228, 1981.

Goupil MT, Steed DL, and Kolodny SC: Hyperbaric oxygen in the adjunctive treatment of chronic osteomyelitis of the mandible: report of case, J Oral Surg 36:138-140, 1978.

Hart GB and Mainous EG: The treatment of radiation necrosis with hyperbaric oxygen, Cancer 37:2580-2585, 1976.

Hashimoto N, Kurihara K, Yamasaki H, et al: Pathological characteristics of metastatic carcinoma in the human mandible, J Oral Pathol 16:362-367, 1987.

High CL, Frew AL, and Glass RT: Osteosarcoma of the mandible, Oral Surg 45:678-684, 1978.

Igo RM, Taylor CG, Scott AS, and Jacoby JK: Coccidioidomycosis involving the mandible: report of case, J Oral Surg 36:72-75, 1978.

Jaffe W, Knapp J, Chaung VP, et al: Osteosarcoma: intra-arterial treatment of the primary with cis-diamine-dichloroplatinum II (CDP), Cancer 51:402-407, 1983.

Kerley TR, Mader JT, Hulet WH, et al: The effect of adjunctive hyperbaric oxygen on bone regeneration in mandibular osteomyelitis: report of case, J Oral Surg 39:619-623, 1981.

Lindquist C, Teppo L, Sane J, et al: Osteosarcoma of the mandible: analysis of nine cases, J Oral Maxillofac Surg 44:759-764, 1986.

Mainous EG, Boyne PJ, and Hart GB: Hyperbaric oxygen treatment of mandibular osteomyelitis: report of three cases, J Am Dent Assoc 87:1426-1430, 1973.

Mansfield MJ, Sanders DW, Heimbach RD, et al: Hyperbaric oxygen as an adjunct in the treatment of osteoradionecrosis of the mandible, J Oral Surg 39:585-589, 1981.

Martinelli C, Melhado RM, and Callestini EA: Squamous cell carcinoma in a residual mandibular cyst, Oral Surg 44:274-278, 1977.

Martis C: Chondrosarcoma of the mandible: report of case, J Oral Surg 36:227-230, 1978.

Marx RE and Ames JR: The use of hyperbaric oxygen therapy in bony reconstruction of the irradiated and tissue-deficient patient, J Oral Maxillofac Surg 40:412-420, 1982.

Milobsky SA, Milobsky L, and Epstein LI: Metastatic renal adenocarcinoma presenting as periapical pathosis in the maxilla, Oral Surg 39:30-33, 1975.

Mizukawa JH, Dolwick MF, Johnson RP, et al: Metastatic breast adenocarcinoma of the mandibular condyle: report of case, J Oral Surg 38:448-451, 1980.

Musser LM, Tulumello TN, and Hiatt WR: Actinomycosis of the anterior maxilla, Oral Surg 44:21-24, 1977.

Nakajima T, Yagata H, Kato H, and Tokiwa N: Surgical treatment of chronic osteomyelitis of the mandible resistant to intraarterial infusion of antibiotics: report of case, J Oral Surg 35:823-827, 1977.

Nishimura Y, Yakata H, Kawasaki T, et al: Metastatic tumors of the mouth and jaws: a review of the Japanese literature, J Maxillofac Surg 10:253-258, 1982.

Nolan R and Wood NK: Central squamous cell carcinoma of the mandible: report of case, J Oral Surg 34:260-264, 1976.

Quinn JH, Kreller JS, and Carr RF: Metastatic renal cell carcinoma to the mandible: report of case, J Oral Surg 39:130-133, 1981.

Rosen G, Caparros B, Huvos AG, et al: Preoperative chemotherapy for osteogenic sarcoma, Cancer 49:1221-1230, 1982.

Rosenquist JB and Beskow R: Tuberculosis of the maxilla, J Oral Surg 35:309-310, 1977.

Sato K, Nukaga H and Horikoshi T: Chondrosarcoma of the jaws and facial skeleton: a review of the Japanese literature, J Oral Surg 35:892-897, 1977.

Shafer WG: Personal communication, 1980.

Shear M: Primary intra-alveolar epidermoid carcinoma of the jaw, J Pathol 97:645-651, 1969.

Sirsat MV, Sampat MB, and Shrikhande SE: Primary intra-alveolar squamous cell carcinoma of the mandible, Oral Surg 35:366-371, 1973.

Trifaud A, Clavel M, Delepine G, et al: Age and dose of chemotherapy as major prognostic factors in a trial of adjuvant therapy of osteosarcoma combining two alternating drug combinations and early prophylactic lung irradiation: French Bone Tumor Study Group, Cancer 61:1304-1311, 1988.

Walker S, Middelkamp JH, and Sclaroff A: Mandibular osteomyelitis caused by Actinomyces israelii, Oral Surg 51:243-244, 1981.

Wannfors K and Hammarstrom L: Infectious foci in chronic osteomyelitis of the jaws. Int J Oral Surg 14:493-503, 1985.

Weaver A, Fleming SM, and Smith DB: Mouthwash and oral cancer; carcinogenic or coincidence? J Oral Surg 37:250-253, 1979.

Yagan R, Bellon EM, and Radivoyevitch M: Breast carcinoma metastatic to the mandible mimicking ameloblastoma, Oral Surg 57:189-194, 1984.

Yakata H, Nakajima T, Yamada H, and Tokiwa N: Actinomycotic osteomyelitis of the mandible, J Oral Surg 36:720-724, 1978.

Zachariades N and Papanicolaou S: Breast cancer metastatic to the mandible, J Oral Maxillofac Surg 40:813-818, 1982.

22

Multiple separate well-defined radiolucencies

NORMAN K. WOOD
PAUL W. GOAZ
MARIE C. JACOBS

The entities that may produce multiple separate cystlike radiolucencies include the following:

Anatomic variations
Multiple cysts or granulomas
Basal cell nevus syndrome
Multiple myeloma
Metastatic carcinoma
Histiocytosis X
Rarities
  Ameloblastomas
  Cherubism
  Craniofacial dysostosis
  Gaucher's disease
  Giant cell granulomas
  Hyperparathyroidism with multiple distinct
    osteolytic lesions
  Lingual mandibular bone depressions
  Lymphomas
  Maffucci's syndrome
  Mucopolysaccharidoses
    Hunter's syndrome
    Hurler's syndrome
    Maroteaux-Lamy syndrome
    Sanfilippo A
    Sanfilippo B
    Sanfilippo C
    Scheie's syndrome
  Multiple dental cysts in arachnodactyly
  Neurofibromatosis
  Neimann-Pick disease
  Nodular cemental masses
  Oxalosis and hyperoxaluria
  Oxycephaly
  Papillon-Lefèvre syndrome
  Pseudotumors of hemophilia
  Scleroderma
  Squamous odontogenic tumors (familial and
    nonfamilial)
  Traumatic bone cysts

The multiple separate cystlike radiolucencies must be distinguished from the multilocular type of radiolucency (which is not made up of

459

numerous distinctly separate lesions but appears to be a single lesion formed of contiguous and coalescent cystic spaces).

ANATOMIC VARIATIONS

As is true of other radiolucent anatomic structures, those that cause multiple separate cystlike radiolucencies may be mistaken for pathoses.

Focal osteoporotic bone marrow defects, discussed in Chapter 19, may produce the radiographic image of a cystlike radiolucency. Occasionally, several such separate marrow spaces are observed on radiographs of a patient's jaw (Fig. 22-1) and the clinician must then decide whether they are marrow spaces or one of the pathologic conditions listed on p. 459.

These defects are discussed in Chapter 16 as periapical radiolucencies and in Chapter 19 as solitary cystlike radiolucencies. On occasion both types may occur in the same individual. In such cases both are usually present bilaterally in the mandible.

If previous radiographs of the jaws are available, the clinician can compare the areas in question to determine whether there has been a change in the pattern. If the radiolucencies were apparent on earlier radiographs, are of the same relative proportions and appearance, and are obviously only casually associated with the crown or root of a tooth (and in the absence of other signs and symptoms), a reasonable assumption would be that they are multiple separate cystlike marrow spaces. If a change in the trabecular pattern of an area in a jaw is evident on a sequence of radiographs, the clinician would do well to determine whether this change is related to a change in function. It is unusual to find such multiple cystlike marrow spaces in the maxilla. Thus, if suspicious images are found there and also in the mandible, they very likely represent a pathologic condition.

Multiple postextraction sockets sometimes appear as separate cystlike radiolucencies and be misdiagnosed as pathoses by the unwary examiner. Although such images are to be expected on radiographs of a jaw after recent tooth extractions, they may persist for years. Radiolucencies representing multiple extraction wounds would, of course, be found in the alveolar portion of the jawbone in edentulous regions (Fig. 22-2). Mandibular sockets are usually much more prominent and well defined than are their maxillary counterparts because the finer architecture of the bone in the upper

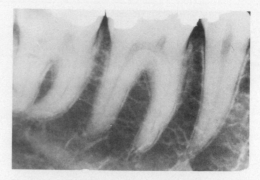

Fig. 22-1. Multiple marrow spaces at the apices of the molar and premolar.

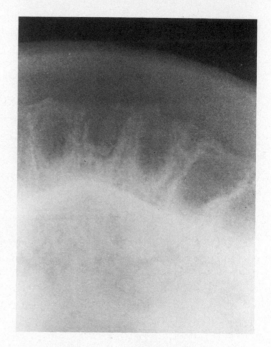

Fig. 22-2. Multiple sockets.

jaw is less likely to silhouette the sockets so clearly.

If the extractions are recent, the clinician is able to identify the sockets readily from the patient's history and by the telltale condition of the alveolar ridge (which clinically shows the depressions on the surface mucosa, each surrounded by an elevation over the crest of the bony socket walls). If, however, the extractions were performed months or years before, only a persistent, stable pattern in the alveolar bone apparent on periodic radiographs indicates the identity of the sockets.

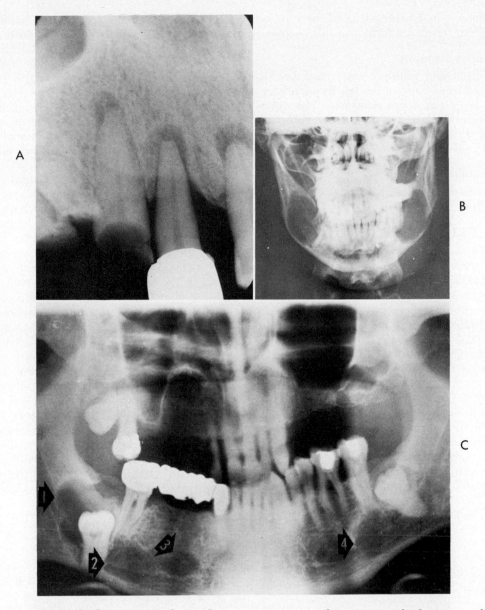

Fig. 22-3. Multiple conventional granulomas or cysts (no syndrome). **A,** Multiple periapical granulomas. **B,** Bilateral cysts. **C,** Orthopantomograph showing multiple cysts. *1,* Follicular; *2* and *4,* radicular; *3,* residual.   (**B** courtesy D. Skuble, DDS, Hinsdale, Ill. **C** courtesy N. Barakat, DDS, Beirut, Lebanon.)

MULTIPLE CYSTS OR GRANULOMAS (CONVENTIONAL TYPE*)

From time to time, multiple conventional cysts or granulomas occur in otherwise healthy patients who do not have any recognizable syndrome. Reports indicate that these cysts may be dentigerous cysts (Norris et al., 1987), radicular cysts, primordial cysts, or keratocysts (Fig. 22-3). There seems to be a familial tendency for multiple odontogenic cysts.

Instances of multiple periapical granulomas have been noted, but they are usually identifiable as sequelae of pulpitis, since they are associated with untreated carious teeth (Fig. 22-3). Solitary examples of these individual entities

---

*In the context of this discussion, the term "conventional" refers to those multiple jaw cysts whose initiation can apparently be attributed to strictly local factors.

are discussed in Chapters 16, 17, and 19, so they are not discussed further in this chapter.

Differential diagnosis

Uncomplicated multiple cysts must be distinguished from those of the less frequently occurring *basal cell nevus syndrome*. This differentiation is developed in the section on the differential diagnosis of the basal cell nevus syndrome (p. 463).

Management

The treatment of cysts is discussed in detail in Chapters 16 and 17.

BASAL CELL NEVUS SYNDROME

The basal cell nevus syndrome is a hereditary complex of abnormalities transmitted as an autosomal dominant trait with a poor degree of penetrance and variable expressivity. The feature that prompts its inclusion in this chapter is the multiple jaw cyst, which may be of the dentigerous, primordial, or radicular variety. The majority of these cysts prove to be keratocysts on microscopic examination.

Features

Characteristic features of the basal cell nevus syndrome embrace varying manifestations of cutaneous and skeletal abnormalities and, frequently, ectopic calcifications.

The syndrome occurs with equal frequency in males and females (autosomal dominant trait)

and usually becomes apparent in patients between 5 and 30 years of age. The most notable and characteristic cutaneous manifestation is the nevoid basal cell carcinomas; these are present as flesh-colored or brownish papules, predominantly on the skin of the face, neck, and trunk but occurring anywhere on the skin surface (Fig. 22-4). The papules frequently appear early in childhood, but additional lesions may occur during the second and third decades.

The majority of these papular basal cell carcinomas are less aggressive than the usual solitary basal cell carcinoma, which characteristically produces a rodent ulcer.

In some cases pits or dyskeratosis or both are present on the palmar and plantar surfaces.

Skeletal abnormalities may include multiple cysts of the jaws, bifid ribs, synostosis of the ribs, kyphoscoliosis, vertebral fusion, polydactyly, frontal and temporoparietal bossing, a mild ocular hypertelorism, and a mild prognathism (Fig. 22-4).

The ectopic calcifications observed most frequently occur in the falx cerebri, the skin, and the jaw cysts. The jaw cysts generally develop at an earlier age than do the basal cell carcinomas. Thus the dental clinician may be the first to encounter and identify this syndrome when he or she discovers the multiple cystlike radiolucencies on radiographs of the jaws.

Pritchard et al. (1982) discussed the variable expressivity of features of this syndrome, ex-

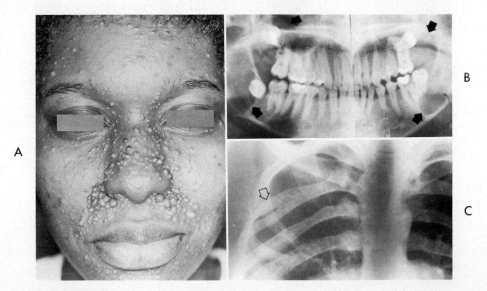

Fig. 22-4. Basal cell nevus syndrome. **A,** Multiple nevoid basal cell carcinomas on the face. **B,** Panograph showing four dentigerous cysts associated with impacted third molars. **C,** Anteroposterior radiograph of the chest depicting a bifid rib. (**A** courtesy D. Bonomo, DDS, Flossmoor, Ill. **B** and **C** courtesy the late J. Ireland, DDS, and J. Dolce, DDS, Mundelein, Ill.)

plaining that no one component of the syndrome is present in all patients.

The jaw cysts, which vary in size from a millimeter or less to several centimeters in diameter, occur more frequently in the mandible and in the premolar and molar region. They may be of the dentigerous, primordial, or radicular type, and a significant number are multilocular (Olson et al., 1981). Woolgar et al. (1987) reported that in some of these cases it is possible that only one cyst is present at any one time but during the lifetime of the patient, multiple cysts occur. These authors also found that the patient age at removal of the first cyst is lower than in cases of nonsyndrome odontogenic keratocysts. On histologic study all types and variations of epithelial linings may occur, but there is a preponderance of the keratocystic type. Frequently microcysts develop in the cyst wall, and peculiar budding of the basal epithelial cells into deeper layers of the wall may be a feature.

The Ellsworth-Howard test is used to differentiate the basal cell nevus syndrome from other disease states that may manifest some of the same clinical characteristics. It evaluates kidney tubular function after parathyroid hormone injection. An absence of significant phosphorus diuresis after an intravenous injection of the hormone is observed in this syndrome.

Differential diagnosis

When most of the features associated with the basal cell nevus syndrome are manifested and apparent, the syndrome does not present a problem in differential diagnosis. Sometimes only two or three features are present, however, and the clinician must then know that early in childhood only the jaw cysts may be apparent, which can cause a diagnostic problem.

In developing a working diagnosis, the clinician should furthermore remember that *multiple conventional jaw cysts* occur more frequently than do those that are a feature of the basal cell nevus syndrome. Consequently, if no other expressions of the disease are present, the clinician may have to proceed with a working diagnosis of multiple conventional jaw cysts while maintaining close posttreatment surveillance to ensure that the additional characteristics of the syndrome do not develop.

Such an occurrence would, of course, be convincing evidence that the case is indeed a basal cell nevus syndrome. The examiner must therefore make the distinction between multiple conventional jaw cysts and the jaw cysts of the basal cell nevus syndrome, since the management of the latter condition is much more complex and difficult.

Usually multiple conventional jaw cysts are well defined and relatively large, so they cannot be confused with *multiple cystlike bone marrow defects* or *multiple postextraction wounds* or *scars*, which are more uniform in shape and arrangement. Should the suspect lesion be associated with an expansion of the buccal plates, however, the diagnosis of either marrow spaces or postextraction sockets would be ruled out.

The multiple radiolucent lesions of *multiple myeloma, metastatic carcinoma*, and *histiocytosis X* can usually be distinguished from multiple conventional jaw cysts and cysts of the basal cell nevus syndrome. The first two former lesions are usually smaller and more numerous, and they affect other bones of the skull and skeleton in addition to the jaws. Lesions of histiocytosis X usually have ragged, vague margins and so are not cystlike.

Multiple radiolucent lesions of *cherubism* may be scattered throughout the jaws of a patient in the first or second decade of life. Contrary to radiolucencies of the multiple cysts of the syndrome, however, these radiolucencies frequently have a multilocular appearance. Although they may be unilocular, they show a more elliptic expansion of the jaws without well-circumscribed or hyperostotic borders.

The abnormal response of a patient with the basal cell nevus syndrome to injections of parathyroid hormone—plus the ectopic calcifications (some of which involve the jaw cysts) and the other skeletal abnormalities—may be confused with such entities as *idiopathic hypoparathyroidism, pseudohypoparathyroidism, pseudo-pseudohypoparathyroidism, basal ganglion calcification syndrome, Turner's syndrome*, and *Gardner's syndrome*. Witkop (1968) has reviewed the differential diagnosis of these entities in detail.

Management

As previously stated, the management of the basal cell nevus syndrome is much more difficult and complex than is management of multiple conventional jaw cysts.

The jaw cysts associated with the basal cell nevus syndrome show a much higher recurrence rate (36.4% in Brannon's series [1976]), possibly because of the phenomena of microcysts, or budding, in the keratocysts. Thus a more vigorous enucleation and more vigilant postoperative surveillance are in order. Treatment of odontogenic keratocysts is discussed in detail in Chapter 19.

The other systemic manifestations and complications (that is, the basal cell carcinomas, the spinal problems, and the increased risk of medulloblastoma in the probands and siblings) require careful evaluation and management by a physician.

MULTIPLE MYELOMA

Multiple myeloma is the most common primary malignant tumor of bone and usually involves a number of bones in the same individual. Although in advanced cases it may appear on radiographic examination as a generalized rarefaction of the skeleton or as numerous radiolucencies with ill-defined, ragged borders, it most frequently occurs as small, circular, multiple, but separate, well-defined (punched-out) radiolucencies; this latter appearance explains the inclusion of the lesion in this chapter.

Features

Multiple myeloma is a malignant plasma cell tumor that is thought to originate from reticulum cells within the bone marrow. It appears with equal frequency in men and women, most commonly affecting patients between 40 and 70 years of age. The bones usually involved are the skull, clavicle, vertebrae, ribs, pelvis, femurs, and jaws (all of which play a prominent role in hematopoiesis); however, any part of the skeleton may be involved. Older studies revealed that in approximately 30% of the cases the jawbones are affected, especially the premolar region and coronoid process. Lambertenghi-Deliliers (1988), in an extensive study of 193 patients with multiple myeloma, found mandibular lesions in 5.18% of patients. These authors indicated that radiographically apparent lesions of the mandible occurred late in the disease.

The patient may complain of pain in the involved bones, which is aggravated by exercise and relieved by rest. When the mandible is involved, paresthesia or numbness of the lip may be a complaint as may looseness and migration of the teeth. Sometimes the myeloma erodes through the buccal plates and produces a rubbery expansion of the jaws. At first the expansion is covered with normal mucosa, but chronic trauma produces an inflamed and eventually an ulcerated necrotic surface. Epstein et al. (1984) reviewed the oral and maxillofacial manifestations of multiple myeloma. Cases, as well as significance, of oral amyloidosis were reported by Salisbury et al. (1983) and Flick

and Lawrence (1980). Examples of oral amyloidosis are shown in Fig. 10-36, A.

Sedimentation rates in multiple myeloma are markedly elevated, and pancytopenias are present. The increased serum gamma globulin produces a reverse in the ratio of albumin to globulin, as well as an elevation in the level of total plasma protein. Plasma cells are usually found in peripheral blood smears.

As occurs in most of the lytic bone diseases that apparently demonstrate alternate active and quiescent phases, the serum calcium values in multiple myeloma may be normal. Hypercalcemia, however, is detected in 20% to 40% of the cases; since the bone resorption rate is generally not rapid enough to cause a rise in the plasma calcium level if the filtration rate is normal, the hypercalcemia is believed to result from an increase in the bone resorption rate combined with a reduction in the glomerular filtration rate.

Although the plasma phosphate value in multiple myeloma is usually normal, a hypophosphatemia is sometimes observed. The serum chemistry levels may resemble those seen in primary hyperparathyroidism, but the serum alkaline phosphatase level is usually normal. In approximately half the cases, Bence Jones proteins* are produced by the abnormal plasma cells making up the multiple tumors.

Complications of multiple myeloma include pathologic fracture (Moriconi and Popowich, 1983), secondary anemia, increased susceptibility to infection, a bleeding tendency, kidney failure, and amyloidosis. Such symptoms as nausea, lethargy caused by the anemia, and vomiting caused in part by the increased serum calcium level are also observed.

The pathologic fractures, which are more frequent than in metastatic carcinoma, result from the myeloma tissue's advancing on adjacent bone, thinning the cortex, and reducing the trabeculae in thickness and number (Moseley, 1963).

The secondary anemia, increased susceptibility to infection, and bleeding tendency result from the overgrowth of myeloma cells in the bone marrow; these cells replace the normal centers of erythrocyte, granulocyte, and megakaryocyte formation.

The kidney failure, which (after pneumonia) is the second most common cause of death in

---

*This protein precipitates when the patient's urine is heated to 50° or 60° C, but the precipitate disappears on boiling and then reappears when the urine is cooled to 60° or 70° C.

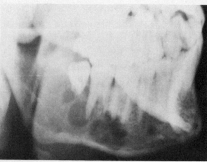

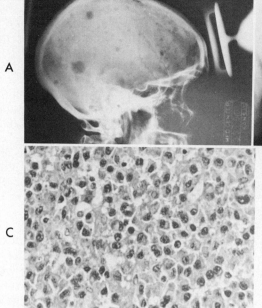

Fig. 22-5. Multiple myeloma. **A,** Numerous punched-out radiolucencies. **B,** Lateral oblique radiograph showing several punched-out radiolucencies in the left mandible. The pulps of the teeth were vital. **C,** Photomicrograph showing sheets of atypical plasma cells.   (**A** courtesy E. Palacios, MD, Maywood, Ill. **B** courtesy O.H. Stuteville, DDS, MD, St. Joe, Ark.)

multiple myeloma, is caused in part by the hypercalcemia, amyloidosis, and blockage of the renal tubules with casts of Bence Jones protein (Nordin, 1973).

As mentioned previously, multiple myeloma may occur with three different radiographic appearances.* The multiple and scattered small, round, well-defined radiolucencies without sclerotic borders, involving several bones of the skeleton, are stressed in this chapter (Fig. 22-5).

The definitive diagnosis is made from a smear of bone marrow aspirate, from a biopsy specimen of an affected region of bone, or from plasma electrophoresis.

The tumors vary greatly in degree of malignancy. They are composed of solid sheets of plasma cells with few or no connective tissue septa (Fig. 22-5). Because of the frequent accumulation of plasma cells in chronic inflammatory proliferations in the oral cavity, differentiation of such lesions from those of solitary myeloma sometimes presents a problem for the pathologist. However, it is generally accepted that lesions consisting of monoclonal plasma cells are neoplastic lesions, whereas lesions with multiclonal plasma cells are inflammatory (Regezi et al., 1983; Wright et al., 1981). These authors described the use of peroxidase and immunofluorescence techniques to determine monoclonicity and polyclonicity in biopsy specimens that were predominantly composed of plasma cells. Results were useful in equivocal cases. Raubenheimer et al. (1987) described in detail the histopathologic characteristics revealed by light and electron microscopy, as well as the results of histochemical tests.

Solitary myeloma lesions of bone are invariably followed by multiple myeloma, although in some cases it may take as long as 20 years for the disseminated disease to become manifest.

Differential diagnosis

The differential diagnosis of multiple myeloma and similar-appearing lesions is discussed with the differential diagnosis of histiocytosis X (p. 469).

Management

Multiple myeloma is a rapidly fatal disease. Approximately half the patients die within 2

---

*Although certain features and locations of lesions on radiographic examination are strongly suggestive of multiple myeloma, none of the bone changes that might be observed in this disease are pathognomonic. At one time, punched-out areas of bone destruction were considered the most common appearance of multiple myeloma. Now there is general agreement that the usual tendency is for the skeleton to be involved by a combination of types of lesions. Also, the degree and extent of bone involvement are directly related to the duration of the disease. The involvement of the skull, coupled with other skeletal lesions, was once considered unequivocal evidence of multiple myeloma; now authorities recognize that the skull is not always involved (Moseley, 1963).

years of the onset of symptoms. The 5-year survival rate is approximately 10%. The primary disease is treated usually by systemic administration of cytotoxic drugs (for example, melphalan, urethan, cyclophosphamide), as well as by steroids and radiation. Alexanian and Dreicer (1984) described improved results from the addition of vincristine and doxorubicin (Adriamycin) to a combination of prednisone and either cyclophosphamide or nitrosourea. Palliative measures are used to control the accompanying pain, bleeding, anemia, and kidney problem.

Inorganic fluoride and phosphate supplements have been used in attempts to relieve the bone pain and reverse some of the abnormal serum electrolyte patterns. Early reports on fluoride therapy were promising, but studies by Harley et al. (1972) and other investigators revealed that fluoride therapy, although effecting some relief of pain, is not as beneficial for resolving bone lesions as it was first considered to be and may even be harmful.

The immune and other defense mechanisms are seriously impaired, so the patient is highly susceptible to infection. Hence any surgical procedure that cannot be postponed should be accompanied by an antibiotic effective against both gram-positive and gram-negative microorganisms.

METASTATIC CARCINOMA

The spread from a primary carcinoma may result in the development of multiple metastases in the skeleton. When this happens, the metastatic bone lesions may assume a variety of radiographic appearances, one of which is multiple small, rounded, and well-defined (punched-out) radiolucencies (Fig. 22-6). Thus metastatic carcinoma is included here.

Features

Metastatic carcinoma is discussed in Chapter 21, so its characteristics are not detailed further here except to indicate that a patient with such a disseminated malignant disease is obviously very ill and may manifest some of the symptoms and problems described for multiple myeloma: fatigue, pancytopenia, bleeding, and ab-

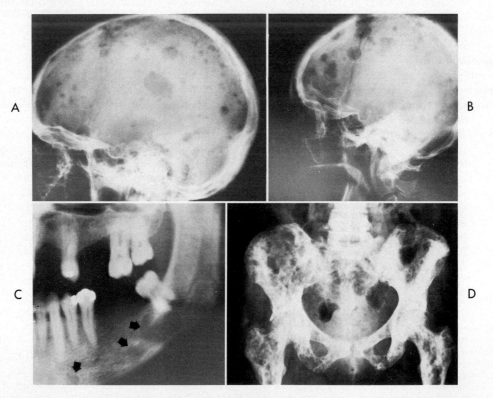

Fig. 22-6. **A** and **B,** Two patients with multiple metastatic carcinomas. **C,** Three distinct mandibular lesions *(arrows)* of metastatic bronchogenic carcinoma in a 58-year-old man. **D,** Another example of metastatic carcinoma. The multiple punched-out lesions in the pelvic bones and femurs are from a renal carcinoma. (**A** and **B** courtesy E. Palacios, MD, Maywood, Ill.)

normal serum calcium, phosphorus, and alkaline phosphatase levels.

Schaffner et al. (1982) described two cases of multiple metastatic lesions to the jaws that closely mimicked periodontal disease. Rohrer and Colyer (1981) described a case of widespread skeletal metastatic adenocarcinoma in which the presenting sign was mental nerve paresthesia.

Differential diagnosis

The differential diagnosis for metastatic carcinoma and similar-appearing lesions is discussed with the differential diagnosis for histiocytosis X (p. 469).

Management

The major considerations determining the management of patients with metastatic carcinoma are enumerated in Chapter 21. Since the presence of multiple metastases is considered a terminal disease, palliative procedures are usually all that can rationally be prescribed.

HISTIOCYTOSIS X

Histiocytosis X is a group of reticuloendothelial diseases that are not well understood. Although agreement is not complete, many authors believe that the three entities making up this group (Letterer-Siwe disease, Hand-Schüller-Christian disease, and eosinophilic granuloma) represent interrelated manifestations of the same basic pathologic process. Histiocytosis X is classified as a nonlipid reticuloendotheliosis and differs from the lipid reticuloendothelioses (for example, Gaucher's disease, Niemann-Pick disease), which are the result of inborn errors of metabolism and in which the reticulum cells produce and store abnormal lipids. Histiocytosis X affects the reticuloendothelial organs such as the spleen, liver, lymph nodes, and bone marrow and may infiltrate mucosa, skin, or viscera.

Two of the entities making up histiocytosis X, Letterer-Siwe disease and Hand-Schüller-Christian disease, may produce multiple lytic lesions in bone that affect several bones simultaneously; the lesion may appear as multiple, small, regular well-defined radiolucencies. Thus these two entities are included in this chapter. Eosinophilic granuloma usually occurs as a solitary radiolucency; however, a significant number of cases have been reported with bilateral involvement (Ragab and Rake, 1975). Lucas et al. (1981) and Granda and McDaniel (1982) described cases of multiple eosinophilic granuloma of the jaws that mimicked advanced periodontal disease.

Features
LETTERER-SIWE DISEASE

Letterer-Siwe disease is the acute, widely disseminated form of histiocytosis X; it may be fatal and occurs almost exclusively in infants under 1 year of age. Numerous enlargements of organs and other swellings caused by accumulations of histiocytes are seen. The patient appears cachectic and frequently has petechiae and necrotic ulcers on the skin and mucous membranes. When there are extensive bony lesions, a severe pancytopenia is produced because of the masses of proliferating histiocytes that displace the hematopoietic marrow. When the skeleton is involved, lesions are usually present in several bones and may appear as multiple small, rounded radiolucencies with well-defined borders (Fig. 22-7). If teeth are present in the affected region, they are frequently mobile and there is gingival bleeding. The features of this disease are described in detail by Zachariades et al. (1987).

HAND-SCHÜLLER-CHRISTIAN DISEASE

In its classic form Hand-Schüller-Christian disease affects children and young adults with three principal manifestations: bony lesions, exophthalmos, and diabetes insipidus. It represents a chronic, disseminated form of histiocytosis X and carries a much more favorable prognosis than does Letter-Siwe disease. The triad of symptoms of Hand-Schüller-Christian disease is not always present in the same patient, however, nor does the presence of additional

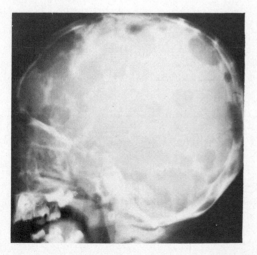

Fig. 22-7. Letterer-Siwe disease in a 15-month-old child.　(Courtesy E. Palacios, MD, Maywood, Ill.)

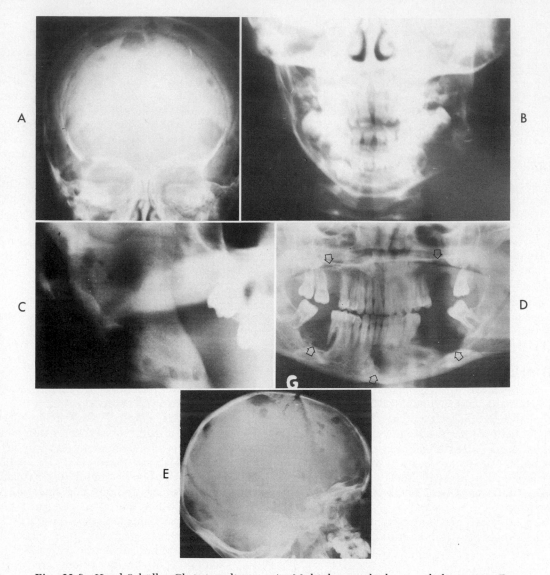

Fig. 22-8. Hand-Schüller-Christian disease. **A,** Multiple punched-out radiolucencies. **B,** Mandibular lesion in the same patient. **C,** Ramus of a 14-year-old boy with Hand-Schüller-Christian disease. Multiple punched-out radiolucencies are evident. **D,** Multiple radiolucent jaw lesions *(arrows)* in a patient with histiocytosis **X. E,** Several punched-out radiolucencies in another patient with histiocytosis X.   (**A, B,** and **E** courtesy E. Palacios, MD, Maywood, Ill. **D** courtesy N. Barakat, DDS, Beirut, Lebanon.)

manifestations rule out the disease. The nature of the symptoms depends on the locations of the histiocytic proliferations.

Frequently the lymph nodes, spleen, and liver are enlarged, and there may be petechial and papular eruptions on the skin and oral mucosa. Ulcerations in the mouth with necrotic lesions and edematous gingivae, as well as loosened teeth, are sometimes seen. Although the most common complaint is a chronic otitis media, loose teeth are frequently one of the initial complaints. Patients with the classic triad of symptoms complain of polydipsia and polyuria resulting from the diabetes insipidus. When there is disseminated bony involvement, a pancytopenia is likely to be present. The bony lesions may appear ragged and patchy and may tend to coalesce, giving a geographic appearance on radiographs of the skull (Fig. 22-8, *A* and *B*); the multiple punched-out lesions also appear fairly frequently on radiographs of the jaws (Figs. 22-8 and 22-9). Hartman (1980) extensively reviewed the findings in 114 cases of histiocytosis that had oral involvement.

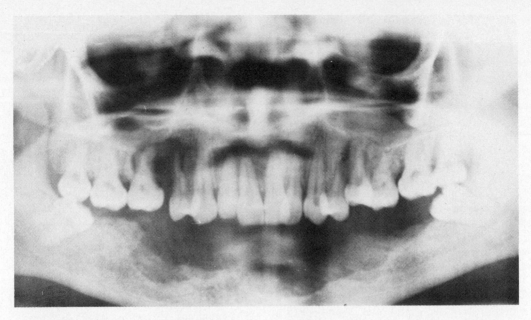

Fig. 22-9. Adult patient with multiple jaw lesions of histiocytosis X.   (Courtesy W. Heaton, DDS, Chicago.)

The histologic appearances are basically similar in Letterer-Siwe disease and Hand-Schüller-Christian disease. Sheets of histiocytes make up the bulk of the enlargements. Scattered accumulations of eosinophils may be seen around areas of necrosis. The histiocytes in Letterer-Siwe disease usually appear more atypical.

Differential diagnosis

When developing the differential diagnosis for the multiple separate well-defined radiolucencies of histiocytosis X, the clinician should divide the pathoses into two groups: large cystlike lesions of the jaws and multiple smaller, punched-out radiolucencies that may occur in the jaws and in several other bones simultaneously.

The large, cystlike lesions are usually characterized by two or more radiolucent areas in the jaws without involvement of other bones. Postextraction sockets, multiple conventional cysts or granulomas, the basal cell nevus syndrome, and cherubism are in this group.

The multiple smaller lesions occurring simultaneously in other bones of the skeleton may be confused with marrow spaces, multiple myeloma, multiple metastatic lesions, and histiocytosis X.

Since the differential diagnosis for the first group is discussed earlier in this chapter (p. 463), only the differentiation for the second group is described here.

CHILDREN

When multiple punched-out, bony lesions are found in children, *histiocytosis X* or *metastatic carcinoma* is the most likely diagnosis. Both diseases would be expected to cause a cachectic condition with many similar systemic manifestations, but the higher incidence of the former in children should lead the watchful clinician to suspect histiocytosis X, as should an inconclusive biopsy report. A history of primary tumor, however, such as medulloblastoma or Wilms' tumor (which usually occur in children), should promote metastatic carcinoma to a higher ranking in the list of possible entities.

ADULTS

Multiple punched-out lesions in several bones of the skeleton in adults should prompt the clinician to rank *multiple myeloma* or *metastatic carcinoma* high in the working diagnosis. Many of the signs and symptoms of these two entities are similar, however, and thus the clinical manifestations are not often beneficial in helping to differentiate between multiple myeloma and metastatic carcinoma. The comparative incidence, however, should lead to the assigning of a higher rank to multiple myeloma than to multiple metastatic carcinoma. Furthermore, if the ratio of albumin to globulin is reversed and Bence Jones proteins are present in the urine, this is almost conclusive proof that the disease in question is multiple myeloma; however, in the absence of definitive serum characteristics, a history of treatment for an earlier primary tumor improves the possibility that the disease is a metastatic tumor. The final decision depends on the microscopic examination of excised tissue or aspirated sample.

Suspect, asymptomatic, multiple, and usually relatively small radiolucencies in the jaw of an apparently healthy adult patient in whom no abnormalities have been disclosed by a general systemic or radiographic examination or both most likely represent multiple distinct *bone marrow defects.*

Management

Letterer-Siwe disease is the more serious variant of histiocytosis X but is no longer considered invariably fatal; with good clinical management some infants and children can live for years in a more chronic phase.

Hand-Schüller-Christian disease, the chronic form of histiocytosis X, has a better prognosis.

There may be a potential for one form of the disease to be transformed into the other, however, and carry with it the coincident prognosis. Radiation therapy and chemotherapy frequently prove helpful and often are palliative. Corrective therapy is necessary to regulate the altered physiology. Zachariades et al. (1987) discuss in detail the prognostic factors for the three forms of histiocytosis.

RARITIES

In unusual cases multiple separate cystlike radiolucencies may prove to be ameloblastomas (Fig. 22-10).

Following is a list of the entities that rarely produce multiple separate well-defined radiolucencies:

Ameloblastomas
Cherubism
Craniofacial dysostosis
Gaucher's disease
Giant cell granulomas
Hyperparathyroidism with multiple distinct osteolytic lesions (Fig. 22-11)
Lingual mandibular bone depressions
Lymphomas
Maffucci's syndrome
Mucopolysaccharidoses
   Hunter's syndrome
   Hurler's syndrome
   Maroteaux-Lamy syndrome
   Sanfilippo A
   Sanfilippo B
   Sanfilippo C
   Scheie's syndrome
Multiple dental cysts in arachnodactyly
Neurofibromatosis
Niemann-Pick disease
Nodular cemental masses (early stage; Fig. 22-12)
Oxalosis and hyperoxaluria
Oxycephaly
Papillon-Lefèvre syndrome
Pseudotumors of hemophilia
Scleroderma
Squamous odontogenic tumors (familial and nonfamilial)
Traumatic bone cysts

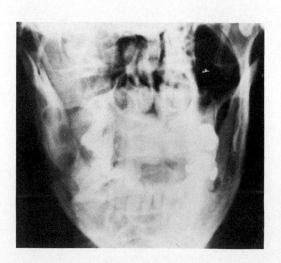

Fig. 22-10. Ameloblastoma showing multiple punched-out radiolucencies in the right ramus. (Courtesy O.H. Stuteville, DDS, MD, St. Joe, Ark.)

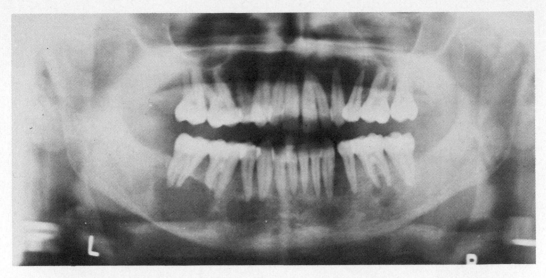

Fig. 22-11. Multiple brown giant cell lesions in the maxilla and mandible in a patient with primary hyperparathyroidism exacerbated by pregnancy. Note also generalized loss of lamina dura and root resorption of lower left first molar tooth. Radiograph has been printed lighter to show detail in rarefied jawbone.   (From Pellegrino SV: J Oral Surg 35:915-917, 1977. Copyright by the American Dental Association. Reprinted by permission.)

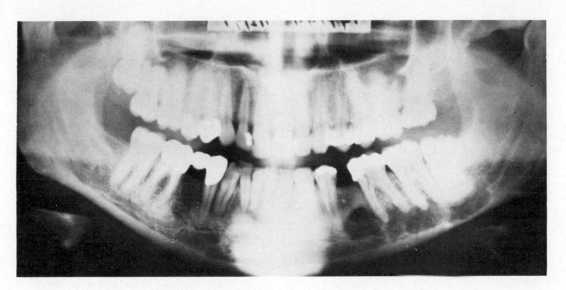

Fig. 22-12. Multiple radiolucent jaw lesions in a 26-year-old woman with sclerosing cemental masses. Some are completely radiolucent, whereas others are in the more radiopaque stage.

The lipid reticuloendothelioses (for example, Niemann-Pick disease and Gaucher's disease) may produce bony lesions that are multiple, well defined, and somewhat round, and there may be a generalized rarefaction.

Cherubism frequently produces multiple radiolucent lesions of the jawbones, but the pattern is usually multilocular. In some instances, however, the pattern is unilocular and the outlines of the radiolucencies may be well defined or poorly defined.

Sometimes multiple well-defined osteolytic lesions (brown giant cell lesions) are seen in hyperparathyroidism (Fig. 22-11), although generalized rarefaction of the skeleton is more commonly produced (see Fig. 23-1).

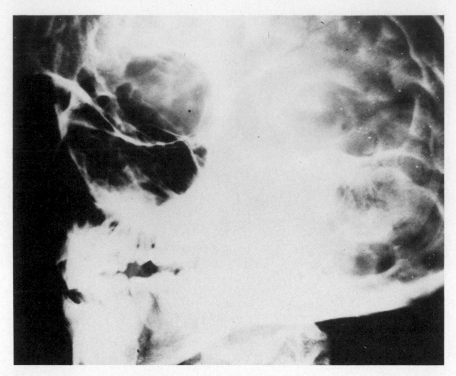

Fig. 22-13. Cranial convolutions in a patient who had early closure of the sutures of the skull. (Courtesy A.C.W. Hutchinson collection, Northwestern University Dental School Library, Chicago.)

Multiple cystic areas are also seen in the jaws of patients with Hunter's or Hurler's syndrome.

Leukemias, especially the acute varieties, may be seen with multiple punched-out radiolucent lesions in the skull and other bones, but seldom are the jawbones thus affected.

Lymphosarcoma rarely may give the same appearance.

Multiple dental cysts have been reported in arachnodactyly.

Radiographs of the skull in craniofacial dysplasia or oxycephaly often reveal multiple radiolucencies (Fig. 22-13), but such radiolucencies are not seen in radiographs of the jaws.

REFERENCES

Alexanian R and Dreicer R: Chemotherapy for multiple myeloma, Cancer 53:583-588, 1984.

Brannon RB: The odontogenic keratocyst, a clinicopathologic study of 312 cases. I. Clinical features, Oral Surg 42:54-72, 1976.

Epstein JB, Voss NJS, and Stevenson-Moore P: Maxillofacial manifestations of multiple myeloma, Oral Surg 57:267-271, 1984.

Flick WG and Lawrence FR: Oral amyloidosis as initial symptom of multiple myeloma, Oral Surg 49:18-20, 1980.

Granda FM and McDaniel RK: Multiple progressive eosinophilic granuloma of the jaws, J Oral Maxillofac Surg 40:174-178, 1982.

Harley JB, Schilling A, and Glidewell O: Ineffectiveness of fluoride therapy in multiple myeloma, N Engl J Med 286:1283-1288, 1972.

Hartman KS: Histiocytosis X: a review of 114 cases with oral involvement, Oral Surg 49:38-54, 1980.

Lambertenghi-Deliliers G, Bruno E, Cortelezzi A, et al: Incidence of jaw lesions in 193 patients with multiple myeloma, Oral Surg 65:533-537, 1988.

Lucas WJ, Smith RG, and Meiselman M: Clinical pathological conference. Part I and Part II. Eosinophilic granuloma of the jaws, J Oral Surg 39:522-525 and 597-598, 1981.

Moriconi ES and Popowich LD: Plasma cell myeloma: management of a mandibular fracture, Oral Surg 55:454-456, 1983.

Moseley JE: Bone changes in hematologic disorders, New York, 1963, Grune & Stratton, p 37.

Nordin BEC: Metabolic bone and stone disease, Baltimore, 1973, Williams & Wilkins, p 17.

Norris LH, Piccoli P, and Papageorge MB: Multiple dentigerous cysts of the maxilla and mandible: report of a case, J Oral Maxillofac Surg 45:694-697, 1987.

Olson RAJ, Stroncek GG, Scully JR, et al: Nevoid basal cell carcinoma syndrome: review of the literature and report of case, J Oral Surg 39:308-312, 1981.

Pritchard LJ, Delfino JJ, Ivey DM, et al: Variable expressivity of the multiple nevoid basal cell carcinoma syndrome, J Oral Maxillofac Surg 40:261-269, 1982.

Ragab RR and Rake O: Eosinophilic granuloma with bilateral involvement of both jaws, Int J Oral Surg 4:73-79, 1975.

Raubenheimer EJ, Dauth J, Van Wilpe E: Multiple myeloma: a study of 10 cases, J Oral Pathol 16:383-388, 1987.

Regezi JA, Zarbo RJ, and Keren DF: Plasma cell lesions of the head and neck: immunofluorescent determination of clonality from formalin-fixed paraffin-embedded tissue, Oral Surg 56:616-621, 1983.

Rohrer MD and Colyer J: Mental nerve paresthesia: symptom for a widespread skeletal metastatic adenocarcinoma, J Oral Surg 39:442-445, 1981.

Salisbury PL III and Jacoway JR: Oral amyloidosis: a late complication of multiple myeloma, Oral Surg 56:48-50, 1983.

Schaffner DL, McKinney RV Jr, Braxton M, et al: Metastatic disease of the jaws simulating periodontal pathologic conditions, J Am Dent Assoc 105:809-812, 1982.

Witkop CJ: Gardner's syndrome and other osteognathodermal disorders with defects in parathyroid functions, J Oral Surg 26:639-642, 1968.

Woolgar JA, Rippin JW, and Browne RM: The odontogenic keratocyst and its occurrence in the nevoid basal cell carcinoma syndrome, Oral Surg 64:727-730, 1987.

Wright BA, Wysocki GP, and Bannerjee D: Diagnostic use of immunoperoxidase techniques for plasma cell lesions of the jaws, Oral Surg 52:615-622, 1981.

Zachariades N, Anastasea-Vlachou K, Xypolyta A, and Kattamis C: Uncommon manifestations of histiocytosis X, Int J Oral Maxillofac Surg 16:355-362, 1987.

23

Generalized rarefactions of the jawbones

NORMAN K. WOOD
PAUL W. GOAZ
ROLLEY C. BATEMAN

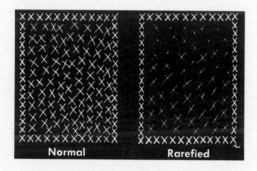

Normal   Rarefied

Following is a list of the generalized rarefactions of the jawbones:

Hyperparathyroidism
  Primary
  Secondary
  Tertiary
Osteoporosis
  Postmenopausal and senile
  Of Cushing's syndrome
  Drug-induced
  Of malnutritional states
  Thyrotoxic
Osteomalacia
Hereditary hemolytic anemia
  Thalassemia
  Sickle cell
Leukemia
Histiocytosis X
Paget's disease
Multiple myeloma
Rarities
  Acromegaly (pseudo-osteoporosis)
  Agranulocytosis
  Burkitt's lymphoma
  Central cavernous hemangioma
  Congenital heart disease
  Cyclic neutropenia
  Diabetes
  Down's syndrome
  Erythroblastosis fetalis
  Gaucher's disease
  Hypervitaminosis D
  Hypogonadism
  Hypoparathyroidism
  Hypophosphatasia
  Hypovitaminosis C
  Lymphosarcoma
  Massive osteolysis (phantom bone disease)
  Multiple metastatic carcinomas
  Multiple sclerosis
  Myelofibrosis
  Osteogenesis imperfecta
  Other diffuse malignant tumors
  Oxalosis and hyperoxaluria
  Polycythemia
  Postradiation rarefaction

Pregnancy—late stages
Progeria
Protein-deficiency states
Rickets
Sarcoidosis
Spherocytosis
Urticaria pigmentosa
XO syndrome
XXY syndrome

HOMEOSTASIS OF BONE

Bones are complex organs consisting of a dense outer cortex covered with a specialized connective tissue of varying thickness, the periosteum. The inner medullary portion comprises small communicating cavities, or marrow spaces, filled with red (hematopoietic) or yellow (adipose) marrow. These marrow spaces and the inner surface of the cortex are lined with a delicate connective tissue, the endosteum.

Osteoblasts, which proliferate from undifferentiated cells, are responsible for the formation of the organic bone matrix (osteoid). Normally the osteoid quickly becomes mineralized.

Osteoclasts actively resorb bone and are thought to form from the coalescence of macrophages and from undifferentiated cells (Little, 1973b).

Maintenance of normal bone density or mass requires normal (mechanical) function along with the interaction of a number of intricate and delicate systems: osseous, endocrine, renal, gastrointestinal, nutritional, hematopoietic, and neurocirculatory.

The endocrine glands play important and often antagonistic roles in maintaining normal bone mass. Hormones such as the following, in physiologic amounts, usually promote the formation of bone: growth hormone, testosterone and other androgens, estrogens, and calcitonin. Hormones such as parathyroid hormone, cortisol, and thyroxine usually promote the resorption of bone.

All the rarefying diseases included in this chapter represent a disruption of bone homeostasis that may result from either an imbalance among the factors just noted or the direct influence of a disease process on the bone itself.

NORMAL VARIATIONS IN THE RADIODENSITY OF BONE

Radiographs reveal a considerable variation in the density of normal jawbones. Men frequently have heavier bones than women because of the more powerful anabolic effects of testosterone. Heavy, vigorous men usually have more osseous tissue, which in turn produces a denser radiographic image. The bones of thin, delicate people (men and women) usually cast a less dense, more fragile-appearing radiographic shadow. This normal variation in radiodensity is in part caused by differences in the size and shape of the marrow spaces and the number and prominence of the trabeculae.

Thus differences in radiodensity are apparent on radiographs of different persons. Furthermore, variations in radiodensity are apparent in the jaws of the same person. For example, bone is frequently denser in the anterior region of the mandible than in the more radiolucent, inferior region superior to the mylohyoid ridges, partly because of the salivary gland depression, which thins the bone in this region. Furthermore, the thickness of soft tissue overlying the bone, the patient's complexion, and the variations resulting from radiographic equipment and the exposure and developing of film all contribute to the apparent differences in the radiodensities of bone.

Functional stress is also closely related to the bony architecture. Usually, within physiologic limits, the greater the applied mechanical forces are, the more radiopaque the image of the bone is. This relationship between structure and function is illustrated by the frequent observation that when teeth are lost, the alveolar bone in the edentulous area becomes relatively radiolucent.

When all the modifying factors are considered, it is not surprising that images that mimic changes seen in rarefying disease are frequently found in radiographs of normal jaws.

HYPERPARATHYROIDISM

Parathyroid hormone plays an important role in maintaining calcium homeostasis. A decrease in the plasma calcium level to below the normal level stimulates the parathyroid gland to secrete additional parathyroid hormone, which in turn causes the plasma calcium to rise until it has been restored to the normal level. When the plasma calcium reaches the normal concentration, the secretion of hormone is reduced.

Although the manner in which parathyroid hormone elevates the level of plasma calcium is the subject of active research (and some controversy), the following sequence of events is well established and serves to provide a useful outline of the reactions promoted by this hormone:

1. The bone and kidneys are the target organs of parathyroid hormone, which mediates the coalescence of macrophages to

form mobile-type osteoclasts; these osteoclasts actively resorb bone (Little, 1973b).

2. When bone is resorbed, calcium is released to the extracellular fluid and the serum calcium level may be elevated.

3. The level of serum phosphorus, unlike that of serum calcium, is not elevated because parathyroid hormone acts on the epithelium of the kidney tubules and causes a phosphorous diuresis while concomitantly inducing an increased calcium reabsorption from the glomerular filtrate.

4. Parathyroid hormone may also increase the absorption of calcium from the intestine, but this has not been definitely established (Jaworski, 1972).

Hence in the healthy person injections of parathyroid hormone produce an elevated plasma calcium level, a decreased plasma phosphorus level, and an increased alkaline phosphatase level. An increase in this serum enzyme is observed whenever there is increased activity in bone.

Hyperparathyroidism is a disease in which there may be a complex of biochemical, anatomic, and clinical abnormalities resulting from the increased secretion of parathyroid hormone. It may occur in primary, secondary, and tertiary forms. It is included in this chapter because all three types may produce a generalized rarefaction of the jawbones, as well as several other changes. Worth (1963, p. 356) stated that this entity is the most common cause of a generalized rarefaction of the jaws.

Although it has become traditional to assume that classic hyperparathyroidism produces marked and predictable changes in the serum chemistry values, as well as loss of the lamina dura, it is important for the clinician to know that such changes do not always occur and indeed have proved to be the exception rather than the rule. This is especially true regarding changes in the lamina dura that have been traditionally described and reputed to be specific for the disease.

With the development of immunoassay techniques for measuring plasma levels of parathyroid hormone, it has been shown that approximately 50% of the detectable cases of primary hyperparathyroidism do not show radiologic, clinical, or biochemical changes other than increased parathyroid hormone levels (Bartter, 1973). Such cases are termed "normocalcemic" hyperparathyroidism. It is evident that in mild or early cases abnormalities are not usually detected, whereas in more advanced cases symptoms may be mild, marked, or variable. Radio-graphic changes in bone are considered to develop and become apparent only in the more advanced stages of the disorder; changes in the jawbones are often late manifestations of the radiographically demonstrable bony disease (Silverman et al., 1968).

The features next discussed are characteristic of all three types of hyperparathyroidism; to emphasize this point, we discuss the disorder itself before we describe the three forms of the disease.

Features

Hyperparathyroidism is a relatively common disease. Jackson and Frame (1972) estimated that one of every 1000 patients examined at a general diagnostic clinic has some form of hyperparathyroidism; however, a significant percentage of these patients are symptomless. These authors aptly described the features of the advanced disease as a composite of "bones, stones, abdominal groans, and psychic moans with fatigue overtones." Patients complain of weakness, anorexia, nausea, vomiting, constipation, abdominal pains, muscular and joint pains, polyuria, polydipsia, and emotional instability.

In addition, a variety of osseous changes may be present, including metastatic calcification, subperiosteal erosion, osteitis fibrosa generalisata, disturbances in the jawbones, brown giant cell lesion, and rarely osteosclerosis.

METASTATIC CALCIFICATION

Ectopic calcification in soft tissue is the most common feature of hyperparathyroidism. A reported 45% to 80% of the patients have nephrolithiasis or nephrocalcinosis. Other soft tissues involved are the subcutaneous tissues, walls of blood vessels, articular cartilages, and joint capsules. Lithiasis frequently develops in the pancreas and the salivary glands.

SUBPERIOSTEAL EROSION

Subperiosteal erosion of bone, especially of the middle phalanges, is considered the radiographic hallmark of hyperparathyroidism (Fig. 23-1). It is also seen frequently in other sites (such as the outer third of the clavicle, distal end of the femur, medial surface of the neck of the femur, and upper end of the tibia). Walsh and Karmiol (1969) considered the loss of lamina dura a type of subperiosteal erosion, likening the periodontal ligament to periosteum. Subperiosteal resorption of bone is the most characteristic radiographic feature of osteitis fibrosa, and when present, it is almost always

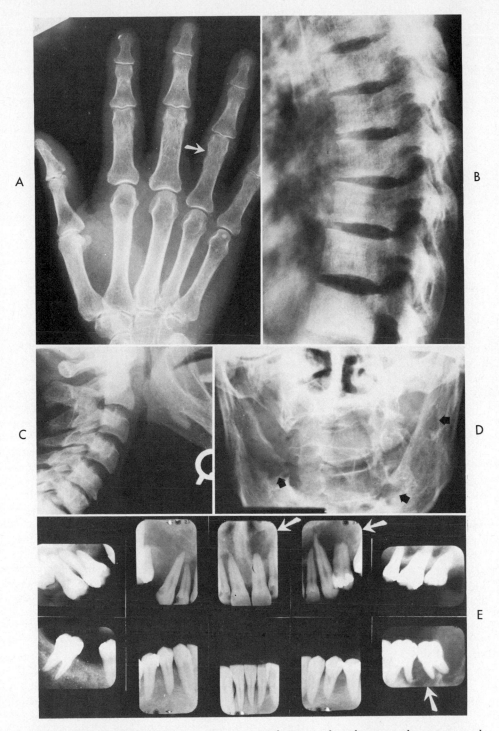

Fig. 23-1. Hyperparathyroidism. **A,** The arrow indicates early subperiosteal erosion on the third phalanx. **B,** Generalized rarefaction and loss of cortical margins in the thoracic vertebrae. **C,** Similar findings in the cervical vertebrae and mandible. **D,** Generalized rarefaction of the maxilla and mandible with thinning or loss of the cortical plates and three brown giant cell lesions *(arrows).* **E,** Generalized rarefaction, loss of lamina dura, and two brown giant cell lesions *(arrows).* Most of these photographs have been printed lighter than normal to elucidate detail in the rarefied bones.   (**A** to **C** courtesy E. Palacios, MD, and J. Adamski, MD, Maywood, Ill. **D** and **E** courtesy O.H. Stuteville, DDS, M.D., St. Joe, Ark.)

pathognomonic for some variety of parathyroid dysfunction (Jackson and Frame, 1972).

OSTEITIS FIBROSA GENERALISATA (CYSTICA)

The older term "osteitis fibrosa cystica" was adopted because osteitis fibrosa lesions often appeared cystlike on radiographs. These areas were later found to be made up of fibrous tissue, however, so the term "cystica" was not appropriate and its use was discontinued. The term "osteitis fibrosa generalisata" refers to the pattern of generalized rarefaction seen in the skeleton as a late change in primary, secondary, or tertiary hyperparathyroidism and occasionally in pseudohypoparathyroidism* (Fig. 23-1). It occurs in approximately 13% of patients with hyperparathyroidism (Bartter, 1973). Early symptoms include vague aches and pains, which may be quite disseminated; later symptoms are severe bone pain and tenderness followed by fractures and the development of deformities.

On radiographs the bones may appear quite radiolucent with thin cortices and hazy, indistinct trabeculae. Some bones may be less homogeneous, presenting a moth-eaten image. Regions in which the trabeculae are completely missing have a cystlike appearance on radiographs.

On histologic examination the radiolucent areas are found to contain sparse, narrow trabeculae scattered throughout a fibrous stroma. A few osteoclasts may be present in Howship's lacunae. Watson (1973) referred to brown giant cell lesions as localized regions of osteitis fibrosa—which prompts us to question whether indeed histologic studies of areas of osteitis fibrosa generalisata in their earlier, more active stages might yield a picture similar to that seen in brown giant cell lesions. Certainly the examiner would expect to see a more vascular and cellular stroma, with an abundance of osteoclasts, in the early stages.

JAWBONE CHANGES

The bone changes of hyperparathyroidism do not occur as frequently in the jawbones as in the long bones and the skull, but hyperparathyroidism is the most common cause of generalized rarefaction of the jaws (Worth, 1963, p. 356).

---

*Pseudohypoparathyroidism with osteitis fibrosa is a rare condition. It is characterized by the serum changes typical of hypoparathyroidism (hypocalcemia, hyperphosphatemia, and normophosphatasia), by increased levels of circulating parathyroid hormone, and by the skeletal changes of hyperparathyroidism.

Generalized rarefaction of the skeleton is not specific for hyperparathyroidism, since identical radiographic changes may be seen in several of the other conditions detailed in this chapter. If the jaws are affected, the complete maxilla and mandible are usually involved. The rarefaction may be of a homogeneous nature in which the normal trabecular pattern is lost and replaced by a granular or ground-glass appearance (Fig. 23-1). Sometimes the rarefaction has a mottled or moth-eaten appearance, showing variation in density. If the alveolus is severely affected, the teeth may be mobile and may migrate (Worth, 1963, p. 357). The radiopaque cortical plates outlining the bones and anatomic regions and features (such as nasal fossa, maxillary sinus, mandibular canal, mental foramen, alveolar crest, crypts of unerupted teeth, and lamina dura) may be thinned or lost entirely (Fig. 23-1). Similarly the oblique and mylohyoid ridges may be less prominent or may not show at all.

The lamina dura is diminished or completely absent in only approximately 10% of the cases. Silverman et al. (1968) stated that the loss of lamina dura is the most overrated characteristic of hyperparathyroidism. The degree of loss depends on the severity and duration of the disease. The teeth are not affected but appear relatively more radiopaque because of the contrast resulting from the loss of the lamina dura and the decrease in density of the surrounding bone (Fig. 23-1).

The clinician should realize that, even though reduced radiopacity of the jaws is a late manifestation of the disease, in some cases the jawbones may be the first to show such a change. Also, since the jawbones are examined radiographically more frequently than any other bones of the skeleton, bone changes in the jaws may be the first indication of the disease.

BROWN GIANT CELL LESION

The brown giant cell lesion of hyperparathyroidism is discussed as a cystlike radiolucency in Chapter 20 and as a multilocular radiolucency in Chapter 21. Although described by some authors as a localized area of osteitis fibrosa, osteitis fibrosa and the brown giant cell lesion are generally considered separate entities.

Giant cell lesions occur slightly less often than osteitis fibrosa generalisata, developing in less than 10% of the patients with hypercalcemia. Although the lesions may occur in the pelvis, ribs, and femurs, they are most common in the jaws, where they may cause radiolucencies that are either peripheral or central and unilocular or multilocular. If they arise in the osteoporotic jaw, their margins are not well defined (Fig. 23-1). Worth (1963, p. 360) maintained that giant cell lesions are not so common in secondary hyperparathyroidism, but other authorities do not mention this distinction. Giant cell lesions may be the only sign of hyperparathyroidism, and when a giant cell lesion recurs after excision, hyperparathyroidism should be suspected.

The gross specimen is moderately soft and reddish brown, and it bleeds readily. On histologic study it has giant cells scattered throughout a fibrovascular stroma in which foci of hemosiderin are present (see Fig. 19-13, *F*). It cannot be distinguished on a histologic basis from the giant cell granuloma. However, giant cell granulomas are more common in younger individuals, whereas the brown giant cell lesion is more common in patients over 30 years of age.

Surgical excision of the giant cell lesion is generally considered unnecessary, since the lesion resolves after the hyperparathyroidism is controlled. Nevertheless, a biopsy is advised for identification.

Primary hyperparathyroidism

Primary hyperparathyroidism is the result of a primary hyperplasia or a benign or malignant tumor of the parathyroid glands. Bartter (1973) reported that 50% of the patients with hyperparathyroidism have a mild form of the disease and do not show clinical, radiographic, or biochemical changes. He referred to this variety as "normocalcemic" hyperparathyroidism. Depending on the level of parathyroid hormone production, any or all of the changes described for hyperparathyroidism may be apparent. In advanced cases the classic serum changes of increased levels of calcium and alkaline phosphatase and a decreased level of phosphorus are usually present.

Secondary hyperparathyroidism

Secondary hyperparathyroidism occurs when the parathyroid glands are stimulated to produce increased amounts of parathyroid hormone to correct abnormally low serum calcium levels. Chronic renal disease and osteomalacia (delayed mineralization of new bone stemming from a lack of or an inability to utilize dietary calcium) are the most common conditions that feature the hypocalcemic state. The low serum calcium levels stimulate increased production and secretion of parathyroid hormone, which then induce bone resorption with the liberation of calcium and phosphate ions. Contrary to the situation in primary hyperparathyroidism, however, there is an inverse relationship in secondary hyperparathyroidism between the levels of serum parathyroid hormone and serum calcium. The increased parathyroid activity and calcium mobilization are reflected not by an increase but by a decrease in the serum calcium level (Rasmussen and Brodier, 1974, p. 150).

In osteomalacia the most common cause of hypocalcemia is an impaired absorption of calcium from the intestine caused by a deficiency of vitamin D.

The cause of hypocalcemia in secondary hyperparathyroidism resulting from kidney disease is more obscure. Although phosphorus excretion is known to be impaired, with a resultant hyperphosphatemia in certain types of chronic kidney disease, what produces the hypocalcemia is not known. Several theories have been proposed but some evidence or observation exists to contradict each one; no theory is free of question. The resultant demand on the parathyroid glands usually produces a hyperplasia of all four glands, and the increased parathyroid hormone secretion causes an increased resorption of bone, which becomes radiographically evident in advanced cases. The classic changes in serum chemistry in secondary hyperparathyroidism are hypocalcemia, hyperphosphatemia, and an increased serum alkaline phosphatase level.

With more patients being managed by dialysis, it is likely that the incidence of secondary hyperparathyroidism will increase. Fletcher et al. (1977) discussed the oral manifestations of secondary hyperparathyroidism related to long-term hemodialysis therapy. Wysocki et al. (1983) described changes in the predentin layer of patients being treated with chronic hemodialysis.

Tertiary hyperparathyroidism

Occasionally, parathyroid tumors develop after a long-standing secondary hyperparathyroidism; this condition is known as "tertiary hyperparathyroidism." In effect, a secondary hyperparathyroidism has developed into a type of primary hyperparathyroidism. The increased parathyroid hormone levels produce increased bone resorption and a resultant hypercalcemia. All the skeletal manifestations of the other types of hyperparathyroidism may be seen in this rather rare variation of the disease.

Differential diagnosis

See the differential diagnosis section at the end of the chapter (p. 496) for a discussion of the basic clinical and biochemical features that help distinguish the disorders presented in this chapter.

Management

Early detection of hyperparathyroidism is necessary, since the advanced disease may cause irreversible kidney damage, hypertension, and death (not to mention the discomfort, pain, fractures, and emotional problems that attend the condition).

Treatment of the primary and tertiary types requires excision of the parathyroid tumors. Patients usually are relieved of back pain within 48 hours after the excision, but improvement may not appear on radiographs for approximately 1 month (Watson, 1973).

In the secondary type complete restoration of kidney function is usually not possible, but a subtotal parathyroidectomy is frequently beneficial. Watson (1973) reported that in secondary hyperparathyroidism the oral administration of adjusted doses of vitamin D restores a normocalcemia by enhancing the absorption of calcium from the intestine. The ingestion of 1 g of calcium daily (equivalent to the calcium in 1 quart of milk) can prevent skeletal demineralization in most cases of severe hyperparathyroidism (Walsh and Karmiol, 1969); the skeletal changes return to normal when the hyperparathyroidism is brought under control.

If the fibrosis is not too severe in advanced cases of osteitis fibrosa generalisata, the radiographic appearance of the bones usually returns to normal 6 months after treatment. If fibrosis is extensive, fibrotic bone may be replaced by sclerotic bone (Stafne, 1969).

OSTEOPOROSIS

Osteoporosis of the skeleton is the most common form of metabolic bone disease. It is not a specific disease entity but represents a nonspecific reaction of the skeleton to several predisposing factors or diseases. It is a generalized rarefaction of the bones resulting from a deficiency of bone matrix rather than a deficit of mineral. The bone is normal but deficient in amount; in other words, there is a reduced volume of bone tissue relative to the volume of anatomic bone.

Osteoporosis develops in disease states in which there is an imbalance between bone formation (anabolism) and bone resorption (catabolism). Such disturbances develop in one of three ways: (1) a slight increase in bone resorption with a slight decrease in formation, (2) a severe increase in bone resorption with a nor-

mal rate of formation, or (3) normal bone resorption with a severe decrease in formation. Osteoporosis may be acquired or congenital, regional or generalized. In the present context the regional (isolated) examples are not considered.

Features

The majority of patients with osteoporosis show no symptoms. In advanced cases the clinical onset is often heralded by an attack of severe pain that is aggravated by movement and occurs after trauma or strenuous muscular effort. Osteoporosis is probably the most common cause of backache in elderly persons (Watson, 1973).

The pathologic bone changes in osteoporosis tend to involve the central axial part of the skeleton (spine, long bones, pelvis, skull, feet) in contrast to the bone changes in osteomalacia, which more frequently involve the peripheral skeleton. Because of shortening of the trunk, the osteoporotic patient may notice a gradual loss of height.

RADIOGRAPHIC CHANGES

Whatever the factor predisposing a patient to the development of an osteoporosis, the radiographic changes are quite similar. Since there must be at least a 30% to possibly a 50% or 60% loss of calcium content from a bone before the loss can be detected on radiographs, much bone tissue is lost before the change becomes radiographically apparent. In general, radiographic changes in osteoporosis can be described as a decrease in the density of the bone; specifically, a loss of the normal trabecular pattern and a thinning of the cortex occur. The skull shows a diffuse decrease in density and assumes a spotty appearance.

Jaws. Although the maxilla and the mandible may become osteoporotic from a number of causes, some diseases and conditions show a greater tendency toward osteoporosis than others. For example, patients with Cushing's syndrome and patients receiving cortisone therapy more frequently have bone changes in the jaws, and although thyrotoxicosis and postmenopausal or senile osteoporosis do not usually involve the jaws (Worth, 1963, p. 360), jaw changes may occur in advanced stages of these diseases.

If osteoporosis is present in the jaws, a generalized rarefaction of the maxilla and the mandible is evident. Individual trabeculae are fine and indistinct, and many are completely obliterated. The overall picture is one of diffuse

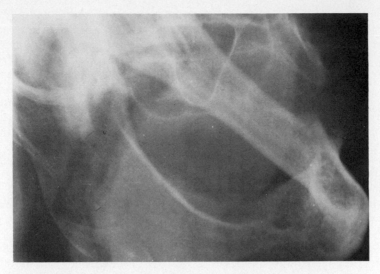

Fig. 23-2. Osteoporosis of the mandible, senile type.

granularity. The cortical borders of the bone and anatomic chambers, such as the nose and maxillary sinus, are thinner and less distinct (Fig. 23-2). The lamina dura characteristically persists longer than in hyperparathyroidism, but it may be indistinct in advanced and severe cases and sometimes may be completely obliterated.

Interestingly, Bras et al. (1982) suggested the use of the mandibular angular cortex as a diagnostic index in metabolic bone loss. These researchers reported that a distinct cortical layer in this location is not present before the fifteenth year of life. After the fifteenth year, however, the thickness of the cortex at the normal angle is relatively constant, although it is thinner in women over 60 years of age. The researchers recommended that the cortex be evaluated especially when metabolic bone disease is being considered in the differential diagnosis of a case.

This description notwithstanding, the jaws have not been adequately studied in most reports of osteoporosis.

BIOCHEMICAL CHANGES

The serum calcium, phosphorus, and alkaline phosphatase levels are within normal limits in osteoporosis unless fractures are present.

HISTOPATHOLOGIC FEATURES

When a section of osteoporotic bone is studied under low-power magnification, a thinned cortex is apparent and the trabecular pattern is irregular. Many of the trabeculae have disap-

peared, and most of those that remain are extremely thin. Otherwise the bone appears normal.

Types of osteoporosis

Numerous predisposing conditions or disease states may induce an osteoporosis, including postmenopausal and senile states, Cushing's syndrome, drug therapy, malnutrition, and thyrotoxicosis. Regardless of the cause, the histologic changes are similar.

POSTMENOPAUSAL AND SENILE OSTEOPOROSIS

Although precise causes have not been identified, the normal aging process in the skeleton of an adult human is known to begin soon after the age of 20 and progress slowly with the advancing years. This aging process is part of a more generalized condition that affects all the tissues of the body. In some persons additional contributing factors may accelerate the process and as a result frank osteoporosis develops.

An overall decrease in the anabolic hormones (particularly estrogen) in postmenopausal women may cause a lag in the formation of bone, and since bone resorption continues at approximately the normal rate, a progressive and extensive resorption of bone results. In this condition, referred to as postmenopausal osteoporosis, the loss of bone substance is limited to the spine, pelvis, and ribs; the skull and extremities remain intact (Snapper, 1957).

The imbalance between the formation and resorption of bone continues for approximately

10 years after the climacteric or menopause. Then the rarefying process levels off. At approximately 60 years of age, a generalized atrophy of the bone—senile osteoporosis—becomes apparent. This atrophy occurs much more frequently and is more marked in women, in whom it probably represents a combination of postmenopausal and senile osteoporotic damage.

In senile osteoporosis the rarefaction involves mainly the spine, ribs, and vertebrae, but a minor amount of rarefaction also involves the peripheral skeleton. Whereas this slight amount in women is the result of senile osteoporosis, the rarefaction of the spine, ribs, and vertebrae is a combination of postmenopausal and senile osteoporoses.

Senile osteoporosis is thought to be caused by a number of factors operating together, but sometimes one factor is dominant and identifiable. For example, a decline in calcium absorption is not uncommon in elderly men and women, partly because absorption or metabolism of vitamin D decreases with increasing age. Also, in the aging process, less bone is formed because of a decrease in the anabolic hormones. There is, furthermore, a decrease in muscle protein, which in turn results in less muscular activity; less muscular activity results in a decreased flow of blood to the bone. Thus the oxygen supply to the bones is decreased, and the resulting hypoxic condition favors bone resorption.

In elderly persons the altered hormonal spectrum, which is part of the aging process, may lead to the formation of (usually) small thrombi; these thrombi plug small vessels in the bone and cause a loss of bone vitality and hence resorption (osteoporosis). The poor nutritional habits of many elderly persons also add to this problem.

When the cause cannot be determined, the osteoporosis is termed "idiopathic." Since no specific agent is available yet to stimulate bone formation, the current treatment for osteoporosis consists mainly of palliative procedures. To this end analgesics are prescribed, and dietary counseling is given to ensure a diet rich in protein with general supplements of calcium and vitamins C and D.

CUSHING'S SYNDROME

Cushing's syndrome is a complex of symptoms, including buffalo torso (adiposity about the upper portion of the trunk and a bump at the base of the neck), moon face (puffiness of the face), altered hair distribution (masculiniz-

ing effects in women, girls, and boys), hypertension, elevated blood glucose levels, increased excretion of 17-ketosteroids in the urine, and osteoporosis. These symptoms are evoked by an increased output of glucocorticoids, especially cortisol.

In children this condition results from hyperplasia or tumors of the adrenal cortex, and in adults most frequently from a pituitary adenoma. The excess cortisol acts to produce osteoporosis in at least two ways:

1. As a catabolic* hormone it contributes to the degradation of protein and severely limits the formation of bone matrix by reducing the amount that each osteoblast synthesizes.
2. It promotes the formation of osteoclasts from the osteogenic undifferentiated cells and thus enhances bone resorption.

Osteoporosis is seen in 64% of the women and 75% of the men with Cushing's syndrome. The pelvis, ribs, vertebrae, long bones, and skull are most commonly involved. The jaws may show changes in advanced cases, with the density or the lamina dura diminished or even completely missing. After the adrenocortical problem is corrected, the osteoporosis usually disappears in young, growing individuals, but the rarefaction appears to be irreversible in adults (Reynolds and Karo, 1972).

DRUG-INDUCED OSTEOPOROSIS
Cortisol and cortisone. Prolonged administration of glucocorticoid drugs often produces a cushingoid syndrome with the accompanying osteoporosis occasioned by the same mechanisms as those described for Cushing's syndrome. Concurrent administration of androgens, estrogens, calcitonin, and fluorides fails to protect the bone from the adverse effects of the corticoids (Duncan, 1972). It has been determined, however, that the endocrine imbalance resulting from the continuous use of cortisol can be minimized if the daily dose is synchronized with the physiologic cortisol peak that occurs in the normal diurnal cycle between 6 and 8 AM.

Contraceptive drugs. There is an interaction between the progestational compounds used as contraceptive agents and the increased levels of cortisol that are occasioned by stress. In addition to the usual effect of cortisol on the he-

---

*In this chapter the nature of the hormones' effects is described in general terms without distinguishing whether indeed the hormones are acting—for example, as catabolic or antianabolic agents—in a particular event.

matopoietic tissue (that is, causing an increase in the number of megakarocytes formed), the combination of the two compounds causes the production of abnormal megakaryocytes, which in turn form abnormal, sticky platelets. These platelets immediately fuse and give rise to multiple small thrombi.

The thrombi occlude small vessels in the tissues, and when the process occurs in osseous tissues, small foci of bone supplied by these occluded vessels die and the dead bone is subsequently resorbed (Little, 1973b). When sufficient bone has been removed, radiographic changes become evident. The levels of cortisol required for thrombus formation vary with each progestational steroid, but they are lowest with the efficient contraceptive agents (Little, 1973a).

MALNUTRITIONAL STATES

Sufficient protein must be absorbed from the intestine to supply the constant need for matrix formation. A deficiency in protein can cause osteoporosis and may result from a protein-poor diet or from gastrointestinal disturbances such as gastric resection (the patient usually eats less), colitis, regional enteritis, and malabsorption syndromes.

A vitamin C deficiency produces an osteoporosis by (1) causing a defective matrix to be formed by the osteoblasts and (2) weakening the sinusoidal vessel walls in medullary bone. The sinusoidal vessels tend to dilate and rupture, resulting in the pooling of blood and hypoxia, which subsequently leads to loss of vitality and the removal of bone by phagocytic osteoclasts.

THYROTOXIC OSTEOPOROSIS

A hyperthyroid patient may have an increased basal metabolic rate, increased temperature, flushing, weight loss, emotional instability, overalertness, tremors, and exophthalmos.

The hyperthyroid state leads to osteoporosis if it remains untreated for several years. Since most patients receive definitive treatment at a relatively early state of their disease, radiographic bone changes are not a usual feature of the condition. This consideration may help to explain the variation in frequency with which osteoporosis has been reported to occur in hyperthyroidism (Koutras et al., 1973).

Agreement is not unanimous concerning the mechanism(s) responsible for the production of osteoporosis in hyperthyroidism; nevertheless, one theory holds that thyroxine mediates the action of cortisol on bone and an excess of thyroxine results in a more efficient utilization of this steroid. Thus there is increased bone resorption. Although the thyroxine appears to increase both the formation and the resorption of bone, the balance of bone activity favors resorption (Rasmussen and Brodier, 1974, p. 192). There is a tendency toward hypercalcemia, but the serum calcium level is generally within normal range and the alkaline phosphatase level is increased—the latter correlating well with the increased bone activity.

Osteoporosis is more often seen in children with hyperthyroidism, and the radiographic picture is similar to that of osteoporosis produced by other causes. The jaws may be involved as a late change, and both the maxilla and the mandible show uniform involvement.

In young patients the treatment of thyrotoxicosis usually results in a restoration of the bone mass. In older patients the osteoporosis usually persists after treatment (Koutras et al., 1973).

Differential diagnosis

For a discussion of the differential diagnosis of osteoporosis, see the differential diagnosis section at the end of the chapter (p. 496).

Management

If a dental clinician observes osteoporosis on radiographs of the jaws, he or she should consult an internist. Treatment and prognosis of osteoporosis are discussed in the sections concerning the individual types.

OSTEOMALACIA

"Rickets" in children and "osteomalacia" in adults embrace a group of disorders characterized by a rarefaction of the skeleton and caused by a deficiency of calcium for the mineralization of normal osteoid. The calcium deficiency responsible for the rachitic or osteomalacic state may be the result of one or a combination of the following: vitamin D deficiency, calcium malabsorption, liver and renal disorders, prolonged anticonvulsive drug therapy, and hypophosphatemic rickets.

Vitamin D acts to promote the absorption of calcium from the intestine and also induces the rapid calcification of osteoid (Bartter, 1973). Thus a deficiency of this vitamin can readily lead to rarefaction of the skeleton.

Calcium-deficient diets, as well as malabsorption states such as those encountered after gastric resection (probably resulting from deficient intake of calcium and vitamin D, since these patients tend to eat less) and in chronic pancreatitis, small bowel ischemia, and gluten enteropathy, may be the cause of the calcium deficiency even if adequate amounts of vitamin D are present. Biliary obstruction may also produce a calcium deficiency by preventing bile salts from reaching the intestine; the presence of bile salts in the intestine is necessary for fat absorption. The resulting impairment of fat absorption causes a deficiency in vitamin D absorption (vitamin D is fat soluble) and hence the decreased absorption of calcium.

Prolonged administration of anticonvulsant drugs (such as phenobarbital and primidone) can result in calcium deficiency because these drugs enhance liver enzyme activity, which leads to an increased breakdown of vitamin D to biologically inert products (Conacher, 1973).

A variety of renal diseases, which may be congenital or may result from a chronic nephritis, are associated with imbalances of serum calcium and phosphorus; as a result an osteomalacia is produced. Such cases are often complicated by a secondary hyperparathyroidism that is consequent to a low level of serum calcium, so both an osteomalacia and an osteitis fibrosa generalisata may be present.

Except that serum calcium level tends to be normal, hypophosphatemic rickets seems to be a specific disease entity showing the features of vitamin D deficiency. These patients require much larger doses of vitamin D to correct the deficiency than would normally suffice to correct an avitaminosis D. Generally there is a familial background, but not invariably. Although the pathogenesis is not clear, the main problem may result from reduced phosphorus absorption or reduced tubular reabsorption of phosphorus or both (Nordin, 1973, pp. 78-80).

Features

The clinical features of osteomalacia include weakness and generalized bone pain. The pain is localized in the bones rather than in the joints, and back pain is not so common as in osteoporosis. Approximately one third of the patients have spontaneous fractures (Conacher, 1973).

Characteristic radiographic features are not apparent in many osteomalacic patients. When a change is evidenced, however, it is often a generalized demineralization of the skeleton such as that seen in osteoporosis. Pseudofractures (or Milkman's fractures) and greenstick fractures are practically pathognomonic for osteomalacia in adults.

Pseudofractures in osteomalacia appear as radiolucent bands extending into the bones from the cortex, usually at right angles to the periosteal margins. These are partial or complete fractures without displacement, in which callus has been deposited but has failed to calcify. The pseudofractures are at sites of entry of the nutrient arteries. In cases of advanced osteomalacia, there are complete fractures and bowing.

Radiographic changes do occur in the jaws of osteomalacic patients and are identical to those found in osteoporosis: a generalized rarefaction, a cortical thinning, and a homogeneous granular appearance throughout the maxilla and mandible. The lamina dura may be less prominent or completely absent.

In osteomalacia caused by a vitamin D deficiency, the serum calcium level is initially decreased. This prompts an increased parathyroid activity, which causes a decrease in serum phosphorus levels by inducing a phosphorous diuresis. Although the parathyroid hormone causes a resorption of bone and the alkaline phosphatase level is concurrently elevated with the increased bone activity,* insufficient calcium is mobilized to maintain calcium homeostasis (Rasmussen and Brodier, 1974, p. 150).

On microscopic examination, overly wide osteoid seams may be observed to surround thinned cortices and trabeculae.

Differential diagnosis

For a discussion of the differential diagnoses of osteomalacia, see the differential diagnosis section at the end of the chapter (p. 496).

Management

Management of osteomalacia is directed toward correcting the basic defect, whether a dietary deficiency of calcium or vitamin D or a gastrointestinal or renal problem.

HEREDITARY HEMOLYTIC ANEMIAS

Hemolytic anemias are discussed in this chapter because they produce a somewhat characteristic type of rarefaction of the bones. The rarefaction is caused by the development of larger than usual marrow spaces as well as,

---

*The elevation in the level of bone serum alkaline phosphatase in osteomalacia, rickets, and certain other bone diseases is generally attributed to increased osteoblastic activity; the osteoblasts are the cells richest in alkaline phosphatase. Whether this is the correct explanation, however, is uncertain. Sometimes serum alkaline phosphatase appears to correlate better with the resorption than with the formation of bone (Nordin, 1973, p. 68).

in some instances, a greater ratio of medullary bone to cortical bone. These changes are the result of a marked hyperplasia of the hematopoietic tissue induced by the increased demand for effective erythrocytes in the anemias.

Since there is a potential to replace fatty marrow with red marrow when a need for more erythrocytes arises, the hyperplastic changes in the hemolytic anemias are not restricted to bones that normally show erythropoiesis.* (The changes are often more pronounced in these bones, however.) Accordingly, the fatty marrow of the adult mandible and maxilla may revert to the hyperplastic hematopoietic variety in response to stress imposed by the anemias. The skeletal changes are directly proportional to the severity of the disease. Although prominent changes may be observed in severe, untreated cases, in mild cases no radiographic changes are evident.

Thalassemia (Mediterranean or Cooley's anemia)

Thalassemia (Greek, *thalassa*, sea) was once considered to be found almost exclusively in people of Mediterranean origin, but it is now recognized to be a relatively common disorder of wide distribution (Moseley, 1963). It occurs in a number of different genetic forms with similar hematologic and clinical features. Although there are several classifications of the thalassemias, the most widely accepted consists of two main categories, major and minor.†

There is a type of thalassemia between these two that has a hazy clinical picture and is sometimes designated as intermediate thalassemia. This entity is not well defined but includes some features of the more severe thalassemia minors and the less severe thalassemia majors.

The basic anomaly in thalassemia is a defective erythrocyte with a deficient amount of structurally normal hemoglobin (Stewart and Prescott, 1976). The individual with thalassemia has a markedly shortened life span.

---

*In the embryo and neonate the cavities of all the bones contain only red marrow. With advancing age the red marrow is gradually replaced by yellow or fatty marrow. In the normal adult the red marrow is found only in the vertebrae, ribs, sternum, diploë, and proximal epiphyses of the femur and humerus.

†Thalassemia major occurs in persons who are homozygous for the autosomal dominant trait. Thalassemia minor occurs in persons who are heterozygous for the condition.

FEATURES

Thalassemia major is a severe disorder of infants and children that usually becomes evident within the first year or two of life. Its clinical picture is of pallor, weakness, severe anemia, irritability, lethargy, and in some cases hepatosplenomegaly. The patient seldom survives beyond adolescence.

Patients with the intermediate type of thalassemia have similar but less severe symptoms.

Patients with the minor type of thalassemia are asymptomatic or have barely perceptible symptoms and show mild changes in the hemogram. Alexander and Bechtold (1977) described a case that demonstrated oral signs of the disease.

On radiographs the skull in thalassemia major is enlarged because of an increase in the width of the diploë. Sometimes, numerous white, hairlike shadows arising from the inner table of the cranial vault appear to protrude from the surface of the bone and produce the hair-on-end effect. The outer plate is displaced externally and may be less prominent or missing completely (Fig. 23-3). In severe cases the maxilla, mandible, and zygoma are markedly increased in size and the paranasal sinuses are reduced, except for the ethmoid because of the lack of red marrow in its bony walls.

Although iron deficiency anemias produce some changes in the skull, the marked enlargement of the facial bones is not usually seen in any anemia other than thalassemia. In fact, the maxillary enlargements resulting in prominent cheek bones and anterior displacement of the incisors produce a characteristic "rodent" facies, which when coupled with the sinus hypoplasia is pathognomonic of thalassemia (Edeiken, 1981).

Although a range of changes may be apparent in the jaws of patients with thalassemia, not all the changes are evident in a particular patient. The cortices may be thinned, and the tooth roots short and spike shaped (Fig. 23-4). In general, there is a blurring of the trabeculae—but with large, circular bone marrow spaces delineated by pronounced trabeculae. The lamina dura about the tooth roots and the opaque lamina around the crypts of developing teeth may be thin. There is a generalized rarefaction (Poyton and Davey, 1968), and occasionally a honeycomb pattern is seen throughout the jaws (Fig. 23-4). Van Dis and Langlais (1986) discussed the oral manifestations and complications of the thalassemias.

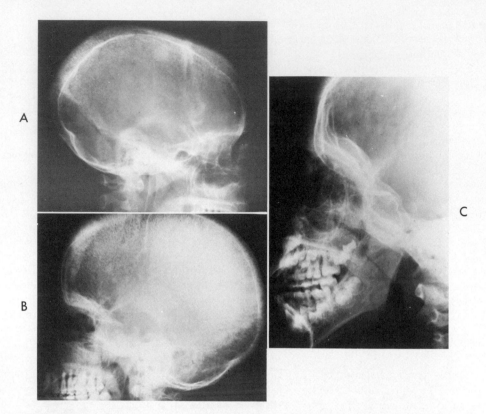

Fig. 23-3. Thalassemia. **A** and **B,** Two patients. Generalized rarefaction, the widening of the inner table, and the hair-on-end effect are evident. **C,** Generalized rarefaction of the skull and jaws in another patient.   (**A** and **B** courtesy E. Palacios, MD, Maywood, Ill. **C** courtesy R. Moncada, MD, Maywood, Ill.)

Aspiration biopsy of the bone marrow reveals a specimen with very active, immature hematopoietic tissue.

DIFFERENTIAL DIAGNOSIS

The radiographic appearance of the thalassemias is distinct from that produced by *osteoporosis, osteomalacia,* and *osteitis fibrosa generalisata* but is similar to what might be seen in other *hemolytic anemias.* The mild changes that may be found in the minor form, however, do not differ greatly from the minor variations expected in normal marrow patterns (Fig. 23-4). The history, clinical features, and blood studies are necessary to identify the general condition as thalassemia and to identify the specific form of it.

MANAGEMENT

Treatment of the thalassemias is limited to administering transfusions and other supportive therapy. The dental clinician must consult the patient's internist before initiating dental procedures because of the potential problems of bleeding and hypoxia and the increased possibility of infection.

Sickle cell anemia

Sickle cell anemia is a hereditary disease affecting blacks almost exclusively. The disease that is apparent on clinical examination occurs in homozygotes; heterozygotes for the character possess only the sickle cell trait, which does not (except in rare instances) produce any clinical manifestations. Approximately 10% of American blacks carry the sickle cell trait, whereas only 0.5% have the disease. The manifestations usually appear early in childhood.

The sickle cell defect lies in the inherited abnormal hemoglobin, which has diminished oxygen-carrying capacity and is less soluble in the reduced state than is normal hemoglobin. The result is that under conditions of low oxygen tension, the reduced abnormal hemoglobin crystallizes from solution within the red blood cells and causes the cells to take on abnormal

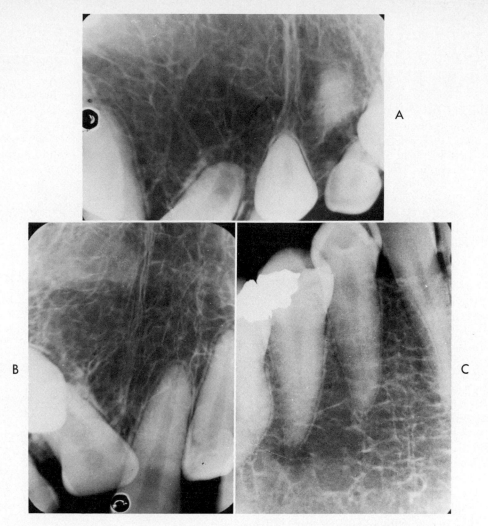

Fig. 23-4. Thalassemia. **A** and **B,** Honeycomb rarefaction in periapical radiographs. The lamina dura is present. **C,** Similar pattern in a healthy person. (**A** and **B** courtesy A.P. Angelopolous, DDS, Athens, Greece.)

shapes (especially crescents or sickles). The episode is termed a "sickle cell crisis"; during these phases the sickled erythrocytes become physically trapped in small vessels, form thrombi, and cause the development of tiny infarctions. Thrombosis of vessels in the brain may cause severe neurologic deficiencies such as stroke, convulsions, coma, and drowsiness, as well as speech, visual, and hearing disturbances. Occlusion of smaller vessels results in headaches and cranial nerve neuropathies, including palsies, paresthesias, and neuralgias. The more minor symptoms are usually transitory and disappear when the thrombus undergoes dissolution. Cox (1984) described oral pain that occurred in sickle cell patients, which evidently was not related to common dental problems. When these infarctions occur in bone, foci of dead bone develop and are then re-

sorbed. Thus the rarefaction related to the anemia-induced erythroblastic hyperplasia is intensified. Repeated infarctions are thought to produce sclerotic regions in the bone.

FEATURES

The patient with sickle cell disease may exhibit pallor, fatigue, weakness, dyspnea, retardation of growth, acute abdominal pain, and joint and muscle pains. A child with sickle cell disease is quite susceptible to infection. Most patients with this disease die before reaching 40 years of age.

The sickle cell patient often has relatively long, gangling extremities, which are particularly striking when contrasted with the short, often rotund torso (Chernoff, 1967).

Oral ulcers may be present, particularly on the gingivae; these oral ulcers represent infarcts that have become secondarily infected (see Fig. 11-11, *A*).

Splenomegaly is present in approximately 30% of adolescents with sickle cell anemia, but by adulthood the spleen has become fibrosed and small. The hemogram shows a mild to severe anemia, increased reticulocyte count, and marked poikilocytosis. A special sickle cell preparation applied to a drop of blood on a glass slide demonstrates the sickling phenomenon (Fig. 23-5). Electrophoretic analysis of hemoglobin is also used to establish the diagnosis.

Although Robinson and Sarnat (1952) reported that 18 of 22 patients with sickle cell disease showed generalized rarefaction of the skeleton, most authors believe that bone changes are not found so frequently and are not so pronounced as those in thalassemia. The skull may show the hair-on-end appearance, which again is usually not so marked as in thalassemia. The following radiographic changes in the jaws, either singly or in combination, have been reported to indicate sickle cell anemia (Sanger and Bystrom, 1977; Sanger et al., 1977).

1. The trabeculae may be reduced in number.
2. The remaining trabeculae appear coarsened and sharply defined.
3. Occasionally, prominent horizontal trabeculae between the teeth have a step-ladder appearance (Figs. 23-5 and 23-6).
4. Although the lamina dura and other cortices are usually normal, a thinning of the inferior border of the mandible and the alveolar crestal cortex may be observed.
5. There may be sclerotic areas in the bone that represent healed infarcts.
6. Changes are more remarkable in children (Sanger and Bystrom, 1977).

In contrast, Mourshed and Tuckson (1974), in their study of the radiographic features of the jaws in sickle cell anemia, reported that similar radiographic appearances may be observed in normal patients (Fig. 23-6). Furthermore, these authors did not observe cortical thinning of the inferior border of the mandible or sclerotic areas in their series of patients with sickle cell disease. Rather, they stressed that radiographic features of the jaws should not be regarded as reliable diagnostic criteria for sickle cell disease. They strongly recommended, however, that if any of these radiographic features are present, the clinician should resort to the appropriate laboratory procedures to determine whether the patient has sickle cell disease.

DIFFERENTIAL DIAGNOSIS

When the radiographic changes described for sickle cell disease are present, they are suggestive of *hemolytic anemia* but may also be found frequently in radiographs of a healthy individual. If the patient is black and has a family history of sickle cell anemia, this prompts a high ranking of sickle cell anemia in the differential diagnosis. If the patient displays sugges-

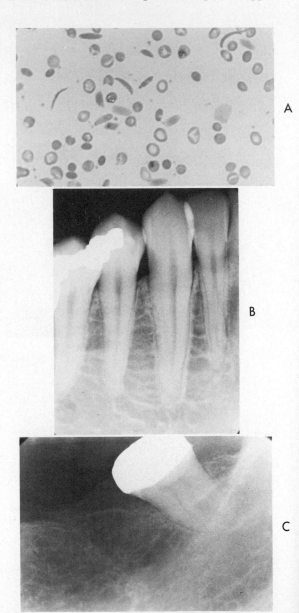

Fig. 23-5. Sickle cell anemia. **A,** Smear of peripheral blood showing sickle-shaped erythrocytes. **B,** Periapical radiograph showing the stepladder pattern. This pattern is also observed in healthy patients. **C,** Spherocytosis. Honeycomb radiolucency and the faint lamina dura are evident.

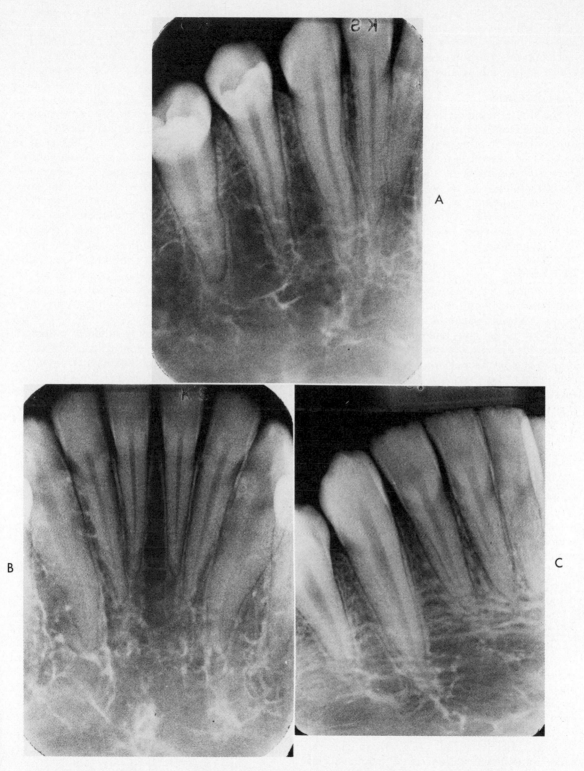

Fig. 23-6. **A** and **B**, Periapical films of a young black with sickle cell anemia. Films show the rarefied appearance of the bone, the generalized decrease in number of trabeculae, and also the sketchy traces of thick opaque trabeculae. **C**, Normal periapical radiograph showing a similar appearance.

tive symptoms, the working diagnosis must be sickle cell anemia. The final diagnosis, of course, depends on a hemoglobin analysis by electrophoresis, hemogram, and a special erythrocyte sickle cell preparation.

MANAGEMENT

The dental clinician and the patient's internist must closely consult before dental work is undertaken for a person with sickle cell disease. Consultation is necessary because of the increased possibility of infection and the possible precipitation of a sickle cell crisis by the stressful situations frequently associated with dental procedures. Girasole and Lyon (1977) reported three cases of sickle cell osteomyelitis of the mandible.

LEUKEMIA

Leukemia is a malignancy of the hematopoietic tissue involving one of the leukocytic cell types. Although cause has not been clearly established in human leukemia, Karpas (1982) discussed the viruses associated with leukemias. Marrow replacement by proliferating cells of the myeloid series causes general rarefactions of bone, so the disease is included in this chapter. The more aggressive the disease is, or the younger the patient, the more likely the bones are to show gross changes. (Van Slyck, 1972).

The radiographic appearance of leukemia may vary from multiple punched-out defects to solitary, moderately well-defined areas of osteolysis to generalized rarefaction. Occasionally osteosclerosis is observed. The maxilla and the mandible in growing persons possess active hematopoietic marrow; thus the clinician is prompted to anticipate that these bones will be involved with a leukemic infiltrate and develop osteolytic lesions.

Features

The onset of leukemia may be insidious or abrupt, and the symptoms are related to the resulting anemia, thrombocytopenia, and tissues that may be infiltrated or infected by the proliferating leukemic cells. The patient may exhibit pallor and weakness, as well as petechiae or ecchymoses in the mucous membrane or skin. Michaud et al. (1977) thoroughly detailed oral manifestations of leukemia in children.

The pallor is noticeable on the oral mucosa, which usually is normal in other respects, except in the case of monocytic leukemia. This type of leukemia frequently causes the devel-

opment of ulcers on the oral mucosa, gingival enlargements, bleeding, and gangrenous stomatitis. The ulcers are often covered with a yellow-gray fibrinous pseudomembrane that bleeds readily (Williamson, 1970). Bressman et al. (1982) described a case of acute myeloblastic leukemia in which the only complaints at the time of the patient's initial visit were pain in two premolar teeth and gingival bleeding.

Occasionally, oral changes are observed in other types of leukemia also. Leukemic infiltration of the oral soft tissues may produce swelling of the palate and other regions of the jaws. Lymph nodes are frequently enlarged (Michaud et al., 1977), and there may be a slight hepatosplenomegaly. Fever is a common symptom, as are abdominal and bone pains. Leukocyte counts in active stages may range from 20,000 to 100,000 per milliliter. In chronic leukemias or in remission phases of acute types, the signs and symptoms are more moderate.

Radiographically discernible osteolytic changes are present in more than 60% of the cases of acute childhood leukemia. Demonstrable bone lesions, however, are not so common in cases of acute adult leukemia*; only approximately 12% of the lymphosarcomas† involve bone (Van Slyck, 1972). The rarefaction may be quite pronounced, with the trabecular architecture of the jawbone almost completely destroyed, the cortices thinned, and the lamina dura missing.

Worth (1966) described the following radiographic changes observed in the jaws of patients with leukemia or lymphosarcoma:

1. The formation of the tooth crowns may be incomplete and delayed.
2. The cortices of the tooth crypts may be partially or completely destroyed.
3. There may be enlargement of the crypts with failure of bone formation about the apical portion of erupting or developing teeth (Fig. 23-7).
4. The developing tooth may assume an asymmetric position within the crypt with or without destruction of some or part of the crypt cortex.

---

*In adults very little hematopoietic tissue remains in the skeleton, so there is much greater reserve space in the fatty marrow cavities for the expansion of the proliferating leukemic cells before they eventually encroach on the bone itself.
†Lymphosarcoma is mentioned here because, although it arises in aggregates of lymphoid tissue, it does occasionally infiltrate and replace bone marrow and may be associated with a blood picture of lymphatic leukemia.

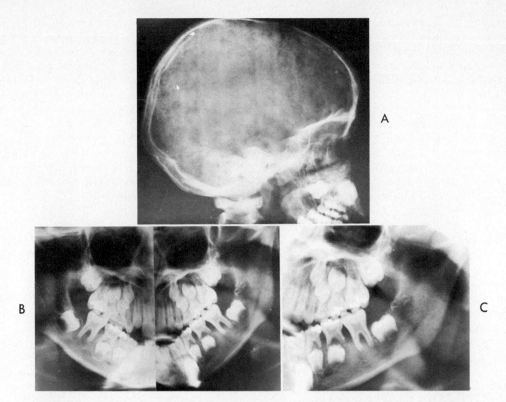

Fig. 23-7. Acute leukemia. **A,** Generalized rarefaction of the skull and ramus. **B,** Generalized rarefaction and diminution or loss of the lamina dura around roots and crypts. The left mandible is more severely affected than the right. **C,** Enlarged view of the left mandible in **B.** Radiographs have been printed lighter than normal to elucidate detail in the rarefied bone. (**A** courtesy R. Moncada, MD, Maywood, Ill. **B** and **C** courtesy T. Emmering, DDS, Maywood, Ill.)

5. Incompletely formed crowns may be situated entirely above the alveolar crest, being completely elevated out of the bone.
6. Partially formed teeth, especially those having incomplete root formation, may be found to have excessively rapid eruption.

In a study of 214 children with acute leukemia, Curtis (1971) reported finding jawbone changes in 65% of the cases of acute lymphatic leukemia and 55% of the cases of acute myelogenous leukemia. He observed that osteoporosis usually commenced with the destruction of the apical portion of the cortex about the most distal crypt of the developing mandibular molar and progressed forward. He indicated that this was the most frequently found abnormality in the jaws. Unilateral changes developed in the jaws of some patients, bilateral changes developed in the jaws of others. The alveolar crests were not usually involved. When changes in the crest were present, however, they were the result of an extension of a medullary lesion, not of the disease process's commencing at the crest. Changes in the lymphatic and myelogenous types were indistinguishable. Remissions were reflected by improvement in the radiographic appearance.

In addition to the osseous defects of leukemia, periosteal apposition of new bone may be discernible; it develops as a reaction to the penetration by the leukemic cells between the cortex and the periosteum (Lichtenstein, 1977, p. 325).

Unlike the lytic changes, osteosclerosis is an occasional finding and is more common in myelogenous leukemia than in the other types (Worth, 1963, p. 371).

Differential diagnosis

For a discussion of the differential diagnosis of leukemia, see the differential diagnosis section at the end of this chapter (p. 496).

Management

Antitumor drugs (such as methotrexate and prednisone) are used for the induction and maintenance of remissions of the leukemias. Palliative measures to counteract anemia, bleeding problems, and infection are necessary, especially in the acute phase of the disease. Cases of acute childhood leukemia carry the poorest prognosis. Because of the significant immunosuppressive effects of the cytotoxic drugs, suprainfections such as candidiasis, herpes, and bacterial infections are common. Actually, more acute oral infections than acute nonoral infections develop in these patients, although most of the acute bacterial infections are associated with granulocytopenia (Peterson and Overholser, 1981).

HISTIOCYTOSIS X

Histiocytosis X is a reticuloendothelial disease that may cause a generalized rarefaction of the jaws, especially in the Letterer-Siwe and Hand-Schüller-Christian varieties. This reticuloendotheliosis is discussed in Chapter 22 as a disease that produces multiple separate radiolucencies that are well defined but without a cortical margin.

Features

The rarefied appearance of the jawbone produced by Letterer-Siwe or Hand-Schüller-Christian disease may closely mimic the leukemic changes. In most cases, however, the bone destruction in histiocytosis X commences at the alveolar crest instead of in the medullary re-

gion of the bone, where it is more typical of leukemia. Extrusion of the teeth, thinning of the cortices and lamina dura, and crypt and tooth involvement (all changes seen in leukemia) may be present in histiocytosis X (Fig. 23-8). New bone formation, however, is not characteristic of the latter disease.

Differential diagnosis

The basic clinical and biochemical features that help distinguish the disorders presented in this chapter are discussed in the differential diagnosis section (p. 496).

Management

Although the acute disseminated form, Letterer-Siwe disease, is the more serious variant of this disease, it is no longer considered invariably fatal; with good clinical management some infants and children can be treated for years, and the disease can enter a more chronic phase (Lichtenstein, 1977, p. 418).

Hand-Schüller-Christian disease, being a chronic form of histiocytosis X, carries a better prognosis. Radiation therapy frequently proves helpful. Often, palliative and corrective measures are also necessary to regulate the altered physiology (diabetes insipidus) and control potentially serious secondary infections. Allard et al. (1978) reported satisfactory results from marrow–cancellous bone grafting of the defects in the alveolar bone.

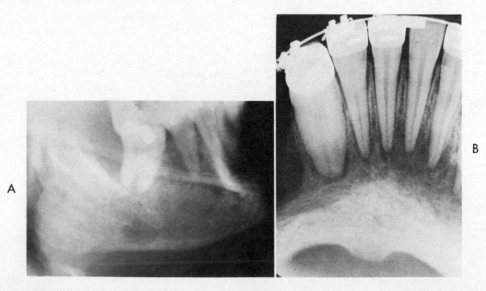

Fig. 23-8. Histiocytosis X. **A,** Generalized rarefaction and a discrete lesion. **B,** Diffuse radiolucency of bone in another patient.   (**A** courtesy R. Goepp, DDS, Zoller Clinic, University of Chicago.)

PAGET'S DISEASE (OSTEITIS DEFORMANS)

The intermediate stage of Paget's disease is discussed in detail in Chapter 25, which emphasizes the mixed radiolucent and radiopaque appearance of the disease. The late stage, with its dense, cotton-wool appearance, is stressed in Chapter 30. The early stage, characterized by a radiographic appearance of rarefaction, is discussed in this chapter.

Features

Inclusive features of Paget's disease are not reviewed here, since they are presented in detail in Chapter 25 and 30.

Clinicians are not as well acquainted with the radiolucent stage of Paget's disease as with the cotton-wool (late) stage. Osteoporosis circumscripta of the skull is an example of this disease in its osteolytic phase (Fig. 23-9) (Anderson and Dehner, 1976). Furthermore, Paget's disease may initially cause a general homogeneous rarefaction of the jawbone and a fine ground-glass appearance identical to that seen in hyperpara-thyroidism. The entire jawbone may be involved, with the cortices thinned and the lamina dura missing (Fig. 23-9, *C*).

Whereas both jaws may be affected, it is not characteristic for the same stage of the disease to be manifested in both simultaneously. (There is a progressive development of the disease from one bone to another.) The maxilla is more frequently involved than the mandible and is almost always affected first (Fig. 23-9).

Paget's disease may also involve the pelvis, vertebrae, and femurs, but the rarefaction stage is less common in these bones. The serum alkaline phosphatase levels are markedly elevated, as high as or higher than those in any other disease (Goldsmith, 1972).

Histopathologic study of the early stage shows active resorption, with osteoclasts present in Howship's lacunae. The trabeculae are small, disorganized, and scattered throughout a fibrous stroma (Fig. 23-9). Bone with the mosaic pattern usually is not present at this stage, being characteristic of a more advanced phase of the disease.

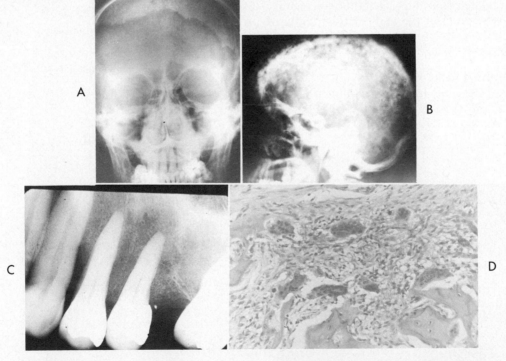

Fig. 23-9. Paget's disease, early stage. **A,** Osteoporosis circumscripta of the skull. **B,** Two stages of Paget's disease: intermediate stage in the skull and early osteolytic stage in the maxilla (which is almost completely radiolucent). **C,** Same patient as in **B.** Generalized rarefaction of the maxilla, loss of lamina dura, and relative increase in radiopacity of the teeth. The mandible was unaffected. **D,** Photomicrograph of early Paget's disease showing the increased amount of fibrous tissue and the numerous osteoclasts resorbing thinned bony trabeculae. (**A** courtesy R. Moncada, MD, Maywood, Ill.)

Differential diagnosis

For a discussion of the differential diagnosis of Paget's disease, see the differential diagnosis section at the end of the chapter (p. 496).

Management

Palliative measures are necessary to alleviate symptoms of the disease (such as early and persistent pain). Various regimens have been used to curb the degenerative advance of Paget's disease; although some have been effective in relieving the pain, most have been disappointing in their effects on bone lesions.

MULTIPLE MYELOMA

Multiple myeloma is a disease characterized by the development of multiple malignant tumors of plasma cells. It originates in the bone marrow and represents the most common primary malignancy of bone. It is discussed in Chapter 22, where its radiographic appearance as multiple punched-out radiolucencies is emphasized.

Features

In advanced cases the gross destruction of the medullary portions of the bones, coupled with resorption of the cortices from within, is so extensive that a generalized osteoporosis is obvious (Fig. 23-10).

Differential diagnosis

For a discussion of the differential diagnosis of multiple myeloma, see the differential diagnosis section at the end of the chapter (p. 496).

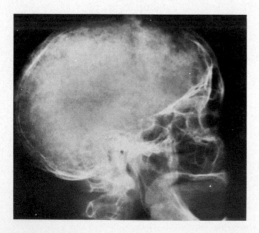

Fig. 23-10. Advanced multiple myeloma. Generalized rarefaction of the skull and jaws is evident. Most of the radiopaque appearance of the skull is produced by the brain. (Courtesy E. Palacios, MD, Maywood, Ill.)

Management

Multiple myeloma is a rapidly fatal disease; about half the patients die within 2 years of the onset of symptoms. The 5-year survival rate is approximately 10%. The disease is treated with cytotoxic drugs (such as melphalan, urethan, and corticosteroids) and radiation. Palliative measures are used to alleviate the accompanying pain, bleeding, anemia, and kidney problems.

RARITIES

As shown in the list of rarities at the beginning of this chapter (and in the list that follows), a varied group of diseases may produce generalized rarefactions of the skeleton, including the jaws (Figs. 23-11 and 23-12).

Either these diseases occur rarely, however, or they seldom produce rarefactions of the bone or jaws. Nevertheless, the clinician must know of them when he or she is developing a differential diagnosis for a particular case. Usually the other symptoms coincidental with the rarefaction direct the clinician to include the appropriate diseases in the working diagnosis.

The following list includes rare generalized rarefactions:

Acromegaly (pseudo-osteoporosis)
Agranulocytosis
Burkitt's lymphoma (Fig. 23-12)
Central cavernous hemangioma
Congenital heart disease
Cyclic neutropenia
Diabetes
Down's syndrome
Erythroblastosis fetalis
Gaucher's disease
Hypervitaminosis D
Hypogonadism
Hypoparathyroidism
Hypophosphatasia
Hypovitaminosis C
Lymphosarcoma (Fig. 23-11)
Massive osteolysis (phantom bone disease)
Multiple metastatic carcinomas (Fig. 23-13)
Multiple sclerosis
Myelofibrosis
Osteogenesis imperfecta
Other diffuse malignant tumors
Oxalosis and hyperoxaluria
Polycythemia
Postradiation rarefaction
Pregnancy—late stages
Progeria
Protein-deficiency states
Rickets
Sarcoidosis
Spherocytosis
Urticaria pigmentosa
XO syndrome
XXY syndrome

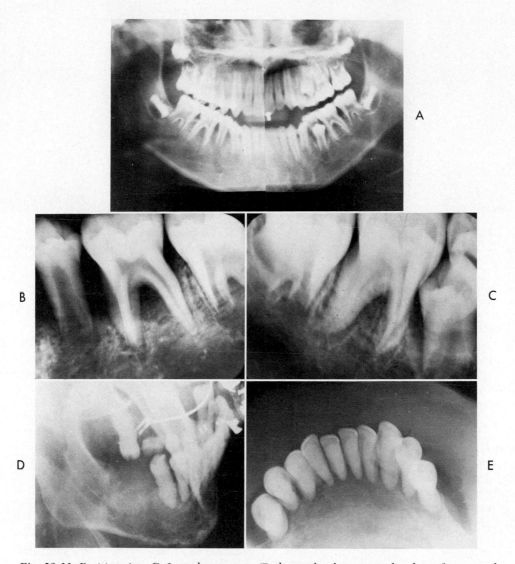

Fig. 23-11. Rarities. **A** to **C**, Lymphosarcoma. (Radiographs show generalized rarefaction and loss of the lamina dura around the roots, **A**, as well as the blurred appearance of bone and loss of lamina dura, **B** and **C**.) **D** and **E**, Diffuse squamous cell carcinoma of the anterior mandible showing loss of lamina dura and generalized rarefaction.

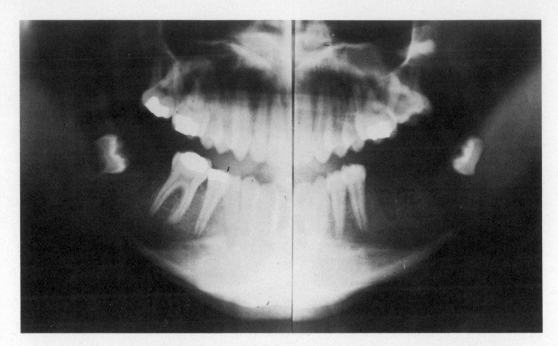

Fig. 23-12. Panorex radiograph of a patient with Burkitt's lymphoma showing gross rarefaction and almost complete loss of the bone in the molar and ramus areas bilaterally.   (Courtesy N. Palm, DDS, Detroit.)

DIFFERENTIAL DIAGNOSIS OF RAREFACTIONS OF THE JAWBONE

Because of the wide range of naturally occurring anatomic variations in healthy bone, distinguishing the radiographic appearance of normal jawbone from changes produced by disease is frequently quite difficult. The jawbones of frail but healthy persons with delicate structures may appear to be more radiolucent than usual. Some persons may normally have relatively large marrow spaces, whereas others normally have a faint lamina dura. As a general rule, if the patient is well and changes are not evident on serial radiographs, the appearance of the bone is most likely within the range of normal variation.

The ensuing discussion, which pertains to the development of a differential diagnosis and a working diagnosis for the disorders included in the present chapter, requires some initial qualification, since it is unique in relation to other discussions of differential diagnosis in this text.

All the pathoses discussed in this chapter are systemic diseases, and, needless to say, the differential diagnosis of bone diseases requires a detailed history and careful physical examination. To describe all the manifest and subtle differences that characterize these entities is an endeavor beyond the scope of this text.

An effort has been made, however, to present sufficient detail that the dental practitioner can appreciate the relationships between the oral and systemic manifestations and thereby be prepared for a consultation with the physician, that is, the dental practitioner can, first, recognize the need for the consultation and, second, be prepared to provide the most appropriate dental therapy when necessary.

In addition to causing rarefactions of the skeleton, the conditions listed here (except two or three of the rarities) produce other systemic changes. These features are identified by the general clinical examination and laboratory tests—supplementing the radiographic findings. Thus, although there are no simple formulas, the clinical and laboratory examinations help the clinician establish the rankings of the probable entities in the differential diagnosis.

Some hints that we have found helpful in specific instances are discussed in the following paragraphs.

There is a tendency to immediately diagnose a rarefaction of the jawbones accompanied by a loss of lamina dura as hyperparathyroidism.

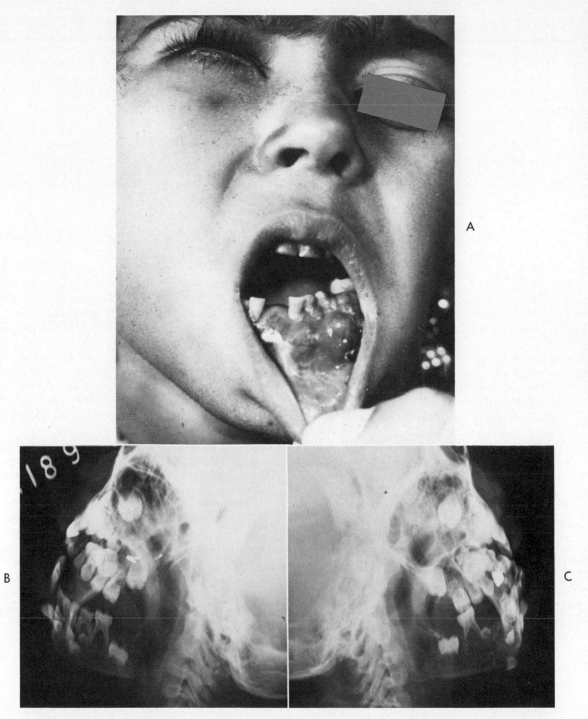

Fig. 23-13. Disseminated metastatic retinoblastoma to the mandible in a 3-year-old girl. **A,** Intraoral view showing the tumorous expansion of the anterior alveolus. **B** and **C,** Right and left lateral oblique radiographs showing the general rarefaction of the mandible with a loss of most of the cortices and disruption of several developing permanent teeth.   (From Perriman AP and Figures KH: Oral Surg 45:741-748, 1978.)

Table 23-1. Comparison of the serum values in metabolic bone diseases

Disease	Calcium	Phosphorus	Alkaline phosphatase
Hyperparathyroidism			
Primary	Increased	Decreased	Increased
Secondary	Normal to decreased	Increased	Increased
Tertiary	Increased	Normal to increased	Increased
Osteoporosis	Normal	Normal	Normal
Osteomalacia			
Vitamin D deficiency	Decreased	Decreased	Increased
Hypophosphatemia	Normal	Decreased	Increased
Paget's disease	Normal	Normal	Increased
Multiple myeloma	Normal to increased	Normal	Increased

True, a hyperparathyroidism may be the most common cause of rarefaction, but when one considers the many and varied disease processes that can produce a similar radiographic appearance, it becomes obvious that all the local and systemic features of a case must be carefully evaluated before an adequate working diagnosis can be developed.

Subperiosteal erosions, especially of the middle phalanges, are almost pathognomonic for hyperparathyroidism, as are the recurrent benign giant cell lesions of the jaws. Another important feature that suggests primary hyperparathyroidism is hypophosphatemia. Except for its occurrence in hyperparathyroidism, hypophosphatemia occurs only in avitaminosis D, hypophosphatemic rickets, and osteomalacia. Unlike primary hyperparathyroidism, however, hypercalcemia is not found in the other conditions (Table 23-1).

The lamina dura is more apt to be deficient in osteoporosis than in osteomalacia (Worth, 1963, p. 360). The lamina dura characteristically appears normal in the hemolytic anemias (especially sickle cell anemia).

Pseudofractures and greenstick fractures in adults are almost pathognomonic for osteomalacia.

Jawbone lesions of histiocytosis X more often commence at the crest of the alveolar ridge. By contrast, those of leukemia characteristically originate in the deeper, medullary portion. Also, bone proliferation is foreign to the former condition but may be a feature of leukemia or lymphoma.

Several diseases that occur primarily in young persons are thalassemia, sickle cell anemia, acute leukemia, and histiocytosis X. *Older persons (over 40 years) are affected primarily by* hyperparathyroidism (especially secondary or tertiary), osteoporosis, osteomalacia, Paget's disease, and multiple myeloma.

Laboratory values may be particularly useful in differentiating among the preceding diseases, but the limitations of these parameters must be kept in mind. The biochemical indices and morphologic characteristics of the diseases may undergo spontaneous and independent variations. Thus a disease that characteristically shows an increased serum calcium level may not show an increase during a regression of symptoms. Furthermore, variable factors—including diet, stress, and degree of physical activity—may influence these parameters, not to mention the day-to-day fluctuations caused by variable technical factors in the laboratory. Then, too, concomitant systemic conditions may present confusing results, so their interactions must be considered.

The serum alkaline phosphatase level is commonly elevated during accelerated bone activity (whether resorption or apposition). It may be higher than normal in obstructive liver disease (jaundice), however, and often is higher than normal in both nonjaundiced patients with liver damage and pregnant women. Thus an increase is not always pathognomonic for increased bone activity. Consequently, although a high serum alkaline phosphatase level may suggest Paget's disease, biliary obstruction, or pregnancy, the history and cursory physical examination help the clinician determine which circumstance was responsible for this change in the patient's biochemistry.

The characteristic changes in the serum chemistry for some of the diseases discussed in this chapter are listed in Table 23-1, at the top of this page.

In 50% of cases of multiple myeloma, Bence Jones protein is present in the urine.

REFERENCES

Alexander WN and Bechtold WA: Alpha thalassemia minor trait accompanied by clinical oral signs, Oral Surg 43:892-897, 1977.

Allard JR, Landino RJ, and Cerami JJ: Autogenous marrow-cancellous bone grafting in a patient with Hand-Schüller-Christian disease, J Oral Surg 36:293-296, 1978.

Anderson JT and Dehner LP: Osteolytic form of Paget's disease, J Bone Joint Surg [Am] 58:994-1000, 1976.

Bartter FC: Bone as a target organ: toward a better definition of osteoporosis, Perspect Biol Med 16:215-231, 1973.

Bras J, van Ooij CP, Abraham-inpign L, et al: Radiographic interpretation of the mandibular angular cortex: a diagnostic tool in metabolic bone loss. I. Normal state, Oral Surg 53:541-545, 1982.

Bressman E, Decter JA, Chasens AI, et al: Acute myeloblastic leukemia with oral manifestations: report of a case, Oral Surg 54:401-402, 1982.

Chernoff AI: The hemoglobinopathies and thalassemia. In Beeson PB and McDermott W, editors: Textbook of medicine, ed 2, Philadelphia, 1967, WB Saunders Co, p 1046.

Conacher WD: Metabolic bone disease in the elderly, Practitioner 210:351-356, 1973.

Cox GM: A study of oral pain experience in sickle cell patients, Oral Surg 58:39-41, 1984.

Curtis AB: Childhood leukemias: osseous changes in jaws on panoramic dental radiographs, J Am Dent Assoc 83:844-847, 1971.

Duncan H: Osteoporosis in rheumatoid arthritis and corticosteroid-induced osteoporosis: symposium on metabolic bone disease, Orthop Clin North Am 3:571-583, 1972.

Edeiken J: Roentgen diagnosis of diseases of bone, vol 2, ed 3, Baltimore, 1981, Williams & Wilkins, p 1069.

Fletcher PD, Scopp IW, and Hersh RA: Oral manifestations of secondary hyperparathyroidism related to long-term hemodialysis therapy, Oral Surg 43:218-226, 1977.

Girasole RV and Lyon ED: Sickle cell osteomyelitis of the mandible: report of three cases, J Oral Surg 35:231-234, 1977.

Goldsmith RS: Laboratory aids in the diagnosis of metabolic bone disease, Orthop Clin North Am 3:545-560, 1972.

Jackson CE and Frame B: Diagnosis and management of parathyroid disorders: symposium on metabolic bone disease, Orthop Clin North Am 3:699-712, 1972.

Jaworski ZFG: Pathophysiology, diagnosis, and treatment of osteomalacia: symposium on metabolic bone disease, Orthop Clin North Am 3:623-652, 1972.

Karpas A: Viruses and leukemia, Am Sci 70:277-285, 1982.

Koutras DA, Pandros PG, Koukoulommati AS, and Constantes J: Radiological signs of bone loss in hyperthyroidism, Br J Radiol 46:695-698, 1973.

Lichtenstein L: Bone tumors, ed 5, St. Louis, 1977, The CV Mosby Co.

Little K: Bone behavior, New York, 1973a, Academic Press, Inc.

Little K: Osteoporotic mechanisms, J Int Med Res 1:509-529, 1973b.

Michaud M, Baehner RL, Bixler D, and Kafrawy AH: Oral manifestations of acute leukemia in children, J Am Dent Assoc 95:1145-1150, 1977.

Moseley JE: Bone changes in hematologic disorders (roentgen aspects), New York, 1963, Grune & Stratton, pp 26-27.

Mourshed F and Tuckson CR: A study of the radiographic features of the jaws in sickle cell anemia, Oral Surg 37:812-819, 1974.

Nordin BEC: Metabolic bone and stone disease, Baltimore, 1973, Williams & Wilkins.

Perriman AO and Figures KH: Metastatic retinoblastoma of the mandible, Oral Surg 45:741-748, 1978.

Peterson DE and Overholser CD: Increased morbidity associated with oral infection in patients with acute non-lymphocytic leukemia, Oral Surg 51:390-393, 1981.

Poyton HG and Davey KW: Thalassemia: changes visible in radiographs used in dentistry, Oral Surg 25:564-576, 1968.

Rasmussen H and Brodier P: The physiological and cellular basis of metabolic bone disease, Baltimore, 1974, Williams & Wilkins.

Reynolds WA and Karo JJ: Radiologic diagnosis of metabolic bone disease: symposium on metabolic bone disease, Orthop Clin North Am 3:521-543, 1972.

Robinson IB and Sarnat SG: Roentgen studies of the maxilla and mandible in sickle cell anemia, Radiology 58:517-523, 1952.

Sanger RG and Bystrom EB: Radiographic bone changes in sickle cell anemia, J Oral Med 32:32-37, 1977.

Sanger RO, Greer RO, and Averbach RE: Differential diagnosis of some simple osseous lesions associated with sickle cell anemia, Oral Surg 43:538-545, 1977.

Silverman S, Ware WH, and Gillooly C: Dental aspects of hyperparathyroidism, Oral Surg 26:184-189, 1968.

Snapper I: Bone disease in medical practice, New York, 1957, Grune & Stratton, pp 201-202.

Stafne EC: Oral roentgenographic diagnosis, ed 3, Philadelphia, 1969, WB Saunders Co, p 264.

Stewart RE and Prescott GH, editors: Oral facial genetics, St. Louis, 1976, The CV Mosby Co.

Van Dis ML and Langlais RP: The thalassemias: oral manifestations and complications, Oral Surg 62:229-233, 1986.

Van Slyck EJ: The bony changes in malignant hematologic disease: symposium on metabolic bone disease, Orthop Clin North Am 3:733-744, 1972.

Walsh RF and Karmiol M: Oral roentgenographic findings in osteitis fibrosa generalisata associated with chronic renal disease, Oral Surg 28:273-281, 1969.

Watson L: Endocrine bone disease, Practitioner 210:376-383, 1973.

Williamson JJ: Blood dyscrasias. In Gorlin RJ and Goldman HM, editors: Thoma's oral pathology, vol 2, ed 6, St Louis, 1970, The CV Mosby Co., pp 943-944.

Worth HM: Principles and practice of oral radiologic interpretation, Chicago, 1963, Year Book Medical Publishers.

Worth HM: Some significant radiographic appearances in young jaws, Oral Surg 21:609-617, 1966.

Wysocki GP, Daley TD, and Ulan RA: Predentin changes in patients with chronic renal failure, Oral Surg 56:167-173, 1983.

Section B   Radiolucent lesions with radiopaque foci or mixed radiolucent-radiopaque lesions

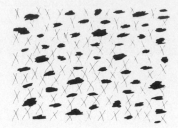

The normal anatomic structures and disease states that produce mixed radiolucent-radiopaque images on radiographs present a particular challenge in that a wide variety of normal and pathologic conditions can produce them.

Several of the radiolucent-radiopaque lesions in this group represent intermediate stages in the development or maturation of more opaque lesions; that is to say, a particular pathologic entity may commence as an osteolytic lesion, which shows as a radiolucency on the radiograph. During its development, foci of calcified material may form within the osteolytic area, and when these foci become large enough and sufficiently mineralized, they become radiographically apparent. Thus the mixed radiolucent-radiopaque condition frequently represents an intermediate stage in the development of the lesion.

Maturation or mineralization often continues until most of the lesion, with the possible exception of a thin radiolucent rim, becomes opaque.

The outstanding feature of this especially interesting group is the close correlation between the radiographic appearance and the microstructure of the individual lesions.

On histologic examination all the lesions in the radiolucent-radiopaque stage contain calcified areas of either hard tooth tissue (or bone) or nondescript mineralized material. In a few instances the radiopacities are hazy and poorly defined and microscopic examination shows that they are not produced by calcified material but by dense composites of fibrous tissue. This effect is even more pronounced when the lesion is large and causes a buccolingual expansion of the mandible (see Fig. 24-15).

The response of bone to some extrinsic state or to frank bone disease may, however, cause a sclerosis without an initial, radiographically apparent osteolytic stage. The influence of the disease state on the bone is then mild, and the primary effect is stimulation of osteoblastic activity, resulting in a bony sclerosis. These sclerosed regions usually appear as radiopacities within (and not sharply demarcated from) normal-appearing bone.

24

Mixed radiolucent-radiopaque lesions associated with teeth

NORMAN K. WOOD
PAUL W. GOAZ
JAMES F. LEHNERT

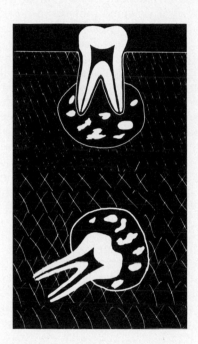

The following are mixed radiolucent-radiopaque lesions associated with teeth:

Periapical mixed lesions
Calcifying crown of developing tooth
Tooth root with rarefying osteitis
Rarefying and condensing osteitis
Periapical cementoma—intermediate stage
Cementifying and ossifying fibroma
Rarities
  Calcifying and keratinizing odontogenic cyst
  Cementoblastoma—intermediate stage
  Foreign bodies
  Generalized (nodular cemental masses; Paget's
    disease)
  Odontoma—intermediate stage
  Osteomyelitis—chronic

Pericoronal mixed lesions
Odontoma—intermediate stage
Adenomatoid odontogenic tumor
Keratinizing and calcifying odontogenic cyst
Ameloblastic fibro-odontoma
Calcifying epithelial odontogenic tumor
Odontogenic fibroma
Rarities
  Ameloblastic fibrodentinoma
  Cystic odontoma
  "Eruption sequestrum"

Periapical mixed lesions

CALCIFYING CROWN OF DEVELOPING TOOTH

The radiographic appearance of crypts containing tooth germs in early stages of development is discussed in Chapter 19, where it is stated that they appear as cystlike radiolucencies. The cusp tips are the first part of the developing tooth to calcify; as soon as sufficient mineral is deposited in the matrix of the cusp tips to make them radiographically apparent, the developing tooth can be recognized as a radiolucency with radiopaque foci (Fig. 24-1). Thus the intermediate stage of tooth formation may be imprudently mistaken for a mixed radiolucent-radiopaque lesion.

Presumably the clinician trained to interpret radiographs of the jaws would not make this error, since he or she would expect to encounter such normal structures in the radiographs of patients under 20 years of age. In unusual cases, however, tooth buds of the third molar may develop in patients over 20 years of age and the development of the maxillary second premolar buds may be delayed until approximately the eleventh year.

Before calcification, permanent tooth buds may appear in the periapical regions of deciduous teeth and in a few months undergo sufficient mineralization to appear as periapical radiolucencies with radiopaque foci. The clinician should therefore be familiar with the normal positions, chronologies, and radiographic appearances of the tooth buds with calcifying crowns. If there is a question, the clinician can compare the appearances of the developing contralateral teeth to confirm the identity of these calcifying crowns.

The radiographic appearance in certain cases may not be definite enough to allow the clinician to make a firm diagnosis of calcifying crown (for example, when the developing tooth's formation or calcification is delayed, when the tooth is not in its normal position, or when the tooth is supernumerary and not immediately identifiable). Subsequent periodic radiographs reveal the nature of the suspect region as the form of the calcifying crown becomes more typical.

TOOTH ROOT WITH RAREFYING OSTEITIS

Retained roots and root tips are the abnormal radiopacities most commonly found in edentulous regions of the jaws. Retained roots may be present in the jaws of one of every four edentulous persons; 80% of these retained roots are in the posterior region of the jaws, and 6% of all retained root tips are associated with radiolucent areas. (This latter statistic is a corollary to the observation that the root canal of a retained root is frequently continuous with the oral cavity at its coronal end.) Thus the root canal may become the channel for infection, with a resulting rarefying osteitis in the periapex and the production of a radiolucent-radiopaque jaw lesion. Such root tips are surrounded by granulation tissue, and they may be totally asymptomatic or the patient may complain of intermittent slight pain or swelling. When the patient's resistance becomes depressed, an acute infection may ensue and produce a fluctuant, painful, smooth-surfaced mass (abscess).

On microscopic examination a section of the lesion shows chronic granulation tissue about a cross section of the tooth root with perhaps a purulent root canal.

The retained root is relatively easy to identify when the shape of the root has persisted

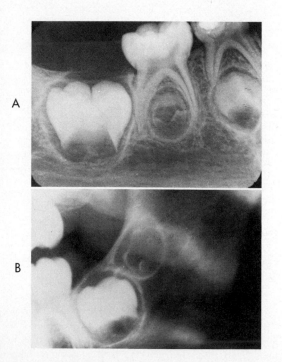

Fig. 24-1. Calcifying crowns of developing teeth. **A,** Mandibular right second premolar. **B,** Mandibular left third molar.

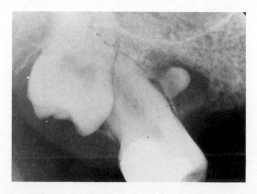

Fig. 24-2. Root tip with accompanying rarefying osteitis.

along with the linear radiolucent shadow of the root canal, a portion of the periodontal membrane space, and the surrounding lamina dura. In other instances, however, when the root fragment has been resorbed to some extent, the root canal is not discernible, the lamina dura is no longer present, and chronic inflammation has produced a rarefaction of the surrounding bone (Fig. 24-2), the clinician's diagnostic problem is more difficult.

Differential diagnosis

Root tips that are atypical in appearance (partially resorbed, with the root canal and lamina dura obscured) and surrounded by rarefying osteitis may be confused with an intermediate-stage cementoma or odontoma, a chronic osteomyelitis, an ossifying fibroma, an osteogenic sarcoma, a chondrosarcoma, or a metastatic osteoblastic carcinoma. If recent preextraction radiographs are available, however, they usually help to identify the lesion as a root tip.

The *metastatic osteoblastic carcinoma, chondrosarcoma*, and *osteogenic sarcoma* may share two characteristics with a retained root tip whose identity is obscured by rarefying osteitis: local discomfort of the patient and a radiolucency with usually ill-defined, ragged margins. The malignant tumors all show moderate to rapid growth, as evidenced by an enlargement of the region that may become apparent on clinical examination within a few weeks. An acute abscess originating from an infected root tip, however, usually enlarges rapidly within a few days and becomes quite painful, inflamed, and perhaps fluctuant. If the infection is chronic, a draining sinus may develop. Of course, a medical history indicating that the patient has a primary malignancy elsewhere or has symptoms that suggest such a tumor prompts the examiner to suspect a metastatic osteoblastic tumor.

If the patient has no predisposing systemic disease and no history of trauma to the area and if the lesion is in the maxilla, *osteomyelitis* may be assigned a low rank in the differential diagnosis. An absence of pain, swelling, or drainage further deemphasizes osteomyelitis in the diagnosis.

If the patient is over 20 years of age, the radiolucent-radiopaque lesion is unlikely to be an *odontoma* that has yet to develop beyond the intermediate stage.

The radiopacities in fibro-osseous lesions of periodontal ligament origin (PDLO) (such as a *cementoma*) are frequently multiple and have a more uneven density and a less well-defined outline than do those of root tips. Thus the clinician would be influenced to assign a low rank to this entity in the list of possible diagnoses. Also, if the lesion is single, asymptomatic, and situated in the maxilla or the molar region of a white man, it is unlikely to be a cementoma. Furthermore, in contrast to the margins of the radiolucency surrounding an infected root tip, which are usually poorly defined and somewhat ragged, the radiolucent margins about a cementoma are well defined and smoothly contoured.

On the basis of incidence alone, the working diagnosis for a relatively small, well-defined, smoothly outlined, homogeneously dense radiopaque image surrounded by an ill-defined, ragged radiolucency in a tooth-bearing area of the jaws would be a root tip surrounded by rarefying osteitis.

Management

Retained root tips that are infected should be removed. If an acute abscess is present, it should be incised, drained, cultured, and irrigated at least twice daily and the patient should be given suitable antibiotic therapy. After the infection has subsided, the root tip and surrounding soft tissue should be removed, the bone defect curetted, and the tissue microscopically examined.

RAREFYING AND CONDENSING OSTEITIS

Frequently a chronic infection in the jawbone, precipitated by a nonvital tooth or a retained root, induces both a rarefying and a condensing osteitis (Fig. 24-3). The chronic infection thus acts as an irritating factor (causing resorption of bone) and as a stimulating factor (producing dense bone)—perhaps as a defense mechanism to contain the local problem.

Bone resorption occurs where the irritating products of the chronic infection are most concentrated (that is, about the apex), whereas bone apposition occurs some distance from this point (at the periphery of the rarefying lesion). The diffusion of the irritating products of the infection through the tissues results in their dilution, and the irritating products then induce osteoblastic activity and sclerosis at the periphery of the osteolytic area.

When the chronic infection has run a steady course, a reasonably well-defined, somewhat homogeneous radiopacity is seen more or less circumscribing the radiolucency around the root end (see Fig. 27-3). When the course of

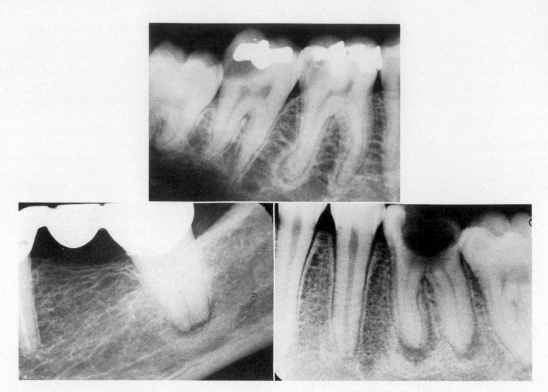

Fig. 24-3. Combined periapical rarefying and condensing osteitis. The teeth in the three cases were nonvital. The rarefying osteitis contacts the root end, and the condensing osteitis (radiopaque halo) is located around the periphery of the rarefied area.

the chronic infection is punctuated by acute exacerbations, however, the radiographic picture is less orderly and the sclerosis more diffuse and less homogeneous.

Features, differential diagnosis, and management

Features, differential diagnosis, and management of rarefying and condensing osteitis are similar to those for a root tip with rarefying osteitis. Marmary and Kutiner (1986) reported an incidence of approximately 9.5% in a randomly selected population. The differential diagnosis is further discussed in this chapter in the differential diagnosis sections concerning benign fibro-osseous lesions (PDLO) and the intermediate stage of odontoma.

PERIAPICAL CEMENTOMA— INTERMEDIATE STAGE

The periapical cementoma is thought to be a reactive phenomenon that arises from elements within the periodontal ligament (Hamner et al., 1968; Waldron, 1985; Waldron and Giansanti, 1973a, 1973b).

The cementoma or periapical cemental dysplasia is discussed in Chapter 16 as a periapical radiolucency, in Chapter 19 as a cystlike radiolucency, and in Chapter 27 as a periapical radiopacity. In this chapter the emphasis is on its intermediate radiolucent-radiopaque stage, which embraces a spectrum of radiographic appearances between the totally radiolucent and the mature radiopaque stage (Figs. 24-4 and 24-5).

Features

Cementomas most often occur in the periapices of vital teeth, but they may also be found elsewhere in either jaw, as a solitary lesion and as multiple lesions. Approximately 90% occur in the mandible, usually in the anterior region. They are seldom if ever found in the anterior maxilla. They have a higher predilection for women (approximately 80%) and for blacks. Neville and Albenesius (1986) found that 5.9% of black women have at least one periapical cementoma. Marmary and Kutiner (1986) reported an incidence of approximately 0.5% in 889 randomly chosen patients at The Hebrew

University–Hadassa Faculty of Dental Medicine. Cementomas may vary from a few millimeters to several centimeters in diameter, and they seldom occur in patients under 30 years of age. They are ordinarily asymptomatic; the usual periapical lesion seldom grows large enough to expand the jaw, but in rare cases some may.

The initial lesion of the cementoma is osteolytic; as it matures, particles or spicules of calcified material develop in the cystlike radiolucency (Figs. 24-4 and 24-5). When these foci of calcification become radiographically apparent, the lesion is considered to be in its intermediate stage of maturation. The size, shape, number, and discreteness of the contained radiopacities vary greatly from lesion to lesion and from patient to patient as the calcified components become larger and coalesce and the lesion becomes more radiopaque.

Regardless of its stage of development, the cementoma usually has well-defined, smoothly contoured radiolucent borders (Figs. 24-4 and 24-5). Sometimes sclerosis is induced in the bone at the periphery of the radiolucent border and appears on the radiograph as a hyperostotic margin.

The microscopic appearance reflects what is seen on the radiograph. At the intermediate stage a cementoma is made up of a fibroblastic-type matrix that is moderately vascular and contains a varied number of calcified zones of cementum or bone, or cementum and bone in varying combinations (Fig. 24-5). The cementum may be distinguished from bone by the differences in width and pattern of the intrinsic collagenous bundles as they appear under polarized light (Waldron and Giansanti, 1973a).

Differential diagnosis

Entities that should be included in the differential diagnosis of the intermediate stage of cementoma are rarefying osteitis in combination with condensing osteitis, chronic osteomyelitis, fibrous dysplasia, calcifying crowns, ossifying and cementifying fibroma, postsurgical calcifying bone defect, odontoma (intermediate stage), juxtaposed pericoronal mixed lesions, osteogenic sarcoma, chondrosarcoma, and metastatic osteoblastic carcinoma.

The cementomas are slow growing, which distinguishes them from the more rapidly growing malignant *metastatic osteoblastic carcinoma*, *chondrosarcoma*, and *osteogenic sarcoma*. Like the cementomas these malignancies may appear as mixed radiolucent-radiopaque

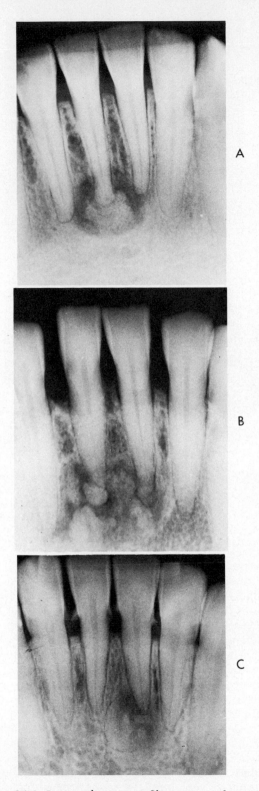

Fig. 24-4. Intermediate-stage fibro-osseous lesions (PDLO). **A** to **C**, Cementomas in periapices of teeth with vital pulps.

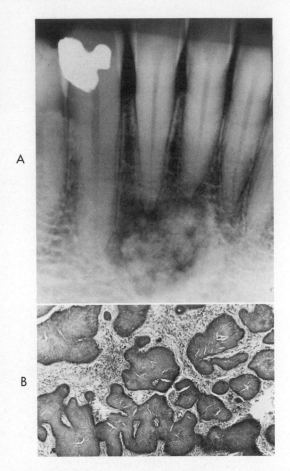

Fig. 24-5. Intermediate-stage fibro-osseous lesions (PDLO). **A,** Cementoma. **B,** Microscopic study showing the small separate masses of acellular cementum characteristic of cementomas. (**A** courtesy M. Smulson, DDS, Maywood, Ill.)

unerupted tooth, sometimes between teeth but seldom in the periapex.

The scattered calcifying foci in a *healing postsurgical bone defect* may be identified by a history of a recent enucleation.

Calcifying crowns, which are present in the jaws of patients under 20 years of age, are easily identified by their anticipated location in the jaw, the radiographically distinguishable tissues of the tooth, and usually the presence of a similar picture in the contralateral jaw.

These considerations narrow the working diagnosis to periapical cementoma, cementifying and ossifying fibroma, rarefying osteitis combined with condensing osteitis, chronic osteomyelitis, and fibrous dysplasia.

The current, generally accepted concept of *fibrous dysplasia* of the jaws supposes several obvious differences between this entity and the fibro-osseous lesions originating from the periodontal ligament (the cementoma and the cementifying and ossifying fibroma):

1. Fibrous dysplasia is slightly more common in the maxilla, whereas 90% of fibro-osseous lesions (PDLO) are found in the mandible.
2. Fibrous dysplasia has a definite tendency to develop during the first and second decades of life, whereas the periapical cementoma is seldom observed in patients under 30 years of age.
3. Fibrous dysplasia affects men and women equally, whereas the cementoma has a high predilection for women.
4. Jaw expansion caused by lesions of fibrous dysplasia is usually of the elongated fusiform type, whereas jaw expansion caused by fibro-osseous lesions (PDLO) is less common and is usually more nodular or dome shaped.
5. The radiographic borders of the lesions of fibrous dysplasia are characteristically poorly defined (that is, they merge imperceptibly with normal bone), whereas the radiographic borders of fibro-osseous lesions (PDLO) are well defined (Waldon and Giansanti, 1973b).

Application of these differences should enable the clinician to distinguish between most of the lesions of fibrous dysplasia and PDLO that he or she encounters.

Fibrous dysplasia containing only mottled areas of calcification is more difficult to differentiate. However, this mottled appearance represents an immature stage seldom seen in persons over 20 years of age; this consideration contributes to the differentiation.

lesions, but unlike the smooth, well-defined fibro-osseous lesions, they are usually irregular and ill defined. Furthermore, these malignancies (together with the chondroma) frequently cause root resorption, whereas the cementomas characteristically do not.

The mass or masses of calcified material within an *intermediate-stage odontoma,* especially of the compound variety, frequently show a somewhat orderly relationship of the radiodense enamel to the dentin and pulp spaces. The *complex odontoma,* on the other hand, is more difficult to recognize because the hard dental tissues may be so disorganized that they appear as irregular masses of calcified material. Even in these lesions, however, the more radiopaque enamel component may be discernible and often provides a clue to the identity of the lesion. In addition, the odontoma is usually located above the crown of an

Of course, if the patient is a young girl with a known case of Albright's syndrome and has jaw lesions, the clinician would have to rank fibrous dysplasia as a likely diagnosis.

If the lesions are periapical and the tooth is vital, the possibility is minimized that a pathosis has resulted from an infection of a root canal, such as might produce the combination of *rarefying* and condensing *osteitis* and *chronic osteomyelitis*. The absence of pain, drainage, inflammation, and tenderness to palpation, as well as the absence of regional lymphadenitis, further prompts the examiner to assign a lower ranking to these entities, which are a direct result of infection. In addition, it is helpful to consider that in cases of combined periapical rarefying and condensing osteitis, the radiolucent zone always lies next to the root end, whereas the radiopaque zone (condensing) forms a halo outside the radiolucency.

It may be difficult to differentiate between a periapical cementoma and a cementifying and ossifying fibroma because both lesions occur at the apices of vital teeth, are basically round with well-defined borders, and mature through the three stages. It is necessary to differentiate between the two lesions because the cementifying and ossifying fibroma is a potentially troublesome lesion requiring excision, whereas the periapical cementoma seldom requires removal.

The following characteristics help the clinician differentiate the two lesions. The periapical cementoma (1) is a common lesion, (2) has a predilection for the lower incisor teeth, (3) has a marked predilection for females, (4) almost invariably occurs in patients over 30 years of age, (5) seldom attains a diameter of more than 1 cm, (6) seldom produces clinically discernible expansion, and (7) often occurs as multiple lesions. In contrast, the ossifying fibroma (1) is an uncommon lesion, (2) has a predilection for the premolar and molar area of the mandible, (3) affects males and females equally, (4) occurs in patients under 30 years of age (average age is 26.4 years), (5) frequently attains a diameter of 2 to 4 cm (Fig. 24-6), (6) frequently produces a clinically discernible expansion, and (7) occurs as a single lesion.

Occasionally, unerupted malposed teeth with a mixed radiolucent-radiopaque lesion are positioned in such a fashion that the mixed image contacts the image of the periapex of neighboring teeth (see Fig. 24-11). The diagnostician then faces the difficulty of deciding whether the lesion was primarily a periapical lesion or a pericoronal lesion. The correct decision in such a case often greatly facilitates the differential diagnosis process. Additional radiographic views frequently separate the lesion either from the periapex or from the crown of the unerupted tooth.

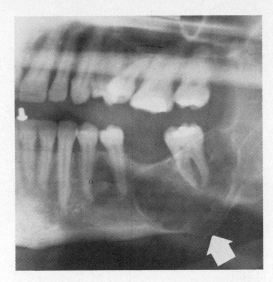

Fig. 24-6. Ossifying fibroma. Arrow shows the large, well-marginated radiolucent lesion with radiopaque foci involving the roots of the mandibular second molar tooth.   (Courtesy W. Schoenheider, DDS, Oak Lawn, Ill.)

CEMENTIFYING AND OSSIFYING FIBROMA

The cementifying and ossifying fibromas are thought to be uncommon neoplastic processes that originate from elements in the periodontal ligament (Hamner et al, 1968; Waldron, 1985; Waldron and Giansanti, 1973a, 1973b). These authors explained that in response to a variety of stimuli, cells of the periodontal ligament are capable of producing lesions comprised of cementum, lamellar bone, fibrous tissue, or any combination of these tissues. If a certain lesion contains only bony spicules and fibrous elements, it traditionally is recognized as an ossifying fibroma. Conversely, if the lesion contains only cemental and fibrous tissue, it is called a cementifying fibroma. If the lesion contains a mixture of cementum and bone in a fibrous tissue stroma, it is recognized as a cemento-ossifying fibroma. It is understood that these are three subclassifications of otherwise identical lesions.

Features

The cementifying and ossifying fibromas usually occur as periapical lesions that are basically

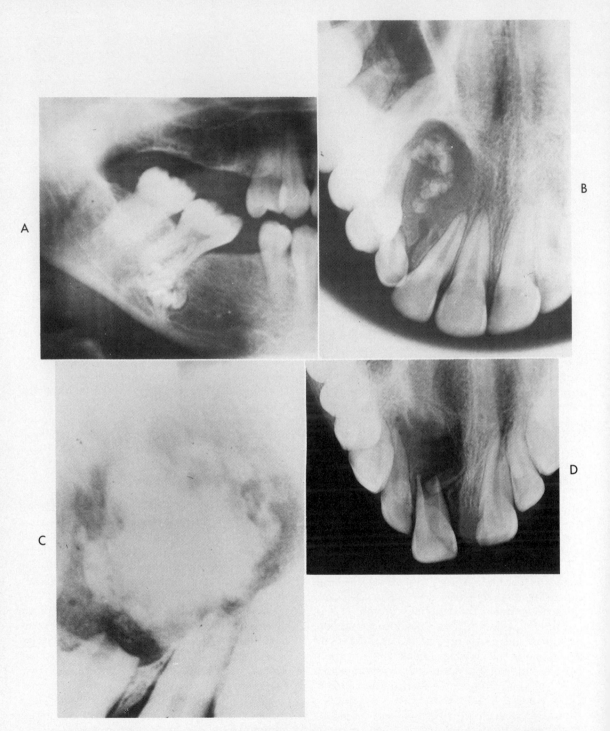

Fig. 24-7. Rare periapical mixed lesions. **A,** Compound odontoma at the apices of a second molar tooth—a most unusual location. **B** and **C,** Calcifying odontogenic cysts. **B,** In the canine region of a 14-year-old girl. **C,** In the maxillary incisor region. The unusually radiopaque lesion has caused root resorption. **D,** A mixed radiolucent-radiopaque lesion at the apex of the nonvital central incisor. The lesion was basically a pulpoperiapical lesion, and the rectangular radiopaque image was the mesial segment of the crown of the other central incisor, which had been broken off in a traumatic incident and driven up into the tissue. **E,** Several radiopaque foci (root canal–filling material) within a periapical radiolucency.   (**B** from Seeliger JE and Regneke JP: J Oral Surg 36:469-472, 1978. Copyright by the American Dental Association. Reprinted by permission. **C** courtesy K. Kennedy, DDS, Chicago. **E** courtesy M. Smulsen, DDS, Maywood, Ill.)   *Continued.*

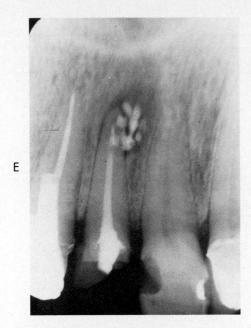

E

Fig.24-7, cont'd. For legend see opposite page.

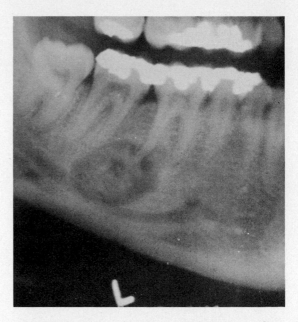

Fig. 24-8. Cementoblastoma in the intermediate stage at the apex of the distal root of the vital first molar tooth.   (Courtesy N. Barakat, DDS, Beirut, Lebanon.)

round and well marginated (Fig. 24-6). Seventy percent occur in the mandible, primarily in the premolar and molar region. The average age of patients with ossifying fibroma is 26.4 years, and the sexes are approximately equally affected (Hamner et al., 1968). These authors stated that the age range of patients was from 7 to 58 years. Eversole et al. (1985) reported on their study of 64 cases. They found a marked predilection for females and for the premolar and molar region of the mandible. The cementifying and ossifying fibromas usually occur as solitary entities, go unnoticed when small, and frequently reach a size of 2 to 4 cm in diameter, expanding the jaws as they grow.

Differential diagnosis

The differential diagnosis of cementifying and ossifying fibromas is discussed with the differential diagnosis of periapical cementomas.

Management

The usual periapical cementoma, which is not large enough to produce an expansion of the jawbone, does not require treatment. Nevertheless, the clinician should periodically examine such lesions radiographically to be certain that the mixed radiolucent-radiopaque area is not enlarging. If a good portion of a lesion has become calcified, this is an indication that the lesion is mature and is not likely to increase in size.

Few fibro-osseous lesions (PDLO) become large enough to produce an expansion of the cortical plate. Those that do should be conservatively enucleated, and the tissue should be microscopically examined to establish the final diagnosis. Attempts should be made to conserve teeth in the region. If an unusually large lesion is permitted to grow, pathologic fracture may become a threat. Sometimes, when the lesion is permitted to grow and expand peripherally until subjected to trauma, the overlying mucosa becomes ulcerated and a secondary osteomyelitis develops in the fibro-osseous lesion. Zachariades et al. (1984) reported on their series of 16 cases of ossifying fibroma that were treated by local excision or resection and bone graft; only one lesion recurred.

RARE PERIAPICAL MIXED LESIONS

There is a vast array of rare lesions and lesions that are common but rarely appear to be primarily associated with the periapex. For instance, a mixed periapical lesion seen at the root end of a tooth in a periapical film could represent a generalized condition such as sclerosing cemental masses or Paget's disease. Figs. 24-7 and 24-8 illustrate some of the rare mixed periapical lesions. Features of mixed radiolucent-radiopaque periapical lesions are shown in Table 24-1 (p. 510).

Table 24-1. Mixed radiolucent-radiopaque periapical lesions

Entity	Predominant sex	Predominant age	Predominant jaw	Predominant region	Distinguishing features
Calcifying crowns	M = F	Under 20	—	Tooth-bearing areas	Compare with appearance in contralateral and opposing arches
Tooth root with rarefying osteitis	M = F	10-60	—	80% posterior	Position of tooth root on preextraction radiograph
Rarefying and condensing osteitis	M = F	20-60	Mandible	Premolar-molar	—
Calcifying postsurgical bone defect	M	—	Mandible	—	History of surgery
Periapical cementoma	F—80%	Over 30	Mandible 90%	Tooth-bearing areas (especially anterior mandible)	Vital teeth; circular; size <1 cm; well-defined margins with radiolucent rim; often multiple
Cementifying and ossifying fibromas	M ~ F	Avg. = 26.4*	Mandible 70%	Premolar-molar	Circular; 2-5 cm; well marginated; solitary

~, Approximately equal.
*For ossifying fibroma.

Pericoronal mixed lesions

ODONTOMA—INTERMEDIATE STAGE

The odontoma is a benign tumor containing all the various component tissues of teeth. It is the most common odontogenic tumor, representing 67% of all odontogenic tumors in the series reported by Regezi et al. (1978). The odontoma seems to result from a budding of extra odontogenic epithelial cells from the dental lamina. This cluster of cells forms a large mass of tooth tissue that may be deposited in an abnormal arrangement but consists of normal enamel, dentin, cementum, and pulp.

The compound odontoma comprises odontogenic tissues laid down in a normal relationship, and the resulting structure bears considerable morphologic resemblance to teeth. When the tooth components are less well organized and toothlike structures are not formed, however, the lesion is termed a "complex" odontoma. Some tumors are a combination of both types (that is, they contain not only multiple toothlike structures but also calcified masses of dental tissue in haphazard arrangement). Such lesions are called "compound-complex" odontomas. Another type, the ameloblastic odontoma, is an uncommon tumor and basically represents what the name implies.

In its development the odontoma passes through the same stages as does a developing tooth. Thus, as the odontogenic tissues are laid down and proliferate, there is a resorption of bone so the lesion is radiolucent. An intermediate stage then follows; because of the partial calcification of the odontogenic tissues, this stage is characterized by a radiolucent-radiopaque image. This process continues to the most radiopaque stage, in which the calcification of the dental tissues is completed.

The early or intermediate stages of the developing odontoma are usually not seen or recognized as often as the late stage is, presumably because the earlier lesions are not clinically apparent. Also, the formation of odontomas begins in children when the natural

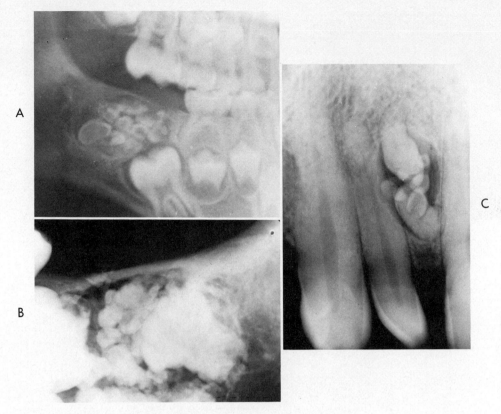

Fig. 24-9. Intermediate-stage odontoma. **A** and **C,** Compound odontoma. **A,** The washer effect is produced by partial calcification of the teeth. **B,** Compound-complex odontoma causing impaction of the molar.   (**A** courtesy M. Dettmer, DDS, Wheaton, Ill. **B** courtesy R. Latronica, DDS, Albany, N.Y.)

dentition is developing, and routine radiographs are rarely made of patients at this age. The intermediate or mixed radiolucent-radiopaque stage in the development of the odontoma is stressed in this chapter (Figs. 24-9 and 24-10). Features of mixed radiolucent-radiopaque pericoronal lesions are shown in Table 24-2 (p. 519).

Features

The most common complaint of a patient with an odontoma relates to the delayed eruption of a permanent tooth. Some odontomas, however, produce no accompanying symptoms and are discovered on routine radiographic examination.

The compound variety is more common than is the complex, and 62% of the compound variety occur in the maxilla, having a predilection for the incisor-canine region but no sex bias (Minderjahn, 1979). The complex odontoma, on the other hand, is more common in the mandible, and approximately 70% of these tumors are located in the first and second molar areas. Approximately 68% of complex odontomas occur in females (Minderjahn, 1979). Or and Yucetas (1987) also found that the compound type is more common (59.2%) but found that both types are more common in the mandible.

The majority of lesions are almost completely radiopaque when discovered in patients in their second and third decades; this consideration has led to the conclusion that the early and intermediate stages appear at a younger age. The lesions are nonaggressive; although most measure between 1 and 3 cm in diameter, occasionally one reaches a much larger size and causes extensive asymmetry of the jaw.

A complex odontoma frequently is situated between the crown of an unerupted tooth and the crest of the ridge, effectively blocking the tooth's eruption. For this reason the clinician should secure radiographs of the area when a tooth's eruption has been delayed. In the intermediate stage the complex odontoma may be seen as a mixed pericoronal lesion (Figs. 24-9 and 24-10).

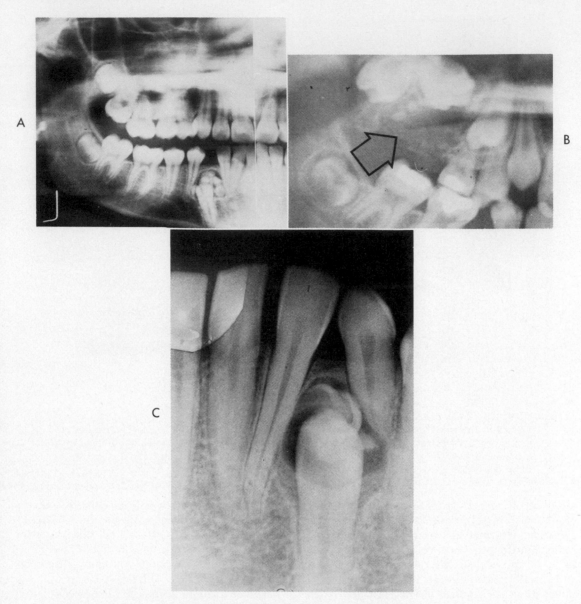

Fig. 24-10. Pericoronal intermediate-stage odontomas associated with an impacted mandibular canine. **B,** Minimal calcification has occurred in this odontoma *(arrow)* located pericoronally in the maxillary first and second molar region.   (**A** courtesy the late J. Ireland and J. Dolce, Chicago. **B** courtesy W. Schoenheider, DDS, Oak Lawn, Ill.)

On radiographs the intermediate-stage compound odontoma appears as a well-defined radiolucent lesion containing varying numbers of radiopaque (washerlike) cross sections of developing teeth and longitudinal, hollow radiopaque shadows of developing teeth (Figs. 24-9 and 24-10). The degree of calcification and opacity varies from stage to stage and from lesion to lesion. The complex odontoma appears on radiographs as a well-defined radiolucency with many radiopaque foci that vary greatly in size, shape, and prominence (Figs. 24-9 and 24-10).

The microscopic appearance of the compound odontoma corresponds to the histologic structure of normal teeth, whereas the intermediate stage of a complex odontoma reveals deposits of dentin, enamel, enamel matrix, cementum, and pulp tissue arranged in a completely haphazard relationship.

Differential diagnosis

The *compound odontoma* seldom presents a problem in differential diagnosis, even in the intermediate stage, because of its characteristic radiographic appearance. Despite this statement, however, on microscopic examination a particular tumor may show areas of ameloblastic proliferation and thus prove to be an *ameloblastic odontoma*. It is impossible to distinguish these two lesions by clinical or radiographic examination or on the basis of the history.

On the contrary, the *complex odontoma* in its intermediate stage may mimic several other lesions: fibro-osseous lesions (PDLO), calcifying odontogenic cyst, adenomatoid odontogenic tumor (intermediate stage), calcifying epithelial odontogenic tumor (CEOT), postsurgical calcifying bone defect, fibrous dysplasia, rarefying osteitis with condensing osteitis, and chronic osteomyelitis.

Chronic osteomyelitis and *rarefying osteitis* with *condensing osteitis* may be initially ruled out because of the absence of pain, tenderness, inflammation, drainage, or regional lymphadenopathy. The radiographic margins of these entities are usually poorly defined and roughly contoured, whereas the radiolucent borders of the complex odontoma are as well contoured and defined as the margins of a crypt about a developing tooth. Periodic radiographs of untreated infectious lesions frequently show the lesions to be increasing in size, whereas the complex odontoma does not increase in size after calcification of the odontogenic tissues has commenced.

Even when *fibrous dysplasia* appears mottled or has a smoky pattern on the radiograph, it has poorly defined borders, so it can be deemphasized as a possible diagnosis.

These comparisons narrow the clinician's working diagnosis to include fibro-osseous lesions (PDLO), calcifying odontogenic cyst, adenomatoid odontogenic tumor, CEOT, and postsurgical calcifying bony defect. All these entities produce well-defined radiolucencies containing radiopaque foci that may be located pericoronally.

The *postsurgical calcifying defect* is easily eliminated from consideration if there is no recent surgical procedure in the patient's history.

The *CEOT* (Pindborg tumor) is the rarest of these conditions. Unlike the odontoma, which develops in the first and second decades of life, the CEOT occurs at an average patient age of 40.41 years (Franklin and Pindborg, 1976). As with the complex odontoma, the molar region of the mandible is the preferred site and a large percentage are associated with unerupted teeth. In view of this information, a radiolucency with radiopaque foci associated with the crown of an unerupted mandibular molar tooth in a child or adolescent is much more likely to be an intermediate-stage odontoma than a CEOT. After a considerable amount of mineralization has taken place in the odontoma, the differentiation is easier to establish because the CEOT does not often produce large, dense masses of calcified tissue.

In its intermediate stage of development, the *adenomatoid odontogenic tumor* is radiographically indistinguishable from the fibro-osseous lesions (PDLO), the calcifying odontogenic cyst, and the complex odontoma; like the odontoma it occurs most often in the first two decades of life. Unlike the complex odontoma, however, which is relatively common and is most often found in the molar region of the mandible, the adenomatoid odontogenic tumor is not common and usually is found in the anterior maxilla.

The *calcifying odontogenic cyst*, like the adenomatoid odontogenic tumor, is not a common lesion. 75% of cysts occur anterior to the first molars; 47% occur in patients under 31 years of age. Like the complex odontoma, it has a predilection for the mandible. The aspiration test is often helpful in differentiating the calcifying odontogenic cyst from the odontoma. Whereas aspiration of a calcifying odontogenic cyst may yield a thick, granular, yellow fluid (keratin), aspiration of an odontoma is nonproductive.

In the intermediate stage of development, a *fibro-osseous lesion (PDLO)* shares several characteristics with a complex odontoma: both usually develop in the mandible, both are asymptomatic (except in unusual instances when they attain a large size), and both may have a similar radiographic appearance at this stage of development. The fibro-osseous lesion (PDLO), however, is usually situated in a more inferior position in the mandible and frequently appears as a periapical lesion, whereas the complex odontoma is usually situated in a more superior position between the crown of a tooth and the crest of the ridge. The periapical cementoma is seen more in women over 30 years of age, and the intermediate-stage complex odontoma is seen in patients under 30 years of age; these characteristics further contribute to the differential diagnosis.

Management

Because of its capsule of peripheral fibrous connective tissue, which is really the follicle or periodontal ligament of the abnormal dental structure, the odontoma is easily enucleated. Such treatment is curative. Nevertheless, suitable periodic postoperative examination is necessary to ensure that complete healing has taken place. Microscopic examination is especially necessary to ensure the diagnosis.

ADENOMATOID ODONTOGENIC TUMOR

The adenomatoid odontogenic tumor is an uncommon odontogenic tumor that may undergo different stages of development. Regezi et al. (1978) reported that it represented 3% of their series of odontogenic tumors. It may occur as a well-circumscribed radiolucency, or it may contain radiopaque foci. The lesion is discussed in detail in Chapter 16, where its peri-

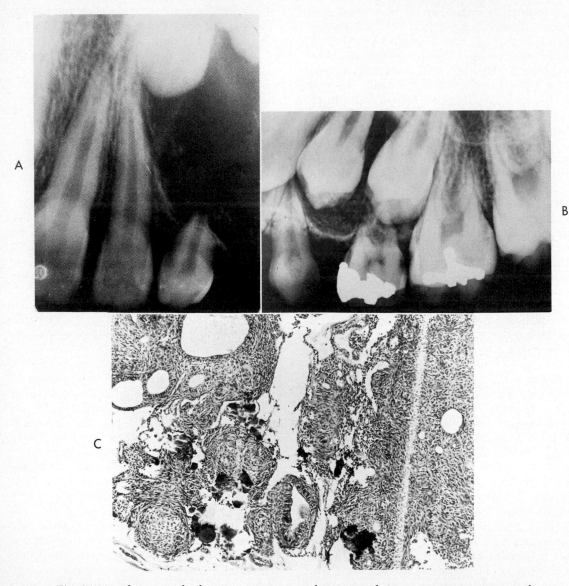

Fig. 24-11. Adenomatoid odontogenic tumors in the intermediate stage seen as pericoronal radiolucencies with radiopaque foci. **A,** In the maxillary canine region. **B,** Different case in the upper premolar region. **C,** Photomicrograph of adenomatoid odontogenic tumor. Dark foci of calcified material are evident. (**A** courtesy K. Giedt, Aberdeen, S.D. **B** from Abrams AM, Melrose JR, and Howell FV: Cancer 22:175-185, 1968.)

coronal radiolucent appearance is stressed. The mixed radiolucent-radiopaque stage is emphasized in this chapter.

Features

The adenomatoid odontogenic tumor is a slow-growing lesion that occurs most often in patients between 10 and 30 years of age. Approximately 95% occur in the anterior regions of the jaws (65% in the maxilla), and 75% are associated with an impacted tooth (most often a canine). Approximately 65% of the lesions occur in women and girls. A delayed eruption of a permanent tooth or a regional swelling of the jaws may be the first symptom. Pain or other neurologic signs are not characteristic.

On radiographs the adenomatoid odontogenic tumor is a pericoronal cystlike radiolucency that mimics the radiographic appearance of a dentigerous cyst. In the maturing stage (which represents 65% of the lesions reviewed by Gargiulo et al. [1974]) sharply defined radiopaque foci are seen within the radiolucency (Fig. 24-11).

On microscopic examination small deposits of calcified material are present and scattered over a background of odontogenic cells that form cords and swirls of ductlike structures and pseudoacini (Fig. 24-11).

Differential diagnosis

The differential diagnosis of the adenomatoid odontogenic tumor is discussed in the section on the differential diagnosis of the odontoma. The lesions most often confused with the adenomatoid odontogenic tumor are the *keratinizing and calcifying odontogenic cyst*, the *intermediate-stage odontoma*, and the *CEOT*.

Management

The adenomatoid odontogenic tumor is readily enucleated; recurrences are rare.

KERATINIZING AND CALCIFYING ODONTOGENIC CYST

The keratinizing and calcifying odontogenic cyst is considered to occupy a position between a cyst and an odontogenic tumor—having some characteristics of both. This entity accounted for 2% of all the odontogenic tumors reported by Regezi et al. (1978). In its early stages of development, this cystic keratinizing tumor is completely radiolucent, but later the radiolucency contains scattered radiopaque foci (Fig. 24-12). When it occurs in a dentigerous cyst position, it appears as a pericoronal radiolucency with radiopaque foci.

Features

The keratinizing and calcifying odontogenic cyst is a slow-growing, completely benign condition. Freedman et al. (1975) found that it occurred with equal frequency in the maxilla and mandible and 54.2% occurred in females. These authors reported that the calcifying odontogenic cyst was much more common in females under the age of 41, whereas in patients over the age of 41 it was much more common in males. Their review of cases showed that 47% occurred in patients under 31 years of age and that 75% of the lesions were situated anterior to the first molar teeth. The cyst may vary in size and enlarge sufficiently to expand the mandible.

Most of the lesions are intrabony, but some occur in the soft tissues and may cause a saucering of the adjacent bone. The lesions are usually cystic, and aspiration may yield a viscous, granular, yellow fluid. Nagao et al. (1983) searched the Japanese literature on the calcifying odontogenic cyst and discovered 23 reported cases. The cysts occurred equally in males and females whose mean age was 21 years. Unerupted teeth and root resorption were observed in about one half of the cases.

The radiographic appearance is of a cystlike radiolucency containing quite distinct radiopaque foci (Figs. 24-7 and 24-12), although a considerable number do not show radiopaque foci because the calcifications are still too small to show on radiographs. Radiolucencies may be unilocular or multilocular, and some are not cystic but solid (McGowan and Browne, 1982).

The microscopic appearance is unique for an oral lesion and has some characteristics of the calcifying epithelioma of Malherbe (which occurs in the skin). The basal cells are low, cuboidal or columnar cells with dark, large nuclei. The cells above the basal layer are irregular in arrangement and surround nests or sheets of large, epithelial ghost cells filled with atypical-appearing keratin. Some of these nests of ghost cells calcify (Fig. 24-12); when they reach a sufficient size, they become recognizable as radiopaque foci in the radiolucent lesion.

Differential diagnosis

Because of its radiographic appearance, the keratinizing and calcifying odontogenic cyst is most frequently confused with the partially calcified odontoma, the calcifying epithelial odontogenic tumor, and an adenomatoid odontogenic tumor. The differentiating features of these lesions are discussed in the section on the differential diagnosis of the odontoma.

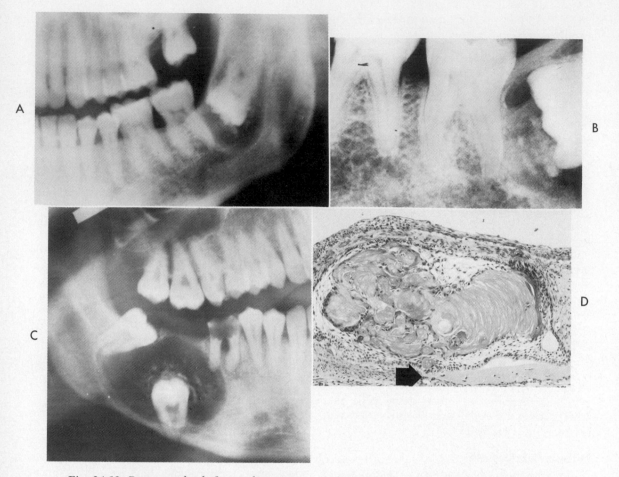

Fig. 24-12. Pericoronal calcifying odontogenic cysts with radiopaque foci within the cystlike radiolucency (**A** and **B** are the same case). **C,** Panograph of different calcifying odontogenic cyst. **D,** Photomicrograph of calcifying and keratinizing odontogenic cyst. Nodular formation of keratin and ghost cells within the epithelium of the cyst wall is evident. Calcified tissue can be observed at the inferior aspect *(arrow).*   (**A** and **B** courtesy R. Latronica, DDS, Albany, N.Y. **C** courtesy W. Schoenheider, DDS, Oak Lawn, Ill. **D** courtesy S.O. Raibley, DDS, Maywood, Ill.)

Management

Since the keratinizing and calcifying odontogenic cyst has a tendency for continued growth, surgical enucleation is the treatment of choice. Recurrences occur on occasion (McGowan and Browne, 1982; Slootweg and Koole, 1980).

AMELOBLASTIC FIBRO-ODONTOMA

Ameloblastic fibro-odontomas are benign mixed odontogenic tumors that contain cords and nests of odontogenic epithelium and also some calcified odontogenic tissue in a myxomatous stroma. Slootweg (1981) considered this lesion an immature complex odontoma. Gardner (1984), although recognizing the difficulty in some cases of differentiating between the true ameloblastic fibro-odontoma and the developing odontoma on a histologic basis, does not believe that these two are the same entity. This tumor represented 2% of the odontogenic tumors reported by Regezi et al. (1978).

Features

Minderjahn reviewed statistics of the ameloblastic fibro-odontoma in 1979 and reported the following: patients in the first two decades of life most commonly had this lesion, with the average patient age being 12 years; a preponderance of the patients were males (63%); the mandible had a slightly higher incidence, and the most commonly affected site was the premolar and molar region.

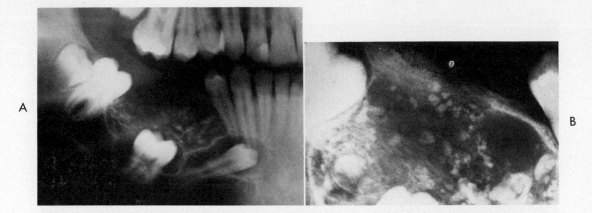

Fig. 24-13. Ameloblastic fibro-odontoma. **A,** Panorex radiograph. **B,** Periapical view. The radiopaque foci within the radiolucency are associated with the crown of the impacted first molar.   (From Curran JB, Owen D, and Lanoway J: J Can Dent Assoc 46:314-316, 1980.)

The ameloblastic fibro-odontoma is frequently located in a position pericoronal to an imbedded tooth and is initially completely radiolucent, but it acquires increasingly prominent radiopaque foci as the hard dental tissues within it become mineralized (Fig. 24-13).

Differential diagnosis

The pericoronal variety of ameloblastic fibro-odontoma must be included in the differential diagnosis of such lesions as the intermediate stage odontoma, the calcifying odontogenic cyst, the adenomatoid odontogenic tumor, and the calcifying epithelial odontogenic tumor.

Management

The ameloblastic fibro-odontoma is a benign, well-encapsulated tumor that should be conservatively enucleated. Even though it does not show a tendency to recur, patient follow-up is necessary.

CALCIFYING EPITHELIAL ODONTOGENIC TUMOR (PINDBORG TUMOR)

The calcifying epithelial odontogenic tumor (CEOT) is considered rare, representing approximately 1% of odontogenic tumors (Franklin and Pindborg, 1976; Regezi et al., 1978). It may have several radiographic appearances: (1) a pericoronal radiolucency, (2) a pericoronal radiolucency with radiopaque foci (Fig. 24-14), (3) a mixed radiolucent-radiopaque lesion not associated with an unerupted tooth, (4) a "driven snow" appearance, and (5) a dense radiopacity (occasionally). In their extensive review, Franklin and Pindborg (1976) reported

that the most common pictures were that of a pericoronal radiolucency and of diffuse radiopacities within radiolucent areas.

Features

From a review of 113 cases, Franklin and Pindborg (1976) reported the following statistics. All but five of the lesions were intraosseous. The intrabony lesion occurred in patients from 9 to 92 years of age, and the mean age at initial diagnosis was 40.41 years. Males and females were equally affected. Sixty-eight percent of the tumors occurred in the mandible, with a marked predilection for the molar region of the mandible (Fig. 24-14). The molar region of the maxilla and the premolar region of the mandible were the next most common sites. Fifty-two percent of the cases were undoubtedly associated with an unerupted tooth. The CEOT commonly occurred as a painless, slowly increasing expansion of the jaws. Small lesions were usually entirely asymptomatic.

Microscopic study shows abundant sheets of polyhedral epithelial cells, which usually have prominent intracellular bridges. A variable amount of pleomorphism is present, but rarely are there mitotic figures (Fig. 24-14, *C*). Circular areas within these epithelial cells are filled with a homogeneous eosinophilic material. This eosinophilic material becomes calcified and follows a pattern of concentric deposition known as Liesegang's rings.

Differential diagnosis

The differential diagnosis of the pericoronal radiolucent-radiopaque image of CEOT is in-

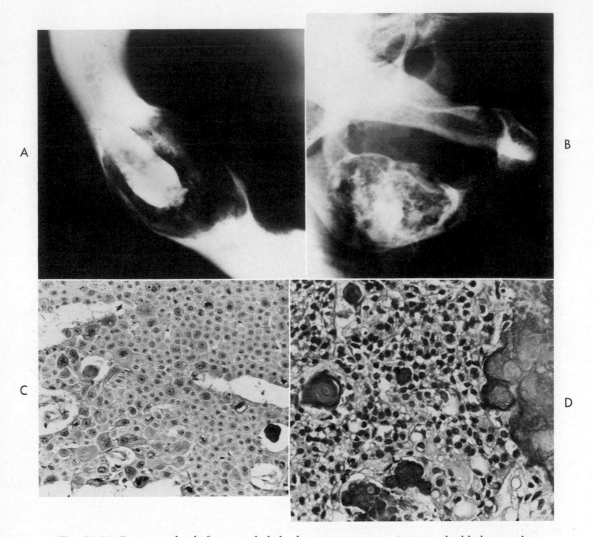

Fig. 24-14. Pericoronal calcifying epithelial odontogenic tumor. **A,** An embedded premolar tooth and small radiopaque foci are seen within the radiolucency in this occlusal view of the mandible of a 57-year-old man. **B,** Lateral oblique radiograph of a 77-year-old woman showing a mixed radiolucent-radiopaque image in association with an embedded molar tooth. **C** and **D,** Photomicrographs of calcifying epithelial odontogenic tumor. The pleomorphism of epithelial cells is evident in **C. D,** Clear epithelial cells and calcified material can be seen. (**A** and **B** from Franklin CD and Hindle MO: Br J Oral Surg 13:230-238, 1976. **D** courtesy S.O. Raibley, DDS, Maywood, Ill.)

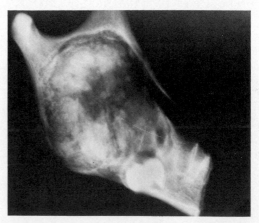

Fig. 24-15. Odontogenic fibroma. Radiograph of a surgical specimen shows the well-defined borders of the fibroma and the displaced third molar. The radiopacities were caused by the density and thickness of the fibrous tumor. No calcifications were present in this lesion.

cluded in the discussion of the differential diagnosis of the odontoma.

Management

Surgical excision that includes a satisfactory border of apparently normal tissue is the recommended treatment for the CEOT. The recurrence rate is considerably lower than that of the ameloblastoma; however, careful patient follow-up is mandatory.

ODONTOGENIC FIBROMA

The central odontogenic fibroma is a rare, poorly understood, benign lesion that is thought to originate from cells of the periodontal ligament or other segments of the odontogenic apparatus. The lesions consist of fibrous tissue containing nests of odontogenic epithelium and, frequently, calcified material that resembles cementum droplets. The hard deposits are apparent as radiopaque foci if they are large enough and adequately mineralized; otherwise the lesion may be completely radiolucent.

Despite the absence of calcification, some central lesions have a hazy radiopaque pattern caused by the areas of dense fibrous tissue in a lesion of considerable buccolingual dimension.

Features

The odontogenic fibroma usually occurs in patients under 40 years of age, shows no sex predilection, and is found more commonly in the mandible. It is a slow-growing lesion and does not cause pain or other neurologic symp-

Table 24-2. Mixed radiolucent-radiopaque pericoronal lesions

Entity	Predominant sex	Predominant age	Predominant jaw	Predominant region	Distinguishing features
Odontoma compound	M ~ F	5-20	Maxilla 62%	Incisor; canine	Radiolucent, smooth contours with well-defined radiopaque washers within
Odontoma complex	F—68%	5-20	Mandible	Molars—70% first, second; usually supracoronal	Radiolucent, smooth contours with well-defined, patternless radiopacities within; unerupted tooth
Adenomatoid odontogenic tumor	F:M = 2:1	Median = 16.5	Maxilla 65%	95% anterior of jaws 65% in canine areas	Pericoronal radiolucency—75%; often, small radiopaque foci
Keratinizing and calcifying odontogenic cyst	Overall— M ~ F F—< age 41 M—> age 41	47% under 31	Maxilla – mandible	75% anterior to first molar	Viscous yellow aspirate
Ameloblastic fibro-odontoma	M—63%	5-20 Avg. = 12	Mandible ~ maxilla	Premolar-molar	
Calcifying epithelial odontogenic tumor	M ~ F	Avg. = 40.41	Mandible 68%	1. Mandibular molar 2. Maxillary molar; mandibular premolar	At least 52% associated with unerupted tooth
Odontogenic fibroma	M = F	Under 40	Mandible	Tooth-bearing regions	

~, Approximately equal.

toms. It may grow large enough to expand or even destroy the cortical plate and cause facial asymmetry.

Central odontogenic fibromas appear as well-defined radiolucencies, perhaps containing radiopaque foci, and may cause spreading and migration of teeth in the region where they occur; characteristically they do not cause root resorption (Fig. 24-15).

Occasionally a completely radiolucent central odontogenic fibroma occurs on radiographs as a pericoronal radiolucency and mimics a follicular cyst. A central odontogenic fibroma with a combined radiolucent-radiopaque appearance, on the other hand, resembles a calcifying odontogenic cyst.

The central odontogenic fibroma may be confused with a calcifying odontogenic cyst, an intermediate-stage odontoma, a benign, inter-mediate-stage fibro-osseous lesion (PDLO), an adenomatoid odontogenic tumor, a CEOT, or a calcifying postsurgical bone defect.

Management

Complete enucleation and microscopic examination of the surgical specimen is the required treatment for an odontogenic fibroma.

RARITIES

Virtually any mixed radiolucent-radiopaque lesion that occurs in the jaw may contact the crown of an unerupted tooth and so appear as a mixed pericoronal lesion. Because of the many unerupted teeth in the jaws of patients under 15 years of age, a greater incidence of such an "accidental" appearance can be expected during these early years. Fig. 24-16 illustrates two examples of the rare cystic odontoma.

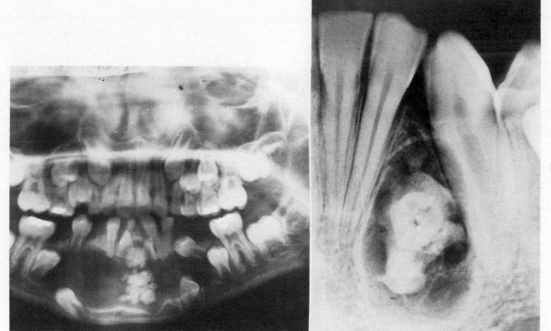

Fig. 24-16. Cystic odontomas. **A,** Orthopantomograph showing an odontoma within a large dentigerous cyst. **B,** Cystic odontoma in an intraradicular location between the lateral incisor and canine tooth.   (**A** courtesy the late M. Kaminski, DDS, and S. Atsaves, DDS, Chicago. **B** courtesy W. Kinsler, DDS, Chicago.)

REFERENCES

Eversole LR, Leider AS, and Nelson K: Ossifying-fibroma: a clinicopathologic study of sixty-four cases, Oral Surg 60:505-511, 1985.

Franklin CD and Pindborg JJ: The calcifying epithelial odontogenic tumor, Oral Surg 42:753-765, 1976.

Freedman PD, Lumerman H, and Gee JK: Calcifying odontogenic cyst, Oral Surg 40:93-106, 1975.

Gardner DG: The mixed odontogenic tumors, Oral Surg 58:166-168, 1984.

Gargiulo EA, Ziter WD, Mastrocola R, and Ballard BR: Odontogenic adenomatoid tumor (adenoameloblastoma): report of case and review of the literature, J Oral Surg 32:286-290, 1974.

Hamner JE, Scofield HH, and Cornyn J: Benign fibro-osseous jaw lesions of periodontal membrane origin, Cancer 22:861-878, 1968.

Marmary Y and Kutiner G: A radiographic survey of periapical jawbone lesions, Oral Surg 61:405-408, 1986.

McGowan RH and Browne RM: The calcifying odontogenic cyst: a problem of preoperative diagnosis, Br J Oral Surg 20:203-212, 1982.

Minderjahn A: Incidence and clinical differentiation of odontogenic tumors, J Maxillofac Surg 7:142-150, 1979.

Nagao T, Nakajima T, Fukushima M, et al: Calcifying odontogenic cyst: a survey of 23 cases in the Japanese literature, J Maxillofac Surg 11:174-179, 1983.

Neville BW and Albenesius RJ: The prevalence of benign fibro-osseous lesions of periodontal ligament origin in black women: a radiographic survey, Oral Surg 62:340-344, 1986.

Or S and Yucetas S: Compound and complex odontomas, Int J Maxillofac Surg 16:596-599, 1987.

Regezi JA, Kerr DA, and Courtney RM: Odontogenic tumors: analysis of 760 cases, J Oral Surg 36:771-778, 1978.

Slootweg PJ: An analysis of the interrelationship of the mixed odontogenic tumors—ameloblastic fibroma, ameloblastic fibro-odontoma, and the odontomas, Oral Surg 51:266-276, 1981.

Slootweg PJ and Koole R: Recurrent calcifying odontogenic cyst, J Maxillofac Surg 8:143, 1980.

Waldron CA: Fibro-osseous lesions of the jaws, J Oral Maxillofac Surg 43:249-262, 1985.

Waldron CA and Giansanti JS: Benign fibro-osseous lesions of the jaws: a clinical-radiologic-histologic review of sixty-five cases. I. Fibrous dysplasia of the jaws, Oral Surg 35:190-201, 1973a.

Waldron CA and Giansanti JS: Benign fibro-osseous lesions of the jaws: a clinical-radiologic-histologic review of sixty-five cases. II. Benign fibro-osseous lesions of periodontal ligament origin, Oral Surg 35:340-350, 1973b.

Zachariades N, Vairaktaris E, Papanicolaou S, et al: Ossifying fibroma, Int J Oral Surg 13:1-6, 1984.

25

Mixed radiolucent-radiopaque lesions not necessarily contacting teeth

NORMAN K. WOOD
PAUL W. GOAZ

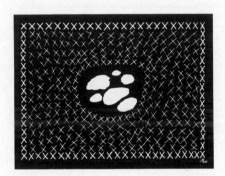

The following list is composed of mixed radiolucent-radiopaque lesions that are not necessarily associated with teeth:

Ossifying postsurgical bone defect
Chronic osteomyelitis
Osteoradionecrosis
Fibrous dysplasia
Paget's disease—intermediate stage
Cementifying and ossifying fibromas
Osteogenic sarcoma
Osteoblastic metastatic carcinoma
Chondroma and chondrosarcoma
Ossifying subperiosteal hematoma
Rarities
  Adenomatoid odontogenic tumor
  Ameloblastic fibrodentinoma
  Ameloblastic fibro-odontoma
  Ameloblastoma (bone-forming component)
  Calcifying epithelial odontogenic tumor
  Central hemangioma
  Ewing's sarcoma
  Intrabony hamartoma
  Keratinizing and calcifying odontogenic cyst
  Lymphoma of bone
  Malignant tumors with superimposed
    osteomyelitis
  Sclerosing cemental masses
  Odontodysplasia
  Odontoma (intermediate)
  Osteoblastoma (intermediate)
  Osteoid osteoma

OSSIFYING POSTSURGICAL BONE DEFECT

Frequently, when central benign pathoses have been enucleated and the surgical wounds closed, primary healing takes place through ossification of the surgically produced hematoma, which is then slowly transformed to normal bone under favorable conditions. A radiograph taken shortly after the surgery shows a well-defined homogeneous radiolucency. If the radiograph is made later when some calcification of the hematoma has taken place, the previously well-defined homogeneous radiolucency contains many poorly defined radiopaque foci (Fig. 25-1).

Sometimes the appearance can be best described as a coarse salt-and-pepper image. At other times the radiopacities seem to concentrate in separate hazy aggregations and may present a puzzling picture if the clinician is not cognizant of the recent surgical procedure (Fig. 25-1, *B*). Later, as the calcification progresses and includes the entire defect, the radiographic image illustrates the unstructured development of the poorly calcified new bone, in contrast to the regular trabecular pattern of the adjacent normal bone. This unordered bone is usually remodeled to a normal architecture under the influence of internal stresses induced by the masticatory forces.

When bone marrow or chips have been implanted as graft material in a postsurgical defect, many radiopaque images of varying shape and size, not unlike those just described for a normally calcifying defect, can be seen in the radiolucent wound (Fig. 25-1, *A*).

Differential diagnosis and management

A recent history of a lesion enucleated in the area in question should establish the identity of postsurgical calcifying defect. Nevertheless, the clinician must always consider the possibility of a recurrent pathosis, especially when the initial lesion was aggressive. If there is any question, frequent and careful periodic clinical and radiographic examinations are in order. This precaution is recommended for all surgical cases but is especially important when the initial lesion was invasive and destructive.

CHRONIC OSTEOMYELITIS

Chronic osteomyelitis is discussed in Chapter 21, which focuses on the totally radiolucent type. In this chapter the mixed radiolucent-radiopaque appearance is emphasized.

Osteomyelitis rarely occurs without the presence of a predisposing condition such as uncontrolled debilitating systemic disease, sclerosing disease of the jawbones in which the vascular supply is compromised (for example, Paget's disease, osteopetrosis, diffuse cementosis, postirradiation stages), and inadequate reduction of jaw fractures or inadequate surgical enucleation of pathoses. The maxilla is rarely affected because of its more fragile bone pattern and richer blood supply.

Features

Clinical examination shows signs of infection, which may include inflammation, tenderness, pain, swelling, a draining sinus, regional lymphadenopathy, leukocytosis, and an increased erythrocyte sedimentation rate. Nonvital bone fragments or sections of jawbone may protrude from an ulcerated mucosal or cutaneous surface.

The radiographic appearance of chronic osteomyelitis is most often a mixed radiolucent-radiopaque image. In many cases the borders

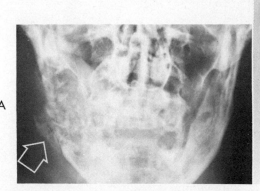
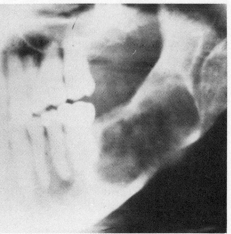

Fig. 25-1. **A,** Enucleated cyst cavity grafted with autogenous bone chips *(arrow)*. **B,** Mixed radiolucent-radiopaque appearance of a residual cyst as the cavity begins to ossify after surgical enucleation. (**A** courtesy O.H. Stuteville, DDS, MD, St. Joe, Ark. **B** courtesy W. Heaton, DDS, Chicago.)

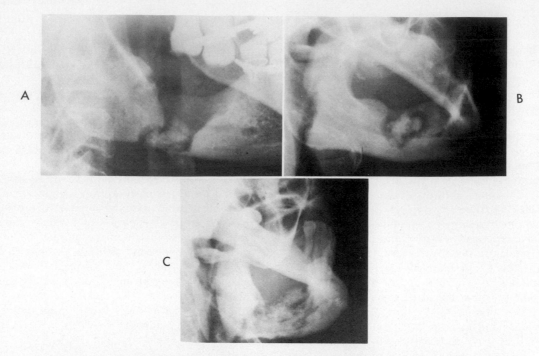

Fig. 25-2. Chronic osteomyelitis showing sequestra. **A,** The patient had a compound fracture. **B** and **C,** The patients had uncontrolled diabetes. (**B** courtesy O.H. Stuteville, DDS, MD, St. Joe, Ark. **C** courtesy E. Palacios, MD, Maywood, Ill.)

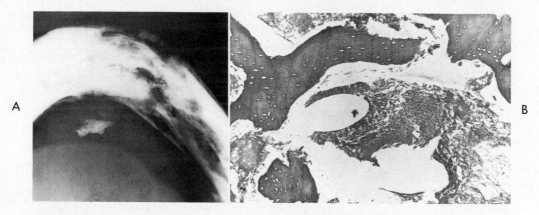

Fig. 25-3. Chronic osteomyelitis. **A,** Lesion in the mandible. **B,** Empty lacunae in nonvital trabeculae surrounded by necrotic material. (**A** courtesy S. Blackman, BDS, Chicago.)

are ragged and poorly defined, but in others they are well defined (Figs. 25-2 to 25-6). The radiolucent areas usually consist of infected granulation tissue containing areas of necrosis or fibrosis or both. The radiopaque areas represent sclerosed, often nonvital bone or sequestra or both (Fig. 25-3). Proliferative periostitis, discussed in Chapter 28, may show an alternating radiolucent-radiopaque. laminated appearance at the surface of the affected bone (Fig. 25-5).

Differential diagnosis

The differential diagnosis of chronic osteomyelitis is covered in the discussion of fibrous dysplasia. The lesions most frequently confused with chronic osteomyelitis are fibro-osseous lesions of periodontal ligament origin (PDLO), mottled-type lesion of fibrous dysplasia, rarefying and condensing osteitis, Paget's disease, malignant tumors that can produce a ragged radiolucent-radiopaque pattern (osteogenic sar-

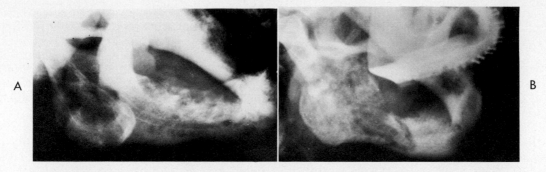

Fig. 25-4. Osteoradionecrosis. Characteristically, a large section of the mandible is involved with the ill-defined destructive process. Both patients had received radiation for squamous cell carcinoma of the oral cavity.   (**A** courtesy R. Kallal, DDS, Chicago. **B** courtesy O.H. Stuteville, DDS, MD, St. Joe, Ark.)

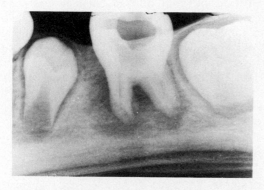

Fig. 25-5. Proliferative periostitis, formerly termed Garré's osteomyelitis, in an 11-year-old child. Rarefaction is evident at the periapices of the first molar. The periostitis at the inferior border of the mandible has produced alternate light and dark (less calcified) laminations.   (Courtesy N. Barakat, DDS, Beirut, Lebanon.)

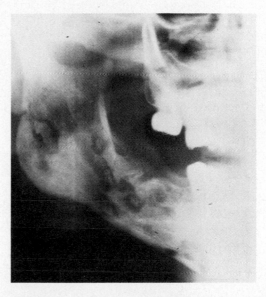

Fig. 25-6. Unusual appearance of the right ramus and body of the mandible produced by osteomyelitis.   (Courtesy A. Indresano, DDS, Cleveland, and P. O'Flaherty, DDS, Chicago.)

coma, chondrosarcoma, osteoblastic metastatic carcinoma, lymphoma of bone, Ewing's tumor), and a secondarily infected bone tumor.

A secondarily infected bone tumor and chronic osteomyelitis are indistinguishable by clinical or radiographical examination or by the patient interview. Incidence alone, however, favors a diagnosis of osteomyelitis.

Management

The management of chronic osteomyelitis is discussed in detail in Chapter 21. Basically it involves controlling the underlying systemic disease (if present), administering the proper antibiotic, performing incision, irrigation, saucerization, and sequestrectomy (if necessary), and possibly giving hyperbaric oxygen treatments (Mainous et al., 1973).

OSTEORADIONECROSIS

Osteoradionecrosis is generally regarded as a disease condition of both hard and soft tissue after irradiation of the region. It is characterized by hypovascular, hypocellular, and hypoxic tissue that has a diminished capacity for normal repair (Holmes et al., 1989; Marx, 1983a, 1983b; Marx and Johnson, 1987). This tissue and its overlying mucosa may break down, leading to superficial infection of the denuded bone.

The disease may be asymptomatic in its early stages if the overlying mucosa remains intact. When ulceration of the surface mucosa occurs, tenderness and pain are a common complaint.

In a full-blown case, radiographs show a mixed radiolucent-radiopaque lesion over a significant region of the jawbone (Fig. 25-4).

Prevention and management

The oral tissues, especially the teeth and the periodontia, should be maintained in excellent health if possible. Most authors recommend the extraction of condemned teeth at least 10 to 14 days before radiographs are made (Beumer et al., 1983a, 1983b; Marciani and Ownby, 1986; Starcke and Shannon, 1977). Hyperbaric oxygenation has been an effective treatment modality because it promotes angiogenesis. Marx et al. (1983a, 1983b, 1985, 1987) recommended hyperbaric oxygenation with aggressive surgery in a progressively staged manner for treating osteoradionecrosis. Epstein et al. (1987) also recommended hyperbaric oxygenation and proposed a classification of osteoradionecrosis.

FIBROUS DYSPLASIA

Fibrous dysplasia is a poorly understood benign disturbance of bone that, although classified as a benign fibro-osseous disease, is currently considered by most oral pathologists to arise from specific bone-forming mesenchyme and to be a separate entity from the benign fibro-osseous lesions of PDLO (Waldron, 1985; Waldron and Giansanti, 1973a, 1973b). Essentially this lesion comprises varying proportions of fibrous tissue and spicules of bone.

The radiographic appearance of fibrous dysplasia varies considerably, and the density of the lesions ranges from relatively radiolucent to quite radiopaque. The lesions are seldom spherical but rather are usually elongated or elliptic, especially in the mandible (Fig. 25-7). The shape of the lesions that extend into the maxillary sinus is influenced by the configuration of this chamber.

The lesions may be unilocular or multilocular, and their borders are usually poorly defined because of the gradual blending of the altered bone with the adjacent normal pattern. This transitional zone is often more than 1 cm wide. The density of the lesion varies with the proportion of fibrous to osseous tissue, which relates to the lesion's stage of development.

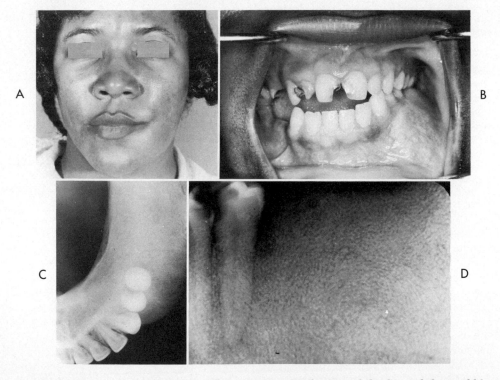

Fig. 25-7. Fibrous dysplasia, intermediate stage. **A,** Deformity of the lower left mandible, producing facial asymmetry. **B,** Smoothly contoured expansion of the left mandible, which caused malocclusion. **C,** Occlusal radiograph showing a fusiform expansion of the left mandible with a ground-glass appearance. Characteristically, the anterior border of the lesion is indistinct. **D,** Periapical radiograph showing the ground-glass pattern.

Three basic patterns are usually described:

1. An early primarily osteolytic fibrous stage that may be completely radiolucent
2. An intermediate stage recognizable by its smoky, hazy, or mottled radiolucent-radiopaque pattern (Fig. 25-8), which is produced by poorly defined aggregates of small spicules of bone distributed throughout the radiolucent area (Occasionally, radiopaque areas in this pattern have a ground-glass appearance or the complete lesion has a moderately opaque ground-glass pattern; Fig. 25-7.)
3. A more mature phase that is variously described as having a salt-and-pepper, ground-glass, or orange peel appearance, and that varies in opaqueness depending on the number, size, and radiographic distinctness of the trabeculae

The lesions with the mottled radiolucent-radiopaque appearance are emphasized in this chapter because they are considered more immature than those having the uniformly opaque, ground-glass appearance.

Features

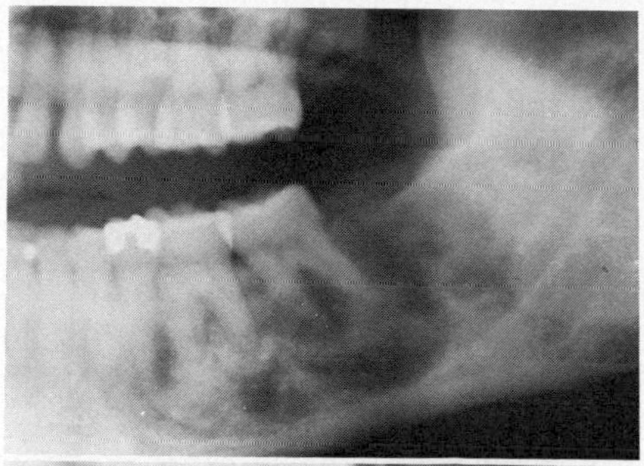

Fibrous dysplasia of the facial bones has characteristics and behavior patterns different from those of fibrous dysplasia involving other bones; consequently it should be considered a separate entity.

Aside from the lesions accompanying Albright's syndrome, fibrous dysplasia usually occurs as a solitary (monostotic) lesion in the mandible but frequently involves the maxilla, zygoma, and sphenoid as a unit (Figs. 25-7 and 25-8). The maxilla is involved by a solitary lesion slightly more often than the mandible. The zygoma and the maxillary sinus may also be affected, but the anterior maxilla and the mandibular symphysis appear to be immune. Men and women are affected equally.

The lesion grows slowly, finally causing a fusiform expansion of the jaw and a nontender facial asymmetry. As a rule the lesion stops growing when skeletal growth ceases as growth hormone declines to adult levels (Hall et al., 1984). Like most benign conditions originating beneath the surface epithelium, the expansion is smooth and covered with normal-appearing mucosa or skin. Surface ulcerations are uncommon but may be seen when the mass intrudes on the occlusion. Pain or paresthesia is unusual. Teeth in the involved segment may show minimal migration or displacement but characteristically are not loosened. Serum chemistry values are within normal limits because of the slow growth.

The region of hazy radiopaque-radiolucent mottling is often somewhat rectangular and is seen in younger patients (Fig. 25-8). Sometimes the radiopaque foci are dense, but usually they will have a ground-glass appearance. Minor displacement of teeth or divergence of roots may be present, and occasionally whole segments of teeth appear to have moved. Root resorption is not a feature.

On microscopic examination the proportions of fibrous tissue and bone vary from lesion to lesion, as do the size and distribution of the bony aggregations. This accounts for the diverse radiographic appearances. Fibrous tissue predominates in the more radiolucent areas, and if bony trabeculae are present, they are too small or inadequately mineralized to show as radiopaque foci. The ground-glass areas consist of small bony trabeculae of approximately equal size, many of which are radiographically appar-

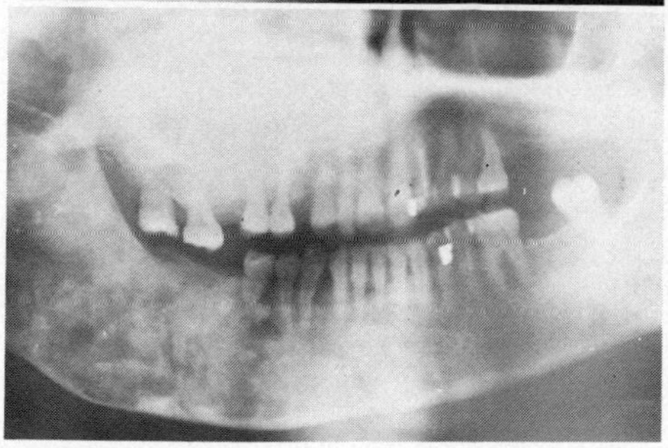

Fig. 25-8. Fibrous dysplasia, intermediate stage. **A,** A smoky or mottled radiopacity (seen also in **B**) is evident within the radiolucency. **B,** The radiograph shows one lesion in the maxilla and one in the mandible. Polyostotic types in the jaws are unusual unless they accompany Albright's syndrome. The mottled pattern seen in the mandibular lesion in **B** is similar to the mottled pattern evident in the skull of a patient with Paget's disease (Fig. 25-9). (**A** courtesy S. Atsaves, DDS, Chicago. **B** courtesy N. Barakat, DDS, Beirut, Lebanon.)

ent. The dense radiopaque areas are made up of larger trabeculae with less intervening fibrous tissue. The fibrous stroma varies in cellularity and amounts of collagen present. The trabecular margins usually show what appears to be a streaming of collagen fiber bundles from the bone into the stroma.

The majority of the bony trabeculae are composed of woven bone (not the lamellar type laid down in haversian systems) on which osteoblastic rimming is not usually seen (Waldron and Giansanti, 1973a). As the lesion becomes more mature, spicules of lamellar bone with osteoblastic rimming appear.

Albright's syndrome occurs in girls and is characterized by precocious sexual development, multiple bones affected with lesions of fibrous dysplasia (polyostotic), and café-au-lait spots on the skin and oral mucosa.

Hall et al. (1984) reported an interesting case in which growth of the bony lesions in a boy became dormant as the patient reached adulthood and were reactivated during the patient's middle thirties because of a pituitary adenoma.

Differential diagnosis

The mottled type of fibrous dysplasia must be differentiated from chronic osteomyelitis, ossifying and cementifying fibromas, Paget's disease, osteosarcoma, osteoblastic metastatic carcinoma, chondrosarcoma, Ewing's sarcoma, and lymphomas of bone. The well-circumscribed entities such as a healing surgical defect, intermediate-stage odontoma, and other odontogenic lesions should not be a differential problem.

Lymphomas of bone are rare and may be seen as poorly defined rarefactions, perhaps with a few septa of bone left intact, which give a multilocular appearance. Other lymphomas may exhibit both osteoblastic activity and bone resorption and hence produce a mixed radiolucent-radiopaque appearance (see Fig. 25-18). The pattern is much more irregular and bizarre than that seen in the mottled lesion of fibrous dysplasia. Also, smooth, well-contoured external bony borders are always maintained in fibrous dysplasia on both clinical and radiographic examination. This is almost never the case in extensive malignancies or osteomyelitis.

Chondrosarcoma is an uncommon malignant tumor of the jaws that usually affects a much older age-group (30 to 60 years) than fibrous dysplasia (5 to 20 years). In addition, chondrosarcomas frequently produce pain whereas fibrous dysplasia rarely does. The typical rectangular, more-ordered radiographic appearance

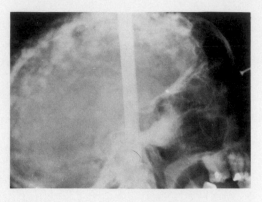

Fig. 25-9. Paget's disease. The mottled pattern is produced by a cotton ball appearance distributed throughout a generalized radiolucency. The jaws were not involved. (Courtesy R. Goepp, DDS, Zoller Clinic, University of Chicago.)

of fibrous dysplasia differentiates this entity from the chondrosarcoma, whose radiolucent-radiopaque image is completely disordered, often invading the cortex.

Osteoblastic metastatic carcinoma also is seldom seen with a pattern as monotonous as that of the mottled type of fibrous dysplasia. A history of either symptoms of or treatment for a primary tumor elsewhere is usually elicited during the history taking. The majority of osteoblastic metastatic carcinomas are found in an older age-group.

Osteosarcoma of the mixed fibroblastic and osteoblastic type produces a radiolucent-radiopaque image. This tumor has a predilection for a younger age-group (average 27 years) and so is more similar in this manner to fibrous dysplasia than most of the other entities in this discussion. However, the radiographic pattern in osteosarcoma is much more disorderly than that seen with fibrous dysplasia (see Figs. 25-11 to 25-13). Generally one of the radiographic features of osteosarcoma is apparent: sunburst appearance, cumulus cloud appearance, Codman's triangle, asymmetric bandlike widening of the periodontal ligament, or onionskin appearance of redundancy of the cortical plate.

The mottled appearance seen in *Paget's disease* may be identical to that seen in fibrous dysplasia (Figs. 25-8, *B*, and 25-9). Classically Paget's disease simultaneously affects several bones of the skeleton; this feature enables the clinician to separate such a case from the single isolated lesion of fibrous dysplasia even if it is large and involves almost all of the jaw. However, in occasional cases of atypical Paget's disease, only the mandible is involved. Such cases are more difficult to differentiate from fibrous dysplasia. The presence of extensive hypercementosis and an age over 40 years prompt the clinician to favor Paget's disease in such a case.

Adding to the difficulty in diagnosis is the possibility of *Albright's syndrome* because two or more of the bones are affected with fibrous dysplasia. Here the presence of café-au-lait spots on the skin as well as precocious puberty in a young girl identifies the disorder as Albright's syndrome. The extremely high serum alkaline phosphatase levels in Paget's disease direct the diagnostician away from a diagnosis of fibrous dysplasia and permit the establishment of a firm diagnosis of Paget's disease when typical bone changes are present.

Cementifying and ossifying fibroma (fibro-osseous lesions [PDLO]) may be seen with a mottled appearance (Fig. 25-10) similar to that seen in fibrous dysplasia. The following differences are now recognized:

1. *Shape.* The cementifying and ossifying fibromas are predominantly round whereas those of fibrous dysplasia are more rectangular.
2. *Jaw expansion.* Jaw expansion caused by cementifying and ossifying fibroma is usually nodular or dome shaped whereas the jaw expansion of fibrous dysplasia is usually of the elongated fusiform type.
3. *Margins.* The cementifying and ossifying fibroma has sharply defined radiographic margins. In contradistinction, the margins of fibrous dysplasia are indistinct, blending imperceptibly with normal bone.
4. *Predominant jaw.* Approximately 70% of cementifying and ossifying fibromas occur in the mandible. Fibrous dysplasia shows a slight predilection for the maxilla.
5. *Predominant age.* The age range for ossifying fibromas is from 7 to 58 years, and the average age is 26.4 years. The majority of active cases of fibrous dysplasia are found in patients under 20 years of age.

Chronic osteomyelitis in its radiolucent-radiopaque appearance can mimic the mottled appearance of fibrous dysplasia. When pain and purulent drainage are present, a diagnosis of osteomyelitis is easy to make. Likewise, the presence of conditions predisposing to the development of osteomyelitis would prompt the clinician to rank this entity higher in the working diagnosis. With the exception of proliferative periostitis, bone infections involve a considerably older age-group. In osteomyelitis radiographs usually show irregular cortices of

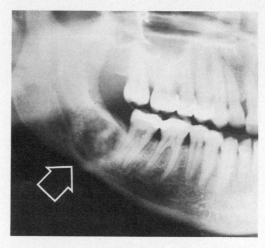

Fig. 25-10. Arrow shows an ossifying fibroma in the third molar region of a 36-year-old woman.

bone at least at one point along the expanded region. This is almost never so in fibrous dysplasia, in which the expanded bony periphery, although thinned, appears smoothly contoured and basically uniform.

Management

The usual course of fibrous dysplasia is for a lesion to appear in a young person, grow slowly for a decade or so, stabilize, and slowly return to normal. Consequently, occlusion and tooth-jaw relation should be observed carefully during the years of bone growth. Occasionally, surgical recontouring is required to improve esthetics or as a preparation for a prosthesis.

PAGET'S DISEASE (OSTEITIS DEFORMANS)—INTERMEDIATE STAGE

Paget's disease is also described in Chapter 23, where its generalized osteolytic stage, producing a generalized rarefaction of the involved bones, is emphasized. The dense, mature, cotton-wool appearance is described in Chapter 30. Like many of the other pathoses discussed in this chapter, Paget's disease may pass through three stages:

1. The initial stage is osteolytic and fibroblastic, causing a generalized radiolucency.
2. The intermediate stage is both osteolytic and osteoblastic, producing some large trabecular clusters, which appear as radiopaque areas within the generalized radiolucency.
3. The mature stage, although still possessing some osteoclastic behavior, is pre-

dominantly osteoblastic and shows as a dense cotton-wool pattern on radiographs.

The intermediate stage of the disease is emphasized in this chapter. The course of Paget's disease suggests that it results from a disorder in the coordination of osteoblastic and osteoclastic activity.

Features

Paget's disease appears to be familial and transmitted as an autosomal dominant trait. It seldom becomes evident before 40 years of age. The bones most frequently involved are the skull, vertebrae, pelvis, femurs, and jaws. The involved bones are thickened, and the foramina are often constricted. Thus pressure is induced on the structures that pass through the foramina, causing neurologic signs.

A spectrum of radiographic features characterizes the intermediate stage of this lesion, from the first indication of a developing radiopacity in the osteolytic stage to the cotton ball appearance of calcified areas interspersed with radiolucent areas, producing the distinctive cotton-wool appearance (Fig. 25-9).

Frequently the affected bones are at different stages of the disease. The skull commonly becomes involved before the maxilla, and the maxilla before the mandible. We have seen patients in whom the skull was almost completely radiopaque, the maxilla was in the mixed radiolucent-radiopaque stage, and the mandible was either uninvolved or in the radiolucent stage. Teeth in the involved jaw may demonstrate spreading, migration, and (characteristically) hypercementosis.

On microscopic examination the intermediate stage of Paget's disease shows areas made up chiefly of fibroblastic tissue containing a few trabeculae of bone with osteoclasts often evident in Howship's lacunae at the periphery. Other areas show many trabeculae with osteoblasts and osteoclasts rimming the bone in closely adjacent areas.

Using low power of the microscope, the clinician may detect a mosaic pattern within the larger trabeculae. This pattern is produced by the many reversal lines caused by the sequences of destruction and repair repeated again and again in the same spicule.

Although the serum chemistry values may vary with lapses and progressions of the disease, the alkaline phosphatase levels are usually very high whereas the calcium and phosphorus levels are within normal limits.

Differential diagnosis

Paget's disease should be suspected in persons who have generalized mixed radiolucent-radiopaque lesions throughout the jaws. If a radiographic survey demonstrates generalized radiolucent, mixed radiolucent-radiopaque, or cotton-wool changes in other bones, the disturbance is almost certain to be Paget's disease. A high serum alkaline phosphatase level strengthens this impression.

None of the other mixed radiolucent-radiopaque lesions discussed in this chapter affect multiple bones and show such complete involvement of the individual bones as does Paget's disease.

Several bones may be involved by *fibrous dysplasia in Albright's syndrome*, but unlike Paget's disease, which is a disturbance in adults over 40 years of age, this disorder affects young girls. If the clinician has only one periapical radiograph of the involved jaw, he or she may easily mistake the radiographic image for many of the other lesions discussed in this chapter. It is inexcusable to attempt a diagnosis without access to radiographs showing the full extent of the lesions.

Management

Paget's disease is a slowly progressive pathosis with no known cure. Palliative procedures to alleviate the neurologic and locomotive problems are indicated. Edentulous patients may require frequent adjustment or the continued fabrication of new dentures because of the constantly expanding jawbones.

As the disease progresses, the involved bones initially become more fragile and thus subject to pathologic fracture. As apposition exceeds resorption, however, and the mature stage of Paget's disease is reached, the bone becomes condensed and avascular and is then predisposed to osteomyelitis. The incidence of osteogenic sarcoma is greatly increased in patients with Paget's disease.

CEMENTIFYING AND OSSIFYING FIBROMA

The cementifying and ossifying fibromas are discussed in detail in Chapter 24, where their mixed periapical appearance and location at the apices of teeth are stressed. These lesions may also occur separately from teeth. Fig. 25-10 illustrates a mixed spherical radiolucency containing a mottled radiopaque appearance in the edentulous third molar area of a 36-year-old woman. Cementifying and ossifying fibromas occur in the tooth-bearing regions of the jaws, particularly the premolar and molar regions of the mandible.

OSTEOGENIC SARCOMA

Osteogenic sarcoma is second only to multiple myeloma as the most common primary malignant tumor of the jawbones. It may display three basically different radiographic images: totally radiolucent, mixed radiolucent-radi-

opaque, or completely radiopaque. Osteogenic sarcoma is discussed in Chapter 21, where its radiolucent picture is stressed. In this chapter the mixed radiolucent-radiopaque appearance is detailed.

Features

Osteogenic sarcoma of the jaws is usually a rapidly growing tumor that may produce pain, paresthesia, or anesthesia. It occurs more often

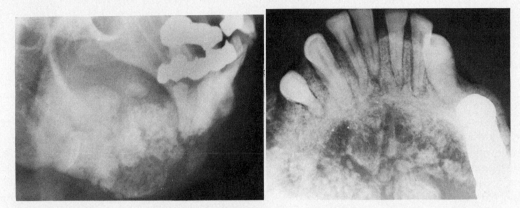

Fig. 25-11. Osteogenic sarcoma. Lateral oblique and occlusal views of the same patient. The gross production of neoplastic bone has produced a cumulus cloud appearance. Increased width of the periodontal ligament may be seen around the roots of the anterior teeth. In some cases the widening is asymmetric. The marked proliferation of neoplastic bone is evident on both radiographs.   (Courtesy R. Goepp, DDS, Zoller Clinic, University of Chicago.)

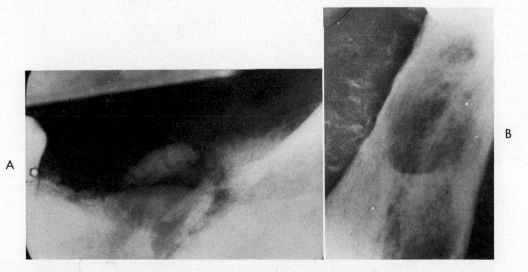

Fig. 25-12. Osteogenic sarcoma. **A,** The ragged borders of the mixed radiolucent-radiopaque lesion are evident. **B,** Bone destruction in the medullary portion of the bone produced by an osteogenic sarcoma in another patient. A sunburst effect at the periphery is shown.   (**A** courtesy R. Goepp, DDS, Zoller Clinic, University of Chicago. **B** courtesy S. Blackman, BDS, Chicago.)

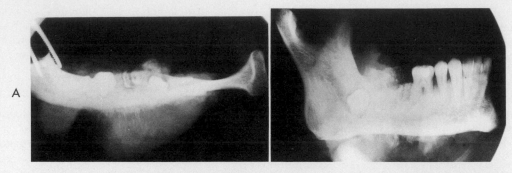

Fig. 25-13. Osteogenic sarcoma. Radiographs of a surgical specimen. The sunburst pattern can be seen emanating from the buccal cortex, especially in **A.** (Courtesy O.H. Stuteville, DDS, MD, St. Joe, Ark.)

in the mandible, and the peak age of incidence falls between 25 and 30 years of age. In the early stages, unless the mass is chronically traumatized, its surface is smoothly contoured and covered with normal mucosa.

The radiolucent-radiopaque lesion usually has ragged, ill-defined borders, and its radiographic pattern is the result of areas of excessive bone production intermingled with radiolucent foci of bone destruction (Figs. 25-11 and 25-12). In some lesions sequestra are formed, and these usually appear as well-defined, dense radiopacities. If the tumor invades the periosteum, many thin irregular spicules of new bone directed outward and perpendicular to the surface of the lesion may develop (Figs. 25-12 and 25-13). They produce the "sunburst" effect, which, although not pathognomonic for osteogenic sarcoma, is highly suggestive of the lesion. Another characteristic appearance is the "cumulus cloud" formation illustrated in Fig. 25-11.

Sometimes two triangular radiopacities project from the cortex and mark the lateral extremities of the lesion. These are referred to as Codman's triangles. Rarely osteogenic sarcoma causes periosteal deposition of bone in an onionskin pattern.

On microscopic examination, fibroblastic tissue occupies the radiolucent areas and contains deposits of osteoid tissue and malignant osteoblasts. The tumor bone in the radiopaque areas is irregular and immature. A transitional type of cartilage may also be present in the tumor.

Differential diagnosis

The lesions most frequently confused with an osteogenic sarcoma are the chondrosarcoma, osteoblastic metastatic carcinoma, ossifying subperiosteal hematoma, peripheral fibroma with calcification, fibrous dysplasia, and chronic osteomyelitis.

Although on radiographic and clinical examination the *peripheral fibroma with calcification* may resemble an osteogenic sarcoma that has originated in the periodontal ligament, the slow, benign growth of the former entity distinguishes it readily from this malignant tumor.

An unwary examiner may easily mistake the *ossifying subperiosteal hematoma* for an osteogenic sarcoma. This entity occasionally develops when trauma to the jawbone produces a sizable subperiosteal hematoma. Such hematomas may calcify and produce a disturbing radiographic appearance, often simulating the sunburst effect. A history of recent trauma to the bone should alert the clinician to the possibility that the ill-defined bony margin is a calcifying hematoma.

An *osteoblastic type of metastatic tumor* may also produce a mixed radiographic image similar to that found in osteogenic sarcoma but without the sunburst effect. The absence of a primary tumor or associated symptoms should prompt a low ranking for this entity in the differential diagnosis.

The *chondrosarcoma* can be tentatively distinguished from the osteogenic sarcoma because it usually affects an older age-group and more often involves the maxilla. Its radiographic and clinical features, however, may closely mimic those of the osteogenic sarcoma.

Differentiating features of fibrous dysplasia and chronic osteomyelitis are discussed in the section on fibrous dysplasia.

Management

The treatment of osteogenic sarcoma is discussed in Chapter 21.

OSTEOBLASTIC METASTATIC CARCINOMA

Metastatic tumors to the jawbone usually produce poorly defined, ragged radiolucencies; they are discussed in Chapter 21. Although any osteoblastic metastasis to the jaws is rare, some secondary tumors from primary lesions in the prostate and occasionally from the breast may be of this type (Figs. 25-14 and 25-15).

Metastatic prostatic tumors to bone may develop as entirely radiolucent, entirely radiopaque, or mixed radiolucent-radiopaque lesions.

Whether a metastatic tumor promotes osteoblastic activity in the tissue or organ involved apparently depends primarily on whether the metastasized tumor cells produce significant levels of acid and alkaline phosphatase.

Other metastatic tumors that are usually osteolytic may induce osteoblastic activity in the tumor or neighboring bone. Such lesions also appear on the radiograph as mixed radiolucent-radiopaque lesions with usually vague, irregular borders. The dissemination may be so great that the resultant picture mimics Paget's disease (Figs. 25-14 and 25-15).

Whether lesions of this type are well circumscribed or not usually depends on the aggressiveness of the tumor: the less aggressively a lesion behaves, the more circumscribed it appears on the radiograph.

When multiple small nests of sclerosing or osteoblastic metastatic tumor have become disseminated throughout the jawbone, a coarse salt-and-pepper pattern may be seen on radiographs (Fig. 25-14).

Features

The clinical features of osteoblastic metastatic carcinoma are similar to those described

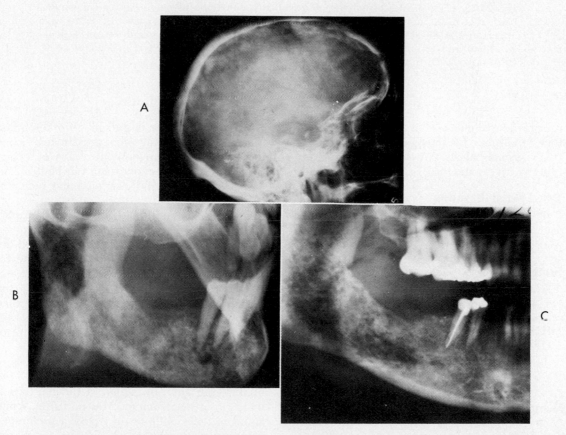

Fig. 25-14. Osteolytic and osteoblastic metastatic carcinoma. **A,** The extensive metastasis of a prostatic carcinoma with both osteoblastic and osteolytic activity is evident. **B,** A metastatic breast carcinoma to the mandible showing a salt-and-pepper appearance. **C,** Another case of metastatic carcinoma from the breast producing a coarse, irregular, salt-and-pepper lesion in the right body and ramus.   (**A** courtesy E. Palacios, MD, Maywood, Ill. **B** courtesy R. Goepp, DDS, Zoller Clinic, University of Chicago. **C** courtesy D. Cooksey, DDS, Los Angeles.)

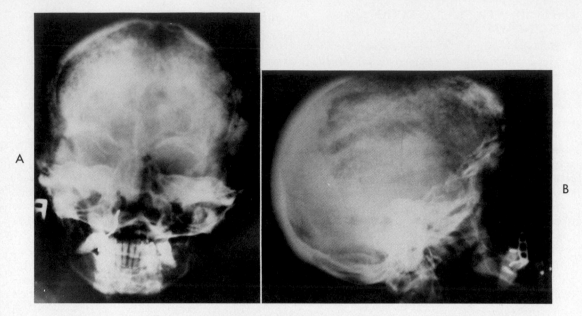

Fig. 25-15. Disseminated osteolytic and osteoblastic metastatic adenoid cystic carcinoma that originated in the oral cavity. **A,** Posteroanterior view of the skull and jaws. A cotton-wool appearance in the skull and large, bilateral radiolucent lesions in the mandible can be seen. **B,** Lateral radiograph of the skull and jaws showing both radiolucent and radiopaque areas. (**B** courtesy O.H. Stuteville, DDS, MD, St. Joe, Ark.)

for central malignancies of the jawbones. A history of surgery for or symptoms of a primary tumor usually alerts the clinician to the possibility of metastatic disease.

Differential diagnosis

The differential diagnosis of osteoblastic metastatic carcinoma is presented in the discussion of osteogenic sarcoma.

Management

The management of patients with metastatic tumors is described in detail in Chapter 20.

CHONDROMA AND CHONDROSARCOMA

Both the chondroma, which is benign, and the chondrosarcoma, which is malignant, originate in cartilage and are uncommon tumors of the jawbones.

Features

The chondroma and chondrosarcoma are considered together in this discussion because, except for the more aggressive behavior and the more irregular clinical and radiographic appearances of a very malignant chondrosarcoma, their features are similar. Frequently an ag-

gressive chondroma is difficult to differentiate from a slow-growing chondrosarcoma, since there are few pathognomonic signs or symptoms by which the chondroma can be differentiated from the chondrosarcoma and radiography is of little help.

Both the chondroma and the chondrosarcoma may cause root resorption of the involved teeth, and both may show as either well-demarcated or ill-defined radiolucencies (the radiolucent type of chondrosarcoma is discussed in Chapter 21). Although the opacities in the chondroma usually appear more orderly than those in the chondrosarcoma, both tumors may also develop a radiopaque pattern in the osteolytic bone cavity.

The chondroma and chondrosarcoma favor males slightly and occur more frequently in the maxilla; the anterior region is the most common site of involvement (Martis, 1978). When found in the mandible they have a preference for the premolar-molar regions, the symphysis, the condyle, and the coronoid process. Like other central tumors in the early stages, they are covered with a smooth, normal-appearing mucosa (Fig. 25-16), which later becomes ulcerated because of trauma. Pain is a frequent symptom of both entities.

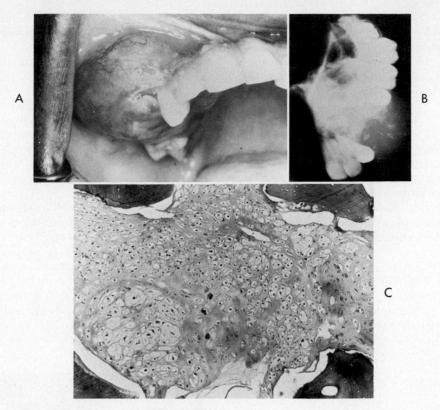

Fig. 25-16. Chondrosarcoma. **A,** Smoothly contoured, nonulcerated swelling in the maxillary premolar region. **B,** Radiograph of the surgical specimen. Radiopaque foci can be seen in the exophytic mass. **C,** Microscopic study of a chondrosarcoma.   (**A** and **B** courtesy R. Nolan, DDS, Waukegan, Ill.)

Sato et al. (1977) reviewed the Japanese literature for chondrosarcoma of the jaws and facial skeleton. These authors reported that this tumor affected the maxilla approximately 1.28 times as frequently as the mandible. The age range of patients with chondrosarcoma was 3 to 78 years, but most occurred between the ages of 30 and 60. The highest incidence occurred in the fourth decade. Chondrosarcoma of the lower jaw occurred twice as often in men as in women. Garrington and Collett (1988a) reviewed selected literature on chondrosarcoma and in a separate paper (1988b) reported on an analysis of 37 cases of this tumor involving the jaws.

On microscopic examination cartilage, chondrocytes, and possibly fibrous or myxomatous tissue are seen in the chondrosarcoma. Areas in which the cartilage has calcified cause the radiopacities. The more aggressive the tumor, the poorer the quality of the cartilage formed and the more atypical the chondrocytes.

Considerable variation occurs in the size of the cells of both tumors, and many cells are bi-nucleated (Fig. 25-16). Osteoid tissue is not seen in a true chondrosarcoma.

These tumors may vary greatly in appearance from area to area, so that large intervening masses of normal-appearing hyaline cartilage may be present in a particular specimen.

Differential diagnosis

The differential diagnosis of the chondroma and the chondrosarcoma is discussed in this chapter with that of osteogenic sarcoma.

Management

Because of the malignant nature of the chondrosarcoma and the difficulty often encountered in differentiating between an aggressive chondroma and a chondrosarcoma, the resection should be wide to ensure the removal of an adequate margin of normal tissue even though the surgeon's working diagnosis is chondroma. Sato et al. (1977) reported that the 3-year survival rate was approximately 50% for chondrosarcoma of the lower jaw but was much lower for tumors of the maxilla.

OSSIFYING SUBPERIOSTEAL HEMATOMA

The ossifying subperiosteal hematoma sometimes occurs when a subperiosteal hematoma of the jawbone is induced by trauma. It may also accompany a jaw fracture.

Features

Usually the ossifying subperiosteal hematoma occurs in people under 15 years of age, in whom the bones are still actively growing. The hematoma ossifies rapidly. The new bone is often formed in perpendicular columns from the cortical plate outward. Such an osseous arrangement gives a sunburst pattern or at times the appearance of an irregularly thickened cortex.

Differential diagnosis

Without a recent history of trauma, the clinical and radiographic appearances of ossifying subperiosteal hematoma may be readily mistaken for such lesions as *osteogenic sarcoma, Ewing's sarcoma, chondrosarcoma,* and *proliferative periostitis.*

Except for the chondrosarcoma, these lesions occur predominantly in younger persons. Although the clinician cannot differentiate between this calcifying phenomenon in the hematoma and the foregoing lesions, such a condition observed soon after a traumatic incident to the jawbone is most likely a calcifying subperiosteal hematoma.

Management

A mass such as the calcifying subperiosteal hematoma should be kept under close observation because (1) the lesion may in reality be a malignant tumor or perhaps proliferative periostitis and (2) the area may have to be surgically excised to improve esthetics and function if the ossified expansion fails to be recontoured by the stresses produced by normal function of the jaws.

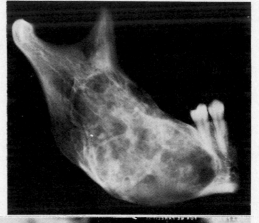

A

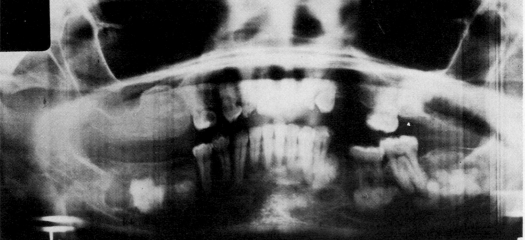

B

Fig. 25-17. **A,** Ameloblastic odontoma of the posterior of the maudible. **B,** Sclerosing cemental masses in a 32-year-old woman. Radiograph shows the mixed radiolucent-radiopaque appearance of these cemental masses, which are in the intermediate stage of maturation. (**A** courtesy O.H. Stuteville, DDS, St. Joe, Ark. **B** courtesy R. Nolan, DDS, Waukegan, Ill.)

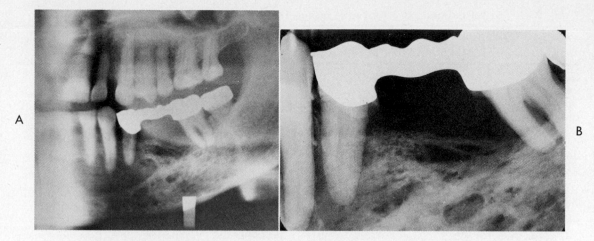

Fig. 25-18. Malignant lymphoma of bone in a man in his fifties. The radiograph shows a radiolucent-radiopaque appearance. **A,** Panograph. **B,** Periapical film. Bone appeared more rarefied in the original radiograph, but this photograph was printed lighter to show more detail.

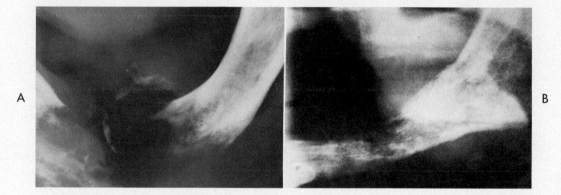

Fig. 25-19. Malignant tumors with superimposed osteomyelitis. **A,** Mandibular occlusal radiograph of a squamous cell carcinoma of the symphysis in a 62-year-old man. The radiopaque sequestrum within the classic radiolucent lesion has ragged, ill-defined borders. **B,** Orthopantomograph of osteoradionecrosis and recurrent squamous cell carcinoma in a 68-year-old man. The ragged, radiolucent-radiopaque appearance is evident.   (**A** courtesy the late M. Kaminski, DDS, and S. Atsaves, DDS, Chicago.)

RARITIES

The following lesions either rarely occur in the jawbones as mixed radiolucent-radiopaque lesions or are more often associated with teeth:

Adenomatoid odontogenic tumor
Ameloblastic fibrodentinoma
Ameloblastic fibro-odontoma (Fig. 25-17, *A*)
Ameloblastoma (bone-forming component)
Calcifying epithelial odontogenic tumor
Central hemangioma

Ewing's sarcoma
Intrabony hamartoma
Keratinizing and calcifying odontogenic cyst
Lymphoma of bone (Fig. 25-18)
Malignant tumors with superimposed osteomyelitis (Fig. 25-19)
Sclerosing cemental masses (Fig. 25-17, *B*)
Odontodysplasia
Odontoma (intermediate stage)
Osteoblastoma (intermediate stage)
Osteoid osteoma

Table 25-1. Mixed radiolucent-radiopaque lesions not necessarily contacting teeth

Entity	Predominant sex	Predominant age	Predominant jaw	Predominant region	Distinguishing features
Ossifying postsurgical bony defect	M	—	Mandible	—	History of surgery
Chronic osteomyelitis and osteoradionecrosis	M > F	40-80	Rare in maxilla	Body of mandible	Predisposing conditions: trauma, diabetes, Paget's disease, previous radiation
Fibrous dysplasia	M = F	5-20	Maxilla > mandible (slightly)	Symphysis and anterior maxilla exempt	Noncircular; borders poorly defined; ground-glass, mottled pattern
Paget's disease	M > F (slightly)	Over 40	Maxilla	Generalized	Cotton-wool; multiple bones involved; elevated serum alkaline phosphatase level
Cementifying and/or ossifying fibroma	M ~ F*	Avg. = 26.4*	Mandible 70%	Premolar-molar	Circular, 2-5 cm, well marginated
Osteogenic sarcoma	M > F	10-40; peak 27	Mandible ~ maxilla	Body of mandible	Sunburst; many radiographic appearances (see Table 22-1); well marginated
Osteoblastic metastatic carcinoma	?	40-80	Mandible	Body of mandible	History of parent tumor in prostate or breast
Chondroma and chondrosarcoma	M > F (slightly)	30-60	Maxilla 1.2 times mandible	Anterior maxilla, mandible; premolar-molar; symphysis; condyle; coronoid	Pain; many radiographic appearances (see Table 22-1)
Ossifying subperiosteal hematoma	M > F	5-20	—	—	Rapid growth after trauma

~Approximately equal.
*For ossifying fibroma.

REFERENCES

Beumer J, Harrison R, Sanders B, et al: Postradiation dental extractions: a review of the literature and a report of 72 episodes, Head Neck Surg 6:581-586, 1983a.

Beumer J, Harrison R, Sanders B, et al: Preradiation dental extractions and the incidence of bone necrosis, Head Neck Surg 5:514-521, 1983b.

Epstein JB, Wong FLW, and Stevenson-Moore P: Osteoradionecrosis: clinical experience and a proposal for classification, J Oral Maxillofac Surg 45:104-110, 1987.

Garrington GE and Collett WK: Chondrosarcoma. I. A selected literature review, J Oral Pathol 17:1-11, 1988a.

Garrington GE and Collett WK: Chondrosarcoma. II. Chondrosarcoma of the jaws: analysis of 37 cases, J Oral Pathol 17:12-20, 1988b.

Hall MB, Sclar AG, and Gardner DF: Albright's syndrome with reactivation of fibrous dysplasia secondary to pituitary adenoma and further complicated by osteogenic sarcoma: report of a case, Oral Surg 57:616-619, 1984.

Hamner JE, Scofield HH, and Cornyn J: Benign fibro-osseous jaw lesions of periodontal membrane origin, Cancer 22:861-878, 1968.

Holmes H, Cousins G, and Gullane PJ: Osteoradionecrosis: its pathophysiology and treatment; a review of new concepts, Oral Health 79:17-24, 1989.

Mainous EG, Boyne PJ, and Hart GB: Elimination of sequestrum and healing of osteoradionecrosis of the mandible after hyperbaric oxygen therapy: report of case, J Oral Surg 31:336-339, 1973.

Marciani RD and Ownby HE: Osteoradionecrosis of the jaws, J Oral Maxillofac Surg 44:218-223, 1986.

Martis C: Chondrosarcoma of the mandible: report of case, Oral Surg 36:227-230, 1978.

Marx RE: A new concept in the treatment of osteoradionecrosis, J Oral Maxillofac Surg 41:351-357, 1983a.

Marx RE: Osteoradionecrosis: a new concept of its pathophysiology, J Oral Maxillofac Surg 41:283-288, 1983b.

Marx RE and Johnson RP: Studies in the radiobiology of osteoradionecrosis and their clinical significance, Oral Surg 64:379-390, 1987.

Marx RE, Johnson RP, and Kline SN: Prevention of osteoradionecrosis: a randomized prospective clinical trial of hyperbaric oxygen versus penicillin, J Am Dent Assoc 111:49-54, 1985.

Sato K, Nukaga H, and Horikoshi T: Chondrosarcoma of the jaws and facial skeleton: a review of the Japanese literature, J Oral Surg 35:892-897, 1977.

Starcke EN and Shannon IL: How critical is the interval between extractions and irradiation in patients with head and neck malignancy? Oral Surg 43:333-337, 1977.

Waldron CA: Fibro-osseous lesions of the jaws, J Oral Maxillofac Surg 43:249-262, 1985.

Waldron CA and Giansanti JS: Benign fibro-osseous lesions of the jaws: a clinical-radiologic-histologic review of sixty-five cases. I. Fibrous dysplasia of the jaws, Oral Surg 35:190-201, 1973a.

Waldron CA and Giansanti JS: Benign fibro-osseous lesions of the jaw: a clinical-radiologic-histologic review of sixty-five cases. II. Benign fibro-osseous lesions of periodontal ligament origin. Oral Surg 35:340-350, 1973b.

26

Anatomic radiopacities of the jaws

THOMAS M. LUND

Anatomic radiopacities of the jawbones include the following:

Common to both jaws
Teeth
Bone
  Cancellous bone
  Cortical plates
  Lamina dura
  Alveolar process

Peculiar to the maxilla
Nasal septum and boundaries of the nasal fossa
Anterior nasal spine
Canine eminence
Walls and floor of the maxillary sinus
Zygomatic process of the maxilla and the
  zygomatic bone
Maxillary tuberosity
Pterygoid plates and the pterygoid hamulus
Coronoid process

Peculiar to the mandible
External oblique ridge
Mylohyoid ridge
Internal oblique ridge
Mental ridge
Genial tubercles

Superimposed radiopacities
Soft tissue shadows
Mineralized tissue shadows

A tissue or object is radiopaque because it does not permit the unrestricted passage of x rays. On properly exposed and developed radiographs it may appear light or white, depending on differential absorption of the rays. This differential absorption is a function of the density or thickness of the tissue or object. Normal radiopacities, then, may be defined as the radiographic images of normal anatomic structures of sufficient density or thickness or both to appear light or white on radiographs. Normal radiopacities of the jawbones may be common to both jaws, or they may represent specific anatomic structures peculiar to the maxilla or mandible.

Common to both jaws

TEETH
The radiopacities produced by teeth and bone are common to both jaws. Tooth enamel, the most dense tissue in the body, casts the whitest shadow (that is, is the most radiopaque). It covers the coronal portion of the tooth, tapering to a thin layer at the cervical margin. Dentin, which makes up the bulk of the tooth, is less radiopaque and thus readily distinguishable from the enamel. The density of the normally thin layer of cementum covering the root of the tooth is similar to that of dentin, so cementum is usually not distinct on the regular periapical radiograph (Fig. 26-1). Enamel and dentin are both distinguishable in the calcifying tooth germ, which is normally completely surrounded by a thin layer of cortical bone until the tooth starts to emerge through the alveolar crest (Fig. 26-2).

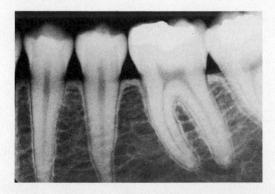

Fig. 26-1. Dense radiopaque shadows of enamel contrast with the less dense shadows of dentin. The continuity of the white line (lamina dura) surrounding the periodontal ligament spaces is apparent. The prominent white shadow of cortical bone delineates the alveolar crest.

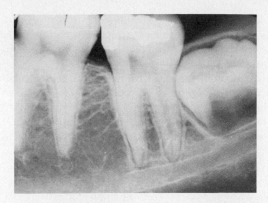

Fig. 26-2. Two linear, radiopaque shadows of cortical bone lining the mandibular canal inferior to the apices of the second molar. The thin white cortex forms the limits of the developing tooth crypt.

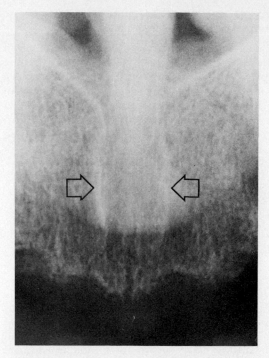

Fig. 26-3. Incisive canal. Two vertical, thin, radiopaque lines *(arrows)* delineate this structure.

BONE
Cancellous bone

The jaws consist chiefly of spongy cancellous (medullary) bone made up of thin strands or trabeculae that cross each other in a seemingly irregular manner. Although irregular, these strands generally assume a network pattern in the maxilla and a parallel pattern in the mandible. Normally the marrow spaces lying between the trabeculae vary widely in size.

Cortical plates

The maxilla and the mandible are covered with thin dense plates of compact bone, called cortical plates, that can be seen on occlusal radiographs of the jaws but do not produce a separate shadow on routine intraoral films. The cortical plates of the mandible are thicker than those of the maxilla, and the plates over the inferior border of the mandible are thickest of all, being readily discernible on radiographs.

Destruction of parts of a cortical plate produces a more radiolucent appearance than does destruction of the cancellous portion of the bone.

Lamina dura

The tooth sockets are normally lined with a thin layer of dense compact bone, which appears on radiographs as a thin white line and is referred to as the lamina dura (Fig. 26-1).

Alveolar process

The alveolar cortical plates, the lamina dura, and the spongy bone lying between them make up the alveolar process. The gingival margin of the alveolar process, termed the alveolar crest, is usually a thin layer of dense cortical bone that is sometimes reproduced as a fine white line on radiographs. This line is frequently discernible on radiographs of the mandibular incisors, where it may appear as a sharply pointed crest if the teeth are close together (see Fig. 26-14).

In the absence of pathoses the alveolar crest may be seen on radiographs of other areas at right angles to the lamina dura (Fig. 26-1).

Other structures, such as the mandibular canal and large nutrient canals in the maxillary alveolus, may be bordered with a thin layer of dense compact bone that shows as a fine white line on radiographs (Fig. 26-2).

The incisive, mental, and mandibular foramina may also be delineated by these white (opaque) lines, as may the edges of the maxillary bones forming the midline suture (Fig. 26-3).

Peculiar to the maxilla

The commonly seen radiopacities of the maxilla are discussed here in the order in which they are encountered, beginning in the anterior region and moving posteriorly.

NASAL SEPTUM AND BOUNDARIES OF THE NASAL FOSSAE

The nasal septum may be seen on films of the central incisors positioned superiorly to the apices of these teeth (Fig. 26-4). It appears as a wide vertical radiopaque shadow and frequently deviates slightly from the midline.

The nasal fossae are lined with compact cortical bone; their floors may be seen extending bilaterally from the inferior limit of the septum as linear radiopacities that curve superiorly when the lateral walls of the fossae are approached (Fig. 26-4).

Also on maxillary premolar and molar periapical radiographs the posterior extension of the floor of a nasal fossa is frequently observed (Figs. 26-5 and 26-6). It usually appears near the upper border of the film and superimposed

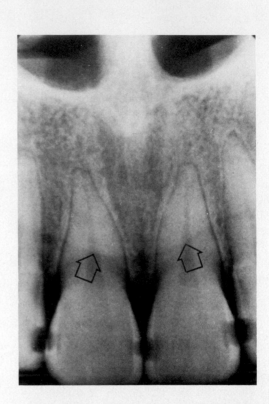

Fig. 26-4. Maxillary incisor region. The arrows denote the soft tissue outline of the tip of the nose. Paired radiolucencies, representing the nasal chambers, are evident at the upper edge of the radiograph. The vertical radiopaque shadow separating them is the nasal septum. The cortical bone forming the floor of the nasal fossa appears as a broad radiopaque line.

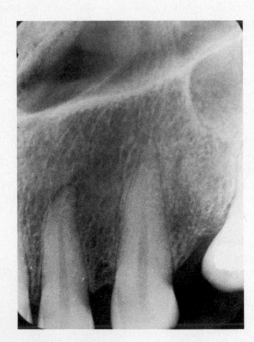

Fig. 26-5. Maxillary sinus Y.

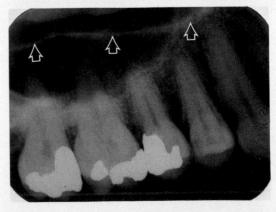

Fig. 26-6. The horizontal radiopaque line (*arrows*) represents the floor of the nasal fossa superimposed with the radiolucent image of the maxillary sinus.

with the image of the maxillary sinus. It may falsely suggest a septum in the maxillary sinus despite its horizontal orientation.

ANTERIOR NASAL SPINE

The anterior nasal spine is a projection of the maxilla at the lower borders of the nasal fossae. It is seen as a small, white, V-shaped, opaque shadow below the nasal septum (Fig. 26-7). The bottom of the V is usually open.

WALLS AND FLOOR OF THE MAXILLARY SINUS (ANTRUM)

The margins or walls of the maxillary sinus are formed by thin layers of dense cortical bone that appear as fine white lines on radiographs of the maxillary teeth. The outline of the sinus can be seen extending from the area of the canine to the tuberosity. When the tube and the film are occasionally fortuitously positioned, an X or an inverted Y is produced on the superior aspect of the canine and first premolar area where the anterior medial wall of the sinus is superimposed with the lateral wall of the nasal chamber (Fig. 26-5). The X is produced when the lines are seen to cross; the inverted Y is produced when the superior portion of the anterior wall of the sinus is indistinguishable.

The floor of the sinus lies above the apices of the maxillary teeth but varies widely as to extent and contour. It is frequently scalloped as it dips between the roots to varying depths, or it may be smoothly curved or flat, especially in edentulous jaws (Fig. 26-8). Sinus septa may or may not be present; when present, they vary widely in number and location.

ZYGOMATIC PROCESS OF THE MAXILLA AND THE ZYGOMATIC BONE

The zygomatic process of the maxilla, which arises above the alveolar process of the first molar, is usually seen on periapical radiographs as a U-shaped radiopaque shadow above the roots of the maxillary first molar. The sinus may extend into this structure, making the borders appear more radiopaque and further emphasizing the U shape (Fig. 26-9).

The inferior border of the zygomatic (malar) bone may appear on the superior aspect of the maxillary molar area as a dense, more or less horizontal radiopacity extending from the zygomatic process posteriorly; it may be mistaken for pathosis. When a greater portion of this structure appears on the radiograph, it is readily identified (Figs. 26-9 and 26-10).

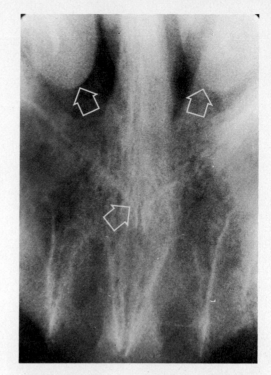

Fig. 26-7. Maxillary midline in an edentulous patient. The two arrows at the upper half of the radiograph identify the inferior turbinates. The lower arrow indicates the anterior nasal spine.

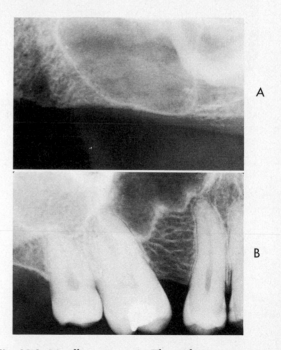

A

B

Fig. 26-8. Maxillary sinus. **A,** The radiopaque cortical line in this edentulous patient delineates a flat sinus floor. **B,** Scalloped appearance of the floor in a dentulous patient.

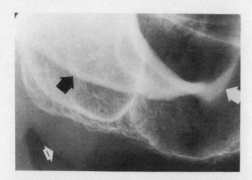

Fig. 26-9. Maxillary molar region. The larger white arrow identifies the zygomatic process of the maxilla. The black arrow indicates the zygomatic bone. The smaller white arrow, *1*, marks the shadow of the fibrous tuberosity. The thin, opaque line in the superior right corner indicates the floor of the nasal fossa.

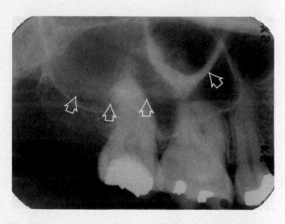

Fig. 26-10. Series of arrows delineates the inferior aspect of the relatively radiopaque shadow that is produced by the zygomatic bone. The anterior arrow indicates the radiopaque **U**, which is the image of the zygomatic process of the maxilla.

MAXILLARY TUBEROSITY

The maxillary tuberosity forms the posterior boundary of the maxillary alveolus. It is a rounded projection, normally of cancellous bone outlined by a thin layer of compact bone (which is a continuation of the alveolar crest). Cancellous bone may extend into the tuberosity, causing this structure to appear on radiographs as a thin shell of cortical bone. On the radiograph the pterygoid plates of the sphenoid bone lie immediately behind the maxillary tuberosity.

PTERYGOID PLATES AND THE PTERYGOID HAMULUS

The lateral pterygoid plate is wider than the medial plate and may be seen on radiographs of the maxillary third molar region (Fig. 26-11).

The medial pterygoid plate, although thinner and rarely seen, gives rise to the hamular process (Fig. 26-11).

The pterygoid hamular process varies in length, thickness, and density, and its tip may be seen lying above or below the level of the alveolar crest on periapical films. It may also be seen on bite-wing radiographs of the molar regions.

CORONOID PROCESS

The coronoid process of the mandible often appears on radiographs of the maxillary third molar region, but it may extend as far forward as the second molar. Although generally cone shaped with its apex pointing upward and forward, it may have varied contours and positions (Fig. 26-12).

Sometimes the radiopaque shadow of the coronoid process has been mistaken for a root fragment in the maxilla.

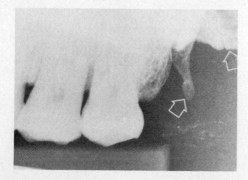

Fig. 26-11. Posterior maxillary region. The hamular process *(lower arrow)* and the lateral pterygoid plate *(upper arrow)* are shown.

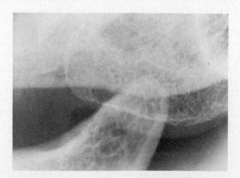

Fig. 26-12. Coronoid process in the posterior maxillary region.

Peculiar to the mandible

This discussion of radiopacities of the mandible commences with the description of those in the most posterior regions and proceeds to those located more anteriorly.

The coronoid process of the mandible has already been discussed as a maxillary radiopaque structure, since it is frequently visible on films of the maxillary third molar region.

EXTERNAL OBLIQUE RIDGE

The external oblique ridge is a continuation of the anterior border of the ramus, which passes forward and downward over the outer surface of the body of the mandible. It is often clearly seen as a prominent radiopaque line passing across the molar region (Fig. 26-13).

In the edentulous mandible, after resorption of the alveolar process, the external oblique ridge may delineate the superior border of the mandibular body in the molar region.

MYLOHYOID RIDGE (INTERNAL OBLIQUE RIDGE)

The mylohyoid ridge originates on the medial portion of the ramus and passes forward and downward over the lingual surface of the mandible, serving as the attachment of the mylohyoid muscle. It is most clearly seen in its posterior portion, where it is most prominent, crossing the retromolar and molar region inferior to and running approximately parallel with the external oblique ridge (Fig. 26-13).

Sometimes the mylohyoid ridge extends along the entire lingual surface of the body of the mandible to the lower border of the sym-physis, and in such cases it may appear on radiographs as a faint narrow radiopaque line extending from the apices of the molars forward to the region below the apices of the incisors.

MENTAL RIDGE

The term "mental ridge" is a misnomer. Two bilateral radiopaque lines are occasionally found to run anteriorly and superiorly from low in the premolar area toward the midline, where they meet (Fig. 26-14, *arrows*). However, there are no ridges on the lower external or internal anterior portion of the mandible that correspond to these white lines on periapical radiographs. This image is seen when the long expanse of cortical bone over the chin is projected by an x-ray beam that is directed tangentially to the cortical surface of the mental tubercle. Its size and prominence depend on how nearly the beam parallels the surface. Only when the beam is directed at an exaggerated negative angle is this artifact produced. It is a hallmark of the bisecting angle technique and probably is never seen when a paralleling technique is used.

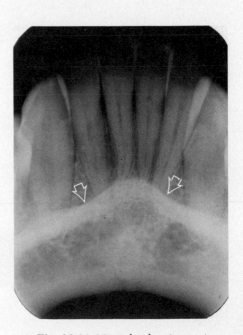

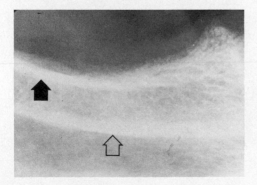

Fig. 26-13. Edentulous right mandibular molar region. The external oblique ridge *(black arrow)* and the mylohyoid ridge *(open arrow)* can be seen.

Fig. 26-14. Mental ridge *(arrow)*.

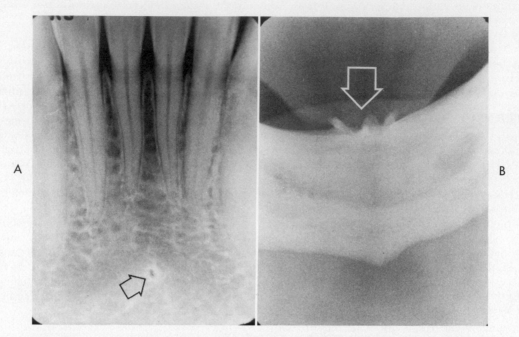

Fig. 26-15. Genial tubercules. **A,** The lingual foramen is encircled by a radiopaque ring *(arrow),* which is produced by the genial tubercles. The lamina dura interdentally forms the pointed alveolar crests. **B,** Occlusal view of the genial tubercles *(arrow).*

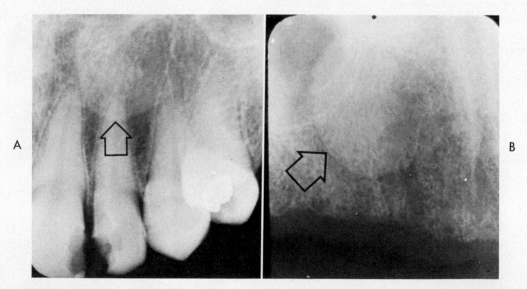

Fig. 26-16. Ala of the nose *(arrows).* **A,** Positioned over the apex of the lateral incisor. **B,** In an edentulous patient.

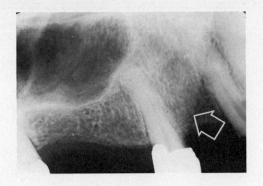

Fig. 26-17. Maxillary premolar region. The nasolabial fold *(arrow)* delineates the anterior border of the cheek.

GENIAL TUBERCLES

The genial tubercles, as many as four, surround the lingual foramen, which is situated on the internal surface of the mandible at the symphysis midway between the superior and inferior borders. They vary in size but usually appear on periapical radiographs as radiopacities in an approximate ring (Fig. 26-15).

On mandibular occlusal films the genial tubercles can be seen as single or multiple protuberances on the medial surface of the mandible in the symphyseal region (Fig. 24-14).

Superimposed radiopacities

SOFT TISSUE SHADOWS

Soft tissue, because of its thickness or density, also casts radiographic shadows that must be identified. As a general rule, the thicker or redder the tissue, the whiter its shadow.

The outline of the lip is often superimposed on the crowns of the teeth in both maxillary and mandibular anterior projections. On radiographs of the maxillary anterior teeth, shadows produced by the soft tissue of the tip of the nose (see Fig. 26-4) and the nasal and alar cartilages are often present; these soft tissue shadows may confuse the examiner if they are not recognized (Fig. 26-16).

The cheeks absorb and scatter x rays, and their outlines may be found on radiographs of the canines and premolars (Fig. 26-17).

Gingival tissue is evident on many routinely exposed films, especially when the soft tissues of the lips and cheeks are superimposed. Fibrous tissue, particularly in the tuberosity area, is readily seen (see Fig. 26-9).

MINERALIZED TISSUE SHADOWS

The radiopaque superimpositions of mineralized tissues, either normal structures or pathologic lesions, must be considered. For example, although not seen on periapical films, the radiopaque outline of the hyoid bone is commonly projected over the body of the mandible on lateral oblique views.

• • •

The foregoing discussion of the many normal anatomic radiopacities illustrates the problem that confronts the uninitiated clinician attempting to identify specific radiopaque shadows. To identify and intelligently interpret the pathologic variations of the anatomic structures, the clinician must have a thorough knowledge of their relative locations and the limits of their normal variations in shape and size.

27

Periapical radiopacities

NORMAN K. WOOD
PAUL W. GOAZ
JAMES F. LEHNERT

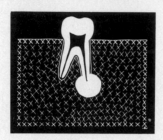

The following entities are periapical radiopacities:

True periapical radiopacities
Condensing or sclerosing osteitis
Periapical idiopathic osteosclerosis
Mature periapical cementoma
Unerupted succedaneous teeth
Foreign bodies
Hypercementosis
Rarities
  Cementifying and ossifying fibromas
  Chondroma and chondrosarcoma
  Hamartoma
  Mature cementoblastoma
  Mature complex odontoma
  Mature osteoblastoma
  Metastatic osteoblastic carcinoma
  Osteogenic sarcoma
  Paget's disease—intermediate and mature
    stages

False periapical radiopacities
Anatomic structures
Impacted teeth, supernumerary teeth, and
  compound odontomas
Tori, exostoses, and peripheral osteomas
Retained root tips
Foreign bodies
Mucosal cyst of the maxillary sinus
Ectopic calcifications
  Sialoliths
  Rhinoliths and antroliths
  Calcified lymph nodes
  Phleboliths
  Arterial calcifications
Rarities
  Calcified acne lesions
  Calcified hematoma
  Calcinosis cutis
  Cysticercosis
  Hamartomas
  Mineralized tumors
  Multiple osteomas of the skin
  Myositis ossificans
  Osteoma cutis
  Pathologic soft tissue masses
  Pilomatrixoma (calcifying epithelioma of
    Malherbe)
  Tonsillolith

SCLEROSING AND SCLEROSED CONDITIONS IN BONE

Since there is some confusion with regard to terminology and causes of sclerosis in bone, a discussion of these aspects is appropriate before the individual periapical lesions are considered. The nomenclature found in the current literature for this spectrum of lesions includes the following terms: *condensing osteitis*, *sclerosing osteitis*, *osteosclerosis*, *enostosis*, *bone whorls*, *bone eburnations*, *hyperostosis*, *focal sclerosing osteomyelitis*, and *sclerosing tumors*.

We prefer to use the following terms to describe specific sclerotic lesions of the jaws:

Condensing or sclerosing osteitis
Idiopathic osteosclerosis
Sclerosing osteomyelitis
Hyperostotic border
Osteosclerosing tumor

The term *condensing* or *sclerosing osteitis* is used when an inflammation (either present or recently past) is likely to be the initiating factor for the sclerosing process; this condition is encountered most frequently in the periapex of a tooth with an infected root canal.

An *idiopathic osteosclerosis* develops during a healing process and is not caused by inflammation; this type of sclerosis is found most frequently in the periapex of a healthy, vital mandibular premolar or molar.

A *sclerosing osteomyelitis* is a chronic osteomyelitis in which there is a sclerosis of either a sequestrum or the surrounding bone. The majority of these lesions show a combination of radiolucent and radiopaque areas.

A *hyperostotic border* is uniformly thin and radiopaque. It frequently surrounds a benign osteolytic process within bone (such as a cyst, a granuloma, a benign tumor, and occasionally a slowly expanding malignancy). It is usually produced in response to the minimal pressures created by a slowly expanding lesion.

An *osteosclerosing tumor* produces an irregular sclerosis. It may result from a primary or secondary malignancy involving bone or from an aggressive benign bone lesion (such as ameloblastoma, another type of odontogenic epithelial tumor, chondroma, myxoma, and hemangioma).

Several different mechanisms have been proposed to account for the osteosclerosis that develops about nests of tumor cells:

1. Chronic inflammation, present in the tissue that surrounds malignant tumor cells, is produced by the reaction of the tissue to the foreign antigens from the tumor cells; the resultant sclerosis is essentially a condensing or sclerosing osteitis.
2. The pressure of either an expanding tumor or blood pulsations (as in an arteriovenous shunt or a hemangioma) initiates a sclerosis that is similar to the hyperostotic border about a cyst but is usually less uniform.
3. Certain tumors possess the inherent ability to induce osteoblastic activity with resultant formation of dense bone, for example, an osteogenic sarcoma, a chondrosarcoma, or a metastatic prostatic carcinoma.

Sclerotic bone may be considered an endpoint of the reaction of the osseous tissue to a mild, chronic mechanical or chemical irritation (it probably represents the bony counterpart of cicatrization in soft tissue).

SCLEROSING OSTEITIS AND IDIOPATHIC OSTEOSCLEROSIS

An area of bony sclerosis is termed "sclerosing or condensing osteitis" if its cause can be associated with an inflammatory process and "idiopathic osteosclerosis" if its cause cannot be readily explained.

Sclerosing and sclerosed lesions of these two types are commonly seen on radiographs of patients over 12 years of age. Approximately 22% of the patients in this age-group have such a sclerotic area in their jaws. Overall incidence is equal in whites and blacks of both sexes (Farman et al., 1978). Basically the lesion is a mass of compact bone within the spongiosa (medullary portion). Its density approximates that of cortical bone. It may be totally enclosed in the medullary portion of the bone, or it may be continuous with one or both of the cortical plates.

Sclerosing osteitis and idiopathic osteosclerosis share a number of characteristics:

1. They are almost invariably painless and do not produce expansion of the cortex.
2. The covering mucosa is normal in appearance.
3. Sinuses are not present, and regional lymph nodes are characteristically asymptomatic.
4. Approximately 85% of the sclerosing and sclerosed areas occur in the mandible of whites, where the first molar region is the predominant site; in blacks approximately 71.6% of focal bony sclerotic areas are in the mandible (Farman et al., 1978).
5. These sclerotic areas may remain unchanged for years (even after successful

treatment of associated infected teeth), they may partially resolve, or they may completely disappear (and the region become radiographically normal again) (Eliasson et al., 1984). Serial radiographs showing any increase in size indicate an active lesion.

Identifying the specific types of sclerosis may not always be possible because the sclerotic area may have been induced by a previous disturbance that is no longer present. In such instances, the clinician who is unable to relate the lesion to any disorder currently apparent then diagnoses the lesion as an idiopathic osteosclerosis.

On radiographs the regions of sclerosis vary from a few millimeters to 2 or 3 cm in diameter. Shape may vary from irregular to round to almost linear. The appearance of the lesions ranges from a slight or prominent accentuation of the normal trabecular pattern in milder cases to a dense, homogeneous radiopacity in more pronounced cases.

Different areas of a sclerotic lesion may also demonstrate variations in density. Margins may be smoothly contoured or ragged, well defined or vague, and the radiodensity of the lesion may tend to blend with that of the adjacent normal bone. Even borders of the same lesion may have variable definition. Bony sclerosis and resorption (rarefaction) may be active in the same lesion and appear on radiographs as a combined radiolucent-radiopaque image (Fig. 27-1).

On histologic study the sclerosing and sclerosed lesions consist of notably thickened trabeculae with a concomitant decrease in size and number of marrow spaces (Fig. 27-2). Vascularity and the number of lacunae present are reduced, whereas incremental lines are numerous and prominent. Chronic inflammation may be present at the periphery of the area, depending on the cause and stage of the lesion's development.

• • •

Periapical radiopacities are a common finding on radiographic surveys of dentulous patients. These entities may be grouped into two divisions: (1) *True* periapical radiopacities are produced by lesions that actually surround the apex or are located in the periapex. (2) *False* (projected) periapical radiopacities are produced by entities that are situated buccally or lingually to the apex and whose radiopaque images are superimposed on the apical region.

Lesions producing false radiopacities are usually situated either at the periphery of the

bone (for example, a torus) or in the soft tissues adjacent to the bone (for example, a sialolith). False radiopaque shadows may be projected away from the apex by changing the horizontal or vertical angulation of the beam, that is, by the Clark tube-shift technique (Clark, 1910). This procedure usually differentiates the false from the true periapical radiopacity; the image of the latter cannot be shifted from the periapex by altering the angle of exposure.

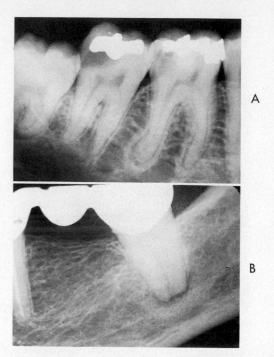

Fig. 27-1. Combined periapical rarefying and condensing osteitis. **A,** At the apex of the distal root of the first molar. The condensing osteitis is evident only at the apex of the mesial root of this molar. **B,** At the apices of the second molar.

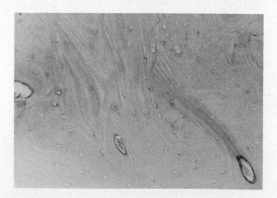

Fig. 27-2. Sclerosis of bone. This high-magnification photomicrograph reveals very dense bone with a few small, fibrovascular spaces and few lacunae; some of the lacunae are empty.

True periapical radiopacities

True periapical radiopacities are a group of lesions that occur in the immediate region of the periapex and are composed of dense bone, cartilage, hard dental tissues, or foreign material.

CONDENSING OR SCLEROSING OSTEITIS

Condensing or sclerosing osteitis is a sclerosis of bone induced by inflammation. It most often occurs as a pulpoperiapical lesion and is the most common periapical radiopacity observed in adults (seen in approximately 8%). In direct contrast to the reaction seen in rarefying osteitis (in which bone resorption is the predominant process), the reaction in this lesion is a proliferation of bone tissue.

Both the condensing and the rarefying lesions occur chiefly at the apex of a pulpless tooth or a tooth with an infected pulp(s) and are produced by an extension of the inflammatory process into the periapical area.

The highly concentrated products of infection are thought to act as irritants and produce bone resorption, whereas the diluted irritants may induce bone proliferation such as that seen in condensing osteitis. This concept is illustrated occasionally when a periapical area of rarefying osteitis is surrounded by a radiopaque halo of condensing osteitis (Fig. 27-1). In such instances bone is resorbed near the apex, where the toxic products from the infected canal are most concentrated; bone proliferation is stimulated at the periphery of the rarefied area, where, because of their diffusion through the tissue, the products from the infected canal are more dilute.

Features

The clinical features of condensing or sclerosing osteitis are discussed with those of sclerosing osteitis and idiopathic osteosclerosis. The pulps of the involved teeth are nonvital, although the sclerosing may have commenced before the complete pulp became nonvital, in which case the tooth may react positively to electrical pulp testing procedures. Jordan et al. (1978) showed that if carious molar teeth were treated with indirect pulp capping, some of these periapical lesions would disappear and the pulps remain vital. Also, since the process is of such a low grade, there is usually no pain, swelling, drainage, or associated lymphadenitis. The radiographic image varies greatly in size, shape, contours, and discreteness of margins (Fig. 27-3).

The vast majority of these lesions are found in the mandible. Eliasson et al. (1984) reported

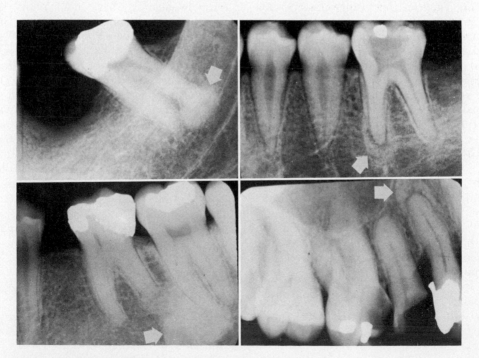

Fig. 27-3. Periapical condensing osteitis *(arrows)*. The pulps of all four teeth tested nonvital. Root resorption is evident on maxillary case.

that 48 of their 49 cases were in the mandible. The ratio of female-to-male incidence in their study was 3 to 2. The teeth most frequently involved were the mandibular premolars and molars. Eliasson et al. (1984) reported that 12% of their cases of condensing osteitis showed root resorption. More than 50% of their cases were found in patients under 30 years of age. If the lesion is in an active stage, careful selection and examination of biopsy material from the periphery show the presence of chronic inflammation. Marmary and Kutiner (1986) reported that 6% of their patients had this lesion and that 84% of the lesions were located in the mandible, principally at the apices of the first molar.

Differential diagnosis

Condensing or sclerosing osteitis must be differentiated from all the other true periapical radiopacities: periapical idiopathic osteosclerosis, periapical cementoma, an unerupted tooth, a foreign body introduced during root canal therapy, hypercementosis, and the rare lesions. In addition, the clinician must rule out the false periapical radiopacities by using the Clark tube-shift technique when exposing additional films.

Hypercementosis can be differentiated from the other true periapical radiopaque lesions by considering that it is the only common lesion that is an integral (hyperplastic) part of the tooth root. Thus on the radiograph it is completely separated from the periapical bone by the shadow of the periodontal ligament.

The radiographic image of a *foreign body introduced during root canal therapy*, along with the history of its insertion, should be diagnostic. The material—whether amalgam, cement, root canal points, or some other substance—usually can be recognized on the radiograph by its shape and density. Thus it is seldom confused with other radiopaque entities that appear in the periapex.

Condensing or sclerosing osteitis may be differentiated from the remaining periapical radiopaque lesions and from *periapical idiopathic osteosclerosis* by considering that in the osteitis the tooth pulp is usually nonvital, whereas in the other associated lesions it is vital (except when there is, rarely, concomitant but unrelated pulp death).

The *periapical cementoma* always has a thin, uniform radiolucent rim in the mature radiopaque stage. This feature differentiates this lesion from condensing osteitis and idiopathic osteosclerosis.

Management

Extraction of the infected tooth or treatment of its root canal is indicated. Approximately 30% of these sclerotic areas do not resolve to normal-appearing bone after adequate treatment. However, Eliasson et al. (1984) reported that a much higher percentage revert to bone that appears normal. These authors further reported that 85% of the lesions of condensing osteitis partially or totally regressed, whereas 15% remained unchanged. The mean observation period was 4.3 years.

PERIAPICAL IDIOPATHIC OSTEOSCLEROSIS (ENOSTOSIS, BONE WHORLS, BONE EBURNATION)

Periapical idiopathic osteosclerosis is a relatively common finding on full-mouth radiographs of dentulous patients over 12 years of age. About 4.3% of the patients within this age-group have at least one such periapical osteosclerotic lesion (Farman et al., 1978). It is second only to condensing osteitis as the most frequently seen periapical radiopacity. The term "idiopathic" emphasizes that the cause of the lesion is not readily apparent or understood.

Features

Most lesions of this type, like those of condensing osteitis, are located in the periapex of the mandibular first premolar and canine (Farman et al., 1978). The associated teeth are invariably healthy, have vital pulps, and are asymptomatic (Figs. 27-4 and 27-5). Since the patient does not complain, the entity is usually discovered on routine radiographs. There is no associated pain, cortical change, softness, expansion, drainage, or lymphadenitis. The overlying alveolar mucosa appears normal.

The radiopacity of periapical idiopathic osteosclerosis may vary from a few millimeters to 2 cm in diameter. Its shape may range from generally round to very irregular, and sometimes a triangular configuration is observed. The degree of density may vary from a slight accentuation of the trabecular pattern to a dense homogeneous radiopaque mass. Borders may be well defined or vague, well contoured or ragged (Figs. 27-4 and 27-5). Occasionally, multiple and bilateral periapical lesions are also discovered.

Differential diagnosis

The entities that are most frequently confused with idiopathic periapical osteosclerosis and must be distinguished from it are condens-

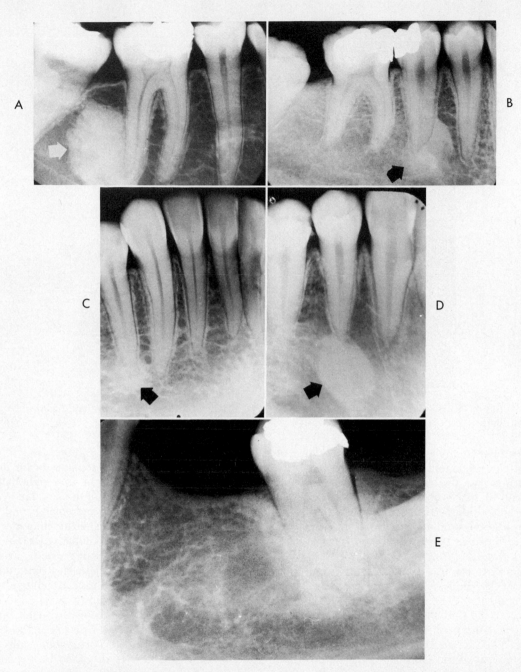

Fig. 27-4. **A** to **D,** Periapical idiopathic osteosclerosis *(arrows).* The pulps of these teeth tested vital. **E,** Dense trabeculation surrounding the roots of a vital molar because of heavy occlusal function.

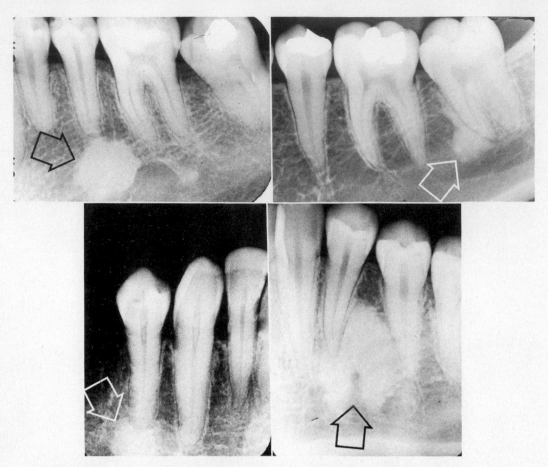

Fig. 27-5. Arrows indicate idiopathic osteosclerotic lesions at the apices of teeth with healthy pulps.

ing osteitis, mature fibro-osseous lesions of periodontal ligament origin (PDLO), hypercementosis, and abnormally dense alveolar bone induced by heavy occlusal stress.

Periapical idiopathic osteosclerosis should be differentiated from the dense trabecular pattern in *alveolar bone induced by heavy masticatory function*. Frequently an isolated tooth is subjected to occlusal trauma, and the sclerosis induced by the abnormal stresses has a more diffuse outline. The sclerosis is usually not localized to the periapical region but involves the entire alveolar process about the tooth (Fig. 27-4, *E*). When forces are not directed in line with the long axis of the tooth, the reactive sclerosis may develop on the side of the root in line with the direction of the excessive force.

Hypercementosis is recognized by the club-shaped appearance of the affected root and by the root's separation from the adjacent normal bone by the periodontal ligament.

In contrast to periapical idiopathic osteosclerosis, the *mature periapical cementoma* is a characteristically rounded radiopacity with a well-defined border and is separated from normal bone and the root by a thin radiolucent halo. If earlier radiographs of the area are available, they may reveal the radiolucent and radiolucent-radiopaque stages of the cementoma.

Because the periapical idiopathic osteosclerosis and *periapical condensing osteitis* are so similar clinically, radiographically, and sometimes histologically, they may be difficult to differentiate. The former entity develops in the periapex of a tooth with a healthy, vital pulp, however, whereas the latter occurs at the apex of a tooth with an infected or nonvital pulp.

The following rarities may also be mistaken for idiopathic periapical osteosclerosis: complex odontoma, Paget's disease, cementoblastoma, osteoblastoma, osteogenic sarcoma, chondrosarcoma, metastatic prostatic carcinoma, and hamartoma.

If the lesion were a *metastatic prostatic carcinoma*, the clinician would expect to find some symptoms of or obtain a history of treatment for primary tumor along with a report of increased serum acid phosphatase.

If the lesion were a *chondrosarcoma* or an *osteogenic sarcoma*, the clinician would find ragged radiolucent areas along with the radiopacities. A mixed radiolucent-radiopaque appearance is not seen in idiopathic periapical osteosclerosis.

The *osteoblastoma* and *cementoblastoma* begin as radiolucent lesions, progress through a mixed radiolucent-radiopaque stage, and are mature as radiopaque images. If earlier radiographs of the area in question are available, they help establish the entity's course of development. Also, the cementoblastoma is usually round, whereas areas of osteosclerosis are less regular in form and outline. (In addition, the former lesion is attached to the root apex but the latter is not.)

If it were located in the periapex, the *complex odontoma*, especially a small lesion, might be difficult to distinguish from an idiopathic periapical osteosclerosis. The complex odontoma, however, occurs much less frequently than idiopathic osteosclerosis and usually is seen over the crown of an unerupted (impacted) tooth or between the roots of teeth. Also it is infrequently situated periapically. Furthermore, the denser, sharper radiopacities caused by the deposits of enamel usually produce greater variations in the degree of radiodensity and thus aid the clinician in differentiating the odontoma from a periapical idiopathic osteosclerosis. Finally, a radiolucent line of more or less uniform width (corresponding to the periodontal ligament space), which rims the odontoma and separates it from the adjacent normal bone, is usually apparent, and this feature is not characteristic of idiopathic osteosclerosis.

Management

Areas of periapical idiopathic osteosclerosis are not of clinical significance except that they should be distinguished from condensing osteitis since teeth associated with the latter lesion require endodontic treatment.

Periodic reexamination of lesions suspected of being periapical idiopathic osteosclerosis is recommended to ensure that this clinical impression is correct. In rare cases, when there is associated root resorption, the affected tooth may require endodontic care or extraction.

MATURE PERIAPICAL CEMENTOMA

The periapical cementoma undergoes maturation from an early radiolucent, osteolytic, fibroblastic stage (Chapter 16), through an intermediate radiolucent stage with radiopaque foci (Chapter 24), to a mature radiopaque stage. In this chapter the mature stage of the lesion is emphasized as a periapical radiopacity.

Features

The features of the cementoma are described in detail in Chapter 16, so only a brief summary is given here. Ninety percent of cementomas occur in the mandible; approximately 80% occur in women; and cementomas have a definite predilection for blacks. Neville and Albenesius (1986) reported a prevalence of 5.9% in black women. This lesion is not commonly found in patients under 30 years of age.

The cementoma occurs at the apex of a vital tooth and is completely asymptomatic except for rare cases, in which the lesion reaches a size sufficient to produce an expansion of the cortical plates with possible subsequent ulceration of the mucosa.

On radiographs the completely mature periapical cementoma is predominantly round or oval with smoothly contoured borders. It varies in diameter from 0.5 to 2 cm and in rare instances may be larger. The mature periapical cementoma is uniformly dense and devoid of trabecular pattern and has a thin radiolucent border (Fig. 27-6).

On histologic study the lesion is made up of a mass of cementum containing few cells (Fig. 27-6). A mixture of cementum or bone may be present, or in some instances the calcified material is entirely bone.

The mature cementoma is particularly interesting because its radiographic features correlate so well with the histologic picture:

1. Very little fibrous or vascular tissue is present, except at the periphery, and shows as the thin radiolucent rim that surrounds the radiopaque mass on the radiograph.
2. A hyperostotic line may be present in the bone adjacent to, and delineating, the radiolucent rim. On histologic study this line is osteosclerotic bone.
3. Root resorption is not characteristic, but on occasion the adjacent root shows hypercementosis.

Differential diagnosis

In the mature stage the periapical cementoma must be differentiated from periapical idiopathic osteosclerosis, condensing osteitis, and hypercementosis.

The periapical, spherical type of *hypercementosis*, which sometimes involves the ante-

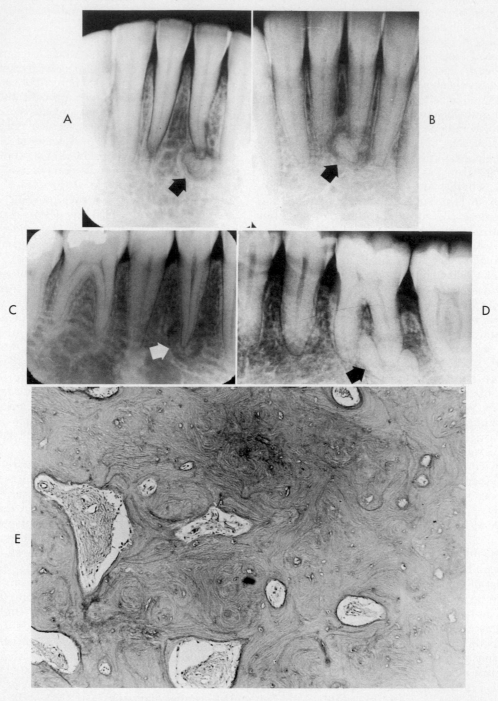

Fig. 27-6. **A** to **D,** Mature periapical cementomas *(arrows).* The pulps of these teeth tested vital. (The lesion in **D** is horseshoe shaped.) **E,** Microscopy of a mature cementoma.   (**A** courtesy M. Smulson, DDS, Maywood, Ill.)

rior teeth, may be confused with the cementoma by the unwary examiner. Careful study of the radiograph, however, reveals that the hypercementosis is attached to a part of the root and is separated from the periapical bone by the radiolucent periodontal ligament space, which surrounds the entire root.

Condensing osteitis may usually be ruled out because it occurs in the periapex of a nonvital tooth, whereas a cementoma usually does not. The tooth that has a cementoma at its apex, however, is equally susceptible to pulp injury by the usual agents; thus the alert clinician may (rarely) find a periapical cementoma at the apex of a pulpless tooth. In addition, condensing osteitis does not have a radiolucent rim, but fibro-osseous lesions (PDLO) do.

Periapical idiopathic osteosclerosis and mature periapical cementomas may be difficult to differentiate because both occur in the periapex of healthy teeth with vital pulps. The cementoma, however, is smoothly contoured and almost always round or oval, whereas periapical idiopathic osteosclerosis is usually quite irregular in shape. Also, the uniformly thin radiolucent border that can be recognized surrounding the cementoma is not present in idiopathic osteosclerosis (Fig. 27-6, *C*).

The rare periapical radiopacities (p. 559) and the false (projected) radiopacities may also be mistaken for mature fibro-osseous lesions (PDLO). The projected group, however, may be immediately eliminated if the clinician cannot shift the radiographic image from the periapex on additional films by altering the angle of exposure.

The *cementoblastoma* affects the periapices of the premolars and molars almost exclusively, whereas 80% of cementomas are seen in the mandibular incisor region.

When systemic symptoms are absent, *Paget's disease* and *metastatic osteoblastic prostatic carcinoma* can be assigned a low rank in the differential diagnosis. Also many radiopaque areas are seen scattered throughout the jaws of most patients afflicted with Paget's disease.

Osteosarcoma, chondroma, and *chondrosarcoma* do not characteristically produce such a solid, uniform radiopaque pattern.

The density of the *complex odontoma* usually is not uniform. The more opaque images of the enamel contrasting with the less opaque images of dentin enable the clinician to differentiate between this lesion and the more homogeneously opaque cementoma. The complex odontoma seldom occurs periapically.

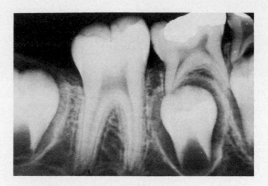

Fig. 27-7. Unerupted second premolar.

Management

The proper management of a periapical cementoma requires continued observation and subsequent verification through periodic radiographic examination. Surgical enucleation and microscopic examination are indicated for the larger lesions that cause expansion of the cortical plate or when the clinician is unsure of the working diagnosis.

UNERUPTED SUCCEDANEOUS TEETH

When the permanent crowns of succedaneous teeth are completely formed and the resorption of the root ends of the corresponding deciduous teeth is initiated, the images of the permanent tooth crowns represent periapical radiopacities (Fig. 27-7). Obviously such shadows occur only on radiographs of persons under 12 or 13 years of age. Since these teeth are easily recognized for what they are, however, this entity is included in the present discussion only for completeness and does not require further consideration.

Impacted teeth are not included in the discussion of true periapical radiopacities; they rarely occur at the apices of other teeth. Although they may appear at these locations, the clinician can usually shift their images in the periapical region by making another radiograph with a different angle of exposure. Impacted teeth are discussed later in this chapter with the false periapical radiolucencies.

FOREIGN BODIES (ROOT CANAL–FILLING MATERIALS)

Radiopaque foreign bodies in the periapex are almost always root canal–filling materials. The images produced by extruded gutta percha, silver points, sealer, or a retrograde amalgam restoration and the filled root canal (Fig. 27-8), coupled with the history of a related pro-

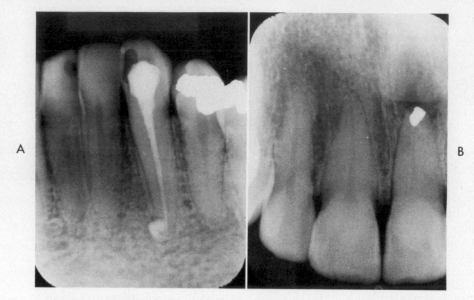

Fig. 27-8. Periapical foreign bodies (endodontic materials). **A,** Gutta percha. **B,** Retrograde amalgam filling. (**B** courtesy F. Weine, DDS, Chicago.)

cedure, contribute to the easy recognition of these periapical radiopacities. Consequently they require no further description.

HYPERCEMENTOSIS (CEMENTAL HYPERPLASIA)

Hypercementosis has been defined by Stafne (1969) as "excessive formation of cementum on the surface of the root of the tooth." The early stages are only microscopically detectable, but as additional layers of cementum are added, the accumulation becomes apparent on the radiograph (Fig. 27-9).

The etiology of hypercementosis is not well understood, but repeated observations seem to indicate that this lesion is sometimes associated with the development of periapical inflammatory conditions, periapical cementoma, and systemic disease (such as Paget's disease, acromegaly, and giantism).

Features

Hypercementosis is completely asymptomatic and is usually discovered on routine radiographic surveys. The premolars are more often affected than are the remaining teeth (6:1), and the first molars are next in order of involvement. The hypercementosis may be confined to just a small region on the root, producing a nodule on the surface, or the whole root may be involved. In multirooted teeth, one or two or all roots may show hypercementosis. Of-

ten teeth are bilaterally involved, and a generalized form with hyperplasia of cementum on all root surfaces has been reported. The teeth affected are usually vital and are not sensitive to percussion.

On radiographs the altered shape of the root is apparent if there has been a reasonable amount of cemental hyperplasia. An isolated nodule or the characteristic club-shaped root may be seen. In either case the root is surrounded by a normal periodontal ligament space* and lamina dura. The different densities of the excess cementum and root dentin are such that the original outline of the dentin root is discernible on the radiograph (Fig. 27-9). Hypercementosis on anterior teeth may appear as a spherical mass of cementum attached to the root end.

On histologic study the cementum may be acellular (primary) or cellular (secondary). It is usually deposited in layers but may be arranged in an irregular fashion with fibrovascular inclusions.

Differential diagnosis

Hypercementosis may be differentiated from the *false radiopaque images* that are projected

---

*Hypercementosis may well be a response to the elongation of a tooth or the loss of supporting bone and is initiated by an inherent tendency for maintenance of the normal width of the periodontal ligament (Shafer et al., 1983).

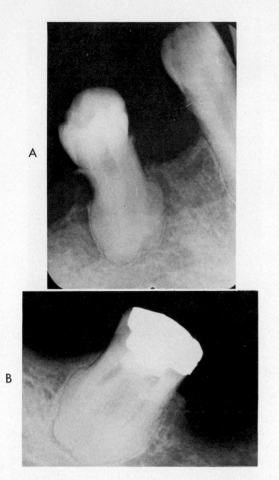

Fig. 27-9. Hypercementosis. **A,** On a mandibular premolar. **B,** On a mandibular molar.

over the apex by two features of the projected images:

1. The projected radiopacities are not delineated by a periodontal ligament space and lamina dura as is the hypercementosis.
2. The projected images may be shifted in relation to the apex by altering the angle at which additional radiographs are exposed.

The true periapical radiopacities are more difficult to differentiate from hypercementosis. They include cementomas, condensing osteitis, periapical idiopathic osteosclerosis, and such developmental anomalies as fused roots, dilacerations, and similar images caused by multirooted teeth.

The club-shaped images cast by *multirooted teeth* and the shadows of *dilacerated roots* can be identified by making successive radiographs exposed from different angles.

Sometimes the *fused roots* of multirooted teeth have a bulbous shape, but these fused roots can be recognized by the apparently expanded region of the root that does not have the relatively lower radiodensity of hyperplastic cementum.

Periapical idiopathic osteosclerosis, condensing osteitis, and *cementomas* lie outside the shadow of the periodontal ligament and lamina dura, whereas hypercementosis forms an integral part of the root surface and is therefore enclosed by a normal periodontal ligament space and lamina dura. Although this distinction contributes to the differentiation, there may be difficulty in differentiating these entities when the periodontal ligament space and lamina dura are indistinct. Differentiation may also be a problem when the clinician is confronted by the spherical type of hypercementosis that is occasionally seen on the anterior teeth. In hypercementosis, continuity with the root surface is discernible if the radiograph is carefully examined.

Management

Hypercementosis does not require special treatment, although the obvious surgical problem is encountered during the removal of the involved tooth. When many teeth show hypercementosis, the patient should be examined for diseases such as Paget's, acromegaly, and giantism.

RARITIES

A number of entities may cause true periapical radiopacities, but since they are rare or are only rarely homogeneous and radiopaque, they are merely listed here:

Cementifying and ossifying fibroma
Chondroma and chondrosarcoma
Hamartoma
Mature cementoblastoma (Fig. 27-10)
Mature complex odontoma
Mature osteoblastoma
Metastatic osteoblastic carcinoma
Osteogenic sarcoma
Paget's disease—intermediate and mature stages (Fig. 27-11)

The complex odontoma is included in this list of rarities because it usually occurs supracoronally or between the roots of adjacent teeth, so it only rarely produces a periapical radiopacity. It is listed with true periapical radiopacities because its image cannot usually be shifted from the apex, since its buccolingual dimension is relatively large.

The reader is directed to the references at the end of the chapter for sources of further information concerning these disorders.

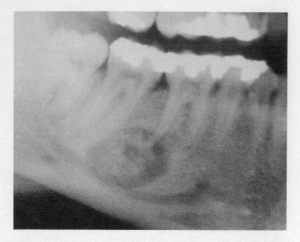

Fig. 27-10. Cementoblastoma at the apices of the distal root of the first molar tooth, which has a vital pulp. The symmetric, round radiopacity and the radiolucent rim are evident.   (Courtesy N. Barakat, DDS, Beirut, Lebanon.)

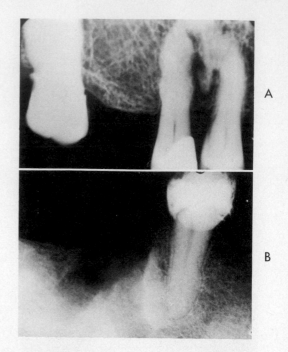

Fig. 27-11. Paget's disease.   (**A** courtesy R. Goepp, DDS, Zoller Clinic, University of Chicago.)

False periapical radiopacities

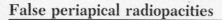

False (projected) periapical radiopacities are produced by a large number of entities, may be categorized into (1) radiodense bodies within the bone, situated either bucally or lingually to the apex, and (2) hard or soft tissue situated on the periphery of the bone or in the adjacent soft tissue.

It is important to emphasize that a normal or pathologic soft tissue mass projected over bone may impart a considerably denser quality to the shadow of the bone.

False periapical radiopacities have a characteristic that is diagnostically useful: their relation to the apex is such that the radiopaque images can be shifted from the apex by altering the angle of projection. Additional views (such as occlusal, lateral oblique, posteroanterior, Waters', and panographic) may be necessary to establish the true location of the entities that produce these radiopacities.

ANATOMIC STRUCTURES

Either soft tissue or bony anatomic structures may be projected as radiopaque shadows over tooth apices. Examples of such configurations include the anterior nasal spine, the ala of the nose, the malar process of the maxilla, the external oblique ridge, the mylohyoid ridge, the mental protuberance, and the hyoid bone (Fig. 27-12).

Identification of these structures depends on an awareness of the regional anatomy, a general understanding of the geometry required to radiographically visualize the area, and usually at least two different radiographic projections of the area.

IMPACTED TEETH, SUPERNUMERARY TEETH, AND COMPOUND ODONTOMAS

Since it is unusual for impacted or supernumerary teeth or those in a compound odontoma to be situated directly at the apex of an erupted tooth, these entities are classified as false periapical radiopacities.

The periapical radiopaque images produced by an impacted or supernumerary tooth or an odontoma are readily identified by their density and shape (Fig. 27-13). In most cases the images can be shifted from the apex by the Clark tube-shift technique.

TORI, EXOSTOSES, AND PERIPHERAL OSTEOMAS

Tori, exostoses, and, less frequently, osteomas are situated at the periphery of the jaws and may vary greatly in size, shape, and location. Although the nature of these bony protuberances is still a matter of debate, the tori and

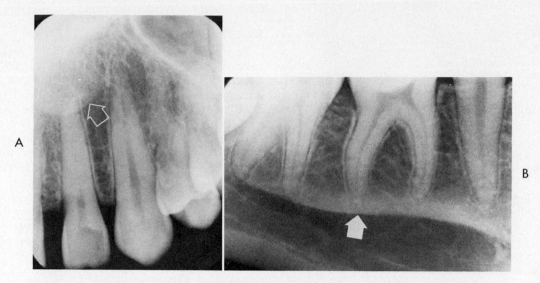

Fig. 27-12. Projected anatomic periapical radiopacities. **A,** Ala of the nose *(arrow).* **B,** Mylo-hyoid ridge *(arrow).*

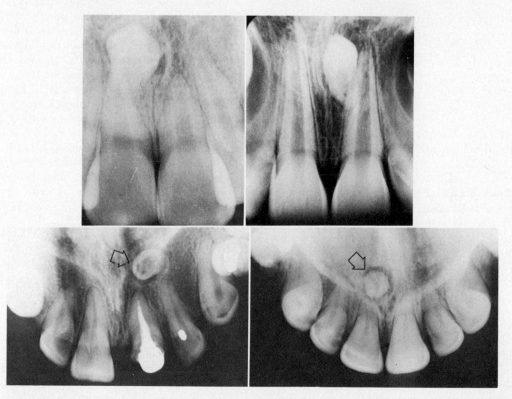

Fig. 27-13. Arrows indicate the impacted supernumerary teeth as projected periapical radio-opacities.

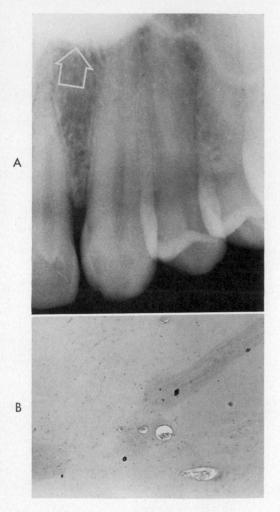

Fig. 27-14. A, Maxillary torus *(arrow)* as a projected periapical radiopacity. **B,** Microscopy of the torus.

exostoses are usually considered developmental lesions and the osteoma is considered a benign neoplasm. They are all discussed in detail in Chapter 10 as examples of exophytic lesions. Because they originate deep to the surface epithelium and are slow growing, they have a smoothly contoured surface.

On radiographic examination, tori, exostoses, and periosteal osteomas may appear as single or multiple, smoothly contoured, somewhat rounded, dense radiopaque masses (Fig. 27-14). Since they are peripheral, if their shadows happen to fall in an apical area on the radiograph, shifting the tube on a subsequent exposure (Clark tube-shift technique) readily demonstrates that these images are false periapical radiolucencies. In addition, these radiopaque images are not circumscribed by a periodontal ligament space and lamina dura.

Such information from the radiographs, corroborated by clinically apparent intraoral bony protuberances, render the diagnosis obvious.

RETAINED ROOT TIPS

Retained root tips, especially in the molar regions, may be so situated that their radiopaque shadows are projected over the apex of an adjacent tooth (Fig. 27-15). When this happens, the root tip's position relative to the apex in question can be demonstrated on subsequent films by the Clark tube-shift technique. If the shapes of the root, its root canal, the surrounding periodontal ligament, and the lamina dura remain, unaltered, the identification is relatively easy; if these features are obliterated, however, the nature of the radiopacity may not be so obvious. Furthermore, a condensing osteitis may develop about the root tip and obscure it on the radiograph.

FOREIGN BODIES

A variety of foreign materials within the jawbone or in the surrounding soft tissue may be projected over apices and cause periapical radiopacities on the radiograph (Fig. 27-16). A list of such objects includes metal fragments, buttons, zippers, hooks, other metal dress accessories, jewelry, and various dental materials and fragments of instruments. Usually the images cast by such items are distinctive and readily identifiable. If there is a history of trauma to the region, the clinician may anticipate finding a foreign body embedded in the tissue and even look for its appearance on the radiograph. Price (1986) discussed the problem presented when dental materials become foreign bodies in the tissue. He proposed a method of determining the standard opacities of dental materials.

MUCOSAL CYST OF THE MAXILLARY SINUS

The mucosal cyst of the maxillary sinus occurs in approximately 2% of the population. This entity represents a retention cyst in the lining mucosa of the maxillary sinus.

Features

The incidence of mucosal cyst of the maxillary sinus, which affects men and women equally and may be bilateral, peaks during the third decade of life. Although most of these cysts are symptomless, a significant number produce accompanying symptoms of a sinusitis.

On radiographs the cyst usually appears as a relatively dense, dome-shaped mass with its

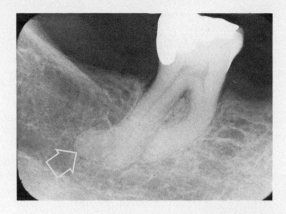

Fig. 27-15. Retained root tip of the mesial root of the third molar *(arrow)* projected onto the periapex of the second molar.

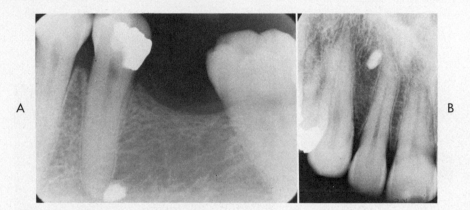

A   B

Fig. 27-16. Metal fragments projected as periapical radiopacities. **A,** This foreign body proved to be in the buccal cortical plate. **B,** This foreign body proved to be in the upper lip.

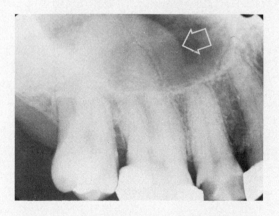

Fig. 27-17. Tentative diagnosis of benign mucosal cyst *(arrow)* of the maxillary sinus projected as a radiopacity over the molar roots.

base on the floor of the maxillary sinus; the apices of the maxillary first and second molars may appear to be within the opaque image of the cyst (Fig. 27-17).

The location and appearance of the dome-shaped radiopaque structure of the mucosal cyst of a maxillary sinus are almost diagnostic. Although the cyst may remain constant in size for a long time, it also may spontaneously

empty either slowly or rapidly; thus periodic radiographic examinations frequently reveal a radiopacity of varying dimensions. This entity is discussed in detail in Chapter 35.

Differential diagnosis

When a mucosal cyst of the maxillary sinus appears as a periapical radiopacity, it must be differentiated from the true radiopacities—a condensing or sclerosing osteitis, a periapical idiopathic osteosclerosis, and a cementoma. Additional radiographic views (such as panographic, Waters', and posteroanterior) usually identify it as a mass situated in the maxillary sinus.

The smooth dome shape of the mucosal cyst of the maxillary sinus often differentiates it from a *malignant tumor of the sinus.*

Occasionally, *fibrous dysplasia* originating on the floor of the maxillary sinus mimics a maxillary sinus retention phenomenon, but the ground-glass appearance of the former entity helps distinguish this lesion from the mucosal cyst. The differential diagnosis of the benign mucosal cyst is discussed further in Chapter 35.

Management

When the clinician discovers what appears to be a mucous retention cyst in the maxillary sinus and it is asymptomatic, periodic radiographs are in order.

ECTOPIC CALCIFICATIONS

Ectopic calcifications* in the soft tissues surrounding the jaw may be mistaken on radiographs for calcified odontogenic structures. Such deposits of abnormal calcific salts may be readily distinguished from calcified odontogenic structures and lesions by considering that

*Pathologic deposits of calcium salts in tissues that are normally uncalcified.

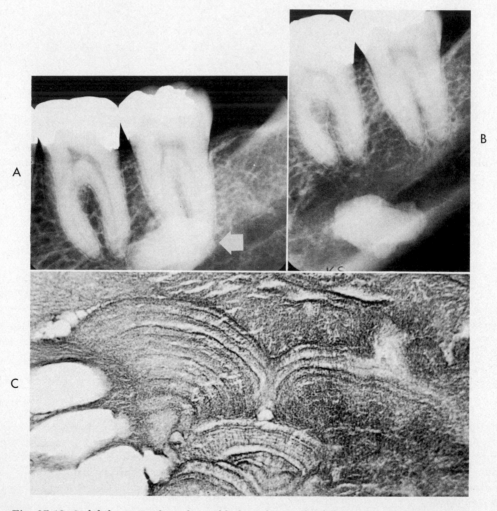

Fig. 27-18. Sialolith. **A,** In the submandibular salivary gland projected over the apex of the mandibular second molar *(arrow).* **B,** The shift in the image of the stone is caused by an altered vertical angle of exposure. **C,** Photomicrograph.

the latter radiopacities are almost always surrounded by a periodontal ligament type of space and a lamina dura, whereas the former do not have such characteristic borders. Also, the location of these ectopic calcifications can be shown to be some distance from the teeth by Clark's tube-shift technique. Katz et al. (1989) discussed these considerations in detail.

Sialoliths (salivary gland calculi)

Sialoliths are calcareous (radiopaque) deposits in the ducts of the major or minor salivary glands or within the glands themselves. They are thought to form from a slowly calcifying nidus of tissue or bacterial debris (organic matrix).

In their early stages the sialoliths may be either too small or insufficiently mineralized to be visible on radiographs. If they are not expelled from the duct, however, they eventually become large enough to be visible as radiopacities (Fig. 27-18).

FEATURES

When sialoliths reach a critical size or position, they effect a partial or complete obstruction of the duct.

This obstruction results in a sialadenitis, which is manifested as a painful swelling of the gland that is most pronounced just before, during, and immediately after meals. The enlargement usually is minimal when the patient awakes in the morning. Often several episodes of sialadenitis occur before the patient seeks professional help. Since the major or collecting ducts are usually completely occluded, milking the gland and duct is nonproductive.

The submaxillary salivary gland and duct are the most frequent sites of sialoliths; some clinicians believe this is because the oral terminus of the duct is superior to the gland and gravity tends to cause secretions to pool in the gland and duct system. Sialoliths vary greatly in size, shape, density, contour, and position, and they may be solitary or multiple (Fig. 27-18). They are frequently seen within the substance of the submaxillary gland and may be one solid mass or many smaller masses.

Although sialoliths in the submaxillary gland and duct may be seen on periapical films, they are best visualized on occlusal, lateral oblique, and panoramic radiographs. They are uncommonly found in the parotid gland or its duct but, when present in the duct, may be seen on periapical films superimposed over the maxillary molars or the posterior maxillary alveoli. Haug et al. (1989) described the successful use of xeroradiography in the diagnosis of nonradiopaque sialoliths.

On histologic examination a sialolith resembles calculus, showing concentric rings of alternating light and dark bands (Fig. 27-18).

Sialoliths occur frequently and may be seen as small, rounded radiopacities on periapical films (see Fig. 28-24). Yamane et al. (1984) reported on 76 cases.

DIFFERENTIAL DIAGNOSIS

The first step in the diagnostic procedure is to obtain another radiographic view of the stone taken at a different angle from the first. This step verifies that the radiopacity in question is actually a false (projected) periapical radiopacity.

Once the radiopacity is established to be a projected radiopacity, the sialolith must be distinguished from several entities—a calcified lymph node, an avulsed or embedded tooth, a foreign body, a phlebolith (calcified thrombus), calcification in the facial artery, myositis ossificans, and an anatomic structure (such as the hyoid bone).

The radiopaque image of the *hyoid bone* is frequently projected over the region of the submaxillary gland, duct, and mandible on lateral oblique radiographs but appears bilaterally on panoramic films. Thus, if the mass is single on both the lateral oblique and the panographic radiograph, it is not likely to be the hyoid bone. The shape of the hyoid bone (V) is actually so diagnostic that clinicians do not mistake this structure for pathosis.

Myositis ossificans is a rare disturbance characterized by the formation of bone in the interstitial tissue of muscle. It has also been observed in the superficial tissues away from muscle, however, even in the skin. When muscles of the face are involved, the masseter muscle is most frequently affected. This results in a restriction of mandibular movements, which should alert the clinician to the possibility of myositis ossificans.

Calcification in the walls of the facial artery may also be projected over the apex of teeth and produce a suspect area. If a significant length of the artery is involved, the resultant serpentine, calcified image is diagnostic, but if there are calcific deposits in just a short section of the vessel, the resultant image may be mistaken for a sialolith, especially if the section of facial artery that courses through the submandibular space is involved.

A *phlebolith* sometimes occurs in the floor of the mouth and may be seen on an occlusal radiograph; it usually accompanies a clinically discernible varicosity. If the clinician finds a radiopacity in the floor of the mouth and there is no sialadenitis, he or she should be inclined to favor phlebolith as a diagnosis. The final differentiation between these two entities may have to await surgery.

A *foreign body* is usually readily diagnosed by its characteristic shape and by the history of a traumatic incident to the region.

Similarly an *avulsed tooth* lying in the soft tissues should be recognized by its shape and relative density, and the clinician should be able to obtain a history of a traumatic incident.

A *calcified submandibular lymph node* may be difficult to distinguish from a sialolith occurring within the submandibular gland, since some of the lymph nodes in the submandibular space rest on the surface of the submandibular gland (some are even inside the capsule of the gland). Also a calcified lymph node and a sialolith would be projected into the same general region on the radiograph. The relative incidences of the two entities, however, favor the diagnosis of sialolith; furthermore, if a painful swelling accompanies a calcified mass in the submandibular space, this strongly indicates a sialolith, since a calcified node represents an old, burned-out, asymptomatic lesion. On the contrary, if the calcified mass has a smooth, rounded contour, it is more apt to be a calcified lymph node than a sialolith. A sialogram may help distinguish between these entities. When painful swelling is not present, the examiner may be able to determine by careful bimanual palpation whether the firm mass is within the submaxillary salivary gland.

MANAGEMENT

When a stone is discovered in the duct or the gland proper, it should always be removed.

If the sialolith is impacted in the duct and the case is complicated by secondary infection, the infection should be eliminated before the stone is surgically removed. If the stone is in Wharton's duct, it may be approached and removed intraorally.

When the sialolith is small and located within the gland, it can ordinarily be removed by simple incision. If it is large, however, the gland must be excised; also when a sialolith is in the gland, the surgery may have to be performed even though there is a concurrent sialadenitis.

Rhinoliths and antroliths

Rhinoliths and antroliths are calcified masses occurring in the nasal cavity and maxillary sinus, respectively. Their development is similar to that of a sialolith—commencing with the calcification of a nidus of tissue debris or concentrated mucus, which continues to grow because of the precipitation of calcium salts in concentric layers.

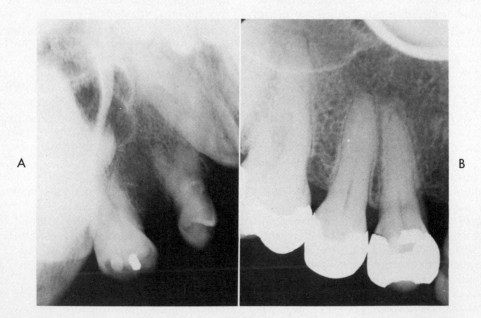

Fig. 27-19. **A,** Large antrolith projected over the roots of a molar. **B,** Lens of the patient's eyeglasses projected as a radiopacity.

Rhinoliths and antroliths are included in this chapter because their images on periapical radiographs may be cast over the apices of adjacent maxillary teeth.

FEATURES

Usually no symptoms accompany the smaller rhinoliths or antroliths, but the larger stones may be associated with a sinusitis or a nasal obstruction.

These calcifications are usually found on routine radiographs of the region and are of various shapes from round to oval to irregular with outlines that may be smooth or ragged (Fig. 27-19). They may appear as a dense, homogeneous radiopacity or may show concentric rings of radiopaque and radiolucent material. In some instances small radiolucent areas are distributed haphazardly throughout the radiopaque mass.

Rhinoliths and antroliths may contain so little mineral that their image is quite faint. On microscopic examination they resemble sialoliths and calculi. Appleton et al. (1988) reported two cases of rhinoliths; one was found to be a pink bead. Damm and Ziegler (1985) reported a case that turned out to be calcification surrounding a button.

DIFFERENTIAL DIAGNOSIS

When solitary radiopacities are seen in the superior aspect of a maxillary periapical film, antroliths and rhinoliths must be considered as possible diagnoses. It is then particularly important to obtain additional maxillary views (such as panoramic, occlusal, Waters', and posteroanterior), as well as several additional periapical views, to facilitate the differential diagnosis, since these projections show the complete lesion or structure and demonstrate whether the mass is in the sinus, nasal cavity, or adjacent maxillary alveolar bone.

Different projections further enable the clinician to determine the relative location of the object as he or she compares its apparent shift in position according to the varying angles of exposure.

A knowledge of the anatomy of the area coupled with the information obtained from a complete radiographic examination enables the clinician to identify and differentiate the following entities, which can be confused with antroliths and sialoliths: a cone cut, eyeglasses, a complex odontoma, a mature cementoma, a periapical condensing osteitis, a buccal exostosis, a palatal torus, an impacted tooth, the ala of the nose, and the malar process of the maxilla.

A *cone cut* in the superior aspect of a periapical film appears as a homogeneous radiopacity containing no detail. However, its contour is convex like that of the rhinolith. Such cone cuts are not likely to be present or similarly positioned on additional films.

Eyeglasses occasionally show on radiographs as a solid, homogeneous radiopacity rather than a radiopaque rim (Fig. 27-19). Although antroliths are not likely to occur bilaterally and with such symmetry, additional radiographs should be taken after the removal of the eyeglasses to determine the identity of the opacities.

The radiopaque images of a *complex odontoma* and a *mature cementoma* may mimic those produced by an antrolith, but the former images have characteristically radiolucent borders. When these odontogenic tumors become large enough to cause a bulge in the floor of the antrum, differentiation from an antrolith may be difficult; fortunately, the complex odontoma and the mature cementoma rarely reach such a size in this location.

Periapical condensing osteitis at the apices of a maxillary premolar may simulate an antrolith on periapical films. However, the adjacent teeth test nonvital in the case of periapical condensing osteitis, and additional films show that the mass is not encroaching on the antrum. These considerations help identify the radiopacity as a periapical condensing osteitis.

The dense, rounded radiopacity produced by a *buccal exostosis* or a *palatal torus* is frequently seen in the superior aspect of a maxillary periapical radiograph and may closely resemble the image produced by an antrolith or a sialolith. Clinical detection of the torus or the exostosis, however, provides the correct diagnosis.

An *impacted tooth* may be confused with an antrolith or a rhinolith, especially when it is projected high on the film or when it is positioned in the jaw so that its image is not characteristic of a tooth. Good-quality films, properly positioned, show the typical clear outlines of the impacted tooth.

The *ala of the nose* may be projected over the periapices of the upper incisors or canines and appear as a partially mineralized rhinolith (see Fig. 27-12, A). Again, additional films and a familiarity with the regional anatomy suggest the correct diagnosis.

The inferior portion of the *malar process of the maxilla* or the zygomatic bone on some periapical films appears identical to an antrolith (see Fig. 28-20). Additional projections enable the clinician to correctly identify this structure.

When a mature cementoma or a complex odontoma produces a bulge in the floor of the maxillary sinus, differentiating it from an antrolith or some other pathosis of the maxillary sinus (such as a mucosal retention cyst, fibrous dysplasia, a tumor, and root tips) is more difficult.

Root tips in the maxillary sinus may be difficult to differentiate from a small antrolith unless the root canal is evident.

Except for the rare osteoma, a *tumor* of the maxillary sinus usually is less radiopaque than an antrolith.

Although possibly quite opaque on a Waters' projection, *fibrous dysplasia* usually has a ground-glass appearance on periapical films.

The dome-shaped appearance of a *mucosal retention cyst* usually distinguishes this phenomenon from the more spherical-appearing antroliths.

MANAGEMENT

Patients with antroliths and rhinoliths should be referred to an otolaryngologist for evaluation and management.

Calcified lymph nodes

Calcified lymph nodes occur in the cervical and submaxillary regions (Fig. 27-20). The majority are calcified tuberculous nodes. On certain radiographic views their images are projected over the mandibular bone and occasionally over the apex of a mandibular tooth.

FEATURES

Calcified lymph nodes are asymptomatic and are usually found on a routine radiographic survey.

The patient may have a history of successful treatment for tuberculosis. Any of the cervical

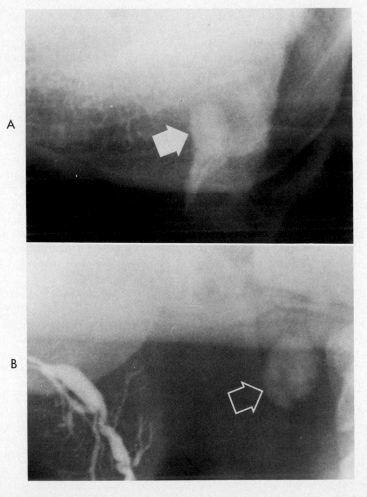

Fig. 27-20. Solitary calcified cervical lymph node *(arrow)*. **A,** Projected over the mandible as a radiopacity. **B,** Another view of the same node showing the image shifted away from the mandible. A sialogram of the submandibular salivary gland proved that the calcified lesion was not a sialolith.   (Courtesy R. Goepp, DDS, Zoller Clinic, University of Chicago.)

and submandibular nodes may be involved. In some cases just an isolated node has been calcified; in others several nodes or perhaps a whole chain of nodes has become calcified.

If the nodes are superficial, they may be palpated as bony, hard, round, or linear masses with variable mobility.

On radiographs a single round, oval, or linear calcified radiopaque mass may be seen (Fig. 27-20). Frequently the outlines are well contoured and well defined, depending on whether the original inflammatory process was contained within the capsule of the lymph node.

DIFFERENTIAL DIAGNOSIS

The differential diagnosis of calcified lymph nodes is discussed with the differential diagnosis of the sialolith (p. 565).

A calcified lymph node is classified as a false periapical radiopacity, and its image may be projected on many views. One feature that helps differentiate it from a sialolith is that the calcified node is invariably asymptomatic, whereas the sialolith is frequently accompanied by a painful sialadenitis of the associated gland. Also the sialolith usually has an irregular outline, whereas the calcified node is most often smoothly contoured.

MANAGEMENT

Calcified lymph nodes do not require treatment.

Phleboliths

Phleboliths are calcified thrombi occurring in venules, veins, or sinusoidal vessels of hemangiomas. They may occur singly or as multiple calcifications, are usually small radiopacities, may be round or oval, and may show concentric light and dark rings (see Fig. 28-22). When they are projected over the mandibular bone or the periapices of mandibular teeth, they may easily be confused with sialoliths.

Arterial calcifications

Calcification frequently accompanies arteriosclerosis, and the facial artery is sometimes affected. When a considerable length of this artery is involved, the serpentine outline and the position of the faint radiopacity are pathognomonic. When just a small segment of the artery is involved, however, and the radiopaque image of this segment is cast over the body of the mandible near the inferior border, the artery may simulate a sialolith within the submaxillary gland or duct or a small, calcified lymph node.

RARITIES

Included among the rarities are soft tissue calcifications that occur as single or multiple entities:

Calcified acne lesions
Calcified hematoma
Calcinosis cutis
Cysticercosis
Hamartomas
Mineralized tumors
Multiple osteomas of the skin
Myositis ossificans
Osteoma cutis
Pathologic soft tissue masses
Pilomatrixoma (calcifying epithelioma of Malherbe)
Tonsillolith

REFERENCES

Appleton SA, Kimbrough RE, and Engstrom HIM: Rhinolithiasis: a review, Oral Surg 65:693-698, 1988.

Clark CA: A method of ascertaining the relative position of unerupted teeth by means of film radiographs, Proc R Soc Med 3:87-90, 1910.

Damm DD and Ziegler RC: Roentgeno-oddities: factitious rhinolith, Oral Surg 59:662, 1985.

Eliasson S, Halvarsson C, and Ljungheimer G: Periapical condensing osteitis and endodontic treatment, Oral Surg 57:195-199, 1984.

Farman AG, Joubert JJ, and Nortje CJ: Focal osteosclerosis and apical periodontal pathosis in "European" and Cape coloured dental outpatients, Int J Oral Surg 7:549-557, 1978.

Haug RH, Bradrick JP, and Indresano AT: Xeroradiography in the diagnosis of nonradiopaque sialoliths, Oral Surg 67:146-148, 1989.

Jordan RE, Suzuki M, and Skinner DH: Indirect pulp-capping of carious teeth with periapical lesions, J Am Dent Assoc 97:37-43, 1978.

Katz JO, Langlais RP, Underhill TE, and Kimura K: Localization of paraoral soft tissue calcifications: the known object rule, Oral Surg 67:459-463, 1989.

Marmary Y and Kutiner G: A radiographic survey of periapical jawbone lesions, Oral Surg 61:405-408, 1986.

Neville BW and Albenesius RJ: The prevalence of benign fibro-osseous lesions of periodontal ligament origin in black women: a radiographic survey, Oral Surg 62:340-344, 1986.

Price C: A method of determining the radiopacity of dental materials and foreign bodies, Oral Surg 62:710-718, 1986.

Shafer WG, Hine MK, and Levy BM: A textbook of oral pathology, ed 4, Philadelphia, 1983, WB Saunders Co, p 334.

Stafne EC: Oral roentgenographic diagnosis, ed 3, Philadelphia, 1969, WB Saunders Co, p 25.

Yamane GM, Scharlock SE, Jain R et al: Intraoral salivary gland sialolithiasis, J Oral Med 39:85-90, 1984.

28

Solitary radiopacities not necessarily contacting teeth

NORMAN K. WOOD
PAUL W. GOAZ

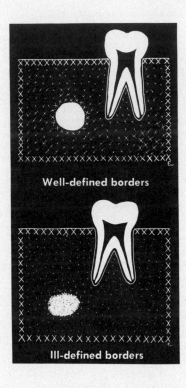

Well-defined borders

Ill-defined borders

Following is a list of radiopacities that may not be in contact with the roots of teeth:

True intrabony radiopacities
Tori, exostoses, and peripheral osteomas
Unerupted, impacted, and supernumerary teeth
Retained roots
Idiopathic osteosclerosis
Condensing or sclerosing osteitis
Mature cementoma
Fibrous dysplasia
Sclerosing osteomyelitis and diffuse sclerosing
  osteomyelitis
Proliferative periostitis (Garrè's osteomyelitis)
Mature complex odontoma
Ossifying subperiosteal hematoma
Rarities
  Cementifying and ossifying fibroma
  Chondromas and chondrosarcomas—
    radiopaque variety
  Mature osteoblastoma
  Metastatic osteoblastic carcinomas—
    radiopaque variety
  Osteoblastoma
  Osteochondroma
  Osteogenic sarcoma—radiopaque variety

Projected radiopacities
Anatomic structures
Foreign bodies
Pathologic soft tissue masses
Ectopic calcifications
  Sialoliths of major and minor salivary glands
  Rhinoliths and antroliths
  Calcified lymph nodes
  Tonsillolith
  Phleboliths
  Arterial calcifications
Rarities
  Calcified acne lesion
  Calcified hematoma (soft tissue)
  Calcinosis cutis
  Hamartoma
  Myositis ossificans
  Peripheral fibroma with calcification
  Pilomatrixoma (calcifying epithelioma of
    Malherbe)

Many of the radiopacities included in this chapter are discussed in Chapter 27. It seems expedient, however, to repeat the listing of these entities in this chapter and reconsider some of them, since they may also occur as solitary radiopacities not contacting the roots of teeth. Such an arrangement is appropriate, since there is a difference in the incidence of these entities, which correlates with their contacting the roots of teeth.

Certainly this consideration affects the development of a valid differential diagnosis. Condensing or sclerosing osteitis is a good case in point: as a periapical radiopacity, the lesion occurs quite commonly, but its occurrence as a solitary radiopacity not contacting the roots of teeth is uncommon. Thus the two entities are discussed in both chapters.

In this chapter solitary radiolucencies not contacting the roots of teeth are discussed as true intrabony radiopacities and projected radiopacities.

True intrabony radiopacities

TORI, EXOSTOSES, AND PERIPHERAL OSTEOMAS

Tori, exostoses, and peripheral osteomas are discussed in Chapter 10 as exophytic lesions and in Chapter 27 as projected (false) periapical radiopacities.

Some authors contend that tori exostoses are developmental lesions, in contrast to osteomas (which they describe as a neoplasm). From the standpoint of clinical diagnosis, however, we consider that these three lesions probably represent one pathologic process and arise on a hereditary basis. This inference is based on the limited information currently available relating to the incidence of osteoma; moreover, all three entities produce similar clinical and radiographic appearances and have almost identical microstructures.

Consequently, although the clinical differentiation of tori, exostoses, and osteomas may be quite arbitrary, those that occur in the midline of the palate or on the lingual aspect of the mandibular ridge (usually in the region of the premolars) are termed palatal and mandibular tori, respectively; those that occur in other alveolar sites are referred to as exostoses; and when a torus or an exostosis becomes unusually large, it is called an osteoma. The tori, exostoses, and osteomas usually become discernible in patients over 16 years of age.

Features

Whether the well-defined radiopaque shadows of these bony protuberances are projected over the images of tooth roots on periapical films depends on which jaw is shown on the radiograph and whether the segment of the jaw most proximal to the bone lesion is dentulous (Fig. 28-1). Usually a torus on the mandible, an

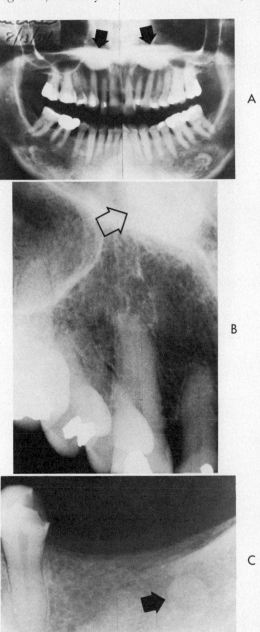

Fig. 28-1. **A,** Palatal torus *(arrows)* appears as bilateral radiopacities in this panograph. **B,** Palatal torus *(arrow)* projected superior to the apex of the canine. **C,** Small lingual mandibular torus *(arrow)* appearing as a rounded radiopacity.

exostosis, and sometimes an osteoma (in either jaw) cast radiopaque shadows over the images of tooth roots if the jaw segments in which they occur are bearing teeth.

King and Moore (1976) compared the incidence of tori in London, England, and Lexington, Kentucky, and found that the percentage of incidence was higher and the maxillary tori were larger in the Kentucky sample. King and King (1981) compared tori incidence in three populations: Florida whites, Florida blacks, and Kentucky whites. They found no significant difference in incidence of maxillary tori among the three groups, but this lesion was twice as common in females. Florida blacks had approximately three fourths as many of these lesions as Florida and Kentucky whites.

Differential diagnosis

Correlating the clinical finding of a smooth, nodular, hard protuberance with the radiographic finding of a smoothly contoured radiopacity establishes the correct diagnosis and eliminates the need for additional radiographs or an extensive differential diagnosis. Nevertheless, as shown in Fig. 28-2, a case of a mature ossifying fibroma can mimic an exostosis. However, in this case periapical films showed a

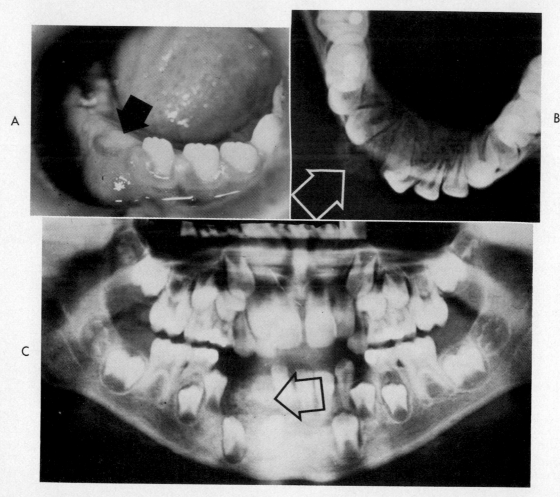

Fig. 28-2. Ossifying fibroma in an 8-year-old boy, which resembled an exostosis both on clinical examination, **A,** and in the occlusal radiograph, **B. C,** Orthopantomograph showing that the radiopaque lesion has blocked the eruption of the lower right permanent incisor and canine tooth.　(Courtesy N. Choukas, DDS, Maywood, Ill.)

thin radiolucent rim surrounding the mature fibro-osseous lesion. In addition, an early osteogenic sarcoma or a small chondrosarcoma can mimic a torus or exostosis.

Management

Tori, exostoses, and peripheral osteomas may not have to be treated, but they may be removed surgically for phonetic, psychologic, or prosthetic reasons or if they are being chronically irritated.

UNERUPTED, IMPACTED, AND SUPERNUMERARY TEETH

Unerupted permanent molars and impacted and supernumerary teeth are the next most common solitary radiopacities after tori, exostoses, and osteomas whose images may not overlap the roots of other teeth. In 1000 panoramic radiographs of patients applying to Dental School Clinic in Australia, Barrett et al.

(1984) found only 17 unerupted teeth. In contrast, Spyropoulos et al. (1981), using similar methods on 368 edentulous dental school patients in Athens, Greece, found 34 unerupted teeth (most were maxillary canines). If good quality radiographs are obtained, the recognizable outline of a tooth and the radiolucent shadows of the pulp canal, periodontal ligament, and follicular space establish the identity of these entities (Fig. 28-3). Bizarre shapes of malformed teeth coupled with technically poor films may complicate the identification of the entities.

RETAINED ROOTS

Retained roots are a common finding in edentulous regions of the jaws, and the images of retained roots usually do not contact those of other roots. Ennis and Berry's survey of edentulous patients (1949) disclosed that approximately 25% of these patients had retained

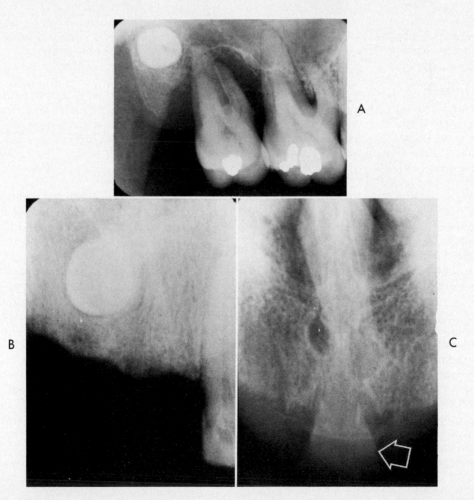

Fig. 28-3. **A** and **B,** Impacted teeth. **C,** Cartilage of the nasal septum *(arrow)* that resembles the crown of a developing incisor.

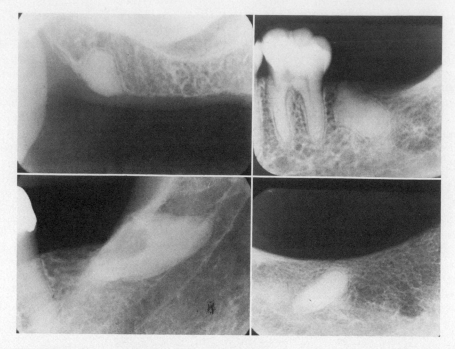

Fig. 28-4. Retained roots. The periodontal ligament space and lamina dura cannot be clearly detected around some of the root fragments. The root canal shadows are not apparent.

roots and 80% of the roots were located in the posterior regions of the alveolar processes. Approximately 6% of the retained roots had an accompanying radiolucency. This last group would be classified as mixed radiolucent-radiopaque lesions, which are discussed in Chapter 24.

In a study completed in London, Ritchie and Fletcher (1979) found that approximately 50% of edentulous patients had a retained root. Interestingly, the vast majority were seen in the upper jaw. Spyropoulos et al. (1981) found 114 root fragments in 368 edentulous patients; 71% of these were also found in the maxilla.

Features

The majority of retained roots are quiescent, asymptomatic, and found on routine radiographs. If they are unaltered, their identification is relatively easy, but if chronic infection has caused the root canals to be obliterated or has resulted in some peripheral resorption or enveloping condensing osteitis, their recognition may be difficult (Fig. 28-4). A careful study of the radiograph, however, usually discloses the homogeneous quality of the root tip's shadow, which is in contrast to the more or less obscure trabecular character of the sclerotic bone. Thus the differentiation is possible.

On occasion, either retained roots become infected or long-standing chronic infection is exacerbated and local swelling, pain, regional lymphadenitis, space infections, and even osteomyelitis ensue.

Differential diagnosis

The differential diagnosis for retained roots is discussed later in this chapter with the differential diagnosis of condensing osteitis.

Management

The management of a retained root tip depends on the circumstances of the individual case. If the root tip is small, asymptomatic, and situated relatively deep so that its removal would require removing a good deal of bone or if it is so close to an important structure that the structure could be severely damaged during the root's removal, it should not be removed unless a serious pathologic condition appears to be associated with it. The patient should simply be apprised of its presence, and its status should be periodically evaluated by serial radiographs.

Roots that are both near the surface and beneath the site of a proposed artificial denture or bridge, roots associated with a pathologic lesion, or roots causing pain should be removed.

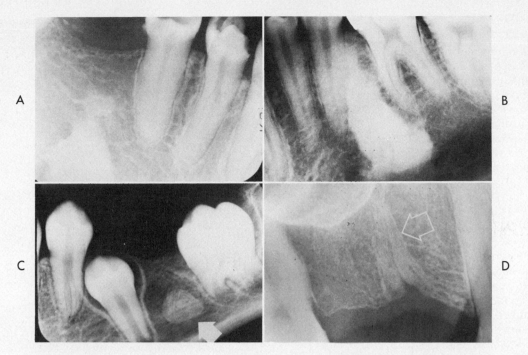

Fig. 28-5. **A** to **C**, Idiopathic osteosclerosis. The second premolar pulp in **B** was vital. **C**, Idiopathic osteosclerosis *(arrow)*. **D**, Socket sclerosis *(arrow)*. The central linear radiolucent shadow resembles a root canal.

IDIOPATHIC OSTEOSCLEROSIS

Idiopathic osteosclerosis is discussed in Chapter 27 as a periapical radiopacity. The objective of its inclusion in this chapter is to emphasize and illustrate that this entity is not always found in association with the roots of teeth.

Features

Idiopathic osteosclerotic lesions may occur in the alveolus, between the roots of teeth, just below the crest of the ridge, or in the body of the mandible (Fig. 28-5).

Usually the cause is obscure. When the lesion is present in the alveolus between the first and second premolars or between the second premolar and the first molar, its occurrence is generally described as a sequela of retained deciduous molar roots. These retained roots are resorbed and replaced by sclerotic bone, or fragments of the roots are completely surrounded and obliterated by the condensed bone.

Because the radiopaque areas of periapical condensing osteitis frequently do not resolve after extraction of a tooth, many such residual areas may be diagnosed as idiopathic osteoscle-rosis if the clinician is unaware that teeth with infected or nonvital pulps have been removed from the area. This possibility should be considered when a suspect area is encountered. Postextraction wounds and other surgical defects may be the site of idiopathic osteosclerosis (Fig. 28-5).

The sclerotic lesion is usually solitary but may be multiple or even bilateral; however, its bilateral occurrence would be only incidental and should not be considered a significant diagnostic feature.

On microscopic examination, thickened trabeculae with few lacunae and greatly reduced marrow and fibrovascular spaces are seen.

Differential diagnosis

The differential diagnosis of idiopathic osteosclerosis is discussed later in this chapter with the differential diagnosis of condensing osteitis.

Management

The identification of idiopathic osteosclerosis is all that is necessary. The clinician should observe the course of the lesion by taking serial radiographs, however.

CONDENSING OR SCLEROSING OSTEITIS

Condensing or sclerosing osteitis is an osteosclerosis that can be explained as a sequela of an inflammatory process.

It occurs much less frequently as a periapical radiopacity in edentulous regions, of course. In edentulous regions it is almost always a residual lesion or limited to reactions around retained roots or root tips. Its appearance as a periapical radiopacity is described in Chapter 27.

Features

On radiographs, condensing or sclerosing osteitis resembles the radiopacity of idiopathic osteosclerosis except that root tips are usually identifiable within the radiopaque lesion or there may be a history or some presumptive evidence that an infected tooth was previously removed from the area. The borders may be ragged or smoothly contoured, vague or well defined (Fig. 28-6).

The microscopic appearance is identical to that of idiopathic osteosclerosis except that, if the lesion is still active, an extensive examination of the specimen discloses restricted areas of chronic inflammation. If the source of infection was removed some time before the specimen was taken, the inflammatory reaction may have completely subsided, with only the dense mass of trabeculae remaining.

Differential diagnosis

Many of the entities discussed in this chapter must be included in the differential diagnosis. The lesions that may be confused with condensing or sclerosing osteitis are a variety of the projected radiopacities that are not attached to or within the alveoli or jawbone under scrutiny: cementoma, retained roots, unerupted tooth, mature complex odontoma, osteoblastic malignant tumor, sclerosing osteomyelitis, tori, exostoses, peripheral osteomas, and idiopathic osteosclerosis.

As discussed in Chapter 27, the *projected radiopacities* can be readily identified by obtaining additional radiographs of the area using Clark's tube-shift technique.

The opacities produced by hard odontogenic tissue, including the *mature cementoma, retained roots, unerupted tooth,* and *mature complex odontoma,* may be recognized by their distinctive shapes and densities and their radiolucent borders. A partially resorbed root tip or root fragment is usually relatively small and, if not surrounded by condensing osteitis, in most

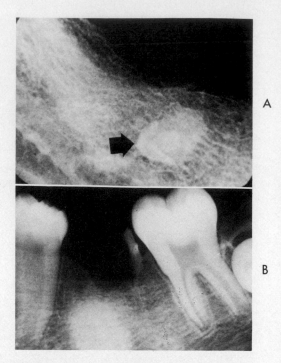

Fig. 28-6. Condensing osteitis. **A,** Surrounding a small, round root tip *(arrow).* **B,** Surrounding the mesial root of a grossly decayed molar.

cases retains enough of its shape to be recognizable. It should be found only in tooth-bearing areas of the jaws.

Although an *osteoblastic malignancy* producing a completely radiopaque lesion in this area is very rare, in the event of such an occurrence, the examining clinician must consider osteogenic sarcoma, metastatic prostatic carcinoma, or metastatic mammary carcinoma. Keyes et al. (1988) reported a case of lymphoma of the mandible that closely resembled a condensing osteitis. In addition to the symptoms of the primary tumor or the history of its treatment, the tumor is usually accompanied by pain, swelling, and frequently paresthesia. Paresthesia, if present, strongly suggests that the lesion is malignant.

Sclerosing osteomyelitis is a moderate proliferative reaction of the bone to a mild type of infection. The patient usually has a history of a prolonged tender swelling with, in some cases, intermittent drainage through a sinus from the body of the mandible. Osteomyelitis seldom becomes established in healthy persons who do not have a history of jaw fracture. Condensing osteitis, by comparison, is usually asymptomatic.

The opacities produced by the *tori, exostoses,* and *peripheral osteomas* can be identified promptly if the characteristic painless, smooth nodular swelling on the jaws is detected during the clinical examination.

Differentiating between condensing or sclerosing osteitis and *idiopathic osteosclerosis* is often difficult if not impossible when the suspect lesion is in an edentulous region and cannot be related to a specific tooth. Of course, if a root tip can be observed within the region of sclerotic bone, the diagnosis is condensing osteitis. Thus, if the sclerotic area does not contain root tips and the lesion has not formed at the apex of a tooth with an infected or nonvital pulp, the diagnosis of idiopathic osteosclerosis is appropriate.

Management

The treatment of condensing or sclerosing osteitis surrounding a root tip must be tailored to the individual situation.

As with root tips, lesions that are in the superficial alveolar crest should be removed to prepare for a prosthesis and to prevent the occurrence of active infection.

Deeper lesions that are asymptomatic are usually not disturbed but are observed with serial radiographs.

Lesions complicated by acute or chronic infection should be enucleated, and the patient should receive appropriate presurgical and postsurgical antibiotic therapy.

MATURE CEMENTOMA

The cementoma that develops from cells of the periodontal ligament is discussed in Chapter 16 as a periapical radiolucency, in Chapter 24 as a mixed radiolucent-radiopaque lesion, and in Chapter 27 as a periapical radiopacity. In this chapter its occurrence as a solitary radiopaque mass in edentulous regions of the jaws is discussed.

Features

When these mature fibro-osseous lesions occur without apparent relation to teeth, they have the following features:

1. They are ordinarily found at the apices of vital teeth but also occur with significant frequency in edentulous regions. Many of these latter lesions are undoubtedly resid-

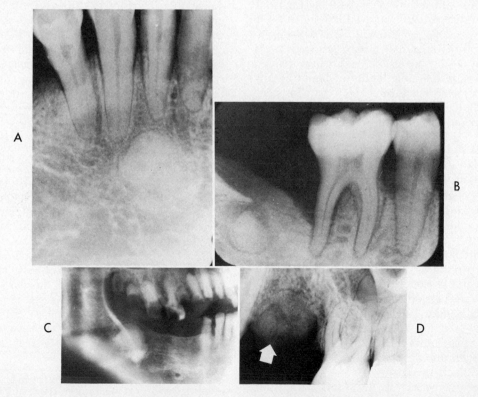

Fig. 28-7. **A** to **C**, Mature cementomas. **D**, Mature ossifying fibroma *(arrow).*   (Courtesy N. Barakat, DDS, Beirut, Lebanon.)

ual (that is, they were left in place when the involved tooth was removed).

2. They may be solitary or multiple, and their radiographic appearance is similar to that of the periapical variety. The mature lesions are uniformly radiopaque and almost invariably have a radiolucent border. Most of the lesions are round to oval but occasionally have irregular shapes (Fig. 28-7).

3. On histologic study they consist almost entirely of varying proportions of dense cementum and bone with few lacunae or vascular spaces. Polarizing microscopy is usually required to differentiate cementum from sclerotic bone.

Differential diagnosis

The differential diagnosis of a mature cementoma is discussed earlier in this chapter with the differential diagnosis of condensing osteitis.

Management

The proper treatment of a mature cementoma entails only its recognition and periodic observation by serial radiographs. It is important to identify the cementoma so that surgical removal is not mistakenly undertaken.

Lesions situated in the crest of the ridge, however, are usually removed if a denture is to be placed over the area (Fig. 28-7, *D*). Lesions that continue to enlarge may produce an expansion of the mandible and cause pain or numbness in the area, so these should be enucleated. This procedure enables the clinician to establish the correct diagnosis by microscopic examination of the tissue removed.

FIBROUS DYSPLASIA (FIBRO-OSSEOUS LESIONS NOT OF PERIODONTAL LIGAMENT ORIGIN)

Much confusion and disagreement have persisted over the years concerning the fibro-osseous lesions. More recently, however, pathologists have recognized that this group should be subdivided, on the basis of a number of features, into fibro-osseous lesions arising from cells of the periodontal ligament (PDLO) and fibro-osseous lesions not derived from elements of the periodontal ligament. The cementomas, cemento-ossifying fibromas, and ossifying fibromas are examples of the former type, whereas fibrous dysplasia of the facial bones is an example of the latter.

Fibrous dysplasia is discussed with ill-defined radiolucencies in Chapter 21 and is dis-

cussed in Chapter 25 as a mixed radiolucent-radiopaque lesion. In this chapter its more radiopaque, classic, ground-glass appearance is emphasized.

Features

Fibrous dysplasia is basically a bony lesion of children, adolescents, and young adults that may involve the jawbones. It occurs in males and females equally and in the maxilla only slightly more often than in the mandible. When it occurs in the maxilla, it may extend into the maxillary sinus, floor of the orbit, and zygomatic process and backward toward the base of the skull (Fig. 28-8).

The lesion is a painless expansion of the jawbone, which grows slowly for some years and then becomes arrested. The jawbone expansion is usually fusiform (low plateau) rather than nodular or dome shaped and is firm, smoothly contoured, and covered with normal-appearing mucosa.

The majority of the enlargements measure between 2 and 8 cm in length.

The radiographic image cast by these lesions is generally uniform and of the classic ground-glass* type (Fig. 28-8). In an earlier stage there may be a mixed pattern with irregular radiodense foci distributed throughout a lesion of ground-glass appearance or through a radiolucent area. As the lesion matures, the foci become more radiopaque. The margins of the lesion are vague on the radiograph because there is a gradual transition between the pathosis and the surrounding normal bone.

Mature lesions on extraoral radiographs often appear to be completely radiopaque, but usually on periapical films the region shows the ground-glass feature.

On histologic study, spicules of woven bone that appear in Chinese letter–like (retiform) patterns are seen scattered throughout a fibrous tissue stroma. Osteoblastic rimming of the bony spicules is usually missing. More mature lesions show a larger proportion of bone to fibrous tissue and frequently contain some lamellar-type bone with osteoblastic rimming. Waldron (1985) summarized the current concepts concerning fibrous dysplasia.

---

*The terms "orange peel," "stippled," and "salt-and-pepper" are also used synonymously with "ground-glass" to describe the image produced by many closely arranged, small trabeculae.

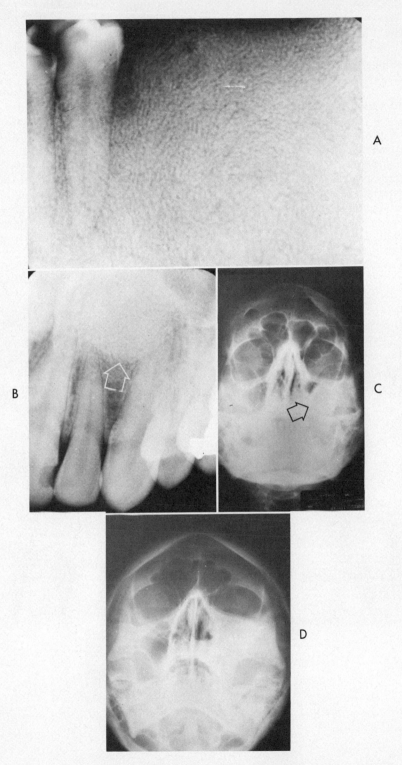

Fig. 28-8. Fibrous dysplasia. **A** and **B**, The ground-glass appearance in two patients. **C** and **D**, Waters' views of two other patients with fibrous dysplasia of the left maxillary sinus. A ground-glass appearance was seen on periapical films. Arrows in **B** and **C** show the lesions. (**D** courtesy E. Palacios, MD, Maywood, Ill.)

Differential diagnosis

A solitary, painless fusiform enlargement is almost certainly fibrous dysplasia when it is firm, smooth, and covered with normal mucosa, has a radiopaque, ground-glass appearance, and occurs in the jawbone of a relatively young person.

Other diseases such as *Paget's disease* in the radiolucent stage and *hyperparathyroidism* may produce a ground-glass appearance of the bone, but the overall effect is one of rarefaction, not of radiopacity. Also, the radiographic pattern in these two diseases is generalized, not localized and solitary as in fibrous dysplasia. Occasionally, radiopaque ground-glass patterns may be seen in both Paget's disease and hyperparathyroidism (Fig. 28-9).

Although several bones may be involved with fibrous dysplasia in *Albright's syndrome,* which occurs in young girls, this syndrome is readily identified by its accompanying features of precocious puberty and café-au-lait spots on the skin.

Occasionally, mature cementifying and ossifying fibromas may assume a radiopaque ground-glass appearance, as may calcifying postsurgical bone defects (Fig. 28-9).

Management

Fibrous dysplasia should be managed by close clinical and radiographic observation, since the lesions may undergo surges of growth during hormonal changes. Recontouring of the bone to correct a deformity is occasionally nec-

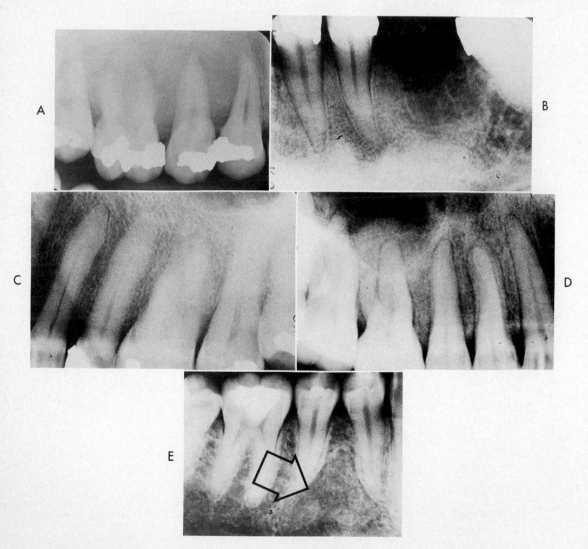

Fig. 28-9. Ground-glass lesions. **A** and **B,** Fibrous dysplasia. **C,** Paget's disease. **D,** Secondary hyperparathyroidism. **E,** Resolving traumatic bone cyst *(arrow).* (**D** courtesy P. O'Flaherty, DDS, Chicago.)

essary for esthetic or prosthetic reasons, but block resection is seldom if ever indicated. Radiation therapy is not recommended because of the possibility of radiation-induced sarcomas.

FOCAL SCLEROSING OSTEOMYELITIS AND DIFFUSE SCLEROSING OSTEOMYELITIS

Osteomyelitis is discussed in Chapter 16 as a periapical radiolucency, in Chapter 21 as a ragged radiolucency, and in Chapter 24 as a mixed radiolucent-radiopaque lesion. The sclerosing variety of osteomyelitis, which represents a reaction to a low-grade infection, is included in this chapter because it sometimes occurs as a totally radiopaque lesion.

Features

The borders of the radiopaque lesions may be ragged or smooth, well defined or vague (Fig. 28-10).

Identification of a focal sclerosing osteomyelitis in the bone usually depends on detecting symptoms of chronic infection such as tenderness, pain, or local swelling. A regional lymphadenitis is a frequent complaint, and a draining sinus may accompany some cases.

On microscopic examination, dense, sclerotic nonvital bone is seen. Acute inflammation is present in some areas and, occasionally, focal collections of pus are found (Fig. 28-10).

Diffuse sclerosing osteomyelitis (DSO) is a different entity from the small, isolated lesions of focal sclerosing osteomyelitis, which have an obvious cause. DSO occurs occasionally and has been recognized for a number of years. This disease is mainly confined to the mandible, and typically a large section of the mandible is involved. Early symptoms are vague and consist of pain, swelling, and mild elevations in systemic temperature. On radiographic examination, changes occur slowly during the course of several years. Osteolytic areas predominate at first and when symptoms are at their worst; they disappear as symptoms regress. Periodically symptoms recur and wane. As episodes become less frequent and less severe, dense bony sclerosis predominates and the radiolucent segments diminish. Generally the lesion persists and recurs, and treatment has been unsatisfactory (Farnam et al., 1984).

Jacobsson et al. (1982) attempted to clarify the obscure cause of DSO of the mandible. Paying special attention to anaerobic culture techniques, they found *Propionibacterium acnes* and *Peptostreptococcus intermedius* to be of etiologic importance in some cases. These authors suggested that DSO is caused by "endogenic, low-grade bacterial infection probably of dental origin, while the chronicity of the disease may depend on different immunologic mechanisms." Van Merkesteyn et al. (1988) reported on 27 cases and concluded that their findings did not support infection as a cause.

Jacobsson and Hollender (1980) discussed the cause, therapy, and prognosis of DSO. These authors made special recommendations for long-range management of these lesions.

Differential diagnosis

The lesions necessarily included in the differential diagnosis for a solitary intrabony area of sclerosis are an osteoblastic or sclerosing malignancy, condensing osteitis, fibrous dysplasia, and diffuse cementosis.

A totally radiopaque *osteoblastic or sclerosing malignancy* is rare—possibly an osteogenic sarcoma or a metastatic osteoblastic prostatic, bronchogenic, or mammary carcinoma. Should one occur, however, rapid growth, frequent

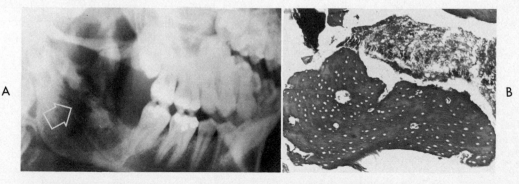

Fig. 28-10. Sclerosing osteomyelitis after a jaw fracture. Some of the radiopaque areas are sequestra. **A,** Radiopaque lesion *(arrow)* in the ramus. **B,** Photomicrograph.   (**A** courtesy O.H. Stuteville, DDS, MD, St. Joe, Ark.)

pain without symptoms of infection, and paresthesia (frequently produced by malignant lesions of bone) help distinguish it from the more common sclerosing osteomyelitis. Nevertheless, a malignant tumor with a superimposed osteomyelitis may be difficult to identify because of the overlapping signs and symptoms. Lesions occurring after radiation may also present a problem in differentiating between a sclerosing osteoradionecrosis and a recurrent tumor.

Condensing osteitis can usually be eliminated from the differential diagnosis by the presence of the more subjective symptoms of infection that frequently accompany a chronic osteomyelitis and are not a feature of condensing osteitis.

Management

The first step in managing sclerosing osteomyelitis is to control the contributing systemic disease, if one is present. A protracted course of antibiotics, judiciously selected and administered, is indicated; however, some cases require incision and drainage and possibly enucleation and saucerization if the antibiotic therapy fails to eliminate the bone infection. The use of hyperbaric oxygen may be beneficial.

PROLIFERATIVE PERIOSTITIS (PERIOSTITIS OSSIFICANS, GARRÈ'S OSTEOMYELITIS, NONSUPPURATIVE OSTEOMYELITIS)

Proliferative periostitis, a particular type of osteomyelitis, is so distinctive that it has been considered a separate entity. For many years this entity has been referred to as Garrè's osteomyelitis. (It is interesting that Wood et al. (1988) reviewed the original paper by Garrè and found not only that Garrè's name has been consistently misspelled in the literature but also that Garrè did not describe this type of osteomyelitis at all.) This condition is characterized by the formation of new bone on the periphery of the cortex over an infected area of spongiosa. The formation of new bone is a response of the inner surface of the periosteum to stimulation by a low-grade infection that has spread through the bone and penetrated the cortex.

Strains of staphylococci and streptococci are the microorganisms most commonly cultured. Periapical odontogenic infection is a frequent cause of proliferative periostitis of the jaws, although an occasional case can be traced to a pericoronitis.

We infer, from the paucity of reports in the dental literature that recount the occurrence of this disease and our own experience, that proliferative periostitis of the jaws is a relatively uncommon dental complication. For this lesion to develop, a peculiar combination of circumstances must coexist:

1. The periosteum must possess a high potential for osteoblastic activity (this requirement is satisfied in young patients).
2. A chronic infection must be present.
3. A fine balance must be maintained between the resistance of the host and the number and virulence of organisms present, so the infection can continue at a low, chronic stage—invasive enough to stimulate new periosteal bone formation but not severe enough to induce bone resorption.

Proliferative periostitis is included in this chapter because it may produce a solitary radiopacity that does not contact the roots of teeth.

Features

Proliferative periostitis is seen almost exclusively in children and rarely occurs in patients over 30 years of age.

The patient may complain of pain caused by odontogenic infection before the intermittent, usually nontender swelling develops at the inferior border or other peripheries of the mandible. The most frequent site is the inferior border of the mandible below the first molar (Fig. 28-11). The maxilla is seldom affected.

Lichty et al. (1980) reviewed 22 reported cases of proliferative periostitis and reported the following: (1) the mean age was 12 years; (2) the female-to-male ratio of prevalence was 1.4:1 (3) an abscessed mandibular first permanent molar was the most common inciting factor; (4) facial asymmetry was present; (5) swelling was bony hard and usually nontender; (6) overlying mucosa and skin appeared normal; (7) treatment consisted of an initial course of antibiotics and extraction of the causative tooth; and (8) regression usually occurred within 2 to 6 months.

Cheng et al. (1984) reported a simultaneous occurrence of proliferative periostitis with cervicofacial actinomycosis. Eisenbud et al. (1981) reported a case of proliferative periostitis that occurred simultaneously in all four quadrants.

If the chronic infection becomes established just beneath the periosteum and is not treated, the swelling persists and soon becomes hard as new bone is laid down. After the infection has

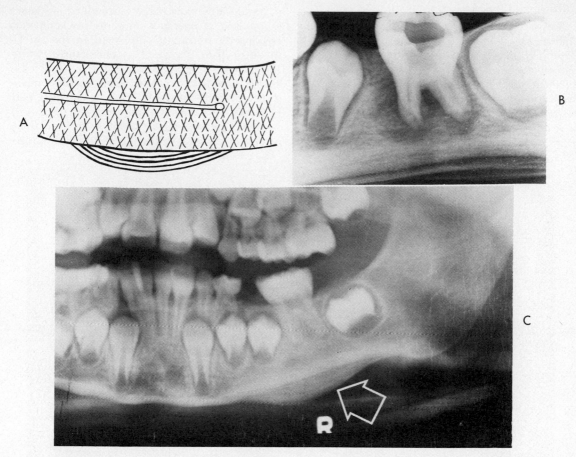

Fig. 28-11. Proliferative periostitis. **A,** Diagram of periosteal new bone formation in a layered or "onion skin" appearance. The integrity of the original cortex is usually maintained. **B** and **C,** Two cases of proliferative periostitis in the first molar region of the mandible. **B,** The definite layering effect and the rarefying osteitis are evident at the apex of the pulpless molar. **C,** The layering effect is not so noticeable in this more radiopaque periostitis *(arrow),* which was caused by a chronically infected second deciduous molar tooth that had been extracted recently.   (**B** courtesy N. Barakat, DDS, Beirut, Lebanon. **C** courtesy J. Baird, DDS, Evanston, Ill.)

been eliminated, the hard elevation usually disappears slowly as the bone is recontoured by the functional forces.

The swelling is characteristically convex, varying in length and depth of bone deposits. It may range from 2 cm to involvement of the whole length of the mandibular body on the affected side. The covering skin or overlying mucosa may appear normal or be moderately inflamed. Occasionally fever and a leukocytosis are present.

On radiographs a smoothly contoured, moderately convex bony shadow can be seen extending from the preserved cortex of the jaw (Fig. 28-11). The space between this new, thin shell of bone and the cortex may be quite radiolucent without images of trabeculae. Later

an alternating light and dark laminated appearance may be seen, and when the whole lesion mineralizes, the lesion may be completely radiopaque (Fig. 28-11). Nortje and Wood (1988) reported on an extensive radiologic analysis of 93 cases in the jaws. These researchers found that the number of separate laminations ranged from 1 to 12.

In most cases the adjacent jawbone appears normal on the radiograph, but sometimes there may be accompanying radiolucent or osteosclerotic osteomyelitis changes.

On histologic examination, dense new bone is seen with minimal vascular spaces. The periosteum is thickened and shows an overactive osteoblastic layer. Scattered regions of chronic inflammation may be present.

Differential diagnosis

Lesions that necessarily are included in the differential diagnosis for a condition that resembles proliferative periostitis are Ewing's sarcoma, fibrous dysplasia, osteogenic sarcoma, infantile cortical hyperostosis, callus, ossifying hematoma, tori, exostoses, and peripheral osteomas.

Ewing's sarcoma may produce a convex peripheral radiopaque lesion quite similar to that of proliferative periostitis, and indeed its classic onion ring appearance mimics the laminated radiopacity frequently observed in the osteomyelitis (Fig. 28-12). This characteristic, the shared predilection for children, and the shared symptom of tender swellings often make distinguishing between Ewing's sarcoma and proliferative periostitis quite difficult. Further, in both diseases the adjacent bone may show osteolytic changes, although a moth-eaten type

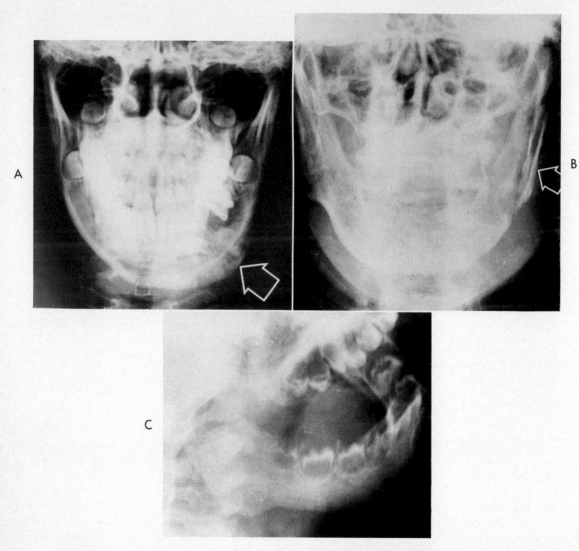

Fig. 28-12. Other lesions that produce cortical duplication. **A,** Posteroanterior radiograph of Ewing's sarcoma in the left mandible of a young girl. The cortical redundancy and layering effect *(arrow)* can be seen at the inferior border of the mandible. (Fig. 21-15 shows the extent of bone destruction of this lesion in a lateral view.) **B,** Posteroanterior radiograph showing a cortical redundancy in the left ramus *(arrow).* This appearance was produced in a 56-year-old man by a large segment of bone being fractured and displaced to the buccal area during a traumatic episode. A chronic osteomyelitis had become established here at the time this radiograph was taken, so the segment represents a large sequestrum. **C,** Redundancy of inferior border of the mandible in a case of cortical infantile hyperostosis.   (**A** courtesy N. Barakat, DDS, Beirut, Lebanon. **C** courtesy R. Moncada, MD, Maywood, Ill.)

of destruction is more typical of Ewing's sarcoma (Eversole et al., 1979). Ewing's sarcoma also shows rapid, unrestricted growth and often produces a paresthesia of the lip.

Fibrous dysplasia may appear to be located on the periphery, but a careful inspection of the radiograph usually reveals that the complete thickness of bone is altered and has the ground-glass appearance.

Osteogenic sarcoma may cause a peripheral radiopacity, and it occurs predominantly in somewhat the same age-group as proliferative periostitis. The radiographic image of this tumor, however, usually appears more irregular, and the sunburst effect (if present) is so characteristic that the two entities are not likely to be confused.

Although *infantile cortical hyperostosis* occurs in the same age-group of children, it differs from proliferative periostitis in that it is a generalized expansion of the cortices of several bones (Fig. 28-12), usually including the mandible, whereas the proliferative periostitis is a single local expansion.

A *callus* developing around a healing fracture may also appear as a peripheral radiopacity, but it is usually not radiodense. A history of trauma and radiographic evidence of the fracture line help identify the callus.

A *hematoma* may develop subperiosteally after trauma to a bone. This collection of extravasated blood occasionally ossifies, resulting in a peripheral radiopaque enlargement of the bone. The hematoma may then be confused with proliferative periostitis, but its radiopacity is not so uniform; rather, a more mottled appearance, coupled with a history of trauma to the suspect area, should identify the ossifying hematoma.

Since *tori, exostoses*, and *peripheral osteomas* also occur at peripheral borders of the mandibular body, they might be confused with proliferative periostitis. These entities are distinguishable from proliferative periostitis, however, since they do not show a predilection for patients under 20 years of age, they are more nodular (even polyploid in some cases), and they require months and years to increase appreciably in size.

Eversole et al. (1979) reviewed six cases of proliferative periostitis and outlined criteria for its differentiation from the other neoperiostoses.

Management

In most cases proliferative periostitis can be successfully treated by simply removing the

source of infection (usually an infected tooth) and administering an appropriate antibiotic. The periosteal lesion then gradually regresses until the original bone contour has been reestablished.

Sometimes the projecting mass is extensive, and surgical contouring for esthetics may be in order. This procedure in turn provides a specimen for microscopic study and a final diagnosis can be established.

McWalter and Schaberg (1984) described what appears to be the first case of a proliferative periostitis to be treated successfully with endodontics instead of by extraction of the causative tooth and a course of antibiotics. These authors reported that during the year after endodontic treatment, the periapical radiolucency filled in with new bone and the peripheral bony expansion was completely resorbed.

MATURE COMPLEX ODONTOMA

The complex odontoma is a developmental anomaly of tooth tissue that, like teeth, is completely radiolucent in the initial stage, passes into a mixed radiolucent-radiopaque stage, and

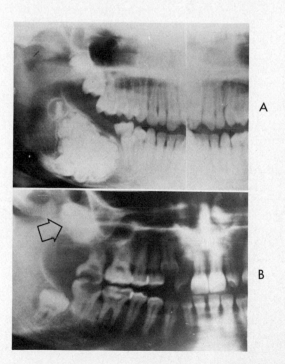

Fig. 28-13. Complex odontoma. **A,** Causing impaction of a mandibular molar. **B,** In the maxillary third molar region *(arrow).* (**A** courtesy V. Barresi, DDS, DeKalb, Ill., and D. Bonomo, DDS, Flossmoor, Ill. **B** courtesy B. Saunders, DDS, Los Angeles.)

may mature as a completely radiopaque lesion surrounded by a radiolucent halo of varying width. The tumor is made up of the three calcified dental tissues, but these are laid down in a disorganized, irregular mass without normal morphologic relationships of one tissue to another.

Odontomas are discussed in detail in Chapter 24, which describes them as radiolucent images containing radiopaque foci.

Features

The mature complex odontoma is seldom seen in patients under 6 years of age. When it occurs, it most commonly affects the first and second permanent mandibular molars, often forming in the alveoli just superior to the crowns of these teeth and effectively preventing their eruption (Fig. 28-13).

Pain or paresthesia is not characteristic of these tumors, which may vary in diameter from 1 to approximately 6 cm and may produce a bulge on the mandible.

On radiographic examination the mature lesion of considerable buccolingual width appears as a homogeneously dense radiopacity; the earlier lesion of less width may show irregular radiodense patterns throughout and may even cast a cotton-wool image on the radiograph. Although the outline of the calcified mass within the odontoma may be quite irregular, the radiolucent rim surrounding the lesion has a well-defined and smooth outer periphery.

On histologic study the lesion is composed of varying proportions of enamel, dentin, cementum, and pulp tissue in a disorganized arrangement.

Differential diagnosis

Because *mature fibro-osseous lesions (PDLO)* (for example, cementomas) are solitary dense radiopacities with radiolucent rims, they are the entities most frequently confused with the mature complex odontoma. Usually, however, a cementoma forms in persons over 30 years of age, whereas an odontoma develops in much younger patients (although both lesions may persist and be found in late adulthood). A cementoma may be situated deep in the alveolar bone, whereas the complex odontoma extends high into the alveolus, even to the crest of the ridge.

Management

Surgical enucleation of the odontoma is the treatment of choice, and the excised material should be microscopically examined.

OSSIFYING SUBPERIOSTEAL HEMATOMA

Occasionally a subperiosteal hematoma sustained as the result of trauma ossifies instead of resolving. Early in the course of its ossification, it appears as a mixed radiolucent-radiopaque lesion, but as ossification is completed, it becomes a dense, radiopaque, smoothly contoured convex expansion on the periphery of the bone (Fig. 28-14). The swelling is nontender.

Differential diagnosis

The differential diagnosis of the ossifying subperiosteal hematoma is discussed earlier in this chapter with the differential diagnosis of proliferative periostitis.

Management

Functional forces reshape the deformed bone and reestablish normal contour if the lesion is subjected to the vectors of these forces. If the bone enlargement persists for a few months, recontouring may be necessary for improved function and esthetics and in preparation for the construction of a prosthetic appliance.

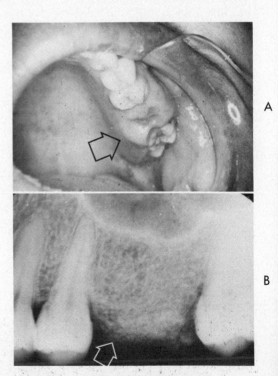

Fig. 28-14. Calcified subperiosteal hematoma (*arrow*) after tooth extraction with primary closure of the mucosa. **A,** Clinical appearance. **B,** Periapical radiograph of the hematoma (*arrow*).

RARITIES

The following entities rarely occur as solitary completely radiopaque lesions:

Cementifying and ossifying fibromas
Chondromas and chondrosarcomas—radiopaque variety
Mature osteoblastoma
Metastatic osteoblastic carcinomas—radiopaque variety
Osteoblastoma
Osteochondroma
Osteogenic sarcoma—radiopaque variety

Projected radiopacities

Radiopaque shadows that may be projected over the roots of teeth are discussed in detail in Chapter 27. The radiopacities that may be projected over the jawbone but not necessarily over a periapex are essentially the same. Consequently, illustrations of these entities are included in this chapter without further discussion. They include the following:

Anatomic structures
Foreign bodies (Figs. 28-15 and 28-23)
Pathologic soft tissue masses (Figs. 28-16 and 28-25)
Ectopic calcifications
    Sialoliths of major and minor salivary glands (Figs. 28-17 and 28-24)
    Rhinoliths and antroliths (Fig. 28-20)
    Calcified lymph nodes
    Tonsillolith
    Phleboliths
    Arterial calcifications (Fig. 28-21)
Rarities
    Calcified acne lesion
    Calcified hematoma (soft tissue)
    Calcinosis cutis
    Hemartoma
    Myositis ossificans
    Peripheral fibroma with calcification
    Pilomatrixoma (calcifying epithelioma of Malherbe)

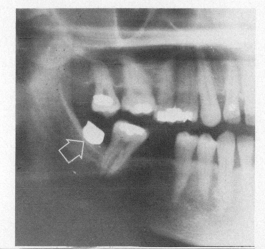

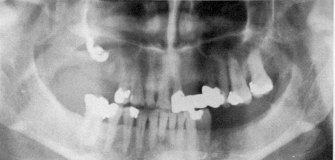

Fig. 28-15. Foreign bodies. **A,** Bullet in the cheek (*arrow*). **B,** Endodontic filling material in the right maxillary sinus. (**B** courtesy N. Barakat, DDS, Beirut, Lebanon.)

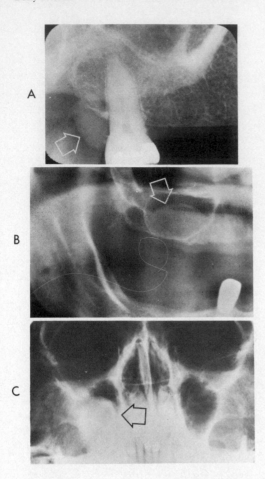

Fig. 28-16. Soft tissue shadows. A, Fibrous tuberosity (arrow) superimposed over the coronoid process. B and C, Retention cysts of the maxillary sinus (arrows). (C courtesy E. Palacios, MD, Maywood, Ill.)

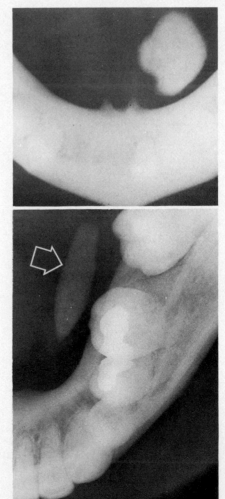

Fig. 28-17. Sialoliths in Wharton's ducts. (Courtesy R. Latronica, DDS, Albany, N.Y.)

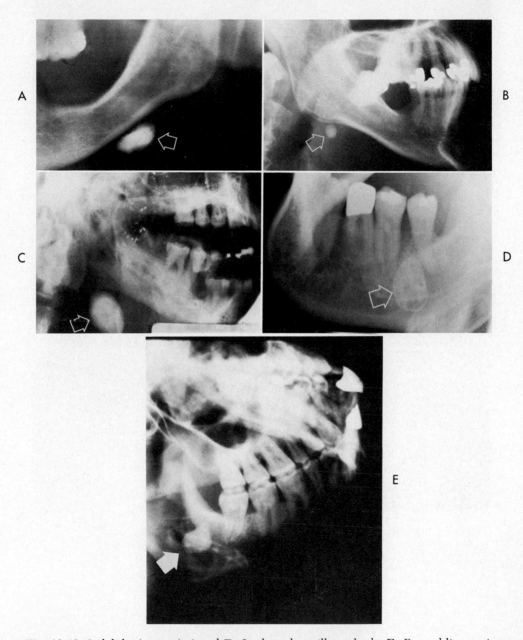

Fig. 28-18. Sialoliths *(arrows).* **A** and **D,** In the submaxillary glands. **E,** Resembling an impacted tooth.   (**B** and **C** courtesy O.H. Stuteville, DDS, MD, St. Joe, Ark. **D** courtesy R. Goepp, DDS, Zoller Clinic, University of Chicago. **E** courtesy D. Bonomo, DDS, Flossmoor, Ill.)

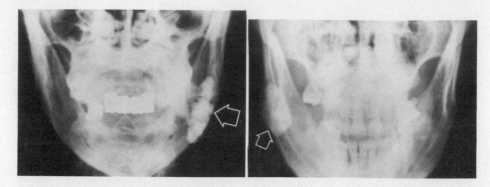

Fig. 28-19. Calcified cervical nodes *(arrows)* projected over the angles of the mandible. Both patients had a history of tuberculosis.   (Courtesy O.H. Stuteville, DDS, MD, St. Joe, Ark.)

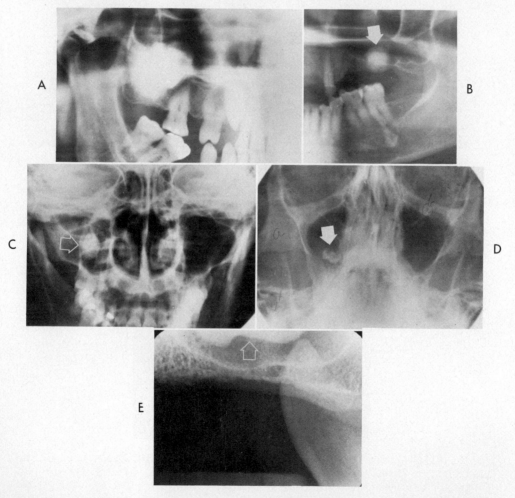

Fig. 28-20. Antrolith. **A,** In the maxillary sinus above the third molar. **B,** In the left maxillary sinus *(arrow)*. **C,** In the maxillary sinus *(arrow)* above the premolar. **D,** Resembling a developing crown of a tooth or a complex odontoma *(arrow)*. **E,** The inferior aspect of the radiopaque zygomatic bone *(arrow)* could be mistaken for an antrolith.   (**B** courtesy the late M. Kaminski, DDS, and S. Atsaves, DDS, Chicago.)

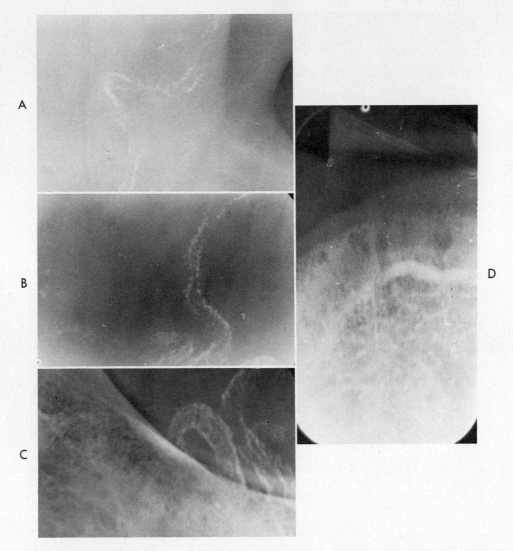

Fig. 28-21. Calcified arteries. **A** to **C**, Three arteriosclerotic facial arteries. **D**, Calcified inferior labial artery projected over the alveolar bone in the anterior mandible.   (**A** to **C** courtesy R. Latronica, DDS, Albany, N.Y. **D** courtesy R. Goepp, DDS, Zoller Clinic, University of Chicago.)

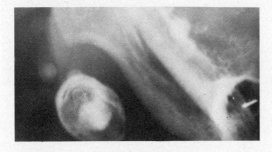

Fig. 28-22. Phlebolith just below the inferior border of the mandible. (Courtesy E. Palacios, MD, Maywood, Ill.)

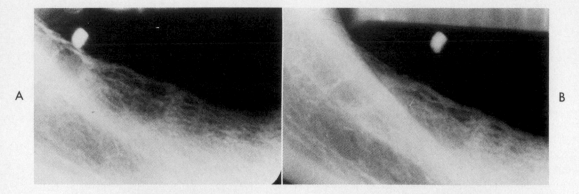

Fig. 28-23. Foreign metallic object in the cheek. The shifting of the image can be seen in the two periapical radiographs, which were taken at different vertical angles.

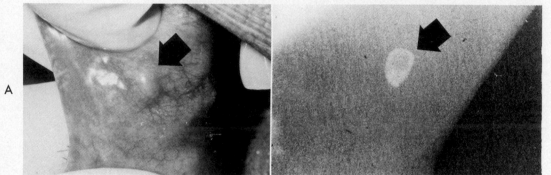

Fig. 28-24. Sialolith of minor salivary gland of the lip near the angle. **A,** Clinical picture showing the small, nodular mass *(arrow)* in the soft tissue, which was very firm to palpation. **B,** Soft tissue radiograph of the lip showing a round, radiopaque sialolith *(arrow)*, which appears to be less dense in the center.   (Courtesy J. Jensen, DDS, Long Beach, Calif.)

Fig. 28-25. Round radiopacity *(arrow)* situated in the soft tissue on the crest of the ridge in the mandibular canine region. Biopsy proved the lesion to be a peripheral fibroma with ossification, which probably developed in the interdental papilla when the patient still had teeth in the region.   (Courtesy P.D. Toto, DDS, Maywood, Ill.)

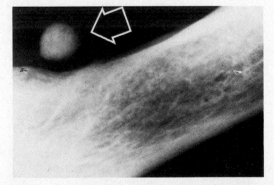

REFERENCES

Barrett AP, Waters BE, and Griffiths CJ: A critical evaluation of panoramic radiography as a screening procedure in dental practice, Oral Surg 57:673-677, 1984.

Cheng K, Werchola O, Sadowsky D, et al: Simultaneous occurrence of Garrè's osteomyelitis with cervicofacial actinomycosis, J Oral Med 39:44-46, 1984.

Eisenbud L, Miller J, and Roberts IL: Garrè's proliferative periostitis occurring simultaneously in four quadrants of the jaws, Oral Surg 51:172-178, 1981.

Ennis LM and Berry HM Jr: The necessity for routine roentgenographic examination of the edentulous patient, J Oral Surg 7:3-19, 1949.

Eversole LR, Leider AS, Corwin JO, and Karian BK: Proliferative periostitis of Garrè's: its differentiation from other neoperiostoses, J Oral Surg 37:725-731, 1979.

Farnam J, Griffin JE, Schow CE, et al: Recurrent diffuse osteomyelitis involving the mandible, Oral Surg 57:374-378, 1984.

Jacobsson S, Dahlen G, and Moller AJR: Bacteriologic and serologic investigation in diffuse sclerosing osteomyelitis (DSO) of the mandible, Oral Surg 54:506-512, 1982.

Jacobsson S and Hollender L: Treatment and prognosis of diffuse sclerosing osteomyelitis (DSO) of the mandible, Oral Surg 49:7-14, 1980.

Keyes GC, Balaban FS, and Lattanzi DA: Periradicular lymphoma: differentiation from inflammation, Oral Surg 66:230-235, 1988.

King DR and King AC: Incidence of tori in three population groups, J Oral Med 36:21-23, 1981.

King DR and Moore GE: An analysis of torus palatinus in a transatlantic study, J Oral Med 31:44-46, 1976.

Lichty G, Langlais RP, and Aufdemorte T: Garrè's osteomyelitis literature review and case report, Oral Surg 50:309-313, 1980.

McWalter GM and Schaberg SJ: Garrè's osteomyelitis of the mandible resolved by endodontic treatment, J Am Dent Assoc 108:193-195, 1984.

Nortjé CJ and Wood RE: Periostitis ossificans versus Garrè's osteomyelitis. II. Radiologic analysis of 93 cases in the jaws, Oral Surg 66:249-260, 1988.

Ritchie GM and Fletcher AM: A radiographic investigation of edentulous jaws, Oral Surg 47:563-567, 1979.

Spyropoulos ND, Patsakas AJ, and Angelopoulos AP: Findings from radiographs of the jaws of edentulous patients, Oral Surg 52:455-459, 1981.

Van Merkesteyn JPR, Groot RH, Bras J, and Bakker DJ: Diffuse sclerosing osteomyelitis of the mandible: clinical radiographic and histologic findings in 27 patients, J Oral Maxillofac Surg 46:825-829, 1988.

Waldron CA: Fibro-osseous lesions of the jaws, J Oral Maxillofac Surg 43:249-262, 1985.

Wood RE, Nortjé CH, Grotepass F, et al: Periostitis ossificans versus Garrè's osteomyelitis. I. What did Garrè really say? Oral Surg 65:773-777, 1988.

29

Multiple separate radiopacities

NORMAN K. WOOD
PAUL W. GOAZ

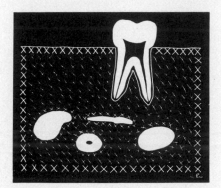

Most of the lesions that appear as multiple but separate radiopacities occur more frequently as solitary radiopacities.

Tori and exostoses
Multiple retained roots
Multiple socket sclerosis
Multiple mature cementomas
Multiple periapical condensing osteitis
Multiple embedded or impacted teeth
Cleidocranial dysplasia
Multiple hypercementoses
Rarities
  Calcinosis cutis
  Cretinism (unerupted teeth)
  Cysticercosis
  Gardner's syndrome (osteomas)
  Idiopathic hypoparathyroidism
  Maffucci's syndrome
  Multiple calcified acne lesions
  Multiple calcified nodes
  Multiple chondromas (Ollier's disease)
  Multiple odontomas
  Multiple osteochondromas
  Multiple osteomas of skin
  Multiple phleboliths
  Multiple sialoliths
  Myositis ossificans
  Oral contraceptive sclerosis
  Paget's disease—intermediate stage
  Sickle cell sclerosis

The majority of the entities included here are discussed in Chapter 27 as periapical radiopacities or in Chapter 28 as solitary radiopacities not contacting the roots of teeth. As described in those two chapters, radiopaque lesions that appear to be within the jaw may actually be in or on the periphery (cortex) of the jawbone or in the adjacent soft tissues. The radiopaque shadows may also represent ghosting or images of multiple artifacts on the film, so it is important to rule out those possibilities (Kaugers and Collett, 1987).

TORI AND EXOSTOSES

Tori and exostoses are described as exophytic lesions in Chapter 10 and as single radiopacities in Chapters 27 and 28. In the context of this chapter, therefore, it remains only to note that tori (especially the lingual mandibular type) frequently develop as multiple nodules that may be contiguous or separate. Exostoses may also be multiple, especially those occurring on the buccal surfaces of the jaws. In either case they appear as relatively dense, smoothly contoured multiple radiopacities on radiographs of the jaws (Fig. 29-1).

Differential diagnosis

Multiple tori or exostoses must be differentiated from any of the other similar-appearing entities included in this chapter. If multiple smoothly contoured radiopacities are present on periapical radiographs and the typical peripheral nodules are palpable on the buccal or lingual alveolar surfaces, the diagnosis is clear-cut.

Rare diseases such as *Maffucci's syndrome*, *Ollier's disease*, and *multiple osteochondromas* should sometimes be considered, but a detailed discussion of these entities is beyond the scope of this text.

Management

Multiple tori and exostoses require surgical excision (1) for psychologic reasons, (2) if they are continually being traumatized, (3) if they are interfering with speech or mastication, or (4) if they will interfere with the fabrication of a prosthetic appliance.

MULTIPLE RETAINED ROOTS

Solitary retained roots are discussed in Chapter 28. Multiple retained roots are usually asymptomatic but may cause pain if they become infected.

A painful ulcer on the crest of a ridge may be the first sign of retained roots, especially if a relatively large root fragment has been present under a denture for a number of years. A periapical radiograph reveals the cause of the ulcer.

Since some patients' roots seem to be prone to fracture during extraction, the clinician occasionally finds several retained root fragments on the radiographs of one person. If the shapes of the roots, pulp canals, and periodontal ligaments have persisted, these multiple well-defined radiopacities are easily identified as root fragments (Fig. 29-2). A low-grade infection and accompanying resorption and condensing osteitis, however, may obscure the diagnosis.

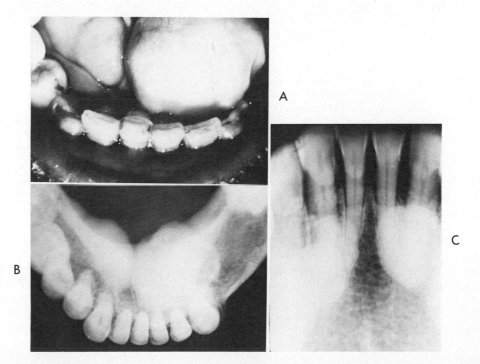

Fig. 29-1. Multiple large tori. **A** and **B,** Clinical and radiographic appearances in one patient. **C,** Periapical radiograph of another patient.   (**A** and **B** courtesy P. Akers, DDS, Chicago.)

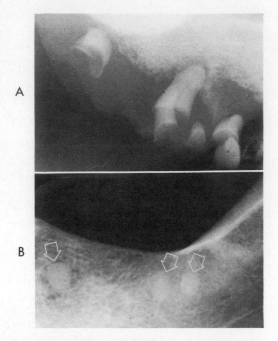

Fig. 29-2. Multiple root fragments. **A,** Readily identified. **B,** Not so readily identified (*arrows*).

Nevertheless, careful study of the radiograph enables the clinician to distinguish a root tip from an area of sclerotic bone on the basis of the texture of the radiopacity: the root fragment has a homogeneous density, whereas the trabeculated nature of the sclerotic bone is usually detectable.

Differential diagnosis

The radiographic appearance of multiple retained roots is diagnostic. If the root fragments have been fractured at the level of the alveolar crest and the radiolucent images of the periodontal ligaments are indistinct, however, multiple retained roots may be difficult to distinguish from *multiple sclerosed sockets.* The study of available radiographs taken shortly after the extractions were performed enables the clinician to distinguish between retained roots and sclerosed sockets.

Retained root tips may not be readily recognized when the root tips are chronically infected and *condensing osteitis* has developed about them. Where there are multiple retained roots, however, all the roots are not likely to be involved with sclerosed bone; one or two fragments retain their typical appearance, and these suggest the correct diagnosis. A more detailed discussion of the differentiation of retain root fragments may be found in the discussion of the differential diagnosis of condensing osteitis in Chapter 28 (p. 576).

Management

Since it is not safe to assume on the basis of radiographic evidence alone that retained roots are free of infection, removal of retained roots should be considered. If the root tips are small, asymptomatic, and apparently free of pathosis, however, and if a relatively large amount of alveolar bone may have to be removed, it is best to leave them undisturbed. Periodic radiographic surveillance is required.

MULTIPLE SOCKET SCLEROSIS

Tooth socket sclerosis is a special form of osteosclerosis that occasionally develops in a socket after tooth removal. Examples of the sclerosis of solitary sockets are described in Chapter 28. Since multiple sclerotic lesions may also occur when a number of tooth sockets are healing after multiple extraction, this entity is included in this chapter as well (Fig. 29-3).

Although the specific cause is unknown, socket sclerosis is believed to be the result of a sudden disturbance of the osteogenic-osteolytic balance in bone metabolism. Burrell and Goepp (1973) reported an increased incidence of socket sclerosis among patients with problems of gastrointestinal malabsorption or kidney disease. In the study, which included both inpatients and outpatients, 2.7% of the patients had one or more sclerosed tooth sockets. The authors calculated that this incidence was much higher than that found in the general population.

Features

Since the development of sclerosed bone in healing sockets is not accompanied by local symptoms, the radiopaque lesion is discovered on routine radiographs. Sclerosis of tooth sockets is found more often in older adults and seldom if ever in persons under 16 years of age. Sequential radiographs made when the sclerosis is active reveal the successive stages of development.

When a socket is healing normally, the lamina dura usually disappears within 4 months and the socket is completely obliterated by 8 months. When socket sclerosis is developing, however, the lamina dura fails to resorb. The deposition of sclerotic bone begins in the depth of the socket and continues along the socket walls. As the lateral walls of sclerotic bone approximate each other, the thin, vertical radiolucent shadow of the void between them re-

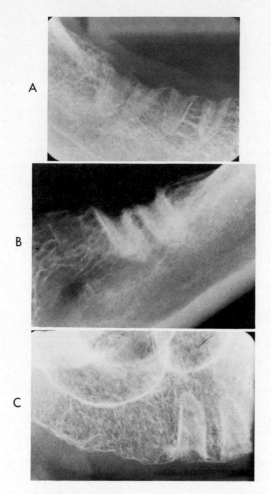

Fig. 29-3. Multiple socket sclerosis.   (**A** courtesy R. Goepp, DDS, Zoller Clinic, University of Chicago.)

sembles the image of a pulp canal on periapical radiographs (Fig. 29-3). At this stage the sclerosed socket can be easily mistaken for a retained, ankylosed root.

On histologic study, socket sclerosis is identical to osteosclerosis that occurs in other locations. Dense, broad trabeculae of bone with few lacunae and few vascular marrow spaces are characteristic of the microscopic appearance.

Differential diagnosis

Socket sclerosis may be mistaken for *retained roots* because both have identical shapes. Differentiating between the two is especially difficult when the socket has not yet completely calcified and a thin, central core resembles a root canal. Since osteosclerosis of a tooth socket usually involves the length of the socket, however, the radiopaque images of

roots fractured well below the alveolar crest are not confused with this dense remodeling of the socket. If the periodontal ligament space is not apparent, the radiopacity should be identified as socket sclerosis. The uncommon ankylosed roots are exceptions. If radiographs of the area are available and were made shortly after the extractions were performed, the identity of the opaque material in the sockets should not be in doubt; the retained root tips are apparent from the time of the extractions, whereas the osteosclerotic healing of the sockets requires months to become obvious.

Management

Once the diagnosis of socket sclerosis has been established (biopsy may be necessary in some cases), consultation with the patient's physician is recommended, since there is reason to suspect that the patient may have a gastrointestinal malabsorption problem or a kidney malady (Burrell and Goepp, 1973).

The sclerosed tooth socket does not require definitive treatment.

MULTIPLE MATURE CEMENTOMAS

Variations in the appearance and nature of cementomas have been discussed in Chapters 16, 21, 24, 25, and 27. In this chapter multiple mature cementomas occurring in the jaws are emphasized (Fig. 29-4).

Although multiple cementomas are most frequently found in the periapices of mandibular incisors, they may occur in the periapices of any of the mandibular teeth and (less frequently) in the maxilla. Tanaka et al. (1987) found that multiple cementomas in Japanese women occurred predominantly in the premolar and molar region of the mandible. Multiple mature cementomas have also been found in edentulous regions; these probably represent residual cementomas that persisted after the removal of the associated teeth. The features of multiple cementomas are similar to those of the solitary cementoma (Chapter 16).

Differential diagnosis

Multiple mature cementomas must be differentiated from the intermediate stage of Paget's disease, sclerotic cemental masses, the complex odontoma, idiopathic osteosclerosis, toris, exostoses, and osteomas, and multiple retained root fragments, as well as some of the rare lesions listed at the beginning of this chapter.

In some cases of intermediate-stage *Paget's disease*, separate round radiopaque areas are seen scattered throughout the jaws. The mar-

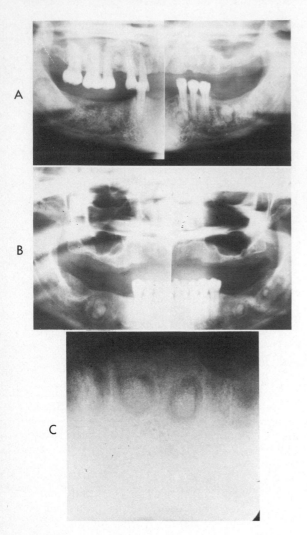

Fig. 29-4. **A** and **B,** Multiple cementomas in two patients. **C,** Two mature cementomas in the mandibular incisor region of another patient. Mature cementomas have radiolucent rims.

gins of these radiopaque osteoblastic areas are not so well defined as the margins of mature cementomas, however, nor do they have uniform radiolucent rims. Further radiographic examination of the patient reveals the deformation of the skull and other bones, and these findings help the clinician recognize Paget's disease.

The features of *sclerotic cemental masses* are quite different from those of mature multiple cementomas. Sclerotic cemental masses are much less common, relatively large, and multiple; they merge together and occupy much of the body of the mandible and maxilla. They appear as large radiopaque masses usually with radiolucent borders and have the cotton-wool appearance often seen in the late stages of Paget's disease. The rate of occurrence of sclerotic cemental masses in families suggests that these tumors are inherited as an autosomal dominant trait. The lesions are most common in black women over 35 years of age.

The *complex odontoma* may resemble a mature cementoma in that it often appears as a dense radiopacity surrounded by a radiolucent border; however, it is usually larger and occurs almost invariably as a solitary lesion. Furthermore, most complex odontomas do not show a homogeneous opacity as the mature cementomas do; instead, they show varying degrees of opacity corresponding to the various densities of enamel, dentin, cementum, and pulp tissue present.

Idiopathic osteosclerotic lesions are frequently solitary, but they may occur bilaterally, usually in the mandibular molar regions. Unlike multiple mature cementomas, the lesions are often irregularly shaped radiopacities without radiolucent rims. In addition, the opacity of the mature cementomas is more homogeneous. Although the images of the osteosclerotic lesions may be dense, a trabecular quality usually is apparent, and in some areas there is a continuity with the adjacent normal trabeculae.

Tori, exostoses, and *osteomas,* like multiple mature cementomas, are radiopaque, but they do not have radiolucent perimeters. Also their identity can be substantiated on clinical examination by the presence of bony hard exophytic nodules.

In contrasting the radiographic images of *multiple retained root fragments* and multiple mature cementomas, the clinician often observes that one or more of the fragments are root shaped and have the appearance of shadows of root canals. In addition, most of the root fragments have some of the radiolucent periodontal ligament still present, and the cementomas are separated from the adjacent normal bone by a thin radiolucent space. Furthermore, the cementomas usually are more rounded than the root fragments and do not have a radiolucent feature suggesting a root canal.

Management

It is usually not necessary to remove multiple mature cementomas unless a rare lesion grows large enough to expand the cortex. Radiographs of cementomas should be taken periodically, so the clinician can observe the course of the lesion and verify the working diagnosis.

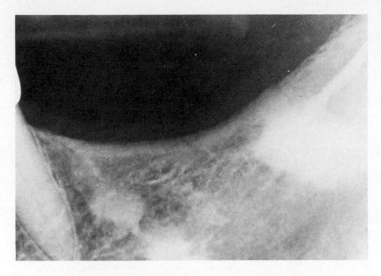

Fig. 29-5. Multiple idiopathic osteosclerosis.

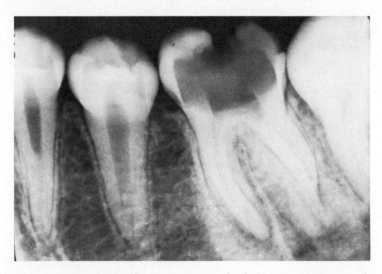

Fig. 29-6. Multiple periapical condensing osteitis. The lesions are present in the periapices of both roots of the first molar.

MULTIPLE IDIOPATHIC OSTEOSCLEROSIS

Idiopathic osteosclerosis is discussed in detail in Chapter 27 as a periapical radiopacity and in Chapter 28 as a solitary radiopacity not contacting teeth. Because this entity sometimes occurs bilaterally and in multiple separate areas in the mandibular molar or premolar region (Fig. 29-5), it is included in this chapter. The lesions are quite dense, irregularly shaped radiopacities, varying from 0.5 to approximately 2 cm in diameter. They are most often found at the periapices of vital teeth.

MULTIPLE PERIAPICAL CONDENSING OSTEITIS

Condensing osteitis is discussed in Chapter 27 as a periapical radiopacity and in Chapter 28 as a solitary radiopacity not contacting the roots of teeth. Since a patient may readily develop pulp pathosis in more than one tooth and since the lesions of condensing osteitis may be found in more than one periapex, it is appropriate to include condensing osteitis in this chapter (Fig. 29-6). Periapical idiopathic osteosclerosis is differentiated from periapical condensing osteitis in that the pulps of the teeth involved with the former are vital, whereas the pulps of the teeth involved with the latter are degenerating or nonvital. Also, multiple lesions of condensing osteitis may be found surrounding multiple root fragments.

MULTIPLE HYPERCEMENTOSES

Hypercementosis, as discussed in Chapter 27, usually occurs as a solitary lesion. Multiple hypercementoses are commonly seen in Paget's disease and occasionally may occur in the absence of systemic disease (Leider and Garbarino, 1987).

MULTIPLE EMBEDDED OR IMPACTED TEETH (NO SYNDROME)

Occasionally the clinical and radiographic examinations of a patient reveal several embedded* or impacted teeth. The particular entity considered here is not the usual impacted third molar or canine but is the more unusual circumstance that occurs when a number of permanent teeth fail to erupt. Some-

times this failure to erupt results from crowding by supernumerary teeth (Kantor et al., 1988). At other times the normal number of permanent teeth are present and there is no apparent mechanical explanation for the lack of eruption.

The inexplicable failure to erupt is caused by a loss or lack of the eruptive force. In contrast to cleidocranial dysplasia, which is characterized by a number of other defects in addition to impacted teeth, this entity is not accompanied by a fixed complex of symptoms. Lateral oblique and posteroanterior radiographs of the jaws of these patients reveal the multiple radiopacities scattered throughout the jaws (Fig. 29-7).

---

*In this discussion the term "embedded" is used to describe a tooth that has failed to erupt because of some imbalance in the coordinated forces responsible for the axial movement of teeth. The "impacted" tooth, in contrast, is prevented from erupting by a physical barrier in the path of eruption.

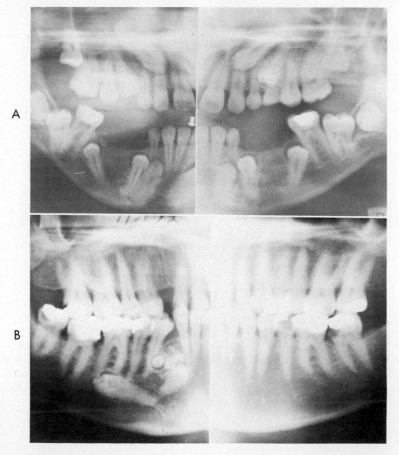

Fig. 29-7. Multiple impacted teeth (no syndrome). **B,** Compound odontoma. The impacted canine and several other teeth are evident. (**A** courtesy W. Schoenheider, DDS, Oak Lawn, Ill.)

Good-quality periapical films enable the clinician to readily identify the radiopacities as unerupted teeth or impacted teeth or both.

Features

During the clinical examination of a patient with no history of tooth extraction, the clinician may encounter one or more edentulous areas in conjunction with malposition and malocclusion of the permanent teeth that are present. When this happens, the clinician should anticipate finding embedded or impacted teeth on the patient's radiographs.

Differential diagnosis

When there is a clinical absence of a number of teeth, three diseases should be included in the differential diagnosis: partial anodontia, cretinism, and cleidocranial dysplasia.

Partial anodontia may be considered during the initial oral screening examination when certain permanent teeth are observed to be absent and the history indicates that they have not been extracted. When radiographs are available, however, and reveal that the missing teeth are in reality present as embedded or impacted teeth, partial anodontia can be rejected.

In some instances, *cretinism* (hypothyroidism in young children) causes crowding (Loevy et al., 1987), delayed eruption, and impaction of permanent teeth. The short stature of the patient, however, combined with a history of hypothyroidism and low serum thyroxine levels, should guide the clinician to the correct diagnosis.

The radiographs of a patient with *cleidocranial dysplasia* demonstrate similar problems of multiple supernumerary and impacted teeth. The accompanying features of cranial and clavicular abnormalities, however, enable the clinician to recognize cleidocranial dysplasia. Multiple embedded or impacted teeth occur more commonly as isolated events than as part of a syndrome.

Management

Impacted teeth should be removed because of the danger of pathologic fracture, odontogenic infection, or development of a follicular cyst. They should also be removed to prepare for a prosthetic appliance. A careful clinical examination should be performed to eliminate from consideration the possibility that these patients may have cleidocranial dysplasia.

CLEIDOCRANIAL DYSPLASIA

Cleidocranial dysplasia is a syndrome of unknown cause. It is usually transmitted as an autosomal dominant trait. One of the features that characterize the disease is the presence of multiple supernumerary and impacted teeth; thus it is included in this chapter.

Features

Usually persons with cleidocranial dysplasia are of shorter than average stature. The syndrome is so named because the two bones that are always involved are the skull and the clavicles.

The skull is enlarged but has a shorter than normal anteroposterior dimension (brachycephaly). Frontoparietal bossing is usually present. There is delayed closing of the fontanelles; occasionally they remain open throughout life. Secondary centers of ossification develop in the suture lines, so an unusual number of wormian bones are formed.

The clavicles are either partially or completely absent (Fig. 29-8), which permits the patient an unusual range of shoulder movements; some patients are able to approximate their shoulders in front of their chests.

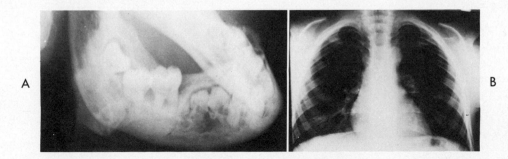

Fig. 29-8. Cleidocranial dyplasia. **A,** Numerous impacted teeth can be seen on this lateral oblique radiograph of the mandible. **B,** The complete absence of clavicles is apparent.   (**A** courtesy R. Goepp, DDS, Zoller Clinic, University of Chicago. **B** courtesy R. Kallal, DDS, Chicago.)

The jaws are also involved. The maxilla is often small and the mandible is usually normal in size, so a pseudoprognathism results. The palate frequently has a high arch and may be cleft. There is a delayed eruption of the permanent dentition because of the presence of many supernumerary teeth, most of which resemble premolars. Thus multiple impactions occur (Fig. 29-8). Follicular cysts may be associated with the impacted teeth.

Often the multiple impactions are the first manifestation of the syndrome to be recognized; the clinician is then prompted to look for other features. The air sinuses may be underdeveloped or absent. The zygoma and lacrimal and nasal bones may show hypoplasia. The nasal bridge may be depressed, and its base broad. Other bones (for example, vertebrae, long bones, pubic bone, and bones of the hands) may show faulty development.

Differential diagnosis

The differential diagnosis of the feature of multiple impaction in cleidocranial dysplasia is discussed earlier in this chapter with the differential diagnosis of embedded and impacted teeth. The differentiation of the remaining features of cleidocranial dysplasia from other craniofacial syndromes is beyond the scope of this discussion.

Management

When the clinician encounters multiple embedded or impacted teeth other than third molars or canines, he or she should pursue the patient's history and clinical examination, paying special attention to any of the other features of cleidocranial dysplasia that may be present. The syndrome must be managed by a team of health professionals, so that all the ramifications of the disease receive adequate treatment. The impacted teeth should be removed in most cases.

RARITIES

Multiple soft tissue calcifications may be projected over the jawbones on radiographs. In addition, radiographs of rare tumors of teeth, bone, and cartilage, as well as the intermediate stage of Paget's disease, may show multiple radiopacities of the jaws. Following is a list of these rarities:

Calcinosis cutis
Cretinism (unerupted teeth)
Cysticercosis (Fig. 29-9)
Gardner's syndrome (osteomas)

Idiopathic hypoparathyrodism
Maffucci's syndrome
Multiple calcified acne lesions
Multiple calcified nodes (Fig. 29-10)
Multiple chondromas (Ollier's disease)
Multiple odontomas
Multiple osteochondromas
Multiple osteomas of skin
Multiple phleboliths (Fig. 29-11)
Multiple sialoliths (Fig. 29-12)
Myositis ossificans
Oral contraceptive sclerosis
Paget's disease—intermediate stage (Fig. 29-13)
Sickle cell sclerosis

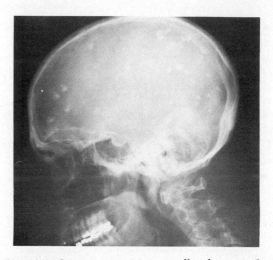

Fig. 29-9. Cysticercosis. Many small radiopaque foci are scattered within the cranium. One small faint radiopacity is present over the mandibular third molar region. (Courtesy E. Palacios, MD, Maywood, Ill.)

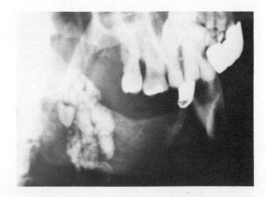

Fig. 29-10. Multiple calcified cervical nodes projected over the ramus. Other radiographic views showed the radiopacities in different positions. The patient had a history of tuberculosis. (Courtesy O.H. Stuteville, DDS, MD, St. Joe, Ark.)

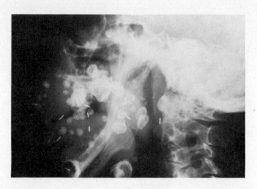

Fig. 29-11. Multiple phleboliths in a patient with large hemangiomas of the face. The short radiopaque rods are radon seeds.   (Courtesy E. Palacios, MD, Maywood, Ill.)

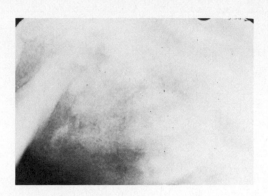

Fig. 29-13. Multiple radiopacities of Paget's disease in the maxillary premolar region.

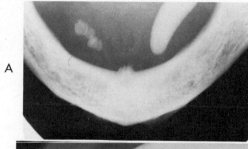

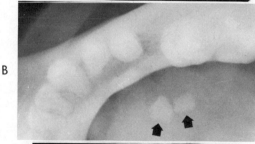

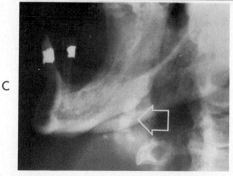

Fig. 29-12. Multiple sialoliths. **A,** Bilateral occurrence. **B,** Two stones in Wharton's duct *(arrows).* **C,** Multiple occurrence *(arrow)* in the submaxillary gland.   (**A** and **B** courtesy R. Latronica, DDS, Albany, N.Y. **C** courtesy E. Palacios, MD, Maywood, Ill.)

REFERENCES

Burrell KH and Goepp RA: Abnormal bone repair in jaws, socket sclerosis: a sign of systemic disease, J Am Dent Assoc 87:1206-1215, 1973.

Kantor ML, Bailey CS, and Burkes DJ: Duplication of the premolar dentition, Oral Surg 66:62-64, 1988.

Kaugers GE and Collett WK: Panoramic ghosts, Oral Surg 63:103-108, 1987.

Leider AS and Garbarino VE: Generalized hypercementosis, Oral Surg 63:375-380, 1987.

Loevy HT, Aduss H, and Rosenthal IM: Tooth eruption and craniofacial development in congenital hypothyroidism: report of case, J Am Dent Assoc 115:429-431, 1987.

Tanaka H, Yoshimoto A, Toyama Y, et al: Periapical cemental dysplasia with multiple lesions, J Oral Maxillofac Surg 16:757-763, 1987.

30

Generalized radiopacities

THOMAS E. EMMERING

A multitude of diseases are capable of causing osseous changes in the jaws and skull. Discussion in this chapter is limited primarily to those that at one stage or another in their development appear as generalized radiopacities of the jawbones.

Sclerotic cemental masses
Paget's disease—mature stage
Osteopetrosis
Rarities
  Albright's syndrome
  Caffey's disease (infantile cortical
    hyperostosis)
  Camurati-Engelmann disease
  Craniometaphyseal dysplasia
  Craniodiaphyseal dysplasia
  Fluorosis
  Gardner's syndrome
  Hyperostosis deformans juvenilis
  Melorheostosis
  Metastatic carcinoma of prostate
  Multiple large exostoses and tori
  Osteogenesis imperfecta
  Osteopathia striata
  Pyknodysostosis
  van Buchem's disease

Diseases of bone that can produce generalized radiopacities are not frequently encountered in the general population. Sclerotic cemental masses, Paget's disease, and osteopetrosis are the most common of these and are listed in order of diminishing frequency. They are discussed, whereas the rarer disorders are only listed.

SCLEROTIC CEMENTAL MASSES OF THE JAWS (GIGANTIFORM CEMENTOMAS, MULTIPLE ENOSTOSES, FLORID OSSEOUS DYSPLASIA)

The terms *sclerosing cemental masses of the jaws, gigantiform cementomas, multiple enostoses,* and *florid osseous dysplasia* refer to the same disease process. Although such a grouping is not accepted by all pathologists, Waldron

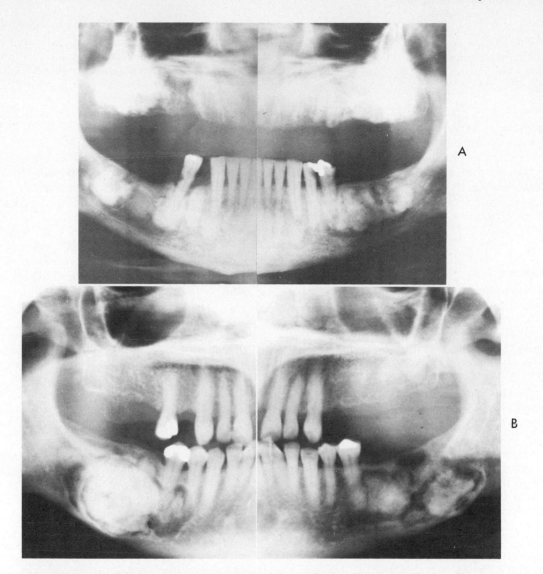

Fig. 30-1. Sclerotic cemental masses. **A,** Nodular, rather well-circumscribed radiopaque masses are distributed throughout the maxilla and mandible. This panograph is of a 45-year-old black woman. **B,** Panograph of nodular masses in another black woman, 42 years of age, showing greater involvement of the mandible than of the maxilla.   (**B** courtesy R. Kallal, DDS, Chicago.)

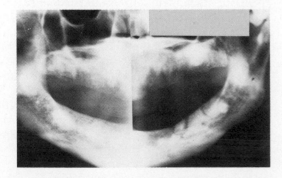

Fig. 30-2. Sclerotic cemental masses in a middle-aged black woman who was asymptomatic. The particular pattern that is prevalent in this case is more diffuse, less nodular, and less well defined than usual.

et al. (1975) prefer to combine these entities under one heading—sclerotic cemental masses of the jaws—because of their obvious similarities. Melrose et al. (1976) suggest the term "florid osseous dysplasia" for this group of lesions.

The large radiopaque masses (cementum*) in sclerotic cemental masses of the jaws frequently become so disseminated that the complete body of the mandible and tooth-bearing regions of the maxilla show a generalized radiopacity (Figs. 30-1 and 30-2).

Our experience is that sclerotic cemental masses represent the most common cause of pathologic generalized radiopacities of the jaws.

Features

Sclerotic cemental masses are apparently inherited as an autosomal dominant trait (Winer et al., 1972).

Bhaskar and Cutright (1968) summarized the characteristics of this disorder as follows:

1. The lesions are restricted to the jaw-bones.
2. The vast majority of the patients are over 30 years of age.
3. There is a marked predilection for women, and the disease is more common in blacks.
4. Mandibular involvement is much more common than maxillary involvement.

Early or mild cases are detected on routine radiographic surveys. More advanced or severe cases, however, may be detected by a painless expansion of the alveolar process of the mandible and, less frequently, of the maxilla. The patient who is wearing dentures complains of the constant need for adjustment of the prosthesis. In extreme cases the surface mucosa over the expanded alveolar process may become ulcerated and a superimposed osteomyelitis may develop. Patients with this complication usually experience tenderness, pain, and possibly purulent drainage from the region. Serum chemistry levels are characteristically within normal limits because of the insidious nature of the bone changes.

Radiographs, at first glance, seem to demonstrate a pagetoid, cotton-wool appearance with multiple irregularly shaped radiopaque areas. On closer examination, well-defined radiolucent rims can be seen surrounding most of the radiopaque areas (Bhaskar and Cutright, 1968; Winer et al., 1972) (Fig. 30-1). The radiopaque patterns vary in size but are usually large and may be either multiple or diffuse and continuous throughout the jaw (Figs. 30-1 and 30-2). As with most odontogenic hard tissue lesions, sclerotic cemental masses commence as radiolucencies and mature through the mixed stage into the radiopaque stage.

Using polarizing microscopy, Waldron et al. (1975) demonstrated that the radiopacities in 34 of 38 cases were of cementum, whereas in the remaining four cases the radiopacities were of bone.

Differential diagnosis

The differentiating features of sclerotic cemental masses are discussed in the differential diagnosis section at the end of the chapter.

Management

Patients with asymptomatic, mild cases of sclerotic cemental masses do not require treatment. The disease must be correctly identified and observed annually with radiographs, however; if the natural dentition is present, every effort must be made to preserve it, since patients with this disease exhibit poor healing and osteomyelitis may develop after tooth loss.

More severe cases or cases in which superficial lesions are located near the crest of the alveolar ridge may require recontouring to accommodate dentures or prevent ulceration.

The management of a superimposed or primary osteomyelitis is discussed in Chapter 21.

PAGET'S DISEASE—MATURE STAGE

Paget's disease is a chronic disease of bone that may occur in three stages: (1) the early osteoclastic stage (generalized rarefaction), (2) the intermediate stage, which demonstrates both osteoclastic and osteoblastic activity (a mixed radiolucent-radiopaque appearance), and (3) the mature stage, in which osteoblastic activity predominates (a generalized cotton-wool radiopacity).

The osteoclastic stage is described in Chapter 23 as a generalized rarefaction, and the intermediate stage is described in Chapter 25 as a mixed radiolucent-radiopaque image. The mature cotton-wool appearance is emphasized in this chapter.

---

*If one considers this condition to be basically a benign fibro-osseous lesion of periodontal ligament origin, one would expect to find cementum or bone or a mixture of these two tissues. In any event the presence of the large aggregations of densely calcified tissues predisposes to a secondary osteomyelitis.

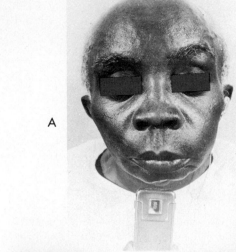

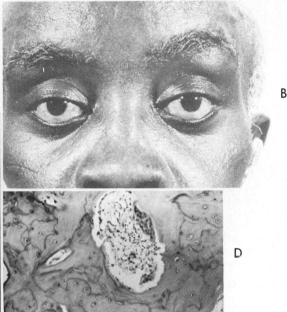

Fig. 30-3. Paget's disease. **A** and **B**, The enlarged skull and maxilla, the marked exophthalmos, and the hearing aid in the left ear are evident. **C**, Lateral radiograph reveals a dense cotton-wool appearance throughout the skull and maxilla. **D**, Photomicrograph depicts the classic mosaic pattern within the bone, which resembles finger painting. The presence of osteoblasts and osteoclasts at the bone margins is evident.

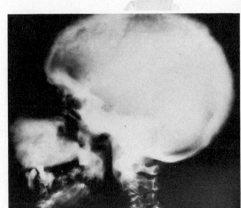

Features

True Paget's disease occurs most often in patients over 40 years of age and may present many clinical signs and symptoms, which are not always obvious until the disease becomes relatively far advanced. The notable features may be enlargement of the skull and jaws (Fig. 30-3), usually the maxilla, although there have been cases of mandibular involvement only (Gee et al., 1972). Prominent involvement of the facial bones (occasionally seen) may produce a leonine appearance sometimes referred to as a leontiasis ossea.

Additional clinical features depend on which other bones are involved. Deformities of the spine, femurs, and tibiae result in shortened stature, broadening of the chest, spinal curvature, and a waddling gait. Involved bones are more easily subject to fracture; some authors claim an incidence of up to 30% as evidenced by the appearances of bone callus on radiographs.

Dental problems become notable as osteoblastic activity creates expansion and progres-

sive enlargement of the maxilla. The alveolar ridge is widened, the palate is flattened, and any teeth present undergo migration, tipping, possible loosening, and increased interproximal spacing. It is difficult for edentulous patients to wear removable prostheses, which must be periodically remade to accommodate alveolar expansion.

Although many authorities believe osteoclastic and osteoblastic activities continue throughout the course of the disease, the radiographic appearance varies according to the stage of the disease. The osteoblastic phase eventually becomes predominant. Osteoblastic areas initially show as small radiopaque foci but coalesce as the disease matures into large radiopaque patches with few residual radiolucent areas (Figs. 30-4 and 30-5). This latter image is often referred to as the cotton-wool appearance.

In patients with jaw involvement, the skull is also affected; sometimes osteolytic activity continues intermittently in these bones even after the predominant activity in the jaws has be-

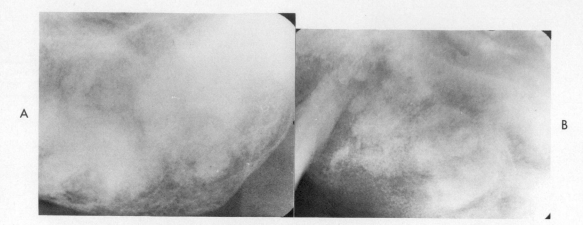

Fig. 30-4. Paget's disease. The cotton-wool appearance can be seen in the edentulous maxillary molar region, **A,** and in the canine and premolar region, **B.** (Courtesy R. Goepp, DDS, Zoller Clinic, University of Chicago.)

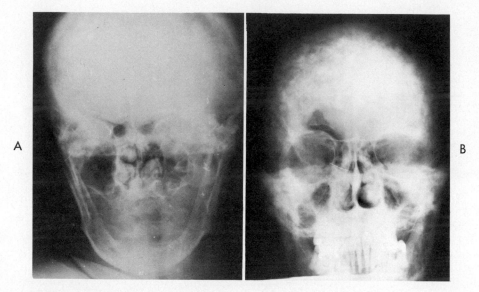

Fig. 30-5. Paget's disease in two patients. **A,** The dense cotton-wool pattern is shown in the skull. The maxilla and mandible are not involved in this patient. **B,** The cotton-wool radiopacities can be seen throughout the maxilla, zygoma, and skull. The mandible is not involved in this patient. (**A** courtesy E. Palacios, MD, Maywood, Ill. **B** courtesy O.H. Stuteville, DDS, MD, St. Joe, Ark.)

come osteoblastic. Dental radiographs of later stages of Paget's disease demonstrate proliferation of bone and hypercementosis of tooth roots, and the hypercementosis may become quite exaggerated. Frequently a loss of definite lamina dura occurs around the teeth and, rarely, some root resorption. On occasion, local areas of the jaw continue to grow at an accelerated rate. Marks and Dunkelberger (1980) cautioned dentists to be alert to the oral changes

because they may be the first clinicians to suspect a diagnosis of Paget's disease. Otis et al. (1986) summarized the etiologic theories and reported a case.

The dental practitioner must also be alert to the presence of areas of bone resorption and apposition, since these areas may signal the development of osteogenic sarcoma and osteogenic sarcoma has an increased incidence in Paget's disease.

Serum alkaline phosphatase values are characteristically markedly elevated, whereas serum calcium and phosphorus levels are usually within normal limits.

The mature stage of Paget's disease produces some distinct microscopic features:

1. The bone is very dense with a few small fibrovascular spaces appearing between massive trabeculae that have resulted from the fusion of smaller trabeculae.
2. The classic mosaic pattern is usually present in the trabeculae and is produced by the many reversal lines that are a result of the increased resorption and apposition of bone.
3. Osteoblasts and some osteoclasts are seen rimming the trabeculae (Fig. 30-3, *D*).

Differential diagnosis

The differentiating aspects of generalized radiopacities of the jawbones are discussed in the differential diagnosis section at the end of the chapter.

Management

The management of patients with Paget's disease is discussed in Chapters 23 and 25. Sofaer (1984) discussed the special problems encountered with extractions in patients with Paget's disease. The clinician must be especially watchful for the development of osteosarcoma in bones affected with Paget's disease.

OSTEOPETROSIS (ALBERS-SCHÖNBERG DISEASE, MARBLE BONE DISEASE)

Osteopetrosis, characterized by overgrowth and sclerosis of bone with resultant thickening of the bony cortices and narrowing of the marrow cavities throughout the skeleton, is an uncommon disease of unknown cause (Figs. 30-6 and 30-7). The resultant generalized radiopacity of the skeleton qualifies this disease for inclusion in this chapter. The disease was first described in 1907 by Albers-Schönberg. A survey of the literature by Cangiano et al. (1972) revealed approximately 300 reported cases. In 1978 Wong et al. identified a total of 450 cases.

Features

Osteopetrosis is generally subdivided into two main types: the clinically benign, dominantly inherited form and the clinically malignant, recessively inherited form (Shafer et al., 1983).

Benign osteopetrosis usually develops later in life than the malignant form of the disease and is considerably less severe, a few cases not being diagnosed until middle age. Although the patient may sustain fractures after minor trauma, the marked symptoms of the malignant form are not characteristic of the benign disorder. Usually benign osteopetrosis is discovered incidentally on routine radiographs. The serum chemistry levels characteristically show normal values in both forms of the disease.

The malignant form of osteopetrosis is present at birth or develops in early childhood. The disease is severe and debilitating, with no known survivors beyond the age of 20 years. Patients with malignant osteopetrosis have symptoms indicative of neurologic and hematologic derangements, which are direct results of the primary bone disorder—severe anemia, blindness, deafness, multiple fractures of the long bones with resulting deformity, hepatosplenomegaly, hydrocephalus, possible mental retardation, and osteomyelitis.

On radiographs osteopetrosis is characterized by an increased density of the entire skeleton, resulting in a diffuse homogeneous, symmetrically sclerotic appearance of all bones (Can-

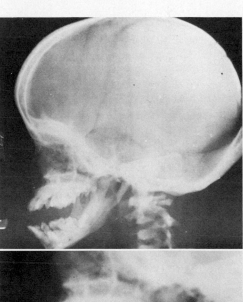

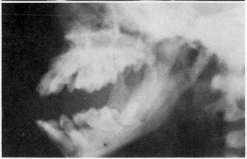

Fig. 30-6. Malignant osteopetrosis of the skull and jaws in a 4-year-old boy. Radiographs show the uniformly dense radiopaque involvement of the bones. (Courtesy R. Moncada, MD, Maywood, Ill.)

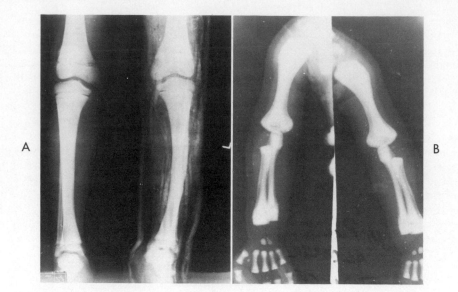

Fig. 30-7. **A,** Osteopetrosis of the lower extremities in an 8-year-old boy. Radiograph shows the almost complete obliteration of the medullary portions of the femurs and tibiae, as well as the cast on the left leg. **B,** Upper extremities of an infant with malignant osteopetrosis. (Courtesy R. Moncada, MD, Maywood, Ill.)

giano et al., 1972). Pathologic fractures are the most common clinical sign to occur (40%).

Marked changes in the radiographic appearance of the skull are evidenced in osteopetrosis: the normal landmarks are lost in the dense, diffuse radiopacity; the diploe is effaced (Fig. 30-6); there is encroachment and narrowing of the cranial foramina, which results in nerve and vessel compression. Hearing loss, impairment of vision, and facial palsy ensue.

The bone may appear so dense on a dental radiograph that the roots of the teeth are obscured. Density is generally homogeneous, with greatly increased thickening of the trabeculae and corresponding reduction of the marrow spaces. The radiographic appearance of the lamina dura is often lost in the overall density, and the presence of possible periapical pathosis is extremely difficult to discern (Fig. 30-6). This factor, coupled with the reduction of marrow spaces, causes a predilection toward osteomyelitis. Younai et al. (1988) reported autopsy findings in the mandible of a 10-year-old girl who died of osteopetrosis.

Differential diagnosis

The differentiating aspects of generalized radiopacities of the jawbones are discussed in the differential diagnosis section at the end of this chapter. Ruprecht et al. (1988) reported a case and offered a differential diagnosis containing rare conditions.

Management

There is no cure for the primary defect in osteopetrosis. Palliative measures are instituted to alleviate the secondary symptoms of the disease. The teeth and periodontal structures should be maintained in good health to minimize the possibility of superimposed osteomyelitis of the jaws. Steiner et al. (1983) discussed the great difficulties of managing osteomyelitis of the mandible in patients with osteopetrosis.

RARITIES

Many rare diseases, some of which are syndromes, may manifest generalized radiopacities of a few or many bones of the skeleton. A list includes the following:

Albright's syndrome
Caffey's disease (infantile cortical hyperostosis) (Fig. 30-8)
Camurati-Engelmann disease
Craniometaphyseal dysplasia
Craniodiaphyseal dysplasia
Fluorosis
Gardner's syndrome (Fig. 30-9)
Hyperostosis deformans juvenilis
Melorheostosis
Metastatic carcinoma of prostate
Multiple large exostoses and tori (Fig. 30-10)
Osteogenesis imperfecta
Osteopathia striata
Pyknodysostosis
van Buchem's disease

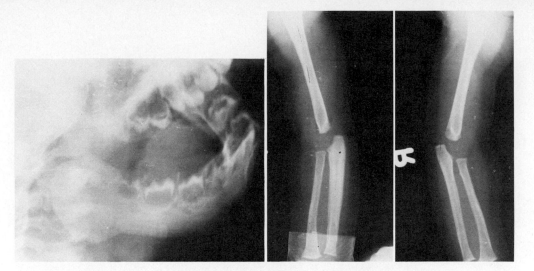

Fig. 30-8. Jaws and arms of a 6-month-old infant with infantile cortical hyperostosis. Proliferation of the cortices has almost completely obliterated the shadows of the medullary cavities. (Courtesy R. Moncada, MD, Maywood, Ill.)

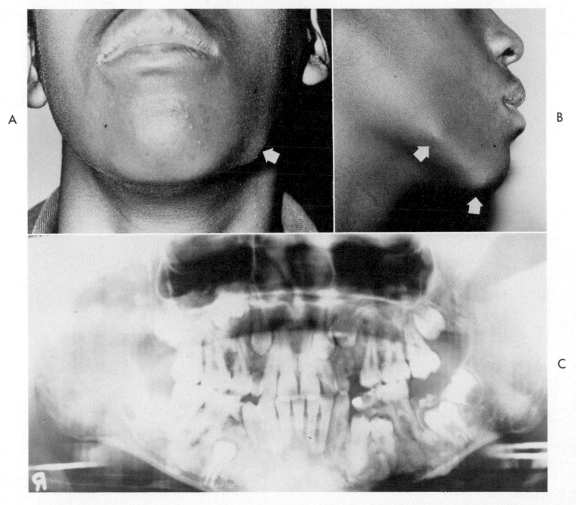

A

B

C

Fig. 30-9. Gardner's syndrome in a young man. **A** and **B,** Facial views showing nodular enlargements *(arrows)* on the inferior aspect of the mandible caused by the multiple osteomas. **C,** Panograph showing the diffuse and nodular radiopacities in the jaws that are produced by the multiple osteomas.   (Courtesy W. Heaton, DDS, Chicago.)

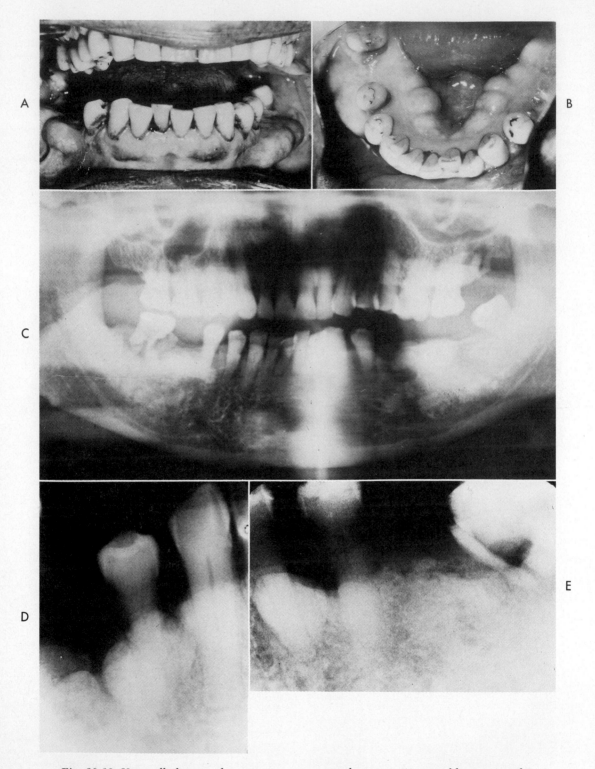

Fig. 30-10. Unusually large and numerous exostoses and tori in a 56-year-old man. **A** and **B**, Intraoral clinical views. **C** to **E**, Panographic and periapical radiographs showing the dense radiopaque pattern throughout the body of the mandible.

DIFFERENTIAL DIAGNOSIS OF GENERALIZED RADIOPACITIES OF THE JAWBONES

When a clinician detects a generalized radiopacity of the jaws, he or she must consider especially these conditions in the differential diagnosis: polyostotic fibrous dysplasia, osteopetrosis, Paget's disease, diffuse cementosis, and normal variations in form and density.

Polyostotic fibrous dysplasia may be confused with Paget's disease because several bones occasionally are involved; however, fibrous dysplasia usually involves a section of a bone rather than the complete bone. Hence the involved bones generally exhibit asymmetric enlargement. Furthermore, serum chemistry changes are slight in fibrous dysplasia.

Malignant osteopetrosis cannot be confused with Paget's disease and diffuse cementosis because it is almost invariably fatal by the age of 20 years, whereas the other entities occur predominantly in patients beyond the fourth decade of life. *Benign osteopetrosis*, however, may be seen in older persons. Osteopetrosis usually involves all the skeletal bones; this feature helps the clinician differentiate it from Paget's disease, which commonly involves five or six bones at most. Diffuse cementosis involves only the mandible and the maxilla.

Paget's disease can be differentiated from diffuse cementosis and malignant osteopetrosis by the classic bones it most often involves: skull, pelvis, vertebrae, femurs, maxilla, and mandible. Also, the serum chemistry measurements show markedly elevated alkaline phosphatase values, which, in combination with diffuse radiopacities for some bones, is practically pathognomonic for Paget's disease. Similarly, advanced hypercementosis of the teeth, in combination with generalized radiopacities of several bones, is often considered pathognomonic.

Sclerotic cemental masses have a strong predilection for black women over 30 years of age. The most salient features of this disease are that (1) only the jaws are affected and (2) radiographs of the jaws reveal radiopaque masses frequently rimmed by a radiolucent border. These two features are unique to sclerotic cemental masses and clearly differentiate them from Paget's disease and osteopetrosis.

Normal variations in form and radiodensity of the jawbones must be considered in the differential diagnosis, and this aspect is discussed in detail in Chapter 23 (p. 475). Dense radiographic images of the jawbones may be seen in patients who have heavy jawbones and ruddy complexions or are overweight. However, such an image may also be related to incorrectly exposed or processed radiographs.

The clinician should also bear in mind the rarer diseases that are capable of causing this condition, but a discussion of these is beyond the scope of this text.

REFERENCES

Albers-Schönberg H: Ein bisher nicht beschriebene Allgemeinerkrankung des Skelettes im Röntgenbild, Fortschr Geb Roentgenstr 11:261, 1907; cited in Thoma KH: Oral pathology, ed 2, St. Louis, 1944, The CV Mosby Co., Chapter 7.

Bhaskar SN and Cutright DE: Multiple exostosis: report of cases, J Oral Surg 26:321-326, 1968.

Cangiano R, Mooney J, and Stratigos GT: Osteopetrosis: report of case, J Oral Surg 30:217-222, 1972.

Gee JK, Zambito RF, Argentieri GW, et al: Paget's disease (osteitis deformans) of the mandible, J Oral Surg 30:223-227, 1972.

Marks JM and Dunkelberger FB: Paget's disease, J Am Dent Assoc 101:49-52, 1980.

Melrose RJ, Abrams AM, and Mills BG: Florid osseous dysplasia: a clinical, pathologic study of 34 cases, Oral Surg 41:62-82, 1976.

Otis LL, Terezhalmy GT, and Glass BJ: Paget's disease of bone: etiological theories and report of a case, J Oral Med 41:214-219, 1986.

Ruprecht A, Wagner H, and Engel H: Osteopetrosis: report of a case and discussion of the differential diagnosis, Oral Surg 66:674-679, 1988.

Shafer WG, Hine MK, and Levy BM: A textbook of oral pathology, ed 4, Philadelphia, 1983, WB Saunders Co., p 684.

Sofaer JA: Dental extractions in Paget's disease of bone, Int J Oral Surg 13:79-84, 1984.

Steiner M, Gould AR, and Means WR: Osteomyelitis of the mandible associated with osteopetrosis, J Oral Maxillofac Surg 41:395-405, 1983.

Waldron CA, Giansanti JS, and Browand BC: Sclerotic cemental masses of the jaws (so-called chronic sclerosing osteomyelitis, sclerosing osteitis, multiple enostosis, and gigantiform cementoma), Oral Surg 39:590-604, 1975.

Winer HJ, Goepp RA, and Olson RE: Gigantiform cementoma resembling Paget's disease: report of case, J Oral Surg 30:517-519, 1972.

Wong ML, Balkany TJ, Reeves J, et al: Head and neck manifestations of malignant osteopetrosis, Otolaryngology 86:585, 1978.

Younai F, Eisenbud L, and Sciubba JJ: Osteopetrosis: a case report including gross and microscopic findings in the mandible at autopsy, Oral Surg 65:214-221, 1988.

Part IV

Lesions by region

31

Masses in the neck

RAYMOND L. WARPEHA

The more common masses occurring in the neck are listed below and are ranked in approximate order of frequency.

Anatomic structures
Benign lymphoid hyperplasia
Acute lymphadenitis
Fibrosed lymph nodes
Sebaceous cysts
Space abscesses
Salivary gland inflammations
Lipomas
Salivary gland tumors
Thyroid gland enlargements
Benign systemic lymph node enlargements
  (infectious mononucleosis and viral diseases)
Epidermoid and dermoid cysts
Metastatic tumors
Thyroglossal cysts
Cystic hygromas
Lymphomas
Branchial cysts
Rarities
  Actinomycosis
  Alcoholism
  Anorexia nervosa
  Burkitt's lymphoma
  Cat-scratch disease
  Cutaneous emphysema
  Ectopic salivary gland tissue
  Laryngocele
  Ludwig's angina
  Plunging ranula
  Mesenchymal tumors
  Mikulicz's disease
  Neural tumors
  Primary tumors of mesenchymal tissue
  Sarcoidosis
  Subcutaneous emphysema
  Tuberculosis (scrofula)

In other chapters lesions are discussed in the same order as they are listed. In this chapter, however, it was considered more useful to group the neck lesions according to the regions where they predominantly occur. Thus the discussion of pathologic masses of the neck is divided into the following segments:

1. Masses of nonspecific location
2. Masses in the submandibular region
3. Masses in the parotid region
4. Masses in the median-paramedian region
5. Masses in the lateral neck region

The identification of a particular mass in the neck involves a reasoning process that combines the information obtained from the medical history and the physical examination of the mass and then evaluates it in relation to the normal structures and their positions in the neck. In addition, further information from laboratory and radiographic studies may be required. After the foregoing information is analyzed, a clinical diagnosis or a group of likely diagnoses *(differential diagnosis)* can be formulated. Although a clinical diagnosis might suffice in some instances, a definitive (microscopic) diagnosis is frequently required for proper treatment. For this determination, tissue for microscopy or material for culture is necessary. Obtaining tissue or tissue products for study may involve certain additional insult and when done ineptly may compromise therapy or perhaps even hinder the cure of a malignant neoplasm. For these reasons the most definitive step in diagnosis—microscopic study—may be reserved for final consideration.

PHYSICAL EXAMINATION AND ANATOMY OF THE NECK

Physical examination of a region involves inspection, palpation, percussion, and auscultation. Palpation plays the major role in the examination of neck masses. Although auscultation of bruits within blood vessels is a necessary part of a complete neck examination, auscultation and percussion are seldom the focal measures in the clinician's evaluation of neck masses.

To detect subtle changes in the contour of the neck, the clinician must know the normal topography of this region. Good lighting and total exposure of the neck with the shoulders bared are necessary for proper visualization. Most visible neck masses cause asymmetries that rapidly attract the examiner's attention.

Certain normal skeletal and soft tissue structures of the neck are readily identified by palpation. Familiarity with the usual size, contour, consistency, and mobility of these structures is necessary both to identify them readily and to distinguish the normal palpable masses from pathologic ones.

Skin and subcutaneous tissues within the neck

The investing cervical fascia is attached to the readily palpable lower border of the mandible, mastoid process, hyoid bone, and clavicles. It forms a heavy membrane over the deep structures of the neck, placing a screen between these structures and the examiner's fingers. The mobile skin and subcutaneous tissues are superficial to the investing fascia. Thus masses arising within this layer exhibit the mobility of the layer unless fibrosis or a malignancy has secondarily fixed the layer to deeper structures.

Specific regions of the neck and their palpable anatomic structures

SUBMANDIBULAR REGION

The boundaries of the submandibular region are easily recognized, with the lower border of the mandible from its angle to the canine region forming the superior margin and the bellies of the digastric muscle constituting the anterior and posterior limits of the inferior border of the region (Fig. 31-1, A). These muscular bellies are palpable only when they are stiffened by function. Therefore the examiner can define the limits of this region by asking the patient to open the jaw against resistance (the examiner holding the jaw shut) while the examiner palpates the rising ridges of the digastric muscle.

The submandibular gland lies within this region on the extremely mobile mylohyoid muscle, which forms a hammock between the hyoid bone and the inner aspect of the mandibular body. Although most of the gland lies superficial to the mylohyoid muscle and consequently occurs in the neck, a small part insinuates itself around the free posterior border of the muscle and lies in the posterior floor of the mouth.

Merely palpating the gland externally gives only a vague impression of its dome. If, however, the patient is asked to push the tongue against the anterior teeth, the gland's circumference can be better defined because the tightening of the floor of the mouth (mylohyoid muscle) creates a rigid base for palpation.

Bimanual palpation offers the greatest opportunity to feel the entire structure and is a mandatory step in any physical examination. The examiner accomplishes this by inserting two or three fingers into the patient's mouth to support the distensible mylohyoid muscle while palpating the submandibular gland externally with the fingers of the opposing hand (see Chapter 3).

The submandibular gland does not occupy the entire submandibular region. Numerous lymph nodes are also found within the areolar tissue of this region but are not ordinarily palpable (Fig. 31-2).

PAROTID REGION

The parotid gland fills the parotid region (Fig. 31-1, B). This is the area bounded anteriorly by the posterior border of the ascending mandibular ramus and posteriorly by the external auditory canal, mastoid process, and upper portion of the sternocleidomastoid muscle. The gland overlaps the mandibular ramus and masseter muscle for a short distance beyond their posterior borders. Also, the inferior tip of the gland extends 1 to 2 cm below the projected line of the inferior border of the mandible (Fig. 31-1, B).

The parotid gland is more difficult to palpate than the submandibular gland because the firm, adherent investing fascia normally prevents precise identification of the normal gland's margins. In addition, bimanual examination is difficult to perform because of the presence of the interposed pharyngeal structures and ramus and because of the gag reflex. In some cases, however, bimanual palpation of the parotid region is mandatory to establish certain clinical findings and may be accomplished by resorting to topical or general anesthesia.

Lymph nodes are found within and superficial to the parotid gland in the subcutaneous tissues of the preauricular area and at the lower pole of the gland (Fig. 31-2). Consequently, pathoses of these structures must also be considered in the differential diagnosis of any mass in the parotid region.

MEDIAN-PARAMEDIAN REGION

The median-paramedian area is bounded superiorly by the lower border of the mandible and laterally by the attachments of the anterior

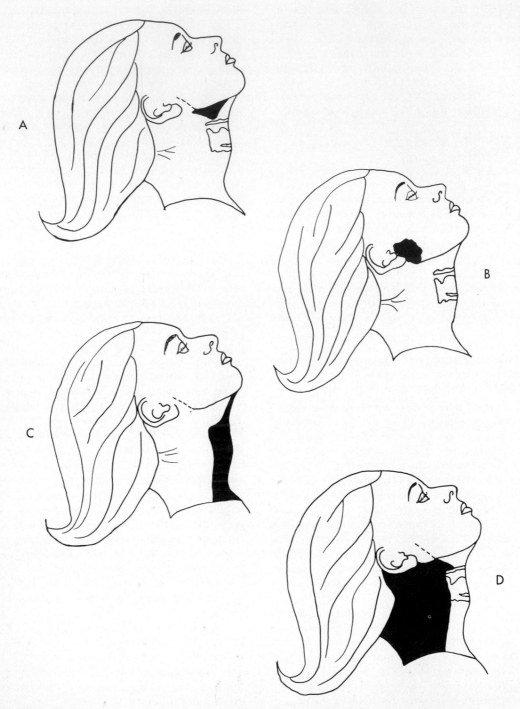

Fig. 31-1. **A,** Submandibular region. **B,** Parotid region. **C,** Median-paramedian region. **D,** Lateral region. See text for the description of the boundaries of each region.

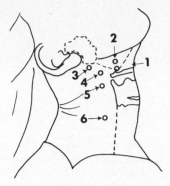

Fig. 31-2. Major cervical lymph node areas. *1,* Submental; *2,* submandibular; *3,* subparotid; *4,* subdigastric; *5,* bifurcation; *6,* jugulo-omohyoid.

bellies of the digastric muscles. The posterior boundary is delineated by the posterior extremities of the hyoid bone and the thyroid and cricoid cartilages. The medial parts of the clavicles and superior margin of the manubrium form the inferior boundaries of the region (Fig. 31-1, *C*).

The most important structure in the median-paramedian region is the butterfly-shaped thyroid gland, which has two lateral lobes connected by a narrow isthmus that crosses the trachea at a variable distance below the palpable ridge produced by the cricoid cartilage. Like the submandibular and parotid glands, the thyroid gland lies deep to the investing cervical fascia, and its features are partially masked from palpation. The lateral lobes of the gland, forming the greater part of its mass, are further concealed by the overlying infrahyoid strap muscles and the bulky sternocleidomastoid muscle. Thus the normal thyroid gland is not palpable in the usual sense but rather is recognized by a feeling of fullness to the touch. The left lobe frequently imparts a greater fullness because it is usually larger than the right.

A mass within or an enlargement of the lateral lobes of the thyroid gland is best appreciated by manipulation of the overlying sternocleidomastoid muscle. While one hand stabilizes the gland by insinuating the fingers behind the posterior border of that muscle, the palpating fingers of the opposite hand determine the features of the lateral lobe. The isthmus is palpated near the midline below the prominent, ringlike cricoid cartilage and is best felt during a swallowing motion, since the gland is attached to the trachea and moves upward with this structure during deglutition.

The presence of a mass in a lateral lobe is similarly verified by palpation while the patient swallows. In such a case the intrinsically attached mass moves with the thyroid gland.

The palpable hyoid bone and thyroid cartilages are also present within the median-paramedian region. The mobility of these structures requires bimanual fixation similar to that used in examining the submandibular and thyroid glands. The greater cornu of the hyoid bone and superior cornu of the thyroid cartilage are occasionally mistaken for stony-hard lymph nodes in the upper cervical chain, which would imply malignant metastasis. The two cornua are normal structures anterior to the cervical node chain, however, and they are identified by their presence bilaterally and their upward displacement during swallowing.

In the median-paramedian region, lymph nodes are found above the hyoid bone in the submental area and in front of the cricothyroid membrane. Normally these nodes are not palpable, and such masses in the neck are considered in the ensuing discussion.

LATERAL REGION

The lateral neck region is the portion of the neck remaining after the preceding regions have been defined. It is the area posterior to the hyolaryngotracheal conduit, below the posterior belly of the digastric muscle and tip of the parotid gland, and extends down to the clavicle (Fig. 31-1, *D*). It is crossed obliquely by the sternocleidomastoid muscle, which obliterates the detail of the central structures in this region.

The contents of this region include the large vessels and nerves of the neck just anterior to the bodies and transverse processes of the cervical vertebrae. The transverse processes of the first and seventh cervical vertebrae are vaguely palpable as immovable hard masses below the tip of the mastoid and in the supraclavicular area, respectively. They become more apparent in the thin and emaciated patient and are prominent in the postsurgical patient after radical neck dissection with removal of the sternocleidomastoid muscle and soft tissues of the lateral neck region.

The carotid pulse can be felt on the prominent bulge marking the carotid bifurcation. This structure lies below the posterior belly of the digastric muscle, level with the angle of the mandible, and is frequently mistaken for a pathologic mass by the unwary examiner. Just as the greater cornu of the hyoid bone, superior cornu of the thyroid cartilage, or transverse processes of either the first or the seventh cervical vertebra may be mistaken for disease, so in the elderly patient, calcification within the arterial wall at the carotid bifurcation may be misinterpreted as a hard node of metastatic cancer. However, careful manipulation of the artery and determination of whether the carotid pulse can be detected through the hard mass identify the mass as part or not part of the artery.

A vertical groove can be felt in the middle third of the neck immediately behind the sternocleidomastoid muscle between the anterior and middle scalene muscles in all patients but the very obese. It contains the cervical and brachial plexus nerve roots after they exit the intervertebral foramina. Although the individual nerve roots cannot be detected by touch, pathologic masses associated with these structures would be found along this line. An example is the amputation neuromas that sometimes form on the nerve stumps after a radical neck dissection.

The lateral neck region carries the greatest number of lymph nodes found in the neck (Fig. 31-2). It is also the most common site of lymph node metastases from head and neck cancer because the lymph from several of the common primary cancer sites drains first to nodes in this area. As in other regions, normal lymph nodes of the lateral neck region are not palpable. The distribution and drainage areas of the nodes in this and other regions of the neck are described next.

Lymph nodes of the neck

A capillary plexus of endothelial tubes is found below the epidermis and oral mucosa of the head and neck. It collects the fluid from the interstitial spaces for return to the large venous trunks at the base of the neck. Between a given capillary plexus and the veins are increasingly larger channels, the lymphatics, with one or more lymph nodes in their course. Within each of these lymph nodes the fluid must again pass capillary-sized channels before proceeding through to the efferent lymphatic channel.

The first lymph node encountered in a channel draining a particular submucosal or subepidermal lymph capillary plexus is called the "first-echelon node" because it is here that pathogenic organisms or free tumor cells within the lymph fluid meet their first resistance to travel.

The first-echelon nodes are also found in the preauricular (superficial to the parotid gland

and investing fascia), postauricular, and suboccipital areas. With the submental and submandibular nodes they form a collar about the face and scalp, filtering the drainage from the subepidermal lymph plexuses of the skin in this region.

GENERAL CHARACTERISTICS OF PATHOLOGIC MASSES

Before the discussion of specific masses by region, it is appropriate to review some of the characteristics of abnormal masses, since the presence or absence of certain features often directs the clinician to the correct disease or group of diseases. These characteristics are common to abnormal masses no matter where the masses are found in the body.

Degree of tenderness

Tenderness usually indicates inflammation or infection or both within the tissues affected. Benign or malignant tumors and cysts are usually nontender. Painful tumors are usually the result of frank invasion of a nerve, but pain may also reflect rapid growth and simple compression of sensory nerves. In other cases a secondary inflammatory process or abscess or both within a tumor or cyst may be the cause of tenderness.

Consistency

Solid masses impart a feeling of firmness, whereas cysts and abscesses are soft to rub-

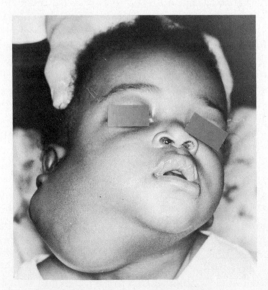

Fig. 31-3. Large lymphoma. This child had a rapidly growing rubbery mass.   (Courtesy O.H. Stuteville, DDS, MD, St. Joe, Ark.)

bery. Fluctuation may be masked by a surrounding zone of inflammation or fibrous tissue, or a fluid-filled mass may be situated so deep in the tissues that fluctuance is not demonstrable. Although other signs of the inflammatory process are generally present, whether an abscess is fluctuant or not depends on its stage of development.

In the early stage before a pool of pus forms, the swelling is due to inflammation only, so the mass is not fluctuant but is firm in consistency. Later, if a pool of pus does form, the swelling becomes fluctuant. Still later, in the regressing stage, the fluctuance disappears as the pus is eliminated.

Malignant tumors and their metastases to lymph nodes are frequently described as stony hard, although lymph nodes involved by lymphoma have a distinctly rubbery feeling (Fig. 31-3). Tuberculosis characteristically produces a caseation necrosis of several nodes, resulting in a matted type of mass.

Degree of mobility

Each structure of the neck has its own range of motion when manipulated. A decrease in mobility may be associated with fixation of the structure to less mobile ones.

Lymph nodes are ordinarily freely movable but become fixed in certain pathologic conditions. Usually fixation of a node is the result of an inflammatory process that has penetrated the node's capsule and caused fibrosis to the surrounding immovable structures. Less frequently, in cases of metastatic spread, the malignant cells penetrate the capsule and invade the surrounding tissue.

PATHOLOGIC MASSES

Aside from masses originating in the skin, the majority of neck masses may be categorized into the following general types: (1) enlarged lymph nodes, (2) enlarged submandibular, parotid, and thyroid glands or masses within these glands, (3) congenital cysts of specific origin and location, and (4) derivatives of vessels and nerves in the lateral neck region. Other distinctive masses in the neck not falling into this classification are discussed with those occurring in specific regions of the neck.

Masses of nonspecific location

Commonly occurring masses, although not specific to the neck region (for example, the lipoma), are not classified or discussed here. Also, it is obvious that some masses are not peculiar to certain regions of the neck but may occur anywhere in the neck; these most frequently originate in the skin or lymph nodes and are referred to as masses of nonspecific location.

ENLARGED LYMPH NODES

Enlarged lymph nodes are by far the most commonly found pathologic masses in the neck. The majority of the enlarged cervical lymph nodes are the result of an acute or chronic response to an infectious organism (lymphadenitis), the growth of a metastatic tumor, or a primary malignant neoplasm (lymphoma). These three main groups of lymph node pathosis are listed according to frequency of occurrence, with the most common group noted first.

A lymphadenitis is by definition an inflammation or infection of a lymph node and frequently occurs when an infection is present in the tissues drained by the particular node's pathway. Pathoses of this type may be divided into acute or chronic, solitary or multiple, local or disseminated, and specific or nonspecific.

As with the same process in other organs and tissues, the sequelae of a lymphadenitis depend on the modifying factors. If the adenitis is short lived, the node may subsequently return to practically normal size and architecture. If, on the other hand, the infection is acute, the node may become painful, necrotic, and liquefied and may lead to a space abscess.

In more chronic cases a permanent hyperplasia of the lymph node may result; such a pathosis is referred to as a benign lymphoid hyperplasia. In some instances of chronic lymphadenitis, scarring replaces the node architecture and the enlarged node remains as a permanently fibrosed mass. Thus two distinct types of benign node enlargement can be found by clinical examination: (1) nontender and (2) tender or painful.

Nontender lymphoid hyperplasia. The majority of nontender benign enlargements of the cervical lymph nodes are nontender lymphoid hyperplasias (Fig. 31-4). At least one or two such enlarged nodes are found in the routine palpation of the neck of almost every patient examined. Nontender lymphoid hyperplasias represent either a persistent chronic lymphadenitis or a permanently enlarged node after an acute or chronic lymphadenitis.

FEATURES. The patient is usually unaware of the enlarged node but in some cases may recount the presence of a previous painful swelling in the region and perhaps identify the primary infection site. The nodes are solitary, discrete, asymptomatic, and usually freely movable. The submandibular, submental, and subdigastric groups are the nodes most frequently affected (Fig. 31-4).

DIFFERENTIAL DIAGNOSIS. The nontender lymphoid hyperplasia is by far the most commonly occurring pathologic mass in the neck.

The painless nature of this benign enlargement differentiates it from the less frequently encountered *acute lymphadenitis.*

As a general rule nontender lymphoid hyperplasia can be differentiated from *secondary carcinoma* by the fact that the carcinoma is bony hard and often fixed whereas the hyperplasia is

firm and usually freely movable. A complete head and neck examination and evaluation are necessary, however, before benign lymphoid hyperplasia can be made the final diagnosis because occasionally a metastatic tumor in an enlarged lymph node has a softer consistency.

MANAGEMENT. If the clinician has any doubt concerning the diagnosis, the patient should be reexamined at 2-week intervals to see whether the mass changes perceptibly. If the mass continues to be asymptomatic and does not enlarge, it is almost certainly a nontender node of lymphoid hyperplasia. If doubt still exists, removal of the node with subsequent microscopic study is advised.

Acute lymphadenitis. Acute lymphadenitis is the second most common pathologic cervical mass and the most common painful enlargement found in the neck. The primary infection may be in the oral cavity, the nasal cavities, the tonsils, or the pharynx. Minor mucosal erosions or shallow ulcers frequently permit the entrance of sufficient bacteria to produce a regional lymphadenitis. Depending on the location of the tooth (Fig 31-5), a periapical abscess, periodontal abscess, or pericoronitis-type infection may cause painful swollen nodes in the submental, submandibular, or subdigastric area (Fig. 31-13, *C*). With tonsillar inflammation the subdigastric node is most commonly involved and has thus become known as the tonsillar node. Rapid regression of the inflammation may result in the node's returning to normal and becoming nonpalpable. In more chronic cases the node becomes fibrosed or

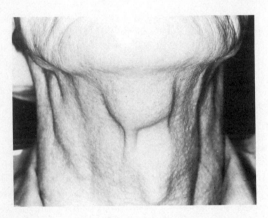

Fig. 31-4. Benign lymphoid hyperplasia. This unusually large example in the submental region was firm, nontender, and freely movable.   (Courtesy S. Svalina, DDS, Maywood, Ill.)

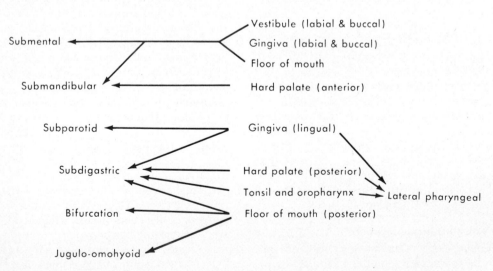

Fig. 31-5. Lymphatic drainage areas of the oral cavity (exclusive of the tongue) and pharynx showing first-echelon lymph nodes for various regions.

persists as an asymptomatic lymphoid hyperplasia. In either circumstance the node is enlarged, firm, and usually freely movable.

FEATURES. Acute lymphadenitis is tender or painful to palpation. Single affected nodes are round, firm, and discrete and may be either movable or fixed. Several nodes in one region may be involved, and in such cases an accompanying inflammation in the adjacent soft tissues causes a firm swelling that prevents palpation of the individual nodes (Fig. 31-13, C). On microscopic examination the node is enlarged, has more numerous germinal centers, and contains acute inflammatory cells. Such a condition is termed a nonspecific adenitis. The architecture of nodes affected by a severe inflammation may be almost obliterated by the inflammatory process, even to the point of necrosis and liquefaction.

DIFFERENTIAL DIAGNOSIS. Acute lymphadenitis must be differentiated from infected cysts and Ludwig's angina.

Ludwig's angina is usually a nonpurulent hemolytic streptococcal infection of the floor of the mouth and submental and submandibular areas. The classic location of this entity, along with the serosanguineous fluid obtained on incision, is almost pathognomonic.

Infected cysts of the neck, except for the sebaceous type, which is very superficial, may be suspected in certain locations; in other words, branchial and thyroglossal cysts characteristically occur in the lateral neck and midline regions, respectively.

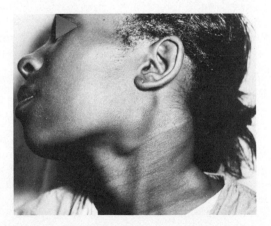

Fig. 31-6. Tuberculous adenitis. The nodular enlargement in the parotid region was tender and moderately soft to palpation. The patient also had pulmonary tuberculosis. (Courtesy O.H. Stuteville, DDS, MD, St. Joe, Ark.)

MANAGEMENT. In most cases, when the primary mucosal infection is eliminated, the secondary acute lymphadenitis soon regresses. Adequate doses of antibiotics administered for at least 5 days are usually employed. Cases of generalized lymphadenitis in which lymph nodes are uniformly and symmetrically enlarged in all accessible areas, such as the axillae, groin, and neck, are not rare, and such a condition usually suggests a viremia. Thus, in cases of multiple and bilateral nodes in the neck, a careful examination of other nodal areas and the spleen, as well as a complete history and physical examination, is necessary to determine whether the enlarged nodes in the neck are a manifestation of a local or a systemic disease.

Rare varieties of specific lymphadenitis. The majority of cases of cervical lymphadenitis result from primary infections by garden-variety bacteria or viruses. Microscopic examination does not show characteristics that relate to these "common" organisms, since only a nonspecific adenitis is seen. Specific diagnostic changes may occur in some rare diseases, however, and the situation is then referred to as a specific adenitis (Robbins, 1967).

The specific lesions within lymph nodes generated by tuberculosis, histoplasmosis, sarcoidosis, and infectious mononucleosis are similar to the lesions in other tissues infected by the organisms causing these diseases. Except for infectious mononucleosis, these are relatively uncommon in the neck, but in some cases lymph node infection that initially appears to be nonspecific (Fig. 31-6) proves on biopsy to be one of the specific infections.

Metastatic carcinoma to cervical nodes. The cervical lymph nodes are more frequently the site of metastatic carcinomas than of primary tumors (lymphomas). The majority of these secondary tumors are the result of metastatic spread from primary tumors in the head and neck, especially those in the oral and pharyngeal cavities. In unusual cases, however, they represent secondary tumors from primary sites below the clavicles.

In addition to the common sites of origin of squamous cell carcinoma of the mouth and oropharynx, other mucosal surfaces, particularly of the larynx and vocal cords, develop tumors that metastasize to regional nodes. The first-echelon nodes for metastatic tumors occurring inferior to the oropharynx are located roughly opposite the primary tumor site in the jugular chain.

Since squamous cell carcinoma constitutes the preponderance of primary malignancies of the head and neck (95% of all oral malignancies are squamous cell carcinomas), it is by far the most common tumor spreading to the cervical nodes (see Fig. 15-9, C). Adenocarcinoma of the salivary glands, occasionally squamous cell carcinoma from the skin, and melanoma are the tumors that next most commonly metastasize to the cervical nodes. Sarcoma characteristically spreads by the blood channels but on a rare occasion involves a lymph node.

The lymphatic trunks draining the upper extremities and the rest of the body below the clavicles converge in the base of the lateral neck region, the supraclavicular area. Hence solitary metastatic nodes in this area are mostly from primary tumors in areas other than the head and neck, such as the breasts, lungs, and stomach. A complete history, physical examination, and specific laboratory studies usually reveal the primary tumor.

FEATURES. Metastatic tumors in lymph nodes are almost always painless and thus are not detected by the patient until they reach considerable dimensions. The smaller nodes are usually detected on routine examination; they characteristically feel stony hard and are freely movable until the tumor cells penetrate the node capsule and invade the surrounding tissue. Then they become fixed, and the expanding tumor may amalgamate surrounding nodes into one larger, stony-hard, fixed mass. In the majority of cases the primary tumor is readily evident, especially if the primary site is in the oral cavity. Small tumors in the nasal cavities, nasopharynx, and larynx, however, may go undetected, the only evidence of their presence being the metastatic tumor. The submandibular and subdigastric nodes are the most frequent sites of early metastatic spread from primary tumors within the oral cavity.

DIFFERENTIAL DIAGNOSIS. The differential diagnosis of metastatic lymph node tumors is considered later in this chapter with the discussion of pathologic masses occurring in specific regions.

Small metastatic nodes may be confused with *fibrosed nodes* or nodes that have undergone *nontender lymphoid hyperplasia* because these entities are firm and may even be fixed to the surrounding tissue by fibrosis resulting from a previous infection. In such cases, however, the history relating to a severe infection in the region would probably direct the clinician to the likely diagnosis of benign lymphoid hyperplasia.

Differentiating between a secondary tumor and a *lymphoma* is also necessary, but the fact that a metastatic tumor is usually stony hard, whereas the lymphoma is more rubbery, is helpful in making this distinction.

MANAGEMENT. Various combinations of resection, radiation, and chemotherapy are used, with inconsistent results. The prognosis for a patient with lymph node metastasis is grave.

Lymphoma. Lymphoma is a neoplastic proliferation within the reticuloendothelial system that occurs as a primary tumor of lymph nodes but is not as common as a metastatic tumor (Batsakis, 1974, p. 346). There are several types of lymphoma, which vary in behavior.

At one time lymphomas were classified as giant follicle lymphoma, reticulum cell sarcoma, lymphosarcoma, and Hodgkin's disease. More recently, disagreement resulting from intensive study has resulted in the development of a more complicated classification, which more accurately reflects the behavior of the specific tumor. A detailed discussion of this newer classification is beyond the scope of the text.

Lymphomas may be solitary or multiple. Although it is generally accepted that they reflect a systemic disease, in about 10% of cases the initial finding is a mass in the neck (Rosenberg et al., 1961).

FEATURES. The nodes involved may be solitary or multiple and unilateral or bilateral; they are usually rubbery and may be a single discrete mass or several nodes joined together (Fig. 31-3). In advanced cases the patient may be quite ill with fever, and the total and differential leukocyte counts may be markedly changed, indicating that the increased production of mononuclear cells has spilled over into the blood. Other node groups such as the axillae, groin, and mediastinum are frequently involved in these advanced cases.

DIFFERENTIAL DIAGNOSIS. Advanced and disseminated lymphomas (Hodgkin's disease) are readily differentiated from other tumors on a clinical basis.

The clinical differentiation between a *metastatic carcinoma* and a lymphoma is described in the differential diagnosis section of the discussion on metastatic carcinoma to cervical nodes.

Multiple and disseminated nodal involvement may also occur with certain *viral diseases* and in *mononucleosis*. In these diseases, however, the nodes are tender and painful, and a Paul-Bunnell heterophil test is positive in infectious mononucleosis.

MANAGEMENT. Radiation and various chemo-toxic drugs as well as steroids are used, with varying results, to treat patients who have malignant lymphoma. Solitary nodes are amenable to surgical excision.

SEBACEOUS CYSTS

Sebaceous cysts occur in hair-bearing areas and are found in the neck with some regularity. They are superficial, dome-shaped masses and are usually detectable on visual examination (see Figs. 31-9, *B*, 31-10, *A*, 31-12, *C*, and 31-13, *B*).

FEATURES. Sebaceous cysts grow slowly and are painless unless secondarily infected. They range from a few millimeters to a few centimeters in diameter. The smaller cysts may have a dimple or enlarged pore on the surface. If situated in the anterior two thirds of the neck, they are movable over the deeper structures because masses arising within the dermis in this area have considerable mobility. The skin of the posterior neck region is more adherent to the underlying fascia, however, and cysts arising in the posterior third of the neck may appear to be fixed to the underlying structures.

Aspiration of a thick material from such a mass is indicative of a sebaceous cyst. Secondary infection is quite common and produces pain, induration, and fixation. Recurrent episodes of infection with periodic painful enlargement of the cyst and purulent drainage are a common sequence of events.

DIFFERENTIAL DIAGNOSIS. Unlike *epidermoid* and *dermoid cysts*, sebaceous cysts most often are superficially located in the skin. Thus they usually cannot be moved independent of skin over the deeper structures. On the other hand, epidermoid cysts are deeper and freely movable unless involved with inflammation and resultant fibrosis.

Although numerous *solid benign* and *malignant tumors* of a primary and occasionally metastatic nature occur in the skin, their firm consistency differentiates them from a sebaceous cyst.

MANAGEMENT. Because of the simplicity of removal and the tendency toward secondary infection, excisional biopsy is recommended. This also identifies the occasional skin tumor that could be mistaken for a cyst on clinical examination. Suitable antibiotics should be administered if the sebaceous cyst is infected.

• • •

The majority of pathologic masses in the neck occur in four regions: submandibular, parotid, median-paramedian, and lateral. Thus the masses are discussed here according to the region in which they occur.

Masses in the submandibular region

The majority of masses in the submandibular region originate in the lymph nodes or the submandibular salivary gland. The first step in diagnosis is to distinguish between submandibular gland and nonsubmandibular gland tissues by careful bimanual, intraoral and extraoral palpation.

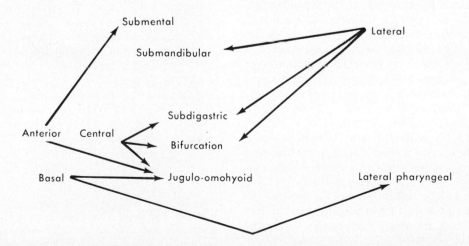

Fig. 31-7. Lymphatic drainage areas of the tongue showing first-echelon lymph nodes.

MASSES SEPARATE FROM THE SUBMANDIBULAR GLAND

A mass may be assumed to be an enlarged lymph node if it is determined not to be the submandibular salivary gland. In such a case all possible sites in the mouth (Figs. 31-5 and 31-7), on the face, and in the nasal vestibule should be carefully examined to detect a source of infection or a primary tumor.

Tender nodes. If the node is tender, whether the constitutional signs of infection such as fever are present or not, and an obvious source of infection such as an abscessed tooth is found, the working diagnosis of lymphadenitis should be made. Such a case is managed by treating the patient with antibiotics or tooth extraction or both. If no primary site of infection can be found, an antibiotic effective against staphylococcal and streptococcal infections should be administered and the patient frequently reexamined to determine whether the size and tenderness of the mass have changed.

If the tender mass subsides, it is assumed to have been an acute nonspecific nonsuppurative lymphadenitis. The specific adenitis of tuberculosis appears in rare cases as a tender mass in children. Such a mass does not respond to ordinary antibiotic treatment, and a general workup, including skin test and chest radiograph, that confirms the presence of tuberculosis should alert the clinician to the possibility of tubercular adenitis. An excisional biopsy establishes the diagnosis if the process is tuberculosis.

If the tender mass expands with or without softening and this change is accompanied by some reduction in pain and tenderness, the mass is assumed to be an abscess forming; incision and drainage are then indicated. In an adult a biopsy of the abscess wall should be performed during the drainage procedure if a primary infection is not found or if the usual signs of inflammation are minimal. Such a precaution is necessary because lymph node metastases from occult carcinomas may undergo necrosis and abscess formation.

A staphylococcal node abscess may be manifested in a fussy neonate or young child as a hard submandibular (or submental or suboccipital) swelling (Fig. 31-8, *A*). A primary infection in the mouth or skin might not be obvious because the hardness of the swelling and the lack of constitutional symptoms suggest that the mass does not have an infectious origin. Usually the abscess matures after a few days, however, and the diagnosis becomes readily apparent.

A submandibular abscess may form by the direct extension of a preexisting infection or abscess in the mouth. This pathosis appears as a diffuse tender fluctuant swelling (Fig. 31-8). The following sequence is typical in the formation of such an abscess:

1. A pericoronitis of a mandibular third molar develops with pus formation.
2. The pus extends into the pterygomandibular space, causing trismus.
3. From the pterygomandibular space the pus breaks through the connective tissue barrier around the anterior margin of the

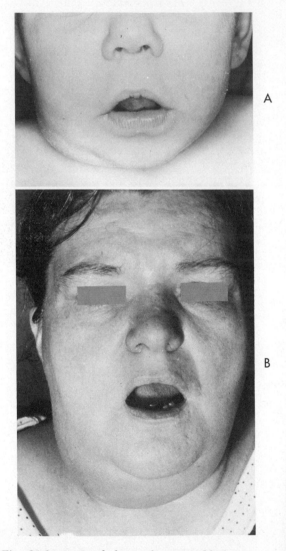

Fig. 31-8. **A,** Staphylococcal submandibular space abscess. This enlarging, hard, tender mass was present for 4 days in a fussy and mildly febrile child. No primary oral or skin infections were found. **B,** Submental and submandibular space abscess secondary to infected mandibular incisors.

medial pterygoid muscle and gains access to the submandibular space.

4. When this happens, a space abscess is produced.

The history and physical findings of an abscess are diagnostic. Hall and Arteaga (1985) discussed the use of computed tomography in the localization of head and neck space infections. Treatment consists of incision, drainage, and irrigation of the abscess and eradication of the primary infection.

Nontender nodes. The majority of nontender nodes in the submandibular region represent either benign lymphoid hyperplasias or fibrosed nodes resulting from a previous oral infection. If a nontender node of short duration is detected, however, especially in a patient over 40 years of age, the clinician must be aware of the increased possibility that it may be a secondary malignant tumor.

Such a case requires a thorough physical and radiographic examination of the head and neck to detect a possible primary malignancy. If a primary tumor is located, a biopsy of the node is performed immediately and a frozen section is examined. If the enlarged node proves to be a typical metastasizing malignancy, a neck dissection of the cervical lymph nodes is performed concurrently with the definitive treatment of the primary lesion. In some institutions a combination of irradiation and surgical resection is used; in others irradiation is the sole method of treatment.

When no primary tumor can be located but the clinician suspects that a submandibular mass may be malignant, an excisional biopsy of the mass should be performed to determine whether it has the stony-hard characteristic of a metastatic tumor. The patient is informed that the mass will be microscopically evaluated for malignancy during the biopsy procedure and that a neck dissection will be completed if the mass proves to be malignant. This policy seems justified, since a substantial increase in the cure rate has been observed when neck resection is undertaken even though the primary site was not detected before removal of the lymph nodes. In over half these patients no primary site is ever discovered (Batsakis, 1974, p. 173).

Multiple nontender nodes occurring unilaterally in the neck without an overt primary cause should be managed the same as a single nontender node.

The occurrence of bilateral multiple nontender cervical nodes with or without generalized lymphadenopathy should prompt a complete medical examination for the detection of systemic disorders.

In the adult, excisional biopsy may be necessary for diagnosis, but it should await the results of other diagnostic tests, which might preclude the necessity for this step.

In the child, multiple enlarged bilateral neck nodes of inflammatory origin are common whereas metastasizing neoplasms are rare. Conversely, lymphomas are more common in children than are secondary tumors. Although biopsies of all asymptomatic nodes in children with multiple and bilateral cervical lymphadenopathy would not be feasible, any unusually large node in a child that shows progressive growth or is rubbery or stony hard should be excised and microscopically examined.

MASSES WITHIN THE SUBMANDIBULAR GLAND

If a mass is within the submandibular gland, the gland should be removed intact and examined histologically at the time of the surgery. A total excision of the gland is required because (1) a high proportion of submandibular tumors are malignant (50%) and (2) the most common tumor in this gland, the pleomorphic adenoma, does not have a restricting capsule (Fig. 31-9, A). Furthermore, a wide local resection of the surrounding tissues and occasionally a radical neck dissection at the time of the excisional biopsy may be necessary. A more complete discussion of salivary gland tumors appears in Batsakis (1974, pp. 1-51).

SUBMANDIBULAR GLAND SIALADENITIS

A painful enlargement of the submandibular gland (sialadenitis) may be produced by two different circumstances: (1) an inflammation or infection of the gland caused by ductal occlusion and (2) an infection not preceded by ductal obstruction.

When the duct is obstructed, eating leads to pain and swelling in the gland because the secretions accumulate behind the obstruction. The pain and swelling tend to subside somewhat between meals and are minimal on waking in the morning. The clinician can determine that the duct is patent if milking the submandibular gland causes the expression of saliva at Wharton's papilla. The clinician may discover a sialolith in the submandibular duct by palpating the floor of the mouth bimanually. In approximately 90% of cases a sialolith is dense enough to show on a radiograph (see Figs. 28-14 and 28-15).

If the results of these examinations are equivocal, sialography with a radiopaque sub-

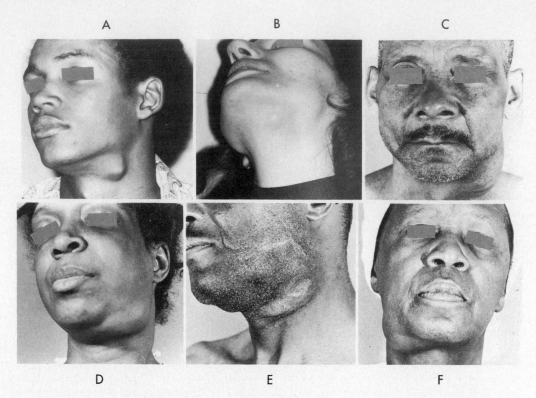

Fig. 31-9. Submandibular masses. **A,** Pleomorphic adenoma of the submandibular salivary gland. **B,** Sebaceous cyst. **C,** Metastatic squamous cell carcinoma to the submandibular and subdigastric nodes. The primary tumor was located in the left floor of the mouth. The mass was painless, firm, and fixed to the surrounding structures. **D,** Metastatic melanoma from a primary lesion on the palate. **E,** Actinomycosis. **F,** Tuberculous adenitis.   (**A** courtesy E. Kasper, DDS, Maywood, Ill.)

stance can be performed to show whether the duct is patent. The advantage of this procedure, however, must be weighed against the hazard of precipitating a retrograde infection. Also, the injection of the disclosing material into the inflamed gland causes the patient additional discomfort.

Obstruction of the duct may also have other causes such as changes in the floor of the mouth produced by a malignant tumor or postoperative scarring. Under these circumstances the obstructive process is frequently insidious, and although the gland is enlarged and firm, tenderness is frequently not a feature.

Elimination of the obstruction by removal of the stone, tumor, or cicatrix is the indicated treatment. Complete removal of the gland may be necessary when much fibrosis is present in a chronic case or when the stone is near or within the gland.

Sialadenitis without prior ductal obstruction. Sialadenitis without prior ductal obstruction is caused by either viral or bacterial infection.

Mumps is the type of viral sialadenitis most commonly occurring in childhood, and although primarily a disease of the parotid glands, it may also affect the submandibular glands. The diagnosis is usually made by confirming a history of contact with an infected person. When such information is lacking, the demonstration of mumps antibodies in the serum establishes the diagnosis.

Other viruses may cause a sialadenitis. Zollar and Mufson (1970) showed the association of coxsackievirus A and echovirus in patients with parotitis whose sera were negative for mumps virus. Although such a viral relationship has not been established in submandibular gland adenitis, such a cause might be considered in uncommon cases of enlarged tender unobstructed glands.

A suppurative sialadenitis is produced almost exclusively by a retrograde bacterial infection in patients with reduced salivary secretion. Such a reduction may be caused by dehydration or the use of parasympathetic blocking drugs and also by partial occlusion of a major duct. The retrograde infection occurs because oral bacteria are able to ascend the duct to the gland in the absence of the duct-cleansing salivary flow.

Pus-producing sialadenitis seldom occurs in the major glands but is more common in the parotid gland. In the submandibular gland it is usually associated with a ductal stone, and the clinical and radiographic examinations previously described should be completed. The use of sialography is contraindicated in suppurative sialadenitis.

Clinically the gland is firm and painful. Pressure over the gland causes the expression of pus from the opening of Wharton's duct if the duct is not completely obstructed. A specimen of pus should be collected and sent for culture and sensitivity tests so an effective antibiotic may be administered. Systemic problems, as well as any local factors causing occlusion of the duct, should be eliminated. Occasionally a child or an adult has recurrent bouts of nonobstructive sialadenitis; such a condition is described as chronic recurrent sialadenitis (Batsakis, 1974, p. 55).

In rare instances a branchial cleft cyst may project into the submandibular region. Also a ranula of the sublingual gland may insinuate itself around the posterior border of the mylohyoid muscle and cause a cystlike mass in this region. These entities must be considered when cystic masses are encountered in this region.

Masses in the parotid region

The numerous masses that commonly occur in the parotid region are similar to those described in the submandibular region. This is to be expected, since the chief structures occupying both regions are the major salivary glands and the lymph nodes. Thus a complete discussion is not repeated for each of the masses dealt with previously; only lesions peculiar to the parotid region are detailed here. Concerning the previously discussed masses, only differences in emphasis are made.

When a mass is discovered in the parotid region, the clinician must first determine whether it is superficial or deep to the investing fascia of the salivary gland. The majority of masses superficial to the investing fascia are enlarged lymph nodes, whereas those masses within the gland are usually either parotid masses or enlarged intraparotid nodes. Masses within the parotid gland are fixed beneath the confines of the investing fascia and capsule of the gland.

ENLARGED MASSES SUPERFICIAL TO THE PAROTID FASCIA

Various lymph nodes are present in the loose connective tissue superficial to the parotid gland and fascia. The preauricular node is found immediately anterior to the external auditory meatus. It is quite mobile unless fixed to the surrounding tissues as a result of penetrating pathoses.

An enlarged *firm, tender,* or *painful mass* that can be moved over the deeper structures in this superficial region is most likely an *acute lymphadenitis* resulting from a furuncle or other infection of the scalp, upper face, conjunctiva, or external auditory canal.

An infected *congenital preauricular cyst* or *sebaceous cyst* must also be considered because either may be found superficial to the parotid fascia (Fig. 31-10, *A*). The rubbery consistency and fluctuance of these masses, however, help to differentiate them from an acute lymphadenitis. Also, erythema and edema of the overlying skin are more characteristic of an infected cyst than of an acute lymphadenitis.

Painless superficial masses are usually benign lymphoid hyperplasias, parotid gland tumors occurring superficial to the gland, or preauricular or sebaceous cysts.

The *preauricular* or *sebaceous cysts* are moderately soft (rubbery) in consistency and fluctuant, whereas the other two entities are firm.

An *extraparotid tumor* cannot be differentiated clinically from a *benign lymphoid hyperplasia* since both may be firm and demonstrate some mobility; however, the former pathosis is rare whereas the latter is common. Should the firm mass continue to grow while remaining painless, it is most likely an extraparotid tumor and should be surgically excised and microscopically studied.

Lymph nodes in the preauricular area are seldom the site of a *lymphoma.* Also rare in this group of nodes is a *metastatic carcinoma,* which may originate from a primary carcinoma or a melanoma in the skin of the region drained.

Whether a mass located at the inferior tip of the parotid lobe is superficial to or within the parotid gland is frequently difficult to determine. In such an instance a primary site for possible tumors or inflammatory lesions is sought on the appropriate skin surfaces of the scalp and face or the mucosal surfaces of the oral cavity, pharynx, and nasal cavities. Because of the distinct possibility that this mass may be a secondary or a salivary gland tumor,

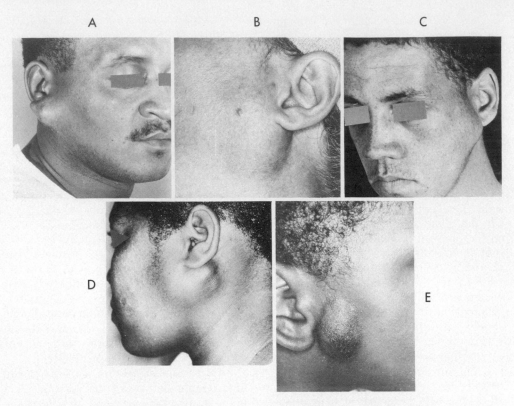

Fig. 31-10. Masses in the parotid region. **A,** Sebaceous cyst. **B,** Benign mixed tumor. The mass was firm and slow growing. **C,** Malignant mixed tumor. This mass was firm and rapidly enlarging. **D,** Parotid space abscess resulting from a dental infection. **E,** Hemangioma.   (**D** courtesy V. Barresi, DDS, DeKalb, Ill.)

if the examination of the frozen section indicates that it is malignant, the mass should be excised and more extensive surgery completed at the same operation.

MASSES WITHIN THE PAROTID GLAND

The majority of masses occurring within the parotid gland are salivary gland tumors. Approximately 70% of these are benign, most being benign mixed tumors that are characteristically slow growing and produce a noticeable firm swelling in the parotid area (Fig. 31-10, *B*). Malignant mixed tumors, on the other hand, usually grow more rapidly, may be stony hard, and may cause a unilateral paralysis of the muscles of facial expression. The types of salivary gland tumors are listed in Chapter 10. Although the clinician may develop an impression of whether the tumor is benign or malignant, the definitive diagnosis must be made by microscopic study in every case.

MANAGEMENT. Besides a parotid gland tumor, a mass within the parotid gland may be an enlarged node, a simple cyst, a cyst of the first

and second branchial arches, or a hamartoma. Although the diagnosis of each of these entities is occasionally suspected on the basis of clinical features, the physical examination is not sufficiently definitive to rule out a tumor. Therefore biopsies must be performed on all masses detected within the parotid gland. Hansson et al. (1988) discussed the benefits of computed tomographic sialography and conventional sialography in the evaluation of parotid gland neoplasms.

If at surgery the mass proves to be a tumor, the complete superficial lobe of the gland is excised, leaving the facial nerve intact. The complete lobe is sacrificed because the most common lesion, the pleomorphic adenoma, frequently penetrates its pseudocapsule and a high recurrence rate results if an attempt is made merely to enucleate the lesion.

When a mass is found to extend into or originate in the deep parotid lobe, the entire gland is removed for pathologic study. A malignant tumor of a type that characteristically metastasizes to the cervical lymph nodes or that shows clinical evidence of metastasis requires resection of the cervical lymph nodes in addition to removal of the primary lesion. Carr and Bowerman (1986) reviewed tumors of the deep lobe of the parotid salivary gland.

In rare instances primary lesions arising in the mouth or oropharynx metastasize to the nodes within the parotid gland, so these regions should be examined carefully before the biopsy procedure. A wide variety of tumors are found within the parotid gland, and these are characterized in detail by Batsakis (1974, p. 433).

SIALADENITIS OF THE PAROTID GLAND

The various types of disturbances causing a sialadenitis have been discussed with regard to sialadenitis of the submandibular gland. The types and characteristics are similar in the parotid gland, so a discussion of these is not repeated for parotid sialadenitis (Fig. 31-11, A). The following points are peculiar to the parotid gland, however:

1. Salivary stones (calculi) in Stensen's duct occur much less frequently than in Wharton's duct, and those that do develop are frequently poorly calcified and radiolucent.
2. Bimanual palpation of much of the duct is impossible because of the ramus of the mandible.
3. The greater susceptibility of the parotid gland to secondary infection frequently prolongs the period of enlargement, pain, and tenderness, in contrast to the short symptomatic attacks characteristic of obstruction of the submandibular duct.
4. Scar tissue, intraductal tumor, and external ductal compression rarely cause obstruction of the parotid duct.

BILATERAL PAROTID ENLARGEMENT

An *asymptomatic* bilateral enlargement of the parotid glands caused by a benign lymphoepithelial lesion with or without enlargement of the submandibular and lacrimal glands has been classically referred to as Mikulicz's disease (Fig. 31-11, B). When a variety of systemic diseases such as lymphoma and sarcoidosis are associated with these findings, the symptom complex is termed Mikulicz's syndrome. The association of symptoms, including xerostomia, combined with conjunctivitis and coupled with a connective tissue disease such as rheumatoid arthritis is called Sjögren's syndrome. In all these disorders the parotid swelling may be bilateral or unilateral. Attempts

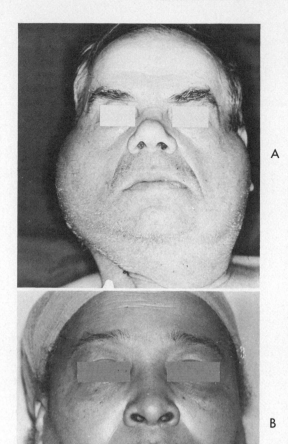

Fig. 31-11. Bilateral parotid swelling. **A,** Painful bilateral suppurative parotitis ("surgical mumps"). There was postoperative staphylococcal infection of the parenchyma of both glands. Pus could be expressed from Stensen's papillae. **B,** Mikulicz's disease. Note the bilateral parotid swelling, which was asymptomatic.   (**A** courtesy O.H. Stuteville, DDS, MD, St. Joe, Ark. **B** courtesy P. Akers, DDS, Chicago.)

have been made to interrelate this group of diseases, but the specific pathogenetic relationships remain unclear.

The identification of an asymptomatic parotid enlargement as one of the aforementioned diseases depends on clinical and laboratory findings. The diagnosis of *Sjögren's syndrome* is strengthened by the demonstration of focal lymphocytic infiltrates in the labial minor salivary glands.

Bilateral parotid swelling has been noted in a variety of nutritional and metabolic disorders (Batsakis, 1974, p. 60). *Enlargement* because of *alcohol* is relatively common, whereas that caused by *drugs* (such as iodine and certain heavy metals) is infrequent but must be considered in the differential diagnosis of parotid swelling. Taylor and Sneddon (1987) reported that parotid enlargement is an early sign of bulimia in a significant number of cases. Finally, swelling of the major salivary glands may occur *after radiation* and is usually painful.

Masses in the median-paramedian region

Pathoses of the thyroid gland and its developmental derivatives account for the majority of pathologic masses in the median-paramedian region.

TENDER ENLARGEMENT OF THE THYROID GLAND

The thyroid gland may undergo inflammatory changes that produce an enlarged tender gland frequently accompanied by dysphagia and voice changes. Suppuration resulting from a bacterial infection is rare; if it occurs, treatment consists of antibiotics and surgical drainage.

An *acute nonsuppurative* form of thyroiditis with persistent signs and symptoms of inflammation occurs. Although the cause of this type of thyroiditis is still obscure, the thyroid glands of these patients usually show a decreased capacity for iodine uptake. Corticosteroids and analgesics have been used to treat the symptoms, but irradiation or surgery is necessary to eliminate the underlying disease (Schwartz, 1969).

Hashimoto's disease is a chronic disorder characterized by an enlarged tender thyroid gland. The disease is thought to be caused by an autoimmune process in which the patient's thyroid gland is sensitive to its own thyroglobulin. The diagnosis is made by laboratory means (Schwartz, 1969, p. 1445). When nodular glands are present in Hashimoto's disease, a complete biopsy may be necessary to rule out thyroid tumor. Treatment of the disease is controversial and ranges from the administration of thyroid hormone to surgical excision of the gland.

NONTENDER ENLARGEMENT OF THE THYROID GLAND

The *simple* goiter is the most common type of diffuse enlargement of the thyroid gland, having a variety of causes, such as familial enzyme defect and iodine deficiency. In some

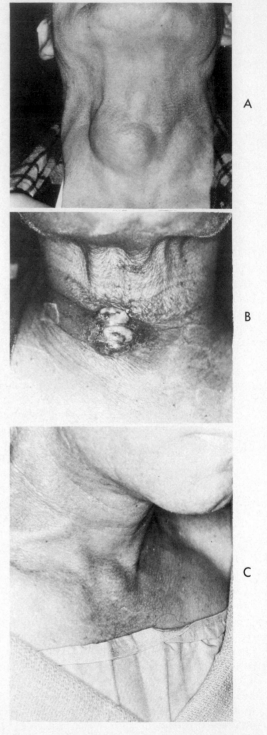

Fig. 31-12. Masses in the inferior aspect of the median-paramedian region. **A,** Benign adenoma of the thyroid gland. The mass was firm and smooth and arose from the right lobe of the gland. Swallowing caused the mass to be elevated. **B,** Anaplastic carcinoma of the thyroid gland. This mass was firm and fixed to the surrounding tissues. **C,** Sebaceous cyst. The cyst was just superficial to the isthmus of the thyroid gland.

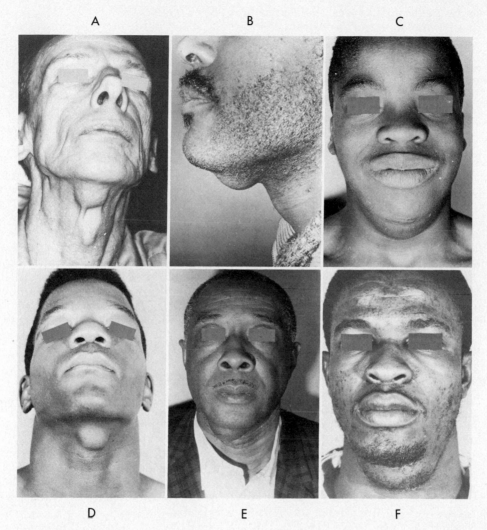

Fig. 31-13. Submental masses. **A,** Unusually large lymphoid hyperplasia. The mass was firm and freely movable. **B,** Sebaceous cyst. The mass was nontender, soft, fluctuant, and obviously attached to the skin. **C,** Diffuse submental acute lymphadenitis secondary to an infection of the lower lip. **D,** Thyroglossal cyst. This soft to rubbery fluctuant mass was elevated as the patient protruded his tongue. **E,** Dermoid cyst. This mass was doughy, fluctuant, and freely movable. **F,** Plunging ranula. This unusual lesion was painless, soft, and fluctuant. (**A** courtesy S. Svalina, DDS, Maywood, Ill. **B** courtesy P. Akers, DDS, Chicago.)

cases multiple nodules accompany the goiter, and this condition presents a dilemma to the clinician, since the nodular architecture could be masking a tumor. Laboratory studies, including radioactive iodine uptake to evaluate thyroid function, are necessary in the diffusely enlarged or nodular glands. Treatment of the goiter may be medical or surgical, depending on the cause, symptoms, and nodularity. For further details the reader is referred to Schwartz (1969, p. 1445).

MASSES WITHIN THE THYROID GLAND

Benign and malignant tumors and cysts occur as masses within the thyroid gland.

If a mass is found within the thyroid gland (Fig. 31-12), it is excised with the lateral lobe of the gland. The excision is performed to determine whether the mass is malignant, and the involved lateral lobe is completely excised to prevent transection of a tumor during the removal of the mass.

An uncommon entity known as *Riedel's thyroiditis* develops as a fixed and hard mass, thus mimicking a malignant neoplasm. If the diagnosis of Riedel's thyroiditis is established, the treatment of choice is thyroid hormone, surgery being reserved for patients who require relief of tracheal and esophageal constriction.

When a thyroid mass is found, careful examination of the cervical lymph nodes is required to detect the infrequent but possible occurrence of metastatic tumor. Furthermore, metastatic tumor from a primary lesion in either the thyroid gland or the lower larynx may be present in an enlarged lymph node located on the cricothyroid membrane. The preoperative diagnostic workup in the patient with a thyroid mass is discussed in detail by Schwartz (1969).

THYROGLOSSAL CYSTS

Cystic masses arising from remnants of the embryonic thyroglossal duct are found in the midline anywhere from the base of the tongue to the sternum (Fig. 31-13, *D*). The duct may persist in postnatal life as a draining tract or a cystic mass. A pathognomonic sign is the upward thrust of the mass when the patient protrudes the tongue, which demonstrates the connection of the thyroglossal duct and the tongue.

A thyroglossal cyst most commonly occurs below the hyoid bone and is usually readily visualized on clinical examination as a dome-shaped mass. These cysts may also be found submentally above the hyoid bone (Fig. 31-13, *D*) and within the musculature of the tongue. On rare occasion, thyroid tumors develop in the walls of these cysts. Van Der Wal et al. (1987) reported their findings in 41 cases. Treatment consists of total excision of the cyst and the entire tract to the base of the tongue.

SUBMENTAL MASSES

As stated in the preceding discussion, a *thyroglossal cyst* in a suprahyoid position is found as a submental mass.

Although it is uncommon, an *epidermoid* or *dermoid* cyst may occur in the submental area (Fig. 31-13, *E*), lying in the midline. Although it is fluctuant, its doughy consistency helps the clinician to differentiate it from the more rubbery thyroglossal cyst.

Excision of submental cystic masses of these two types with subsequent microscopic study establishes the diagnosis and is the recommended treatment.

Submental lymph nodes drain the regions of the lips and are subject to all the acute, chronic, inflammatory, and neoplastic changes described for nodes of the submandibular and parotid regions (Fig. 31-13, *A* and *C*). The differential diagnosis and management of submental lymph node pathoses are dictated by the same considerations as discussed for such conditions in the submandibular and parotid regions.

Masses in the lateral neck region
LYMPH NODES

Most masses in the neck are enlarged lymph nodes extending along the linear path of the internal jugular vein from the angle of the mandible to the clavicle. The information concerning lymph nodes in other regions is especially pertinent to those in the lateral neck region, since the preponderance of cervical nodes occur in this segment.

First-echelon nodes for the common cancer sites of the tongue, floor of the mouth, tonsil, and larynx are distributed along the jugular vein from the digastric to the omohyoid muscle (Figs. 31-5 and 31-7). In cancer patients the alternate lymphatic chain of nodes residing along the course of the accessory nerve, posterior to the posterior border of the sternocleidomastoid muscle, must also be carefully examined for lymphadenopathy. Diagnostic and therapeutic measures for dealing with the masses presumed to be enlarged lymph nodes in the region follow the general principles detailed in the previous sections.

MASSES DISPLACING THE UPPER REGION OF THE STERNOCLEIDOMASTOID MUSCLE

The normal structures lying deep to the upper section of the sternocleidomastoid muscle are lymph nodes that drain large submucosal plexuses, the carotid artery, the internal jugular vein, the vagus nerve, and the cervical sympathetic trunk.

A bulging mass in this area may represent a metastatic carcinoma to the jugulodigastric and bifurcation nodes (Fig. 31-14, *A*), a branchial cyst of the second arch (Fig. 31-14, *B*), a carotid body tumor (Fig. 31-14, *D*), or a neurogenic tumor of vagus nerve or cervical sympathetic trunk origin.

Lymph node metastasis in this region is usually from a primary lesion at the base of the tongue or elsewhere in the oropharynx. As the mass enlarges, it displaces the superior aspect of the sternocleidomastoid muscle laterally. If necrosis occurs, the mass may become fluctu-

ant and painful, causing the inexperienced clinician to misdiagnose it as a primary abscess; however, a clinical diagnosis of primary abscess should not be considered likely without a history of an antecedent oropharyngeal infection. To further ensure the detection of a possible malignancy in such a case, a biopsy should be performed at the time the mass is drained to identify the presence of a possible metastatic tumor. If the primary tumor is discovered, the primary and secondary lesions are treated simultaneously.

Branchial cleft cyst. Cystic masses in this area usually prove to be of branchial cleft origin. Branchial cleft cysts may occur at any level in the neck and frequently lie under the sternocleidomastoid muscle (Fig. 31-14, *B*).

If a sinus is present, its opening usually occurs at the anterior border of the sternocleidomastoid muscle. If a cyst and sinus of the second branchial cleft are present, the tract leads

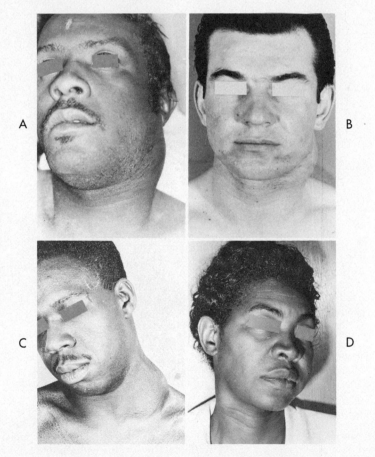

Fig. 31-14. Masses in the lateral neck. **A,** Metastatic squamous cell carcinoma in the subdigastric lymph nodes. This mass was stony hard and fixed. The primary tumor was located in the left side of the nasopharynx. **B,** Branchial cleft cyst. **C,** Cystic hygroma. **D,** Carotid body tumor. The mass was movable only in a lateral direction.

to the tonsillar fossa. Complete excision of the cyst is the indicated treatment.

Frequently microscopic lymph node follicles are seen in the walls of a branchial cyst. Secondarily infected cysts are often mistaken for abscesses, and if these cysts are incised and drained, a cutaneous sinus usually persists.

Carotid body tumors and neurogenic tumors. Carotid body tumors and to a lesser extent neurogenic tumors of cervical sympathetic origin occur under the anterosuperior aspect of the sternocleidomastoid muscle as solid masses (Fig. 31-14, *D*).

Because the masses are affixed to the nerves and vessels, they characteristically are mobile in a lateral direction but not in a vertical direction. Excision of these slow-growing and usually benign tumors is the required treatment, and the final diagnosis is made from the biopsy. For further details on these tumors, the reader is referred to Batsakis (1974, pp. 280-286).

MISCELLANEOUS MASSES OF THE LATERAL NECK REGION

Pan-neck infection. When all or most of the potential spaces of the neck are abscessed, the patient is said to have a pan-neck infection (Fig. 31-15). In such a patient two grave complications may develop: respiratory obstruction and spread of the infection to the mediastinum.

Much has been written about the grave complication of a dental or tonsillar infection reaching the mediastinum through the neck. Although fascial planes play a prominent role in the passage of pus from one potential space in the head and neck to another, it appears more likely that the transmission of infection from the upper neck to the mediastinum is through the areolar tissues in general. The virulence of the organism and the resistance of the patient are frequently more important considerations for the prognosis of the infection than is the size or extent of the abscess.

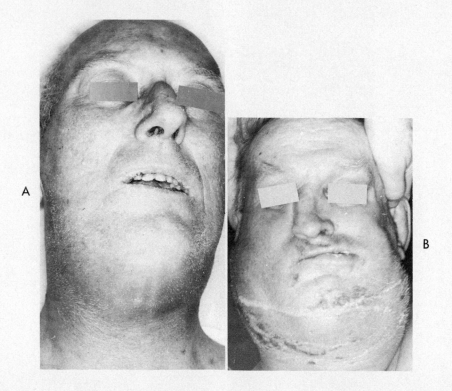

Fig. 31-15. Pan-neck infection. **A,** Elderly man with an infected left upper molar of 5 days' duration and only moderate upper neck swelling. The swelling subsequently became generalized. A chest radiograph showed gas in the mediastinum, and a culture of the region revealed *Bacteroides*. The infection traveled from the upper neck into the mediastinum through the areolar connective tissues. **B,** Pan-neck infection of dental origin. The patient had severe diabetes.   (Courtesy O.H. Stuteville, DDS, MD, St. Joe, Ark.)

This means that the patient with a pan-neck infection may be at the brink of death even when the swelling is minimal (Fig. 31-15, *A*). The key to the gravity of the case is the degree of systemic sepsis, which is reflected in the patient's vital signs. Radiographs of the neck and chest may provide clues as to the type of infection; for example, when a gas-forming organism such as *Bacteroides* is responsible for the infection, radiographs may reveal the presence of gas in the tissues.

The treatment for pan-neck infections is the wide surgical opening of all the planes at the base of the neck and drainage of the mediastinum when involved. Specific antibiotic therapy is unquestionably lifesaving in advanced infections.

Cystic hygroma. A cystic hygroma is a developmental benign cystic dilation of lymphatic vessel aggregates at variable ages after birth. The characteristically soft swelling may occur at any point in the neck from the base of the skull down to the mediastinum (Fig. 31-14, *C*), and frequently it enlarges at an alarming rate. The cystic mass may be solitary or multiple and may infiltrate into and around muscle and nerve, making excision extremely difficult and hazardous.

Few other entities occur in the child as soft compressible masses of indistinct dimensions, so recognition of the cystic hygroma is seldom in question. Also, fluid aspirated from the mass froths readily on agitation—indicative of a cystic hygroma because lymph fluid has a high fat content.

A cystic hygroma frequently occurs at an age when respiratory complications from the mass or from the surgical excision carry a high mortality. Unfortunately, there is also a danger in the infant of sudden enlargement with obstruction of the airway. Thus management in the small child presents a dilemma: whether to remove the cystic hygroma to prevent a possible airway obstruction and risk death resulting from the surgery, or to wait until the child is older and risk that in the interim the mass will suddenly enlarge and cause death by suffocation.

REFERENCES

Batsakis JG: Tumors of the head and neck, Baltimore, 1974, Williams & Wilkins.

Carr RJ and Bowerman JE: A review of tumors of the deep lobe of the parotid salivary gland, Br J Oral Maxillofac Surg 24:155-168, 1986.

Hall MB and Arteaga DM: Use of computed tomography in the localization of head and neck space infections, J Oral Maxillofac Surg 43:978-980, 1985.

Hansson LG, Johansen CC, and Biorklund A: CT sialography and conventional sialography in the evaluation of parotid gland neoplasms, J Laryngol Otol 102:163-168, 1988.

Robbins SL: Textbook of pathology, ed 3, Philadelphia, 1967, WB Saunders Co, p 665.

Rosenberg SA, Diamond HD, Jaslowitz B, and Craver LF: Lymphosarcoma: a review of 1,269 cases, Medicine 40:31-84, 1961.

Schwartz SI: Principles of surgery, New York, 1969, McGraw-Hill, Inc.

Taylor VE and Sneddon J: Bilateral facial swelling in bulimia, Br Dent J 163:115-117, 1987.

Van Der Wal JD, Wiener RHB, Allard SC, et al: Thyroglossal cysts in patients over 30 years of age, Int J Oral Maxillofac Surg 16:416-419, 1987.

Zollar LM and Mufson MA: Parotitis of non-mumps etiology, Hosp Pract 5:93-96, 1970.

32

Lesions of the facial skin

JERALD L. JENSEN
RONALD J. BARR

The following cutaneous diseases are discussed:

Premalignant and
  malignant epidermal
  lesions
  Actinic keratosis
  Bowen's disease
  Squamous cell carcinoma
  Keratoacanthoma
  Basal cell carcinoma
Benign tumors of
  epidermal appendages
  Trichoepithelioma
  Senile sebaceous
    hyperplasia
  Syringoma
  Dermal cylindroma
Miscellaneous tumorlike
  conditions
  Seborrheic keratosis
  Epidermal cysts
Tumors of the melanocytic
  system
  Junctional nevus
  Intradermal nevus
  Compound nevus
  Dysplastic nevus
  Blue nevus
  Nevus of Ota
  Malignant melanoma
Vascular tumors
  Juvenile hemangioma
  Nevus flammeus
  Pyogenic granuloma
  Nevus araneus
  Kaposi's sarcoma
  Angiosarcoma
Miscellaneous tumors
Connective tissue diseases
  Discoid lupus
    erythematosus

Systemic lupus
  erythematosus
Dermatomyositis
Scleroderma
Papulosquamous
  dermatitides
  Psoriasis
  Seborrheic dermatitis
Cutaneous reactions to
  actinic radiation
  Photosensitivity
    dermatitis
  Phototoxic dermatitis
  Photoallergic dermatitis
  Porphyria cutanea tarda
Drug eruptions
  Dermatitis
    medicamentosa
  Dermatitis venenata
Acne and acneiform
  dermatoses
  Acne vulgaris
  Rosacea
  Rhinophyma
  Perioral dermatitis
Dermatologic infections
  Bacterial infections
    Impetigo
    Sycosis barbae
    Erysipelas
  Viral infections
    Herpes zoster
    Viral warts
Miscellaneous conditions
  Xanthelasma
  Amyloidosis

Every patient seeking consultation from a dentist should receive a thorough oral examination. As part of this examination, the dentist should look for and be able to recognize abnormalities of exposed skin, especially facial skin.

Ideally, after such an abnormality has been recognized, the dentist should be able to de-velop a reasonable differential diagnosis. If the lesion requires treatment, or if the diagnosis is in doubt, the patient should be referred to a dermatologist.

This chapter is not intended to be an encyclopedic work on diseases of facial skin. Rather, it is an attempt to present diagnostic aspects of skin diseases that the dentist is likely to encounter in practice. We do not attempt to present a detailed discussion of the management of the conditions presented, since we believe that treatment is the province of the dermatologist.

PREMALIGNANT AND MALIGNANT EPIDERMAL LESIONS
Actinic keratosis

Actinic keratoses are common lesions arising on sun-exposed skin of light-complexioned individuals in response to irradiation, usually solar. The skin in which the keratoses develop is characteristically dry, scaled, wrinkled, atrophic, and sometimes focally hypopigmented.

Features. The lesions are commonly multiple and most frequently involve the face, lower lip, back of the hands, forearms, neck, and bald scalp. The individual lesions are round or irregular, scaly, keratotic, vary from gray to deep brown, and measure 0.1 to 1 cm or more in diameter (Fig. 32-1). The keratotic scale is adherent and may be very thick, producing a cutaneous horn (Domonkos et al., 1982).

The histopathologic appearance of actinic keratosis is characteristic. The epidermis reveals epithelial dysplasia with overlying parakeratosis that is responsible for the scale or horn seen clinically. The dermis exhibits solar elastosis, and frequently a chronic inflammatory infiltrate is present.

If actinic keratoses are not treated, they slowly enlarge, and according to Graham and Helwig (1972) squamous cell carcinoma develops in up to 13% of patients. Signs of malignancy include progressive enlargement, inflammation of the base, ulceration, and increasing induration. Electrodesiccation, curettage, and cryotherapy with liquid nitrogen are all effective forms of therapy.

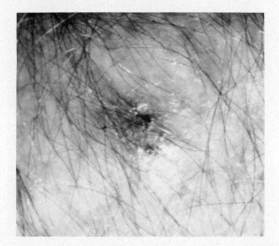

Fig. 32-1. Actinic keratosis. This lesion is a nonspecific, erythematous, slightly scaling or crusted small plaque on sun-damaged skin of this patient's dorsal forearm. (Courtesy the Upjohn Co., Kalamazoo, Mich.)

Differential diagnosis. Lesions that should be included in the differential diagnosis include seborrheic keratoses, arsenical keratoses, and squamous cell carcinomas. Seborrheic keratoses are greasy, elevated, brown or black lesions; arsenical keratoses are seen mainly on the palms and soles; and squamous cell carcinomas have the features described previously.

Bowen's disease

Bowen's disease is an intraepidermal carcinoma (squamous intraepidermal neoplasia) that has its highest incidence in older age-groups and is most common in white men with fair complexions. Chronic sun exposure and exposure to inorganic arsenicals are thought to be important in the etiology of the disease.

Features. The typical lesions of Bowen's disease are round to irregular plaques with thickened keratotic surfaces (Fig. 32-2). Occasionally the lesions are fissured and eroded. The plaques are usually sharply demarcated from the surrounding skin. They are distributed over sun-exposed and covered skin and may be solitary or multiple. Graham and Helwig (1972) stated that 5% of patients with Bowen's disease showed clinical and microscopic evidence of invasive carcinoma occurring in their lesions. This type of carcinoma is much more aggres-

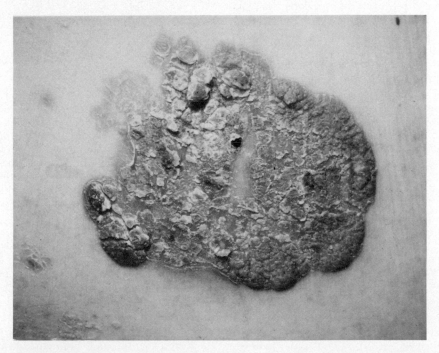

Fig. 32-2. Bowen's disease. The clinical appearance of Bowen's disease may vary significantly. This lesion presents as an erythematous, crusted, and scaly plaque that involves the patient's cheek.

sive than carcinoma arising in actinic keratosis. According to Graham and Helwig (1972) up to 37% of patients with carcinoma arising in Bowen's disease have metastases unless early adequate treatment is given. Moreover, these authors showed that patients with this disease have an increased incidence of primary extracutaneous cancers. As these findings demonstrate, the importance of early diagnosis and treatment of Bowen's disease cannot be overemphasized.

Surgical excision is generally considered the most effective form of treatment for Bowen's disease.

Differential diagnosis. Lesions to be considered in the differential diagnosis include superficial basal cell carcinoma, actinic keratosis, and psoriasis. In patients with psoriasis the lesions are usually more widely distributed and characteristically involve the elbows, knees, and scalp. Microscopic features help to differentiate Bowen's disease from actinic keratosis and superficial basal cell carcinoma.

Squamous cell carcinoma

Squamous cell carcinoma of the skin is more common in men than in women and increases in frequency with age. The etiologic factors known to be important in its development are solar irradiation, x-ray exposure, inorganic arsenic ingestion, chronic skin lesions such as burn scars and long-standing granulomas, local carcinogens such as tars and oils, and hereditary factors (Caro and Bronstein, 1985).

Features. Squamous cell carcinoma of the skin is seen most commonly on exposed areas, especially the face. When arising de novo (without evidence of a precursor lesion or insult), the tumor usually appears as a slowly enlarging, firm nodule with an indurated base. A central crust and ulceration eventually develop (Fig. 32-3). Squamous cell carcinoma arising in actinic keratosis is usually a slowly growing tumor with little or no tendency to metastasize (Graham and Helwig, 1972). In contrast, de novo squamous cell carcinoma is a biologically aggressive neoplasm. Graham and Helwig (1972) estimated that at least 8% of these neoplasms show evidence of regional or distant metastases or both.

The treatment of choice for squamous cell carcinoma depends on the location, size, and depth of penetration of the tumor. Curettage and electrodesiccation are effective for small lesions that are not deeply invasive. Large, deeply invasive tumors are probably best treated by surgical excision.

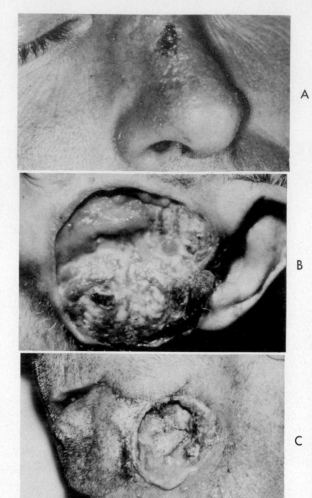

Fig. 32-3. Squamous cell carcinoma. These tumors of the skin of the face may clinically resemble basal cell carcinoma. **A,** Small lesion on the bridge of the nose in a male patient. **B,** Large ulcerated and necrotic lesion originating in the skin of the left cheek in this elderly male. **C,** Advanced lesion that originated in the buccal mucosa and has eroded through onto the face. (**A** Courtesy John Wright, DDS, Dallas; **B** Courtesy Upjohn Co., Kalamazoo, Mich.)

Differential diagnosis. The differential diagnosis includes basal cell carcinoma, keratoacanthoma, other skin tumors, and granulomas. A definitive diagnosis can be made on the basis of characteristic histologic features.

Keratoacanthoma

Keratoacanthoma is a benign, self-limited epithelial lesion that closely resembles squamous cell carcinoma. The lesion can be classified into a number of clinical types, including solitary, multiple, and eruptive (Baer and Kopf, 1963). We consider only the solitary type, since it is the most common.

Features. Solitary keratoacanthomas occur primarily on exposed skin, especially on the central face, in patients over 45 years of age. The typical lesion begins as a firm, erythematous papule that rapidly enlarges over 2 to 8 weeks. The fully developed lesion typically reaches 1 to 2 cm in diameter and is firm, raised, dome shaped, and flesh colored or slightly pink. Its borders are rolled and firm. The center of the lesion exhibits a large keratotic plug that may drop out, leaving a dry crater (Fig. 32-4). After reaching its maximum size, the lesion remains static for approximately 2 to 8 weeks and then spontaneously regresses. During the period of regression the mass gradually shrinks, the keratin plug is expelled, and the lesion heals, leaving a scar. The total duration of the lesion is usually 2 to 8 months (Caro and Bronstein, 1985). Some of these lesions become large and aggressive, invading and destroying adjacent tissue.

Differential diagnosis. The differential diagnosis includes squamous cell carcinoma and basal cell carcinoma. Since distinguishing between keratoacanthoma and squamous cell carcinoma is frequently difficult on clinical examination, and since the ultimate size and aggressiveness of keratoacanthoma cannot be predicted, early diagnosis is indicated. Surgical excision, intralesional injection of 5-fluorouracil, or radiation therapy may be indicated depending on the size and location of the lesion.

Basal cell carcinoma

Basal cell carcinoma is a malignant epithelial tumor of the skin that usually arises from basal cells of the epidermis or from the external root sheath of hair follicles. The most susceptible individuals are those with blue eyes, light hair, and minimal skin pigmentation. Sun exposure plays an important role in the development of basal cell carcinoma. Other carcinogenic influences that have been implicated include chronic ingestion of inorganic arsenicals, x-ray exposure, and burns (Caro and Bronstein, 1985).

Basal cell carcinoma is more common in men than in women, and it is uncommon before 40 years of age. Childhood onset does occur, however, in the nevoid basal cell carcinoma syndrome (Fig. 32-5), in association with xeroderma pigmentosum, and rarely in otherwise normal children (Milstone and Helwig, 1973).

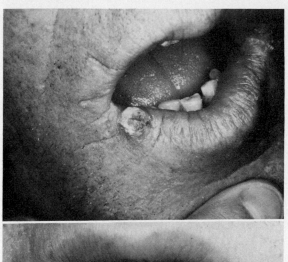

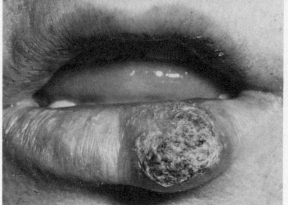

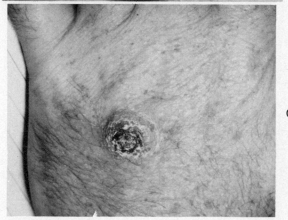

A

B

C

Fig. 32-4. Keratoacanthoma. A well-circumscribed crateriform lesion with a central keratotic plug and a raised, rolled border is typical for keratoacanthoma. These lesions cannot be differentiated from squamous cell carcinoma on the basis of clinical appearance. **A,** Lesion on the lower lip of a 44-year-old male. **B,** Lesion on the lower lip of a 20-year-old male. **C,** Lesion on the dorsal surface of the hand. (**A** and **B,** From Bass KA: J Oral Surg 38:53-55, 1980. Copyright by the American Dental Association. Reprinted by permission.)

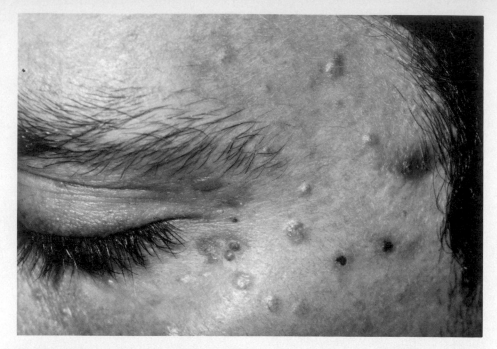

Fig. 32-5. Multiple small, nodular basal cell carcinomas and two crusted biopsy sites on the face of a young man with the basal cell nevus syndrome.

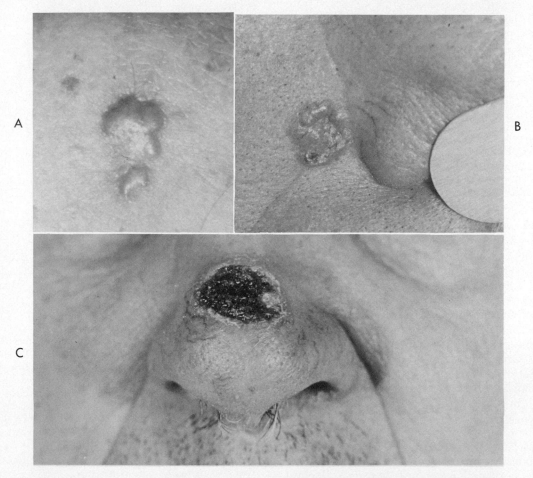

A

B

C

Fig. 32-6. Basal cell carcinoma. These three photographs illustrate stages in the development of basal cell carcinoma. **A,** Typical early lesion characterized by bosselated, irregular nodule. **B,** Small ulcerated lesion under the ala of the nose. **C,** Larger ulcerated lesion on the nose. **B** and **C,** Raised, rolled borders surround the ulcers. The borders are pearly in color and have fine telangiectasias. (**A** Courtesy the Upjohn Co., Kalamazoo, Mich.)

Features. Several clinical forms of basal cell carcinoma are recognized, the most common of which is the noduloulcerative type. This type is most common on the face. As a general rule it occurs on the face above a line drawn from the tragus of the ear to the angle of the mouth. The early lesion is a small translucent papule that may be flesh colored, pale, or erythematous. It enlarges slowly and eventually exhibits a central depression and a firm elevated border (Fig. 32-6). If left untreated, the tumor eventually ulcerates and may result in extensive local tissue destruction. Although metastasis may occur, it is uncommon (Mikhail et al., 1977).

Occasionally, basal cell carcinomas are heavily pigmented and may be mistaken for melanomas or other melanocytic lesions.

A second and less common form of basal cell carcinoma that may be seen on the head and neck is the sclerosing variant. This tumor presents as a yellowish white, sclerotic plaque without a distinct border. The clinical appearance is similar to a small patch of scleroderma, hence the name morphea-like basal cell carcinoma.

Differential diagnosis. The noduloulcerative basal cell carcinoma may be confused clinically with squamous cell carcinoma, malignant melanoma, intradermal nevus, sebaceous gland hyperplasia, and adnexal carcinoma. Characteristic histologic features differentiate these lesions.

In general, treatment for basal cell carcinoma is similar to that for squamous cell carcinoma.

BENIGN TUMORS OF EPIDERMAL APPENDAGES

Benign tumors of epidermal appendages are so classified because they display similarities to apocrine or eccrine glands, hair follicles, or sebaceous glands. Lesions in this group are usually not clinically distinctive. It should be noted, however, that the eccrine spiradenoma is characteristically tender or spontaneously painful (Kersting and Helwig, 1956), whereas other tumors in this group are usually asymptomatic. Three entities in this group, all of which may be multiple and involve the face, are discussed.

Trichoepithelioma

Trichoepithelioma is a benign tumor that recapitulates the structure of hair follicles. These tumors may be multiple or solitary. Multiple trichoepitheliomas, also called epithelioma adenoides cysticum, is a disorder inherited as an

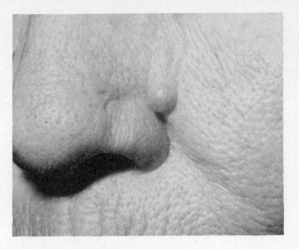

Fig. 32-7. Trichoepithelioma. This lesion presents as a flesh-colored, dome-shaped nodule immediately adjacent to the nose.

autosomal dominant trait (Gray and Helwig, 1963). These tumors begin to appear at puberty, mainly on the face where they are concentrated in the nasolabial folds, over the nose, and on the forehead, upper lip, and eyelids. The individual tumors are flesh-colored, firm papules usually 0.2 to 0.5 cm in diameter. The larger lesions may contain telangiectatic vessels on their surfaces and resemble basal cell carcinomas. Simple excision is curative.

Solitary trichoepithelioma usually has no hereditary tendency and occurs in early adult life as a nondescript, flesh-colored papule on the face (Fig. 32-7).

Senile sebaceous hyperplasia

Senile sebaceous hyperplasia occurs chiefly on the forehead and nose in persons past middle age. One or several elevated, soft, yellowish nodules 0.2 to 0.3 cm in diameter are present. The surfaces of these nodules are frequently umbilicated (Fig. 32-8). On microscopic examination the lesion is characterized by a large, multilobulated sebaceous gland emptying into an enlarged sebaceous duct.

Syringoma

Syringomas typically occur as multiple skin-colored or slightly yellowish, firm papules, 0.1 to 0.3 cm in diameter on the face (especially the eyelids), the neck, and the anterior chest (Fig. 32-9). These tumors usually appear during adolescence and occur primarily in women. Histochemical and electron microscopic observations suggest that syringoma is an adenoma of eccrine ducts (Hashimoto et al., 1966).

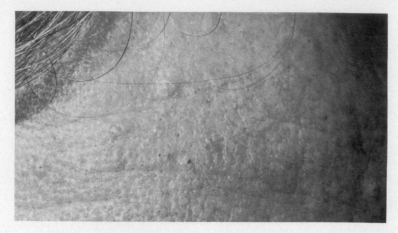

Fig. 32-8. Senile sebaceous hyperplasia. Several lesions seen here on the forehead are flesh-colored to yellow papules with a central punctum.

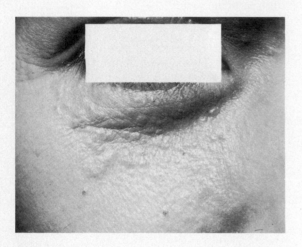

Fig. 32-9. Syringoma. Numerous small, flesh-colored papules are present on both the upper and lower eyelid and the cheek.

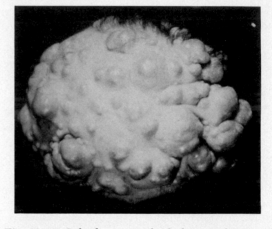

Fig. 32-10. Cylindroma. Multiple large, solitary and confluent nodules replacing most of the scalp are responsible for this lesion being known as a turban tumor.

As with multiple trichoepitheliomas and senile sebaceous hyperplasia, treatment is not indicated except for cosmetic reasons.

Dermal cylindroma

Cylindromas of the skin should not be confused with cylindromas or adenoid cystic carcinomas of salivary gland origin, since the biologic behavior of these entities is markedly different.

Dermal cylindroma is a benign tumor that differentiates in the direction of apocrine or eccrine structures (Lever and Schaumburg-Lever, 1983). Multiple cylindromas have an autosomal dominant mode of inheritance (Lever and Schaumburg-Lever, 1983). In these cases the tumors are most commonly on the scalp.

They may cover the scalp like a turban and then are referred to as turban tumors (Fig. 32-10). Individual lesions are round to oval, firm, pink to red nodules with smooth surfaces. The tumors begin to appear in early adulthood and gradually increase in size and number throughout life.

Individual lesions can easily be excised; however, removal of multiple lesions may require extensive skin grafting.

The association of multiple cylindromas and multiple trichoepitheliomas is well known (Gottschalk et al., 1974). Cases of multiple dermal cylindromas and salivary dermal analogue tumors have been reported by Batsakis and Brannon (1981), Headington et al. (1977), Luna et al. (1987), and Reingold et al. (1977).

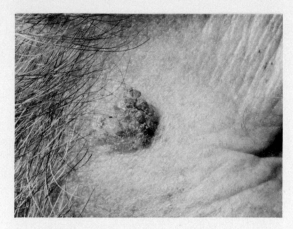

Fig. 32-11. Seborrheic keratosis. This lesion on the patient's temple is hyperpigmented, well circumscribed, and covered by a greasy scale.

MISCELLANEOUS TUMORLIKE CONDITIONS
Seborrheic keratosis

Seborrheic keratoses are benign epidermal tumors seen most commonly in older individuals. Although no specific etiologic factors have been identified, the growth and depth of pigmentation bear a direct relationship to sun exposure.

Features. Seborrheic keratoses are usually multiple and commonly occur on the face, as well as in other areas such as the scalp, proximal extremities, chest, back, and abdomen. Early lesions tend to be sharply defined, light brown to yellowish, flat lesions with a fine verrucous surface. With time they become thicker and appear to be stuck onto the skin surface. Fully developed lesions are usually covered by a greasy scale and are often deeply pigmented (Fig. 32-11). Seborrheic keratoses around the eyes may be pedunculated.

Sudden appearance and rapid increase in number and size of seborrheic keratoses have been noted in association with internal malignancy. This occurrence is known as the Leser-Trélat sign (Liddell et al., 1975).

Seborrheic keratoses can be effectively treated by curettage or freezing with liquid nitrogen.

Differential diagnosis. The differential diagnosis includes malignant melanoma, pigmented basal cell carcinoma, verruca, and skin tag.

Epidermal cysts

Epidermal cysts are also known by a number of other names including follicular cyst, epidermal inclusion cyst, and wen. Clinicians fre-

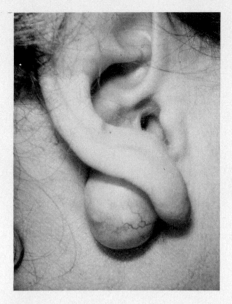

Fig. 32-12. Epidermal cyst. Although most often presenting as subcutaneous nodules, occasional cysts such as this one are superficial and very thinly-walled, so the yellowish white contents can be easily identified. (Courtesy R.J. Herten, MD, San Luis Obispo, Calif.)

quently and incorrectly refer to them as sebaceous cysts. As the name suggests, epidermal cysts are lined by keratinizing stratified squamous epithelium. Most of these lesions are thought to arise from occluded pilosebaceous follicles. The remainder probably arise from traumatically displaced epidermal cells. These lesions are tumors only in the sense that they produce a swelling or mass.

Features. Epidermal cysts occur most commonly on the face, scalp, neck, and back. They are slow-growing, elevated, round, firm dermal or subcutaneous nodules (Fig. 32-12). They vary in diameter from 0.2 to 5.0 cm and are asymptomatic unless they become secondarily infected, in which case they have a glossy red surface. Most patients have only one or a few epidermal cysts; however, in Gardner's syndrome, numerous epidermal cysts occur, especially on the face and scalp (Gardner, 1962).

Differential diagnosis. The differential diagnosis includes other cysts, lipomas, and subcutaneous nodular tumors.

TUMORS OF THE MELANOCYTIC SYSTEM
Melanocytic nevi

Melanocytic nevi are tumors composed of nevus cells. They include junctional, intrader-

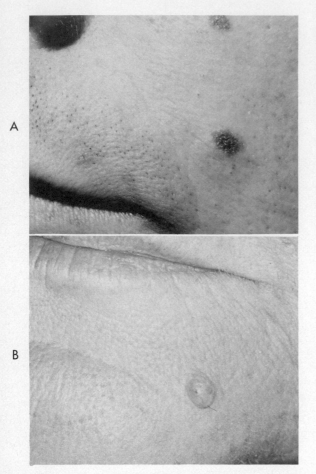

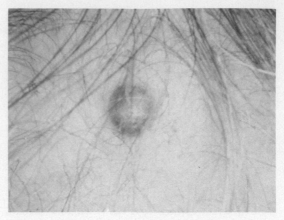

Fig. 32-14. Blue nevus. This lesion on the patient's forehead is dome shaped, well circumscribed, and blue brown. (Courtesy R.J. Herten, MD, San Luis Obispo, Calif.)

Fig. 32-13. Benign nevi. **A,** The upper lesion is a junctional nevus and is homogeneously brown, well demarcated, and flat. The lower lesion is a compound nevus and, because of nevus cells within the dermis, is slightly elevated and has a papillated surface. **B,** Intradermal nevus showing more elevation.

mal, compound, and dysplastic types. In junctional nevi the nevus cells are in the epidermis, in intradermal nevi they are in the dermis, and in compound nevi they are in both the epidermis and the dermis.

Features. Melanocytic nevi are rarely present at birth but begin to appear during the early years of life and reach their greatest incidence in young adults. In pregnancy, new nevi may appear and existing nevi may darken. The vast majority of nevi in young individuals are junctional and tend to be flat or slightly elevated (Fig. 32-13). In adults most nevi are of the intradermal type (Fig. 32-13) and tend to be polypoid, dome shaped, sessile, or papillomatous (Shaffer, 1955).

Nevi characteristically are small, exhibit an orderly array of color and a regularity of pat-

tern, and remain constant in appearance over the years.

Certain nevi have the capacity to transform into malignant melanoma. Although such an event is uncommon, the clinician should be familiar with the features that suggest such a transformation. These changes include ulceration, bleeding, enlargement and darkening, spread of pigment from the lesion into the surrounding skin, pigmented satellite lesions, unexplained inflammatory changes, and pain and itching.

Dysplastic nevi are distinctive lesions that usually are fairly large (greater than 5 mm in diameter), irregular in outline, and colored with a haphazard mixture of tan, brown, and black on a pink to red background. On microscopic examination they exhibit features of dysplasia. These nevi are frequently multiple and may involve the head and neck. However, they most commonly occur on the trunk and proximal extremities. Recognizing these distinctive nevi is important because they indicate an increased risk of malignant melanoma if there is a family history of this disease. (Dixon and Ackerman, 1985; Elder, 1985).

Differential diagnosis. The differential diagnosis includes freckles, lentigines, blue nevi, warts, skin tags, seborrheic keratoses, pigmented basal cell carcinomas, and melanomas.

Blue nevus

The blue nevus represents a localized proliferation of dermal melanocytes.

Features. Blue nevi are usually solitary and are common on the head and neck. Typically

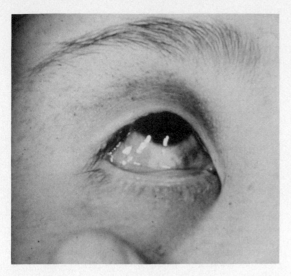

Fig. 32-15. Nevus of Ota. Not only is the periorbital skin blue because of the presence of deep pigment, but also the sclera is characteristically involved. (Courtesy G.W. Cole, MD, Long Beach, Calif.)

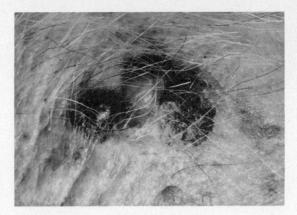

Fig. 32-16. Malignant melanoma. This lesion on the patient's forehead has an irregular border and surface. The color is typically variegated red, white, blue, and brown.

the lesion is a slightly elevated, dark blue-gray nodule with a regular outline and is less than 0.5 cm in diameter. The nodule is easily palpated, and the overlying epidermis is unaltered (Fig. 32-14).

Differential diagnosis. The differential diagnosis includes traumatic tattoo, pigmented basal cell carcinoma, and melanoma.

Nevus of Ota

Nevus of Ota represents a unilateral proliferation of dermal melanocytes in the distribution of the first and second branches of the trigeminal nerve. The lesion is most common in Japanese people, approximately 80% of affected individuals are female, and in about half of cases the lesions are present at birth.

Features. The lesions tend to be macular, to be brown, bluish, or slate to black, and to have ill-defined margins (Fig. 32-15). The ocular and oral mucosa, the auditory canal, and the tympanic membrane may be involved in addition to the skin (Caro and Bronstein, 1985).

Malignant melanoma

Cutaneous melanoma is a malignant tumor of the melanocytic cellular system. On the basis of gross and microscopic features, melanomas are classified into five major types: superficial spreading melanoma, nodular melanoma, lentigo maligna melanoma, acral lentiginous melanoma, and melanoma with an unclassifiable in-

traepidermal component. We discuss only the first three types.

Superficial spreading melanoma and lentigo maligna melanoma each have a biphasic growth pattern (Clark et al., 1976). The first phase is characterized by radial growth in which the malignant cells are confined to the epidermis or to the epidermis and papillary dermis. In this growth phase the lesions are enlarging pigmented macules that are either not palpable or only faintly palpable and have little or no tendency to metastasize. In the second phase, the vertical growth phase, the tumor cells deeply invade the dermis and the characteristic clinical lesion is a palpable nodule. There is a significant propensity for metastasis once the tumor has entered the vertical growth phase. This risk increases with increasing tumor thickness.

Nodular melanoma has a monophasic growth pattern. Its direction of growth is vertical from the beginning (Clark et al., 1976). This tumor occurs as a palpable mass or nodule.

Recently, clinical criteria have been developed that permit the early detection of most primary cutaneous melanomas by visual inspection with the unaided eye. Physicians, dentists, nurses, and even the patient can be taught to recognize early lesions. However, a small percentage of melanomas lack distinguishing features and can be diagnosed only by microscopic examination.

The signs of melanoma in a pigmented lesion as given by Sober et al. (1980) are as follows:

1. Variegated color. The colors that suggest malignancy in a pigmented lesion are

shades of red, white, and blue. Shades of blue are the most ominous. White, pink, and gray shades have been related to the ability of melanomas to undergo spontaneous regression. Reds and pinks reflect inflammation.

2. An irregular border, frequently with a notch or irregular identation. These features are especially common in the superficial spreading and lentigo maligna types of melanoma.
3. An increase in size or change in color.
4. Irregular elevations of the surface (Fig. 32-16). This feature is characteristic of many, but not all, melanomas.

When the preceding features are present, the diagnosis of melanoma can be made in the majority of cases. However, these features are occasionally present in other types of lesions such as pigmented basal cell carcinomas, seborrheic keratoses, compound melanocytic nevi, and some vascular lesions. Microscopic examination helps the clinician to differentiate among these entities. Excisional biopsy, if possible, is the method of choice for obtaining diagnostic material.

VASCULAR TUMORS

Hemangiomas are benign tumors composed of blood vessels. They may be classified as capillary or cavernous. Capillary hemangiomas may be further subdivided into juvenile (strawberry), senile (cherry), nevus flammeus, and pyogenic granuloma.

Juvenile hemangioma

Juvenile hemangiomas are the most common type of capillary hemangioma. The majority of these tumors occur on the head and neck and are noted shortly after birth. Characteristically they undergo a period of rapid growth and then begin to regress after about a year.

Features. The fully developed juvenile hemangioma is elevated, lobulated, sharply circumscribed, and bright red (Fig. 32-17). Most of these lesions require no treatment, since they have a marked tendency to regress (Bowers et al., 1960).

Senile hemangioma

Senile hemangiomas may start appearing in early adulthood, and the number of lesions increases with age. The lesions are bright red and vary in diameter from 1 mm to several millimeters. The larger lesions are soft and dome shaped.

Nevus flammeus

Nevus flammeus lesions, also known as port-wine stains, are present at birth, are unilateral, and are located on the face and neck.

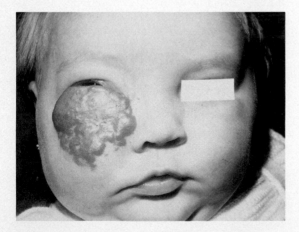

Fig. 32-17. Strawberry hemangioma (juvenile hemangioma). Because this large, red, spongy lesion interfered with the patient's vision, it was necessary to treat it with systemic corticosteroids.

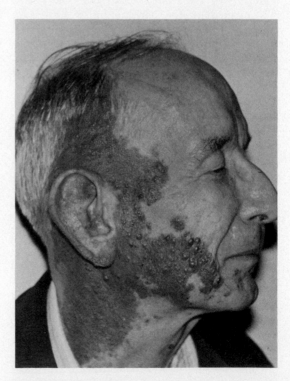

Fig. 32-18. Nevus flammeus. Extensive involvement of the upper portion of the right side of this patient's face was associated with an underlying vascular malformation of the brain consistent with Sturge-Weber syndrome.

Features. Port-wine stains are sharply circumscribed and range from small, red macules to large, red, flat patches that are blanched by pressure. The color ranges from pink to dark or bluish red. The surface is usually smooth; however, small nodular outgrowths may be present.

Nevus flammeus of the face, roughly in the distribution of the trigeminal nerve (Fig. 32-18), leptomeningeal nevus flammeus, cortical calcification of the brain in variable association with contralateral hemiplegia, eye involvement, and mental retardation constitute the Sturge-Weber syndrome (Bluefarb, 1949).

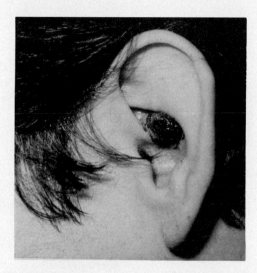

Fig. 32-19. Pyogenic granuloma. This lesion has a nonspecific presentation consisting of a well-circumscribed, blue-black hemorrhagic nodule. It is friable and bleeds easily.

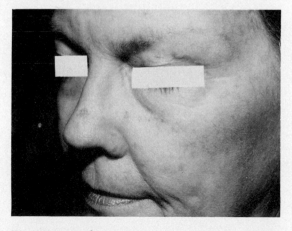

Fig. 32-20. Spider angioma. This patient has numerous typical dilated, tortuous capillaries with a radial configuration.

Pyogenic granuloma

Pyogenic granuloma is composed of lobules of proliferating capillary-sized blood vessels. Mills et al. (1980) suggested the name lobular capillary hemangioma for this lesion. On the skin, pyogenic granulomas commonly involve the hands, forearms, and face. They may occur at any age but are most often seen in children and are thought to be caused by minor trauma.

Features. Pyogenic granulomas typically begin as small red papules that rapidly enlarge to become pedunculated, raspberry-like nodules (Fig. 32-19). With the passage of time the nodules become ulcerated and crusted and may appear yellow, brown, or black. These lesions are usually friable, and minor trauma may cause considerable bleeding.

Differential diagnosis. The differential diagnosis of pyogenic granuloma includes hemangioma, amelanotic melanoma, and metastatic carcinoma.

Nevus araneus

Nevus araneus is commonly called spider angioma; it results from dilation and ramification of superficial arterioles and capillaries. Although it often arises spontaneously, pregnancy and cirrhosis of the liver are conditions predisposing to its appearance.

Features. Arterial spiders are found most frequently over the face, anterior neck, and upper anterior chest. The lesions are bright red and show a central, slightly elevated red spot from which blood vessels radiate (Fig. 32-20). These radiating vessels have been likened to the legs of a spider.

Kaposi's sarcoma

Kaposi's sarcoma is a malignant neoplasm composed of spindle cells and vascular elements. On the basis of epidemiologic and clinical data, the disease can be classified into classic, endemic, and epidemic types. The classic or sporadic type typically arises in older persons of Eastern European or Jewish origin, most commonly involves the skin of the lower extremities, and usually pursues an indolent course. Oral mucosal involvement is rare in this variant. The endemic type of Kaposi's sarcoma occurs in the native black population of equatorial Africa. Epidemic Kaposi's sarcoma occurs in persons with acquired immunodeficiency syndrome (AIDS) and other immunologic disorders. In these individuals the lesions are usually widely distributed over the skin. Moreover, the mucosa and lymph nodes are commonly involved, and response to treatment is poor. The histomorphologic features are similar in all types of the disease.

Features. Epidemic Kaposi's sarcoma is characterized by multifocal, widespread lesions at the onset of the disease. These lesions may involve the skin, oral mucosa, lymph nodes, and visceral organs, and new lesions appear throughout the course of the disease. In rare cases the patient has a single cutaneous lesion, often on the head or neck (Fig. 32-21). In the earliest, or patch, stage the lesions are small, flat, and macular and may be reddish, pink, purplish, or brown. These lesions may be so inconspicuous that they are easily overlooked. As they evolve, they enlarge and develop into papules or plaques (plaque stage). The plaque stage lesions may eventually enlarge and become nodules (nodular stage). The plaque and nodular stage lesions may be red, violet, pink, brown, or various combinations of these colors.

In approximately 26% of homosexual men with AIDS, Kaposi's sarcoma is present at the time of diagnosis or develops during the course of the disease. In contrast, Kaposi's sarcoma develops in only about 3% of heterosexual intravenous drug abusers with AIDS. The incidence of the disease is equally low in persons who have acquired AIDS by other means (Krigel and Friedman-Kien, 1988).

Differential diagnosis. The differential diagnosis of patch stage Kaposi's sarcoma includes hemangiomas, venous lakes, purpura, nevi, and melanomas. Plaque and nodular stage lesions may be confused clinically with AIDS-related angiomatosis (Axiotis et al., 1989), hemangiomas, pyogenic granulomas, nevi, melanomas, cutaneous lymphomas, and angiosarcomas.

Management. Patients with localized, epidemic Kaposi's sarcoma are treated with local modalities such as surgical excision, electrocautery, and curettage or radiation therapy. Patients with disseminated disease may be treated with immunomodulators and single-agent or combination chemotherapy (Krigel and Friedman-Kien, 1988).

Angiosarcoma

Angiosarcomas are malignant tumors that arise from the endothelial cells of blood vessels. They occur in various organs, including skin.

Features. Cutaneous angiosarcomas characteristically involve the scalp and face of elderly persons. They are bluish or violaceous plaques and nodules. These tumors have a marked tendency to spread locally, and according to Rosai et al. (1976), one third eventually give rise to

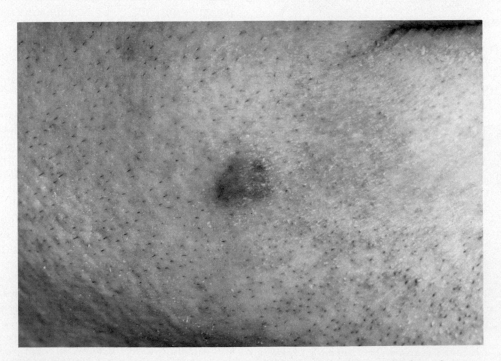

Fig. 32-21. Kaposi's sarcoma manifested as a reddish purple nodule on the face of a young homosexual man.

distant metastases, particularly to cervical lymph nodes. The prognosis is poor with or without treatment.

MISCELLANEOUS TUMORS

Tumors arising in the dermis or subcutaneous tissue of the face may be benign or malignant. Benign tumors are usually well circumscribed, grow slowly, and have been present for a long time when brought to medical attention. Usually these lesions cannot be differentiated accurately on the basis of clinical findings. However, when the tumors are spontaneously painful, traumatic neuromas, multiple leiomyomas, glomus tumors, and eccrine spiradenomas should be considered. Neurofibromas tend to be pedunculated and may be multiple. Vascular tumors, as previously described, usually have a characteristic color.

Malignant tumors in the dermis and subcutaneous tissue characteristically infiltrate and are bound to adjacent tissue. In addition, malignant tumors typically grow more rapidly than their benign counterparts. Recent rapid growth in a previously static tumor suggests malignant transformation.

CONNECTIVE TISSUE DISEASES
Discoid lupus erythematosus

Discoid lupus erythematosus is a relatively benign, chronic skin disease. It occurs in all races, has a worldwide distribution, is more common in women than in men, and is most often seen in patients in their thirties (Gilliam et al., 1985).

Features. Typical mature lesions /of discoid lupus consist of sharply outlined papules and plaques that in the early stages are erythema-

tous and edematous. As the plaques enlarge, the centers become atrophic and scarred while the edges remain red and edematous (Fig. 32-22). Telangiectasia is often present in the active margin of the lesions. With progression the plaques often exhibit thick scales and plugged follicles. The end-stage lesion is a white atrophic plaque that occasionally exhibits areas of hyperpigmentation.

The areas most commonly affected are the malar areas of the face, the nose, the scalp, and the external ears. The vermilion border of the lips and the oral mucosa may also be involved.

Differential diagnosis. The differential diagnosis includes chronic polymorphous light eruption, seborrheic dermatitis, psoriasis, superficial basal cell carcinoma, and systemic lupus erythematosus. Characteristic histologic and immunopathologic features are usually present in discoid lupus erythematosus (Lever and Schaumburg-Lever, 1983).

Management. The topical use of fluorinated steroids is usually effective in the treatment of discoid lupus. Other forms of therapy include intralesional injections of corticosteroids, orally administered antimalarials, and occasionally, systemically administered corticosteroids.

Systemic lupus erythematosus

Systemic lupus erythematosus is a multisystem disease of unknown cause characterized by multiple autoantibodies that participate in immunologically mediated tissue injury. The disease may be acute or insidious in its onset and runs a chronic remitting and relapsing course. The skin, joints, kidneys, and serosal membranes are characteristically involved. Adoles-

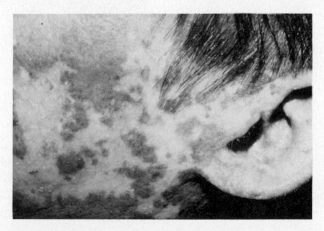

Fig. 32-22. Discoid lupus erythematosus. The lesion is well circumscribed, atrophic, and highlighted by fine follicular plugs and telangiectasias. Involvement of the earlobe is typical. (Courtesy Upjohn Co., Kalamazoo, Mich.)

cent girls and women in their twenties are predominantly affected.

Features. The most common clinical findings in patients with systemic lupus erythematosus are (1) constitutional symptoms such as fever, weight loss, and fatigue; (2) arthralgia or arthritis; (3) renal disease; (4) lymphadenopathy; (5) serositis involving the lungs and heart; (6) gastrointestinal symptoms such as anorexia, nausea, and vomiting; (7) psychoses, convulsive seizures, and peripheral neuropathy; and (8) skin changes (Gilliam et al., 1985). In this discussion we are concerned only with the cutaneous manifestations of the disease.

An erythematous rash is the most frequent cutaneous manifestation of systemic lupus erythematosus. This rash is characteristically present on both cheeks and across the bridge of the nose (Fig. 32-23). Not uncommonly the rash is the first manifestation of the disease, and it frequently occurs after sun exposure. In fact, the patient may mistake this erythematous blush for a sunburn.

The second most common cutaneous lesion seen in systemic lupus erythematosus is a maculopapular rash. Again, this rash frequently follows sun exposure. Facial lesions identical to those seen in discoid lupus erythematosus may occur in about 15% of patients with the systemic form of the disease (Estes and Christian, 1971). Periorbital edema occurs in some patients with an acute onset of lupus nephritis.

Criteria for the classification of systemic lupus erythematosus have been proposed by the American Rheumatism Association (Tan et al., 1982). Definitive diagnosis generally rests on a combination of characteristic clinical and immunologic features, especially antinuclear antibody and antinative DNA antibody tests.

Differential diagnosis. The differential diagnosis includes sunburn, rosacea, discoid lupus erythematosus, seborrheic dermatitis, dermatomyositis, and drug eruption.

Management. Systemic corticosteroid therapy is the treatment of choice for critically ill patients.

Dermatomyositis

Dermatomyositis is an inflammatory disease of the skin, the skeletal muscle, and occasionally the blood vessels. It may be acute, subacute, or chronic. The disease may occur at any age; however, the greatest incidence is in the forties and fifties. Women are affected twice as often as men.

Features. In the majority of cases the first symptoms are soreness and weakness of muscles. The muscle involvement is usually dif-

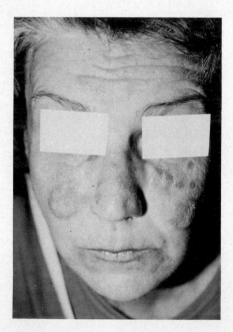

Fig. 32-23. Systemic lupus erythematosus. This patient exhibits a characteristic butterfly distribution of the eruption. Some of the plaques involving the cheek are similar to plaques of discoid lupus.

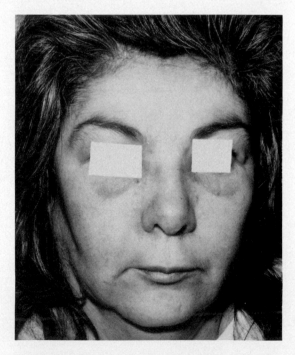

Fig. 32-24. Dermatomyositis. This patient has a heliotrope (violet) discoloration in a classic periorbital distribution.

fuse, bilateral, and symmetric and involves the pelvic and shoulder girdles and neck muscles.

Cutaneous involvement, which may precede or follow the muscle involvement, usually begins with erythema and swelling of the eyelids. The eyelids become pinkish and violet (heliotrope erythema) and may be tender to the touch (Fig. 32-24). Other areas of the skin may be involved; for example, periungual erythema with telangiectasia and violaceous, flat-topped papules on the dorsum of the interphalangeal joints are characteristic (Gilliam et al., 1985).

Dermatomyositis has been associated with internal malignancy in adult patients. However, the value of an extensive evaluation for malignancy is controversial (Callen, 1982).

Differential diagnosis. The differential diagnosis of the skin lesions includes systemic lupus erythematosus, erysipelas, and photosensitivity reactions. The diagnosis of dermatomyositis depends on the findings of elevated serum enzyme levels derived from muscle, excessive creatinuria, electromyographic evidence of muscle disease, and characteristic histologic changes.

Management. The systemic administration of corticosteroids is the major form of therapy.

Scleroderma

Scleroderma is a chronic disease that may occur in a localized form, morphea, or systemically. Systemic scleroderma is a progressive

and often fatal disorder characterized by involvement of the connective tissue of the skin and various internal organs.

In systemic scleroderma the initial complaints are usually related either to Raynaud's phenomenon (paroxysmal vasospasm in the fingers and hands and, less frequently, in the feet and nose) or to chronic, usually nonpitting edema of the hands and fingers. As the disease progresses, the trunk, the face, and eventually the lower extremities are involved. Diffuse involvement of the face results in a characteristic expressionless, pinched, masklike appearance (Fig. 32-25). The patient cannot wrinkle the skin of the face, and radial furrows may be present around the mouth. In this late stage, opening of the mouth is restricted. Characteristic changes also seen on the face are telangiectasias, either alone or in small matlike configurations (Gilliam et al., (1985). Involvement of the fingers may result in tapering with shiny hidebound skin (sclerodactyly). Recurrent, painful ulcerations of the knuckles and fingertips are common. Generalized hyperpigmentation resembling Addison's disease may occur.

Differential diagnosis. The clinical and microscopic features of advanced scleroderma are characteristic.

Management. No specific therapy is curative; however, corticosteroids, cytotoxic agents, and penicillamine have all been used with variable success.

PAPULOSQUAMOUS DERMATITIDES
Psoriasis

Psoriasis is a common chronic, recurrent, scaly, erythematous disease of the skin. It occurs equally in males and females, and all age-groups are affected, although the onset of the disease is less common in the very young and in the elderly.

Features. Typical lesions of psoriasis are bright red patches with sharp, well-defined borders and silvery white scales (Fig. 32-26). The sharp border reflects epidermal hyperplasia, the bright red color is caused by dilated superficial vessels in the papillary dermis, and the silvery white scale results from dramatically shortened epidermal turnover time (Weinstein and Van Scott, 1965) with its attendant incomplete keratinization. The dilated capillaries in the apices of the elongated dermal papillae are so close to the surface that removal of the scale frequently produces fine bleeding points (Auspitz sign).

One of the special features of psoriasis is the capacity to reproduce skin lesions at sites of lo-

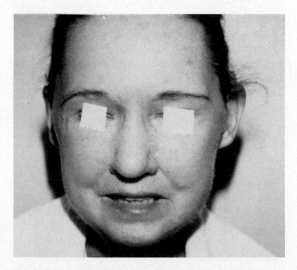

Fig. 32-25. Scleroderma. This patient exhibits a typical sclerodermoid facies with tense, bound-down, shiny skin, which accounts for the loss of the lines of expression. In addition, there are numerous matted telangiectasias, particularly over the central third of the face including the lips.

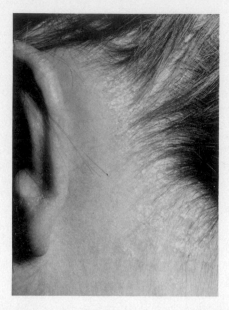

Fig. 32-26. Psoriasis. This patient has a well-circumscribed plaque with micaceous scales involving the scalp and nape of the neck.

cal injury. This is known as the Koebner or isomorphic phenomenon. This phenomenon also occurs in other skin diseases, including lichen planus and Darier's disease.

The most frequently affected areas are the elbows, knees, scalp, and lumbosacral skin. Pitting or punctate dimpling of the nail plate is seen in at least 30% of cases (Ramsay and Hurley, 1985). The prevalence of arthritis is increased in patients with psoriasis (Leczinsky, 1948).

Differential diagnosis. The differential diagnosis includes seborrheic dermatitis and atopic eczema.

Management. Treatment of psoriasis consists of topical corticosteroids, tars, keratolytics, ultraviolet light, and in severe cases, methotrexate.

Seborrheic dermatitis

Seborrheic dermatitis is a chronic inflammatory condition of the skin that cannot be cured; however, remissions of varying duration do occur.

Features. Seborrheic dermatitis is frequently associated with an oily skin and has a predilection for the scalp, eyebrows, eyelids, nasolabial crease, lips, ears, sternal area, axillae, submammary folds, umbilicus, groin, and gluteal crease. The characteristic appearance is dry, moist, or greasy scales and pinkish yellow patches of various sizes and shapes. The margins of the patches are indistinct. Mild involve-

ment of the scalp is commonly known as dandruff. Chronic worry and loss of sleep frequently appear to aggravate this condition.

Seborrheic dermatitis is seen in association with certain other skin diseases, for example, severe acne and psoriasis. It is also seen with certain general diseases such as Parkinson's disease and endocrine states with obesity (Soloman, 1985) and AIDS.

Topical corticosteroids are effective in the treatment of seborrheic dermatitis.

CUTANEOUS REACTIONS TO ACTINIC RADIATION

Exposure to actinic radiation is known to have a number of harmful effects in the skin. These include the sunburn reaction, photoaging, and carcinogenesis. Adverse cutaneous reactions may also occur after simultaneous exposure to chemicals and actinic radiation. These reactions are known as phototoxic and photoallergic reactions.

Phototoxic reactions

A phototoxic reaction is a nonimmunologic reaction that develops within a few hours after the skin has been exposed to a photosensitizing agent and light of proper wavelength and intensity. This reaction usually occurs with the first exposure to the agent (Epstein, 1983).

Features. The most common clinical finding is a sunburned appearance that is followed by hyperpigmentation. One well-known example of phototoxic dermatitis is berlock (berloque, perfume) dermatitis. In women it is seen in areas where perfume is applied, such as the sides of the neck and behind the ears. In men this type of dermatitis is most common on the bearded area where after-shave lotion is applied. Perfumes and after-shave lotions containing furocoumarin, bergamot oil, or related substances are chiefly responsible for this reaction. Other photosensitizing substances include coal tar and its derivatives, which may be found in cosmetics, dyes, insecticides, and disinfectants, and plants containing furocoumarins.

Most systemic photosensitizers tend to produce phototoxic reactions. Frequent offenders are tetracyclines, sulfonamides, chlorothiazides, sulfonylureas, phenothiazines, griseofulvin, and halogenated salicylanilides (Domonkos et al., 1982).

Photoallergic dermatitis

The majority of cases of photoallergy develop after contact with photosensitizing chemicals. Such a reaction is known as a photoallergic

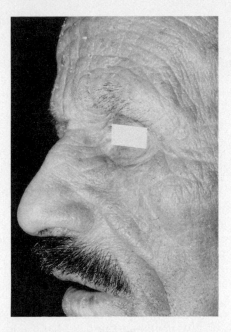

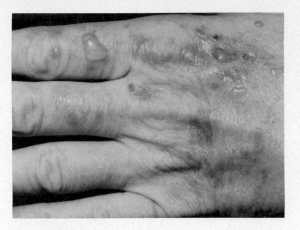

Fig. 32-28. Porphyria cutanea tarda. The backs of this patient's hands are covered by numerous tense, noninflammatory vesicles, one of which is hemorrhagic. The skin is also thin, friable, and irregularly pigmented.

Fig. 32-27. Chronic photoallergic eruption (persistent light reactor). This patient exhibits extensive erythematous, confluent plaques characterized by thickening of the skin and accentuation of skin lines (that is, lichenification). Periorbital sparing is evident. This is an area that is, in part, protected from the sun.

contact dermatitis. These reactions occur only in sensitized persons and are out of proportion to the amount of exposure received. The most common etiologic chemicals are found in bar soaps and cosmetics (Willis, 1974). The initial signs and symptoms are oozing, weeping, and crusting of the affected areas along with intense pruritus. The reaction begins 24 to 48 hours after combined chemical and light exposure. A small number of patients with photoallergic contact dermatitis continue to experience photosensitivity in the apparent absence of continuing exposure to the offending chemical or to a cross-reacting chemical. Such individuals are known as persistent light reactors. They exhibit erythematous, confluent, thickened plaques (Fig. 32-27).

Management. Treatment of photoallergic dermatitis consists of the identification and elimination of the photosensitizing chemical or chemicals. In addition, broad-spectrum sunscreens and antimalarials may be of value.

Porphyria cutanea tarda

Photosensitivity may be of endogenous origin. Examples of this phenomenon are the porphyrias (except for acute intermittent porphyria), in which photosensitivity is caused by the presence of circulating porphyrin molecules (Epstein, 1983). The most common porphyria with cutaneous manifestations is porphyria cutanea tarda.

Features. Individuals with porphyria cutanea tarda are usually over 40 years of age and often drink excessive amounts of alcohol. Cutaneous lesions include bullae and erosions on sun-exposed parts and hyperpigmentation on the face, neck, and hands (Fig. 32-28). Hypertrichosis of the face, especially over the cheekbones, may be seen. In addition, changes in hair color, frequently from red to black, may occur.

The diagnosis is made by demonstrating greatly elevated urinary uroporphyrin excretion. Treatment includes phlebotomy and abstinence from alcohol.

DRUG ERUPTIONS (DERMATITIS MEDICAMENTOSA)

Drug eruptions are unintended reactions that occur after administration of diagnostic or therapeutic agents. Almost any drug administered systemically is capable of causing a dermatitis.

Features. Drug eruptions are often marked by a sudden onset, wide and symmetric dissemination, and pruritus. These eruptions may simulate a wide variety of cutaneous diseases (VanArsdel, 1982). The lesions may be maculopapular, erythematous, vesiculobullous, urticarial, and purpuric or pustular and may be accompanied by constitutional signs and symptoms. Fixed drug eruptions occur persistently at the same site each time the drug is given.

They are often bullous and eczematous initially and later are hyperpigmented.

When trying to elicit a drug history from a patient, the clinician should remember that the patient may be unaware of exposure. For example, the offending agent may be used as a preservative or flavoring agent in food or may be an antibiotic present in milk or meat. Moreover, the patient may forget to say that he or she is taking vitamins or laxatives, either of which may be responsible for the eruption.

Contact dermatitis (dermatitis venenata)

Contact dermatitis can be divided into two types: irritant contact dermatitis, which is caused by a nonallergic reaction, usually from exposure to an irritating substance, and allergic contact dermatitis, which is an acquired immunologic response to a substance that has come in contact with the skin.

Features. Most allergic contact reactions and many irritant contact reactions are of the eczematous type; that is, the primary lesions exhibit any of the stages from erythema and swelling to oozing or vesiculation or both (Fig. 32-29). The secondary lesions exhibit crusting, excoriation, lichenification, and hyperpigmentation.

Certain substances commonly affect certain skin areas. Substances that commonly affect the face and neck are cosmetics, soaps, perfumes, hair sprays, fingernail polish (eyelids), hatbands (forehead), nickel (earlobes), and industrial oil. As might be expected, lesions of contact dermatitis begin in areas of contact, and the shape of the lesions reflects the localization of exposure.

Differential diagnosis. The differential diagnosis includes seborrheic dermatitis, nummular dermatitis, lichen simplex chronicus, and other types of inflammatory lesions.

Management. Therapy for drug eruptions consists of eliminating the offending agent and providing symptomatic and supportive measures.

ACNE AND ACNEIFORM DERMATOSES
Acne vulgaris

Acne vulgaris is a chronic inflammatory disorder of pilosebaceous structures and is seen primarily in the adolescent age-group. The disorder of acne vulgaris is characterized by comedones, papules, pustules, nodules, and cysts, and it tends to occur in areas of the skin where sebaceous glands are well developed (Fig. 32-30), including the face, back, and upper arms.

Acneiform eruptions may be produced by various drugs. The best-known examples are the corticosteroid hormones and the simple salts of iodine and bromine. Many oils, waxes, and chlorinated hydrocarbons produce acneiform eruptions when they come in contact with the skin. This type of acne is known as occupational acne.

Management. Treatment of acne includes topical anticomedogenic agents and antibiotics, either topical or systemic.

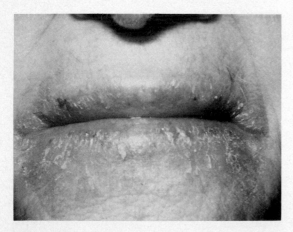

Fig. 32-29. Contact dermatitis. The extensive erythema, fissuring, and crusting involving both lips was caused by neomycin present in a cream that was used for chapped lips. (Courtesy R.J. Herten, MD, San Luis Obispo, Calif.)

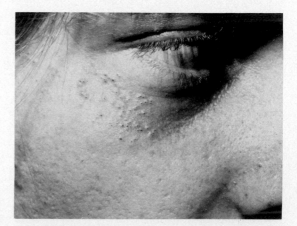

Fig. 32-30. Comedonal acne. The bulk of this patient's lesions are small blackheads. There are a few inflammatory papules and pustules.

Rosacea

Rosacea is a chronic acneiform disorder of the flush area of the face and especially the nose. The condition is seen most commonly in women between the ages of 20 and 60 years.

Features. In the mildest form of the disease, there is slight erythema of the nose and cheeks. As the disease progresses, the lesions become red or purplish red with edema, papules, pustules, and telangiectasia (Tolman, 1985). Treatment consists of oral tetracycline, nonfluorinated, low-potency, topical steroids, and avoidance of factors that cause flushing. Fluorinated steroids may exacerbate the condition or even cause periorificial dermatitis.

Differential diagnosis. The differential diagnosis includes lupus erythematosus, bromoderma, and iododerma.

Rhinophyma

Rhinophyma is a condition characterized by overgrowth of sebaceous glands and connective tissue of the distal half of the nose. This condition is seen almost exclusively in men over 40 years of age (Domonkos et al., 1982).

Features. The tip and wings of the nose are involved by large, lobulated, hyperemic masses that may become pendulous.

Perioral dermatitis

Perioral dermatitis is a distinctive dermatitis confined symmetrically around the mouth with a clear zone between the vermilion border and the affected skin. It is seen primarily in young women and occasionally in men (Epstein, 1972).

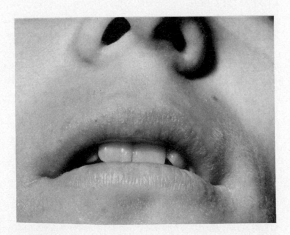

Fig. 32-31. Perioral dermatitis. Very subtle, slightly erythematous papules surround the patient's mouth. There is a thin zone of uninvolved skin most noticeable along the lower lip.

Features. The primary lesion is a pinhead-sized papule or papulovesicle, either flesh colored or red (Fig. 32-31). Eventually the papules are replaced by a more diffuse redness capped by a dry, fissured, yellow-red scale. An uncomfortable burning sensation may be present.

The cause of perioral dermatitis is unknown, but sensitivity to sunlight, atopy, rosacea, demodicidosis, candidiasis, the prolonged use of fluorinated corticosteroid creams, and fluoride dentrifrices have all been blamed.

Differential diagnosis. The differential diagnosis includes acne vulgaris, seborrheic dermatitis, and contact dermatitis. The symmetric distribution around the mouth and the clear zone around the lips help differentiate perioral dermatitis from other entities.

Management. Treatment consists of systemically administered tetracycline along with elimination of the etiologic agent, for example, fluorinated corticosteroids.

DERMATOLOGIC INFECTIONS
Bacterial infections

Bacterial infections of the skin may be either primary or secondary. Primary infections arise on normal skin, are initially caused by a single organism, and tend to have a characteristic appearance. Secondary infections occur on diseased skin. This discussion is limited to selected primary infections in which involvement of facial skin is a prominent feature.

IMPETIGO

Impetigo is a highly communicable infection caused most commonly by group A streptococci. The disease occurs mostly in preschool-age children during the late summer and early fall. Poor hygiene, crowding, and minor trauma contribute to the spread of the infection. In the absence of complications the general health of affected individuals is excellent.

Features. The disease begins with small reddish macules that soon develop into vesicles or bullae. The lesions are very superficial (subcorneal) in location and consequently have thin roofs that rupture easily, discharging a thin, straw-colored seropurulent exudate. This exudate then dries to form a crust, which may become quite thick and has a "stuck-on" appearance. These golden yellow crusts are the hallmark of impetigo (Fig. 32-32).

Individual lesions rarely exceed 1 to 2 cm in diameter. The face, especially around the mouth and nose, is the usual location; however, the lesions may occur anywhere (Dillon,

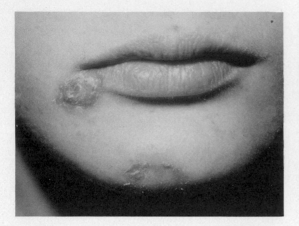

Fig. 32-32. Impetigo contagiosa. Both lesions are characterized by a honey-colored crust with some surrounding erythema.

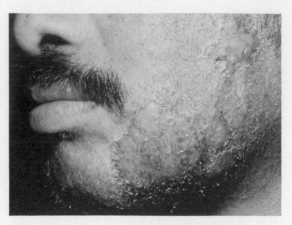

Fig. 32-33. Sycosis barbae. This patient has extensive weeping, crusted, purulent erythematous lesions involving the entire bearded area.

1968). If untreated, the disease may last for many weeks. Glomerulonephritis is an uncommon, but feared, complication of impetigo.

Differential diagnosis. The differential diagnosis includes contact dermatitis caused by poison ivy, tinea infections, and herpes simplex infections. The thick yellow crusts with loose edges should differentiate impetigo from tinea infections and herpes simplex infections. Linear lesions are not characteristic of impetigo but are clearly seen in contact dermatitis resulting from poison ivy. Moreover, impetigo vesicles are more crusted and pustular.

Management. Treatment includes scrupulous cleansing of the area along with antibiotic therapy.

SYCOSIS BARBAE

Sycosis barbae or barber's itch is a deep folliculitis of the beard, usually bacterial.

Features. The primary lesion in sycosis barbae is a follicular pustule. Initially, there is erythema and a burning or itchy sensation. Lesions commonly appear first on the upper lip near the nose. The pustules rupture after washing or shaving, leaving an erythematous area that is later the site of a new crop of pustules (Fig. 32-33). In this way the infection gradually spreads. The hairs of the involved follicles are usually not retarded in their growth and usually do not fall out; however, they may be readily epilated (Maibach et al., 1985).

Differential diagnosis. The differential diagnosis includes contact dermatitis, tinea of the beard, and ingrown hairs (pseudofolliculitis barbae). In contact dermatitis the involved areas are vesicular and crusted, and there are no follicular pustules. Tinea barbae is a slowly

spreading, often annular superficial fungus infection with broken off hairs, and a deeper, nodular type of inflammation may be present. Moreover, tinea barbae rarely affects the upper lip. Pseudofolliculitis barbae manifests 1 to 3 mm papules at sites of ingrowing hairs in black men. The anterior neckline and chin are the areas commonly affected. Bacterial and fungal culture studies should be performed and are helpful in differential diagnosis. Most cases of sycosis barbae are caused by *Staphylococcus aureus*.

Management. Treatment consists of systemic and locally applied antibiotics. In addition, shaving should be light and infrequent, and a new razor blade should be used each day. Infected hairs should be manually epilated daily.

ERYSIPELAS

Erysipelas is an uncommon type of superficial cellulitis caused most commonly by group A streptococci (Schwartz and Weinberg, 1987). A preexisting skin wound or pyoderma can frequently be found and is a predisposing condition. The upper respiratory tract is commonly the source of the organism.

Features. The basic lesion of erysipelas is a red, warm, raised, sharply circumscribed plaque that enlarges peripherally. Vesicles and bullae may form on the surface of the plaque. The process evolves rapidly, with constitutional signs and symptoms that include malaise, chills and fever, headache, vomiting, and joint pains. This disease most commonly involves the face, scalp, and area around the ear, but no area is exempt (Maibach et al., 1985). When the face is involved, the process may extend into the orbit and can be life threatening.

Untreated cases last for 2 to 3 weeks, but response is rapid with antibiotic treatment. Recurrences are common and tend to be in the same location.

Differential diagnosis. Erysipelas may be confused with contact dermatitis and with angioneurotic edema, but fever is absent in these latter conditions. A butterfly pattern on the face may suggest lupus erythematosus, and ear involvement may suggest polychondritis; in addition, herpes zoster may mimic erysipelas.

Viral infections
HERPES ZOSTER

Herpes zoster (shingles) and varicella (chicken pox) are caused by the same virus. Varicella is regarded as the primary manifestation of varicella-zoster virus exposure. The virus is then thought to lie dormant in dorsal root ganglia to later recur as zoster.

Features. Herpes zoster is characterized by groups of vesicles or crusted lesions on an erythematous and edematous base situated unilaterally along the distribution of a spinal or cranial nerve (Fig. 32-34). The cranial nerves most frequently involved are the fifth and seventh. The lesions appear 1 to 7 days after onset of pain and hyperesthesia. New crops of vesicles can appear for 3 to 5 days and then dry up and form crusts that take about 3 weeks to disappear. Severe lancinating pain is common but not invariable. Severe postherpetic neuralgia may occur, especially in older patients.

An increased incidence of herpes zoster in patients with lymphoma and leukemia has been recognized for many years. However,

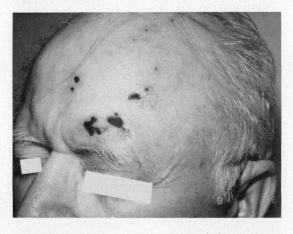

Fig. 32-34. Herpes zoster. Several hemorrhagic crusts with a few small, intact vesicles are present in the skin along the distribution of the ophthalmic branch of the trigeminal nerve. (Courtesy J.A. Klein, MD, Long Beach, Calif.)

Ragozzino et al. (1982) have shown that patients with herpes zoster are not at increased risk for the subsequent development of cancer. Their findings suggest that there is no need to search for an occult cancer or to increase surveillance for cancer after the diagnosis of herpes zoster is made.

Differential diagnosis. The unilateral distribution of painful, grouped vesicles in a dermatomal pattern is typical of herpes zoster.

At present, antiviral therapy for acute herpes zoster in the immunologically normal host is the subject of investigation (Hirsch and Schooley, 1983; Dolin, 1985).

A simple and reliable way of confirming the diagnosis is to demonstrate giant cells with multiple nuclei and acidophilic intranuclear inclusions in Giemsa- or Wright-stained cytologic smears of scrapings from the base of a vesicle (Barr et al., 1977).

VIRAL WARTS

Human papillomaviruses can cause a variety of lesions, including verruca vulgaris (common wart), verruca plana (flat wart), verruca plantaris (plantar wart), and condyloma acuminatum (venereal wart).

Features. Up until the last 15 years, all warts were thought to be caused by the same human papillomavirus, a DNA virus. However, studies have shown that different subtypes of virus are associated with different clinical lesions (Lutzner, 1983). For example, common warts are associated with types 2 or 4, flat warts with type 3, plantar warts with type 1, and venereal warts with type 6. Predisposition to the development of extensive wart disease may reflect a select inherited immunodeficiency or acquired immunodeficiency such as accompanies immunosuppressive drug therapy.

Verruca vulgaris is manifested as one or more irregularly shaped, vegetative, hyperkeratotic, tan to brown papillomas that can occur anywhere but have a predilection for the hands. A variant that occurs on the face is the filiform wart, which is characterized by longer, thinner projections as the name implies. Flat warts are most common in children and frequently occur in large numbers on the face. They are flat, flesh-colored to tan, finely papillated papules, 0.2 to 0.5 cm in diameter (Fig. 32-35). Plantar warts are located on the soles, particularly the ball of the foot. They are usually endophytic and painful. Multiple plantar warts are referred to as mosaic warts. Condyloma acuminatum occurs on the genitalia but has also been reported perianally, on the oral

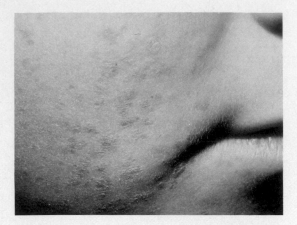

Fig. 32-35. Flat warts. Numerous individual and confluent, flesh-colored to slightly tan, flat-topped papules are typical.

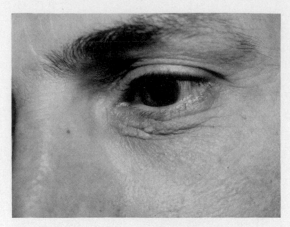

Fig. 32-36. Xanthelasma. Yellow plaques are present on the patient's lower eyelids.

mucosa, and even on the laryngeal mucosa. They are elevated, keratotic, mulberry-like growths. All warts, but particularly veruccae vulgares, may spread to traumatized skin. This is the Koebner phenomenon previously discussed in the section on psoriasis. Although a rare event, malignant transformation can occur in some warts (Lynch, 1982).

Differential diagnosis. Usually the diagnosis is straightforward. Seborrheic keratosis or epithelial nevus may be confused with verruca vulgaris. Biopsy is helpful because veruccae display cytopathic changes of human papillomavirus infection such as vacuolation, hypergranulosis, and even occasional intranuclear inclusions. Flat warts should be distinguished from multiple syringomas or trichoepitheliomas, condylomata acuminata from condylomata lata (syphilitic warts), and plantar warts from callosities or clavi (corns). Paring down a plantar wart with a scalpel blade usually demonstrates punctate hemorrhage or punctate thrombi associated with multiple superficial capillaries. These are not present in callosities or clavi.

Management. Treatment of warts varies, and numerous remedies have been described. Verrucae vulgares frequently respond to liquid nitrogen freezing or keratolytic agents, which usually contain salicylic acid and lactic acid. If possible, facial warts in children should not be treated, since like most warts they spontaneously resolve without scarring in 6 months to 2 years. If treatment is necessary, light liquid nitrogen freezing to a few lesions or the use of topical antiacne medication such as 2.5% to 5% benzoyl peroxide can be effective. Podophyllin is the treatment of choice for venereal warts,

and plantar warts may be treated with salicylic acid plasters, liquid nitrogen freezing, or in selected cases, superficial x-ray therapy.

MISCELLANEOUS CONDITIONS
Xanthelasma

Xanthomas are tumors characterized by collections of lipid-laden macrophages. In many cases these tumors occur in association with acquired or familial disorders leading to hyperlipidemia. Xanthelasma is the most common type of xanthoma.

Features. Xanthelasmas occur mainly on the upper eyelids but may also involve the lower eyelids (Fig. 32-36), especially in the inner canthus area. The lesions are soft, chamois to light yellow-gray, oblong plaques. They vary from 0.2 to 3.0 cm in length. The lesions are seen in adults and rarely in children and adolescents.

Individuals with xanthelasmas should have a workup for the presence of hyperlipidemia, since such an association is frequently present. Pedace and Winkelmann (1965) found hypercholesterolemia in 33% of men and 40% of women with these tumors.

Management. Treatment of individual lesions is probably best accomplished by surgical excision.

Amyloidosis

Primary amyloidosis is associated with cutaneous lesions in about 30% of cases (Rubinow and Cohen, 1978).

Features. Amyloid infiltrates of the skin in primary amyloidosis are characteristically asymptomatic, translucent, waxy, amber papules that have the appearance of translucent

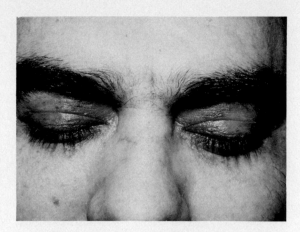

Fig. 32-37. Primary systemic amyloidosis. This patient exhibits typical periorbital hemorrhage secondary to rupture of blood vessels infiltrated by amyloid. A few small, infiltrative papules can be seen along the free margin of the upper eyelids.

vesicles. These papules coalesce to form plaques of various sizes. Amyloid deposition in blood vessels results in purpuric lesions and ecchymoses. The hemorrhagic lesions, as well as the papules and plaques, involve the periorbital areas (Fig. 32-37), the sides of the nose, and the regions around the mouth. In addition, these patients may have oral lesions (Schwartz and Olson, 1975).

Localized amyloidosis may occur in the skin. Amyloid also is occasionally deposited in the stroma of certain epithelial tumors. Cutaneous amyloid deposits are not seen in secondary amyloidosis.

The diagnosis of amyloidosis is established by demonstration of the characteristic emerald-green birefringence of tissue specimens stained with Congo red and examined by polarization microscopy.

Management. There is no specific therapy for primary amyloidosis.

REFERENCES

Axiotis CA et al: AIDS-related angiomatosis, Am J Dermatopathol 11:177-181, 1989.

Baer RL and Kopf A: Keratoacanthoma. In Yearbook of dermatology, Chicago, 1962-63 Series, Year Book Medical Publishers, Inc.

Barr RJ, Herten RJ, and Graham JH: Rapid method for Tzanck preparations, JAMA 237:1119-1120, 1977.

Batsakis JG and Brannon RB: Dermal analogue tumors of major salivary glands, J Laryngol Otol 95:155-164, 1981.

Bluefarb SM: Sturge-Weber syndrome, Arch Dermatol Syph 59:531-541, 1949.

Bowers RE, Graham EA, and Tomlinson KA: The natural history of the strawberry nevus, Arch Dermatol 82:667-680, 1960.

Callen, JP: The value of malignancy evaluation in patients with dermatomyositis, J Am Acad Dermatol 6:253-259, 1982.

Caro WA and Bronstein BR: Tumors of the skin. In Moschella SL and Hurley HJ editors: Dermatology, vol 2, Philadelphia, 1985, WB Saunders Co.

Clark WH Jr et al: The developmental biology of primary human malignant melanoma, Semin Oncol 2:83-103, 1976.

Dillon HC Jr: Impetigo contagiosa, Am J Dis Child 115:530-541, 1968.

Dixon SL and Ackerman AB: Some observations, reflections and questions about dysplastic nevi, Am J Dermatopathol 7(suppl):A18-A25, 1985.

Domonkos AN, Arnold HL Jr, and Odom RB: Andrews' diseases of the skin: clinical dermatology, Philadelphia, 1982, WB Saunders Co.

Dolin R: Antiviral chemotherapy and chemoprophylaxis, Science 227:1296-1303, 1985.

Elder DE: An exchange of ideas about dysplastic nevi and malignant melanomas, Am J Dermatopathol 7(suppl):102-105, 1985.

Epstein JH: Phototoxicity and photoallergy in man, J Am Acad Dermatol 8:141-147, 1983.

Epstein S: Perioral dermatitis, Cutis 10:317-321, 1972.

Estes D and Christian CL: The natural history of systemic lupus erythematosus by prospective analysis, Medicine 50:85-95, 1971.

Gardner EJ: Follow-up study of a family group exhibiting dominant inheritance for a syndrome including intestinal polyposis, osteomas, fibromas, and epidermal cysts, Am J Hum Genet 14:376-390, 1962.

Gilliam JN, Cohen SB, Sontheimer RD, and Moschella SL: Connective tissue diseases. In Moschella SL and Hurley HJ, editors: Dermatology, vol 2, Philadelphia, 1985, WB Saunders Co.

Gottschalk HR, Graham JH, and Aston EE: Dermal eccrine cylindroma, epithelioma adenoides cysticum of Brooke, and eccrine spiradenoma, Arch Dermatol 110:473-474, 1974.

Graham JH and Helwig EB: Premalignant cutaneous and mucocutaneous diseases. In Graham JH, Johnson WC, and Helwig EB, editors: Dermal pathology, New York, 1972, Harper & Row, Publishers, Inc.

Gray HR and Helwig EB: Epithelioma adenoides cysticum and solitary trichoepithelioma, Arch Dermatol 87:102-114, 1963.

Hashimoto K, Gross BG, and Lever WF: Syringoma: histochemical and electron microscopic studies, J Invest Dermatol 46:150-166, 1966.

Headington JT et al: Membranous basal cell adenoma of parotid gland, dermal cylindromas and trichoepitheliomas, Cancer 39:2460-2469, 1977.

Hirsch MS and Schooley RT: Treatment of herpesvirus infections, N Engl J Med 309:963-970, 1983.

Kersting DW and Helwig EB: Eccrine spiradenoma, Arch Dermatol 73:199-227, 1966.

Krigel RL and Friedman-Kien AE: Kaposi's sarcoma in AIDS: diagnosis and treatment. In DeVita VT, Hellmann S, and Rosenberg SA, editors: AIDS: etiology, diagnosis and treatment, Philadelphia, 1988, JB Lippincott Co.

Leczinsky CD: The incidence of arthropathy in a ten year series of psoriasis cases, Acta Dermatol Venereol 82:483-487, 1948.

Lever WF and Schaumburg-Lever G: Histopathology of the skin, Philadelphia, 1983, JB Lippincott Co.

Liddell K, White JE, and Caldwell JW: Seborrheic keratosis and carcinoma of the large bowel: three cases exhibiting the sign of Leser-Trelat, Br J Dermatol 92:449-452, 1975.

Luna MA, Tortoledo ME, and Allen M: Salivary dermal analogue tumors arising in lymph nodes, Cancer 59:1165-1169, 1987.

Lutzner MA: The human papillomaviruses: a review, Arch Dermatol 119:631-635, 1983.

Lynch PJ: Warts and cancer: the oncogenic potential of human papillomavirus, Am J Dermatopathol 4:55-60, 1982.

Maibach HI, Aly R, and Noble W: Bacterial infections of the skin. In Moschella SL and Hurley HJ, editors: Dermatology, vol 1, Philadelphia, 1985, WB Saunders Co.

Mikhail GR et al: Metastatic basal cell carcinoma, Arch Dermatol 113:1261-1269, 1977.

Mills SE, Cooper PH, and Fechner RE: Lobular capillary hemangioma: the underlying lesion of pyogenic granuloma; a study of 73 cases from the oral and nasal mucous membranes, Am J Surg Pathol 4:471-479, 1980.

Milstone EB and Helwig EB: Basal cell carcinoma in children, Arch Dermatol 108:523-527, 1973.

Pedace FJ and Winkelmann RK: Xanthelasma palpebrarum, JAMA 193:893-894, 1965.

Ragozzino MW et al: Risk of cancer after herpes zoster: a population based study, N Engl J Med 307:393-397, 1982.

Ramsay DL and Hurley HJ: Papulosquamous eruptions and exfoliative dermatitis. In Moschella SL and Hurley HJ, editors: Dermatology, vol 1, Philadelphia, 1985, WB Saunders Co.

Reingold IM, Keasbey LE, and Graham JH: Multicentric dermal-type cylindromas of the parotids in a patient with florid turban tumors, Cancer 40:1702-1710, 1977.

Rosai J et al: Angiosarcoma of the skin: a clinicopathologic and fine structural study, Hum Pathol 7:83-109, 1976.

Rubinow A and Cohen AS: Skin involvement in generalized amyloidosis, Ann Intern Med 88:781-785, 1978.

Schwartz HC and Olson DJ: Amyloidosis: a rational approach to diagnosis by intraoral biopsy, Oral Surg 39:837-843, 1975.

Schwartz MN and Weinberg AN: Infections due to gram-positive bacteria. In Fitzpatrick TB et al, editors: Dermatology in general medicine, vol 2, New York, 1987, McGraw-Hill, Inc.

Shaffer B: Pigmented nevi, Arch Dermatol 72:120-132, 1955.

Sober AJ, Fitzpatrick TB, and Mihm M: Primary melanoma of the skin: recognition and management, J Am Acad Dermatol 2:179-197, 1980.

Soloman LM: Eczema. In Moschella SL and Hurley HJ, editors: Dermatology, vol 1, Philadelphia, 1985, WB Saunders Co.

Tan EM et al: The 1982 revised criteria of systemic lupus erythematosus, Arthritis Rheum 25:1271-1277, 1982.

Tolman EL: Acne and acneiform dermatoses. In Moschella SL, Pillsbury DM, and Hurley HJ Jr, editors: Dermatology, vol 2, Philadelphia, 1985, WB Saunders Co.

VanArsdel PP Jr: Allergy and adverse drug reactions, J Am Acad Dermatol 6:833-845, 1982.

Weinstein GD and Van Scott EJ: Autoradiographic analysis of turnover times of normal and psoriatic epidermis, J Invest Dermatol 45:257-262, 1965.

Willis I: Photosensitivity. In Moschella SL, Pillsbury DM, and Hurley HJ Jr, editors: Dermatology, vol 1, Philadelphia, 1974, WB Saunders Co.

33

Lesions of the lips

BRUCE F. BARKER

Colored lesions
White lesions
  Candidiasis
  Squamous cell papilloma
  Verruca vulgaris
  Condylomata
  Lichen planus
  Lichenoid drug eruption
  Actinic keratosis
  Squamous cell carcinoma
  Snuff dipper's lesion
  Cigarette smoker's lip
  Focal epithelial
    hyperplasia
Red lesions
  Hemangioma
  Sturge-Weber syndrome
  Thrombocytopenic
    purpura
  Rendu-Osler-Weber
    disease (hereditary
    hemorrhagic
    telangiectasia)
  Kaposi's sarcoma
  Plasma cell cheilitis
Brown lesions
  Nevus
  Labial melanotic macule
  Melanoma
  von Recklinghausen's
    disease
  Albright's syndrome
  Peutz-Jeghers syndrome
  Addison's disease
  Hemochromatosis
  Kaposi's sarcoma

Yellow lesions
  Lipoma
  Fordyce disease

Ulcerative lesions
  Traumatic ulcers
  Aphthae
  Herpes simplex virus
  Erythema multiforme
  Keratoacanthoma
  Syphilis

Elevated lesions
  Fibromas (fibrous
    hyperplasia)
  Mucocele
  Angioedema
  Melkersson-Rosenthal
    syndrome
  Lipoma
  Salivary gland tumors
  Minor salivary gland
    calculi
  Hemangioma
  Nasolabial cyst
  Plasma cell cheilitis
  Cheilitis glandularis
  Cheilitis granulomatosa
  Squamous cell papilloma

*Developmental
  abnormalities*
  Cleft lip
  Double lip
  Lower lip sinuses
  Commissural pits

A careful examination of the lips is often neglected by members of both the medical and dental professions, yet the lips reveal a heterogeneous group of lesions ranging from congenital abnormalities to benign and malignant neoplasms. The lower lip for instance is a common site for squamous carcinoma; the early signs of the dysplastic changes are often present for years before the development of cancer. In addition, easily observed lip lesions may help the clinician recognize more obscure lesions of the skin and mucosa as well as systemic diseases. It

therefore behooves the dental practitioner to perform a thorough examination of the lips.

This chapter describes the common lesions of lips and, in addition, explores some uncommon conditions that may have manifestations on the lips.

The lesions are arranged in four categories: colored lesions, ulcerative lesions, elevated lesions, and developmental abnormalities. This chapter covers only a small number of the multitude of conditions that may appear on the lips, since almost any skin or mucous membrane disease and almost any soft tissue neoplasm may occur here.

Colored lesions

WHITE LESIONS
Candidiasis

Except for angular cheilosis, *Candida* infections of the lip are not well documented. Angular cheilosis, also called perlèche, occurs at the commissures as a white, red, or more often a red and white fissured lesion (Figs. 33-1 and 33-2). It is most often seen bilaterally, and the major predisposing factor is a decreased vertical dimension. This is usually caused by the nonuse of dentures or by poorly made prosthetic appliances. Vitamin B deficiencies often blamed for this lesion are probably a rare cause. Those who drool or have lip-licking habits are at increased risk, as are those who are undergoing radiation therapy or chemotherapy. Candidiasis can affect any of the oral mucosal surfaces. Fig. 33-2 shows a case affecting the labial mucosa.

An entity that researchers called cheilo-candidosis has occurred in the literature described by Reade et al. (1982). They reported five cases of chronic candidiasis of the lower lip that were often of months' duration and exhibited painful, swollen, erythematous, and keratotic lesions with focal ulcerations and crusting. It was suggested that these uncommon *Candida* infec-

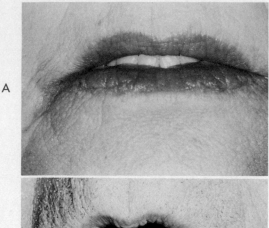

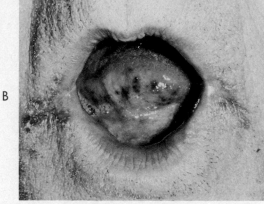

Fig. 33-1. Candidiasis as angular cheilosis. **A,** Lips in more or less closed position in an elderly woman who has loss in vertical dimension. **B,** Lips in open position in an elderly man.

tions of the lip were initiated by chronic irritation resulting from solar or mechanical factors.

Candida infections of the lip are successfully treated by appropriate antifungal medications such as nystatin, ketoconazole, or imidazole derivatives, unless the patient has underlying medical problems that cause a predisposition to fungal infections.

Squamous cell papilloma

The papilloma is a common benign growth that may occur on the lips but is more frequently encountered within the oral cavity. The lesion is classically an exophytic papillary mass, either white or a normal mucosal color (Fig. 33-3). Papillomas occur as single lesions or more uncommonly as multiple lesions. They may be either sessile or pedunculated and may occur at any age but are most common in adults. They are not premalignant but do not spontaneously regress. Surgical excision is the treatment of choice. Studies have identified human papillomavirus (HPV) in more than 50% of oral papillomas. Whether all squamous papillomas are of viral origin is unknown.

DIFFERENTIAL DIAGNOSIS

On clinical examination the papilloma is almost identical to verruca vulgaris, condyloma acuminatum, condyloma latum, and even an early verrucous or papillary squamous carcinoma. Microscopic evaluation should be performed on all papillomas removed.

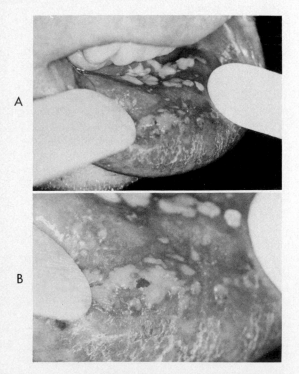

Fig. 33-2. Candidiasis. Diffuse lesions of the lip and labial mucosa.

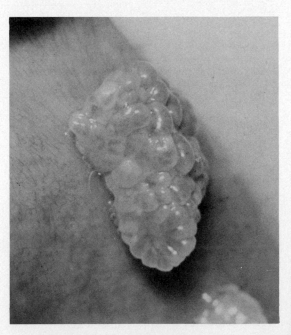

Fig. 33-3. Papilloma on mucosal surface of upper lip in a child who had multiple papillomas.

Verruca vulgaris

Verruca vulgaris is the common wart of the skin; however, it may also occur in the oral cavity, often the result of self-inoculation. Its cause is HPV, subtypes 2 and 4. The exact relationship to oral squamous papillomas is unknown; however, type 2 HPV has been identified in oral papillomas. Identification of HPV is necessary for a definitive diagnosis. The virus cannot be identified with the light microscope without specialized immunofluorescence or immunoperoxidase techniques. DNA probes are more specific.

Condylomata

Condylomata are divided into two types: condyloma acuminatum (Fig. 33-4) of viral origin (HPV 6 and 11) and condyloma latum, which is a lesion of secondary syphilis. Both may be sexually transmitted and may occur on the lips. Diagnosis is determined by an accurate history and microscopic evaluation.

Carcinoma

Either verrucous or exophytic squamous carcinoma may appear identical to papillomas. Most papillomas do not exceed a diameter of 1 cm, whereas carcinomas have unlimited growth potential. Again a biopsy is the only sure way to establish an accurate diagnosis.

Other considerations

Multiple papillomas do occasionally occur but should be differentiated from those in either Cowden's syndrome (multiple hamartoma and neoplasia syndrome) or Goltz-Gorlin syndrome (focal dermal hypoplasia).

Lichen planus

Lichen planus is a mucocutaneous disease of unknown cause that may appear anywhere on skin and mucosa. The buccal mucosa is the most commonly involved intraoral location, but the lips are occasionally involved. A more in-depth discussion of the clinical features and

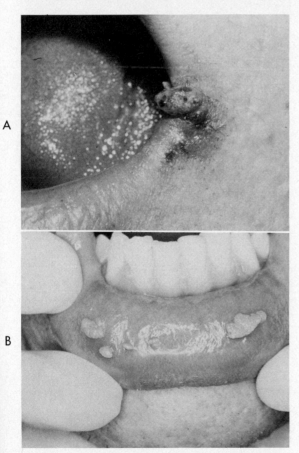

A

B

Fig. 33-4. Condyloma acuminatum. **A,** Exophytic lesion at angle. **B,** Multiple lesions on the mucosal surface of the lower lip.   (**A** courtesy Robert Hiatt, DDS, Kansas City, Mo. **B** courtesy Steven Smith, DDS, Chicago.)

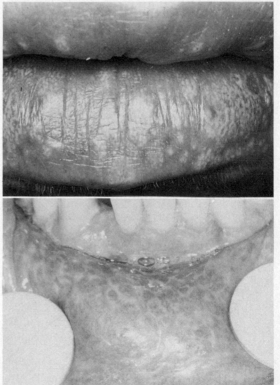

A

B

Fig. 33-5. Lichen planus. White reticular type of lesions on the vermilion border in **A** and on the mucosal surface of the lower lip in **B.**   (**A** courtesy Matt Hourigan, DDS, Kansas City, Mo.)

treatment is found in Chapter 8. The lip lesions usually exhibit the typical white striations (erroneously referred to as striae of Wickham), which are asymptomatic (Fig. 33-5). The lesions, however, may become erosive, red, and painful. If suspect lesions are noted on the lips, the patient should be examined for intraoral lesions or skin lesions, especially on the arms or legs, which help confirm the diagnosis. Occasionally the lesions occur as plaques; however, the edge often demonstrates the typical striae. Patients should be followed closely in view of the potential for malignant transformation. Although the subject is still controversial, malignant change probably occurs in less than 1% of lichen planus cases (Silverman et al., 1985).

DIFFERENTIAL DIAGNOSIS

The conditions that must be differentiated from lichen planus are lichenoid drug eruption, lupus erythematosus, and actinic keratosis. Lupus may appear identical to lichen planus, complete with linear lines (Fig. 33-6); however, it more commonly occurs as a red area. Biopsy with immunofluorescence studies is usually diagnostic.

Lichenoid drug eruptions may also appear identical to lichen planus (Fig. 33-6); in addition, the two are histologically similar. Many drugs and chemicals may cause these reactions, but the most common appear to be nonsteroidal anti-inflammatories, thiazide diuretics, methyldopa, phenothiazines, and gold. An article by Finne et al. (1982) reported that patients with lichen planus had a high contact allergy to mercury. If the offending medications or chemicals can be identified and removed, the lesions may disappear in 3 to 4 weeks. Months may be required in other cases.

Actinic keratosis can be differentiated by the lack of other skin or mucosal lesions; also, striae should not be present. Biopsy, however, is the sure way to a correct diagnosis.

Actinic keratosis (solar keratosis)

Actinic keratosis is a premalignant lesion of the lips that occurs almost exclusively on the lower lip. The etiologic factor responsible for the dysplastic changes seen in the epithelium is actinic radiation from the sun. Collagen and elastic fibers of the underlying connective tissue are also broken down by the same process, leading to a smudged microscopic appearance often referred to as basophilic degeneration. Usually, long-term exposure to sunlight is necessary to induce dysplastic changes; however, as with other skin cancers, fair-complexioned

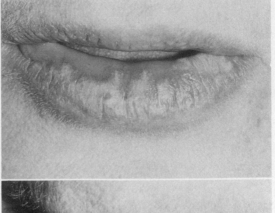
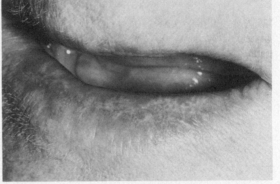

Fig. 33-6. A, Discoid lesion on vermilion border of a patient with systemic lupus erythematosus. This appearance is similar to that seen in keratotic types of lichen planus and lichenoid drug reactions. **B,** Lichenoid drug reaction to an antihypertensive drug in an elderly woman. The white reticular pattern is identical to that seen in lichen planus.

persons are at greater risk. These changes are most often encountered in adults whose occupations require extensive outside work such as farmers, sailors, painters, and construction workers. "Sun worshippers," as would be expected, are not immune.

The typical early lesions are filmy white or even striated, but with continued exposure the tissues may become slightly elevated, crusted, or red and ulcerated (Fig. 33-7). Lesions may be localized or involve the entire lip. Sunscreen lip balm or shading of the lips by protective headgear may prevent progression to squamous carcinoma.

DIFFERENTIAL DIAGNOSIS

No reliable method is available to distinguish actinic changes from severe dysplasia or carcinoma. Therefore, periodic biopsies may be necessary. If severe dysplasia or early carcinoma is detected, it is most often treated by lo-

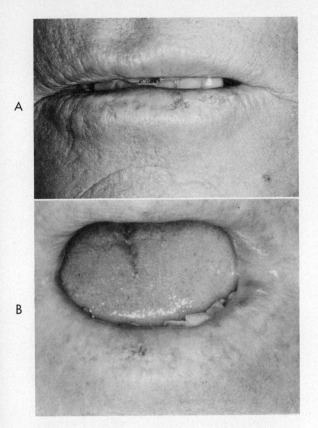

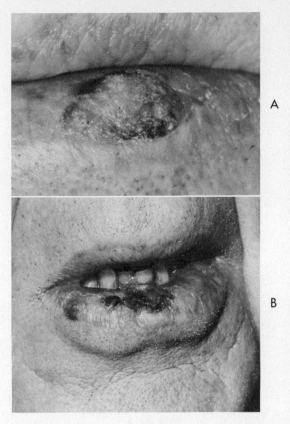

Fig. 33-7. Actinic keratosis. **A** and **B,** Indistinct vermilion border, filmy white areas, and crusting.   (**A** courtesy Brian Brungardt, DDS, Topeka, Kan. **B** courtesy Matt Hourigan, DDS, Kansas City, Mo.)

Fig. 33-8. Squamous cell carcinoma. **A,** Solitary squamous carcinoma of the lower lip. **B,** Numerous eroded and ulcerated lesions that would not heal.

cal excision or, if more diffuse, by a lip shave (vermilionectomy).

Advanced carcinoma must be treated with more extensive surgery or radiation therapy. Actinic changes must also be differentiated from lichen planus, lichenoid drug reaction, lupus erythematosus, and chronic lip biting.

Squamous cell carcinoma (epidermoid carcinoma)

The lip is the most common site of squamous carcinomas in some surveys of oral cancers. However, in many studies lips are excluded from consideration because of their quasiextraoral location and closeness to the skin.

The clinical appearance varies considerably depending on the stage. As pointed out by La Riviere and Pickett (1979), early lesions may be subtle and identical to actinic keratosis; however, crusting, flaking, and ulceration remain as more serious prognostic factors. An advanced lesion is usually an indurated mass with

a cratered, crusted, central area (Fig. 33-8). It is currently believed that actinic rays are the major cause and that most cancers develop in preexisting actinic keratoses. These beliefs are supported by statistics showing that lip carcinomas are seen almost exclusively on the lower lips of older, white (fair-skinned) men. In addition, most patients have had extensive outdoor activities often relating to their occupations. Women have been less affected, possibly because of the use of lipstick and the limited exposure to actinic rays of women who have traditional (indoor) occupations.

Douglass and Gammon (1984) discussed the epidemiologic features of lip cancer in detail. They concluded that (1) any risk factors considered to be causally related to lip cancer must be congruent with factors such as geographic distribution and secular disease trends and (2) although sunlight and smoking are very likely risk factors, genetic predisposition must be reassessed.

Controversy still exists as to the cause of squamous cell carcinoma of the lip; as in most cancers, it is probably caused by different factors. Several studies in the 1940s showed a strong association between lip carcinoma and the use of tobacco, especially the use of pipes. This has been overshadowed in most recent studies by the apparent importance of actinic radiation.

Treatment of choice is either surgery or radiation therapy. Both are very effective in controlling early lesions. As in advanced actinic keratoses, a lip shave or vermilionectomy is widely used with excellent cosmetic effects. The 5-year survival for patients with well-differentiated lesions that have not metastasized is above 90%. The positive prognosis diminishes considerably for anaplastic lesions and for those that have metastasized. Large cratered or indurated lesions may require more extensive surgery or radiation therapy or both. Metastases are uncommon but must be ruled out only after a thorough neck examination. Prophylactic neck dissections are not usually indicated.

DIFFERENTIAL DIAGNOSIS

Because early lesions may look like persistent chapped lips or asymptomatic actinic keratosis, a biopsy is absolutely necessary for diagnosis. Most advanced cratered lesions must be differentiated from a keratoacanthoma. Basal cell carcinomas may appear identical on clinical examination, but most agree that these arise only on the skin surface and extend to mucosa. Tomich and Shafer (1974) described a probable traumatic lesion called *squamous acanthoma* that may appear similar. One in eight of these squamous acanthomas occurred on the lower lip.

Snuff dipper's lesion

Snuff dipper's lesion appears to be on the increase, mainly because of the widespread use of smokeless tobacco products in the younger generation. Greer and Poulson (1983) reviewed this trend in Denver adolescents. Snuff or chewing tobacco is typically held in the mandibular vestibule with the incisor area as a favorite location. The lesions vary slightly in appearance depending on the frequency and duration of the habit; however, the pattern of the lesion is quite characteristic. Most have a folded or wrinkled appearance (Fig. 33-9). This appearance is caused by a wavy hyperkeratosis that usually completely disappears several weeks after the habit is discontinued. Long-

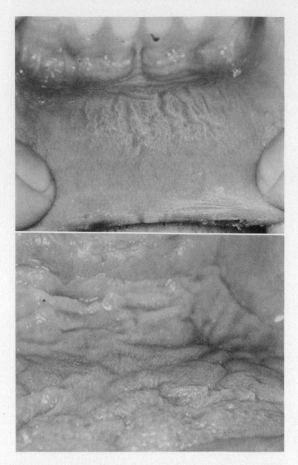

Fig. 33-9. Typical white, corrugated appearance of snuff dipper's lesion.

term exposure of the mucosa may induce dysplasia or carcinoma, either verrucous or squamous. This is especially disquieting considering the widespread use of smokeless tobacco among junior high school students today. Fortunately, years of contact are usually necessary to produce a carcinoma. Winn et al. (1981) showed that there was an approximately 50-fold increased risk of carcinoma in women who had used such tobacco products chronically.

DIFFERENTIAL DIAGNOSIS

The appearance of the lesions is quite characteristic and lends itself to easy diagnosis, especially when a history of smokeless tobacco use is known. Biopsy, however, is the only sure method to determine if dysplastic changes have occurred. A compromise to a biopsy would be to have the patient refrain from using the smokeless tobacco or switch usage to another location to see if the lesion disappears.

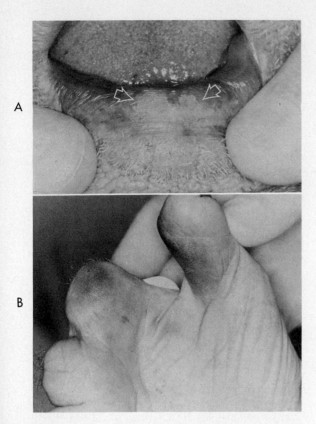

Fig. 33-10. **A,** Cigarette smoker's lip. This white lesion has been present for some months. **B,** Burns are evident on the patient's amputated fingers where he has held his cigarette.   (**A** and **B** courtesy Brian Brungardt, DDS, Topeka, Kan.)

Cigarette smoker's lip

Cigarette smoker's lip is a localized, usually well-defined flat or slightly elevated lesion of the lips that corresponds to the area where the patient holds cigarettes. The lesion usually begins as a reddened area but becomes more white with time (Fig. 33-10). This was first reported by Berry and Landwerlen (1973) and is usually seen in neuropsychiatric patients as a result of thermal injury. A high percentage of patients also had burns on their fingers corresponding to where they held their cigarettes. This should be a diagnostic clue. Another aid is that the lesions are confined to the mucosal aspect of the lip and almost never cross the vermilion border. It is postulated that the patient's psychiatric medications increase their pain threshold, thereby allowing the tissues to be burned. Lesions may involve one or both lips. Malignant transformation has not been reported despite years of smoking by some patients.

Focal epithelial hyperplasia (Heck's disease)

In 1965 Archard et al. first described focal epithelial hyperplasia (FEH) in Navajo children. Since that time it has been described in numerous countries throughout the world. Prevalence in American Indians and Greenlandic Eskimos has been shown to be 32% to 39%, whereas the condition is rare in whites (Praetorius-Clausen, 1973). It is characterized on clinical examination by multiple sessile, white papules that are most commonly seen on the lower lip (see Fig. 10-36), with occurrences also reported on the upper lip, buccal mucosa, tongue, gingiva, and tonsillar pillars. The lesions are soft to palpation, infrequently larger than 0.5 cm in diameter, and most commonly seen in children and young adults. Spontaneous regression has been reported; therefore no treatment is necessary. Although the cause remains uncertain, reports indicate association with human papillomavirus (HPV 13 and HPV 32) (Beaudenon et al., 1987).

DIFFERENTIAL DIAGNOSIS

Multiple squamous papillomas and verrucae are most commonly confused with FEH. On microscopic examination these are easily differentiated from FEH, since, as the name implies, FEH exhibits squamous hyperplasia and hyperkeratosis but not typical papillomatosis. Similarly, dysplastic lesions should not be confused on microscopic examination. Cowden's syndrome, a rare condition, may be manifest as multiple similar lesions and must be ruled out. Other conditions that should be excluded include focal dermal hypoplasia (Goltz-Gorlin syndrome) and oral manifestations of Darier's and Crohn's disease.

BROWN AND RED LESIONS
Nevus (mole)

The nevus is a neuroectodermal lesion that occurs on both skin and mucosa; skin lesions are far more common. Oral nevi have been reviewed by Buchner and Hansen (1979) with total reported cases numbering about 100. Nevi are macular or papular and usually brown-black or blue (see Fig. 12-19). The pigment is derived from melanin produced within the nevus cells. Nevi may be congenital or acquired later in life, reaching their peak occurrence in the late twenties. Clark et al. (1979) postulated that the number of nevi a person has is genetically determined. Nevi may vary considerably in size; however, most lesions occurring on the lips are less than 1 cm in diameter.

Nevi have been divided into several common types, (1) intradermal, (2) junctional, (3) compound, (4) spindle cell, and (5) blue. Histologic evaluation is necessary for differentiation. All types except the spindle cell nevus occur in the oral cavity, with more than one half being the intradermal type. Although junctional nevi have long been implicated as having the potential to undergo malignant change, this theory has been challenged by Clark et al. (1969). They believed that junctional nevi and melanomas are biologically different entities and that most malignant changes are actually the result of misdiagnosis of the original lesion. Congenital nevi, however, are known to undergo malignant change and become melanomas.

DIFFERENTIAL DIAGNOSIS

Histologic examination is mandatory for a definitive diagnosis, since nevi may appear similar to melanomas on clinical examination. Other lesions of possible confusion include amalgam tattoo, labial melanotic macule, incontinence of pigment, and vascular lesions.

Labial melanotic macule (freckle, ephelis)

First described by Weathers et al. (1976) and later reviewed by Buchner and Hansen (1979), a labial melanotic macule usually occurs as a single brownish black, sharply circumscribed lesion of the lower lip (Fig. 33-11). The macules are found most frequently toward the midline in those having a fair complexion and have been detected most frequently in people between the ages of 30 and 45. The macules rarely exceed 0.5 cm in diameter. The cause is unknown, but it has been postulated that these macules may represent three separate entities: a deposition of pigment as a result of trauma or inflammation (postinflammatory), true freckles or ephelides, and a unique lesion that has no cutaneous counterpart. Biopsies of the lesions should be performed for a definitive diagnosis. If lesions have existed for 5 years without change, periodic observation is acceptable.

DIFFERENTIAL DIAGNOSIS

Differential diagnosis of pigmented lesions is presented in Chapter 12 in the discussion of the oral melanotic macule (p. 233).

Melanoma

Melanoma is a malignant tumor of melanocytes. It occurs infrequently in the oral cavity, accounting for approximately 1% of all melanomas. The anterior maxillary gingiva and palate are the most common intraoral locations, with

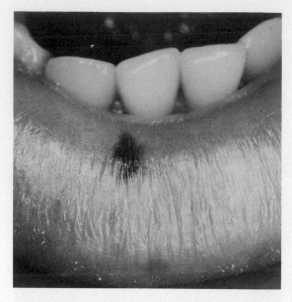

Fig. 33-11. Labial melanotic macule. (Courtesy Matt Hourigan, DDS, Kansas City, Mo.)

the lips being a less frequent site (see Fig. 12-17, C). The reader is referred to the more thorough discussion of melanomas in Chapter 12 and to the articles by Clark et al. (1969, 1979) for an in-depth discussion. All three types of melanoma may occur on the lips: (1) lentigo maligna, (2) superficial spreading melanoma, and (3) nodular melanoma. Since lentigo maligna occurs only on sun-exposed tissues, the lips are the only oral site for this type of melanoma. Lesions of the oral mucosa that resemble lentigo maligna on histologic study have been designated acral lentiginous melanoma and behave more aggressively than lentigo maligna.

Preexisting melanotic lesions may be present for years in the area where melanomas develop. Some of these represent superficial spreading melanomas in the radial growth phase, and excision of lesions at this stage results in an excellent prognosis. For this reason pigmented lesions are better removed than watched. Prognosis for melanomas of the oral cavity has generally been poor. Other lesions easily confused with melanoma include labial melanotic macule, amalgam tattoo, nevus, and vascular lesions. Pigmented lesions that change in configuration or color should be highly suspected of being melanoma.

Hemangioma

The hemangioma is a benign proliferation of blood vessels that occurs in the head and neck region in more than 50% of the cases. On his-

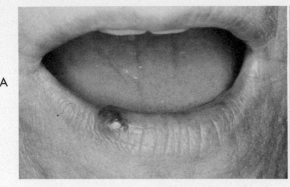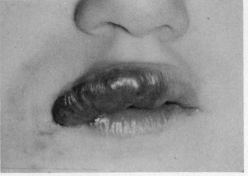

Fig. 33-12. Hemangioma. **A**, Small, nodular lesion on vermilion border of lower lip. **B**, Large, diffuse lesion of the upper lip in a child.   (**B** courtesy James Lowe, DDS, Kansas City, Mo.)

tologic study they are usually divided into cavernous (large vessels) and capillary (small vessels). Most are congenital or occur at a young age and show limited growth potential. Some lesions even undergo spontaneous regression, which has led many to believe that hemangiomas are not true neoplasms but rather hamartomas. To support the claim of neoplastic potential in hemangiomas, one can point to those lesions that exhibit unlimited growth with extensive involvement of soft tissues and bone. Some even lead to fatal hemorrhage.

On clinical examination, hemangiomas appear as either flat or elevated, red or bluish lesions, which usually blanch under pressure (Fig. 33-12). The lips, buccal mucosa, tongue, and palate are common oral locations. The borders of the lesions are not usually well demarcated; therefore what appears to be a small, superficial lesion may have the bulk of the "iceberg" beneath the surface. Large lesions are often pulsatile.

Small lesions are usually successfully treated with surgery, but such procedures should not be attempted before careful evaluation of the extent of the tumor. Other forms of therapy include radiation, sclerosing agents, cryotherapy, and embolization with various materials.

DIFFERENTIAL DIAGNOSIS

Hemangiomas must be differentiated by histologic examination from other vascular lesions such as Kaposi's sarcoma, hemangioendothelioma, hemangiopericytoma, angiosarcoma, arteriovenous malformation, pyogenic granuloma, and varices. Mucoceles may also be a possible differential diagnosis, but they fail to blanch under pressure, which should eliminate them from consideration in most cases.

Multiple pigmentations

Several conditions include pigmentation of the lips as a partial expression of the disease. These conditions include the following:

1. Peutz-Jeghers syndrome
2. Addison's disease
3. Sturge-Weber syndrome
4. Rendu-Osler-Weber disease (hereditary hemorrhagic telangiectasia)
5. Thrombocytopenic purpura
6. Kaposi's sarcoma
7. von Recklinghausen's disease (neurofibromatosis)
8. Albright's syndrome
9. Hemochromatosis

Multiple brown or black lesions may occur with Peutz-Jeghers syndrome, von Recklinghausen's disease, Addison's disease, Albright's syndrome, and hemochromatosis. Almost all of these may present as multiple macular lesions; however, Addison's disease and hemochromatosis may be a diffuse pigmentation. The diagnosis depends on the other manifestations of these conditions rather than biopsy of the lip lesions. A biopsy can determine whether the pigmentation is melanin, which is of little help, since all the lesions just listed have melanin deposition. Hemochromatosis exhibits iron deposits in the tissues, as well as melanin. Von Recklinghausen's disease, Albright's syndrome, and hemochromatosis are discussed in Chapter 12.

PEUTZ-JEGHERS SYNDROME (HEREDITARY INTESTINAL POLYPOSIS)

The major manifestations of Peutz-Jeghers syndrome are the intestinal polyps that are found throughout the intestinal tract but most commonly in the ileum. The syndrome is in-

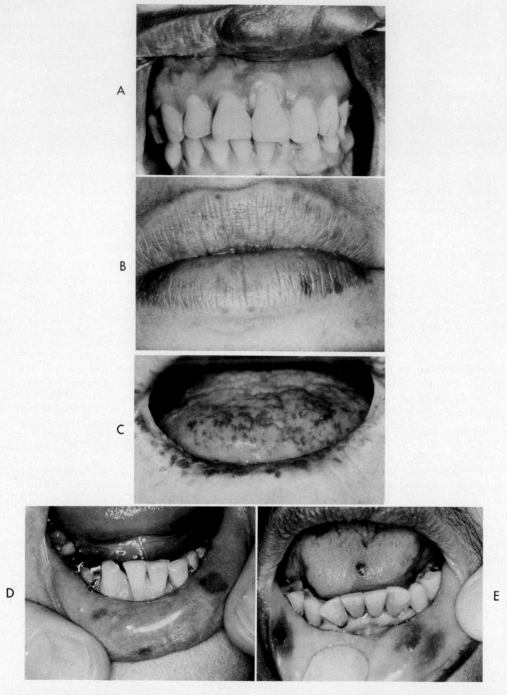

Fig. 33-13. Multiple pigmentation of the lips. **A,** Sturge-Weber syndrome showing nevus flammeus of left side of upper lip and gingiva. **B,** Peutz-Jeghers syndrome. Many pigmented macules are present on both upper and lower lips. **C,** Rendu-Osler-Weber syndrome. Multiple small red macules represent dilated end capillaries. **D,** Three pigmented macules on lower lip resulting from Addison's disease. **E,** Multiple ecchymotic areas of a patient with thrombocytopenia.   (**C** courtesy John Bellome, Kansas City, Mo. **D** courtesy Steven Smith, Chicago.)

herited as an autosomal dominant trait; however, sporadic individual cases have been reported. The polyps are usually benign, but malignant transformation occurs. Despite the benign nature of the polyps, significant morbidity is caused by obstruction and intussusception.

The oral manifestations of this syndrome are melanin pigmentations of the oral mucosa, especially of the lips and perioral skin (Fig. 33-13, *B*). These macular lesions appear at birth or soon after and are usually multiple. Most are small, less than 0.5 cm in diameter, and asymptomatic. The lesions are of clinical significance only as a diagnostic clue to the more serious intestinal problems.

ADDISON'S DISEASE

Addison's disease is caused by adrenal cortical insufficiency and is characterized by melanin pigmentation of skin and mucous membranes (Fig. 33-13, *D*), anemia, diarrhea, nausea, vomiting, lethargy, and poor heart function. Discussion of the physiology of Addison's disease is beyond the scope of this text.

The pigmentation of the lips is usually multifocal but may be diffuse. Pigmentations have been observed on the buccal mucosa, gingiva, and tongue, as well as the lips. These pigmentations may be the first manifestation of Addison's disease. A biopsy is not diagnostic.

STURGE-WEBER SYNDROME

Sturge-Weber syndrome consists of multiple venous angiomas that most commonly occur in the head and neck region following the distribution of the trigeminal nerve and in the leptomeninges. It is much easier to remember the manifestations of this disease by using the descriptive name, encephalotrigeminal angiomatosis, rather than the eponym. The disease is congenital and is therefore initially diagnosed at birth. Extensive angiomas in the leptomeninges may cause neurologic manifestations including seizures. Hemangioma-like lesions may occur throughout the oral cavity including the lips (Fig. 31-13, *A*). Dentists should be cautious of performing surgery in such areas, since significant bleeding may occur. Patients may seek dental care for the gingival enlargement associated with the anticonvulsant drugs used to control the associated seizures.

RENDU-OSLER-WEBER DISEASE

Rendu-Osler-Weber disease is probably better known in the medical field as hereditary hemorrhagic telangiectasia. This is an inherited autosomal dominant condition that is character-

ized by multiple angiomatous lesions of the skin and mucosa. The individual lesions are usually small—hence the term "telangiectasia." Bleeding from the lesions, however, is common and is often one of the symptoms that brings attention to the disease. Lesions appear to increase in number with patient age. In the oral region the lips are one of the most frequently involved locations (Fig. 33-13, *C*). There is no treatment, and if bleeding occurs, it may be difficult to control. The hereditary nature of the disease is important in making a diagnosis.

THROMBOCYTOPENIC PURPURA

A reduction of the number of circulating platelets results in multiple focal areas of bleeding on both the skin and mucous membranes. Platelet count must usually be below $50,000/mm^3$ before spontaneous bleeding occurs. Several types of thrombocytopenia have been described, including primary, which is probably autoimmune in origin, and secondary, which is related to a multitude of other conditions including infections, tumors, certain drugs, and lupus erythematosus. The reader is referred to a current hematology text for a complete list of possible causes. In primary thrombocytopenia, patients have been discovered to have antibodies to their own platelets.

Significant bleeding may result if the lesions are ecchymotic rather than petechial (Fig. 33-13, *E*). Splenectomy and administration of systemic steroids have been successful in treating many cases; however, fatalities still occur. Spontaneous remissions are also reported.

KAPOSI'S SARCOMA

Kaposi's sarcoma was once considered a rare lesion in the United States, but with the discovery of acquired immunodeficiency syndrome (AIDS) it has become a much more frequent diagnosis (Chapter 12). This disease was reviewed by Eversole et al. (1983) and Silverman et al. (1986). This disease traditionally was a type of angiosarcoma that was most frequently seen in elderly Jewish males. In parts of Africa, however, it constitutes 10% of all malignancies and occurs mainly in black children. In Africa the disease is quite aggressive and has a high mortality; in other areas of the world, including the United States, it traditionally has had a prolonged course. The Kaposi's sarcoma that develops with AIDS behaves in a much more aggressive manner than the traditional cases in the United States. For a detailed discussion of AIDS, see Appendix D.

Ulcerative lesions

Ulcers of the lip are common. Some are manifestations of a specific disease, whereas others are consequences of a particular treatment or injury. Traumatic lesions are far more common.

TRAUMATIC ULCERS

By definition, these ulcers are caused by some type of trauma. The trauma may be self-inflicted (factitial), caused by someone in the medical profession (iatrogenic), or the result of any other conceivable injury. Probably the most common cause of lip ulceration is lip biting (morsicatio labiorum) (Fig. 33-14). Poorly fitting dental appliances, sharp malaligned teeth, or perhaps just a momentary lapse of concentration are the most common causes; however, psychogenic factors may also be responsible. A clinical and epidemiologic study has been published by Sewerin (1971). A rare cause is the Lesch-Nyhan syndrome, in which patients have some insensitivity to pain and uncontrollable, jerky movements, which in turn may cause massive self-mutilation of the lips (LaBanc and Epker, 1981). Similar mutilation may occur in patients who unknowingly bite their lips following the administration of local anesthetic related to dental procedures.

The dentist may cause inadvertent ulcerations to patients' lips (iatrogenic) through the use of instruments, appliances, and compounds in various procedures. Examples include rotary instruments, caustic agents, hot compounds, and even a dry cotton roll or gauze pad stuck to the mucosal surface and pulled loose.

DIFFERENTIAL DIAGNOSIS

Traumatic ulcers may appear identical to ulcers of any other cause such as aphthous or even ulcerated tumors. History of an immediately preceding traumatic episode may help in a diagnosis; however, this should not be an absolute criterion. If the ulcer does not begin to heal in a 2-week period, a biopsy should be performed to rule out a more ominous cause. Consideration should be given to the possibility of delayed healing time resulting from diabetes, medications, continuous irritation, or immunodeficiencies.

APHTHAE (CANKER SORES, RECURRENT APHTHOUS STOMATITIS)

Aphthae are discussed more completely in Chapter 11, but they deserve attention here because of their commonness. For a more detailed discussion, articles by Antoon and Miller (1980), Rennie et al. (1985), and Rogers (1977) are recommended. Aphthae occur either as single or multiple ulcers of the mucosal surface of the lips. They do not occur on the skin. This is in contrast to recurrent herpes labialis, which is found almost exclusively on the vermilion border or skin surface of the lips. Aphthae of the lip are similar in appearance and behavior to those of other intraoral locations (Fig. 33-15). They are recurrent, with the intervals be-

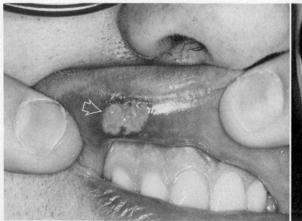
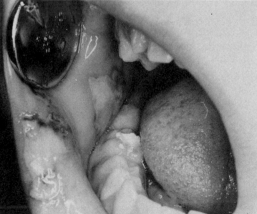

Fig. 33-14. Traumatic ulcer. **A,** A blow to the lip of the patient resulted in a painful ulcer with ragged borders. **B,** Multiple ulcerations from cheek and lip biting during mandibular block anesthesia.   (**B** courtesy James Lowe, DDS, Kansas City, Kan.)

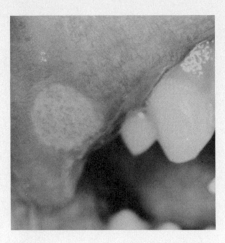

Fig. 33-15. Large aphthous ulcer on mucosal surface of the upper lip.

tween episodes varying from weeks to years. Most ulcers heal within a 2-week period. Healing may be accelerated with the topical application of a corticosteroid, although systemic prednisone may be necessary for large or persistent lesions.

DIFFERENTIAL DIAGNOSIS

Aphthae are most commonly confused with herpes labialis. Herpes begins as groups of vesicles on the vermilion border or skin, whereas aphthae begin as a reddish mucosal macule that undergoes ulceration without vesiculation. Differentiation from other diseases and traumatic ulcers is best accomplished by a history of recurrent lesions. In the absence of this history, a biopsy should be performed if healing does not begin within 2 weeks.

HERPES SIMPLEX VIRUS (HSV)

The lesions of both the initial and recurrent infections with herpes simplex virus may occur on the lips. This highly contagious disease has reached epidemic proportions in the last decade and is only one of several conditions caused by the herpesvirus group. There are two types of HSV, usually called type 1 and type 2. HSV-1 classically affects tissues above the waist, and HSV-2 affects those below the waist, mainly the genitalia. The lip is the most common location for HSV-1 infections, and the genitalia are the most common site for type 2; however, each virus may be found in either location. Corey and Spear (1986) and Straus et al. (1985) reviewed herpes simplex infections.

Primary HSV (gingivostomatitis)

Infections that occur before the development of antibodies against the virus are called primary and occur most commonly in children. This one-time infection occasionally is severe and is accompanied by systemic manifestations including fever, headache, sore throat, malaise, and regional lymphadenopathy. The oral lesions are diffuse and multiple; swollen red gingival tissues are often the initial manifestation. Within several days numerous vesicles develop, and the lips are often involved diffusely. These vesicles rupture quickly, leaving shallow ulcers (see Fig. 6-2). The mucosal ulcers have a raw or membranous covering, whereas those on the skin are crusted. These are contagious lesions, especially during the early phases of the disease (the first 6 days). They heal spontaneously without scarring in 10 to 14 days.

Recurrent HSV (herpes labialis, fever blisters)

Recurrent HSV occurs only in those who have antibodies to HSV. These antibodies may be the result of a known episode of gingivostomatitis, but more often they are the result of a previous unknown, subclinical infection with HSV. It is estimated that 90% of the adult population of the United States have HSV antibodies. The recurrent lesions are not new infections but the reactivation of virus already present in the tissues. The virus does not remain at the site of original infection but follows nerves to the ganglion supplying the area. Here the virus may remain latent until reactivated. Some believe that the virus continuously travels up and down the same nerve pathways until reactivation occurs. The method of reactivation is unclear, but many factors have been implicated. These include fever, hormonal influence, emotional stress, trauma, and sunshine.

The lips are the most common site for recurrent oral lesions. Recurrent herpetic lesions are not as common within the mouth and are usually on the hard palate or gingiva. Patients have a tingling or burning sensation at the site of the developing lesion before any lesion can be seen on clinical examination. Vesicles then develop, usually in small groups, rupture quickly, and ulcerate (Figs. 33-16 and 33-17). On the lips a crust often covers the ulcers. Pain varies considerably but is usually minor. The lesions heal without scarring in 7 to 10 days.

In contrast to primary herpes, recurrent lesions, as the name implies, may repeatedly re-

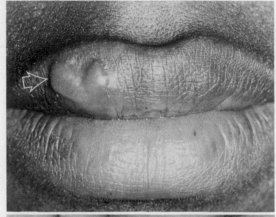

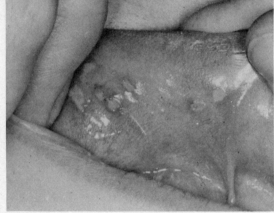

Fig. 33-16. Recurrent herpes. **A,** Two large vesicles on upper lip. A tingling sensation accompanied their formation. **B,** Recurrent herpes on mucosa of upper lip showing the characteristic clustering of small, discrete ulcers. (**B** courtesy of A.C.W.H. Hutchinson Collection, Northwestern University Dental School, Chicago.)

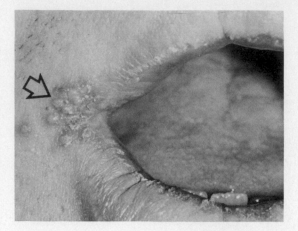

Fig. 33-17. Recurrent herpes. Multiple smaller vesicles at the angle.

DIFFERENTIAL DIAGNOSIS

Many other conditions may be confused with HSV. Despite many clinical differences an aphthous ulcer is a frequent misdiagnosis. Aphthae do not start as vesicles. Several vesiculobullous diseases may also be difficult to distinguish from herpes labialis. These include erythema multiforme, pemphigus, and pemphigoid. Allergic lesions and even burns may appear similar. The cytologic smear is a diagnostic aid. During the early days of a herpes infection a characteristic multinucleated giant cell (polykaryon) can be identified, which is diagnostic of the herpesvirus. Immunofluorescence and immunoperoxidase techniques can also identify the virus in fluid or tissue samples. Biopsy is seldom necessary for diagnosis because of the clinical characteristics of HSV.

ERYTHEMA MULTIFORME (STEVENS-JOHNSON SYNDROME)

This self-limiting disease may involve both the skin and all areas of the oral mucosa, with the lips being a classic location. The disease is characterized by rapid development of lesions with the skin showing the typical "target," "iris," or "bull's eye" lesions. These are discussed in Chapter 6. Mucous membrane lesions are usually multiple red macules, papules, vesicles, or bullae that ulcerate or rupture quickly, leaving raw, painful lesions. The lips are often extensively involved and crusted at the vermilion borders (Fig. 33-18). Most patients have both mucous membrane and skin lesions; however, Lozada and Silverman (1978) reported patients who had involvement only of the oral cavity.

turn. The intervals between recurrences vary from weeks to years even in the same individual. The lesions are most contagious in the first several days. Viral shedding has decreased dramatically when crusting occurs.

MANAGEMENT

Treatment is mainly symptomatic, for there is no cure for HSV. Antiviral medication (acyclovir) shows some promise in shortening the course of primary lesions and reducing viral shedding, but it has minimal effects on recurrent lesions (Douglas et al., 1984; Raborn et al., 1987). Topical interferon has also been shown to reduce the symptoms and severity of the disease in some patients (Glezerman et al., 1988).

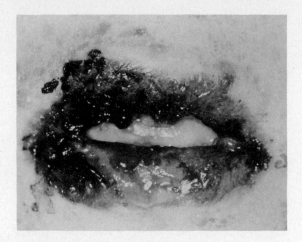

Fig. 33-18. Erythema multiforme. These lesions developed in the child following antibiotic therapy for an ear infection. Skin lesions were also present.

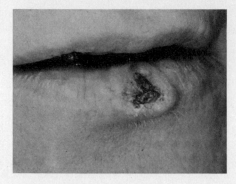

Fig. 33-19. Keratoacanthoma of the lower lip in a 38-year-old man showing typical appearance of central keratin plug in a central depression that is surrounded by smooth, rolled borders. This lesion is clinically indistinguishable from squamous cell carcinoma. (From Bass KD: J Oral Surg 38:53-55, 1980, Copyright by the American Dental Association. Reprinted by permission.)

Although the cause remains unknown, many cases occur several weeks after episodes of herpes simplex. Other triggering agents include numerous drugs including antibiotics, birth control pills, and barbiturates. Radiation therapy and diseases such as ulcerative colitis have precipitated attacks. In approximately one half the cases, no precipitating factors can be identified. Lesions usually heal spontaneously in several weeks, although some cases may persist longer. Recurrences are common unless precipitating factors can be identified and avoided.

Stevens-Johnson syndrome is a more severe form of the disease and includes lesions of the skin, mucous membrane, eyes, and genitalia. Fatalities do occur, but most patients recover. Scarring is not a feature.

There is no specific treatment or cure, but a search for the precipitating factors should be initiated nonetheless. When no etiologic factors are found, analgesics and anesthetics are palliative. Corticosteroid therapy has been shown to alter both the severity and the length of the disease in some patients.

DIFFERENTIAL DIAGNOSIS

Many diseases can be confused with erythema multiforme including recurrent aphthous, Behçet's syndrome, Reiter's syndrome, pemphigus, pemphigoid, herpetic stomatitis, and toxic epidermal necrolysis (Lyell's disease). Herpetic stomatitis may appear quite similar but can be differentiated by initial gingival involvement, lack of "iris" skin lesions, positive cytologic smear, and no history of previous episodes. Aphthae and Behçet's and Reiter's syndromes do not have vesicles or bullous mucosal lesions as features.

KERATOACANTHOMA (SELF-HEALING CARCINOMA)

Keratoacanthoma is best known by dermatologists, since the majority of cases occur on sun-exposed tissues of the face. Oral lesions are rare, with the lips being the most common site. It resembles a squamous carcinoma on both clinical and microscopic examination but is a benign lesion. It is a lesion of adults, predominantly older males. The lesion begins as a sometimes painful nodule that slowly increases in size and develops a central crater (Fig. 33-19). After reaching maximal growth, which rarely exceeds 1.5 cm in diameter, the lesion begins to regress and heals. The entire process may take 3 to 4 months; however, some lesions have been reported to last as long as several years. Because of the close clinical and histologic resemblance to squamous carcinoma, the keratoacanthoma should be treated by surgical excision.

The cause of the keratoacanthoma is unknown; however, considerations include viruses and chemical carcinogens.

DIFFERENTIAL DIAGNOSIS

The most important consideration is squamous carcinoma. Keratoacanthoma usually shows a much more rapid initial growth than squamous carcinoma; however, this is not a reliable criterion. Biopsy is necessary for a diagnosis. Another consideration in a differential diagnosis is the squamous acanthoma as described by Tomich and Shafer (1974).

SYPHILIS

The primary lesion of syphilis occurs at the site of inoculation. This site is most commonly on the genitalia; however, the oral cavity and especially the lips are possible locations. The initial lesion or chancre usually begins as a papule at approximately 3 weeks after contact with the spirochete *Treponema pallidum*. The papule eventually ulcerates, leaving a lesion similar to an aphthous or traumatic ulcer (Fig. 33-20). The chancre heals spontaneously within several months and is highly contagious during this period. Regional lymphadenopathy may also be present.

The classic lesions of secondary syphilis in the oral cavity, called mucous patches, are single or multiple plaques that are gray or white overlying an ulcerated base. These patches actually represent macerated papules, which because of the moisture are covered with a soft, boggy membrane. They are teeming with organisms and are highly contagious. Secondary lesions of syphilis usually develop approximately 6 weeks after initial contact; however, the time is greatly variable. Serologic tests for syphilis are usually positive during the secondary stages of syphilis, in contrast to primary syphilis. Macular or papular skin lesions usually accompany the mucous patches.

Condyloma latum is another lesion of secondary syphilis that may occur on the lip. This is a papular, wartlike lesion, which may be either red or white. It could easily be confused with a papilloma, wart, or condyloma acuminatum. These later lesions usually have individual elevated fingerlike processes, whereas syphilis is more likely to be lobulated.

Treatment of either primary or secondary syphilis is with the appropriate antibiotic, usually penicillin.

DIFFERENTIAL DIAGNOSIS

Chancres may be difficult to distinguish from other, more innocuous lesions, since results of serologic study are usually normal. Dark-field microscopy is not recommended for the examination of intraoral lesions because of the presence of other intraoral spirochetes; however, those lesions located on the vermilion border would be amenable. It is probable that many chancres go undiagnosed or are cured unknowingly with antibiotic therapy.

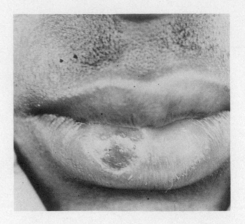

Fig. 33-20. Syphilitic chancre of the lower lip in a young man. (Courtesy Matt Hourigan, DDS, Kansas City, Mo.)

Positive serologic findings may aid in the diagnosis of mucous patches and condyloma latum. The presence of accompanying skin lesions is also helpful. Mucous patches might also be confused with candidiasis.

Elevated lesions

FIBROMAS (TRAUMATIC OR IRRITATION FIBROMA, NODULAR FIBROUS HYPERPLASIA)

A true fibrous neoplasm of the oral mucosa is an extremely rare entity, and the ensuing discussion deals with the extremely common nodular fibrous hyperplasia, which is often erroneously called a fibroma. This nodular lesion of normal color is the most common soft tissue lesion encountered in the oral cavity and occurs commonly on the lips. (Fig. 33-21). Other intraoral locations commonly involved are the gingiva, tongue, buccal mucosa, and soft palate. Since the lesion is a fibrous hyperplasia, usually initiated by trauma such as lip biting, it is not a true neoplasm and has limited growth potential, rarely exceeding a centimeter or two in diameter. The lesion typically grows slowly and varies in consistency from very soft to firm. Very soft lesions often show some degree of adipose tissue on microscopic evaluation—hence the term *fibrolipoma*. Most have a broadly based attachment and are therefore sessile rather than pedunculated. On histologic study the bulk of the nodular mass consists of hyperplastic fibrous connective tissue with minimal inflammation. If considerable inflammation is present, the term *inflammatory fibrous hyperplasia* is used. Another variety, a giant cell fi-

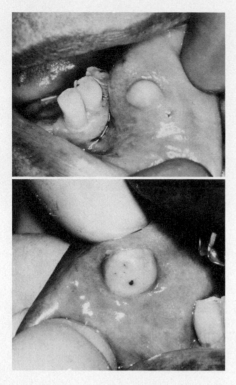

Fig. 33-21. Traumatic fibromas. Typical fibrous hyperplasia lesions of lower lip associated with chronic lip biting in both cases.

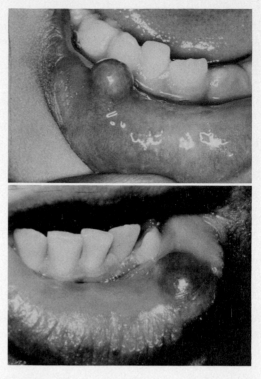

Fig. 33-22. Mucoceles of the lower lip in two different patients.

broma, is characterized by proliferation of stellate and multinucleated fibroblasts (Weathers and Callihan, 1974).

Although occasional fibrous hyperplasias may regress or disappear when the offending irritant is eliminated, most must be surgically removed. Recurrence is rare.

DIFFERENTIAL DIAGNOSIS

All soft tissue tumors, mucoceles, and salivary gland tumors must be ruled out. Multiple recurrences or variation in size favor a mucocele; however, a biopsy with histologic evaluation is the only way to obtain a definitive diagnosis.

MUCOCELE (MUCOUS RETENTION ESCAPE PHENOMENON)

More than 80% of all mucoceles are estimated to occur on the lower lip; however, this lesion may develop in any location where minor salivary glands exist. Most mucoceles occur as the result of severance of a minor salivary gland duct with resultant escape of mucous secretions into the surrounding tissues. Occlusion or partial obstruction of a duct can also re-

sult in a marked dilatation of that duct. This is termed a *mucous retention cyst*, since the mucus-filled cavity is lined with epithelium (in contrast to mucoceles, which have no epithelial lining).

Some type of trauma, such as lip biting, is the usual cause of mucoceles. Since this type of trauma most commonly occurs on the lower lip, the upper lip is an infrequent location. A characteristic of mucoceles is fluctuation in size. Multiple fluctuations may occur as the mucin is phagocytosed, carried off, and replaced by newly secreted mucin.

Mucoceles appear suddenly and reach maximal size within several days. The typical lesion appears as an elevated vesicular or bullous lesion, which often has a slightly bluish or translucent appearance (Fig. 33-22). However, if the lesions are situated more deeply in the tissues, they may be of normal color. The lesion is soft to palpation and often fluctuant. The treatment of choice is surgical excision including the glands from which the mucin is escaping. Recurrence of the mucocele is possible despite surgery, since adjacent salivary gland ducts may be severed during the surgical procedure.

DIFFERENTIAL DIAGNOSIS

The sudden appearance and the fluctuation in size is almost diagnostic of the mucocele; however, biopsy is necessary for a definitive diagnosis. Lesions that may be confused with mucoceles include neurofibroma, lipoma, salivary gland tumors, varix, vascular tumors, and nodular fibrous hyperplasia. Vascular lesions should blanch under pressure, which aids in the differential diagnosis. Salivary gland tumors, such as mucoepidermidal carcinoma, may be identical.

ANGIOEDEMA (ANGIONEUROTIC EDEMA)

Angioedema often involves the lips and is characterized by a sudden diffuse swelling. The swelling, although edematous, is usually somewhat firm and nonpitting (Fig. 33-23). Any tissue may be involved, and multiple lesions have also been reported. Usually only one lip is involved; however, the whole face occasionally may be swollen. Of special concern is swelling of areas such as the tongue, uvula, and larynx, which may lead to respiratory distress.

Angioedema is currently divided into two types, hereditary and nonhereditary. The latter is much more common; unfortunately, in more than 70% of the cases the cause is unknown. Food and drugs can occasionally be incriminated by allergen testing, whereas such causes as psychologic problems and endocrine imbalance have little supportive evidence. Buckley and Mathews (1982) classified the etiologies as follows: IgE mediated, complement mediated, idiosyncratic reactions, and idiopathic. The uncommon hereditary form fits into the complement-mediated group and results from a quantitative or functional defect of C1 inhibitor (Stoppa-Lyonnet et al., 1987). This type of angioedema is inherited as an autosomal dominant trait.

In all types of angioedema the clinical manifestations are similar. In some cases the swelling may last only several hours, but in others it may last as long as 3 days. Accompanying generalized urticaria may be present in approximately 50% of the cases. Recurrence is common, and the intervals are greatly variable, probably depending on exposure to the precipitating factors.

After clinical swellings develop, the standard drug of choice for treatment has been the antihistamine. Obviously, for the nonhereditary type the offending allergen should be identified if possible and eliminated. Hereditary angioedema is often precipitated by trauma; dental

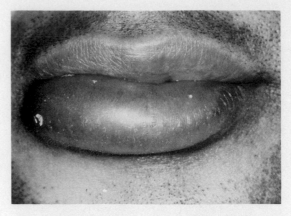

Fig. 33-23. Angioedema. The swelling developed quickly and was present for only 2 hours before this photograph was taken.

extractions frequently are implicated. Since not all trauma can be eliminated, several types of drugs have been effective as prophylactics. Antifibrinolytic agents such as epsilon aminocaproic acid are one type, whereas the other agents are androgens. Danazol, a synthetic androgen, was tested in clinical trials with excellent results (Gelfand et al., 1976).

DIFFERENTIAL DIAGNOSIS

Infections, sarcoidosis, Melkersson-Rosenthal syndrome, cheilitis glandularis, and cheilitis granulomatosa are the conditions likely to be confused with angioedema. The sudden onset and a history of recurrent episodes are major differentiating features. The diffuse character of the swelling should also help rule out smaller, well-demarcated mucoceles.

LIPOMA

Lipoma is a rather rare lesion of the oral cavity, but it occasionally occurs on the mucosal aspect of the lips (Zussman et al., 1988). It is a neoplasm composed of mature adipose tissue. It may occur as a sessile or pedunculated mass covered by atrophic epithelium with the underlying adipose tissue often giving the lesion a yellowish appearance. Lipomas are soft and sometimes almost fluctuant to palpation; therefore they are often confused on clinical examination with cystic lesions or mucoceles. Excisional biopsy is the treatment of choice. Recurrence is rare.

DIFFERENTIAL DIAGNOSIS

Soft traumatic fibromas and mucoceles are the most common lesions to be confused with a

lipoma. Variation in size may indicate a mucocele, but a biopsy is necessary to distinguish a
lipoma from a traumatic fibroma. Other soft tissue neoplasms and salivary gland tumors are
usually more firm to palpation. Malignant tumors of adipose tissue (liposarcomas) may also
appear yellowish and must be ruled out.

SALIVARY GLAND TUMORS

As discussed in other areas of this text, tumors of the minor salivary glands occur most
commonly on the palate, buccal mucosa, and
tongue. Occurrence on the lips appears to account for approximately 5% of these tumors,
with most of these occurring on the upper lip.
Almost all types of both benign and malignant
salivary tumors have been reported to occur on
the lips with little difference in their clinical
appearance.

Salivary gland tumors appear as either soft or
firm masses, with most having a nodular, exophytic component (Fig. 33-24). Ulceration of
the nodular mass may occur, but the presence
of the ulcer gives no clues as to the benign or
malignant nature of the tumor. Those that are
soft to palpation usually have large cystic cavities and an abundance of mucin. The more
solid tumors, both benign and malignant, and
especially benign mixed tumors with large
amounts of bone and cartilage, are firm to palpation.

One salivary gland tumor, monomorphic adenoma, deserves special discussion in relation
to its frequent location on the upper lip. Almost 90% of monomorphic adenomas, especially the canalicular adenoma, occur on or
near the upper lip, and the majority of the
cases are near the midline (Daley et al., 1984;
Nelson and Jacoway, 1973).

Most salivary gland tumors grow slowly and
often exist for years before treatment is sought.
Rapid growth or a sudden change in growth are
more consistent with malignant tumors or benign tumors that have undergone malignant
change. Since there is no good method of clinically differentiating salivary gland tumors from
other soft tissue tumors, cysts, or reactive lesions of the lip, biopsy is mandatory for diagnosis.

MINOR SALIVARY GLAND CALCULI

Sialolithiasis of the major salivary glands is a
well-known entity; however, similar mineral-
izations may occur in ducts of minor glands and
are thought to be more common than reported
in the literature. Anneroth and Hansen (1983)
reviewed 49 cases and found them to occur pri-

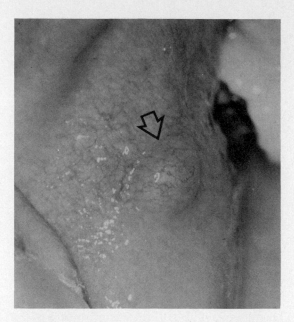

Fig. 33-24. Benign mixed tumor on the labial mucosa near the commissure.

marily in the upper lip of patients in the fifth to
seventh decades. Most appeared as firm to
hard, movable, submucosal nodules (see Fig.
28-17). The lesions varied from 3 to 15 mm in
diameter; the majority were less than 5 mm in
diameter. Etiologic factors include morphologic
features of the involved duct and local trauma.
Excisional biopsy is the treatment of choice,
since on clinical examination alone a submucosal nodule could represent a variety of soft
tissue tumors.

NASOLABIAL CYST (NASOALVEOLAR CYST)

The nasolabial cyst is a nonodontogenic fissural cyst found in the upper lip or soft tissues
of the face inferior to the nose in the nasolabial
fold. It is developmental in origin and thought
to be derived either from epithelial remnants
of the nasolacrimal duct or from entrapment of
epithelial rests during the fusion of the globular
portion of the medial nasal process and the
maxillary process. Therefore the cyst lies entirely within soft tissue and exhibits no radiographic abnormalities. It appears to be slightly
more common in females, with no preference
for right or left sides. Occasionally it is found
bilaterally.

On clinical examination the cyst appears as a
fullness of the nasal vestibule. If it enlarges inferiorly, it may appear to be originating in the
lip, whereas in other instances it may appear as

a swelling in the floor of the nose. The cyst is usually asymptomatic and rarely recurs following surgical removal. On histologic study the lining epithelium may range from cuboidal to squamous to respiratory.

DIFFERENTIAL DIAGNOSIS

In the lip this lesion must be distinguished from lesions of pulpal origin, for example, periapical cyst, granuloma, or abscess. Vitality tests of adjacent teeth help in the differential diagnosis. Radiographs should also aid in ruling out pulp-related or odontogenic cysts. Epidermal inclusion cysts, sebaceous cysts, and salivary gland tumors must be ruled out by biopsy.

PLASMA CELL CHEILITIS

Plasma cell cheilitis is an uncommon entity that deserves brief mention as a possible cause of a diffuse erythematous swelling of the lip. Baughman et al. (1974) reported such a case in a 65-year-old woman and found four other, similar cases in the literature. All were in elderly patients, and all had extensive plasma cell infiltrates in the lesions. Plasmacytoma and multiple myeloma were ruled out, leaving a benign inflammatory lesion with an abundance of plasma cells. Similar lesions of the gingiva had previously been investigated by Kerr et al. (1971) and were found to be caused by ingredients in chewing gum. Baughman's patient, however, exhibited no contact allergy with patch testing and elimination programs. The authors postulated that mechanical irritation or actinic damage acted as a stimulant to the immune system, thus provoking the plasma cell response. The lip lesions are analogous to balanitis of Zoon.

CHEILITIS GLANDULARIS

Cheilitis glandularis is a relatively rare inflammatory disease affecting the lower lip. In the early stages the mucosal surface reveals numerous dilated salivary duct orifices surrounded by a red macular area. Patients occasionally note a mucous secretion at the orifice of the ducts. As the condition progresses, the labial glands may become enlarged, which may cause the lip to become everted (Fig. 33-25). There may be either a superficial inflammatory process or a deep-seated infection. These variations have caused authors to divide this disease into three types, simple, superficial suppurative (Baelz's disease), and deep suppurative (cheilitis glandularis apostematosa). The latter two may cause the lip to become crusted and ulcerated with resultant scarring. The con-

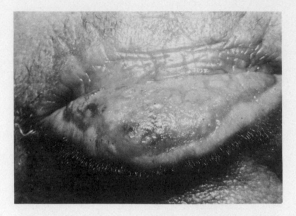

Fig. 33-25. Cheilitis glandularis. The elderly patient had persistent swelling and drainage of the lower lip.

dition is reported to occur most commonly in adult white men; however, occasionally cases are reported in children, blacks, and women.

Although the cause is not completely understood, it is thought that chronic exposure to sun or the elements induces inflammation of the labial salivary glands (Swerlick and Cooper, 1984). Other proposed etiologic factors include bacteria, tobacco, poor oral hygiene, hereditary factors, and even emotional disturbances. Cases of squamous carcinoma arising in cheilitis glandularis have been reported, but the condition is still not considered premalignant. Because of the potential for malignant transformation, surgical stripping or vermilionectomy is the recommended treatment in advanced cases (Oliver and Pickett, 1980).

Differential diagnosis includes angioedema, sarcoidosis, and cheilitis granulomatosa.

CHEILITIS GRANULOMATOSA (MIESCHER'S SYNDROME)

Cheilitis granulomatosa is characterized by a diffuse, soft swelling that develops slowly and may persist for months or years. It is seen most commonly on the lower lip, which is usually of normal color and asymptomatic (Fig. 33-26). Cheilitis granulomatosa may occur alone or in association with facial paralysis and fissured (plicated) tongue. This is referred to as the Melkersson-Rosenthal syndrome. Oliver and Pickett (1980) and Greene and Rogers (1989) reviewed the syndrome; Worsaae and Pindborg (1980) have included gingival enlargement as an occasional occurrence.

Histologic examination reveals the presence of noncaseating granulomas complete with Langhans giant cells. It has not been possible to identify any specific organism or to demon-

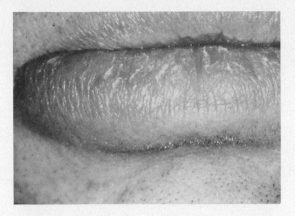

Fig. 33-26. Cheilitis granulomatosa. This patient had persistent swelling of the lower lip for 1 month. Biopsy revealed granuloma formation.

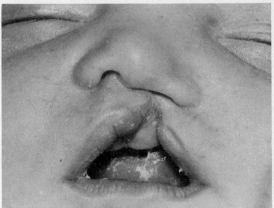

A

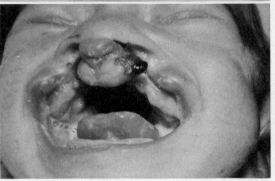

B

Fig. 33-27. Cleft lip. **A,** Unilateral incomplete cleft. **B,** Bilateral complete clefts. (**A** courtesy James Lowe, DDS, Kansas City, Mo. **B** courtesy Matt Hourigan, DDS, Kansas City, Mo.)

strate a relationship to sarcoidosis, which it resembles histologically. Radiation therapy, corticosteroids, and surgery have been used as a treatment with limited success. Recent studies have shown that elimination of infections, such as periodontitis, may reduce the swelling or cause it to disappear.

Differential diagnosis includes angioedema and sarcoidosis. Angioedema usually appears more suddenly and possibly has a history of repeated episodes. Sarcoidosis may be excluded by the absence of any of its other manifestations or by a negative Kveim test. A paper by Brook et al. (1983) investigated a case of granulomatous cheilitis in a patient with Crohn's disease of the lower intestinal tract. He believed that the lip lesions in granulomatous cheilitis are part of wider disease process, which in some cases includes Crohn's disease.

Developmental abnormalities

CLEFT LIP

Cleft lip is a relatively common defect that occurs in approximately 1 in 655 to 1200 births. The cleft is limited to the upper lip, where it represents failure of complete fusion of the maxillary, lateral nasal, and medial nasal processes. Animal studies have shown that there is inadequate mesodermal penetration in the areas of the clefts, which results in destruction of the overlying ectoderm.

Clefts may be unilateral or bilateral (Fig. 33-27). Unilateral clefts are much more common and have a predisposition for the left side. They are also slightly more common in males. Cleft lips occur more frequently in association

with cleft palate than alone. When the clefts extend through the lip and nostril and toward the palate, they are termed *complete.*

Incomplete clefts do not extend into the nostril. Complete clefts are more common in both the unilateral and bilateral types.

The cause of clefts of the lip and palate remains unknown; however, heredity is probably the single most important factor. No single gene has been identified, and most believe that the defect is polygenic. Numerous animal studies have shown that nutritional deficiencies and administration of certain drugs induce clefts. Nutritional deficiencies probably do not cause clefts in humans; however, some studies support the drug theory. Steroids (hydrocortisone) have long been suspected to cause clefts in humans. It has been postulated that emotional stress during pregnancy releases hydrocortisone from the adrenal cortex, which crosses the placental barrier and induces clefts. This has been refuted in a study by Fraser and Warburton (1964). Numerous drugs have also been implicated, including diazepam (Valium), one of

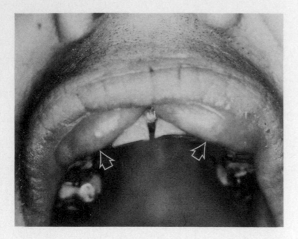

Fig. 33-28. Double lip.

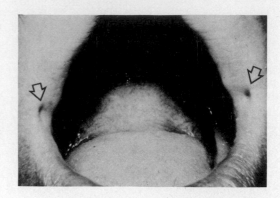

Fig. 33-29. Commissural lip pits.

the most widely prescribed medications. Local factors, such as a decreased blood supply or infections, have also been postulated.

Treatment is complex, especially in complete clefts with palatal involvement. Such cases are usually handled by a team of specialists from dentistry, plastic surgery, speech therapy, and psychology. Incomplete cleft lips are usually corrected surgically; surgery often begins as soon as the baby has regained original birth weight.

DOUBLE LIP (ASCHER'S SYNDROME)

Double lip is a developmental abnormality usually seen on the upper lip; however, both lips may be involved (Fig. 33-28). It consists of redundant tissue and is of no serious consequence other than having cosmetic considerations. It may occur alone or in association with other oral clefts. Rintala and Ranta (1981) discussed confusion of the double lip with developmental grooves.

Ascher's syndrome includes a double lip associated with thyroid enlargement and drooping of the upper eyelid (blepharochalasis).

LOWER LIP SINUSES (LIP PITS, COMMISSURAL PITS AND FISTULAS)

Lower lip sinuses are congenital or developmental defects that occur as singular anomalies or more often in conjunction with cleft lip or cleft palate. These entities are also discussed in Chapter 13. The defects appear as a unilateral depression or more frequently as bilateral depressions or grooves. They are found at the vermilion border of the lower lip (lip pits) or at the commissures (commissural pits) (Fig. 33-29). The upper lip is infrequently affected. The pits or sinuses are thought to represent embryonic remnants of sulci and fissures. Autosomal dominant transmission has been reported in some studies. Rintala and Ranta (1981) brought attention to transverse sulcuslike grooves in the lip, which may be interpreted as a double lower lip. They interpreted this as a variant of the lip sinus. The sinuses or pits end as blind tracts and usually require no surgical intervention. The commissural pits are considerably more common than lip pits, which occur in 1 of 2 million births according to Gorlin et al. (1976).

REFERENCES

Anneroth G and Hansen LS: Minor salivary gland calculi: a clinical and histopathological study of forty-nine cases, Int J Oral Surg 12:80-89, 1983.

Antoon JW and Miller RL: Aphthous ulcers—a review of the literature on etiology, pathogenesis, diagnosis and treatment, J Am Dent Assoc 101:803-808, 1980.

Archard HO, Heck JW, and Stanley HR: Focal epithelial hyperplasia: an unusual oral mucosal lesion found in Indian children, Oral Surg 20:201-212, 1965.

Baughman RD, Berger P, and Pringle WM: Plasma cell cheilitis, Arch Dermatol 110:725-726, 1974.

Beaudenon A et al: A new type of human papillomavirus associated with oral focal epithelial hyperplasia, J Invest Dermatol 88:130-135, 1987.

Berry HH and Landwerlen JR: Cigarette smoker's lip lesion in psychiatric patients, J Am Dent Assoc 86:657-662, 1973.

Brook IM, King DJ, and Miller ID: Chronic granulomatous cheilitis and its relationship to Crohn's disease, Oral Surg 56:405-408, 1983.

Buchner A and Hansen LS: Melanotic macule of the oral mucosa: a clinicopathologic study of 105 cases, Oral Surg 48:244-249, 1979.

Buchner A and Hansen LS: Pigmented nevi of the oral mucosa: a clinicopathologic study of 32 new cases and review of 75 cases from the literature. I. A clinicopathologic study of 32 new cases, Oral Surg 48:131-142, 1979.

Buckley RH and Mathews KP: Common "allergic" skin disease, JAMA (Primer on allergic and immunologic diseases) 248:2611-2622, 1982.

Clark WH, Jr, From L, Bernardino EA, and Mihm, MC: The histogenesis and biologic behavior of primary human malignant melanomas of the skin, Cancer Res 29:705-715, 1969.

Clark WH, Jr, Goldman LI, and Mastrangelo MJ: Human malignant melanoma, New York, 1979, Grune & Stratton, Inc.

Corey L and Spear PG: Infections with herpes simplex viruses, N Engl J Med 314:686-691, 749-757, 1986.

Daley TD, Gardner DG, and Smout MS: Canalicular adenoma: not a basal cell adenoma, Oral Surg 57:181-188, 1984.

Douglass CW and Gammon MD: Reassessing the epidemiology of lip cancer, Oral Surg 57:631-642, 1984.

Douglas JM et al: A double-blind study of oral acyclovir for suppression of recurrences of genital herpes simplex virus infection, N Engl J Med 310:1551-1556, 1984.

Eversole LR et al: Oral Kaposi's sarcoma associated with acquired immunodeficiency syndrome among homosexual males, J Am Dent Assoc 107:248-253, 1983.

Finne K, Goransson K, and Winckler L: Oral lichen planus and contact allergy to mercury, Int J Oral Surg 11:236-238, 1982.

Fraser F and Warburton D: No association of emotional stress or vitamin supplement during pregnancy to cleft lip or palate in man, Plast Reconstr Surg 33:395, 1964.

Gelfand JA, Sherins RJ, Alling DW, and Frank MM: Treatment of hereditary angioedema with danazol: reversal of clinical and biochemical abnormalities, N Engl J Med 295:1444-1448, 1976.

Glezerman M et al: Placebo-controlled trial of topical interferon in labial and genital herpes, Lancet 8578:150-152, 1988.

Gorlin RJ, Pindborg JJ, and Cohen MM, Jr: Syndromes of the head and neck, ed 2, New York, 1976, McGraw-Hill Book Co.

Greene RM and Rogers III RS: Melkersson-Rosenthal syndrome: a review of 36 patients, J Am Acad Dermatol 21:1263-1270, 1989.

Greer RO, Jr, and Poulson TC: Oral tissue alterations associated with the use of smokeless tobacco by teenagers. I. Clinical findings, Oral Surg 56:275-284, 1983.

Kerr DA, McClatchey KD, and Regezi JA: Allergic gingivostomatitis (due to gum chewing), J Periodontol 42:709-712, 1971.

LaBanc J and Epker BN: Lesch-Nyhan syndrome: surgical treatment in a case with lip chewing, J Maxillofac Surg 9:64-67, 1981.

La Riviere W and Pickett AB: Clinical criteria in diagnosis of early squamous cell carcinoma of the lower lip, J Am Dent Assoc 99:972-977, 1979.

Lozada F and Silverman S, Jr: Erythema multiforme: clinical characteristics and natural history in fifty patients, Oral Surg 46:628-636, 1978.

Nelson JF and Jacoway JR: Monomorphic adenoma (canalicular type): report of 29 cases, Cancer 31:1511-1513, 1973.

Oliver ID and Pickett AB: Cheilitis glandularis, Oral Surg 49:526-529, 1980.

Praetorius-Clausen F: Geographical aspects of oral focal epithelial hyperplasia, Path Microbiol 39:204-213, 1973.

Raborn JS et al: Oral acyclovir and herpes labialis: a randomized double-blind, placebo-controlled study, J Am Dent Assoc 115:38-42, 1987.

Reade PC et al: Cheilo-candidosis—a possible clinical entity, Br Dent J 152:305-308, 1982.

Rennie JS et al: Recurrent aphthous stomatitis, Br Dent J 159:361-367, 1985.

Rintala AE and Ranta R: Lower lip sinuses: epidemiology, microforms and transverse sulci, Br J Plast Surg 34:26-30, 1981.

Rogers RS III: Recurrent aphthous stomatitis: clinical characteristics and evidence for an immunopathogenesis, J Invest Dermatol 69:499-509, 1977.

Sewerin I: A clinical and epidemiologic study: morsicatio buccarum/labiorum, Scand J Dent Res 79:73-80, 1971.

Silverman S Jr, Gorsky M, and Lozada-Nur F: A prospective follow-up study of 570 patients with oral lichen planus: persistence, remission, and malignant association, Oral Surg 60:30-34, 1985.

Silverman S Jr et al: Oral findings in people with or at high risk for AIDS: a study of 375 homosexual males, J Am Dent Assoc 112:187-192, 1986.

Stoppa-Lyonnet D et al: Altered C1-inhibitor genes in type I hereditary angioedema, N Engl J Med 317:1-6, 1987.

Straus SE et al: Herpes simplex virus infection: biology, treatment, and prevention (NIH conference), Ann Intern Med 103:404-419, 1985.

Swerlick RA and Cooper PH: Cheilitis glandularis: a re-evaluation, J Am Acad Dermatol 10:466-472, 1984.

Tomich CE and Shafer WG: Squamous acanthoma of the oral mucosa, Oral Surg 38:755-759, 1974.

Weathers DR et al: The labial melanotic macule, Oral Surg 42:196-205, 1976.

Weathers DR and Callihan MD: Giant-cell fibroma, Oral Surg 37:374-384, 1974.

Winn DM et al: Snuff dipping and oral cancer among women in the southern United States, N Engl J Med 304:745-749, 1981.

Worsaae N and Pindborg JJ: Granulomatous gingival manifestations of Melkersson-Rosenthal syndrome, Oral Surg 49:131-138, 1980.

Zussman KM, Correll RW, and Schott TR: Large nonpainful swelling of the lower lip, J Am Dent Assoc 117:849-850, 1988.

34 Intraoral lesions by anatomic region

DANNY R. SAWYER
NORMAN K. WOOD

One of the purposes of this textbook is to teach the student and fledgling clinician how to arrive at a logical differential diagnosis when a lesion or condition is encountered in everyday practice. The text has done this, in part, by helping the reader arrange his or her knowledge of lesions by grouping disease entities according to clinical or radiographic appearance. This chapter, in addition to those that discuss the lip, face, and neck, attempts to aid the student and clinician in arriving at a sound differential diagnosis by considering that certain lesions have a predilection for specific anatomic sites. This approach has been found to be helpful in the past and has been incorporated in other textbooks. In listing lesions by anatomic sites, an attempt has been made to rank lesions according to frequency. On occasion this may be objectionable to some experts in the various fields of dentistry, and we certainly claim no inerrant authority. In developing the list of lesions by areas according to frequency we have consulted many sources including other textbooks, journal articles, computer-determined statistical rankings, and several authorities. The lists are not exhaustive, and the very rare lesions are listed only as "Rarities." It should be recognized in surveying this listing that certain common lesions or, particularly, variations of common lesions may be more commonly seen by a clinician in general practice than by an oral pathologist who bases observations of the frequency of lesions primarily on his or her biopsy service. Further, the frequency of specific lesions is known to vary from one geographic location to another. Thus any particular lesion may be very common in New York City, less common in Foyet, Ontario, Canada, and rare in Ogbomosho, Nigeria. With this in mind, in the remainder of this chapter we present first a brief listing and discussion of the normal ana-

tomic structures of one of the several areas into which the intraoral environment has been divided for the purpose of this encounter. This is followed by a brief list of the more common pathologic lesions of this anatomic location. For the purpose of this book the intraoral environment has been divided into the following anatomic locations:

1. Labial and buccal mucosa and vestibule
2. Gingiva and alveolar mucosa
3. Palate (hard and soft)
4. Oropharynx (fauces, pharynx, and retromolar region)
5. Tongue (dorsal and lateral surfaces)
6. Tongue (ventral surface)
7. Floor of the mouth

LABIAL AND BUCCAL MUCOSA AND VESTIBULE
Anatomic structures
1. Frenum attachments—midline and lateral (labial and vestibular mucosa)
2. Stensen's (parotid) papilla (buccal mucosa)
3. Linea alba (buccal mucosa)
4. Fordyce's granules (labial and buccal mucosa)

Normally the texture of the labial mucosa is smooth, soft, and resilient. The color of this mucosa is normally pink to brown depending on the presence of racial pigmentation. This area is well endowed with vascularity and minor salivary glands. This labial mucosa is commonly traumatized. Thus because of the rich minor salivary gland component, mucoceles are seen with some degree of frequency. Cheek biting or chewing is also rather common. These last two statements are apropos because the student and fledgling clinician must keep in mind what structures are contained in the mucosa of the area of a lesion, as well as the patient's habits, since they may relate to a lesion presented for diagnosis. The texture of the buccal mucosa is similar to that of the labial mucosa, being soft and smooth to granular. It may feel granular because of a rich supply of sebaceous glands, as well as minor salivary glands, in this mucosa. The buccal fat pad may appear prominent, especially in young patients. In whites the color of the buccal mucosa is normally pink, but in persons of the dark-skinned races it may appear blue to blue gray. In blacks there may be a patchy distribution to the pigmentation and the coloration may be more brown to black than blue to blue gray. The oral mucous membrane of the vestibule is thin, and the many small vascular channels are easily observed. The more common lesions of the labial and buccal mucosa and vestibule are listed below; detailed discussions of them are found elsewhere in the text.

Common lesions

1. Fordyce's granules (may be considered a normal variation)
2. Leukoedema (may be considered a normal variation)
3. Cheek biting or chewing
4. Recurrent aphthous ulcers
5. Traumatic ulcers
6. Inflammatory hyperplastic lesions (pyogenic granulomas, fibrous hyperplasias)
7. Leukoplakia and snuff dipper's lesion
8. Lichen planus
9. Mucous retention phenomenon (mucocele)
10. Varix
11. Epulis fissuratum (of denture wearers)
12. Draining sinus of periapical abscess
13. Amalgam tattoo
14. Aspirin burn
15. Hemangioma
16. Squamous cell carcinoma
17. Salivary gland neoplasms
18. White sponge nevus
19. Traumatic neuromas
20. Benign mesenchymal lesions
21. Rarities

GINGIVA AND ALVEOLAR MUCOSA
Anatomic structures
1. Retrocuspid papillae
2. Frenum attachments

The oral mucous membrane continues from the vestibular sulcus over the tooth-supporting bone. This portion of the oral mucosa may be divided into (1) the alveolar mucosa, which is the zone adjacent to the vestibule and (2) the zone adjacent to the teeth, which is the gingiva. The gingiva may be subdivided into the attached gingiva and the free gingiva. The surface of the attached gingiva is generally stippled in healthy patients, although the degree of stippling varies. The free gingival margins and borders of the interdental papillae are smooth. The alveolar mucosa is more delicate in texture, more mobile, and darker red than the gingiva because of a greater vascular supply and because the covering epithelium is nonkeratinized. The alveolar mucosa, unlike the stippled gingival mucosa, is smooth. The normal color of the attached and free gingivae is pink in whites, but again darker pigmentation may be observed in persons of the dark-skinned races. Normally, no minor salivary glands are present in the gingiva. Thus the clinician would not consider a salivary gland lesion of the gingiva at the top of the list in a differential diagnosis.

Common lesions

1. Gingivitis
   a. Localized (localized with periodontitis)
      (1) Related to poor oral hygiene
         (a) Microorganisms
         (b) Calculus
         (c) Food impaction
      (2) Related to restorations or appliances
      (3) Related to mouth-breathing
      (4) Related to tooth alignment
      (5) Related to drugs or chemicals
   b. Generalized (generalized with periodontitis)
      (1) Nonspecific (related to poor oral hygiene and plaque)
      (2) Acute necrotizing ulcerative gingivitis (ANUG)
      (3) Nutrition-related (scurvy)
      (4) Drug-related (phenytoin [Dilantin])
      (5) Hormonal (pregnancy, diabetes, endocrine dysfunctions)
      (6) Allergy-related
      (7) Hereditary (fibromatosis gingivae, although not always hereditary)
      (8) Related to psychotic phenomenon
      (9) Specific granulomatous disease
      (10) Neoplastic (leukemia)
      (11) Desquamative gingivitis and vesiculobullous disease(s)
2. Tori and exotoses
3. Amalgam tattoo
4. Recurrent herpes
5. Pyogenic granuloma
6. Fibrous hyperplasia or fibroma
7. Periodontal abscess

8. Periapical abscess
9. Parulis
10. Peripheral giant cell granuloma
11. Eruption cyst, dental lamina cyst, or gingival cyst
12. Leukoplakia, speckled leukoplakia, or erythroplakia
13. Squamous cell carcinomas
14. Congenital epulis
15. Plasma cell gingivitis
16. Rarities

PALATE (HARD AND SOFT)
Anatomic structures
1. Palatine midline raphe
2. Palatine papilla
3. Rugae
4. Fovea palatinae
5. Small nodules of tonsillar tissue

The mucous membrane covering the anterior hard palate is orthokeratinized and firmly attached to the underlying bone. On the posterior hard palate lateral to the raphe the submucosa contains numerous nerves, blood vessels, and mucous salivary glands. It is in this portion of the hard palate that one would expect to see the majority of minor salivary gland tumors arising, and this holds true. These lateral areas of the posterior hard palate may be soft to palpation because of the presence of fat and mucous glands. The hard palate is normally light pink but may have a bluish gray hue. The soft palate begins posterior to an imaginary line running laterally near the fovea palatinae, which are openings for the common ducts of groups of minor salivary glands in this region. The soft palate extends posteriorly into a thick pendant of mucous membrane known as the uvula. This mucosa of the soft palate is thin and nonkeratinized. The mucosa is quite vascular and may give a slightly darker red color to the soft palate than one sees in the hard palate. There is considerable fat tissue in the soft palate, and if this tissue is prominent, the mucosa may take on a pale yellow color. The texture is generally smooth but punctuated by the openings from numerous salivary glands. Again, as with the posterior lateral aspect of the hard palate, these mucous salivary glands may give rise to occasional salivary gland tumors.

Common lesions
1. Torus
2. Draining sinus from periapical abscess
3. Traumatic ulcers
4. Nicotine stomatitis
5. Candidiasis
6. Inflammatory papillary hyperplasia
7. Herpes (hard palate)
8. Recurrent aphthous ulcers (soft palate)
9. Minor salivary gland tumors (posterior hard palate)
10. Cleft palate or bifid uvula
11. Leukoplakia, speckled leukoplakia or erythroplakia
12. Squamous cell carcinoma (soft palate)
13. Oroantral fistula
14. Median anterior maxillary cyst
15. Median palatal cyst
16. Exophytic bony lesions of the hard palate
17. Benign mesenchymal tumors
18. Necrotizing sialometaplasia
19. Atypical lymphoproliferative disease
20. Rarities

OROPHARYNX (FAUCES, PHARYNX, AND RETROMOLAR REGION)
Anatomic structures
1. Retromolar pad
2. Pterygomandibular raphe
3. Tonsillar pillars
   a. Palatoglossal arch—anterior
   b. Palatopharyngeal arch—posterior
4. Tonsillar fossa
5. Posterior wall of pharynx
6. Waldeyer's ring (adenoids, nasopharyngeal tonsils, pharyngeal bands, palatine tonsils, and lingual tonsils)

The oropharynx and fauces show remarkable variation in size and form. The amount of lymphoid tissue in Waldeyer's ring and the size of this tissue vary among people and from time to time in the same person. Lymphoid tissue not only enlarges in response to such things as infections but also tends to gradually decrease in size with age. The mucosal surface of this area is normally soft, moist, and smooth with small elevations that represent the scattered aggregates of lymphoid tissue that are seen in this location. The mucosa is normally bright pink because of the prominent vascularity. Vascular dilation may give the mucosa a red appearance.

Common lesions
1. Nonspecific viral inflammatory disease
2. Nonspecific bacterial inflammatory disease
3. Enlarged tonsils
4. Recurrent aphthous ulcers
5. Traumatic ulcers
6. Inflammatory fibrous hyperplasias or fibroma

7. Leukoplakia, speckled leukoplakia, or erythroplakia
8. Squamous cell carcinoma
9. Herpes
10. Herpangina
11. Pemphigus or other dermatologic disorders
12. Rarities

TONGUE (DORSAL AND LATERAL SURFACES)
Anatomic structures
1. Fungiform papillae
2. Filiform papillae
3. Foliate papillae
4. Circumvallate papillae
5. Median sulcus
6. Terminal sulcus
7. Lingual tonsil tissue

The dorsal surface of the tongue has an oral mucous membrane that is thick and keratinized and contains papillae, some of which bear taste buds. Mucous and serous glands are present, as is lymphoid tissue (lingual tonsil). Posteriorly there is rich innervation, and vascularity is prominent throughout the surface. The dorsal surface is fairly uniform in appearance, soft and pinkish, and shows little or no racial variation. The lateral border of the tongue usually shows a rather sharp contrast in texture and color to the dorsal and ventral surfaces. The color is normally a deeper red on the lateral aspect than on the dorsal surface.

Common lesions
1. Geographic
2. Fissured
3. Traumatic ulcer
4. Recurrent aphthous ulcers
5. Inflammatory hyperplasias
6. Hemangioma
7. Leukoplakia, speckled leukoplakia, or erythroplakia
8. Median rhomboid glossitis—*Candida*
9. Lichen planus
10. Herpes
11. Hyperplastic lingual tonsil
12. Hairy tongue
13. Bald tongue—vitamin, iron deficiency
14. Squamous cell carcinoma (lateral border)
15. Granular cell myoblastoma
16. Neurofibromatosis
17. Syphilis
18. Macroglossia—amyloid, hypothyroidism, angioneurotic edema
19. Lingual thyroid nodule
20. Rarities

TONGUE (VENTRAL SURFACE)
Anatomic structure
1. Lingual frenum

The mucous membrane of the ventral surface of the tongue is thin and smooth. It is closely adherent to the musculature of the tongue. The normal color varies from red to pink. On this lingual surface the veins may be large and prominent, imparting a bluish color to the ventral surface.

Common lesions
1. Lingual varices
2. Ankyloglossia
3. Traumatic ulcer
4. Leukoplakia, speckled leukoplakia, or erythroplakia
5. Squamous cell carcinoma
6. Benign mesenchymal tumors
7. Mucous retention phenomenon
8. Rarities

FLOOR OF THE MOUTH
Anatomic structures
1. Sublingual folds or ridges—sublingual glands and ducts of the submandibular glands cause these elevations.
2. Sublingual caruncles—these papillae contain openings for the flow of saliva from Wharton's duct.
3. Openings from the ducts of numerous minor salivary glands
4. Genial tubercles
5. Mylohyoid ridge

The oral mucosa of the floor of the mouth is nonkeratinized, soft, and smooth. The mucosa is normally pink in this location. Racial differences are nonexistent to minimal. The degrees of vascularity and prominence vary.

Common lesions
1. Traumatic ulcers
2. Recurrent aphthous ulcers
3. Abscess
4. Leukoplakia, speckled leukoplakia, or erythroplakia
5. Mucous retention phenomenon (ranula)
6. Squamous cell carcinoma
7. Sialolithiasis and sialadenitis
8. Dermoid cyst
9. Salivary gland tumors
10. Lymphoepithelial cyst
11. Ludwig's angina
12. Rarities

A

Lesions of bone that may have two or more major radiographic appearances

	Completely radiolucent	Radiolucent and radiopaque	Completely radiopaque
Adenomatoid odontogenic tumor	Yes	Yes	No
Ameloblastoma and variants	Yes	Yes	No
Calcifying epithelial odontogenic tumor	Yes	Yes	No
Cementoblastoma	Yes	Yes	Yes
Chondroma	Yes	Yes	No
Chondrosarcoma	Yes	Yes	No
Ewing's sarcoma	Yes	Yes	No
Fibro-osseous lesions (PDLO)	Yes	Yes	Yes
Fibrous dysplasia	Yes	Yes	Yes
Giant cell granuloma	Yes	Yes	No
Hemangioma	Yes	Yes	No
Lymphosarcoma	Yes	Yes	No
Metastatic carcinoma	Yes	Yes	Yes
Odontogenic fibroma	Yes	Yes	No
Odontoma	Yes	Yes	Yes
Osteitis	Yes	Yes	Yes
Osteoblastoma	Yes	Yes	Yes
Osteomyelitis	Yes	Yes	Yes
Osteosarcoma	Yes	Yes	Yes
Paget's disease	Yes	Yes	Yes
Postsurgical bone defect	Yes	Yes	Yes
Proliferative periostitis	Yes	Yes	Yes
Reticulum cell sarcoma	Yes	Yes	No
Subperiosteal hematoma	Yes	Yes	Yes
Teeth	Yes	Yes	Yes

B

Normal values for laboratory tests*

I. Hematologic blood values (whole blood [EDTA])
   A. Red blood cell values
      1. Red blood cell count
         a. Male—4.5 to 6.0 million/mm^3
         b. Female—4.0 to 5.5 million/mm^3
         c. During pregnancy—greater than 3.6 million/mm^3
      2. Hemoglobin (Hbg) content
         a. Male—13.5 to 17.5 g/dl
         b. Female—12 to 16 g/dl
      3. Packed cell volume (PCV), or hematocrit
         a. Male—41% to 53%
         b. Female—36% to 46%
      4. Mean corpuscular volume (MCV)
         a. Male—82.2 to 100.6 μg^3
         b. Female—81.9 to 100.7 μg^3
      5. Mean corpuscular hemoglobin (MCH) content
         a. Male—28.4 to 32.0 pg
         b. Female—28.3 to 32.1 pg (MCH)
      6. Mean corpuscular hemoglobin concentration (MCHC)
         a. Male—32.7% to 35.1% (g/dl)
         b. Female—32.5% to 34.7% (g/dl)
   B. White blood cell values
      1. White blood cell count
         a. Infants—6000 to 17,500/mm^3 (first day of life—9400 to 34,000/mm^3)
         b. Adolescents—4500 to 13,500/mm^3
         c. Adults—4500 to 11,000/mm^3
      2. Differential white blood cell count
         a. Neutrophils—35% to 73%; 1680 to 7884/mm^3
         b. Lymphocytes—23% to 33%; 1500 to 3000/mm^3
         c. Monocytes—2% to 6%; 100 to 900/mm^3
         d. Eosinophils—1% to 3%; 50 to 450/mm^3
         e. Basophils—0% to 1%; 50 to 200/mm^3
   C. Bleeding and clotting abnormalities
      1. Platelets (whole blood [EDTA])—150,000-400,000/mm^3
      2. (Ivy) bleeding time (blood from skin)—2 to 7 min
      3. (Lee-White) clotting time (whole blood [no anticoagulant])—5 to 8 min
      4. Prothrombin time (one stage) (whole blood [no citrate])—12 to 14 sec
      5. Partial thromboplastin time (whole blood [no citrate])—25 to 30 sec
      6. Fibrinogen (whole blood [no citrate])—200 to 400 mg/dl
      7. Specific factor analysis (plasma [no citrate])
         a. Factor II assay—60% to 150% of normal, or 0.5 to 1.5 U/ml
         b. Factor V assay—60% to 150% of normal, or 0.5 to 2.0 U/ml
         c. Factor VII assay—65% to 135% of normal, or 60 to 135 AU
         d. Factor VIII assay—60% to 2145% of normal, or 60 to 145 AU
         e. Factor IX assay—60% to 140% of normal, or 60 to 140 AU
         f. Factor X assay—60% to 130% of normal, or 60 to 130 AU
      8. Prothrombin consumption test (whole blood [no anticoagulant])—greater than 30 sec

*Prepared by Paul W. Goaz. Compiled from: Wyngarden JB and Smith LH Jr: Cecil text book of medicine, ed 18, vol 2, Philadelphia, 1988, WB Saunders Co; Ravel R: Clinical laboratory medicine: Clinical application of laboratory data, Chicago, 1989, Year Book Medical Publishers, Inc; Halsted JA and Halsted CH: The laboratory in clinical medicine, ed 2, Philadelphia, 1981, WB Saunders Co.

9. Thrombin time (whole blood [no citrate])—control time (9 to 10 sec) ≠ 2 sec

II. Serum enzymes (serum)
   A. Serum glutamic oxaloacetic transaminase—15 to 40 U/L
   B. Serum glutamic pyruvic transaminase—15 to 35 U/L
   C. Lactate dehydrogenase—45 to 90 U/L
   D. Creatine phosphokinase—0 to 170 U/L
   E. Alkaline phosphatase
      1. Male—62 to 176 U/L
      2. Female—56 to 155 U/L
   F. Acid phosphatase
      1. Male—0.01 to 0.56 U/L
      2. Female—0.13 to 0.63 U/L
   G. Amylase—80 to 180 (Somogyi) U/dl
   H. Lipase
      1. Under 60 years of age—10 to 150 U/L
      2. Over 60 years of age—18 to 180 U/L
   I. Leucine aminopeptidase—8 to 200 (Goldbarg-Rutenbuirg) U/ml
   J. Cholinesterase—0.65 to 1.00 pH units or more per hour

III. Blood chemistry (serum)
   A. Calcium (total)—8.4 to 10.2 mg/dl
   B. Phosphorus—2.7 to 4.5 mg/dl
   C. Glucose
      1. Under 60 years of age—70 to 105 mg/dl
      2. Over 60 years of age—81 to 115 mg/dl
   D. Blood urea nitrogen—7 to 18 mg/dl
   E. Uric acid
      1. Male—3.5 to 7.2 mg/dl
      2. Female—2.6 to 6.0 mg/dl
   F. Cholesterol (plasma [no citrate] or serum) (EDTA)
      1. 20 to 29 years of age
         a. Male—Greater than 194 mg/dl
         b. Female—Greater than 184 mg/dl

      2. 30 to 39 years of age
         a. Male—Greater than 218 mg/dl
         b. Female—Greater than 202 mg/dl
      3. 40 to 49 years of age
         a. Male—Greater than 231 mg/dl
         b. Female—Greater than 223 mg/dl
      4. Over 50 years of age
         a. Male—Greater than 230 mg/dl
         b. Female—Greater than 252 mg/dl
   G. Protein (total)—6 to 8.4 g/dl
      1. Albumin—3.5 to 5.0 g/dl
      2. Globulin—2.3 to 3.5 g/dl
   H. Bilirubin (total)—0.5 to 1.2 mg/dl
      1. Conjugated (direct)—Up to 0.2 mg/dl
      2. Unconjugated (indirect)—0.1 to 1.0 mg/dl

IV. Serum electrolytes and blood gas
   A. Sodium—136 to 146 mEq/L
   B. Potassium—3.5 to 5.1 mEq/L
   C. Chloride—98 to 106 mEq/L
   D. Bicarbonate—18 to 23 mEq/L
   E. Po_2 (whole blood, arterial [heparin])—83 to 100 mm Hg
   F. Pco_2 (whole blood, arterial [heparin])—95 to 100 mm Hg
   G. pH (whole blood, arterial [heparin])—7.35 to 7.45

V. Urinalysis (random sample)
   A. pH—4.7 to 8.0 (mean 6.3)
   B. Specific gravity—1.016 to 1.022
   C. Protein—40 to 150 mg/24 hr (2 to 8 mg/dl)
   D. Ketones—Negative
   E. Bilirubin—0.02 mg/dl
   F. Blood—Negative
   G. Erythrocytes—0 to 1/HPF (high-power field)
   H. Leukocytes—0 to 5/HPF

C

Viral hepatitis

JAMES F. LEHNERT

Viral hepatitis is of particular concern to the dental practitioner because of the potential for infection of the dentist and his or her staff. In fact, dentists in the United States have been shown to be approximately three to five times (oral and maxillofacial surgeons approximately six times) more likely to be exposed to hepatitis B virus than is the general population (West, 1984). There are also reports of dentists transmitting hepatitis B to their patients (Ahtone and Goodman, 1983). Consequently, the practitioner must fully understand the epidemiologies and clinical courses of the various types of viral hepatitis, so that he or she can fully assess each patient who gives a positive history of having had hepatitis A, hepatitis B, hepatitis C, hepatitis D, or hepatitis non-A, non-B.

ACUTE VIRAL HEPATITIS

The majority of symptomatic cases of viral hepatitis fit into a classic pattern, which is described here as acute viral hepatitis. However, the range of clinical manifestations, laboratory findings, histopathologic changes, and sequelae of acute viral hepatitis is broad. Most cases resolve completely within 4 months after the onset of symptoms, but some end in fulminant disease and others progress to chronic hepatitis. This latter sequela may lead to cirrhosis or predispose the patient to primary hepatocellular carcinoma. For every clinically apparent case of acute viral hepatitis, there are several subclinical cases that remain undetected.

Symptoms and signs

Following exposure to viral hepatitis, a variable period of time ensues before the onset of symptoms. Depending on the infecting agent, this incubation period varies; for type A hepatitis it ranges from 2 to 6 weeks, for type B hepatitis, from 1 to 6 months, and for type non-A, non-B hepatitis, from 2 weeks to 6 months.

The onset of nonspecific symptoms marks the beginning of the prodromal or preicteric phase. These symptoms are often described as systemic, flulike complaints and may include malaise, nausea, vomiting, anorexia, myalgia, and right upper quadrant pain. In some patients there is a serum sickness–like reaction with fever, skin rash, and arthralgia; this reaction is more likely to occur with hepatitis B. The prodromal phase may last but a few days or as long as 2 weeks.

The icteric phase starts with the appearance of jaundice. The degree of jaundice varies with the severity of the disease but is usually moderate in acute viral hepatitis. Other symptoms include darkening of the urine and whitish stools. Physical findings at this time may include jaundice, an enlarged, tender liver, and splenomegaly. Usually some of the nonspecific symptoms start to resolve and the patient begins to feel better within a couple of weeks after the onset of jaundice (Hoofnagle, 1981). The icteric phase lasts about 4 to 6 weeks.

The disappearance of jaundice marks the beginning of the convalescent or recovery phase. The signs and symptoms of the prodromal and icteric phases gradually disappear, and abnormal laboratory findings (discussed in the next section) return to normal levels. Complete recovery usually occurs within 4 months after the onset of jaundice.

Laboratory tests

Several laboratory tests are available to aid in the diagnosis of acute viral hepatitis and to monitor hepatic dysfunction during the course of the disease. The abnormal laboratory findings reflect injury to the hepatocytes by the ongoing inflammatory process with subsequent disturbance of bilirubin metabolism.

Bilirubin is a breakdown product of hemoglobin that is metabolized in the liver and excreted in the bile. The normal plasma bilirubin level is less than 1 mg/dl. Jaundice, or yellowish staining of tissues, occurs when the plasma bilirubin level exceeds 3 mg/dl.

Liver function tests of particular concern are the serum aminotransferases. Alanine aminotransferase (ALT, formerly SGPT) and aspartate aminotransferase (AST, formerly SGOT) are specific, sensitive indicators of hepatocyte injury. In acute viral hepatitis their levels are usually elevated to 10 times normal. Other liver enzymes that may show mild elevations are alkaline phosphatase and lactic dehydrogenase.

The prothrombin time (PT), measurement of the extrinsic coagulation pathway, may be slightly prolonged in acute viral hepatitis. A significantly prolonged PT (greater than 20 seconds) is indicative of severe liver disease with extensive hepatocellular injury.

The white blood cell count may show leukopenia, leukocytosis, or atypical lymphocytes.

Tests to identify the specific serum antigens and antibodies associated with type A hepatitis and type B hepatitis are available. These tests are usually necessary to definitively diagnose hepatitis A or hepatitis B; they have also been used to aid in establishing the diagnosis of type non-A, non-B hepatitis by excluding the other two viral agents. The development of an assay for measuring antibodies to the blood-borne virus of non-A, non-B hepatitis has been reported (Kuo et al., 1989).

HEPATITIS A
Epidemiology

Type A hepatitis (infectious hepatitis) is caused by the hepatitis A virus (HAV). Transmission occurs via the fecal-oral route, usually through contaminated food or water. Thus hepatitis A is often associated with poor personal hygiene or overcrowded living conditions and has been shown to occur two to three times more frequently within the lower social classes (Szmuness et al., 1976). Although this disease may occur at any age, it is common in children, particularly those of primary and nursery school age (Balistreri, 1988). Type A hepatitis may occur as localized outbreaks or epidemics, and it accounts for approximately 20% to 30% of the sporadic cases (that is, no known exposure) of viral hepatitis.

Type A hepatitis is usually a mild, self-limiting disease that spontaneously resolves within a month. In some cases the clinical course is so mild and nonspecific that the patient does not seek medical treatment and the disease goes undiagnosed. Overall the mortality for type A disease is very low. The antibody response to the HAV infection confers lasting immunity. There are no chronic carriers or chronic disease states associated with type A hepatitis.

Serology

The average incubation period for hepatitis A is 4 weeks. Late in the incubation period, hepatitis A antigen (HA Ag) appears in the stool but usually disappears by the time, or shortly after, jaundice develops. During this time the disease is highly contagious. Serum aminotransferase (ALT and AST) levels rise rapidly during the prodromal phase, peaking in the early icteric phase, and then decline, returning to normal in the early convalescent phase. Although HAV is usually not detectable in the serum, shortly after the appearance of clinical symptoms there is a rising titer of hepatitis A antibody (anti-HAV). The anti-HAV initially

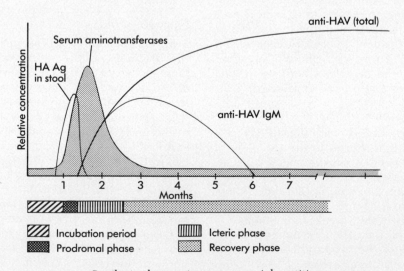

Serologic changes in acute type A hepatitis.

consists mainly of IgM, but after approximately 6 months it is replaced by IgG. Thus the presence of anti-HAV IgM is indicative of acute HAV infection. The figure on p. 694 illustrates these changes.

HEPATITIS B
Epidemiology

Type B hepatitis (serum hepatitis) is caused by the hepatitis B virus (HBV). The major mode of transmission of HBV is the parenteral route (for example, blood, blood products, and contaminated needles). However, it can also be transmitted through close personal contact, since HBV can be found in the saliva, semen, and vaginal secretions of an infected individual (Bernstein, 1980). The different modes of transmission may account for the wide range in the incubation period for type B hepatitis, 1 to 6 months, depending on its route of infection and the size of the inoculating dose. Unlike hepatitis A, type B disease is more common in adults. Groups considered at increased risk for HBV infection include health care professionals who work with blood, blood products, or body secretions; intravenous (IV) drug users; individuals with congenital coagulopathies (for example, factor VIII or IX deficiency); and sexually promiscuous individuals (for example, male homosexuals). Hepatitis B accounts for approximately 50% to 60% of the sporadic cases of viral hepatitis.

The HBV has three distinct antigens that elicit the production of corresponding antibodies in the infected individual. These antigen-antibody systems serve several purposes: (1) to establish or exclude the diagnosis of HBV as the etiologic agent, (2) to aid in determining whether the disease process is acute or chronic, (3) to serve as a prognostic indicator, and (4) to indicate a relative degree of infectivity.

Hepatitis B surface antigen (HBsAg, Australia antigen) is derived from the outer coating of the complete HBV, the Dane particle. The presence of HBsAg is indicative of either intact HBV or incomplete viral particles composed of HBsAg in the serum. Any individual whose test results are positive for HBsAg should be considered potentially infectious. Hepatitis B surface antibody (anti-HBs) is produced in response to HBsAg. The presence of serum anti-HBs, then, indicates prior HBV infection. Hepatitis B core antigen (HBcAg) is derived from the inner core of the complete HBV. HBcAg is not detectable in the serum. However, antibodies to HBcAg (anti-HBc) are, and

they consist of IgM and IgG subclasses (IgM initially, IgG later). Thus the presence of anti-HBc IgM is an indication of acute infection. The third antigen-antibody system associated with HBV infection is HBeAg and anti-HBe. The HBeAg is thought to be related to core antigen. The presence of HBeAg is associated with high viral activity, indicative of active liver disease and increased potential for infectivity. HBeAg is always found in association with HBsAg. During acute type B disease, the seroconversion of HBeAg to anti-HBe usually signals the onset of resolution of the disease (this seroconversion does not occur when acute hepatitis progresses to chronic hepatitis).

The onset of symptoms in acute type B hepatitis is usually more insidious than in type A disease. However, the course of the disease in hepatitis B is usually more severe and prolonged, and fatalities may range from 1% to 3% (Hoofnagle, 1981). Anti-HBs confers lifelong immunity to HBV infection.

Inapparent and chronic hepatitis

Two important features of type B hepatitis should be mentioned. Up to this point acute, symptomatic viral hepatitis has been considered. However, approximately 50% of the cases of type B hepatitis are asymptomatic throughout their course. Thus, despite a negative history for viral hepatitis or jaundice or both, an individual may be infectious during the subacute state associated with inapparent type B disease.

Second, as many as 10% of adults with type B hepatitis, inapparent or symptomatic, later have either the chronic carrier state or chronic hepatitis. Both sequelae are characterized by the persistence of serum HBsAg (for more than 6 months) with variable degrees of infectivity. The chronic HBsAg carrier is asymptomatic and has no clinical or biochemical evidence of liver disease. In addition to HBsAg, other antigens and antibodies associated with the HBV are also present. The chronic HBsAg carrier state may last for years, decades, or a lifetime. Chronic hepatitis B virus infection is characterized by continued mild to moderate symptoms and abnormal laboratory findings (for example, elevated serum aminotransferase levels). Depending on the infection's severity, physical findings may be present. The HBsAg is usually accompanied by HBeAg and anti-HBc. Chronic type B disease may be either chronic persistent or chronic active hepatitis. The former is more common than the latter, but a liver biopsy is often necessary to make the diagnosis. Chronic persistent hepatitis has a benign course with mild symptoms and only slightly elevated ALT and AST levels. It has a good prognosis and has not been shown to progress to chronic active hepatitis or cirrhosis. Chronic persistent hepatitis may eventually resolve, continue on indefinitely, or revert to the chronic HBsAg carrier state. Chronic active hepatitis, on the other hand, is a progressive, destructive inflammatory disease with fibrosis, which proceeds at a variable rate and may result in cirrhosis and, possibly, end-stage liver disease. Chronic active hepatitis may last for months or years, or it may revert to chronic persistent hepatitis.

Delta hepatitis

A potential complication of HBV infection is the development of delta hepatitis. Type D hepatitis is caused by the hepatitis delta virus (HDV), a defective RNA agent that requires the presence of HBsAg to replicate (Rizzetto et al., 1988). Development of screening tests for the delta antigen and its associated antibody has contributed to a better understanding of delta hepatitis. Acute delta hepatitis can occur as either a coinfection with acute hepatitis B or a superinfection, that is, an infection superimposed on the chronic HBsAg carrier state or chronic hepatitis B. The combined effects of HBV infection and acute delta hepatitis are associated with an increased mortality rate. Chronic delta hepatitis superimposed on chronic hepatitis B has been associated with severe, progressive liver disease (Rizzetto, 1983). Recovery from hepatitis B, with loss of HBsAg, also signals recovery from delta hepatitis. Individuals with anti-HBs are also immune to HDV infection.

Serology
ACUTE HEPATITIS B

The average incubation period for HBV infection is 75 days. Approximately 4 to 6 weeks before the onset of symptoms, HBsAg appears in the serum, followed by HBeAg, and their titers begin to rise. Shortly thereafter the serum aminotransferase levels start to increase. Late in the incubation period, anti-HBc appears and rises in titer. Usually the HBsAg titer and the serum aminotransferase levels continue to climb through the prodromal phase and peak in the early icteric phase. HBeAg titers peak earlier and begin to fall with seroconversion to anti-HBe occurring around the height of clinical symptoms. During the icteric phase, levels of HBsAg and serum aminotransferases begin to decrease. Generally HBsAg is no longer detectable in the serum within 4 months after the appearance of symptoms. In the convalescent phase, liver enzymes return to normal and seroconversion from HBsAg to anti-HBs occurs. During this seroconversion there is a variable period of time after HBsAg is no longer detectable before the appearance of anti-HBs. This time is referred to as the "window" period.

In inapparent type B hepatitis, HBsAg and HBeAg may appear in the serum for a short time. Serum aminotransferase levels are mildly elevated but soon return to normal. High titers of anti-HBs and variable titers of anti-HBc and anti-HBe develop. The figure on this page, *below*, illustrates these changes.

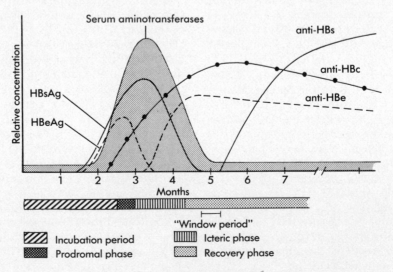

Seologic changes in acute type B hepatitis.

CHRONIC HBsAg CARRIER STATE

In the chronic HBsAg carrier state, the serologic changes seen in acute type B hepatitis are the same except for the persistence of HBsAg (therefore there is no anti-HBs). Liver enzyme levels are normal and the patient is asymptomatic. The figure on this page, *top*, illustrates these changes.

CHRONIC HEPATITIS B

In chronic hepatitis B the serologic changes seen in acute type B disease are the same. However, there is a failure of HBsAg and HBeAg to seroconvert to anti-HBs and anti-HBe. Anti-HBc rises to high titers. Serum aminotransferase levels remain elevated, though usually less than 10 times normal (Hoofnagle, 1981). Mild to moderate symptoms may exist. These findings change as liver disease progresses. The figure on this page, *bottom*, illustrates these changes.

TYPE NON-A, NON-B (TYPE C) HEPATITIS
Epidemiology and clinical features

Non-A, non-B (NANB) hepatitis is caused by at least two viruses, which can be separated

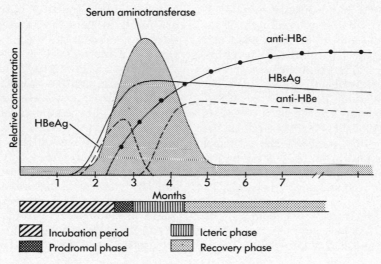

Serologic changes in the chronic HBsAg carrier state.

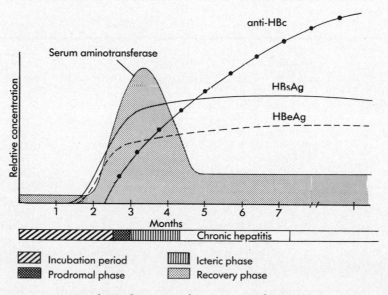

Serologic changes in chronic type B hepatitis.

into two groups based on their epidemiologic characteristics. One type of NANB hepatitis is caused by a blood-borne agent; the other is caused by an agent that, like hepatitis A virus, is transmitted by the fecal-oral route. The enterically transmitted NANB hepatitis has no chronic disease states and is primarily associated with epidemic cases of acute hepatitis that occur in developing countries (Alter, 1989). The remainder of this discussion refers to the blood-borne type.

Recently an agent for blood-borne NANB hepatitis was characterized as an RNA virus (Choo et al., 1989). This agent is now referred to as the hepatitis C virus (HCV); its associated disease is hepatitis C. However, more than one agent is suspected, since multiple episodes of NANB disease have been observed in the same individual (Holland and Alter, 1981; Dienstag, 1983a, 1983b). Experimental results in chimpanzees lead to different conclusions: that there are two distinct agents in posttransfusion non-A, non-B hepatitis (Bradley et al., 1983), and that there is only a single class of agents (Brotman et al., 1985). Further research is necessary to answer this question. The principal mode of transmission for the HCV is the parenteral route. Currently, 90% to 95% of the cases of posttransfusion hepatitis are hepatitis C. Type C disease, then, occurs more frequently in many of the same groups as hepatitis B: recipients of blood or blood products, renal dialysis patients, certain health care professionals,

and IV drug users. Hepatitis C also accounts for about 20% of sporadic cases of acute viral hepatitis, and in many of these cases there is no history of parenteral exposure. Thus modes of transmission other than the parenteral route are assumed. One such route, also paralleling type B hepatitis, is through sexual contact. Promiscuous male homosexuals (Dienstag, 1983a) and spouses of individuals with NANB disease (Holland and Alter, 1981) appear to be at increased risk for infection, but the incidence is low. Other modes of person-to-person transmission are not clear; intrafamilial spread of hepatitis from an individual with NANB disease is infrequent (Holland and Alter, 1981), and saliva on a CPR manikin used by a person in the prodromal phase of NANB hepatitis did not result in infection (Perras et al., 1980). However, a recent study cited personal contact and sexual transmission as significantly associated with acquiring this type of hepatitis (Alter et al., 1989a). Another report suggested that saliva from a chimpanzee infected with NANB hepatitis might contain infectious agent of NANB disease (Abe et al., 1987). A more thorough understanding of the epidemiology of type C hepatitis will come with the information learned from the newly licensed blood test for anti-HCV and with the identification of additional specific serologic markers and the subsequent development of screening tests for them.

The clinical features of acute type C hepatitis are usually less severe than those of hepatitis A

Table C-1. Summary of epidemiologies of acute viral hepatitis

	Hepatitis A	Hepatitis B	Hepatitis C
Agent	HAV	HBV	RNA virus, others (?)
Antigens	HA Ag	HBsAg, HBcAg, HBeAg	
Antibodies	anti-HAV	anti-HBs, anti-HBc, anti-HBe	anti-HCV
Modes of transmission	Fecal-oral	Primarily parenteral but also by contact	Primarily parenteral and probably by contact
Incubation period	2 to 6 weeks	1 to 6 months	2 weeks to 6 months
Clinical course	Symptomatic or inapparent	Approximately 50% inapparent	As many as 75% inapparent
Mortality	Rare	1% to 3%	1% to 2%
Asymptomatic carrier state	No	0.1% to 0.2% of the population	May be as high as 3% to 7% of the population
Chronic hepatitis	No	5% to 10%	40% to 60% following transfusion; <10% of sporadic cases
Postexposure prophylaxis	IG usually effective	HBIG, occasionally IG	IG may be effective
Preexposure prophylaxis (vaccine) available	No	Yes	No

IG, Immune globulin; *HBIG*, hepatitis B immune globulin.

or hepatitis B. After the incubation period (which averages approximately 8 weeks for posttransfusion hepatitis), acute hepatitis C often has insidious prodromal and icteric phases. Symptoms and physical finding, if present, are usually mild. Symptomatic disease with jaundice may occur in 25% of all cases (Holland and Alter, 1981). Serum aminotransferase levels are elevated but usually less than in hepatitis B. These biochemical abnormalities have been associated with viremia and suggest that the patient is potentially infectious throughout the period of enzyme elevation (Czaja and Davis, 1982). Until recently the diagnosis of hepatitis C was by exclusion of other possible causes (for example, other viral agents, hepatotoxins, or congestive heart failure). Now there is a screening test for the hepatitis C antibody. This antibody is usually detectable 10 to 39 weeks (average, 21.9 weeks) after infection via transfusion and was found following transfusion in 15 patients (100%) with chronic hepatitis C and in three patients (60%) with acute resolving hepatitis C (Alter et al., 1989b). The antibody persisted in 14 of the 15 patients with chronic hepatitis C (mean follow-up, 6.9 years) but disappeared in the three patients with acute resolving hepatitis C after an average of 4.1 years (Alter et al., 1989b). Spontaneous resolution usually occurs within 10 to 12 weeks after the onset of symptoms. Mortality associated with acute NANB hepatitis ranges from 1% to 2% (Hoofnagle, 1981).

Despite its mild acute course, type C hepatitis often progresses to the chronic disease state. Chronic hepatitis occurs at a rate of 40% to 60% in posttransfusion cases and less than 10% in sporadic cases (Dienstag, 1983a). Furthermore, most of the posttransfusion cases have histopathologic changes consistent with chronic active hepatitis, but the disease is relatively benign in most of these cases. Spontaneous remission occurs in about half of these cases within 3 years, whereas in other cases the disease either reverts to chronic persistent hepatitis or is progressive. Cirrhosis develops in 10% to 20% of the cases.

Acute type C hepatitis is also associated with an asymptomatic chronic carrier state. The frequency of the hepatitis C carrier state appears to be many times greater than the 0.1% to 0.2% reported for the chronic HBsAg carrier and may be as high as 3% to 7% (Dienstag, 1983a, 1983b).

Table C-1 on p. 698 summarizes the epidemiologies of hepatitis A, hepatitis B, and hepatitis C.

MEDICAL MANAGEMENT

Most patients with acute viral hepatitis are treated at home. Medical management includes bed rest (as necessary), instructions to prevent further spread of the disease, ensuring an adequate diet, and treatment of symptoms (for example, an antiemetic for vomiting). Corticosteroids are contraindicated in treatment of acute viral hepatitis because they may predispose the patient to relapse or to progression to chronic hepatitis (Orland and Saltman, 1986, p. 261). Prednisone, azathioprine, and interferon are used in the treatment of chronic active hepatitis.

Patients with severe disease, those who cannot care for themselves, or patients who cannot maintain an adequate oral intake may require hospitalization. Again, treatment is primarily supportive and palliative. For the majority of cases of acute viral hepatitis, complete recovery usually occurs within 3 to 4 months after the onset of symptoms.

Chronic persistent hepatitis requires no specific therapy, since it is a relatively benign disease with a good prognosis. Chronic active hepatitis may be treated with corticosteroids and azathioprine.

PROPHYLAXIS AND THE HEPATITIS B VACCINE

Hepatitis prophylaxis is often initiated after exposure to viral hepatitis through contact (for example, household, sexual, or close personal contact), accidental needle stick, or transfusion with contaminated blood products. Preexposure prophylaxis may also be warranted before traveling to an area where viral hepatitis is endemic.

Individuals exposed to HAV are protected against hepatitis A (more than 90% of the time) by receiving immune globulin (IG) within 2 weeks after exposure. IG contains anti-HAV and appears to act by conferring temporary, passive immunity or by a passive-active mechanism. In the latter, IG antibodies prevent clinical disease but a subclinical or inapparent infection occurs and results in autogenous anti-HAV production and lifelong immunity. A vaccine for hepatitis A is reported to be in the developmental stages (Mao et al., 1989).

Postexposure prophylaxis following accidental contact or innoculation with HBsAg-positive products in a susceptible individual (that is, unvaccinated, test for anti-HBs is negative) uses both hepatitis B immune globulin (HBIG) and the hepatitis B vaccine (Centers for Disease Control, 1985). HBIG contains high titers of anti-HBs and confers temporary, passive immunity. The single dose of HBIG should be given as soon as possible following exposure, preferably within 24 hours but no later than 7 days after exposure. The first dose of the hepatitis B vaccine should be given at a separate site within 7 days following exposure; the schedule for the remaining doses is unchanged (the immunization regimen is discussed later in this section). The vaccine stimulates production of autogenous anti-HBs, thus enhancing or initiating an active immune response against HBsAg. Individuals who are not given the hepatitis B vaccine should receive a second dose of HBIG 1 month after the first. However, the use of only HBIG or the hepatitis B vaccine for postexposure prophylaxis is not as effective in preventing HBV infection as is their use in combination (Centers for Disease Control, 1985).

In other instances, when the relative risk for HBV infection is lower or unlikely, postexposure prophylaxis may require only HBIG (following sexual exposure) or the hepatitis B vaccine.

IG has been recommended in postexposure prophylaxis for type C hepatitis (Orland and Saltman, 1986, p. 260), but this recommenda-tion appears to be an empirical judgment at this time.

The first hepatitis B vaccine (Heptavax B*), licensed in 1981, is a highly purified, noninfectious preparation of hepatitis B surface antigen (Martin, 1983), which is derived from the pooled plasma of HBsAg-positive carriers. Numerous reports document the safety and efficacy of the vaccine (Gregory, 1984; Krugman, 1982; Martin, 1983). In general, Heptavax B stimulates the production of anti-HBs in 91% to 100% of adults with normal immune systems, with no associated serious side effects or long-term adverse reactions (Seeff and Koff, 1984). Recombivax HB* is the second hepatitis B vaccine. It was licensed in 1986 and contains HBsAg produced by yeast cells. Its immunogenicity and safety are comparable to those of the plasma-derived vaccine, but the recombinant vaccine may be associated with the production of lower levels of HBs in a recipient (Centers for Disease Control, 1987). The current immunization regimen for healthy adults using either vaccine consists of three intramuscular injections, with the second and third doses given at

*Merck Sharp & Dohme.

Table C-2. Interpretation of serologic profiles seen in viral hepatitis

		Test results				
HBsAg	anti-HBs	anti-HBc	HBeAg	anti-HBe	anti-HAV	Comments
−					+IgM	Acute or recent hepatitis A
+						Acute or chronic hepatitis B
+		+IgM	+			Acute hepatitis B
−	−	+IgM		+		"Window" period following acute hepatitis B
+		+IgG		+		Asymptomatic chronic HBsAg carrier or, possibly, chronic type B hepatitis
+		+IgG	+			Chronic hepatitis B
	+	+IgG		+/−		Recovery from hepatitis B
	+	−		−		Prior immunization with the hepatitis B vaccine or, possibly, long after hepatitis B infection
−	−				−	Possible type NANB hepatitis
					+IgG	Past HAV infection

▨ Test not ordered.

1 month and 6 months, respectively, after the initial dose. Since the titer of anti-HBs initially produced in response to the vaccine decreases over time, a booster dose may be required at a later date.

Preexposure prophylaxis with the hepatitis B vaccine is recommended for dentists and auxiliary personnel (Cottone and Goebel, 1983; Czaja, 1984). However, if prior exposure to HBV is equivocal, a screening test for anti-HBs should be performed to establish the need for the vaccine.

DENTAL IMPLICATIONS

Dental practitioners must take every precaution to protect themselves and their staffs from viral hepatitis. A comprehensive medical history is important for identifying patients with a history of viral hepatitis or may elicit symptoms of acute disease. Furthermore, understanding the epidemiologies can aid in determining what type of viral hepatitis the patient had (for example, perhaps at summer camp there was a localized outbreak, associated with IV drug abuse, or perhaps the viral hepatitis followed multiple blood transfusions). But the comprehensive medical history does have its limitations. As one study reported, 50% of the detected HBsAg carriers gave no history of ever having hepatitis, 58% of the patients who gave a history of hepatitis A actually had type B hepatitis, and only 56% of the patients who gave a history of hepatitis B had serologic evidence of type B disease (Goebel, 1979). Therefore a positive history of hepatitis usually necessitates consultation with the patient's physician to determine the type and rule out a chronic carrier or disease state (not applicable with hepatitis A). If a past history of type B hepatitis is suspected, and the patient's medical records are not available, a screening test for HBsAg should be ordered (see Table C-2 on p. 700).

In a patient with an unremarkable past medical history and nonspecific symptoms of malaise, anorexia, weight loss, and fever, regional examination of the sclera and oral mucosa, particularly the lingual frenum, may reveal mild jaundice. If acute viral hepatitis is suspected, no elective dental treatment should be performed until after medical consultation and resolution of the acute disease state.

The dental practitioner should be aware of the various groups considered at high risk for the different types of viral hepatitis. These groups are listed in the box on this page.

Close communication between dentist and physician is essential for the patient with

---

High-risk patients or conditions for viral hepatitis

HEPATITIS A

Individuals from lower social classes or of lower socioeconomic status

Institutionalized persons (e.g., mentally retarded or prisoners) and staff

Military personnel stationed in areas where the disease is endemic

Male homosexuals

Past history of hepatitis B

HEPATITIS B

Health care workers exposed to blood, blood products, or body secretions

Hemodialysis patients and staff

Renal transplant (immunosuppressed) patients

Congenital coagulopathies and other conditions requiring transfusion of blood products

Recipients of multiple blood transfusions

Drug addicts

Institutionalized persons (e.g., mentally retarded or prisoners) and staff

Past history of hepatitis

Sexually promiscuous individuals (male homosexuals and female prostitutes)

Patients from areas where disease is endemic (e.g., Southeast Asia, Haiti, and regions of Africa)

HEPATITIS NANB

Recipients of multiple blood transfusions

Congenital coagulopathies and other conditions requiring transfusion of blood products

Drug addicts

Hemodialysis patients and staff

Renal transplant (immunosuppressed) patients

---

chronic hepatitis and cirrhosis. Potential complications include altered drug metabolism, anemia, bleeding abnormalities secondary to deficiency of clotting factors or thrombocytopenia, circulatory changes, and ascites. Antibiotic prophylaxis may be required for patients with vascular and surgical shunts.

When performing dental treatment on a patient with acute or chronic viral hepatitis, several treatment modifications should be considered. The use of gloves, mask, and protective eyeglasses is mandatory. Aerosol production should be minimized by using a slow-speed handpiece as much as possible, working under a rubber dam, using high-speed evacuation, and judiciously using the air syringe. Strict aseptic technique is essential and should include sterilization of all instruments and handpieces, thorough postoperative disinfection of the operatory, use of disposable smocks and drapes, and proper disposal of contaminated materials. Scheduling these patients late in the day eliminates immediate use of the operatory by another patient. Other considerations for these patients include: obtaining a preoperative prothrombin time before dental surgery (a platelet count may also be necessary if splenomegaly is a complicating factor), modifying chair position to the sitting or semireclining position for patients with ascites, and avoiding use of drugs metabolized by the liver.

REFERENCES

Abe K, Shikata T, Sugitani M, et al: Experimental transmission of non-A, non-B hepatitis by saliva, J Infect Dis 155:1078, 1987.

Ahtone J and Goodman RA: Hepatitis B and dental personnel: transmission to patients and prevention issues, J Am Dent Assoc 106:219-222, 1983.

Alter MJ: Non-A, non-B hepatitis: sorting through a diagnosis of exclusion, Ann Intern Med 110:583-585, 1989.

Alter MJ, Coleman PJ, Alexander J, et al: Importance of heterosexual activity in the transmission of hepatitis B and non-A, non-B hepatitis, JAMA 262(9):1201-1205, 1989a.

Alter MF, Purcell RH, Shih JW, et al: Detection of antibody to hepatitis C virus in prospectively followed transfusion recipients with acute and chronic non-A, non-B hepatitis, N Engl J Med 321(22):1494-1500, 1989b.

Balistreri WF: Viral hepatitis, Pediatr Clin North Am 35(3):637-669, 1988.

Bernstein LM, Koff RS, Siegel ER, et al: The hepatitis knowledge base (short form), Ann Intern Med 93:183-222, 1980.

Bradley DW, Maynard JE, and Popper H: Posttransfusion non-A, non-B hepatitis: physicochemical properties of two distinct agents, J Infect Dis 148:254-265, 1983.

Brotman B, Prince A, and Huima T: Non-A, non-B hepatitis, is there more than a single blood-borne strain? J Infect Dis 151:618-625, 1985.

Centers for Disease Control: Recommendations for protection against viral hepatitis, MMWR 34:313-335, 1985.

Centers for Disease Control: Update on hepatitis B prevention, MMWR 36:353-360, 1987.

Choo Q-L, Kuo G, Weiner AJ, et al: Isolation of a cDNA clone derived from a blood-borne non-A, non-B viral hepatitis genome, Science 244:359-361, 1989.

Cottone JA and Goebel WM: Hepatitis B: the clinical detection of the chronic carrier dental patient and the effects of immunization via vaccine, Oral Surg 56:449-454, 1983.

Czaja AJ: Hepatitis and the dentist, JADA 108:286-287, 1984.

Czaja AJ and Davis GL: Hepatitis non A, non B: manifestations and implications of acute and chronic disease, Mayo Clin Proc 57:639-652, 1982.

Dienstag JL: Non-A, non-B hepatitis. I. Recognition, epidemiology, and clinical features, Gastroenterology 85:439-462, 1983a.

Dienstag JL: Non-A, non-B hepatitis. II. Experimental transmission, putative virus agents and markers, and prevention, Gastroenterology 85:743-768, 1983b.

Goebel WM: Reliability of the medical history in identifying patients likely to place dentists at an increased hepatitis risk, JADA 98:907-913, 1979.

Gregory DH, II: Hepatitis B vaccine: key to the era of preventive control, Postgrad Med 75:199-211, 1984.

Holland PV and Alter HJ: Non-A, non-B viral hepatitis, Hum Pathol 12:1114-1122, 1981.

Hoofnagle JH: Perspective on viral hepatitis: types A and B viral hepatitis, Abbott Park, Ill, 1981, Abbott Laboratories Diagnostic Division.

Krugman S: The newly licensed hepatitis B vaccine: characteristics and indications for use, JAMA 247:2012-2015, 1982.

Kuo G, Choo Q-L, Alter HJ, et al: An assay for circulating antibodies to a major etiologic virus of human non-A, non-B hepatitis, Science 244:362-364, 1989.

Mao JS, Dong DX, Zhang HY, et al: Primary study of attenuated live hepatitis A vaccine (H2 strain) in humans, J Infect Dis 159:621-624, 1989.

Martin CM: Hepatitis B vaccine—what to expect, Oral Surg 56:455-459, 1983.

Orland MJ and Saltman RJ: Manual of medical therapeutics, Boston, 1986, Little, Brown & Co, Inc.

Perras ST, Poupard JA, Byrne EB, et al: Lack of transmission of hepatitis non-A, non-B by CPR manikins, N Engl J Med 302:118-119, 1980.

Rizzetto M, Ferruccio B, and Verme G: Hepatitis delta virus infection of the liver: progress in virology, pathobiology, and diagnosis, Semin Liver Dis 8(4):350-356, 1988.

Rizzetto M: The delta agent, Hepatology 3(5):729-737, 1983.

Rose LF and Kaye D: Internal medicine for dentistry, ed 2, St Louis, 1990, The CV Mosby Co.

Seeff LB and Koff RS: Passive and active immunoprophylaxis of hepatitis B, Gastroenterology 86:958-981, 1984.

Szmuness W, Dienstag JL, Purcell RH, et al: Distribution of antibody to hepatitis A antigen in urban adult populations, N Engl J Med 295:755-759, 1976.

West DJ: The risk of hepatitis B infection among health professionals in the United States: a review, Am J Med Sci 287:26-33, 1984.

D

Acquired immunodeficiency syndrome

DANNY R. SAWYER

In June 1981, acquired immunodeficiency syndrome (AIDS) first became apparent to those at the Centers for Disease Control (CDC) with the reports that five previously healthy young male homosexuals in Los Angeles and New York had become ill with *Pneumocystis carinii* pneumonia and an aggressive form of Kaposi's sarcoma. Since that time, AIDS has become recognized worldwide as a fatal and increasingly prevalent disease. AIDS exhibits a wide spectrum of clinical manifestations, the classic appearance being opportunistic infections and Kaposi's sarcoma but also including an asymptomatic state that gives only laboratory evidence of the disease and a prodromal state characterized by fever, weight loss, and lymphadenopathy.

AIDS is characterized by an irreversible suppression of the body's immune system, specifically, a suppression of the lymphocytes responsible for modulating the system, the helper T-cell lymphocytes. The causative agent was identified in 1983 and 1984 to be a retrovirus and was given several names including human T-cell lymphotropic virus (HTLV-III), AIDS-associated retrovirus (ARV), and lymphadenopathy virus (LAV) (Gallo et al., 1983; Barre-Sinoussi et al., 1983). More recently, almost universal agreement names this virus the human immunodeficiency virus (HIV).

The disease appears to have originated in Africa, where serologic evidence suggests that it has been present for at least two decades. A related strain of human immunodeficiency virus, called HIV-2, has been reported in cases of AIDS in Africa (Clavel et al., 1987). However, the epidemiologic characteristics of AIDS in Africa are quite different from those in the United States; this difference may be related to a difference in the pattern of HIV transmission, which in Africa occurs more frequently by heterosexual contact or the reuse of medical needles.

Epidemiology

AIDS was originally defined by the CDC as a "disease at least moderately predictive of a defect in cell-mediated immunity, occurring in a person with no known cause for diminished resistance to that disease." Although this definition still has some value for epidemiologic studies, it does not take into account either the established role of human immunodeficiency virus (HIV) in the pathogenesis of AIDS or the variety of other clinical manifestations that the HIV may present, which are not included in the CDC's initial definition.

In an attempt to provide uniformity to the diagnosis of AIDS and other HIV-related syndromes, the CDC proposed a revised classification in 1987. This revised classification divided the HIV infections into the following categories (Centers for Disease Control, 1987):

Group I. HIV infection with specified secondary infections or malignant neoplasms. This includes full-blown cases of AIDS. (See box on p. 704.)

Group II. HIV infection with other specified manifestations but no evidence of the secondary infections and neoplasms included in group I. This includes cases previously referred to as pre-AIDS and AIDS-related complex (ARC).

Group III. HIV infections not classified in groups I or II.

Some secondary infections and neoplasms associated with HIV infection

BACTERIAL INFECTIONS

Mycobacteriosis
Salmonella infections
Nocardiosis

VIRAL INFECTIONS

Cytomegalovirus infections
Herpes simplex infections
Varicella infections

FUNGAL INFECTIONS

Candidiasis
Cryptococcosis
Histoplasmosis
Coccidioidomycosis
Other opportunistic fungal infections

PROTOZOAL AND HELMINTHIC INFECTIONS

Pneumocystosis
Cryptosporidiosis
Toxoplasmosis

MALIGNANT NEOPLASMS

Kaposi's sarcoma
Burkitt's lymphoma
Other lymphomas

With further research and clinical experience, modifications to this already revised classification will no doubt continue.

AIDS has now been reported from more than 100 countries worldwide; approximately 70% of the cases occur in the United States (Piot et al., 1988). Epidemiologic studies in the United States have identified the following groups of persons who are at risk for the development of AIDS:

1. Homosexual or bisexual men constitute by far the largest group and represent slightly more than 70% of all cases, including the 7% of patients in this group who are intravenous (IV) drug users (Centers for Disease Control, 1988).
2. IV drug users with no history of homosexuality form the second largest group, representing almost 20% of all cases.
3. Patients with hemophilia constitute approximately 1% of all cases; AIDS is more prevalent in those who received factor VIII concentrates before 1985.
4. Blood and blood component recipients who do not have hemophilia represent approximately 2% to 3% of the cases.
5. Heterosexual men and women who have contacts with members of the other high-risk groups constitute almost 4% of the cases of AIDS.

The HIV-1 virus has been isolated from serum, saliva, breast milk, semen, vaginal secretions, tears, urine, lymphoid cells, and the cerebrospinal fluid (CSF) of patients with AIDS and those at risk of developing AIDS. The virus has never been isolated from a healthy donor.

Transmission

Transmission of HIV-1 virus can occur via three routes: sexual contact, passage of the virus from infected mothers to their newborns, and parenteral inoculation. Venereal transmission is by far the predominant route of infection in the United States. As previously stated, most cases of AIDS in the United States occur as the result of homosexual contact. The male to female ratio of cases of AIDS in the United States is 12:1, whereas in Africa, where most cases are transmitted by heterosexual contact, the ratio is 1:1. Although male to female transmission has been firmly established in both Africa and the United States, the frequency and risk of female to male transmission is not as well understood. HIV transmission parenterally occurs in IV drug users, in hemophiliacs who receive factor VIII concentrates, and in rare cases in recipients of blood transfusions. Perinatal transmission could possibly occur during pregnancy or during the immediate postpartum period. In utero infection via the transplacental route is well documented (Lapointe et al., 1985).

Health care workers, as well as the public, have been concerned about the spread of HIV-1 outside the high-risk group because of the uniformly fatal outcome of AIDS at this time. However, many studies indicate that AIDS cannot be spread by casual contact even within a family group using shared household facilities. Similarly, the risk of acquiring AIDS by occupational exposure is extremely small. By the middle of 1988, the CDC had reported that only 15 health care workers with none of the nonoccupational risk factors had developed

HIV infection. Needlestick injury or open-skin contact with infected blood accounted for most of these cases. The CDC (Centers for Disease Control, 1988) estimated that the risk of sero-conversion after accidental needlestick exposure is approximately 0.5% and less with other forms of exposure.

Laboratory tests

Antibody to HIV in the blood can be detected by enzyme-linked immunosorbent assay (ELISA). Blood banks use antibody tests to screen donated blood for contamination with the HIV. If the ELISA test is positive, a confirmatory Western blot test is performed; this test identifies antibodies to HIV proteins and glyco-proteins. A positive test provides evidence of previous HIV exposure. A negative test indicates either no previous exposure or that the antibody has not had sufficient time to develop. A serum HIV antigen test is available and probably will be used widely in the near future.

Individuals infected with HIV usually develop antibody to the virus in 6 to 12 weeks. Alarmingly, some individuals have been known to be infected with HIV for several years before becoming serologically positive for the antibody (Imagawa et al., 1989). Thus these individuals have the potential to transmit HIV for years before an antibody test indicates infection.

Oral manifestations of AIDS

Hairy leukoplakia
Candidiasis
Kaposi's sarcoma
Squamous cell carcinoma
Lymphoma
Gingivitis and periodontitis
Xerostomia
Herpes simplex
Aphthous stomatitis

Oral manifestations

A number of conditions involving the oral cavity and perioral region have been associated with HIV infection. The oral manifestations of AIDS include those listed in the box on this page. Hairy leukoplakia is one of the unique and unusual oral manifestations associated with HIV infection. It is a white lesion that occurs along the lateral borders of the tongue predominantly in male homosexuals (see figure, *below*). On microscopic examination this particular form of leukoplakia is filamentous. The lesion may spread to cover the tongue completely and can extend onto the buccal mucosa. Evidence suggests that hairy leukoplakia repre-

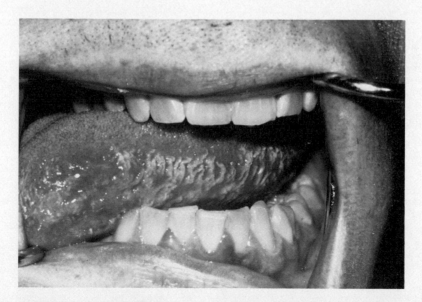

Hairy leukoplakia on the lateral border of the tongue in a man with AIDS. (Courtesy J. Epstein, DMD, MSD, Vancouver, B.C.)

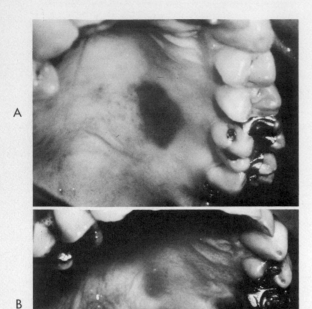

A and B, Solitary and multiple Kaposi's sarcomas on the palates of patients with AIDS. (A and B courtesy J. Epstein, DMD, MSD, Vancouver, B.C.)

sents an opportunistic infection related to the presence of Epstein-Barr virus (Corso et al., 1989). Patients with hairy leukoplakia often are otherwise asymptomatic, and the lesion has been suggested as a significant clinical marker for HIV infection.

Kaposi's sarcoma is another common manifestation of AIDS within the oral cavity (see figure, *left*). The pattern of Kaposi's sarcoma associated with HIV infections and full-blown cases of AIDS presents several features which differ from that of the classic and African types of Kaposi's. Kaposi's sarcoma associated with AIDS is seen more frequently in younger adult men residing in metropolitan areas and may appear as skin lesions (which can occur at any site) or oral lesions or both. Kaposi's sarcoma associated with AIDS normally behaves in an aggressive fashion, and the prognosis is typically poor.

Also characteristic of HIV infection are a distinctive form of gingivitis and a rapidly progressive form of periodontitis currently known as HIV gingivitis and HIV periodontitis, respectively. A rapid, often irregularly destructive horizontal bone loss with only moderate inflammation characterizes the HIV periodontitis (Rosenstein et al., 1989; Winkler and Murray, 1987).

Candidiasis is also frequently seen in patients with HIV infection (see figure, *below*).

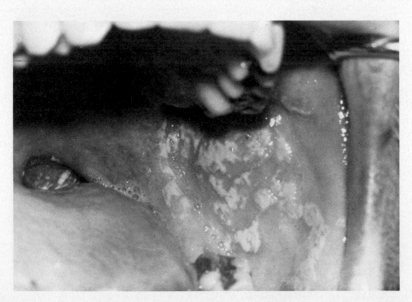

Candidiasis in a patient with AIDS. Several of the oral surfaces, as well as the pharynx, were involved. (Courtesy J. Epstein, DMD, MSD, Vancouver, B.C.)

The candidiasis may appear as a stomatitis or an angular cheilitis. Several types of candidiasis have been described in these patients, including pseudomembranous, atrophic, and hyperplastic. Several investigators have reported cases of herpes simplex infection and aphthous stomatitis in their patients with HIV infection (Epstein and Silverman, 1988; Roberts et al., 1988).

Several reports have observed that xerostomia is not an infrequent complaint of patients with HIV infection (Schiodt and Pindborg, 1987; Silverman et al., 1986; Roberts et al., 1988). Six cases of oral hyperpigmentation in HIV-infected patients have been reported (Langford et al., 1989). The oral manifestations associated with HIV infection and AIDS are described in greater detail in a number of reports (Epstein and Silverman, 1988; Greenspan et al., 1987; Robertson and Greenspan, 1988; Silverman, 1987).

Risk of HIV transmission to the dental community

In one study of 1309 dentists, dental hygienists, and dental assistants, of whom many worked in areas with a high prevalence of HIV infection, only one dentist (0.08%) had HIV antibody (Klein et al., 1988). This dentist had a history of sustaining needlesticks and trauma to his hands. As previously discussed, needlestick injuries and open wounds account for most cases of occupational HIV transmission. The dentist in this study also did not routinely wear gloves when providing dental care. Gloves should be worn for all dental procedures by all dental personnel involved in patient care because of asymptomatic HIV virus carriers and because the virus can be found in both blood and saliva.

In another study of 255 dentists, dental hygienists, and dental assistants, none were found to have antibody to HIV, even though these workers were known to have frequent contact with patients infected with HIV (Flynn et al., 1987). Proper dental management and infection control should make the risk of acquiring AIDS by occupational exposure extremely small.

Dental management

Most cases of HIV infection can and should be treated in the dental office. Historically, dentists have had the right in most situations to refuse to provide treatment in their offices to new patients. Recent court cases indicate that a dentist's right to refuse to provide treatment to a patient with AIDS will be restricted. The American Dental Association's stated policy is that individuals with HIV infection should be treated with dignity and compassion, and the Council on Ethics, Bylaws and Judicial Affairs states that "a decision not to provide treatment to an individual because the individual has AIDS or is HIV seropositive, based solely on that fact, is unethical."

Infectious control procedures as recommended by the Centers for Disease Control and the American Dental Association should be carefully followed in the treatment of patients with HIV infection.

Identification, diagnosis, and treatment of cases of AIDS or infection with HIV should be carried out in consultation with the patient's physician.

Infection control

The Centers for Disease Control and the American Dental Association have published recommendations for infection control in the dental office and laboratory; the very latest recommendations may be obtained from these organizations. Strict adherence to these recommendations will prevent transmission of HIV during and after dental treatment.

Prevention of the transmission of HIV begins before treatment. A thorough medical history is an important first step. During treatment, *all* patients should be treated as potentially infectious. Gloves, mask, protective eyewear or face shields, and clinic or laboratory coats or gowns should be worn by all personnel. The rubber dam and high-volume vacuum evacuation should be used. The dental worker should attempt to minimize droplet formation, splashes, and spatters. Contaminated packets of x-ray film should be touched only with gloved hands, and the film should not be contaminated. The hands should be washed both before and after gloving, preferably with an antimicrobial soap. Gloves should be used for only one patient; torn, cut, or punctured gloves should not be used. It is important to avoid injuries to the hands and skin, so sharp instruments and needles must be handled carefully. Disposable needles should not be bent or broken; if needles are recapped, one of the techniques that minimize accidental needlesticks should be used. Sharp instruments should be placed in puncture-proof containers. Disposable sharp instruments and needles should be placed in puncture-resistant containers, labeled, and disposed of properly.

After providing treatment, while wearing heavy-duty rubber gloves, the clinician should thoroughly clean all instruments. All instruments should be sterilized, if at all possible, and the sterilizer should be monitored with biologic monitors to ensure proper sterilization. All handpieces, dental units, and ultrasonic scalers should be cleaned, flushed, and disinfected. All environmental surfaces should be decontaminated. Disposable coverings can be used to prevent contamination, and these should be discarded properly and replaced. Areas of contact outside the immediate environment of treatment should also be cleaned and disinfected, such as light handles, light switches, heads of x-ray units, and similar areas. Supplies and dental materials must also be decontaminated; that is, impressions, bite registrations, and dental appliances should be cleaned and disinfected. Contaminated liquid wastes (such as blood and suctioned saliva) should be disposed of properly, as should contaminated solid wastes. Local government regulations concerning the disposal of human waste material should be closely followed.

Infection control is paramount in handling patients with a disease that currently has no cure.

Treatment, prognosis, and the future

Since the discovery of AIDS in 1981 and the discovery of its etiologic agent in 1983 and 1984, there have been significant advances in our understanding of this disease. Despite these rapid advances, the prognosis for patients with AIDS is dismal. Recently a 5-year mortality of 85% has been reported, and without a cure the disease no doubt will have a mortality that approaches 100% (Rothenberg et al., 1987).

Research in the area of AIDS treatment is concentrating on the development of three types of drugs: (1) drugs that inhibit HIV multiplication, (2) drugs used to treat opportunistic infections and neoplasms, which are the ultimate killers in cases of AIDS, and (3) drugs used to boost the body's immune system. Although the virus has been identified, it has been found to be an extremely complex one. Molecular analyses have recently revealed a high degree of variability in the extracellular envelope of HIV, even in isolates obtained from the same patient. This high degree of variability has profound clinical implications.

Many antiviral drugs are being tested but only azidothymidine (AZT), which has also been called zidovudine (Retrovir), has received FDA approval at the time of this writing. As an inhibitor of reverse transcriptase, AZT inhibits the replication of HIV. It has caused some reduction in morbidity and mortality in clinical trials but has some serious adverse side effects. Anemia, neutropenia, and leukopenia have been major hematologic abnormalities. Adverse drug reactions involving the oral mucosa have also been reported with AZT. These reactions have been variously reported as glossitis, ulcerative stomatitis, taste perturbation, Stevens-Johnson syndrome, toxic epidermal necrolysis, erythema multiforme, and oral herpes virus ulcers (Arrowsmith, 1989). AZT appears to increase survival times but is not curative.

The most prevalent opportunistic infection in AIDS patients is *Pneumocystis carinii* pneumonia. Pentamidine and sulfamethoxazole-trimethoprim have been shown to be useful in treating *P. carinii* pneumonia. However, adverse side effects do occur frequently, including oral lesions (Arrowsmith, 1989). Studies are being made of the effectiveness of interleukin-2 in boosting the body's immune system and the effectiveness of interferon as an agent for treating Kaposi's sarcoma and other malignant neoplasms in patients with AIDS.

The candidiasis of patients with AIDS can be treated with antifungal agents such as nystatin, clotrimazole, or ketoconazole. Fluconazole has been shown to be effective in treating oropharyngeal candidiasis (FDA Drug Bulletin, 1989). Topical or systemic antiviral agents such as acyclovir have been used successfully in treating herpetic lesions in patients with HIV infection. Antimicrobial mouth rinses have been useful in decreasing pain and preventing secondary infections in patients with candidiasis or herpetic lesions. Scaling and root planing have been used in the treatment of HIV periodontitis. Rinsing with chlorhexidine has been reported to be an effective adjunct to conventional therapy (Grassi et al., 1988).

Although a priority in AIDS research is the development of an effective vaccine to HIV, to date this work has succumbed to the variable nature of the HIV.

Much is known about HIV and AIDS. However, this scourge of modern life remains a lethal epidemic disease of immense magnitude. Because research on AIDS is progressing rapidly, some of the information presented here will be outdated by the time it is published but there is hope for a cure tomorrow.

REFERENCES

Arrowsmith JB: AIDS therapy and the detection of adverse drug effects in dental practice, JADA Suppl:465-485, November, 1989.

Barre-Sinoussi R et al: Isolation of a T-lymphotropic retrovirus from a patient at risk for acquired immunodeficiency syndrome (AIDS), Science 220:868-871, 1983.

Centers for Disease Control: Human immunodeficiency virus (HIV) infection classification, MMWR 36(Suppl 7):1-20, 1987.

Centers for Disease Control: Update: acquired immunodeficiency syndrome and human immunodeficiency virus infection among health care workers, MMWR 37:229-234, 1988.

Clavel F et al: Human immunodeficiency virus type 2 infection associated with AIDS in West Africa, N Engl J Med 316:1180-1185, 1987.

Corso B, Eversole LR, and Hutt-Fletcher L: Hairy leukoplakia: Epstein-Barr virus receptors on oral keratinocyte plasma membranes, Oral Surg 67:416-421, 1989.

Epstein JB and Silverman S: Oral manifestations of human immunodeficiency virus infection: recognition and diagnosis, Can Dent Assoc J 54:413-419, 1988.

Food and Drug Administration: FDA Drug Bul 20(1):6-7, 1989.

Flynn NM et al: Absence of antibody among dental professionals exposed to infected patients, West J Med 146:439-442, 1987.

Gallo RC et al: Isolation of human T-cell leukemia virus in acquired immune deficiency syndrome (AIDS), Science 220:865-867, 1983.

Grassi M et al: Management of HIV-associated periodontal disease. In Robertson P and Greenspan JS, editors. Prospectives on oral manifestations of AIDS: diagnosis and management of HIV-associated infections, Littleton, Mass, 1988, PSG Publishing Co, Inc.

Greenspan D, Greenspan JS, Pindborg JJ, and Schiodt M: AIDS and the dental team, Chicago, 1987, Year Book Medical Publishers, Inc.

Imagawa DT et al: Human immunodeficiency virus type I infection in homosexual men who remain seronegative for prolonged periods, N Engl J Med 320:1458-1462, 1989.

Klein RS et al: Low occupational risk of human immunodeficiency virus infection among dental professionals, N Engl J Med 318:86-90, 1988.

Langford A et al: Oral hyperpigmentation in HIV-infected patients, Oral Surg 67:301-307, 1989.

Lapointe N et al: Transplacental transmission of HTLV-III virus, N Engl J Med 312:1325-1326, 1985.

Piot P et al: AIDS: an international perspective, Science 239:573-579, 1988.

Roberts MW, Brahim JS, and Rinne NF: Oral manifestations of AIDS: a study of 84 patients, J Am Dent Assoc 116:863-866, 1988.

Robertson PB and Greenspan JS, editors: Perspectives on oral manifestations of AIDS: diagnosis and management of HIV-associated infections, Littleton, Mass, 1988, PSG Publishing Co, Inc.

Rosenstein DI et al: Rapidly progressive periodontal disease associated with HIV infection: report of case, J Am Dent Assoc 118:313-314, 1989.

Rothenberg R et al: Survival with the acquired immunodeficiency syndrome: experience with 5833 cases in New York City, N Engl J Med 317:1297-1302, 1987.

Schiodt M and Pindborg JJ: AIDS and the oral cavity, Int J Oral Surg 19:1-14, 1987.

Silverman S: AIDS update: oral findings, diagnosis, and precautions, J Am Dent Assoc 115:559-563, 1987.

Silverman S et al: Oral findings in people with or at risk for AIDS: a study of 375 homosexual males, J Am Dent Assoc 112:187-192, 1986.

Winkler JR and Murray PA: Periodontal disease: a potential intraoral expression of AIDS may be rapidly progressive periodontitis, Calif Dent Assoc J 15:20-24, 1987.

Index